ESTHETIC REHABILITATION IN FIXED PROSTHODONTICS

PROSTHETIC TREATMENT
A SYSTEMATIC APPROACH TO ESTHETIC, BIOLOGIC, AND FUNCTIONAL INTEGRATION

VOLUME 2

ESTHETIC REHABILITATION IN FIXED PROSTHODONTICS

PROSTHETIC TREATMENT | VOLUME 2

A SYSTEMATIC APPROACH TO ESTHETIC, BIOLOGIC, AND FUNCTIONAL INTEGRATION

MAURO FRADEANI, MD, DDS

Private Practice
Pesaro and Milan, Italy

Visiting Associate Professor
Louisiana State University
School of Dentistry
New Orleans, Louisiana (USA)

GIANCARLO BARDUCCI, MDT

Master Dental Technician
Private Laboratory
Ancona, Italy

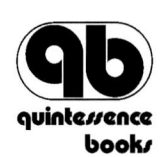

Quintessence Publishing Co, Inc

Chicago, Milan, Berlin, Tokyo, London, Paris, Barcelona,
Istanbul, São Paulo, Mumbai, Moscow, Prague, and Warsaw

First published in Italian in 2007 by Quintessenza Edizioni Srl, Milan.
La Riabilitazione estetica in protesi fissa
Volume 2. Trattamento protesico: Approccio sistematico all'integrazione estetica, biologica, e funzionale

British Library Cataloguing in Publication Data

Fradeani, Mauro
  Esthetic rehabilitation in fixed prosthodontics
  Vol. 2: Prosthetic treatment : a systematic approach to
  esthetic, biologic, and functional integration
  1. Prosthodontics 2. Dentistry - Aesthetic aspects
  I. Title II. Barducci, Giancarlo
  617.6'9

  ISBN-13: 9781850971719

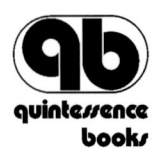

quintessence books

© 2008 Quintessence Publishing Co, Inc

Quintessence Publishing Co, Inc
4350 Chandler Drive
Hanover Park, IL 60133
www.quintpub.com

All rights reserved. This book or any part thereof may not be reproduced, stored in a retrieval system, or transmitted in any form or by any means, electronic, mechanical, photocopying, or otherwise, without prior written permission of the publisher.

Production: Ina Steinbrück, Quintessenz Verlags-GmbH, Berlin
Fotolito: Jens Höpfner, Quintessenz Verlags-GmbH, Berlin
Printing: Bosch-Druck GmbH, Landshut

Printed in Germany

*To **Alessandra** and **Giorgia***

*To **Dalila** and **Stefano***

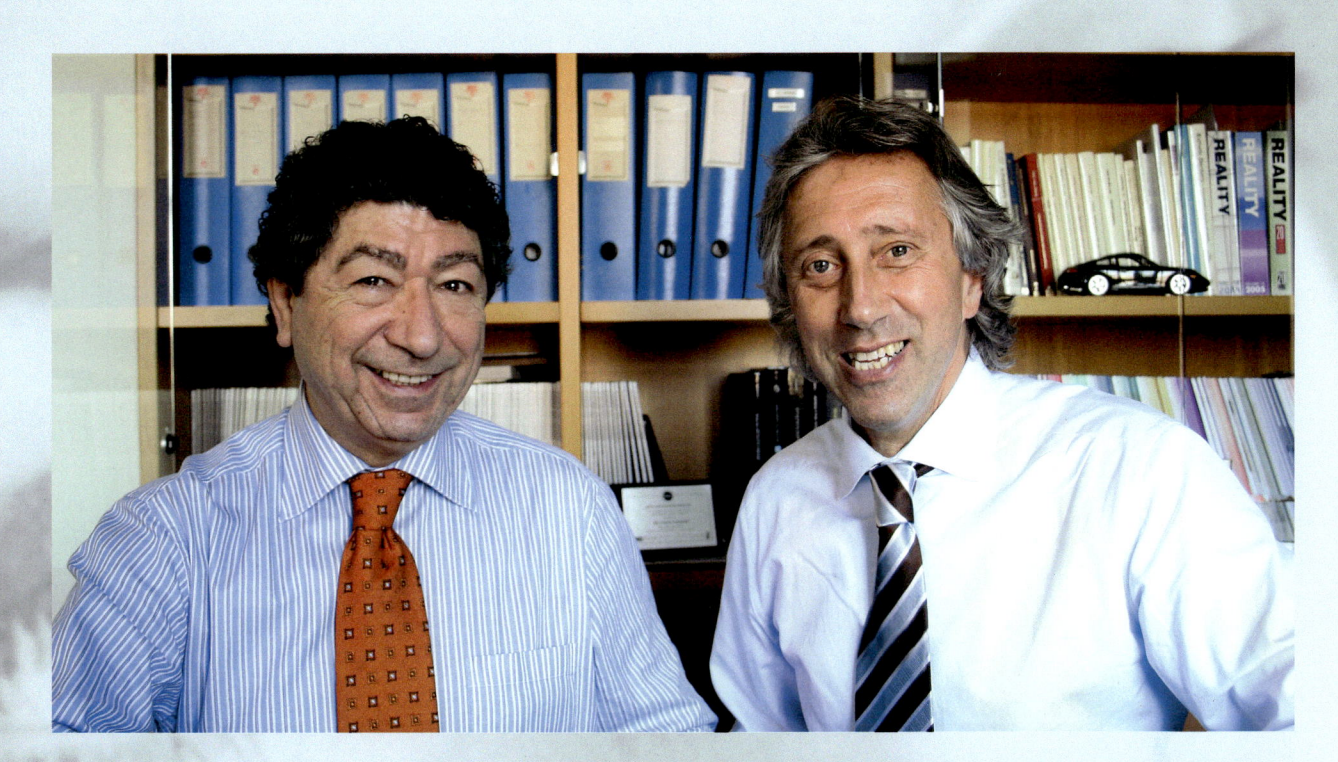

MAURO FRADEANI

After earning degrees in medicine and surgery in 1979, Dr Fradeani completed a specialization in dentistry at the University of Ancona in 1983. He is a Visiting Associate Professor in prosthetics at Louisiana State University, New Orleans, Louisiana (USA). He is also a Past President of the European Academy of Esthetic Dentistry (2003-2004) and of the Italian Academy of Prosthetic Dentistry (1999-2000); Associate Editor of the *European Journal of Esthetic Dentistry*; a member of the editorial boards of *Practical Periodontics and Aesthetic Dentistry* and the *Journal of Esthetic and Restorative Dentistry*; and a member of numerous international academies. Dr Fradeani is the author of Volume 1 in this series, entitled *Esthetic Rehabilitation in Fixed Prosthodontics: Esthetic Analysis* (Quintessence, 2004), which has been translated into 9 languages, and of numerous articles in international journals. He maintains an intense schedule of teaching activities, in Italy and abroad, in the field of prosthetics on natural teeth and implants, with special reference to esthetics. He runs a private practice limited to prosthetics in Pesaro and Milan, Italy.

GIANCARLO BARDUCCI

Mr Barducci started his career in 1974 by establishing his own dental laboratory. He is a member and speaker of ANTLO; an active member of the Italian Academy of Prosthetic Dentistry as well as Past President of the technical dentistry section (1999-2000); and a frequent speaker at national and international conferences. Mr Barducci co-authored (with Dr Mauro Fradeani) chapter 5 of Volume 1 in this series, *Esthetic Rehabilitation in Fixed Prosthodontics: Esthetic Analysis*. He also created all of the prosthetic restorations featured in that book. He has substantial experience in prosthetic rehabilitations on both natural teeth and implants, combined with in-depth knowledge of all-ceramic systems. He practices in Ancona, Italy.

FOREWORD

Esthetic dentistry has become a widespread treatment modality throughout the world, and consequently it is evolving into a more extensive level of "esthetic rehabilitation." In order to treat the ever-growing number of patients in need of extensive esthetic treatment, esthetic dentistry must be combined with an in-depth knowledge of occlusion, implant dentistry, and full-mouth rehabilitation principles. Therefore, it comes as no surprise that so many clinicians are seeking a comprehensive reference textbook that simultaneously covers all of these complex areas in great depth.

In his first textbook, Dr Fradeani laid the scientific and artistic foundation for achieving predictable esthetic dentistry, and, together with Mr Barducci, the authors are now contributing their lifetime expertise in esthetic rehabilitation, allowing the clinician and the laboratory technician to confidently address comprehensive treatment involving veneers, crowns, and implant restorations as well as full-mouth reconstructions.

The common denominator underlying this entire textbook is the integration of the most meticulous, rigorous, and uncompromising functional and esthetic standards, regardless of the initial preoperative condition. With such a wealth of clinical and laboratory material available, the authors have clearly resisted the temptation to produce a show-and-tell conceptual book that might have been a significant contribution in itself. Instead, they are providing the clinician and the dental technician with a very clearly written and most didactic textbook, in which every technique is thoroughly illustrated and meticulously detailed step by step. These authors display a constant desire to share their vast knowledge and their innovative technical tips with an "over the shoulder" feel. This is especially evident in the final section on large-scale rehabilitations, where this practical approach sets the standard for modern, comprehensive dentistry integrating esthetics, implants, and occlusion.

With each case presented, the authors keep reminding us to "keep the end result in mind," and with this common thread, there is maximum emphasis on laboratory techniques and communication with the dental laboratory, with myriad practical applications to preparation design and provisional management. Ultimately, in areas as diverse as esthetic preview, occlusal instrumentation, provisional restorations, biologic management, and impressions, the authors are providing the reader with a true step-by-step approach for maximum predictability with a sound scientific background.

We have greatly benefited over the past years at Louisiana State University from the great teachings of Dr Fradeani and Mr Barducci and we are very pleased to see them contribute to our profession a textbook of such monumental proportion, which will be enjoyed worldwide.

Gerard J. Chiche, DDS
Helmer Professor and Chairman
Department of Prosthodontics
School of Dentistry
Louisiana State University
New Orleans, Louisiana

PREFACE

The aim of this book is to outline a systematic approach to prosthetic rehabilitation on natural teeth and implants, in the anterior sector alone as well as the complete arches. The application of a tried and tested system, experimented with over a period of 25 years, represents, especially for complex rehabilitations, an indispensable means of achieving optimal final results, from the esthetic as well as biologic and functional viewpoints. To this end, after filling in the esthetic checklist (extensively covered in Volume 1), the laboratory checklist is employed, a device as functional as it is indispensable for communicating with the dental technician in an exhaustive and effective manner. The scrupulous compilation of this checklist will allow the clinician to specify clearly any request and modification, in order to create an ideal diagnostic wax-up. Containing all of the variations necessary for optimizing the results of the rehabilitation, the laboratory checklist will consequently ensure the development of a provisional restoration that can be fitted into the mouth in the same position as the technician intended it in the articulator. Perfectly integrated in this way, the proposed system will allow the provisional restoration to be faithfully replicated in the definitive rehabilitation which, thanks in part to the wide range of techniques and restoration materials currently available, will be ideally integrated. This itinerary develops through a series of stages, both clinical and technical, which we have tried to illustrate in as full and exhaustive a manner as possible, with the aid of illustrations and concise diagrams set out to summarize and exemplify the points explained in the text. To this end, we have also selected three cases, illustrating them step by step along the way throughout the chapters. The most significant clinical cases referred to in the text have furthermore been presented again at the end of the book in what we are calling a "case gallery," designed to help the reader obtain an overall organic view through demonstration of the repeatability of the systematic approach proposed.

ACKNOWLEDGMENTS

The production of this book has been made possible through the assistance and collaboration of numerous people who have, either directly or indirectly, contributed to its completion. We consider it fitting to offer our thanks to every one of these people, for the time they have given and for the commitment they have made, in the name of the sentiments that bind us together and the common enthusiasm held for our profession.

Our families first and foremost, for the patience shown and for always being there to offer support and encouragement at times when creating the book demanded much in terms of energy.

Heartfelt thanks to our friends, more than colleagues, and reviewers of the text: Augusto Aquilano, Riccardo Becciani, Tiziano Bombardelli, Mauro Busi, Marco Corrado, Michele D'Amelio, Stefano Gori, and Marco Redemagni, who, with their precious contributions, have actively participated in this project and whose advice has been especially appreciated.

A dutiful mention also to our respective staff members, for their daily commitment and important contribution to bringing our work to fruition.

Special thanks to Franca Baioni, for her fundamental role in the text preparation and editing phase and for her continual dedication to correcting the manuscript. Thanks also to Stan Bailey, who provided an extremely accurate English translation, to Paola Facchin, who assisted me in the revision of the text, and to Luca Meloni, creator of all the illustrations contained in the book.

Thanks again to everyone, because without their contribution this book may still have remained unpublished.

Mauro Fradeani and Giancarlo Barducci

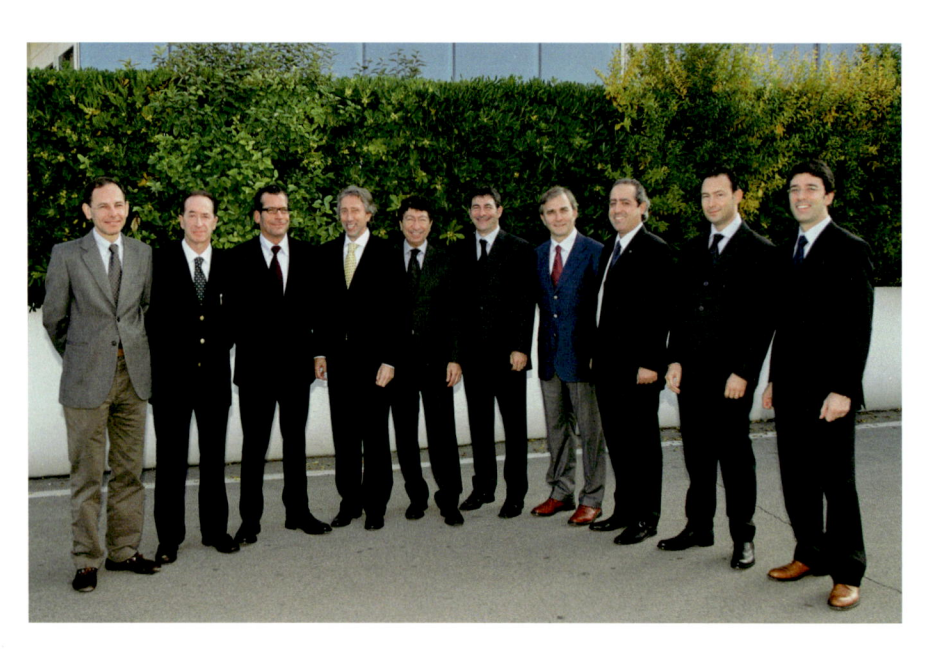

Advanced Continuing Education (ACE) Reviewers
From left:
Dr Tiziano Bombardelli,
Dr Riccardo Becciani,
Dr Stefano Gori,
Dr Mauro Fradeani,
Tech Giancarlo Barducci,
Dr Marco Corrado,
Tech Mauro Busi,
Dr Michele D'Amelio,
Dr Marco Redemagni,
Dr Augusto Aquilano

ESTHETIC REHABILITATION IN FIXED PROSTHODONTICS

PROSTHETIC TREATMENT — VOLUME 2
A SYSTEMATIC APPROACH TO ESTHETIC, BIOLOGIC, AND FUNCTIONAL INTEGRATION

TABLE OF CONTENTS

FOREWORD	8
PREFACE	9
ACKNOWLEDGMENTS	10
INTRODUCTION	26

Chapter 1 — COMMUNICATING TO THE LABORATORY – DIAGNOSTIC WAX-UP
Mauro Fradeani, Giancarlo Barducci — 29

MEDICAL CASE HISTORY	30
DENTAL CASE HISTORY	32
RADIOGRAPHIC EXAMINATION	32
CLINICAL EXAMINATION	34
EXTRAORAL EXAMINATION	34
INTRAORAL EXAMINATION	36
DIAGNOSIS	38
TREATMENT PLAN – PROGNOSIS	40
NATURAL TEETH OR IMPLANTS AS PROSTHETIC ABUTMENTS	42
REPLACING INDIVIDUAL TEETH	42
REPLACING TWO OR MORE TEETH	42
APPROACH WITH THE PATIENT	44
OPERATIONAL SEQUENCE	44

ANTERIOR REHABILITATION

ESTHETIC PREVIEW	48
DIAGNOSTIC SUPPORT	48
DIRECT MOCKUP	48
INDIRECT MOCKUP	52

EXTENSIVE REHABILITATION
TREATMENT PLAN – DIAGNOSTIC WAX-UP 56
LABORATORY CHECKLIST 58

LABORATORY CHECKLIST
ESTHETIC INFORMATION 60
PHOTOGRAPHS 60
FACE 60
SMILE 60
TEETH 60
OCCLUSAL PLANE 62
COLOR 62
SHAPE AND POSITION 64
OVERJET AND OVERBITE 64

LABORATORY CHECKLIST
FUNCTIONAL INFORMATION 66
STONE CASTS 66
OCCLUSAL REGISTRATIONS 66
MAXIMUM INTERCUSPATION 66
CENTRIC RELATION 66
VERTICAL DIMENSION OF OCCLUSION 70
PROTRUSIVE INTEROCCLUSAL RECORD 70
FACEBOW 72
ORIENTING THE CASTS 72
POSTERIOR REFERENCE POINTS 72
ANTERIOR REFERENCE POINT 72

FACEBOW
REFERENCE PLANES – LATERAL VIEW 74
FRANKFORT PLANE 74
ORBITAL-AXIS PLANE 74
ARBITRARY PLANE 74
CAMPER'S PLANE 74
ESTHETIC-FUNCTIONAL IMPLICATIONS 76

FACEBOW
REFERENCE PLANES – FRONTAL VIEW 80
ESTHETIC-FUNCTIONAL IMPLICATIONS 80

FACEBOW – REFERENCE: HORIZON
HORIZONTAL INCISAL PLANE 82
CORRECT REGISTRATION 82

FACEBOW – REFERENCE: HORIZON
HORIZONTAL INCISAL PLANE 84
INCORRECT REGISTRATION 84

FACEBOW – REFERENCE: HORIZON
INCLINED INCISAL PLANE — 88
CORRECT REGISTRATION — 88

FACEBOW – REFERENCE: HORIZON
INCLINED INCISAL PLANE — 90
INCORRECT REGISTRATION — 90

FACEBOW – REFERENCE: INCLINED
OBLIQUE FACIAL INCLINATION — 94
CORRECT REGISTRATION — 94

CLINICAL–PRACTICAL SUGGESTIONS — 96

MOUNTING THE CASTS ON THE ARTICULATOR — 98
FULLY ADJUSTABLE ARTICULATORS — 98
SEMI-ADJUSTABLE ARTICULATORS — 98

ADJUSTMENTS — 100

DIAGNOSTIC WAX-UP — 104
OCCLUSAL ADJUSTMENT OF STONE CASTS — 106

ADDITIVE DIAGNOSTIC WAX-UP — 112

Chapter 2

CREATING AND INTEGRATING THE PROVISIONAL RESTORATION

Mauro Fradeani, Giancarlo Barducci

OBJECTIVE	124
REQUIREMENTS	126
PROVISIONAL RESTORATIONS	
MATERIALS	128
ACRYLIC RESINS – METHYL METHACRYLATE	128
ACRYLIC RESINS – ETHYL METHACRYLATE	128
RESIN COMPOSITES	128
PROVISIONAL RESTORATIONS – PROSTHETIC REHABILITATION	
TOOTH PREPARATION	130
PLANNING THE PROSTHETIC ABUTMENT	130
PRELIMINARY PREPARATION	130
FABRICATING THE PROVISIONAL RESTORATION	
DIRECT TECHNIQUE	134
CHAIRSIDE FABRICATION	134
ACETATE MATRIX	134
FABRICATING THE PROVISIONAL RESTORATION	
INDIRECT TECHNIQUE	138
FABRICATION IN THE LABORATORY	138
PROVISIONAL RESTORATIONS FOR UNPREPARED TEETH	138
PROVISIONAL RESTORATIONS FOR PREPARED TEETH	138
INDIRECT TECHNIQUE	
FAILED INSERTION—UNPREPARED TEETH – CAUSES	140
INDIRECT TECHNIQUE	
FAILED INSERTION—PREPARED TEETH – SOLUTIONS	144
INDIRECT TECHNIQUE	
DIFFICULT INSERTION—PREPARED AND UNPREPARED TEETH – CAUSES	148
UNSATISFACTORY MARGINAL PRECISION	150
INDIRECT TECHNIQUE	
DIFFICULT INSERTION—PREPARED AND UNPREPARED TEETH – SOLUTIONS	
MODIFIED INDIRECT TECHNIQUE	154
PROVISIONAL RESTORATION WITH FACILITATED INSERTION	154
FITTING	154
PRECISION	156

FABRICATING THE PROVISIONAL RESTORATION – MIT – LABORATORY
ANTERIOR REHABILITATION

POURING IN THE SILICONE MATRIX (PSM)	160
TECHNIQUE	160
TECHNICAL CONSIDERATIONS	162

MIT – PSM – CLINIC
ANTERIOR REHABILITATION – POSITIONING IN THE ORAL CAVITY — 166

FABRICATING THE PROVISIONAL RESTORATION – MIT – LABORATORY
REHABILITATION OF ONE OR TWO ARCHES

PRESSING ON THE STONE CAST (PSC)	170
TECHNIQUE	170
TECHNICAL-CLINICAL CONSIDERATIONS	174

MIT – PSC – CLINIC
REHABILITATION OF ONE ARCH
POSITIONING IN THE ORAL CAVITY — 178

MIT – PSC – CLINIC
REHABILITATION OF TWO ARCHES
POSITIONING IN THE ORAL CAVITY — 182

MIT – PSC – CLINIC
CENTERING DEVICE

FACILITATED INSERTION GUIDE	188
RELINING	192
FINISHING	196
RE-MARGINING	200
SALT AND PEPPER TECHNIQUE	200
FLOW COMPOSITES	200
COLORING AND GLAZING	202
CEMENTATION	206

PARTIAL-COVERAGE RESTORATIONS
SHORT-TERM PROVISIONAL RESTORATIONS — 210

POSTERIOR SECTORS	210
PROVISIONAL INLAYS	210
PROVISIONAL ONLAYS AND OVERLAYS	212
ANTERIOR SECTORS	214
PROVISIONAL VENEERS	214
LONG-TERM PROVISIONAL RESTORATIONS	220
FIRST PROVISIONAL RESTORATION	220
SECOND PROVISIONAL RESTORATION	220
SECOND REINFORCED PROVISIONAL RESTORATION	222

CAST REINFORCEMENT	224
FABRICATION TECHNIQUE	224

LONG-TERM PROVISIONAL RESTORATIONS
THE PROVISIONAL RESTORATION
IN PROSTHETIC IMPLANT THERAPY — 226

NON–IMPLANT-SUPPORTED PROVISIONAL
RESTORATIONS — 226
REMOVABLE PROSTHESIS — 226
FIXED PROSTHESIS — 226

PROVISIONAL RESTORATION ON NATURAL TEETH	226
RESIN-BONDED PROSTHESIS	228
ORTHODONTIC PROVISIONAL RESTORATION	230

LONG-TERM PROVISIONAL RESTORATIONS – FIXED PROSTHESIS
IMPLANT-SUPPORTED PROVISIONAL RESTORATION — 232

IMPLANT-SUPPORTED PROVISIONAL RESTORATIONS
DELAYED LOADING – PROVISIONAL RESTORATION — 236

PROVISIONAL RESTORATION ON DEFINITIVE ABUTMENTS	236

IMPLANT-SUPPORTED PROVISIONAL RESTORATIONS
DELAYED LOADING – FIRST AND
SECOND PROVISIONAL RESTORATIONS — 240
COMPLEX REHABILITATIONS AND
ANTERIOR PARTIAL CASES — 240

FIRST PROVISIONAL RESTORATION ON TEMPORARY ABUTMENTS	240
SECOND PROVISIONAL RESTORATION ON DEFINITIVE ABUTMENTS	240

IMPLANT-SUPPORTED PROVISIONAL RESTORATIONS
IMMEDIATE LOADING — 248
SINGLE IMPLANT – IMMEDIATE FUNCTION — 248
REHABILITATING ONE OR TWO ARCHES –
IMMEDIATE LOADING — 254

PROVISIONAL RESTORATIONS – CONCLUSIONS — 266

ESTHETIC INTEGRATION	266
FUNCTIONAL INTEGRATION	268

Chapter 3
BIOLOGIC INTEGRATION OF THE PROVISIONAL RESTORATION AND DEFINITIVE PREPARATIONS
Mauro Fradeani   277

SOFT TISSUES	**278**
PERIODONTAL BIOTYPE	278
ANATOMIC STRUCTURES	278
GINGIVAL SULCUS	278
PROSTHETIC PROCEDURE AND ASSOCIATED BIOLOGIC RISK	**278**
BIOLOGIC INTEGRATION	
PROVISIONAL RESTORATION	**280**
RISK FACTORS	**280**
BIOLOGIC INTEGRATION – PROVISIONAL RESTORATION	
GINGIVAL MARGIN STABILITY	**284**
MARGINAL CLOSURE	**284**
RESTORATION CONTOUR	**286**
INTERPROXIMAL CONTOUR	286
BUCCAL CONTOUR	288
SURFACE CHARACTERISTICS OF THE RESTORATIVE MATERIAL	290
EXCESS CEMENT	290
BIOLOGIC INTEGRATION - PERIODONTALLY HEALTHY PATIENTS	
PREPROSTHETIC SURGERY	**294**
CLINICAL INDICATIONS	**294**
EXPOSURE OF HEALTHY TOOTH STRUCTURE	294
CLINICAL CROWN LENGTHENING	294
SURGICAL THERAPY	**296**
POSTOPERATIVE MONITORING	**296**
AVERAGE TISSUE MATURATION TIMES	298
TISSUE REGROWTH VARIABLES	300
INDICATORS OF TISSUE MATURATION	302
RELINING AND PROSTHETIC FINALIZATION	302
BIOLOGIC INTEGRATION - PERIODONTALLY COMPROMISED PATIENTS	
PROSTHETIC-PERIODONTAL THERAPY	**312**
POSTERIOR SECTORS	**312**
RELINING AND PROSTHETIC FINALIZATION	312
ANTERIOR SECTOR	**316**
RELINING AND PROSTHETIC FINALIZATION	316
FINAL TOOTH PREPARATION	**324**

TOOTH PREPARATION
PREPARATION THICKNESS 326
ANTERIOR SECTOR 326
ANTEROSUPERIOR SECTOR 328

TOOTH PREPARATION
MARGINAL CONFIGURATION 330

TOOTH PREPARATION
RESPECTING BIOLOGIC INTEGRITY 332
PARTIAL PREPARATIONS 332
COMPLETE PREPARATIONS 332

TOOTH PREPARATION - RESPECTING BIOLOGIC INTEGRITY
PULP INTEGRITY 336

TOOTH PREPARATION - RESPECTING BIOLOGIC INTEGRITY
GINGIVAL INTEGRITY 338
SUPRAGINGIVAL MARGIN 338
MARGIN AT THE GINGIVAL CREST 338
SUBGINGIVAL MARGIN 342
VIOLATION OF BIOLOGIC INTEGRITY 342

SUBGINGIVAL MARGIN
INTRASULCULAR PREPARATION 344
RESPECT OF BIOLOGIC INTEGRITY 344
CLINICAL STEPS 344
MAPPING THE SULCUS 344
PREPARATION AT THE GINGIVAL LEVEL 346
INSERTING THE CORD 346
PREPARATION AT THE NEW GINGIVAL LEVEL 346
FINISHING 348
REMOVING THE CORD AND RELINING THE PROVISIONAL RESTORATION 348

BIOLOGIC INTEGRATION
IMPLANT-PROSTHETIC THERAPY 352
PERI-IMPLANT SOFT TISSUES 352
BIOLOGIC IMPLICATIONS 354
CLINICAL BEHAVIOR 354

Chapter 4

FROM THE PROVISIONAL RESTORATION TO THE DEFINITIVE PROSTHESIS: IMPRESSIONS AND DATA TRANSFER

Mauro Fradeani — 373

IMPRESSIONS AND DATA TRANSFER	374
INTEGRATED PROVISIONAL RESTORATION	374
OBJECTIVE	374
PROVISIONAL RESTORATION **VERIFYING THE INTEGRATION**	376
PROVISIONAL RESTORATION IN SITU	376
ESTHETIC PARAMETERS	376
PHONETIC PARAMETERS	378
FUNCTIONAL PARAMETERS	378
BIOLOGIC PARAMETERS	380
PROVISIONAL RESTORATION IN SITU **DATA TRANSFER**	382
IMPRESSION OF THE PROVISIONAL RESTORATION AND OF THE OPPOSING ARCH	382
PROTRUSIVE INTEROCCLUSAL RECORD	382
FACEBOW	382
DATA TRANSFER **FINAL IMPRESSIONS**	384
REMOVING THE PROVISIONAL RESTORATION	384
FINAL IMPRESSIONS	384
POLYVINYL SILOXANES AND POLYETHERS	388
DATA TRANSFER - FINAL IMPRESSIONS **IMPRESSION TECHNIQUE**	390
ONE STEP–DOUBLE MIX	390
RECOMMENDATIONS	390
DATA TRANSFER - FINAL IMPRESSIONS **VISUALIZING THE FINISH LINE**	392
MAPPING THE SULCUS	392
CORDS	392
INSERTION FORCE	392
MECHANICAL ACTION	394
MECHANICAL-CHEMICAL ACTION	394
FINAL IMPRESSIONS **PREPARATION AT THE GINGIVAL CREST – SINGLE-CORD TECHNIQUE**	396
IMPRESSION WITH THE CORD INSERTED	396

FINAL IMPRESSIONS
INTRASULCULAR PREPARATION -
TWO-CORD TECHNIQUE 398
INSERTING THE FIRST CORD 398
INSERTING THE SECOND IMPREGNATED CORD 400
REMOVING THE SECOND CORD AND TAKING THE IMPRESSION 400

IMPRESSION MATERIALS AND TECHNIQUES
VENEERS AND INLAYS-ONLAYS 408
PROBLEMS 408
VENEERS 408
INLAYS-ONLAYS 408

IMPRESSION MATERIALS AND TECHNIQUES
IMPLANTS 410
TAKING THE IMPRESSION ON THE HEAD OF THE IMPLANTS 410
TAKING THE IMPRESSION ON THE ABUTMENTS 410

DATA TRANSFER
OCCLUSAL REGISTRATION -
ANTERIOR REHABILITATION 412
OCCLUSAL REGISTRATION IN PARTIAL CASES 412
ANTERIOR REHABILITATION 412
REGISTRATION BETWEEN ABUTMENTS AND OPPOSING ARCH 412

DATA TRANSFER
OCCLUSAL REGISTRATION -
REHABILITATION OF ONE ARCH 414
REGISTRATION BETWEEN PREPARED TEETH AND OPPOSING ARCH 414

DATA TRANSFER
OCCLUSAL REGISTRATION -
REHABILITATION OF TWO ARCHES 416
CROSS-MOUNTING OF THE MAXILLARY AND MANDIBULAR CASTS 416
REGISTRATION BETWEEN MAXILLARY AND MANDIBULAR ABUTMENTS 416

DATA TRANSFER
RECORDING AND TRANSMITTING THE COLOR 418
RECORDING THE COLOR 418
TRANSMITTING THE COLOR 420

DATA TRANSFER
DEFINITIVE RESTORATION -
LABORATORY CHECKLIST 424

Chapter 5

PRODUCING AND FINALIZING THE PROSTHETIC REHABILITATION

Mauro Fradeani, Giancarlo Barducci   435

PRODUCING THE DEFINITIVE RESTORATION	436
CLINIC	436
LABORATORY	436

PRODUCING THE DEFINITIVE RESTORATION – LABORATORY
MASTER CAST (MC)   438

REMOVABLE ABUTMENTS	438
DIE SPACER	438

PRODUCING THE DEFINITIVE RESTORATION – LABORATORY
SECONDARY CAST (SC)   442

REPLICATING GINGIVAL TISSUES	442
OPTIMIZING THE RESTORATIVE CONTOUR	442
DESIGN OF THE CONNECTING AREAS	442

LABORATORY
CROSS-MOUNTING TECHNIQUE – ANTERIOR REHABILITATION   446

MOUNTING THE CAST OF THE PROVISIONAL RESTORATION WITH THE CAST OF THE OPPOSING ARCH	446
MOUNTING THE MASTER CAST WITH THE CAST OF THE OPPOSING ARCH	446

LABORATORY
CROSS-MOUNTING TECHNIQUE – SINGLE-ARCH REHABILITATION   448

MOUNTING THE CAST OF THE PROVISIONAL RESTORATION WITH THE CAST OF THE OPPOSING ARCH	448
MOUNTING THE MASTER CAST WITH THE CAST OF THE OPPOSING ARCH	448

LABORATORY
CROSS-MOUNTING TECHNIQUE FOR TWO-ARCH REHABILITATIONS   450

MOUNTING THE CASTS OF THE MAXILLARY AND MANDIBULAR PROVISIONAL RESTORATIONS	450
CROSS MOUNTING OF THE MAXILLARY AND MANDIBULAR CASTS	450
CHECKING CROSS MOUNTING WITH MAXILLARY MC AND MANDIBULAR MC	450

ADJUSTING THE ARTICULATOR – LABORATORY
CUSTOMIZED ANTERIOR GUIDANCE   454

CONSTRUCTING THE DEFINITIVE RESTORATION – LABORATORY
SILICONE INDEX — 458

OCCLUSOPALATAL INDEX — 458

BUCCAL INDEX — 462

SUBSTRUCTURE — 466

DESIGN — 466

CHOOSING THE RESTORATIVE MATERIAL — 466

METAL-CERAMIC — 466

ALL-CERAMICS — 468

SILICATE-BASED CERAMICS — 468

FELDSPATHIC CERAMICS — 468

GLASS-CERAMICS — 468

HIGH-STRENGTH CERAMICS — 470

ALUMINA — 470

ZIRCONIUM — 472

SUBSTRUCTURE – FIXED PARTIAL DENTURES — 474

METAL-CERAMIC — 474

ALL-CERAMICS — 474

SUBSTRUCTURE
METAL-CERAMIC, ALL-CERAMICS — 478

CLINICAL CONSIDERATIONS — 478

CONSTRUCTING THE SUBSTRUCTURE
CASE 1, CASE 2, CASE 3 — 480

CASE 1 — 480

CASE 2 — 480

CASE 3 — 480

CLINIC
SUBSTRUCTURE TRY-IN — 482

MARGINAL ADAPTATION: FIXED PARTIAL DENTURES — 482

MARGINAL ADAPTATION: SINGLE RESTORATION — 482

CLINICAL CHECK OF THE MOUNTING
SUBSTRUCTURE – PREVENTIVE SIMULATION (PS) — 484

CONSTRUCTING THE DEFINITIVE RESTORATION - LABORATORY
TREATING THE SUBSTRUCTURE — 488

METAL-CERAMIC — 488

ALL-CERAMICS — 488

CONSTRUCTING THE DEFINITIVE RESTORATION - LABORATORY
LAYERING THE CERAMIC — 490

CONSTRUCTING THE DEFINITIVE RESTORATION - CLINIC

BISCUIT TRY-IN   494

ESTHETIC PARAMETERS   494

FUNCTIONAL PARAMETERS   496

BIOLOGIC PARAMETERS   498

GLAZING   500

POSTSOLDERING   500

DELIVERING THE DEFINITIVE RESTORATION   502

LUTING   504

TEMPORARY LUTING   504

DEFINITIVE LUTING   504

MAINTENANCE   518

CLINICAL CASE GALLERY   524

INDEX   595

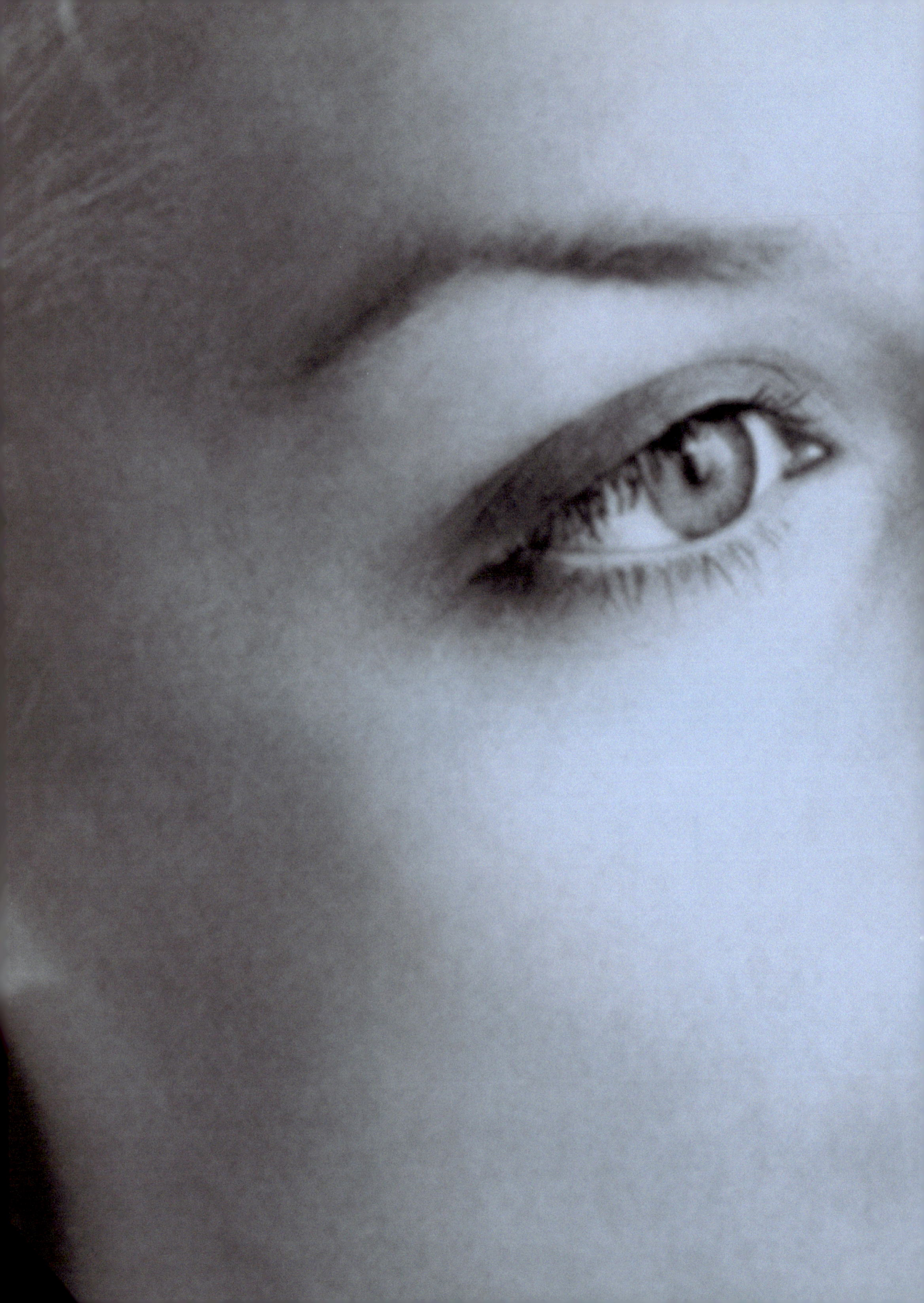

ESTHETIC REHABILITATION IN FIXED PROSTHODONTICS

PROSTHETIC TREATMENT
A SYSTEMATIC APPROACH TO ESTHETIC, BIOLOGIC, AND FUNCTIONAL INTEGRATION

VOLUME 2

PROSTHETIC TREATMENT

The ideal treatment plan must be drawn up following careful esthetic, functional, and structural analysis and with the aid of radiographic examinations and stone casts mounted on the articulator by means of correct use of the facebow. The variations necessary for optimizing the case must be transferred to the technician by carefully filling in the laboratory checklist, to create the diagnostic wax-up that will have to incorporate all of the modifications requested by the clinician (Chapter 1). Fabricating the provisional restoration by the MIT technique, aside from ensuring a correct fit in the oral cavity, will give the clinician the opportunity to evaluate the effectiveness and the validity of the variations made, making it possible to achieve adequate esthetic-functional integration (Chapter 2) and a perfect state of health of the gingival tissues, before proceeding with the definitive preparations (Chapter 3). The final impressions, the impressions of the provisional restorations, all of the occlusal registrations, and record of the facebow will place the technician in a position of being able to finalize the prosthetic rehabilitation correctly (Chapter 4). Cross mounting the casts, creating the silicone indices and the preventive simulation (PS) of the definitive result will make it possible to faithfully replicate all of the characteristics of the functionalized provisional restoration, regardless of the type of restorative material selected (Chapter 5).

PROSTHETIC TREATMENT

VOLUME 2

Chapter 1 — COMMUNICATING TO THE LABORATORY – DIAGNOSTIC WAX-UP

To create, by means of correctly filling in the laboratory checklist, a diagnostic wax-up which, in idealizing the esthetic-functional modifications set as the objective of the treatment, represents a preview of the definitive work.

Chapter 2 — CREATING AND INTEGRATING THE PROVISIONAL RESTORATION

To construct a provisional restoration that, correctly fitted into the oral cavity, will allow the adequacy of the modifications incorporated into the diagnostic wax-up to be verified.

Chapter 3 — BIOLOGIC INTEGRATION OF THE PROVISIONAL RESTORATION AND DEFINITIVE PREPARATIONS

To achieve and maintain, in all therapeutic phases, a perfect state of health of the gingival tissues by means of ideal biologic integration of the provisional restoration.

Chapter 4 — FROM THE PROVISIONAL RESTORATION TO THE DEFINITIVE PROSTHESIS: IMPRESSIONS AND DATA TRANSFER

To transfer accurately to the laboratory the registrations necessary to replicate in the definitive restorations the esthetic-functional characteristics present in the provisional restoration.

Chapter 5 — PRODUCING AND FINALIZING THE PROSTHETIC REHABILITATION

To achieve perfect integration of the prosthetic rehabilitation thanks to a systematic approach and a careful selection of techniques and materials.

VOLUME 2 | PROSTHETIC TREATMENT

ESTHETIC REHABILITATION IN FIXED PROSTHODONTICS

Chapter 1

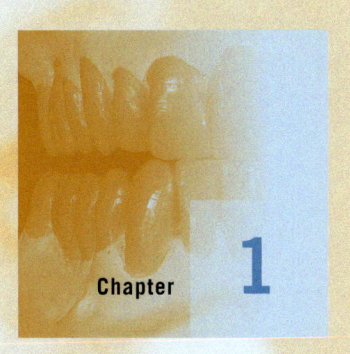

COMMUNICATING TO THE LABORATORY—DIAGNOSTIC WAX-UP

While a correct diagnosis and the resulting treatment plan are essential to the success of a prosthetic rehabilitation, efficient communication to the laboratory is critical as well. After compiling the esthetic checklist, the clinician can complete the laboratory checklist, noting the esthetic-functional changes needed to create the diagnostic wax-up. Simultaneous transfer of the functional registrations, including an accurate recording of the facebow, allows the technician to realize what the clinician has formulated in the treatment plan.

OBJECTIVE _ To transfer to the technician, by means of the laboratory checklist, all of the information gathered in the esthetic-functional analysis, so that the diagnostic wax-up can be made.

COMMUNICATING TO THE LABORATORY—DIAGNOSTIC WAX-UP

A close, mutual collaboration between clinician and technician is essential to achieve a correct fixed prosthetic rehabilitation, providing the two work in synergy and within their own specific disciplines. Facial, dentolabial, phonetic, dental, and gingival analyses, all recorded on the esthetic checklist, together with the necessary functional examination (static and dynamic), provide all of the basic elements for developing an accurate treatment plan, finalization of which often demands a multidisciplinary approach. The esthetic-functional information, carefully collected and compiled, can be transferred to the technician clearly and completely by means of a laboratory checklist. This checklist guides the technician in creating a correct diagnostic wax-up and the subsequent provisional restoration. In this way, important decisions that can be made only by the clinician, based on a careful esthetic and functional analysis of the patient, are not delegated to the technician.

Esthetic rehabilitation in fixed prosthodontics involves substitution and/or restoration of natural teeth with artificial elements fixed to the natural teeth or to osseointegrated implants. The objective is the restoration of biologic integrity, correct function, and optimum esthetics. Treatment may involve just a single tooth or the entire arch (Figs 1-1a to 1-1c), and its success depends on the formulation of a correct diagnosis based on nothing less than careful and meticulous collection of data. Before starting the actual clinical examination, the medical case history and then the dental case history are taken.

MEDICAL CASE HISTORY

Planning any type of therapy must necessarily be preceded by the collection of information about the patient's general state of health.[1,2] Standard printed questionnaires, completed by the patient, provide a general medical history that should then be discussed in more detail during the visit. The patient is asked if he or she has any drug or other allergies; about any recent dental anesthesia and whether it produced any allergic reactions, cardiovascular problems, or even simple lipothymic episodes; and about the existence of any chronic illnesses and therapies currently in progress. Any conditions requiring preventive antibiotic treatment are checked against the risk of bacteremia. The absence of any illnesses that could cause hemorrhagic diathesis must be confirmed, and it is ascertained whether any medicines that alter hemostasis (aspirin, heparin, etc) are being taken. A careful investigation is carried out to exclude all infectious diseases (eg, HBV, HCV, HIV) that could be transmitted to the dental team during the various clinical procedures.

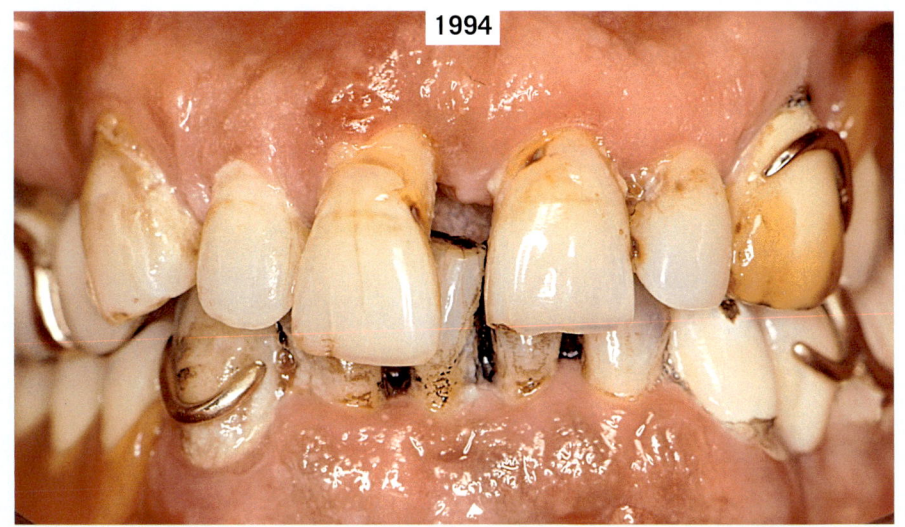

> Fig 1-1a

> Fig 1-1b

> Fig 1-1c

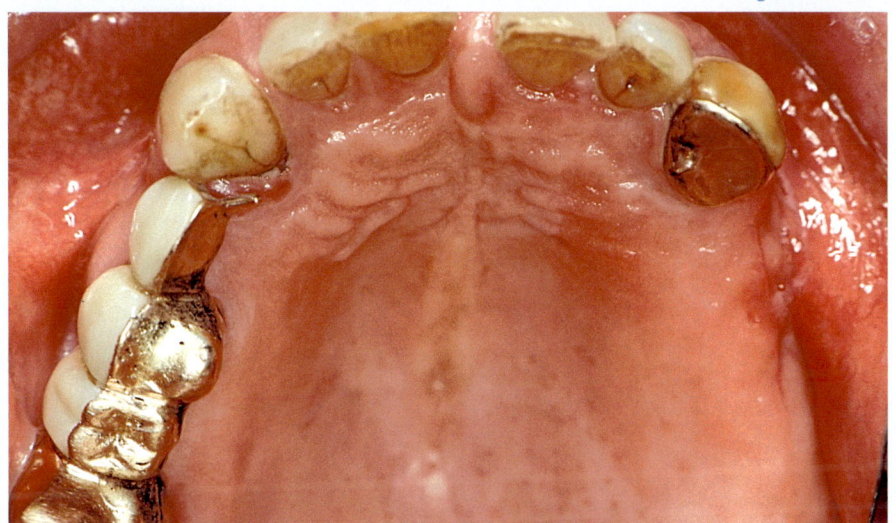

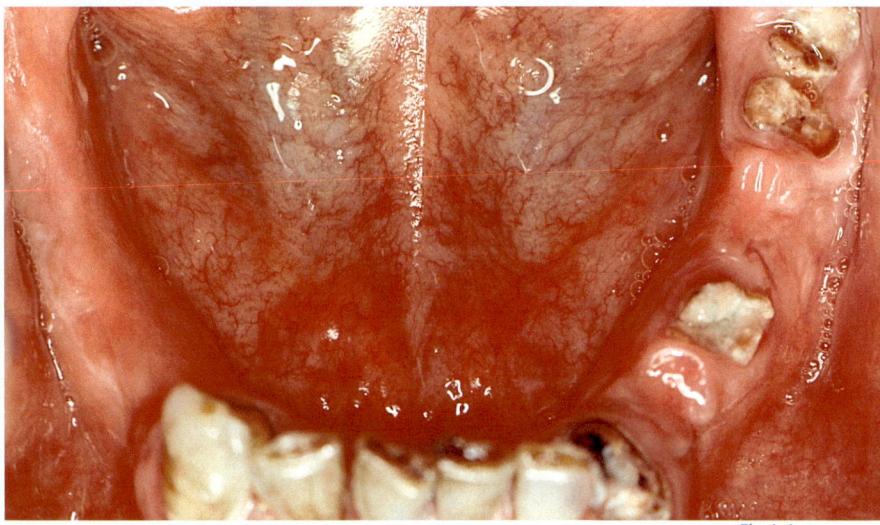

FIG 1 *(a)* The patient, who wears a fixed partial denture in the right maxillary quadrant and a removable partial denture in both the maxillary arch and mandibular arch, came to the office complaining of a large gap between the maxillary central incisors and general dissatisfaction with the prosthetic work carried out. An initial examination showed poor hygiene maintenance. *(b)* On taking out the removable partial dentures, an incongruity was evident on the right side of the maxillary arch between the fixed prosthesis and the large edentulous area on the left, *(c)* while some remaining roots on the left and an extensive edentulous area in the contralateral side were evident in the mandibular arch.

DENTAL CASE HISTORY

Restorative case history The presence of a significant number of restorations and their frequent turnover can indicate a marked carioreceptivity and inadequate oral hygiene at home. The longevity of the restorations aids in the assessment of the prognosis of the planned prosthetic rehabilitation.

Endodontic case history Existing radiographs of previous root canal treatments, compared with those taken in the office, can indicate the progress or stability of any endodontic lesions. Their disappearance and the absence of sensitivity, pain, fistulae, and/or abscesses provide crucial information about the predictability of the tooth as a prosthetic abutment.

Orthodontic case history A radiographic examination must be carried out to assess whether any previous orthodontic treatment has caused root resorption and hence an altered crown-root relationship, which could complicate the process of choosing which teeth to use as prosthetic abutments.

Periodontal case history The patient's report of gingival bleeding, either spontaneous or during brushing, or of dental migration and mobility leading to the development of diastemata should alert the clinician to inflammation and the possible loss of periodontal support. The patient is also asked about frequency of professional oral hygiene care and about any history of periodontal surgery.

Craniofacial case history Patients must be asked whether they experience any pain in the masticatory muscles or in the temporomandibular joints (TMJs). If so, evaluation of the manner in which the symptoms occur, their frequency, and their progress over time is needed to make a differential diagnosis between muscular and articular pain. The patient must also be asked whether any changes have taken place in mandibular movements, resulting in the onset of noise, clicking, or joint locking.

RADIOGRAPHIC EXAMINATION

The full-mouth series, which provides a detailed picture of the root morphology and levels of the osseous ridge, integrates the individual examinations, particularly the periodontal assessment (Figs 1-1d and 1-1e).[3,4] The panoramic radiograph allows efficient assessment of the overall dental situation. It provides information on the position of the third molars and proves useful in the pre–implant planning stage, although it is not valid for the purposes of a periodontal investigation (Fig 1-1f). The computed tomography (CT) scan is useful for evaluating the implant sites, especially in the posterior sectors. By providing a three-dimensional image of the site, it enables clear identification of the anatomic structures to be avoided (eg, nasal fossae, maxillary sinus, inferior alveolar nerve) during implant placement (Fig 1-1g). Oblique transcranial radiographs[5] are useful for identifying any structural and postural variations of the TMJs and can be integrated with data collected from other studies, such as serial tomography, arthrography,[6] and magnetic resonance imaging (MRI).[7–9]

> Fig 1-1d

> Fig 1-1e

> Fig 1-1f

> Fig 1-1g

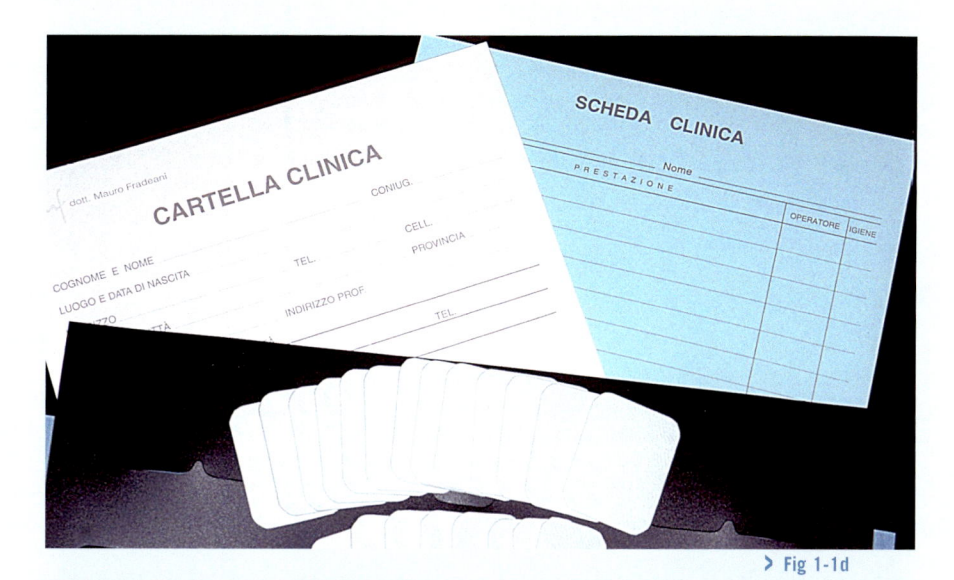

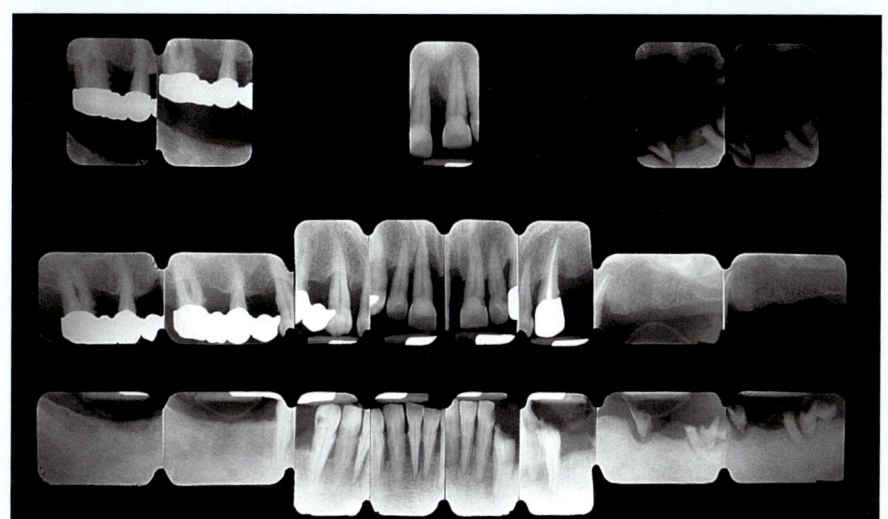

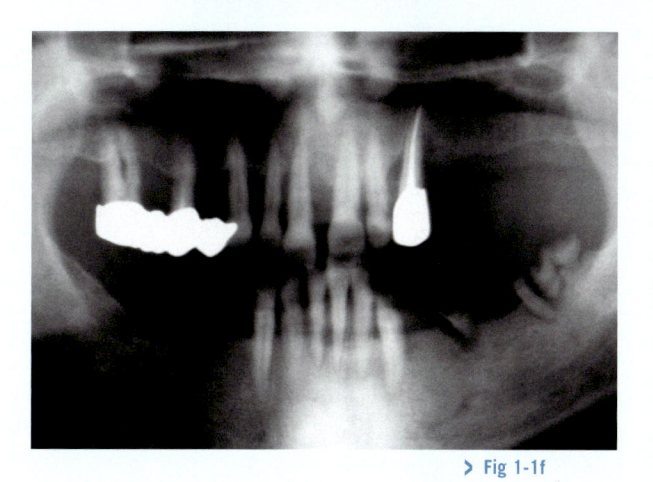

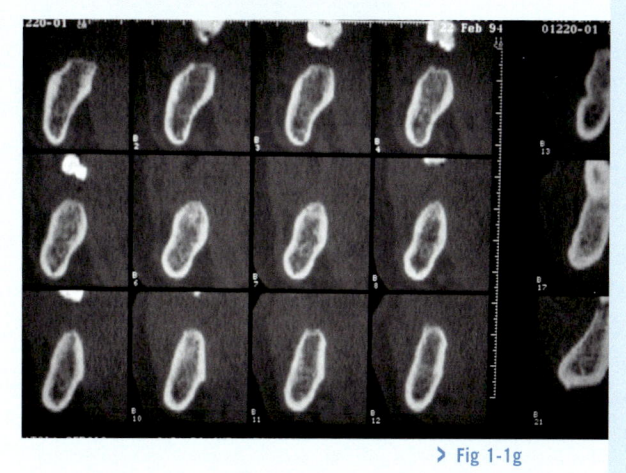

FIG 1 *(d)* The patient's case history is recorded on a medical history form. At the same time, arrangements are made for a full-mouth radiographic series. *(e)* The full-mouth series, which consists of 21 periapical radiographs taken using the long-cone paralleling technique with film-holding instruments, confirms the complexity of the case already made clear during the clinical examination. *(f and g)* Orthopantomography can prove useful for an overall dental assessment and for implant planning, while the CT scan is indispensable for obtaining, through a three-dimensional view, a clear identification of the anatomic structures (maxillary sinus, mandibular canal, etc) to be taken into account when placing the implants.

CLINICAL EXAMINATION

EXTRAORAL EXAMINATION

Facial analysis The extraoral examination begins with facial analysis to identify any asymmetry or disharmony in the face (see volume 1, chapter 2).[10,11] The analysis of the patient's face, with the head in the natural postural position, must be carried out using horizontal and vertical reference lines that allow the face and teeth to be spatially correlated. The frontal view of the patient allows assessment of the contour of the horizontal reference lines (interpupillary and commissural) and of the midline, which serves as the main vertical reference line. The lateral view is used to analyze the patient's profile and the shape and size of the lips.

Dentolabial and phonetic analyses These analyses are essential for evaluating the relationship between the teeth and the lips during the various phases of speech and smiling (see volume 1, chapters 3 and 4) (Fig 1-1h).[10,11] They are performed by the clinician while talking to the patient in an informal and relaxed atmosphere. The results of the study must be noted in the appropriate section of the laboratory checklist (Fig 1-1i), including the correct tooth position as well as the suitability of the occlusal plane and vertical dimension of occlusion (VDO).

Craniofacial evaluation The TMJs are examined by the clinician by pressing on either side of the area medial to the tragus with the patient in maximum intercuspation (MI), on opening, closing, protrusion, and lateral movement. Manual bilateral palpation of the TMJs and of the masticatory muscles[12,13] (masseter, temporalis, external and internal pterygoids, mylohyoid, and digastrics) is used to assess the severity of any pain or increase in muscle tone. Auscultation of the TMJ allows for differential diagnosis between articular clicking, generally an expression of anterior disc dislocation, and crepitation, indicating osteoarthrosis. When assessing the mandibular movements, the clinician should remember that the physiologic values of the mandible opening normally exceed 50 mm.[13,14] A reduced opening (ie, 35 mm or less), its deviation from the sagittal medial plane, or the onset of pain, all oblige the clinician to formulate a differential diagnosis between occlusomuscular pain and intra-articular dysfunction and to normalize the condition of the stomatognathic system before undertaking any prosthetic therapy.

FIG 1 (h) The dentolabial analysis shows the considerable difference in height of the incisal edge and the visible anterior gap that has opened over the years between the maxillary central incisors.

FIG 1 (i) Every part of the esthetic checklist is filled in to provide the clinician with sufficient information to assess the necessary esthetic and functional changes to be made.

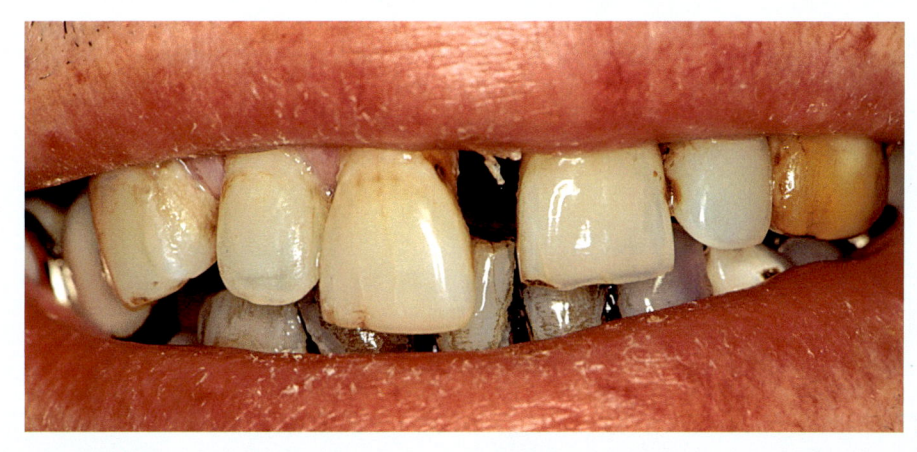

> Fig 1-1h

> Fig 1-1i

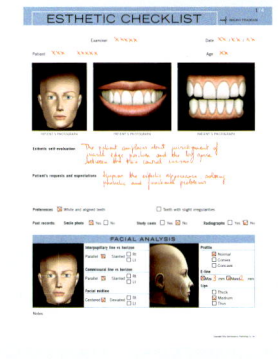

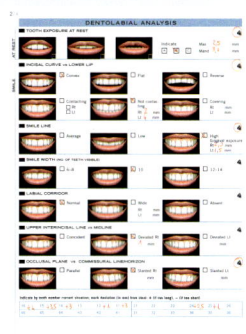

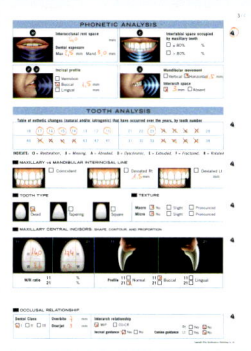

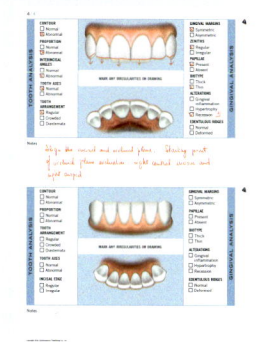

EXTRAORAL EXAMINATION

FACIAL ANALYSIS	■ Frontal view	■ Horizontal reference lines
	■ Lateral view	■ Profile—lips
DENTOLABIAL ANALYSIS	■ Tooth exposure at rest	
	■ Position of the incisal edge	
	■ Smile line	
	■ Width of smile	
	■ Buccal corridor	
	■ Interincisal line versus midline	
	■ Occlusal plane versus commissural line	
PHONETIC ANALYSIS	■ Position of the incisal edge	
	■ Tooth length	
	■ Vertical dimension	
CRANIOFACIAL EVALUATION	■ Palpation of masticatory muscles	
	■ TMJ palpation and auscultation	
	■ Mandibular opening	■ Size
		■ Direction
		■ Painfulness

INTRAORAL EXAMINATION

Evaluation of tooth structure Assessments are made of the amount of residual tooth structure and, where necessary, the possibility of a conservative reconstruction of the prosthetic abutment. If any endodontic treatment or re-treatment has been carried out and a valid apical seal achieved, it may be possible to use the root lumen as an anchor for bonding a post upon which to base the reconstruction of the prosthetic abutment. An evaluation must also be made of whether the residual tooth structure is sufficient to guarantee an adequate ferrule effect for the restoration (> 1.5 mm) (Fig 1-1j). If it is not, the clinician can resort to orthodontic extrusion treatment with fiber resection or to a crown-lengthening procedure. If neither of these options is practical, then the tooth must be extracted and replaced with an implant.

Orthodontic evaluation Correct tooth position and composition are checked in both arches, along with the presence of all permanent teeth. Also noted are any anomalies in tooth arrangement (eg, crowding or diastemata) or in form and contour (eg, conoid) or changes in interdental gaps (eg, mesializations, distalizations, supra-eruptions, or intrusions). Often in the latter case, and especially in an edentulous area, orthodontic therapy must precede prosthetic therapy to re-establish adequate space for the finalization of a traditional partial denture anchored to natural teeth and for correct implant positioning.

Periodontal assessment Some epidemiologic studies have demonstrated that 90% of the population analyzed show, to varying degrees, signs of periodontal disease.[15–17] A careful periodontal evaluation is therefore essential before any treatment plan is formulated. This examination must assess the patient's level of oral hygiene in addition to the following: probing depth, presence/absence of bleeding during probing, level of gingival recession, any mucogingival defects, deep angular lesions, furcation involvement in the posterior teeth, and tooth mobility. In the case of a periodontally compromised dentition (Fig 1-1k), intraoral radiographic examinations should be carried out along with a clinical assessment of the loss of attachment[18,19] to more accurately define the amount of support lost. In such cases, the patient should be involved in a therapeutic intervention aimed at the following:

- Arresting the progression of the disease
- Correcting, where necessary, the defects created by the disease
- Preventing the recurrence of the disease

Before undertaking prosthetic therapy, the clinician must also make sure that the following parameters are observed:

- Probing depth ≤ 3 mm
- Bleeding Index (BI) = 0
- Correct tissue morphology

FIG 1 (j) During prosthetic finalization of the mandibular arch, the residual dental structure of the prosthetic abutment is satisfactory in the two mandibular incisors, but it seems to be critical in the left canine, where the ferrule of the abutment beneath the gold post and core appears to be merely sufficient.

FIG 1 (k) During periodontal examination of the maxillary arch, the substantial distal probing depth (10 mm) and the discharge of purulent exudate demonstrate a considerable periodontal compromise of the left maxillary canine.

EVALUATION OF TOOTH STRUCTURE

- Intact abutment
- Residual abutment
  - Ferrule effect
    - ≥ 2 mm
      - Partial reconstruction of abutment → composite
      - Extensive reconstruction of abutment
      - Endodontic treatment
      - Endodontic post
    - < 2 mm
      - Surgical crown lengthening
      - Orthodontic extrusion with fiber resection
      - Extraction

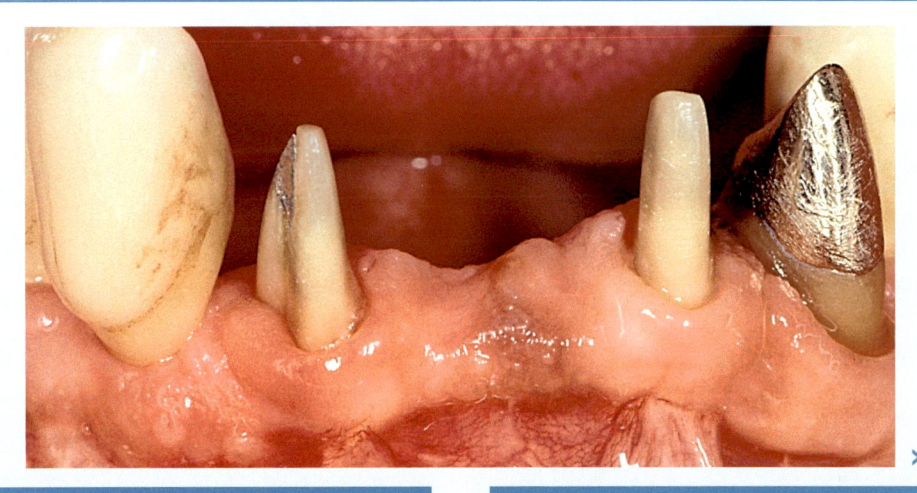

> Fig 1- 1j

ORTHODONTIC EVALUATION

- Tooth position and composition
- Arrangement
  - Crowding
  - Diastemata
- Space modifications
  - Distalization
  - Mesialization
  - Extrusion
  - Intrusion

PERIODONTAL EVALUATION

- Plaque index
- Bleeding on probing
- Probing depth
- Level of attachment
- Mucogingival defects
- Deep angular lesions
- Involvement of the furcations
- Tooth mobility

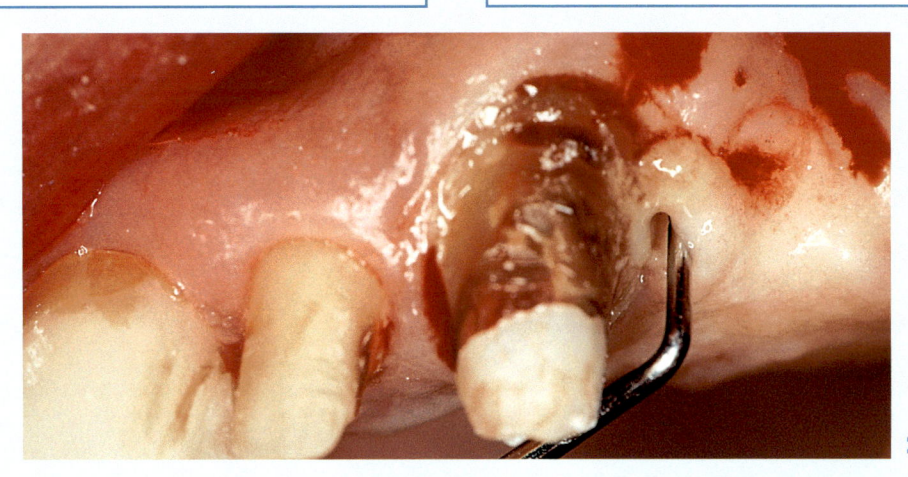

> Fig 1-1k

Occlusal evaluation When the case demands a large-scale prosthetic rehabilitation, it is useful to carry out an analysis of the occlusion directly on the patient, in both the static and dynamic phases. A clinician must *(1)* check for adequate occlusal stability, with well-distributed contacts in the posterior sectors; *(2)* measure any discrepancy between maximum intercuspation (MI) and centric relation (CR), noting the extent and direction; and *(3)* assess the congruity of the vertical dimension of occlusion (VDO). Analyses must also be carried out on the contacts in both normal occlusion and during protrusive and lateral movements of the mandible, the amount of horizontal and vertical overlapping (overjet and overbite), and the presence or absence of anterior guidance, noting any working or nonworking interferences. Any worn facets or other evidence of parafunction must also be noted. The indirect occlusal analysis, based on casts of the dentition mounted on a semi-adjustable articulator, allows a more detailed study of any edentulous spaces, malpositioned teeth, supra-eruptions, and the compensating curves (Spee and Wilson).

DIAGNOSIS

The diagnosis is the synthesis of all data collected during the medical and dental case history, the radiographic examination, and the extraoral and intraoral clinical examinations (Figs 1-1l to 1-1n). Analysis of stone casts of the dental arches, correctly mounted on a semi-adjustable articulator by means of accurate recording of the facebow and the occlusal registrations (Fig 1-1o), is useful in completing the static and dynamic occlusal analysis. The casts guide the technician in developing a diagnostic wax-up based on the indications provided by the clinician on the laboratory checklist (Figs 1-1p to 1-1r). Radiographs and/or stone casts from previous dental treatments also prove useful for diagnosis, as do photographs documenting the changes that have occurred in the esthetic-functional appearance over the course of time. When compared with the current clinical situation, this documentation can be of considerable use because it provides fundamental elements for evaluating the progression or the substantial stability of the pathologies found.

OCCLUSAL EVALUATION

- OCCLUSAL STABILITY
- MI–CR DISCREPANCY
- VERTICAL DIMENSION EVALUATION
- ANTERIOR GUIDANCE EVALUATION
  - Amount of overjet and overbite
  - Posterior sector disocclusion
  - Working-nonworking interferences
- PARAFUNCTIONS
  - Clenching
  - Bruxism

> Fig 1-1l

> Fig 1-1m

> Fig 1-1n

> Fig 1-1o

> Fig 1-1p

> Fig 1-1q

> Fig 1-1r

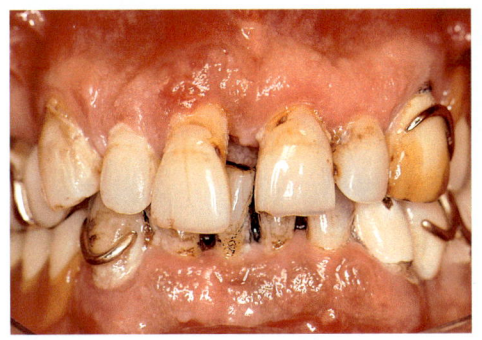

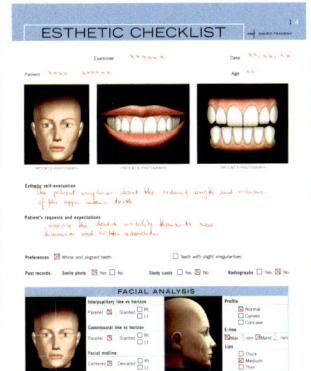

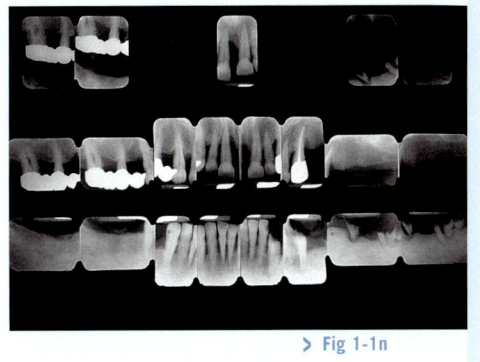

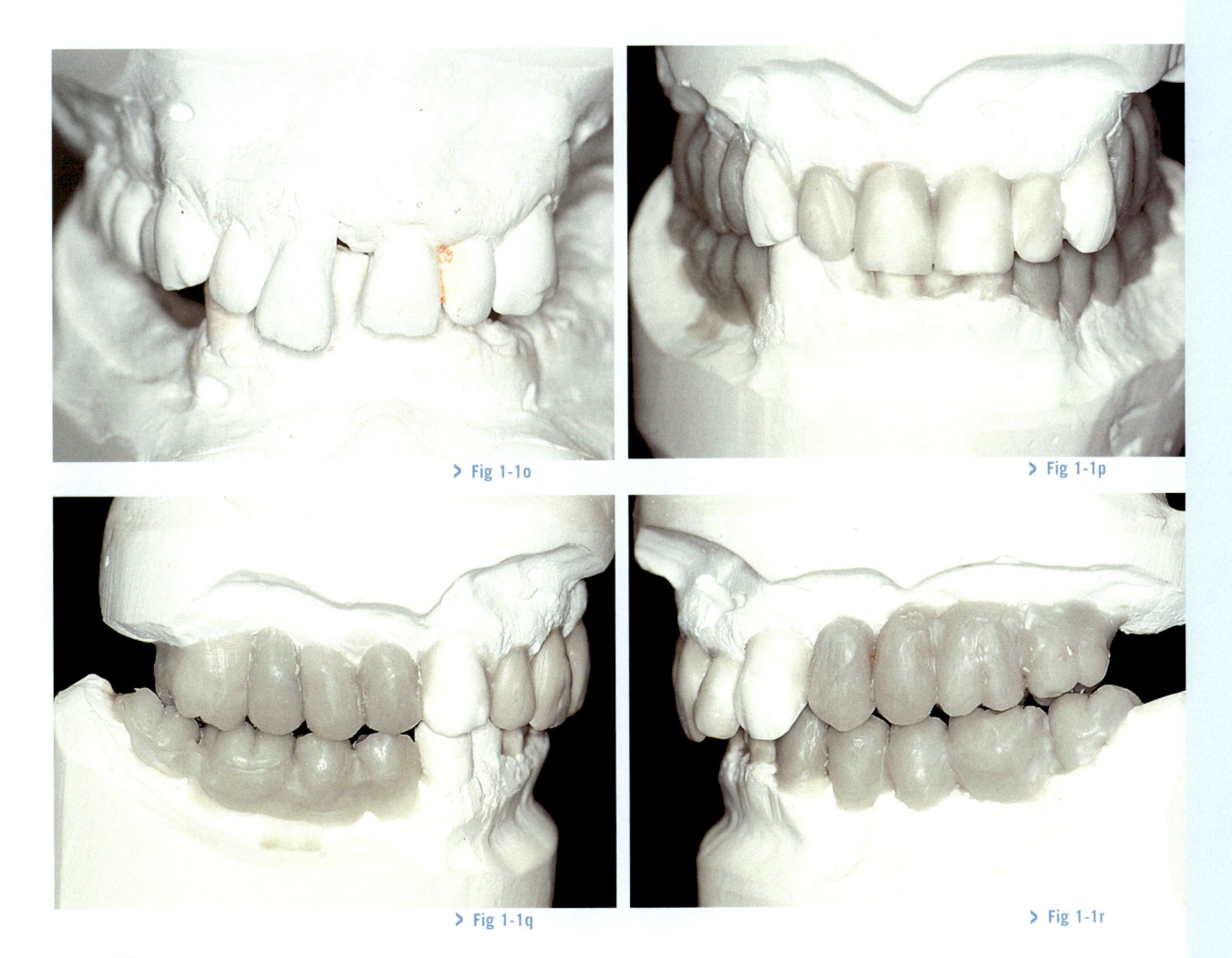

FIG 1 *(l to n)* The clinical examination, accompanied by the completed esthetic checklist and a full-mouth radiographic series, allows the clinician to formulate an accurate diagnosis.

FIG 1 *(o to r)* The stone casts mounted on the articulator show the patient's initial situation. Note the increased gap between the anterior teeth and the significant loss of VDO. The indications provided by the clinic allowed the technician to reproduce in the diagnostic wax-up the necessary increase in VDO and a correct occlusal relationship in the posterior sectors as well as in the anterior ones.

TREATMENT PLAN—PROGNOSIS

Based on the formulated diagnosis, an adequate treatment plan with the relative prognosis must be drawn up. Before any therapy is initiated, the pulpal vitality of the teeth to be used as prosthetic abutments needs to be analyzed by assessment of their response to heat and electrical stimuli. Any teeth whose pulpal health seems dubious should be treated endodontically. If the use of endodontic posts is necessary for reconstruction purposes, teeth that are already devitalized should be re-treated endodontically to guarantee an optimal apical seal, even though no periapical lesions may be noted on the radiographs. For the purposes of a good prognosis, an adequate ferrule (> 1.5) is necessary to minimize the risk of fracturing the prosthetic abutment.[20–25]

It has been suggested that when a fixed partial denture is planned, the root surface area of the potential abutment teeth should be evaluated to ensure that it is not less than that of the missing teeth (Ante's Law).[26–29] This concept has been questioned, however, by several authors[30–32] who have demonstrated that teeth with extremely low periodontal support are able to support fixed prostheses, guaranteeing a good long-term prognosis for the prosthetic rehabilitation.

As shown in these cases, the most important factor is meticulous control of plaque and the correct occlusal design of the prosthesis.[33,34] The prognosis can also be affected by other factors of a more general nature. For example, the onset of periodontal disease will lead to a decidedly less favorable prognosis in a young patient than in an adult patient, just as patients with uncontrolled diabetes are more prone to develop periodontal and implant problems than healthy patients.[35] Whether or not an individual smokes can also influence the success or the prognosis of a rehabilitation, especially in implant cases.[36–42] Other determining factors are the motivation of patients to maintain hygiene at home and the consistency with which they attend periodic professional oral hygiene sessions, both before (Figs 1-1s and 1-1t) and after the periodontal surgical and implant therapy[43–48] (Figs 1-1u to 1-1y).

Worn facets or even more significant tooth abrasions hint at an elevated muscle tone, which is concrete evidence that the prosthetic work will be at risk. To decrease any parafunctional activity or excessive activity of the masticatory muscles, it is a good idea to have the patient wear an occlusal device before starting treatment.[49,50] A similar device worn upon completion of the work will help safeguard the integrity of the restorations.

> Fig 1-1s

> Fig 1-1t

> Fig 1-1u

> Fig 1-1v

> Fig 1-1w

> Fig 1-1x

> Fig 1-1y

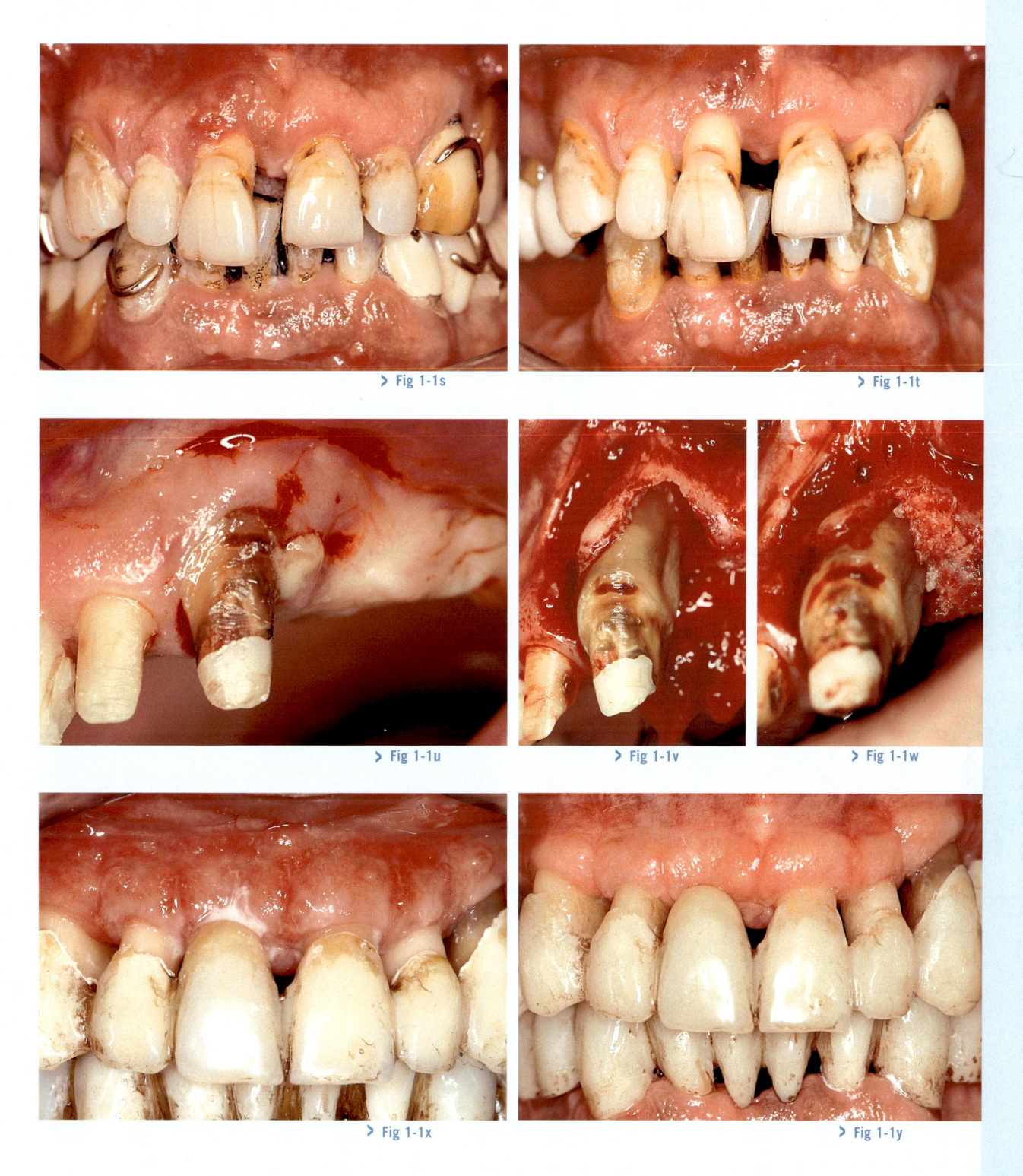

FIG 1 *(s and t)* The patient, a heavy smoker, underwent numerous oral hygiene sessions in the office and was motivated to achieve correct hygienic maintenance at home before embarking upon the periodontal surgery. The discharge of purulent exudate from the left maxillary canine is related to the deep periodontal pocket. *(v)* During surgery, in addition to positioning implants in the posterior sectors, etiologic therapy was carried out on the distal aspect of the root of the left maxillary canine, where a large infraosseous defect is evident. *(w)* Following careful debridement, the defect was filled with autogenous particulated bone taken from the implant site using a bone-cutting forceps. (Surgery by Dr Stefano Parma Benfenati.) The provisional restorations, fitted prior to periodontal surgery, allow the remaining teeth to be stabilized and the occlusal trauma in the postoperative phase to be controlled. *(x and y)* The photographs, taken 2 weeks and 8 weeks after resective surgery, show a gradual healing of the soft tissues. However, a longer period (6 to 9 months) must elapse to allow complete tissue maturation before the final prosthetic phases are begun.

NATURAL TEETH OR IMPLANTS AS PROSTHETIC ABUTMENTS

REPLACING INDIVIDUAL TEETH

It is sometimes possible to replace a single tooth by anchoring it to just one prosthetic abutment with a cantilever in place of the traditional three-element fixed partial denture. This solution does not offer a very favorable prognosis, however, especially in the posterior sectors and in the presence of devitalized teeth.[51-53] Today, the clinician and patient are more inclined to adopt a more conservative implant-prosthetic solution rather than use a traditional fixed prosthesis involving natural teeth that often do not require restoration. However, despite the development of implants and ever-more-advanced techniques, achieving an optimal esthetic result remains difficult to predict, especially in the anterior sector. (see chapter 2, pages 240–265 and chapter 3, pages 352–365).

REPLACING TWO OR MORE TEETH

In cases where there are large edentulous spaces, the use of traditional fixed partial dentures with numerous pontic elements on natural teeth does not offer a satisfactory prognosis.[54] In the posterior sectors, moreover, preserving the natural abutments can sometimes be particularly problematic due to the loss of periodontal support that often leads to involvement of the interradicular areas in the molars. The resective surgical-periodontal therapy required in these cases can necessitate root amputation and result in the presence of hemisections. A prosthodontic-periodontal approach is possible provided that the preserved roots have primary stability, adequate residual support (> 50%), minimal probing depth (3 mm), and a reduced extension of the edentulous area.[55] In the posterior sectors, implant therapy may be the easiest solution. Implantology has substantially altered the prosthetic treatment plan, considerably improving the risk-benefit ratio in many clinical situations.[43-48] The tendency therefore is to replace each missing tooth with an implant, a solution that can produce a more favorable prognosis in large edentulous areas (Figs 1-1z to 1-1ee and 1-1ff to 1-1ll). Nevertheless, some authors[56,57] point out that patients who have undergone tooth extractions due to periodontal disease are more prone to bone loss around the implants and therefore more frequently experience implant failure. In patients whose loss of dentition is the result of large caries lesions, however, treatment with implants has a decidedly more favorable prognosis, indicating that carioreceptivity, unlike periodontal disease, does not affect so-called artificial roots. The choice to treat with implants and the length of the implants used also prove to be strongly influenced by anatomic structures such as the maxillary sinus above and the mandibular canal below. It should also be emphasized that, proceeding toward the posterior regions of the mouth, the implants are subjected to greater occlusal forces because of their proximity to the TMJs. These forces can lead to failure of the prosthetic components. In the posterior sectors, the bone is both qualitatively and quantitatively less suitable for implant positioning.[58] If it is not possible to position implants

> Fig 1-1z

> Fig 1-1aa

> Fig 1-1bb

> Fig 1-1cc

> Fig 1-1dd

> Fig 1-1ee

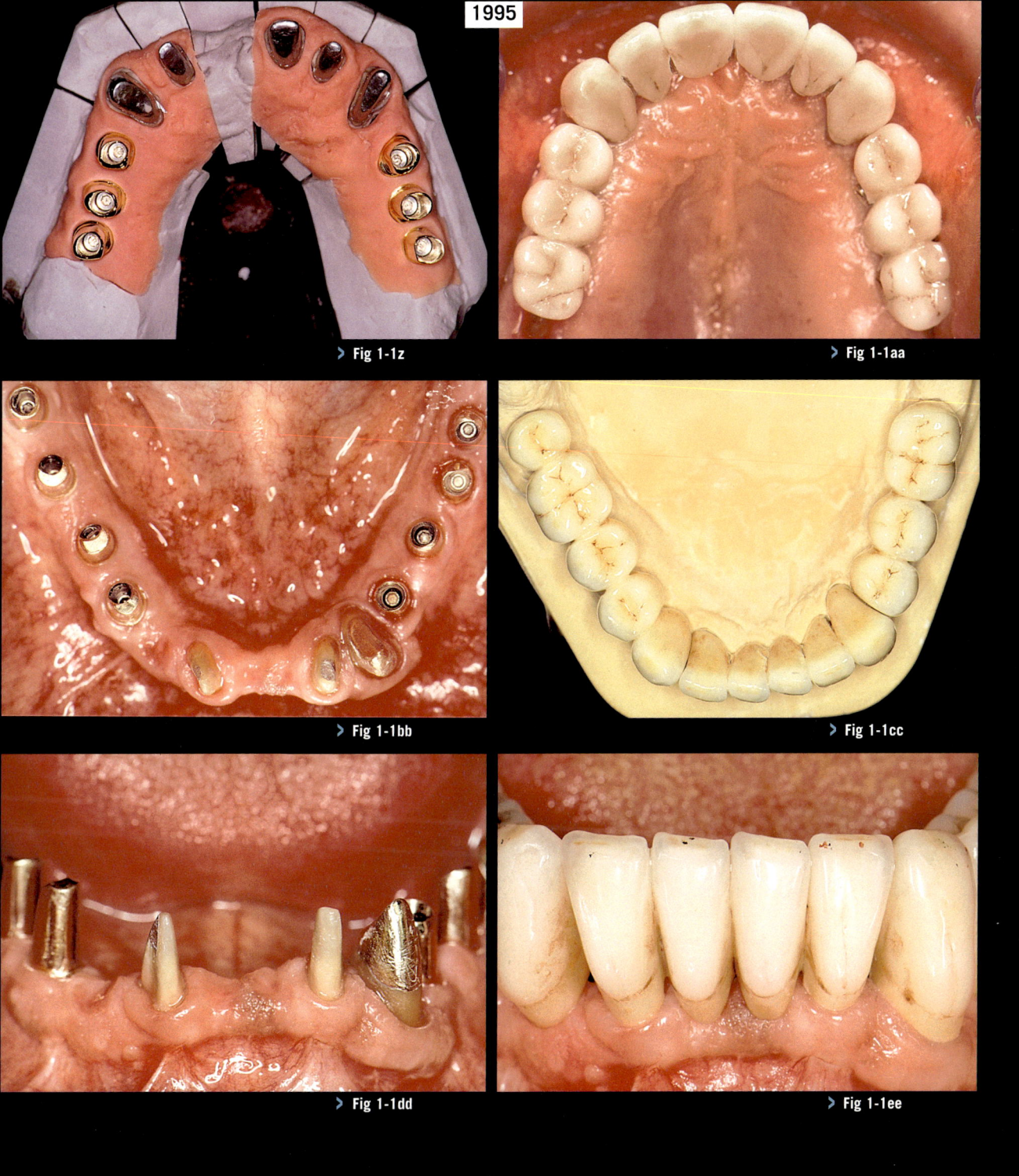

FIG 1 *(z)* The occlusal view of the maxillary cast shows six implants in the posterior sectors and five natural abutments preserved in the anterior sector. *(aa)* In the maxillary arch, the case was finalized by creating an anterior fixed partial denture from one canine to the other on natural teeth, while in the posterior sectors two fixed partial dentures were anchored to implants. *(bb and cc)* In the mandibular arch, due to the placement of implants in the posterior sectors and the preservation of specific natural teeth, it was possible to divide the prosthetic rehabilitation into three parts: two posterior fixed partial dentures on implants and one anterior fixed partial denture on natural teeth. *(dd and ee)* A comparison between the photograph of the natural teeth and the implant abutments and the photograph of the definitive restorations shows that satisfactory esthetic and biologic integration have been achieved.

in the molar region, and there are no natural abutments in this area, shortening the dental arches to the second premolars, though not the ideal solution, does not seem to significantly compromise masticatory capacity[59–61] or function in most patients.[62–65] Nevertheless, the absence of molars—and even the absence of contacts in the posterior area when teeth are present—tends to excessively stress the TMJs[66] and the remaining teeth, thus representing a risk to the entire stomatognathic system. The use of a removable denture, aimed at restoring the occlusal scheme up to the molars, does not seem to be an ideal solution for guaranteeing either adequate occlusal stability or the comfort of the patient.[67–69]

APPROACH WITH THE PATIENT

In creating the treatment plan, the clinician must consider the esthetic and functional needs of the patient and try to comply with requests that are not prohibited by therapeutic contraindications or technical limitations. In most cases the patient does not actually realize how many and which operative phases will be necessary and tends to underestimate the professional commitment required. Although the patient may take the prosthetic treatment for granted, success often can be achieved only by means of a multidisciplinary approach involving the combined efforts of several specialists. It is necessary to point out to the patient the array of different therapeutic options and, where possible, to adapt these not just to specific requests but also to the patient's general condition, psychologic profile, and financial capabilities. Once the ideal therapeutic approach for the patient is established, it is the clinician's duty to clarify every detail of the treatment, while attempting to earn the patient's complete confidence, before embarking upon any operational phase.

OPERATIONAL SEQUENCE

Once the patient understands the treatment plan and has accepted the estimated cost, it is the task of the dental team to schedule and explain the therapeutic sequence and the likely duration of the appointments. Efficient session organization and meticulous respect for the patient are fundamental, especially in complex prosthetic cases that require a multidisciplinary approach. In order to avoid prolonging the operating times unnecessarily, a good chronologic sequence of appointments allows the clinician to monitor the patient and assess healing and maturation of the gingival tissues in cases where periodontal or implant surgery are involved. At the same time, it is necessary to ensure that the patient carefully follows the oral hygiene techniques at home and endeavors to attend periodic professional oral hygiene sessions, which are indispensable for guaranteeing long-term maintenance of the case.

DIAGNOSIS

- **MEDICAL CASE HISTORY**

- **DENTAL CASE HISTORY**
  - Restorative case history
  - Endodontic case history
  - Orthodontic case history
  - Periodontal case history
  - Craniofacial case history

- **EXTRAORAL CLINICAL EXAMINATION**
  - Facial analysis
  - Dentolabial analysis
  - Phonetic analysis
  - Craniofacial evaluation

- **INTRAORAL CLINICAL EXAMINATION**
  - Tooth structure evaluation
  - Orthodontic evaluation
  - Periodontal evaluation
  - Occlusal evaluation

- **RADIOGRAPHIC EXAMINATION**
  - FMS – orthopantomography – CAT – arthrography

- **STONE CASTS**
  - Mounting on articulator

TREATMENT PLAN

- **MULTIDISCIPLINARY EVALUATION** (endodontics, restorative, orthodontics, periodontics, implantology)

- **COMMUNICATION WITH THE PATIENT**

- **OPERATIONAL SEQUENCE**

- **COMMUNICATION WITH THE LABORATORY**

OPERATIONAL SEQUENCE

- Facebow
- Occlusal registrations
- Stone casts mounted on the articulator
  - Diagnostic wax-up → **CH 1**

- Fabrication and integration of provisional restorations
- Any collateral therapies
  (endodontics, reconstructive, orthodontics, periodontology, implantology) → **CH 2**

- Clinical and radiographic re-evaluation
- Choice of restorative material
- Preparations and final impressions → **CH 3**

- Transfer of esthetic-functional information to the laboratory → from provisional to definitive restoration → **CH 4**

- Preventive simulation → biscuit try-in → finalization
- Restorative techniques and ceramic materials → **CH 5**

> Fig 1-1ff

> Fig 1-1gg

> Fig 1-1hh

> Fig 1-1ii

> Fig 1-1jj

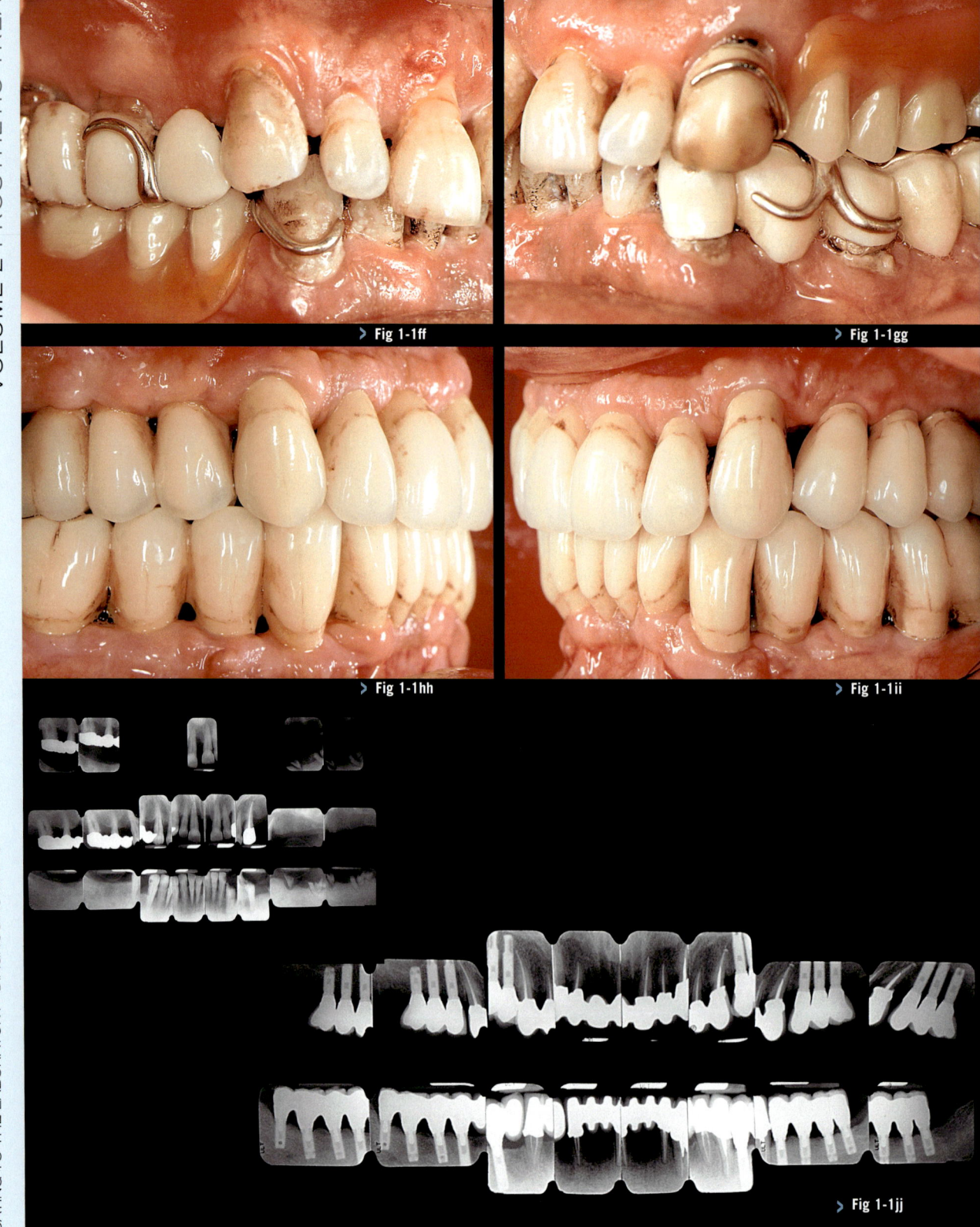

FIG 1 *(ff to ii)* The initial and final intraoral photographs demonstrate the considerable esthetic and functional improvements and the good overall integration achieved on both the natural teeth and the implants. *(jj)* The full-mouth series at the end of treatment, compared with that from the start, shows the success of the treatment carried out. *(kk)* A comparison between the patient's before and after treatment smiles underlines the pleasing harmony achieved. *(ll)* The prosthetic rehabilitation appears to be satisfactorily completed, from the esthetic as well as the biologic and functional viewpoints.

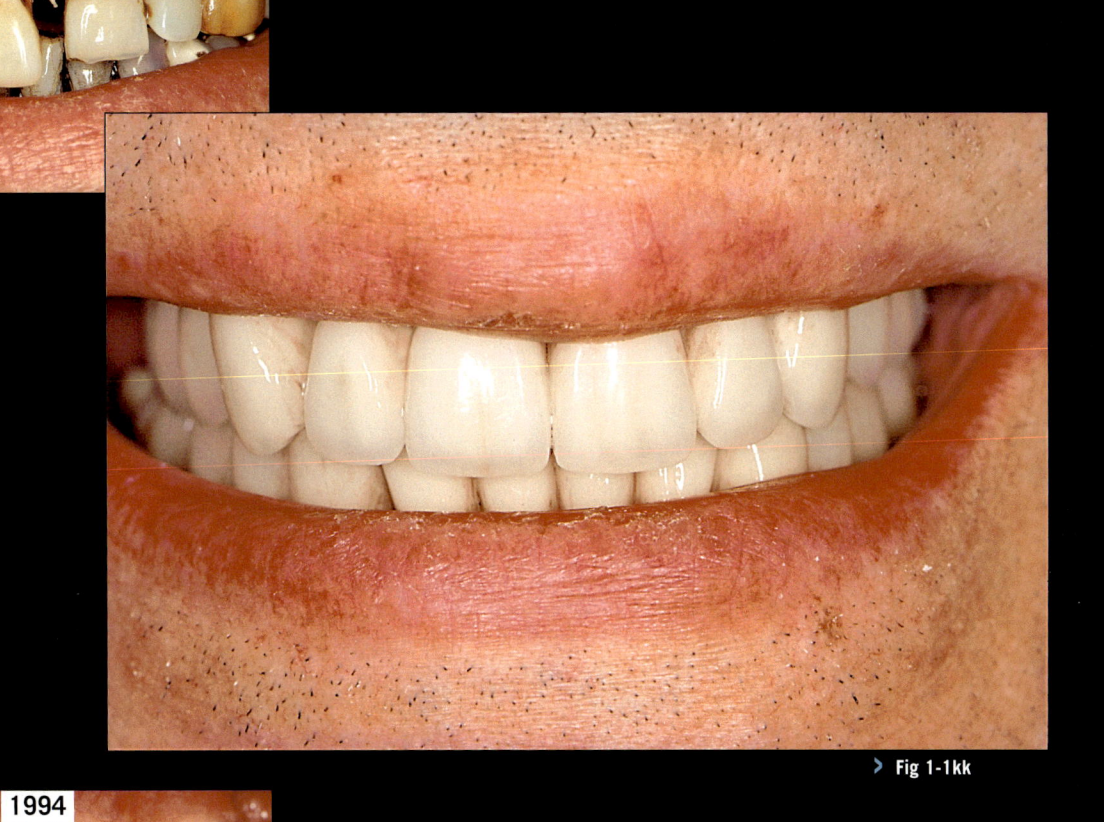

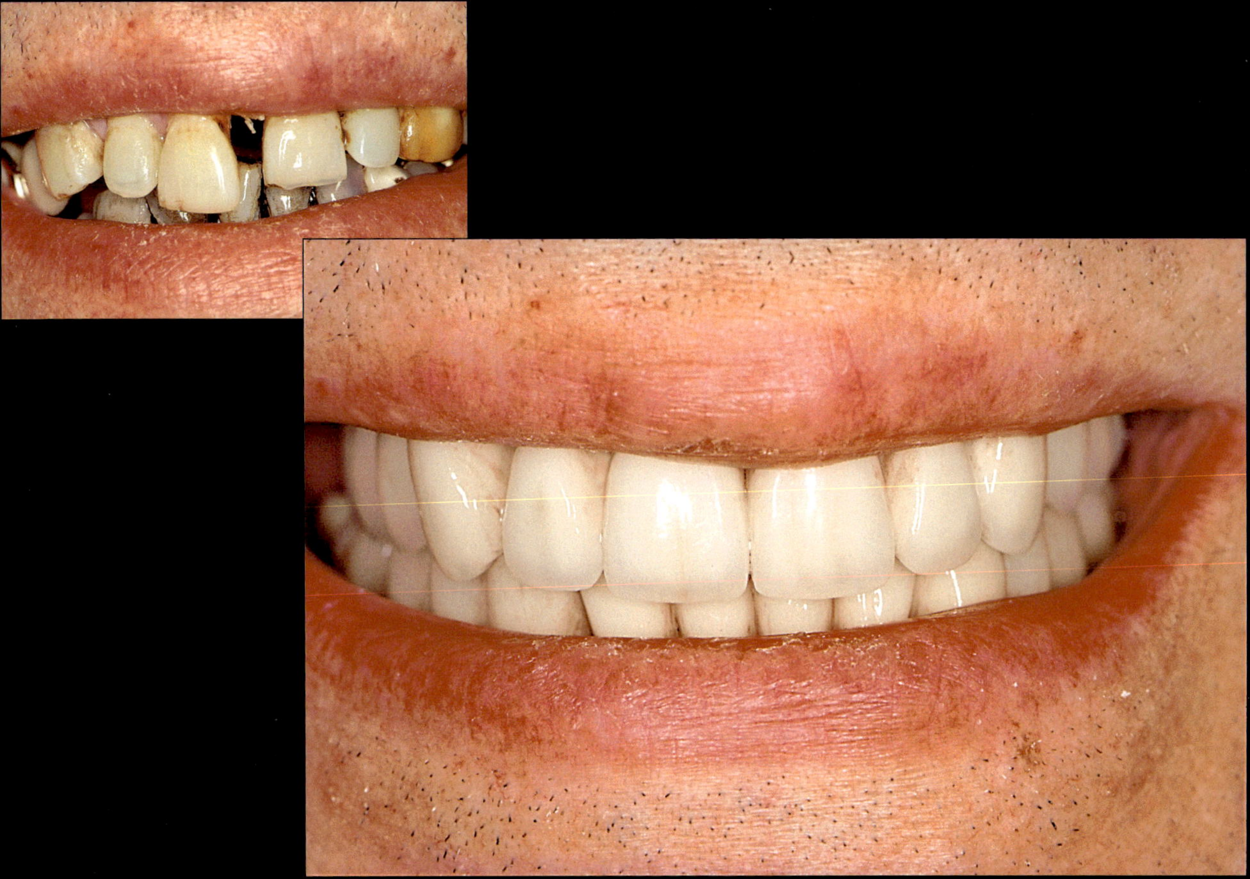

1994

1995

> Fig 1-1kk

> Fig 1-1ll

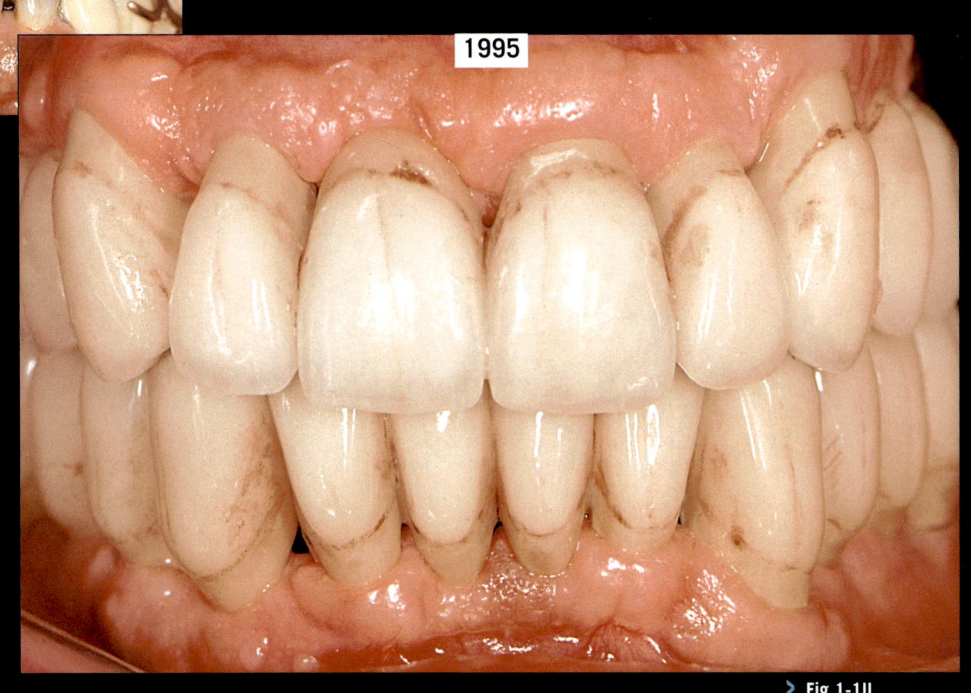

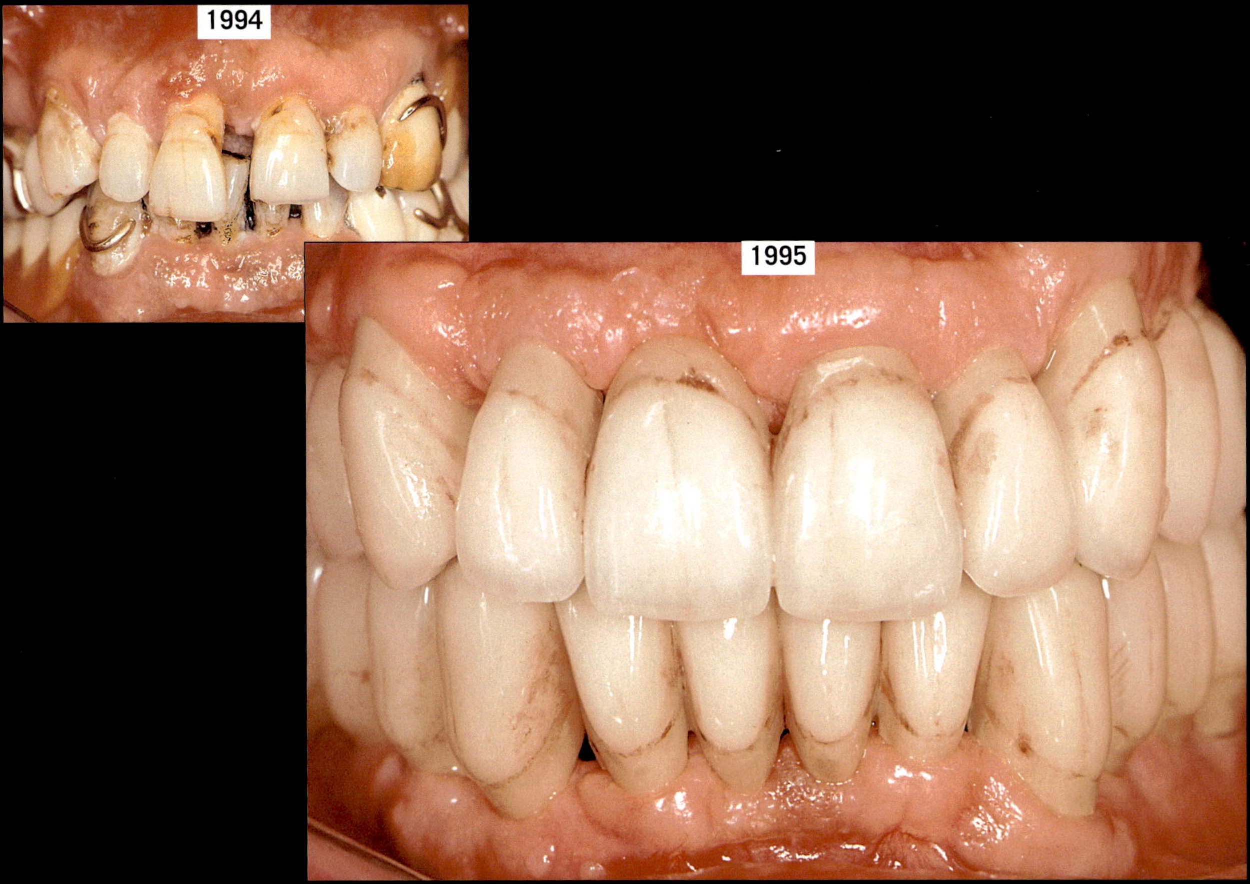

ANTERIOR REHABILITATION
ESTHETIC PREVIEW

DIAGNOSTIC SUPPORT

After the esthetic checklist (Figs 1-2a to 1-2d) has been completed and before any irreversible operative phase (eg, tooth preparations) have been started, it is useful to ask the technician for a diagnostic wax-up and casts derived from it to clinically verify the validity of the planned changes to tooth position and length in the anterior region. Even more immediate, for diagnostic purposes, is the need for preview techniques such as applying composite material (direct mockup) or creating an acrylic resin shell (indirect mockup). Apart from giving the patient the opportunity to see the final esthetic result in advance and thus better comprehend the treatment goals, these techniques give the clinician an important diagnostic confirmation before the final treatment plan is made and the operating methods are established. Computerized imaging representing the possible restorative solutions can also be used along with an explanation to the patient that the clinical outcome may not always correspond exactly.

DIRECT MOCKUP

In cases where anterior teeth must be increased in size or length, or positioned more buccally, a direct mockup can be used. This additive technique makes use of composites added to the surfaces of the involved teeth[70,71] (Figs 1-2e to 1-2m). The clinician adds composite coarsely and then quickly molds and refines it with a bur, taking care not to interfere with the underlying tooth structure. It is not bonded in order to ensure easy removal.

Though the technique applies only to cases involving an increase in size, the direct mockup offers clinicians a quick and effective means of giving the patient an immediate idea of the proposed changes to tooth length and position.

Once the patient has agreed to the proposed changes, an impression of the direct mockup is made before the composite is removed. From this impression, a cast can be made to transfer information to the technician. This cast will then be used to create a correct wax-up for construction of the provisional restoration.

Chapter 1 COMMUNICATING TO THE LABORATORY—DIAGNOSTIC WAX-UP

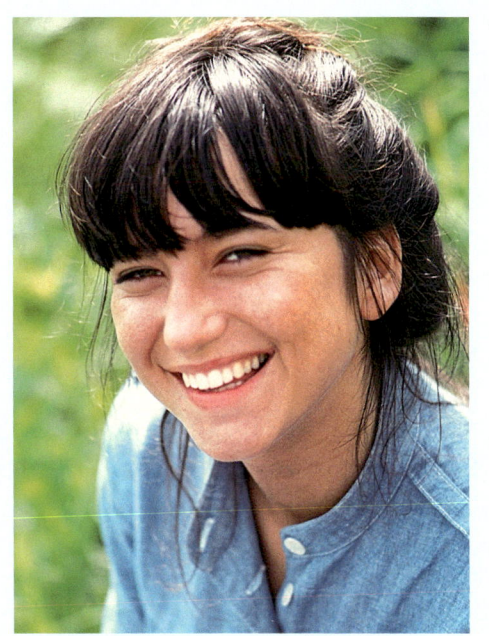

> Fig 1-2a

> Fig 1-2b

> Fig 1-2c

> Fig 1-2d

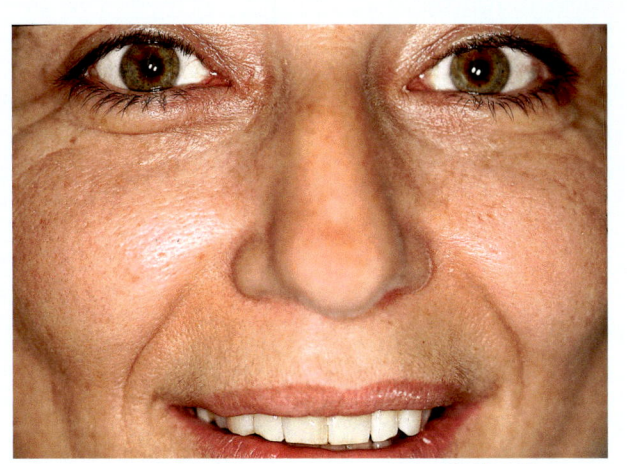

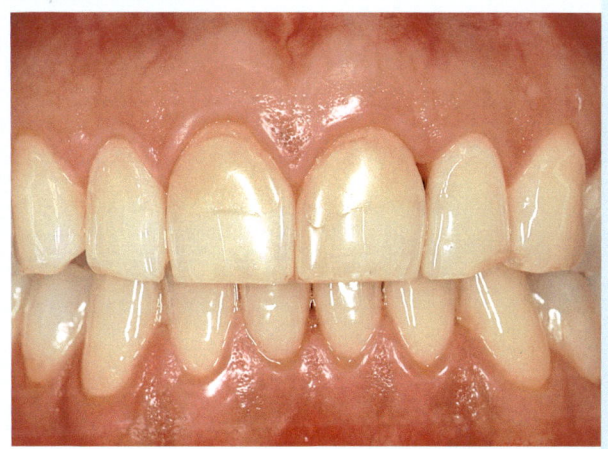

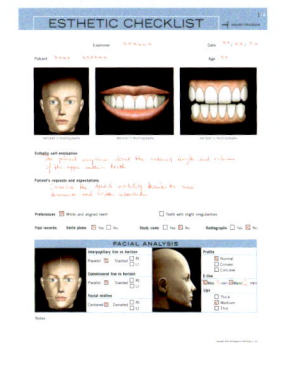

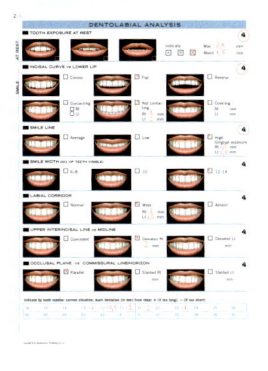

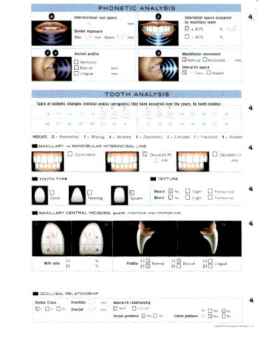

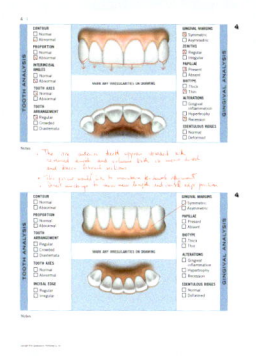

FIG 2 *(a)* At her first visit, the patient showed a photograph from years earlier in which the esthetic harmony of her smile is obvious. *(b and c)* She requested restorative treatment after dental abrasion had compromised the esthetic appearance of her smile by reducing the length and volume of her anterior teeth. *(d)* All parts of the esthetic checklist were filled in to provide the clinician with sufficient information to assess the modifications needed in terms of esthetic appearance.

> Fig 1-2e

> Fig 1-2f

> Fig 1-2g

> Fig 1-2h

> Fig 1-2i

> Fig 1-2j

> Fig 1-2k

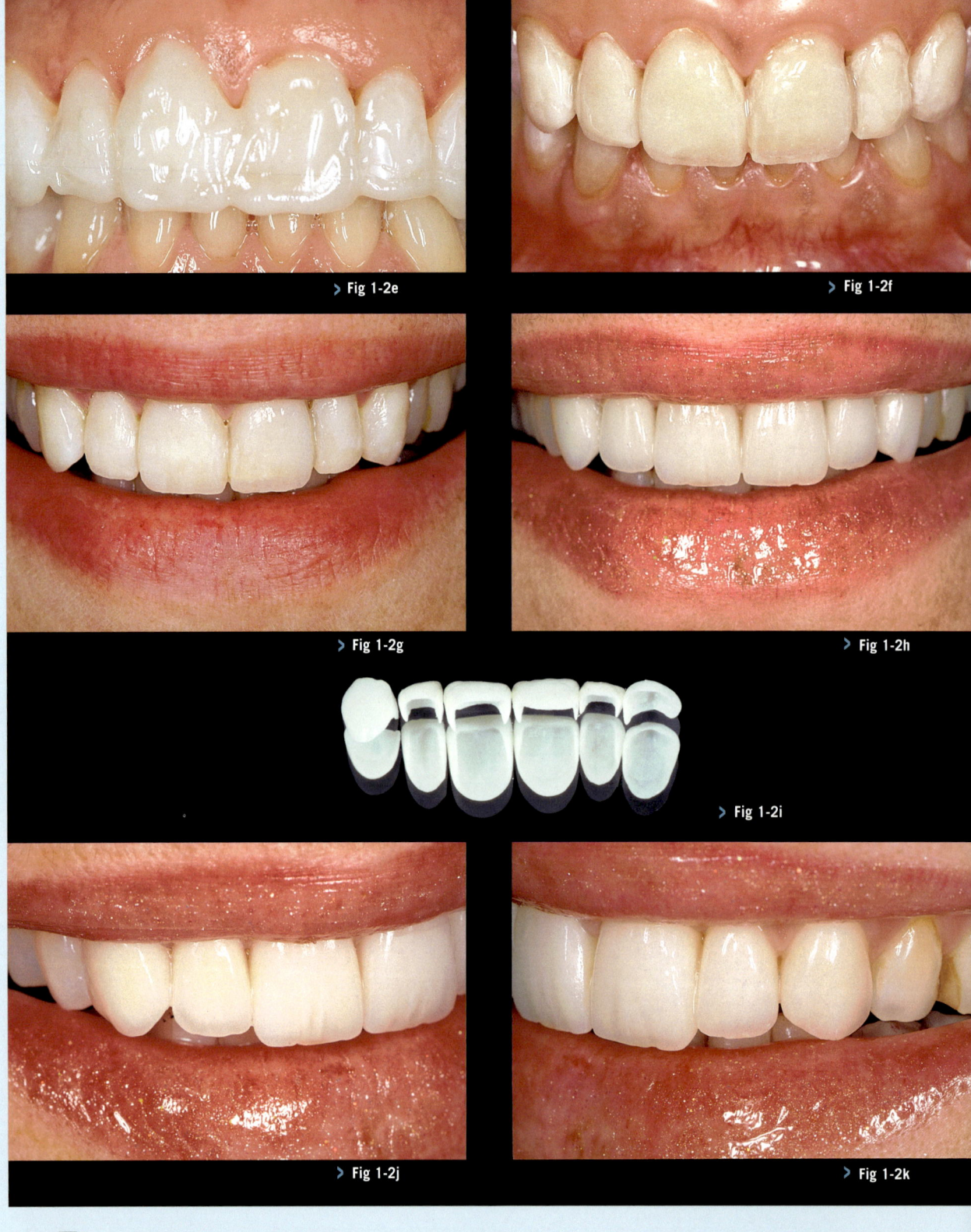

FIG 2 *(e and f)* Even at the first visit, composite was roughly applied to the abraded teeth (direct mockup) and then refined with burs to quickly reach the required tooth shape and length. This gave the patient a tangible idea of the proposed modifications. *(g to i)* After patient consent was obtained, the modifications previewed in the direct mockup were faithfully reproduced in the definitive work with six ceramic veneers. *(j and k)* Upon closer view of the restorations, greater dentolabial harmony can also be seen.

> Fig 1-2l

> Fig 1-2m

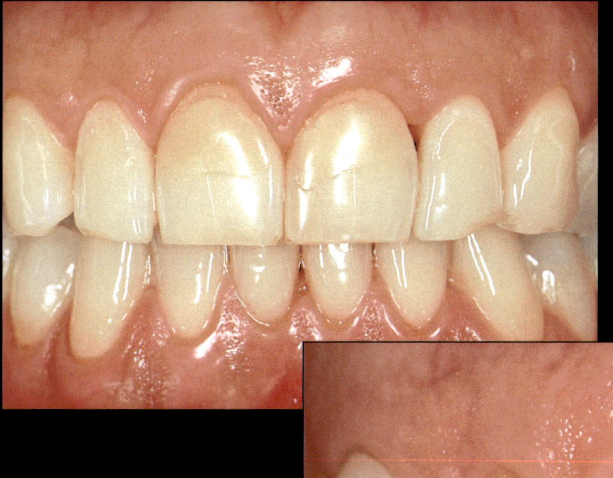

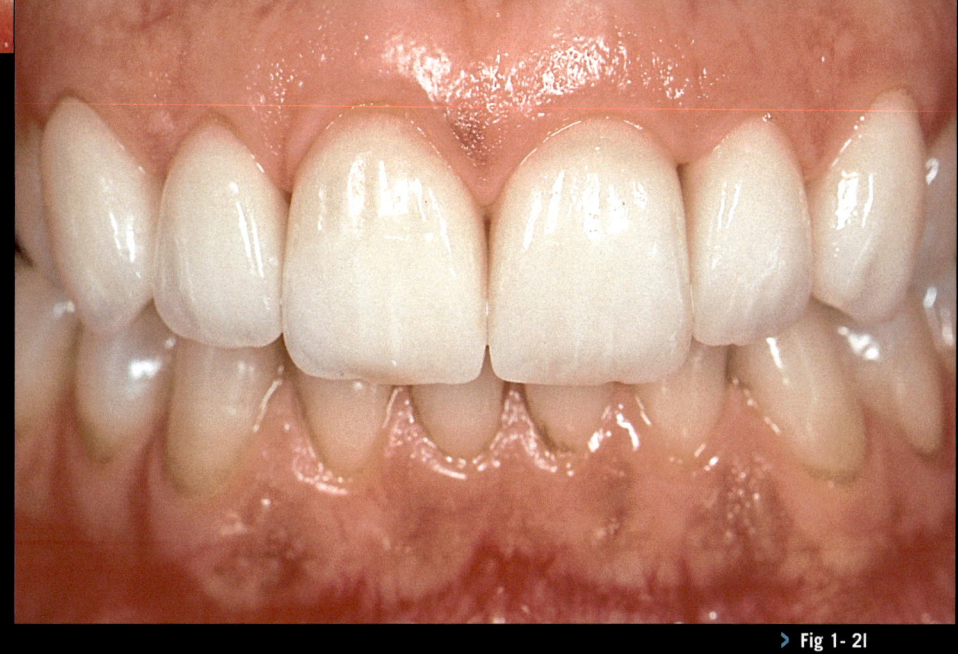

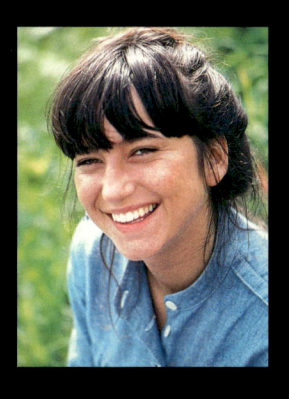

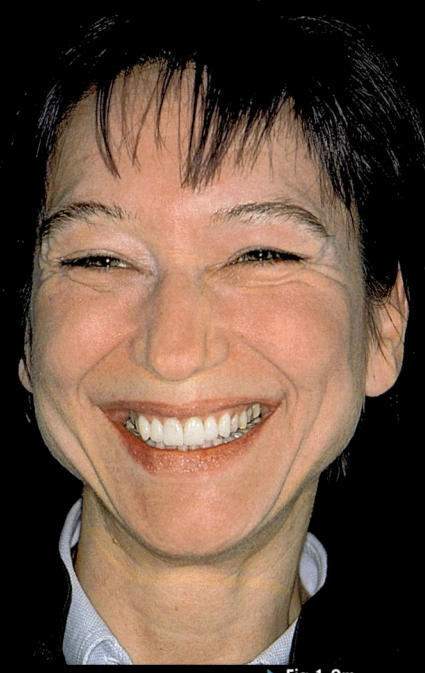

FIG 2 *(l and m)* The treatment made a significant esthetic improvement, giving the patient a pleasing smile once again by means of restored tooth lengths and more congruous proportions between consecutive teeth.

INDIRECT MOCKUP

Like the direct mockup, the indirect mockup is an additive rather than an invasive technique that can prove very useful for diagnostic purposes. It has the single disadvantage, however, of having to be made in the laboratory, with the inevitable additional costs and time involved. Once the technician has completed the diagnostic wax-up based on the clinical information (Figs 1-3a and 1-3b), a stone cast is made (Fig 1-3c). From this cast, a silicone matrix is then created, which can be positioned over the original cast for producing an acrylic resin (indirect) mockup (Figs 1-3d and 1-3e). An acetate matrix can also be molded on the stone cast of the wax-up; representing the ideal volume of the restoration, this transparent matrix proves useful for calculating the thicknesses of the tooth preparations (Figs 1-3f and 1-3g). If necessary, this index can also be used to create a direct mockup by the simple insertion of self-curing or light-curing resin composite.

Like the direct mockup, the indirect mockup technique can be used in cases that involve an increase in dental volume, and it can be created without damaging the underlying teeth. The indirect mockup is easily positioned in the mouth and, despite its inevitable slight oversizing, is invaluable for testing out the esthetic results of the planned treatment before any irreversible procedures are initiated[64,65] (Figs 1-3h to 1-3m).

Any further variations to be made are discussed with the patient to ensure that his or her expectations coincide with possible outcomes. The changes reproduced in the mockup may not meet with the immediate approval of the patient or, even more likely, with that of friends or family. This is especially true for patients who have severely abraded anterior teeth that wore away gradually over time, or for patients who have diastemata dating back to adolescence. If the prosthetic treatment goes ahead, the suitably lined and finished acrylic resin mockup can be used as a provisional restoration.

FIG 3 *(a and b)* The patient had a substantial gap between the maxillary anterior teeth and unattractive tooth shapes, which can also be seen in the preoperative plaster casts. *(c)* The casts derived from the diagnostic wax-up show a considerable esthetic improvement in the anterior tooth composition. *(d and e)* The indirect mockup, fabricated in the laboratory on the original stone cast from a silicone index derived from the plaster cast of the wax-up, reproduces the increase in tooth volume and length made by the technician on the diagnostic wax-up. *(f and g)* An acetate matrix can also be fabricated on the cast of the diagnostic wax-up to reproduce the tooth shape and position exactly. When positioned over the patient's original cast, the transparent matrix makes it possible to evaluate the large space available to finalize the ceramic veneers. In this case, the tooth preparations were kept to a minimum, preserving an ideal amount of enamel for the adhesive cementation.

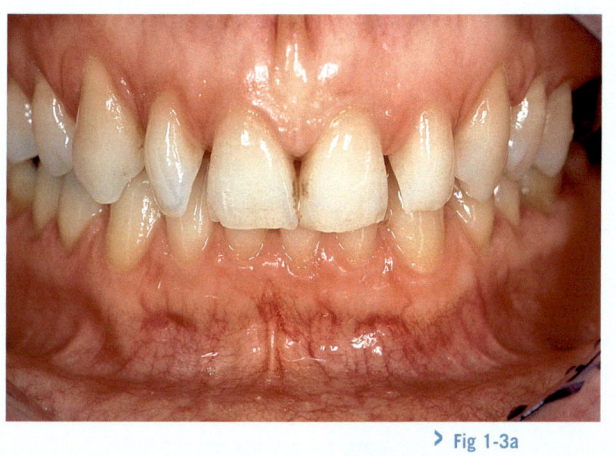

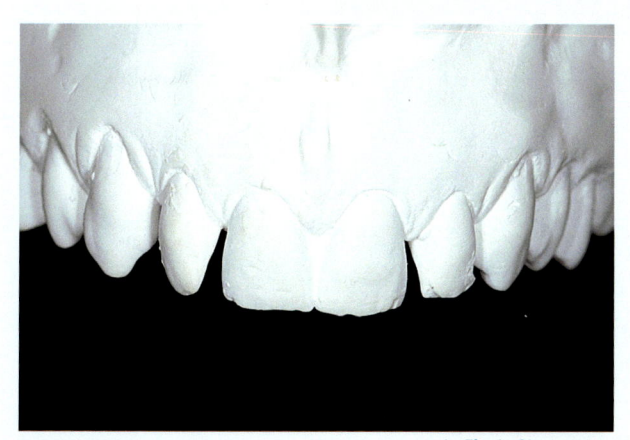

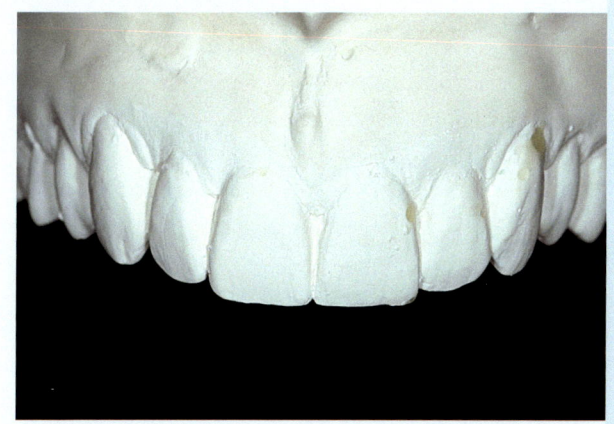

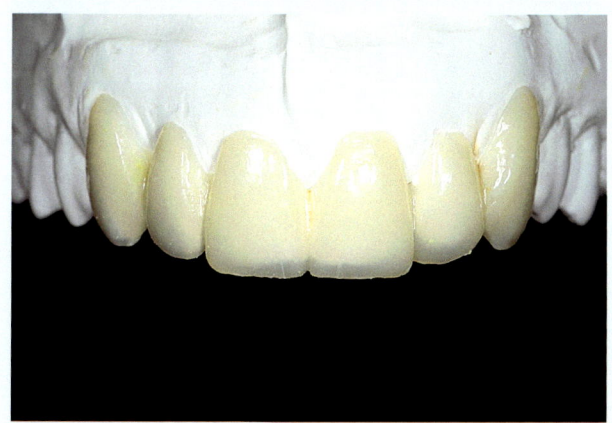

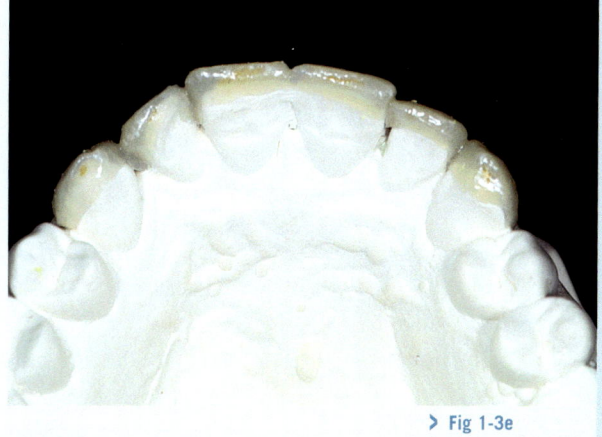

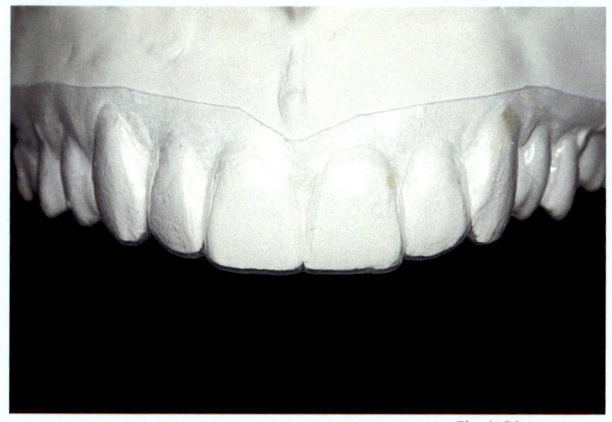

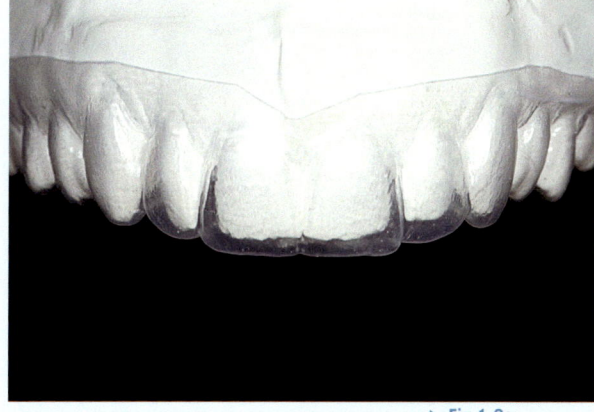

> Fig 1-3a

> Fig 1- 3b

> Fig 1-3c

> Fig 1-3d

> Fig 1-3e

> Fig 1-3f

> Fig 1-3g

> Fig 1-3h

> Fig 1-3i

> Fig 1-3j

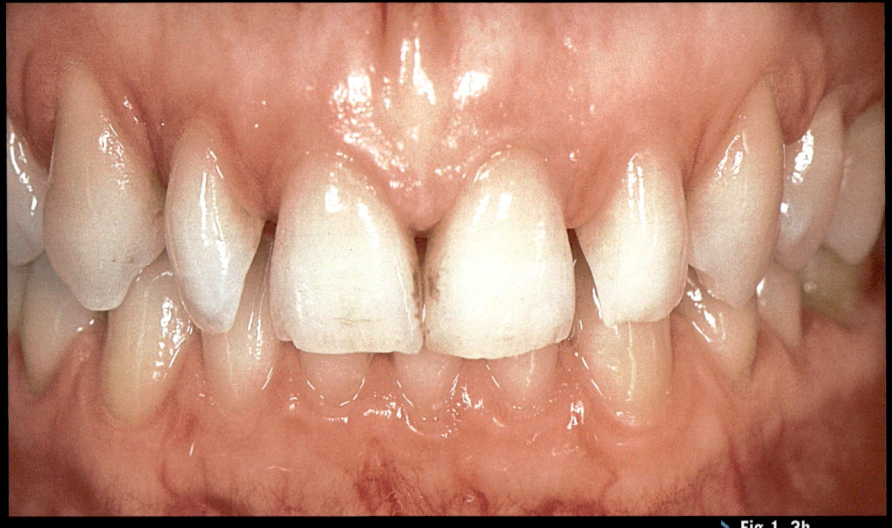

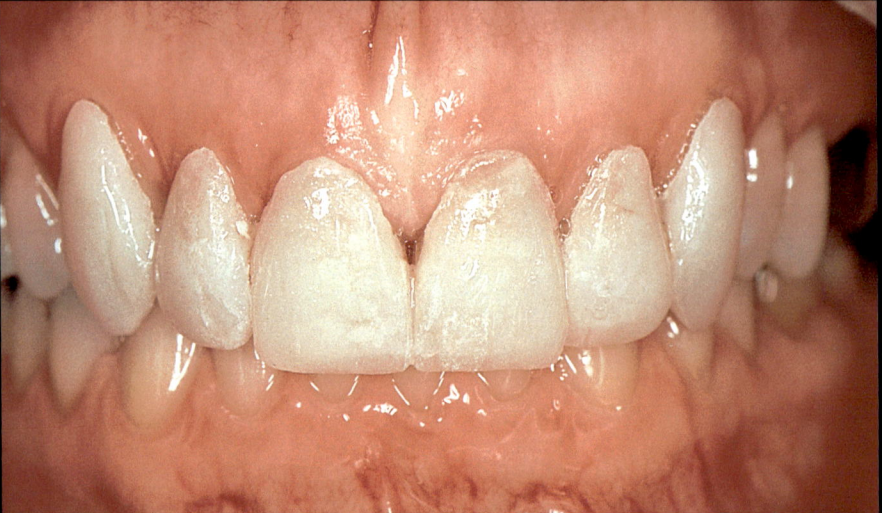

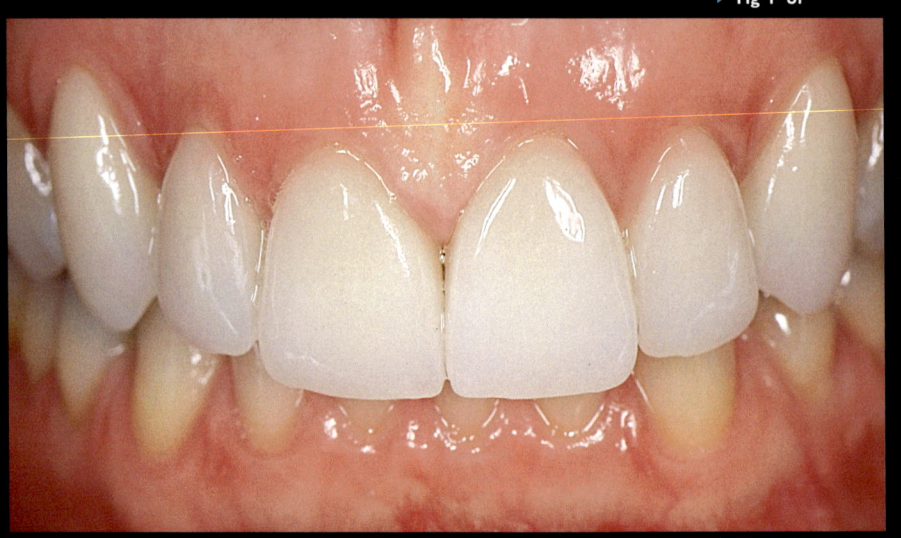

FIG 3 *(h to j)* A comparison between the original situation, the indirect mockup, and the six veneers after cementation shows the progression of changes and the confirmation of the initial plans from the mockup to the definitive work.

> Fig 1-3k

> Fig 1- 3l

> Fig 1-3m

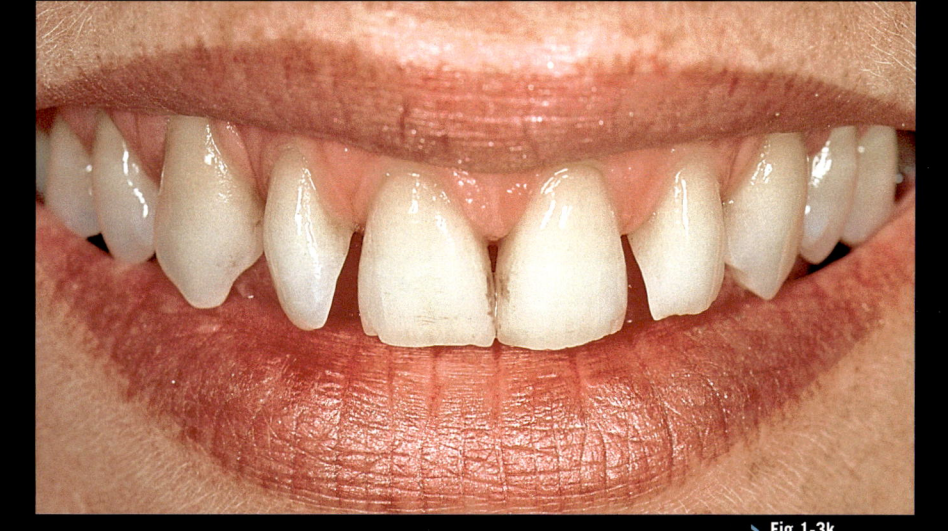

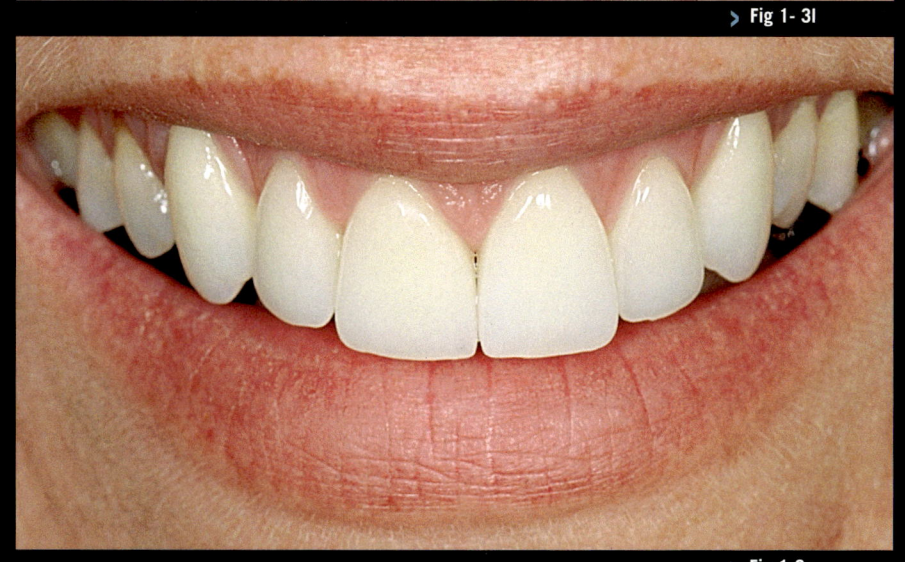

FIG 3 *(k and l)* The unsatisfactory esthetic appearance of the original smile was significantly improved right from the fitting of the indirect mockup. *(m)* After the six anterior veneers were cemented, the overall harmony can be appreciated.

EXTENSIVE REHABILITATION

■ TREATMENT PLAN ■
↓
DIAGNOSTIC WAX-UP

The following clinical case, illustrated step by step (Figs 1-4a to 1-4d), describes the essential phases leading to the diagnostic wax-up. The esthetic checklist (Fig 1-4e), followed by the laboratory checklist (Fig 1-4f), will assist the clinician and the technician along this path, based on the ideal data transfer from the dental clinic to the laboratory.

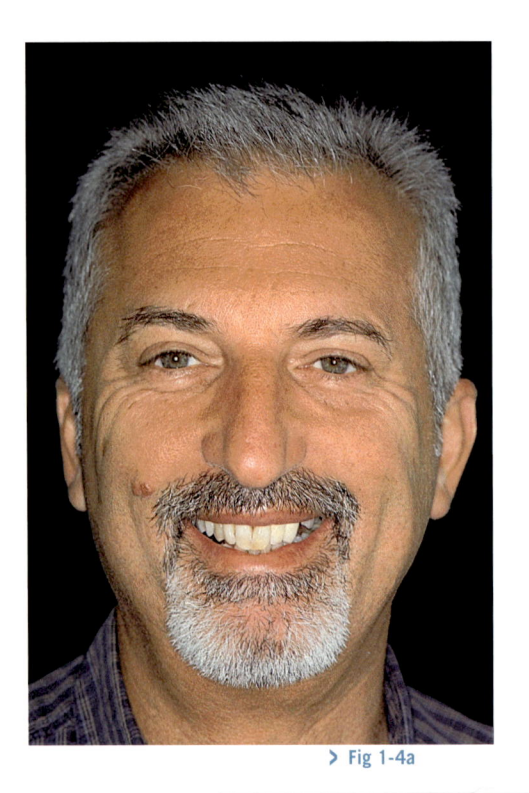

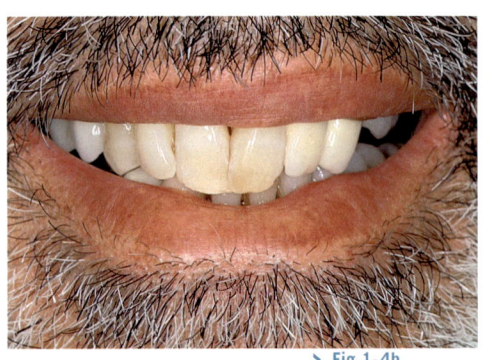

> Fig 1-4a

> Fig 1-4b

> Fig 1-4c

> Fig 1-4d

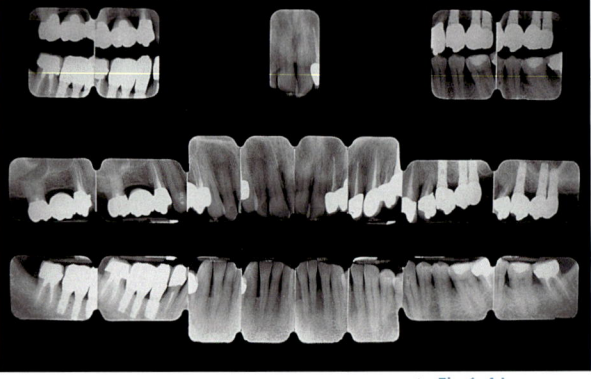

FIG 4 *(a)* The patient has an average smile line. *(b)* Apart from a recently extracted left maxillary first premolar, the patient complains that the two maxillary central incisors overlap and have excessive buccal positioning. *(c)* He would also like to reduce the length of the right mandibular canine and the discrepancy between the anterior mandibular teeth and the right mandibular quadrant. *(d)* The full-mouth radiographic series carried out 2 months earlier still shows the left maxillary first premolar, subsequently extracted by the referring dentist, as well as fixed prostheses on implants and natural dentition.

Chapter 1 COMMUNICATING TO THE LABORATORY—DIAGNOSTIC WAX-UP

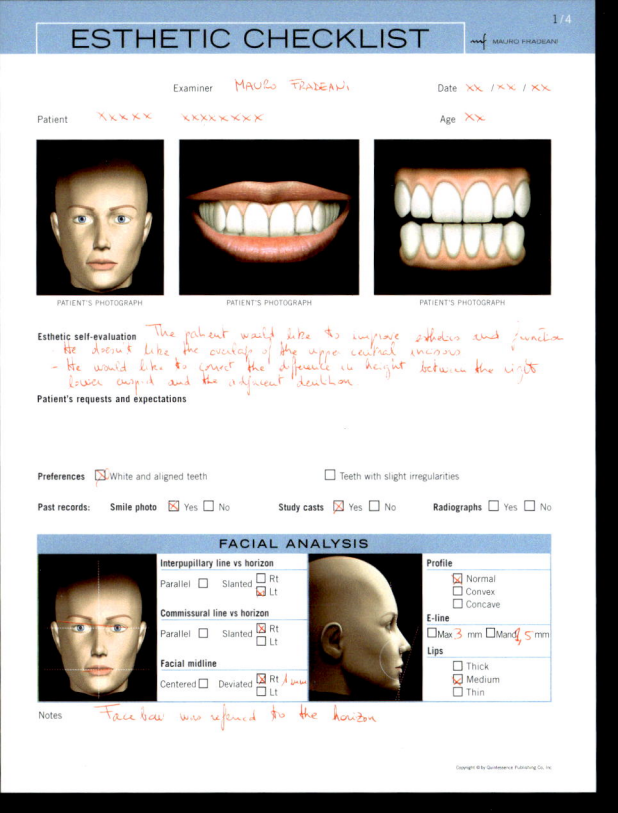

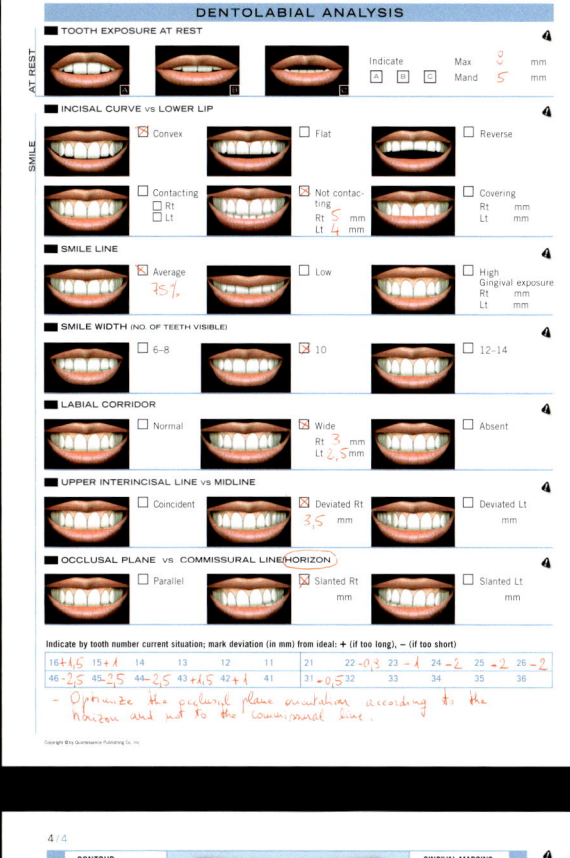

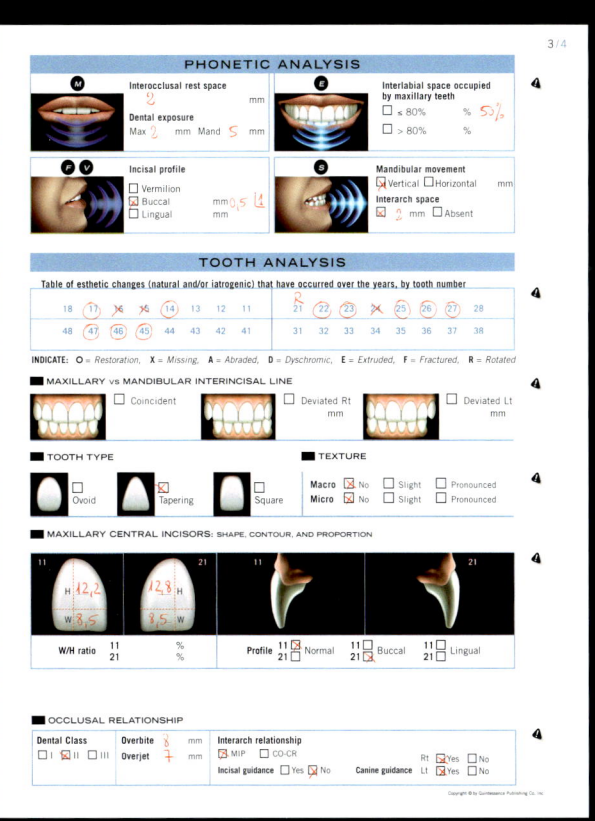

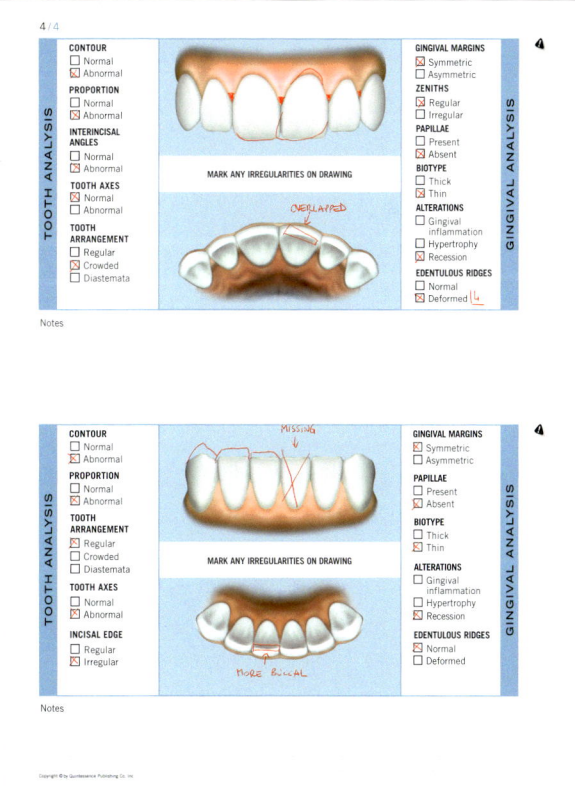

FIG 4 *(e)* All parts of the esthetic checklist are completed to provide the clinician with sufficient information to assess what modifications are necessary from esthetic and functional viewpoints.

LABORATORY CHECKLIST

After filling in the esthetic checklist, the clinician transfers to the technician, by means of an individualized laboratory checklist (Fig 1-4f), all of the esthetic and functional information for the creation of the diagnostic wax-up and subsequently the provisional restoration. The same form should carry a detailed description of any changes to shape and arrangement necessary in the anterior teeth and indicate to the laboratory the type of prosthetic work required and specific materials to be used. A separate space is set aside for noting any corrections to be made to the prosthetic work during the clinical trials.

A second checklist for the laboratory, identical to the first, is compiled by the clinician when carrying out the definitive work and used to transfer all of the esthetic and functional information collected during the provisional phase.

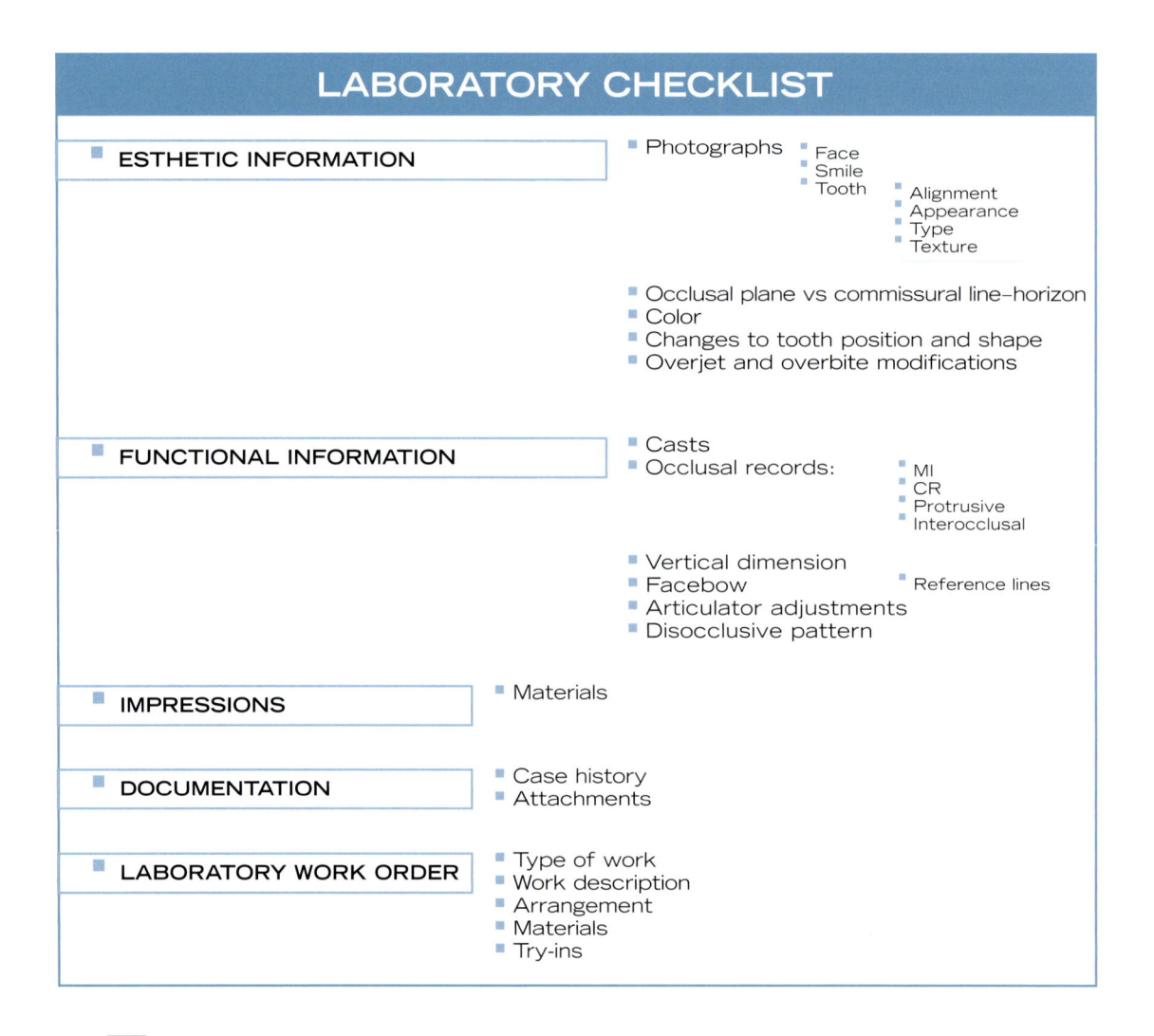

LABORATORY CHECKLIST

- **ESTHETIC INFORMATION**
  - Photographs
    - Face
    - Smile
    - Tooth
      - Alignment
      - Appearance
      - Type
      - Texture
  - Occlusal plane vs commissural line–horizon
  - Color
  - Changes to tooth position and shape
  - Overjet and overbite modifications

- **FUNCTIONAL INFORMATION**
  - Casts
  - Occlusal records:
    - MI
    - CR
    - Protrusive
    - Interocclusal
  - Vertical dimension
  - Facebow
  - Articulator adjustments
  - Disocclusive pattern
    - Reference lines

- **IMPRESSIONS**
  - Materials

- **DOCUMENTATION**
  - Case history
  - Attachments

- **LABORATORY WORK ORDER**
  - Type of work
  - Work description
  - Arrangement
  - Materials
  - Try-ins

Chapter 1 COMMUNICATING TO THE LABORATORY—DIAGNOSTIC WAX-UP

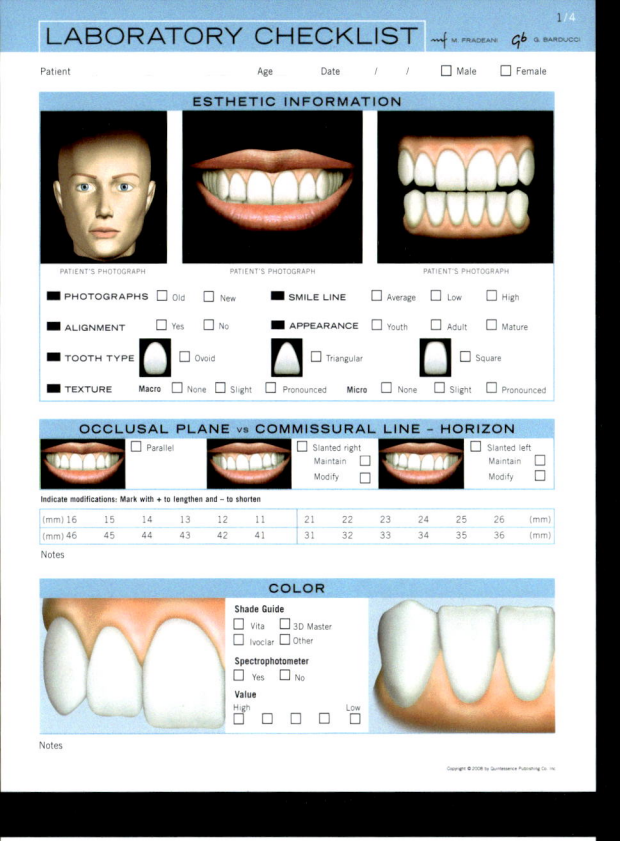

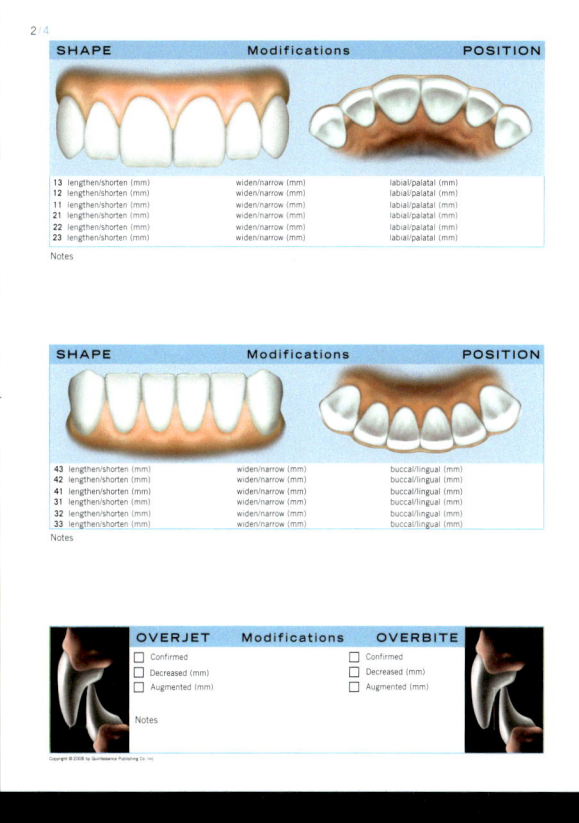

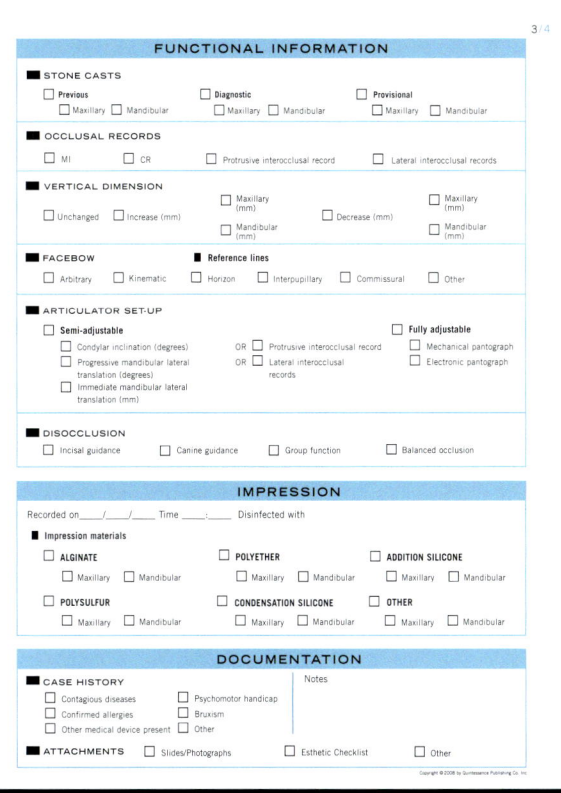

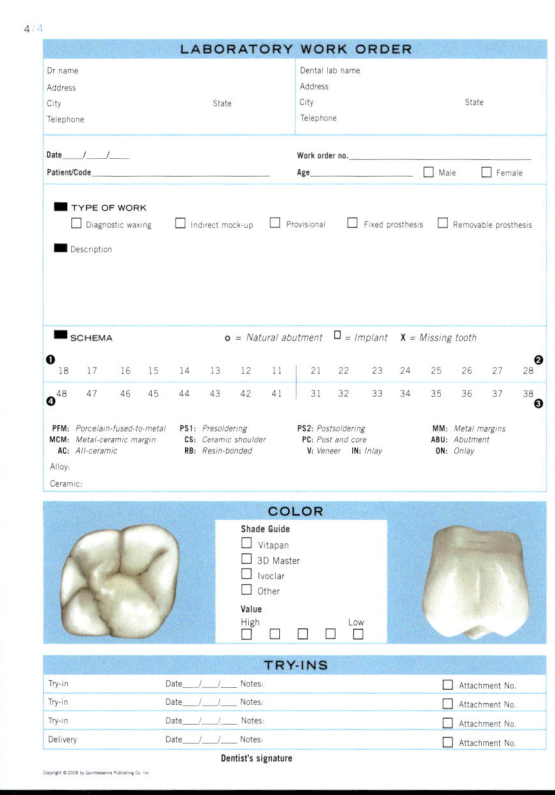

> Fig 1-4f

FIG 4 *(f)* Meticulous completion of the laboratory checklist provides the technician with all of the information necessary to create the diagnostic waxing, provisional restorations, and definitive restoration.

LABORATORY CHECKLIST

ESTHETIC INFORMATION

PHOTOGRAPHS

Although all of the esthetic information is transferred to the technician in the appropriate section of the laboratory checklist, in the interest of ensuring a correct understanding of the case it may also be useful to supply a few photographs that visually support the clinician's notes. It is essential that both the clinician and the technician have the same photographs, in either print or digital format, which allows them to discuss the clinical case even if they are in different locations.

FACE

A photograph of the face allows the technician to gain an overall view of the patient, to assess parallelism between the reference lines and the horizon, to distinguish any vertical disharmony, and to evaluate the proportion between the thirds of the face. It is, however, the clinician's task to decide whether to take any lack of parallelism or disharmony into consideration, employing choices dictated by an overall assessment based on results of the esthetic-functional analysis and the esthetic checklist.

SMILE

The photograph of the smile allows the technician to make out the smile line (average, low, high), the width of the smile (number of teeth displayed), and the presence and size of the buccal corridor (normal, wide, absent). However, because it represents the static expression of a dynamic act, the photograph may not correspond with the patient's natural expressions.[72] The clinician therefore must select the most suitable images for the purpose. The photograph of the smile also allows evaluation of the shape and dimension of the lips, which can suggest the ideal shape and dimensions of the restorations (see volume 1, chapter 2).

TEETH

By means of the intraoral photographs sent with the laboratory checklist, the technician can glean important information regarding tooth type and texture and also confirm the validity of the variations requested by the clinician in terms of tooth position and/or morphology.

LABORATORY CHECKLIST

1/4

M. FRADEANI   G. BARDUCCI

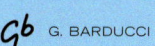

Patient X×××× X×××××××   Age ××   Date ×× / ×× / ××   [X] Male   [ ] Female

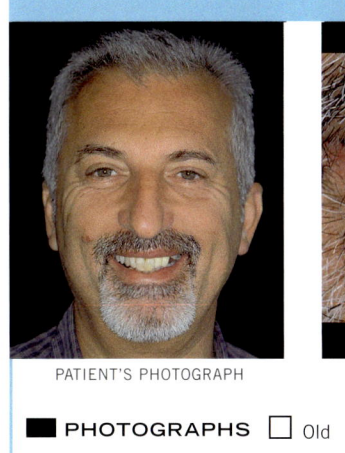

ESTHETIC INFORMATION

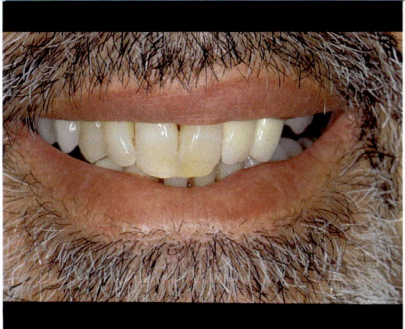

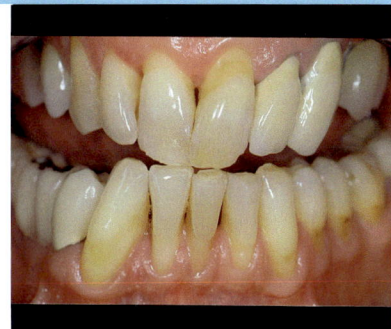

PATIENT'S PHOTOGRAPH   PATIENT'S PHOTOGRAPH   PATIENT'S PHOTOGRAPH

- **PHOTOGRAPHS** [ ] Old [X] New
- **SMILE LINE** [X] Average [ ] Low [ ] High
- **ALIGNMENT** [X] Yes [ ] No
- **APPEARANCE** [ ] Youth [X] Adult [ ] Mature
- **TOOTH TYPE** [X] Ovoid [ ] Triangular [ ] Square
- **TEXTURE** Macro [X] None [ ] Slight [ ] Pronounced   Micro [ ] None [X] Slight [ ] Pronounced

OCCLUSAL PLANE vs COMMISSURAL LINE – HORIZON

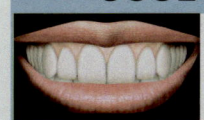

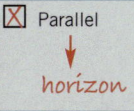

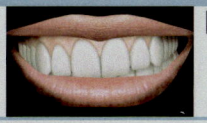

[X] Parallel → horizon   [ ] Slanted right Maintain [ ] Modify [ ]   [ ] Slanted left Maintain [ ] Modify [ ]

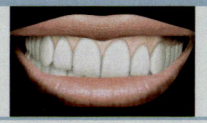

Indicate modifications: Mark with + to lengthen and – to shorten

(mm)	16 -1.5	15 -0.8	14 ___	13 ___	12 ___	11 ___	21 ___	22 +0.8	23 +1.0	24 +2.0	25 +2.0	26 +2.0 (mm)
(mm)	46 +2.5	45 +2.5	44 +2.5	43 -1.5	42 -1.0	41 ___	31 +0.5	32 ___	33 ___	34 ___	35 ___	36 ___ (mm)

Notes • Re-establish the occlusal plane by making it parallel to the horizon
       • Maintain tooth nos. 33 to 36 and use as plane of reference

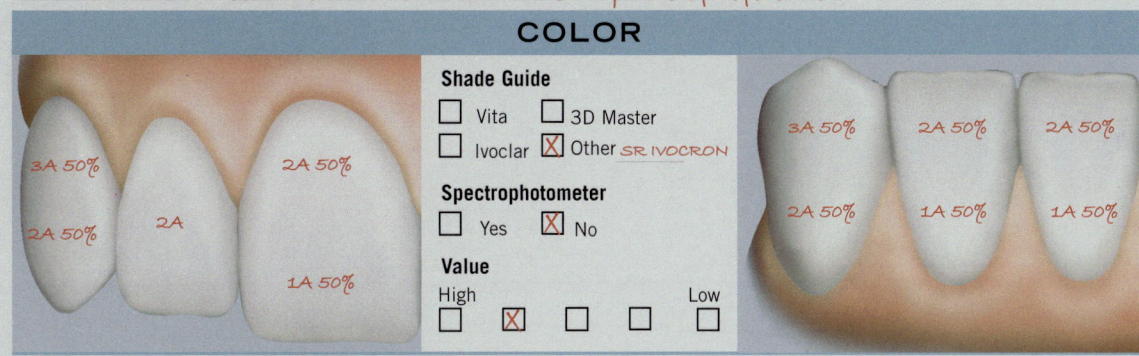

COLOR

3A 50% 2A 50% 2A 1A 50% 2A 50%

Shade Guide
[ ] Vita [ ] 3D Master
[ ] Ivoclar [X] Other SR IVOCRON

Spectrophotometer
[ ] Yes [X] No

Value
High [ ] [X] [ ] [ ] [ ] Low

3A 50% 2A 50% 2A 50%
2A 50% 1A 50% 1A 50%

Notes • Provide adequate translucency in the incisal one third
       • Do not add too many characterizations

Copyright © 2008 by Quintessence Publishing Co. Inc

OCCLUSAL PLANE

If necessary, the clinician may request a variation in the occlusal plane to re-establish parallelism with the chosen reference line. The size of the variation for each tooth is specified on the laboratory checklist, preferably accompanied by a photograph that confirms the necessity of this procedure by highlighting the discrepancy between the two planes (Figs 1-4g to 1-4j).

COLOR

To construct the provisional restoration, the laboratory can be sent only the basic color, with minimal color saturation. The color can be changed in the chair not only by the use of superficial colors, but also by virtue of the reduced thickness of the shell of the provisional restoration (see page 202), which allows the resin used for the relining to affect the final shade.

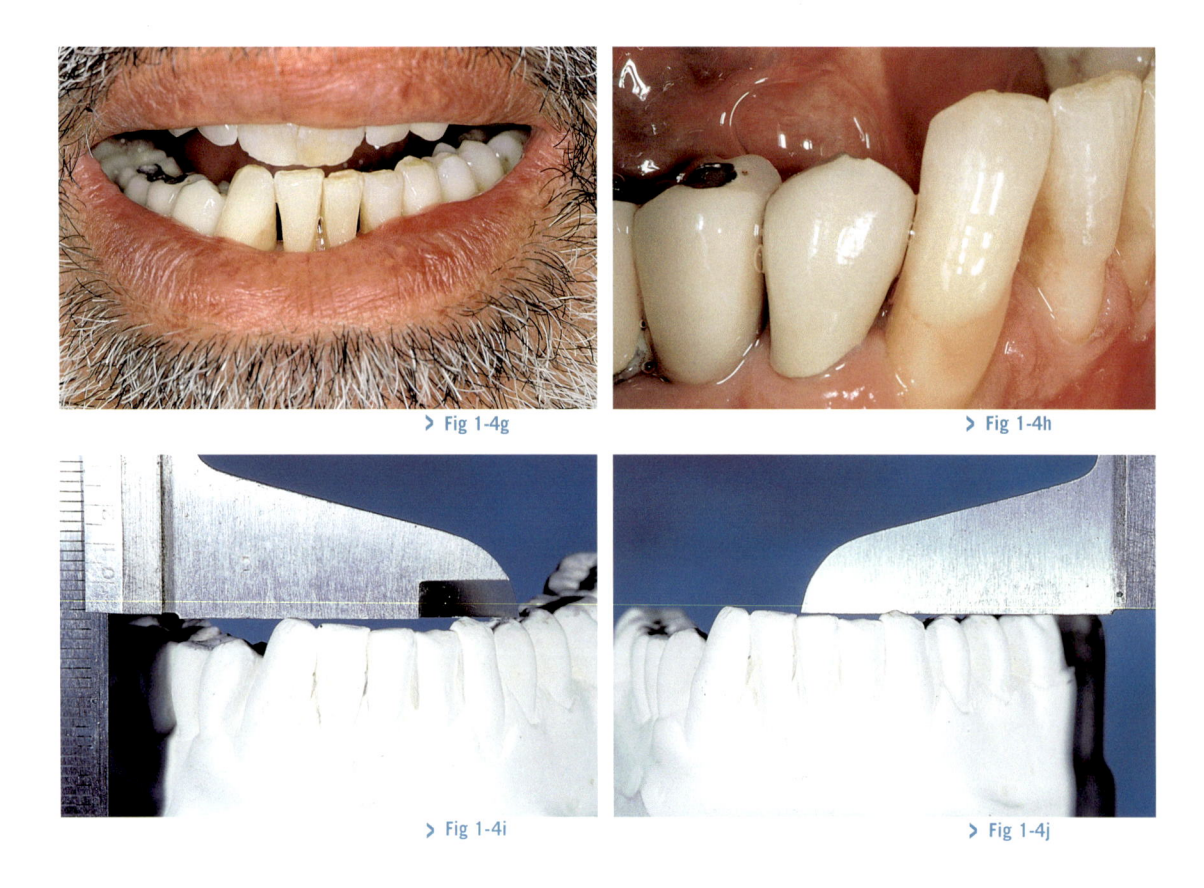

> Fig 1-4g

> Fig 1-4h

> Fig 1-4i

> Fig 1-4j

FIG 4 *(g and h)* When the patient speaks, a significant discrepancy in the mandibular occlusal plane is apparent, as is the sizable difference in level between the canine and the right mandibular premolars (better visualized in the close-up of the mandibular right sector). The plaster cast of the mandibular arch, properly oriented by correct use of the facebow, makes it easy to see the disharmony of the mandibular occlusal plane. *(i and j)* The arm of a caliper used to compare the two mandibular quadrants highlights an intrusion of the right quadrant, compared with the contralateral quadrant, of approximately 4 mm.

LABORATORY CHECKLIST

1/4

M. FRADEANI G. BARDUCCI

Patient **Xxxxx Xxxxxxxx** Age **xx** Date **xx / xx / xx** [X] Male [ ] Female

ESTHETIC INFORMATION

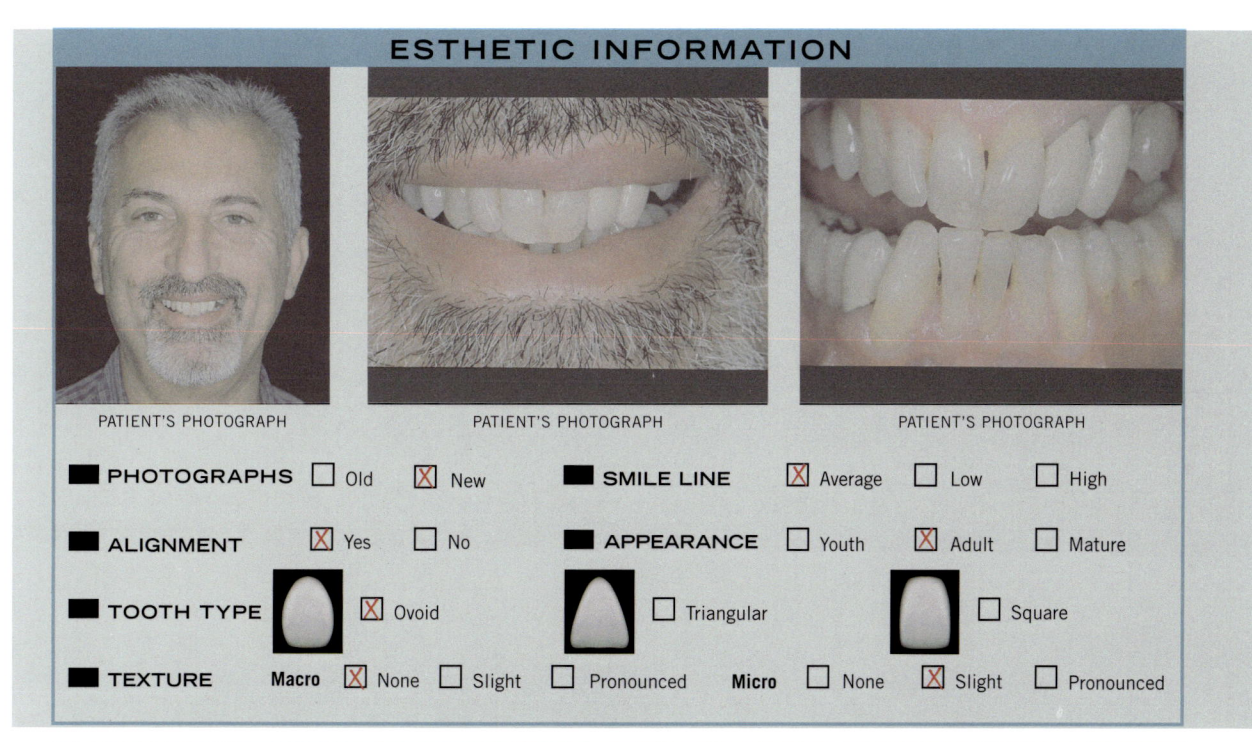

PATIENT'S PHOTOGRAPH | PATIENT'S PHOTOGRAPH | PATIENT'S PHOTOGRAPH

- **PHOTOGRAPHS** [ ] Old [X] New
- **SMILE LINE** [X] Average [ ] Low [ ] High
- **ALIGNMENT** [X] Yes [ ] No
- **APPEARANCE** [ ] Youth [X] Adult [ ] Mature
- **TOOTH TYPE** [X] Ovoid [ ] Triangular [ ] Square
- **TEXTURE** Macro [X] None [ ] Slight [ ] Pronounced   Micro [ ] None [X] Slight [ ] Pronounced

OCCLUSAL PLANE vs COMMISSURAL LINE – HORIZON

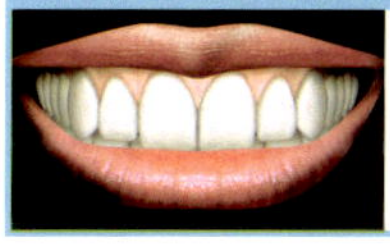

[X] Parallel → horizon   [ ] Slanted right Maintain [ ] Modify [ ]   [ ] Slanted left Maintain [ ] Modify [ ]

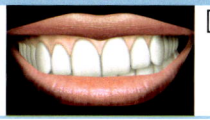

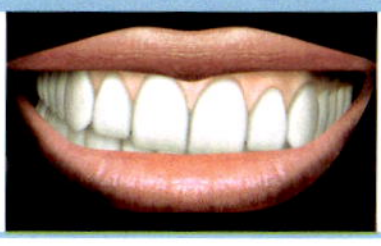

Indicate modifications: Mark with + to lengthen and – to shorten

(mm)	16 **-1.5**	15 **-0.8**	14	13	12	11	21	22 **+0.8**	23 **+1.0**	24 **+2.0**	25 **+2.0**	26 **+2.0**	(mm)
(mm)	46 **+2.5**	45 **+2.5**	44 **+2.5**	43 **-1.5**	42 **-1.0**	41	31 **+0.5**	32	33	34	35	36	(mm)

Notes
- Re-establish the occlusal plane by making it parallel to the horizon
- Maintain tooth nos. 33 to 36 and use as plane of reference

COLOR

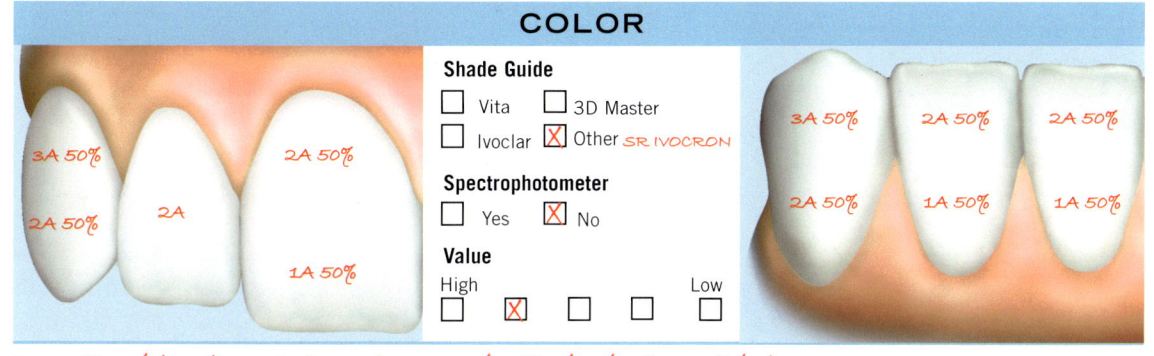

3A 50% 2A 50% 2A 1A 50% 2A 50%

Shade Guide
[ ] Vita [ ] 3D Master
[ ] Ivoclar [X] Other **SR IVOCRON**

Spectrophotometer
[ ] Yes [X] No

Value
High [ ] [X] [ ] [ ] [ ] Low

3A 50% 2A 50% 2A 50%
2A 50% 1A 50% 1A 50%

Notes
- Provide adequate translucency in the incisal one third
- Do not add too many characterizations

Copyright © 2008 by Quintessence Publishing Co. Inc

SHAPE AND POSITION

Modifications The changes to be made to the maxillary anterior sextant (Figs 1-4k and 1-4l) and to the mandibular anterior sextant (Figs 1-4m and 1-4n) are noted on the relevant drawings and specified in the diagrams to provide the technician with precise references for the variations in tooth position, shape, and length necessary for optimal esthetic and functional appearance of the patient.

OVERJET AND OVERBITE

Modifications The changes to shape and position of the anterior teeth, both maxillary and mandibular, directly affect overjet and overbite (Figs 1-4o and 1-4p). They are not therefore merely of esthetic value, but are essential for re-establishing or optimizing the anterior guide, thereby improving the patient's function.

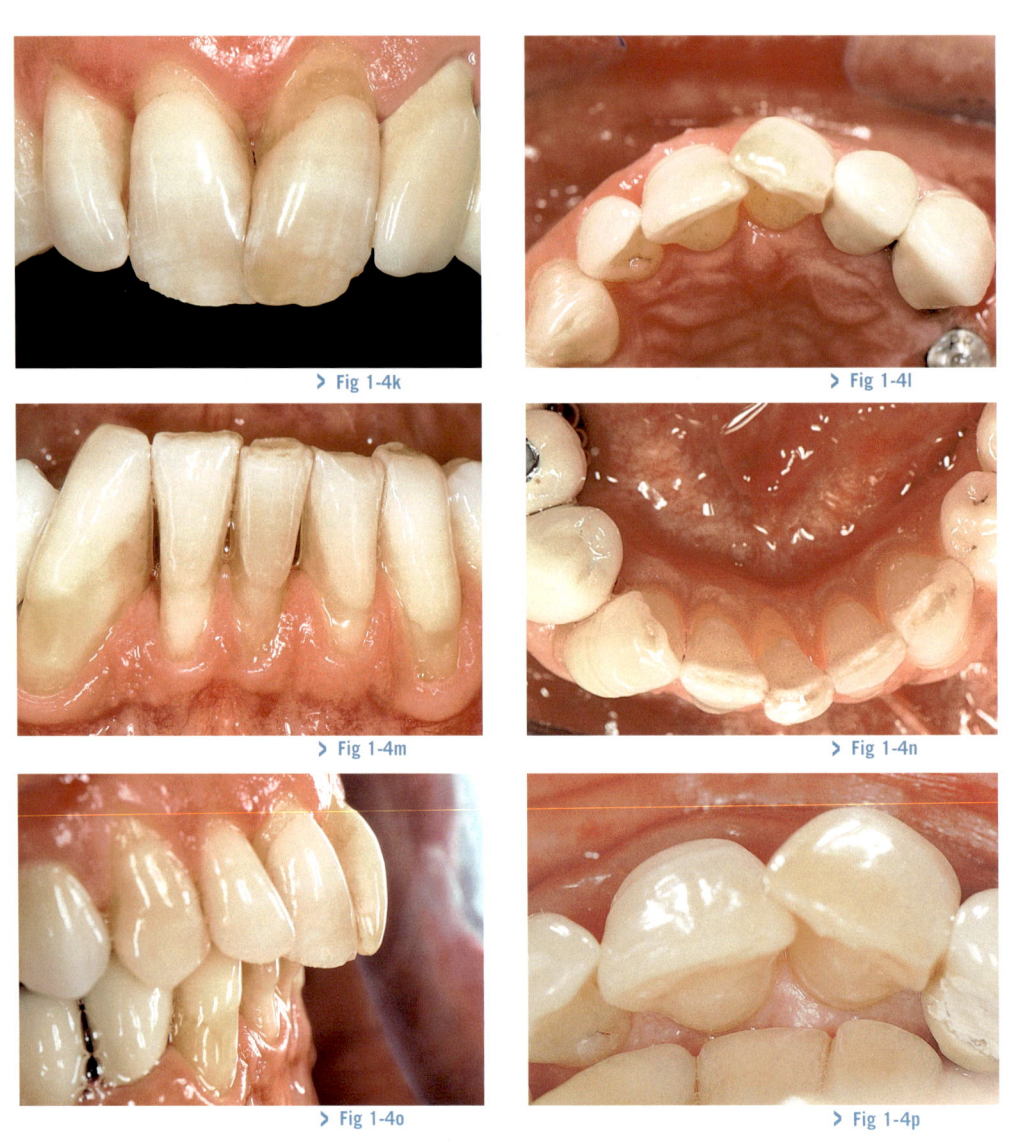

> Fig 1-4k

> Fig 1-4l

> Fig 1-4m

> Fig 1-4n

> Fig 1-4o

> Fig 1-4p

FIG 4 *(k and l)* The frontal and occlusal views of the anterior maxillary sextant show the overlapping of the left central incisor and incongruous restorations on the left lateral incisor and canine. *(m and n)* The frontal and occlusal views of the anterior mandibular sextant show only three incisors and the clear supraeruption of the right canine. *(o and p)* In the lateral and occlusal views of the two arches in occlusion, the considerable amount of overjet and overbite is visible.

Chapter 1 COMMUNICATING TO THE LABORATORY—DIAGNOSTIC WAX-UP

SHAPE — Modifications — POSITION

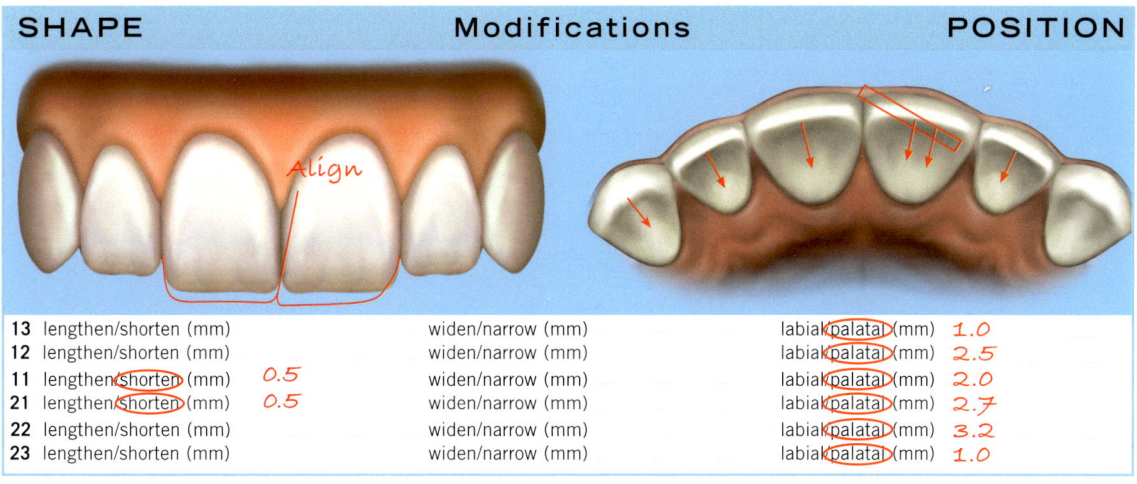

Tooth	Shape	Width	Position (mm)
13	lengthen/shorten (mm)	widen/narrow (mm)	labial/**palatal** (mm) 1.0
12	lengthen/shorten (mm)	widen/narrow (mm)	labial/**palatal** (mm) 2.5
11	lengthen/**shorten** (mm) 0.5	widen/narrow (mm)	labial/**palatal** (mm) 2.0
21	lengthen/**shorten** (mm) 0.5	widen/narrow (mm)	labial/**palatal** (mm) 2.7
22	lengthen/shorten (mm)	widen/narrow (mm)	labial/**palatal** (mm) 3.2
23	lengthen/shorten (mm)	widen/narrow (mm)	labial/**palatal** (mm) 1.0

Notes
- Align the two central incisors
- Slightly overlap the two central incisors with the two lateral incisors
- Shorten the two central incisors by 0.5 mm
- Move the anterior sextant palatally as indicated

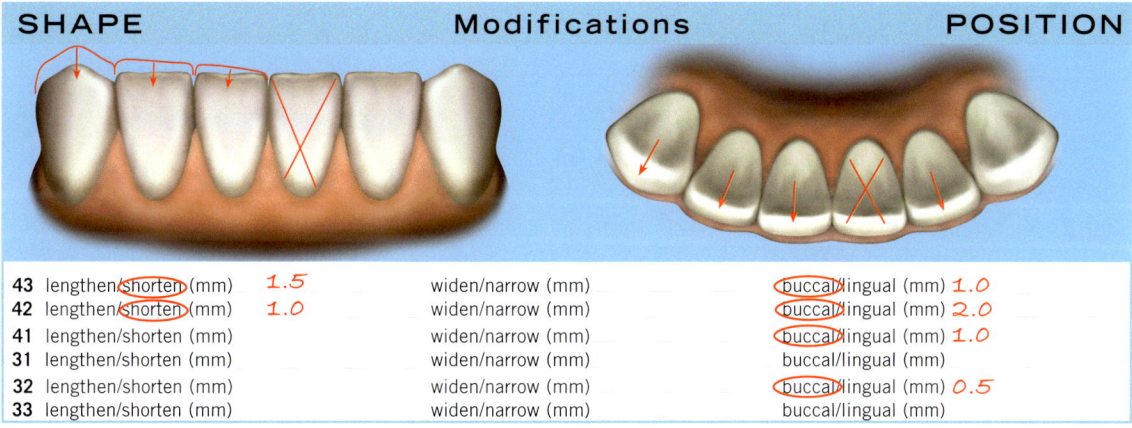

SHAPE — Modifications — POSITION

Tooth	Shape	Width	Position (mm)
43	lengthen/**shorten** (mm) 1.5	widen/narrow (mm)	**buccal**/lingual (mm) 1.0
42	lengthen/**shorten** (mm) 1.0	widen/narrow (mm)	**buccal**/lingual (mm) 2.0
41	lengthen/shorten (mm)	widen/narrow (mm)	**buccal**/lingual (mm) 1.0
31	lengthen/shorten (mm)	widen/narrow (mm)	buccal/lingual (mm)
32	lengthen/shorten (mm)	widen/narrow (mm)	**buccal**/lingual (mm) 0.5
33	lengthen/shorten (mm)	widen/narrow (mm)	buccal/lingual (mm)

Notes
- One central incisor is missing
- Shorten tooth nos. 42 and 43 as indicated
- Move the anterior sextant buccally as indicated

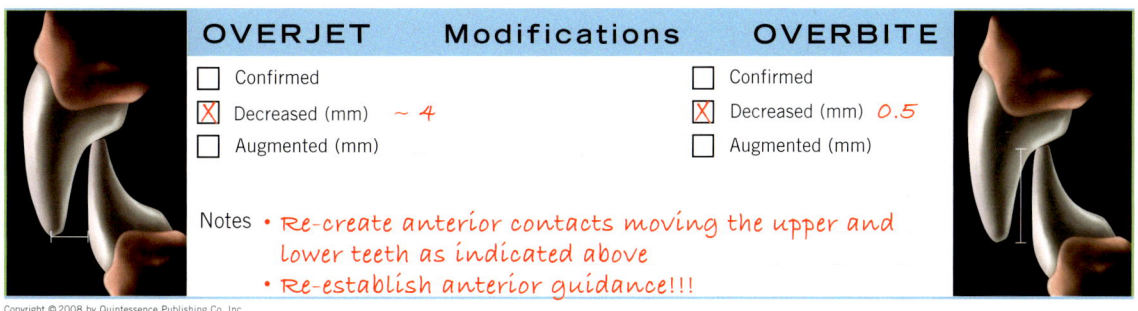

OVERJET — Modifications — OVERBITE

- ☐ Confirmed
- ☒ Decreased (mm) ~4
- ☐ Augmented (mm)

- ☐ Confirmed
- ☒ Decreased (mm) 0.5
- ☐ Augmented (mm)

Notes
- Re-create anterior contacts moving the upper and lower teeth as indicated above
- Re-establish anterior guidance!!!

Copyright © 2008 by Quintessence Publishing Co. Inc

LABORATORY CHECKLIST

FUNCTIONAL INFORMATION

STONE CASTS

The stone casts must be accurate (free from bubbles and streaking) and sufficiently detailed to cover the anatomic areas (palate, tuberosities, retromolar trigone, and fornices). Mounting the casts on the articulator is essential for planning the prosthetic treatment, since it is possible to see even occlusal aspects that are not always easily seen directly in the mouth, such as the interocclusal space of the edentulous areas, the appropriateness of the compensating curves of Spee and Wilson, and the accuracy of the occlusal plane.

OCCLUSAL REGISTRATIONS

The occlusal registration must be as precise as possible to allow accurate positioning of the casts. The material used should be sufficiently ductile not to give any resistance at the moment of registration, but should be rigid and dimensionally stable once hardened. Hard wax (Beauty Pink X-Hard Dental Wax, Moyco Union Broach-Thompson) is still widely used today because of its practical properties. For greater registration precision it is advisable to reline the wax with zinc oxide–eugenol paste (Superbite, Bosworth).[73,74] Silicone materials can be used as an alternative, but because of their resilience they do not guarantee the same accuracy of cast positioning.[75,76]

MAXIMUM INTERCUSPATION

If only a few teeth need to be reconstructed, MI is generally the elected occlusion *(conformative approach)* (see volume 1, chapter 5). The occlusal registration must be taken only between prepared and opposing teeth; placement of the registration material on teeth not involved in the treatment, which would impair correct cast positioning, should be avoided. It is not necessary to record the occlusion if the intercuspal relationship is guaranteed by an adequate number of stable dental contacts in the teeth adjacent to those treated.[77]

CENTRIC RELATION

The occlusal registration in CR should be taken when several quadrants or an entire arch are to be rehabilitated or in the absence of adequate occlusal stability *(reorganizational approach)* (see volume 1, chapter 5). The CR defines the articular relationship between the maxilla and mandible in which the condyles are articulated, with the articular discs interposed in the anterosuperior position (glenoid fossae against the articular eminences). This position is independent of the tooth contacts.[78]

If there are no articular problems, painful symptoms, or significant limitations of mandibular movement, Dawson's bimanual manipulation method has proven to be the most reliable for repeatedly locating the articular position of CR[79–81] (Fig 1-5a).

FUNCTIONAL INFORMATION

■ STONE CASTS
- ☐ Previous
  - ☐ Maxillary ☐ Mandibular
- ☒ Diagnostic
  - ☒ Maxillary ☒ Mandibular
- ☐ Provisional
  - ☐ Maxillary ☐ Mandibular

■ OCCLUSAL RECORDS
- ☐ MI
- ☒ CR
- ☒ Protrusive interocclusal record
- ☐ Lateral interocclusal records

■ VERTICAL DIMENSION
- ☒ Unchanged
- ☐ Increase (mm)
  - ☐ Maxillary (mm)
  - ☐ Mandibular (mm)
- ☐ Decrease (mm)
  - ☐ Maxillary (mm)
  - ☐ Mandibular (mm)

■ FACEBOW
- ☒ Arbitrary
- ☐ Kinematic

■ Reference lines
- ☒ Horizon
- ☐ Interpupillary
- ☐ Commissural
- ☐ Other

■ ARTICULATOR SET-UP
- ☒ Semi-adjustable
  - ☒ Condylar inclination (degrees)
  - ☒ Progressive mandibular lateral translation (degrees)   *10*
  - ☒ Immediate mandibular lateral translation (mm)   *0*
  - OR ☒ Protrusive interocclusal record
  - OR ☐ Lateral interocclusal records
- ☐ Fully adjustable
  - ☐ Mechanical pantograph
  - ☐ Electronic pantograph

■ DISOCCLUSION
- ☒ Incisal guidance
- ☒ Canine guidance
- ☐ Group function
- ☐ Balanced occlusion

IMPRESSION

Recorded on **xx/xx/xx** Time **xx:xx** Disinfected with *glutaraldehyde*

■ Impression materials
- ☒ **ALGINATE**
  - ☒ Maxillary ☒ Mandibular
- ☐ **POLYETHER**
  - ☐ Maxillary ☐ Mandibular
- ☐ **ADDITION SILICONE**
  - ☐ Maxillary ☐ Mandibular
- ☐ **POLYSULFUR**
  - ☐ Maxillary ☐ Mandibular
- ☐ **CONDENSATION SILICONE**
  - ☐ Maxillary ☐ Mandibular
- ☐ **OTHER**
  - ☐ Maxillary ☐ Mandibular

DOCUMENTATION

■ CASE HISTORY
- ☐ Contagious diseases
- ☐ Confirmed allergies
- ☐ Other medical device present
- ☐ Psychomotor handicap
- ☐ Bruxism
- ☐ Other

Notes

■ ATTACHMENTS
- ☒ Slides/Photographs
- ☒ Esthetic Checklist
- ☐ Other

Copyright © 2008 Quintessenza Edizioni S.r.l.

Positioning of the mandible in CR can be achieved only after the stomatognathic musculature has been deconditioned.[82,83]

Indeed, in a patient who has not been sufficiently deconditioned, any attempts at manipulating the mandible can cause defensive neuromuscular reflexes that in turn could induce an involuntary protrusion. At this point, attempting to force the mandible into a more retracted position, as well as excessively compressing the posterior ligament of the disc (Fig 1-5b), can cause an involuntary translation of the condyles into a lower position, with possible hyperocclusion of the prosthetic restorations. If the patient feels pain in the articular area, a differential diagnosis between intra-articular and muscular problems must be made. If positioning of a deprogrammer (cotton rolls or a Lucia jig) between the anterior teeth for 10 to 15 minutes diminishes or eliminates the discomfort, the origin of the problem is muscular (contracted lateral pterygoid). If the pain persists or even increases, it indicates instead that the condyle is compressing the richly innervated retrodiscal tissue. In this case, a complete acrylic resin occlusal device needs to be used for 4 to 6 weeks for stabilization. If, despite these articular problems, no painful symptomatology is found during the articular loading test, the patient's jaws can be maneuvered into the anterosuperior-most position, relying on what Dawson defines as the *adapted centric posture*.[84,85]

The ability to reproduce the mandibular position is fundamental for transmitting the data from the clinic to the laboratory, in cases of both CR and adapted centric posture. Having the confidence that the same occlusal relationship can be found at every step of the procedure allows the technician to create the prosthetic rehabilitation in the correct spatial position and allows the clinician to minimize the refinements necessary at the time of testing and work completion.

In rehabilitation cases, before embarking upon any prosthetic phase, it is a good rule for the clinician to make a preliminary occlusal adjustment in CR, which deconditions the stomatognathic system musculature and provides good intercuspation. Where selective grinding is not performed on the patient, an occlusal registration in CR must be taken. The wax must be of minimum thickness but, above all, must not be perforated because it will be used by the technician to make the occlusal adjustment on the articulator. Its integrity proves that the registration has not been affected by any dental contact that might have caused translation of the mandible following neuromuscular reflexes produced by the periodontal mechanoreceptors.[86]

FIG 5 *(a)* Correct manipulation of the mandible guides the condyles, with interposition of the articular discs, into the most anterosuperior position of the glenoid fossae against the articular eminences. CR is usually recorded by interposing a rigid wax layer between the two arches that does not extend to the anterior teeth, avoiding any instinctive protrusive movement. Despite the minimum thickness, the wax will not have to be perforated. *(b)* Forcing the mandible into a retruded position produces a compression of the posterior ligament that, because of defensive neuromuscular reflexes, can cause the condyles to translate into a lower position and produce a consequent protrusion of the mandible, thus resulting in an incorrect occlusal registration.

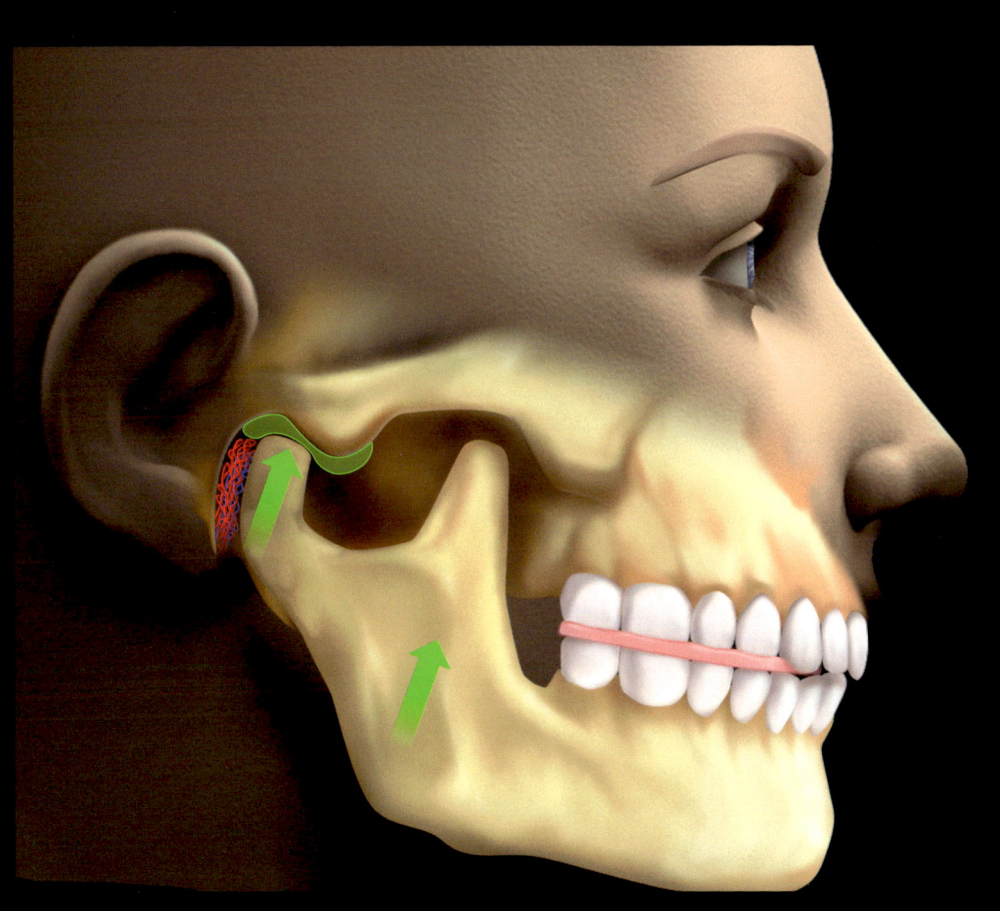

> Fig 1-5a

> Fig 1-5b

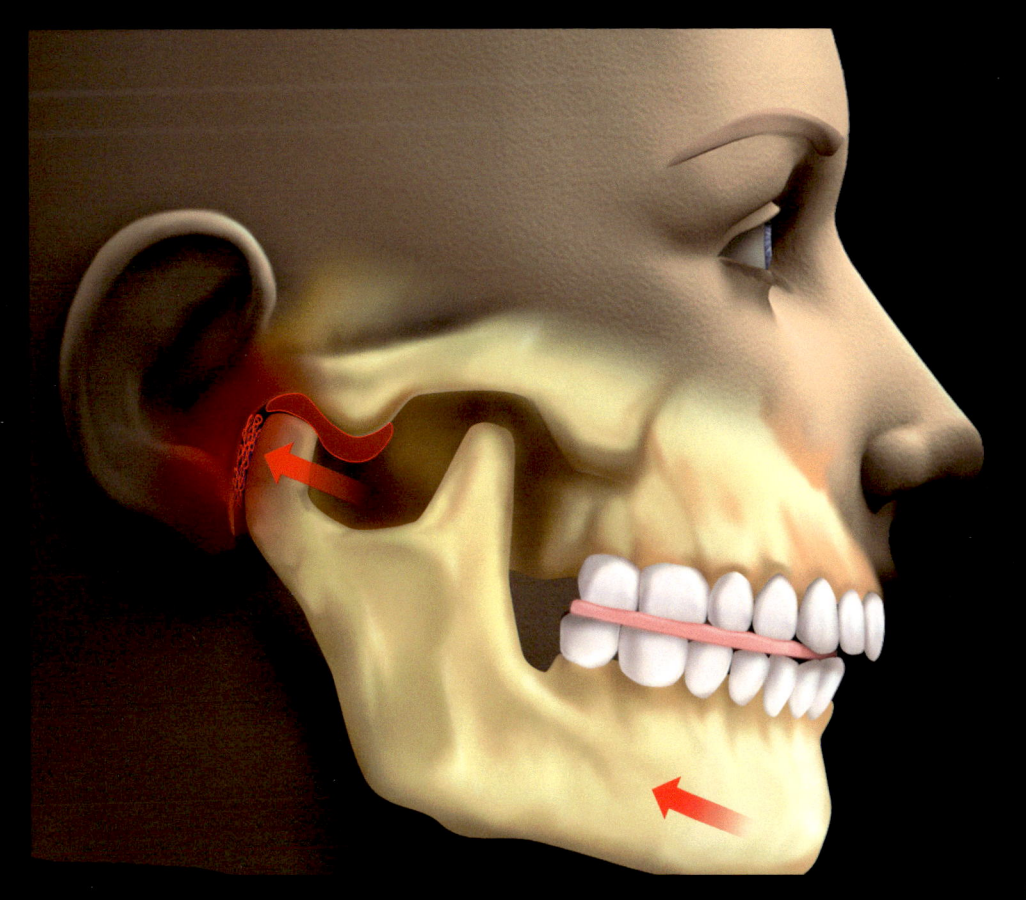

VERTICAL DIMENSION OF OCCLUSION

The VDO is, as Dawson[87] maintains, the intermaxillary space where the teeth erupt until establishing contact; its size is determined by the length of contraction of the elevator muscles. Where there are severe tooth abrasions in both arches, the clinician should increase the VDO to create restorations of adequate length. In such cases, although its increase is necessary from a prosthodontic perspective, the patient's original VDO can nevertheless remain unchanged. The loss of dental substance at the occlusal level may have been compensated for by simultaneous tooth eruption and by osseous addition in the alveolar processes, a phenomenon governed by the ideal length of contraction of the elevator muscles.[87] However, the ideal length of muscular contraction could mean that any increase in the VDO carried through the prosthetic rehabilitation would tend to cancel itself out within the space of a few months because of the phenomenon of dental intrusion.[88] Despite the frequent compensation phenomena described above, calculation of the planned increase in VDO is guided purely by clinical needs that satisfy the structural, functional, and esthetic objectives of the case. Each variation must be checked by testing the patient's adaptation to the new height during the provisional phase. The VDO increase also makes it possible to improve the overbite and overjet values and give the disocclusive path a shallower angle, thereby reducing stress on the masticatory muscles.[89] An increase in the VDO should be indicated to the technician by specifying the amount of variation for each arch. One parameter to help determine which arch should be used to modify the VDO is the location of the position of the incisal margin of the mandibular teeth. This should be found where the upper and lower lips meet when the lips are closed and the teeth are in contact.[90] In cases of prosthetic rehabilitation where it is necessary to alter the VDO, it is usually registered with the same wax used to take the CR, at the height believed to be most clinically appropriate. In this case, the clinician should specify on the laboratory checklist that the registration taken in CR also includes the necessary amount of VDO (Figs 1-6a to 1-6c). One of the most commonly used clinical parameters for testing the validity of the changes made to the VDO is having the patient pronounce the letters M[91–95] and S[90,96–100] (see volume 1, chapter 4).

PROTRUSIVE INTEROCCLUSAL RECORD

Disocclusion of the posterior teeth is ensured by means of anterior guidance, which, together with the degree of condylar inclination, allows them to avoid any interference during protrusive and lateral movements, on both the working and the nonworking sides.[101–103] To establish the correct degree of condylar inclination in the articulator (Figs 1-6d and 1-6e), wax placed between the posterior teeth is used to register the relationship between the two dental arches when the patient closes in the edge-to-edge position. Alternatively, an arbitrary condylar inclination value (20 degrees) can be established that allows interference to be avoided in the posterior teeth.[104] Lateral interocclusal records are not normally registered, since it is preferable to assign a value of 10–15 degrees to the progressive mandibular lateral translation, enough to avoid contact in the posterior teeth.

> Fig 1-6a

> Fig 1-6b

> Fig 1-6c

> Fig 1-6d

> Fig 1-6e

→ continues on page 104

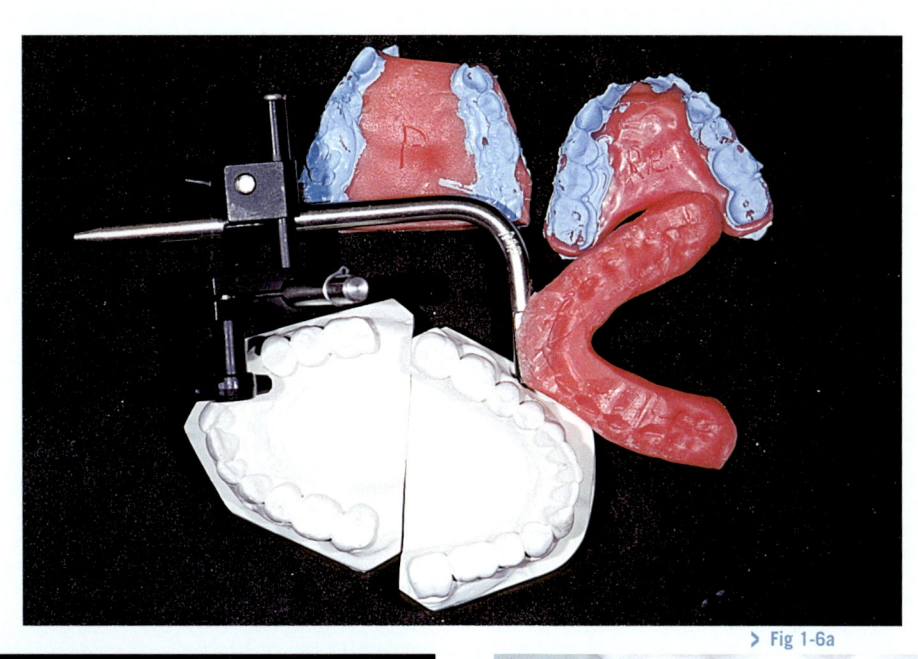

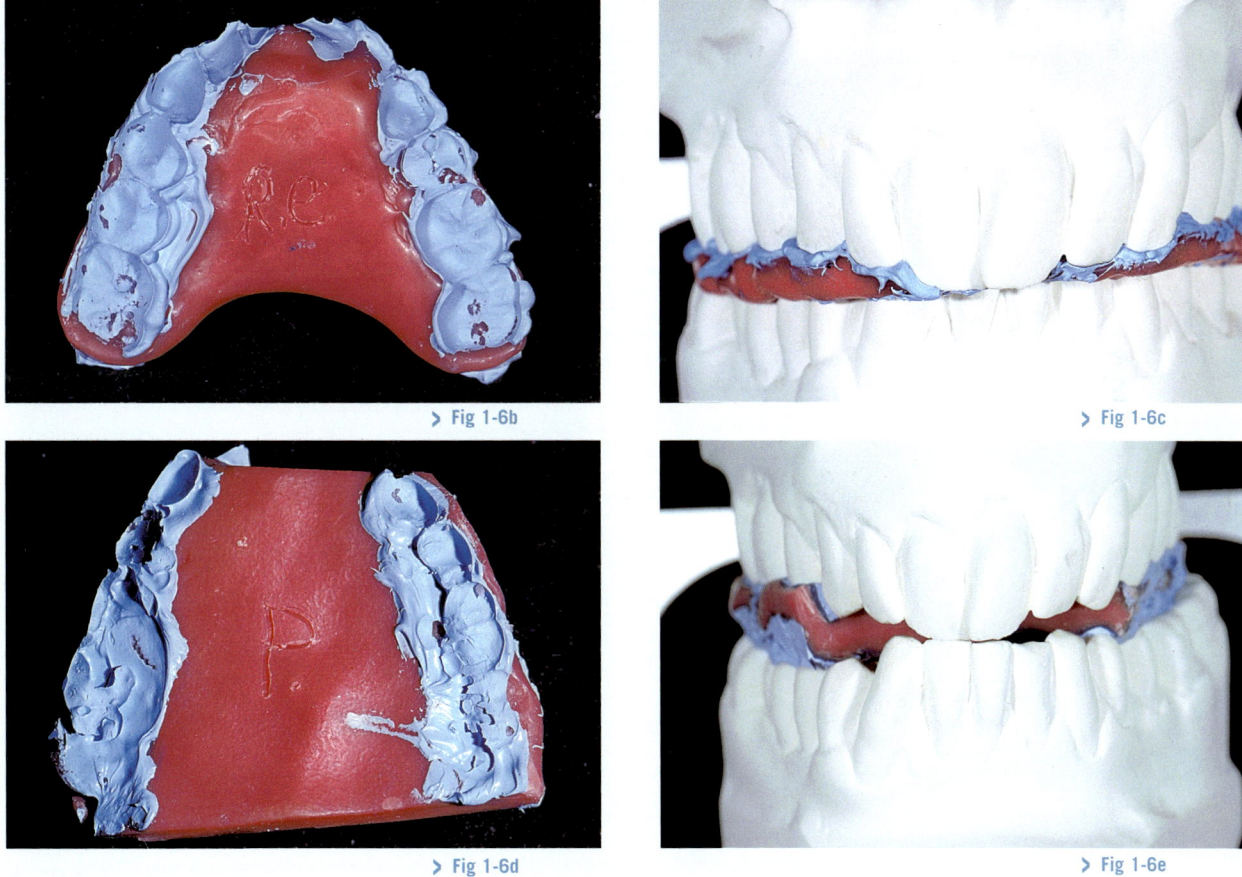

FIG 6 *(a)* The first phase of transferring the information to the laboratory consists of developing the stone casts, correct recording of the facebow, and of the occlusal registration in CR and protrusion. *(b and c)* The CR registration allows the technician to mount the casts on the articulator and is taken using a hard wax relined with a zinc oxide–eugenol paste. The registration must not contain any holes or any excess relining paste because this could impair correct positioning of the casts.

FIG 6 *(d)* By making the patient close in the edge-to-edge position and placing wax between the posterior teeth, the patient's "protrusiveness" is recorded. *(e)* This is actually the end point of the patient's disocclusive pattern, which makes it possible to adjust the condylar inclination of the articulator and to assess the amount of separation of the posterior teeth.

FACEBOW

The masticatory system, comprising the TMJs, the dental arches, and the neuromuscular system, is a complex dynamic mechanism in which various movements can be defined, including opening, closing, protrusion, lateral movements, and translation. When a case is being prepared, the exact interrelationship of the two arches and their arrangement in the three spatial planes should be communicated to the laboratory for appropriate mounting of the casts. The instrument that allows adequate reproduction of the static and dynamic relationship of the masticatory system is the *articulator*[105]; the apparatus that makes it possible to transfer the position of the arches from the patient to the articulator is the *facebow*.

ORIENTING THE CASTS

The facebow is used for mounting the maxillary cast on the articulator. To achieve its correct spatial orientation, three reference points must be selected: two posterior points that detect the hinge axis and one anterior point.

POSTERIOR REFERENCE POINTS

The position of the posterior reference points can be found arbitrarily (arbitrary facebow) or individually (kinematic facebow).

Arbitrary facebow Locating the hinge axis point in this case takes place arbitrarily, using porion or the acoustic meatus as a reference (Fig 1-7a). In the latter case, the use of a facebow equipped with ear inserts is sufficiently reliable, so much so that the arbitrary axis determined with this method proves to be, in most instances, within 6 mm of the true hinge axis point.[106–111]

Kinematic facebow The kinematic facebow allows the patient's terminal hinge axis points (Fig 1-7b) to be taken as a reference, using axiography or pantography. The correct location of the registration points is proven purely by their rotational movement. The difficulty that can be encountered in locating the hinge axis has been the subject of much debate,[112–116] to such an extent as to cast doubt upon the clinical reliability of this method. Its use can be advocated in cases of prosthetic rehabilitation where a significant variation in the VDO is involved.[117]

ANTERIOR REFERENCE POINT

Whether using the arbitrary or kinematic facebow, location of the anterior reference point is determined arbitrarily,[118–121] using the following references:

- Orbitale (lower border of the orbit)
- A point located 23 mm below nasion (same position as orbitale) (Fig 1-7c)
- An arbitrary point located 43 mm above the incisal edge of the maxillary lateral incisor (Fig 1-7d).

POSTERIOR REFERENCE POINTS

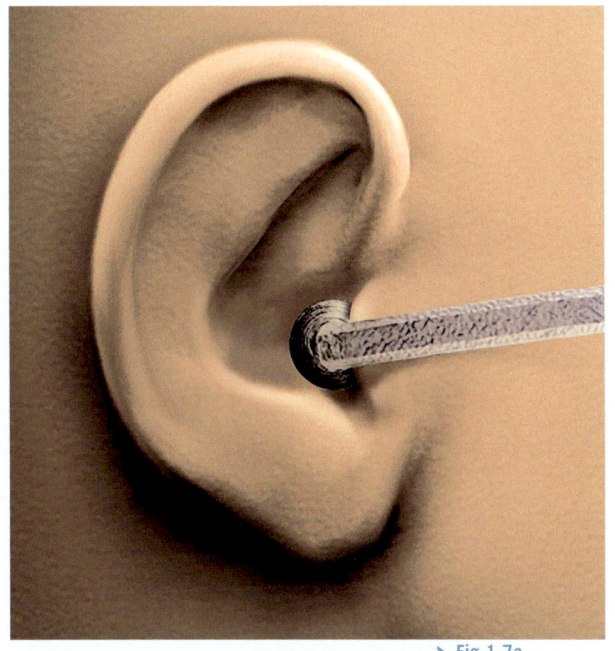

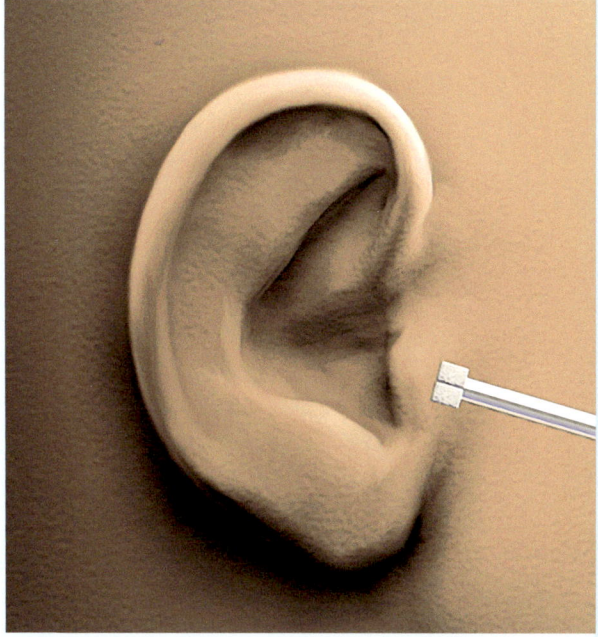

> Fig 1-7a

> Fig 1-7b

ANTERIOR REFERENCE POINT

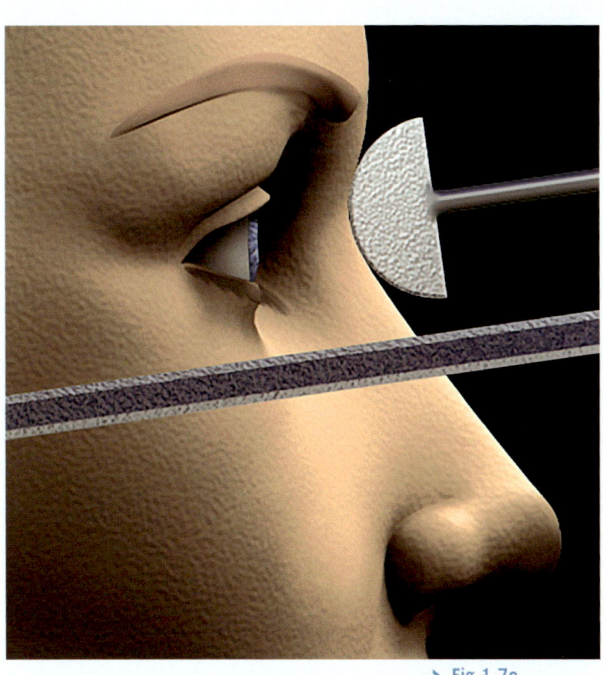

> Fig 1-7c

> Fig 1-7d

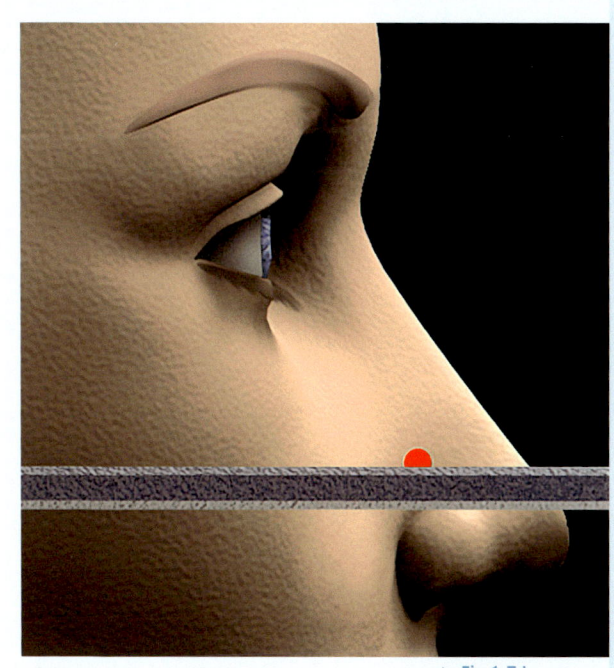

FIG 7 *(a)* The posterior reference points of the arbitrary facebow are usually determined by the ear inserts positioned in the acoustic meatuses. *(b)* The position of posterior reference points using the kinematic facebow is determined by recording the hinge axis with axiography or pantography.

FIG 7 *(c)* The anterior reference point can be the inferior border of the orbit (orbitale) or nasion. In the latter case, the arms of the facebow are practically at the same height as orbitale, so the result is an orientation parallel to the Frankfort plane.
(d) Some systems using both arbitrary and kinematic facebows locate as an anterior reference a point located 43 mm from the margin of the maxillary lateral incisor or from the lower border of the top lip, which corresponds to the ala of the nose.

FACEBOW

REFERENCE PLANES   lateral view

The choice of reference plane, determined by joining the posterior reference points to the anterior one found by means of the facebow, has a direct influence on the orientation of the casts on the articulator, affecting both the esthetic and functional aspects of the restorations. To investigate this problem further we will now consider the implications of choosing between the different reference planes that can be used for the prosthetic rehabilitation (Figs 1-8a and 1-8b).[120]

FRANKFORT PLANE
Posterior reference: porion
Anterior reference: orbitale
The Frankfort plane is identified by the line that joins porion (upper border of the tragus) to the infraorbital point (orbitale).

ORBITAL-AXIS PLANE
Posterior reference: hinge axis
Anterior reference: orbitale
The orbital-axis plane is identified by the line that joins the individual intercondylar axis, found using the pantograph or the axiograph, to the infraorbital point (orbitale).

ARBITRARY PLANE
Posterior reference: acoustic meatuses
Anterior reference: arbitrary point
The arbitrary plane is identified by the line that joins the acoustic meatuses, or other arbitrary posterior reference points, to an arbitrary point identified 43 mm above the incisal border of the maxillary lateral incisor.

CAMPER'S PLANE
Posterior reference: tragus
Anterior reference: ala of the nose
Camper's plane is the line that joins the upper border of the tragus to the lower border of the ala of the nose. It is normally parallel with the occlusal plane, forming an angle of roughly 10 degrees with the Frankfort plane.

The *Frankfort plane* represents by definition the horizontal plane, even if, using orbitale as the anterior reference point, it is actually only parallel with the horizon when the patient bends the head slightly (Fig 1-8a). When the patient holds the head erect, the Frankfort plane lifts upward at the front to form an angle of roughly 8 degrees with the arbitrary horizontal plane, commonly defined as the *esthetic plane*[119] (see volume 1, chapter 2, page 50) (Fig 1-8b). The angle of the orbitale-axis plane is even greater: The terminal hinge axis point is at an average of 7 mm below porion, so joining it to orbitale creates a plane angled at roughly 13 degrees in relation to the esthetic plane.[122] The arbitrary plane, because the anterior reference point that identifies it is roughly 10 mm below orbitale, proves to be the most parallel with the esthetic plane when the patient's head is held in the erect position and the eyes are focused on the horizon.[119-121]

Orbital-axis plane
Frankfort plane

Arbitrary plane

Camper's plane

Occlusal plane

> Fig 1-8a

Orbital-axis plane
Frankfort plane
Arbitrary plane
Esthetic plane

Camper's plane

Occlusal plane

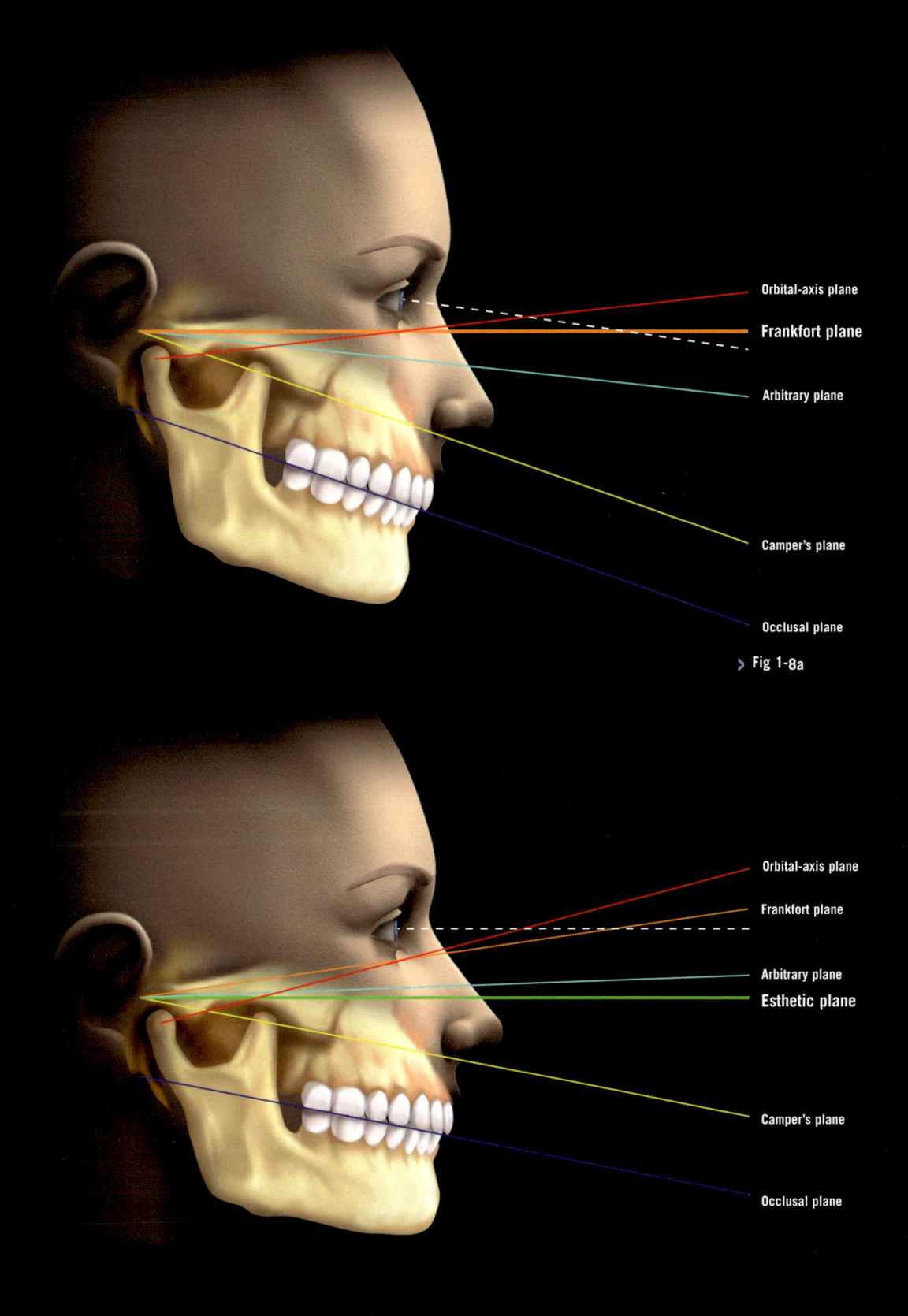

> Fig 1-8b

FIG 8 *(a)* The Frankfort plane is parallel to the horizon when the patient bends the head slightly. *(b)* When the patient holds the head in the erect position, the Frankfort plane is instead inclined upward, forming an angle of roughly 8 degrees with the esthetic plane.

ESTHETIC-FUNCTIONAL IMPLICATIONS

Mounting the casts with a facebow that references the Frankfort plane (Figs 1-9a and 1-10a to 1-10d) or the orbital-axis plane results in an excessive anteroposterior tilting of the occlusal plane in the articulator[119,123] as well as an unnatural buccolingual tilting of the anterior teeth.[119,122-125]

In the absence of precise indications, this could lead the technician, in an attempt to correct it, to incorrectly modify the arrangement of the anterior teeth, with inevitable esthetic and functional repercussions. In addition to the anomalous inclination of the casts, the use of the Frankfort plane or the orbital-axis plane will position the two dental arches in the articulator at a lower level in relation to the condyles than is found in the true clinical situation. This marked positioning error in the vertical direction can produce nonworking occlusal interferences.[126] As Pitchford[119] finds, some manufacturers of articulators have tried to remedy this disadvantage by modifying the orbitale indicator to correct the mounting error in the articulator and to allow a similar orientation of the facebow to the one that uses the arbitrary plane (ie, the one as parallel as possible to the esthetic plane of reference). The use of a facebow that takes the arbitrary plane (Figs 1-9b and from 1-10e to 1-10h) as a reference is therefore to be considered the most clinically suitable because it allows an inclination of the occlusal plane, and therefore of the anterior teeth, to be reproduced in the articulator. This is similar to what the clinician sees when looking at a patient who is holding the head in the erect position.

FIG 9 *(a)* If the facebow employed takes the Frankfort plane as its reference plane and the patient keeps the head erect, the arms of the facebow lift up at the front to form an angle of 8 degrees with the horizontal plane. *(b)* If the facebow instead takes the arbitrary plane as a reference plane and the patient keeps the head erect, the arms of the facebow are more or less parallel to the horizon.

FACEBOW—FRANKFORT PLANE

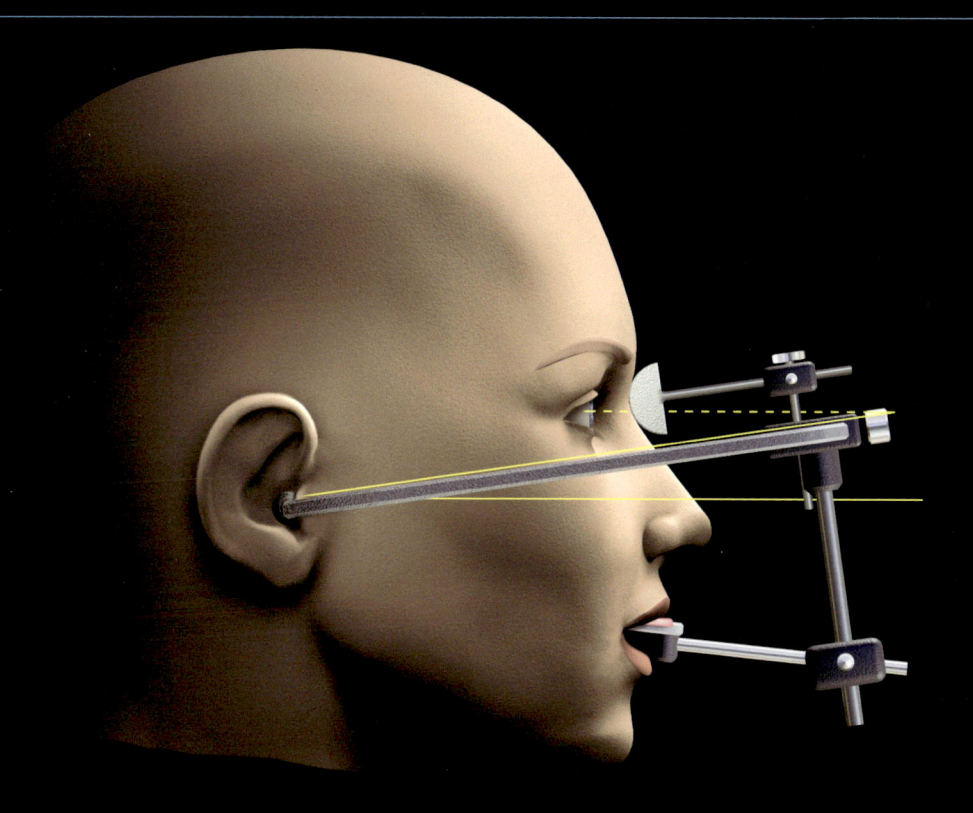

> Fig 1-9a

FACEBOW—ARBITRARY PLANE

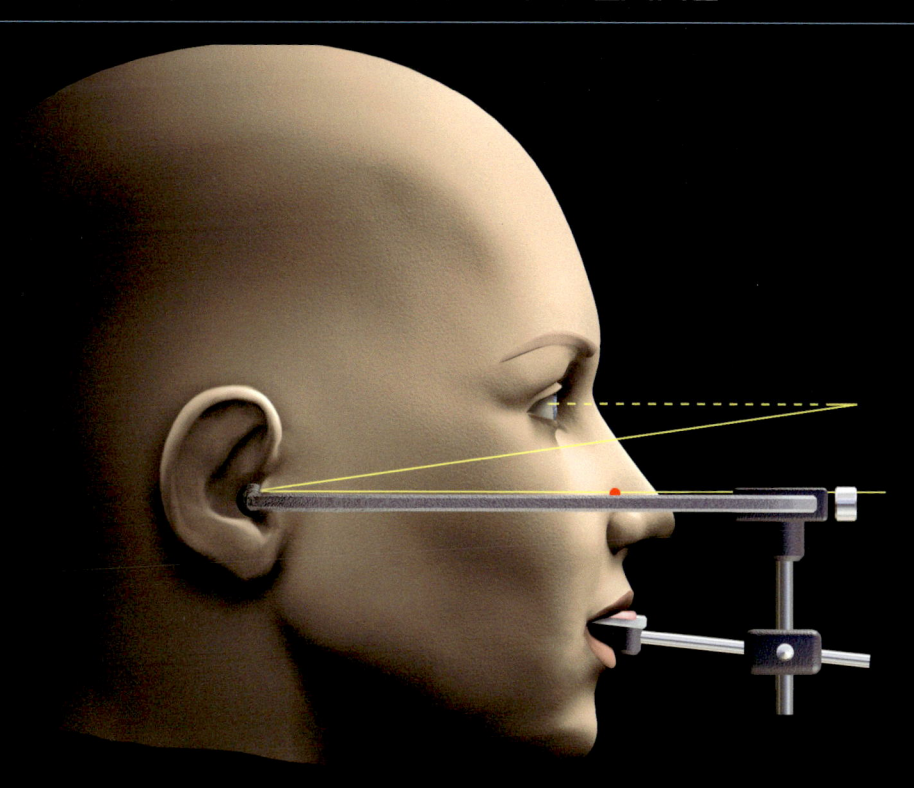

> Fig 1-9b

FACEBOW—FRANKFORT PLANE

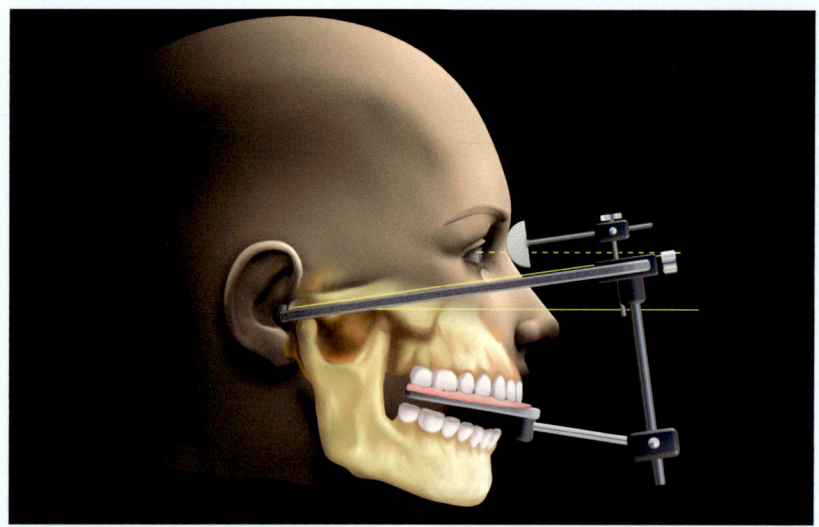

> Fig 1-10a

> Fig 1-10b

> Fig 1-10c

> Fig 1-10d

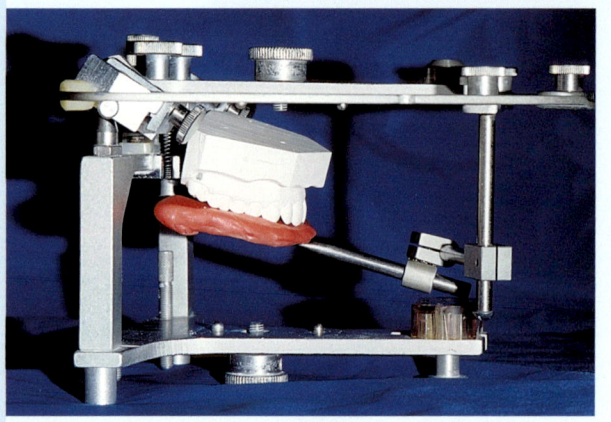

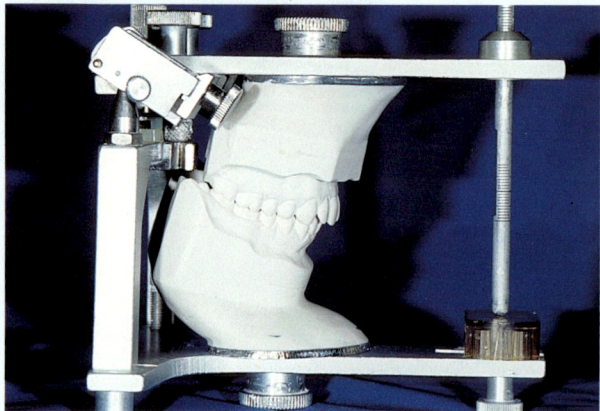

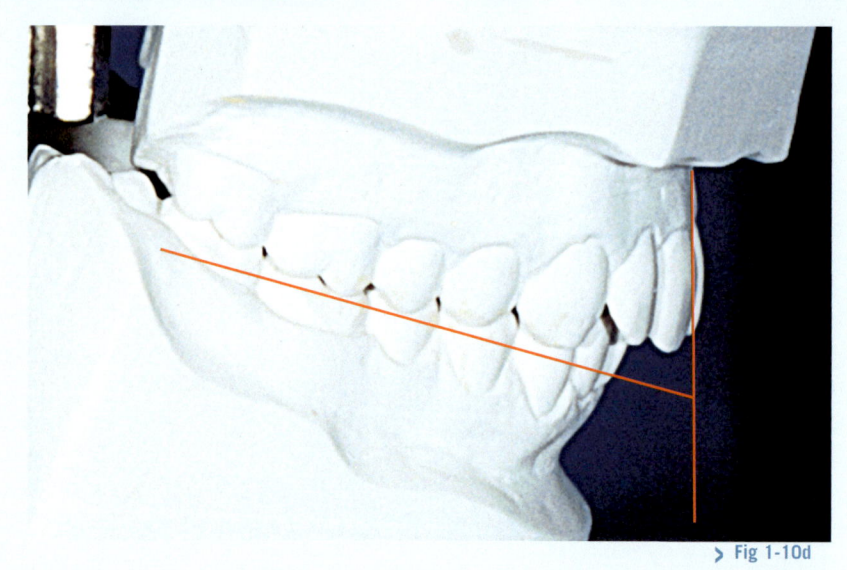

FIG 10 *(a to d)* If using a facebow that takes the Frankfort plane as a reference, the casts mounted on the articulator appear significantly rotated downward, with a pronounced inclination of the occlusal plane in the anteroposterior direction.

FACEBOW—ARBITRARY PLANE

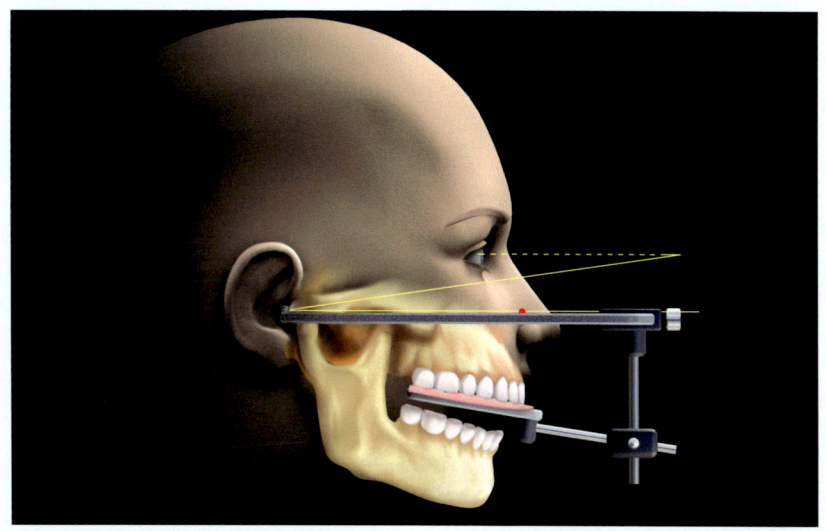

> Fig 1-10e

> Fig 1-10f

> Fig 1-10g

> Fig 1-10h

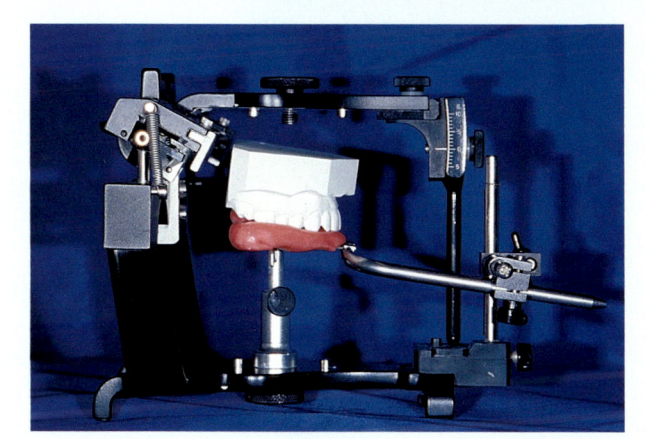

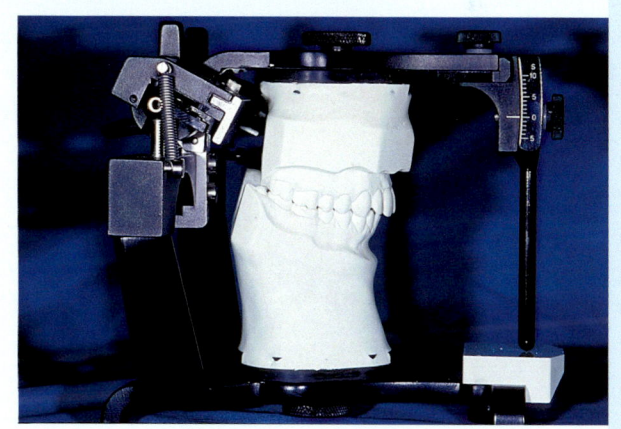

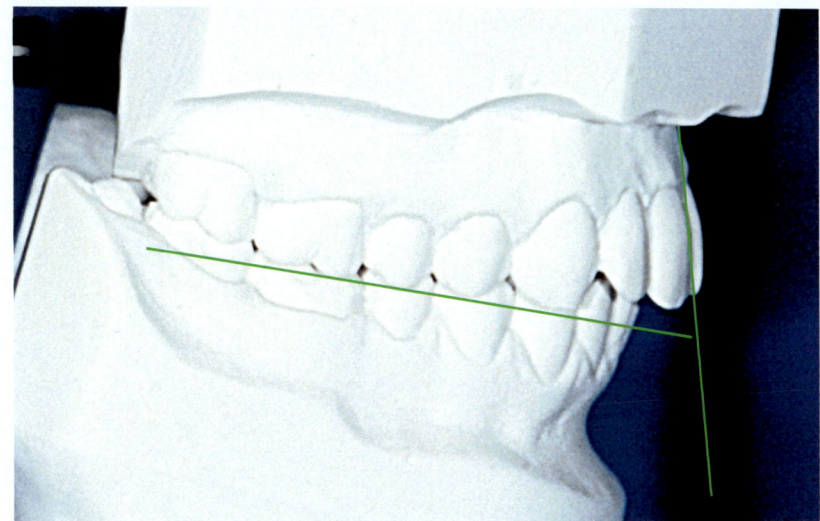

FIG 10 *(e to g)* If a facebow that takes the arbitrary plane as its reference is used, the inclination in the anteroposterior direction of the stone casts mounted on the articulator is much less prominent. *(h)* Consequently, less inclination of the occlusal plane is seen along with a more buccal position of the anterior teeth.

FACEBOW
REFERENCE PLANES frontal view

In a harmonious face, certain horizontal and vertical lines can be identified that map out a sort of regular harmony. The most important are the following:

- *Interpupillary line:* passing through the center of the eyes
- *Commissural line:* passing through the corners of the lips
- *Midline:* passing through glabella and the tip of the chin

The interpupillary line generally identifies the horizontal reference plane.[95] It is usually parallel with the commissural line and perpendicular to the midline, creating an ideal overall harmony (Fig 1-11).[95,125,127–130]

The eyes and lips are not always aligned with the horizontal plane, but one or both may lack parallelism with the horizon. In these situations the horizon is taken as an ideal reference plane for the prosthetic rehabilitation (Fig 1-12).[121]

Correct evaluation of the reference planes is carried out, as shown previously (see volume 1, chapter 2), with the observer positioned facing the patient, who holds the head in a natural posture.[117,131–134]

ESTHETIC-FUNCTIONAL IMPLICATIONS

Before initiating the prosthetic therapy, the clinician's goal is to transfer, by correct use of the facebow, the true position of the patient's occlusal plane to the laboratory, regardless of whether it is parallel or inclined in relation to the horizon (Fig 1-13). In the latter case the technician will read the angle on the articulator and, based on the indications from the clinician in the relevant section of the laboratory checklist, will make any corrections necessary to realign the incisal plane with the horizon.

Ideal facial harmony is strictly connected to parallelism between the occlusal plane and the horizon; any lateral inclination is immediately noticeable[135] and esthetically displeasing (Fig 1-13). However, if the interpupillary line and the commissural line are inclined but parallel to each other (giving a general obliquity of the face in relation to the horizon), the plane described by them could be taken as the reference plane for the prosthetic rehabilitation, thereby following the general oblique trend of the face.

> Fig 1-11

> Fig 1-12a > Fig 1-12b > Fig 1-12c

> Fig 1-12d > Fig 1-12e > Fig 1-12f

> Fig 1-13a > Fig 1-13b > Fig 1-13c

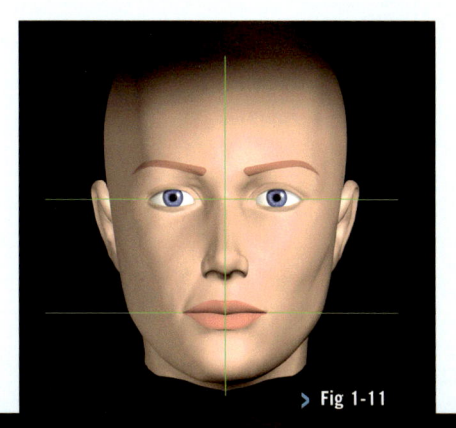

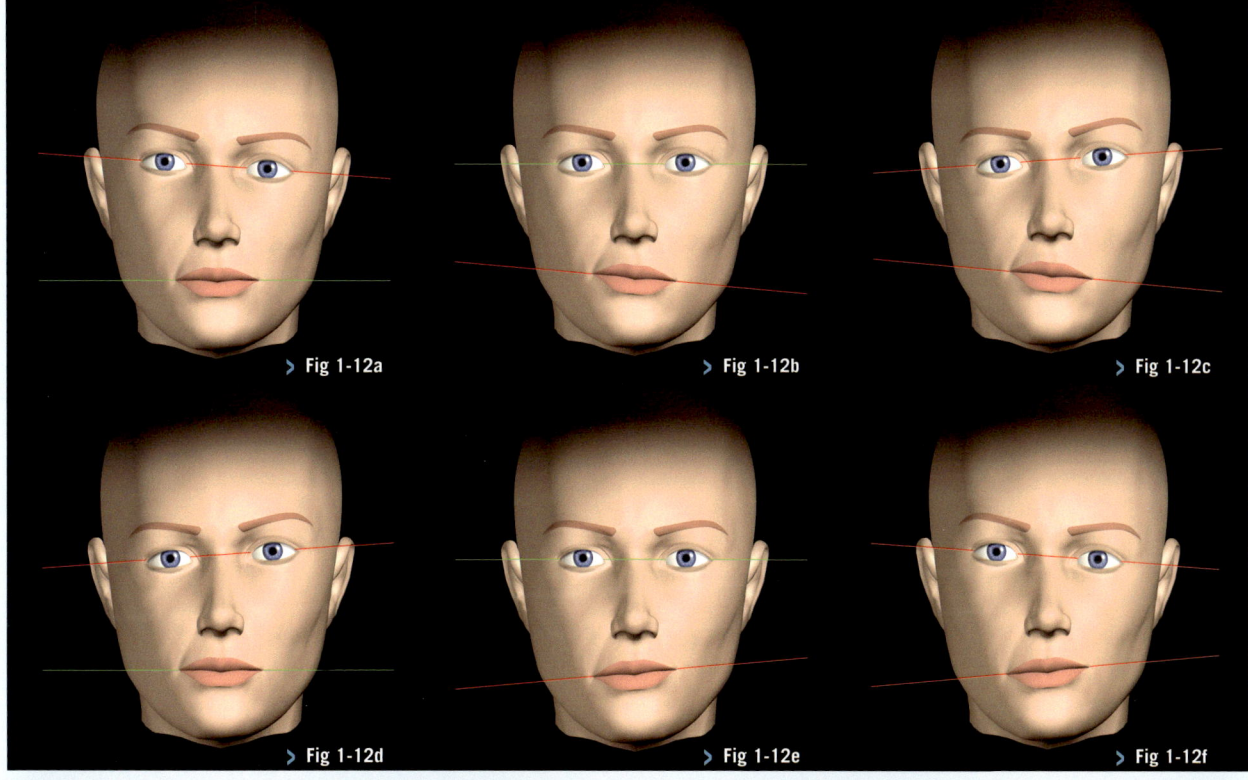

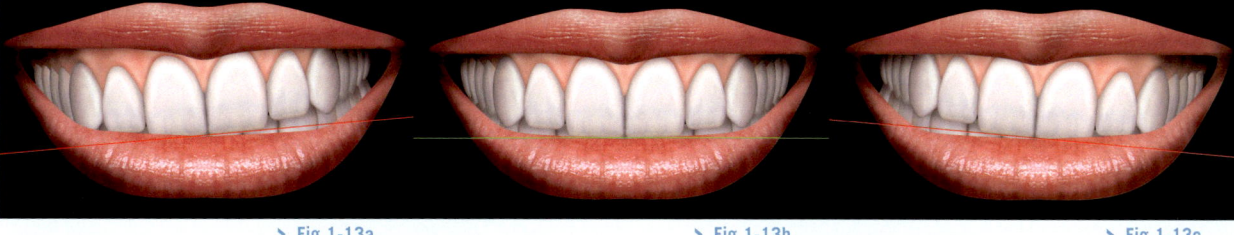

FIG 11 In a harmonic face, certain lines can be identified that between them map out a regular geometry. The parallelism of the main horizontal lines (interpupillary and commissural) relative to the horizon and the perpendicularity of the midline contribute to the sense of overall facial harmony.

FIG 12 *(a to f)* Nature does not always provide the ideal symmetry and parallelism between the interpupillary line, the commissural line, and the horizon. The first two lines can deviate in a variety of ways.

FIG 13 *(a to c)* The incisal plane should ideally be parallel to the commissural line and the horizon, even if it is not uncommon to find significant lateral inclination in nature and, unfortunately, in cases of incongruous prosthetic rehabilitation.

FACEBOW   REFERENCE: HORIZON

HORIZONTAL INCISAL PLANE

CORRECT REGISTRATION

Correct use of a facebow allows the clinical situation to be accurately replicated in the laboratory and the casts to be positioned correctly on the articulator.[117,129,134,136]

A great deal of care must therefore be taken in registering the facebow, whose orientation can only be evaluated by standing in front of the patient. Although this suggestion may appear obvious, according to several authors[115,117,129,136,137] the failure to observe the necessary parallelism between the arms of the facebow and the horizon is one of the errors encountered most frequently during the prosthetic rehabilitation of the anterosuperior teeth.

When using an arbitrary facebow with ear inserts, any inclination of the facebow relative to the horizontal plane is not always due to an anatomic alteration (eg, a lack of alignment of the condyles and/or acoustic meatuses with the horizontal plane) but more frequently is caused by inaccuracy and failure to ensure the correct positioning of the ear inserts.

If the patient's incisal plane is parallel with the horizontal plane, the clinician needs only to orient the arms of the facebow parallel with the horizon, even in cases where the condyles or the acoustic meatuses are not parallel with it (Figs 1-14a and 1-14b). This allows the patient's clinical situation to be correctly reproduced in the articulator, keeping horizontal orientation of the incisal plane (Figs 1-14c and 1-14d).

Where the meatuses and/or condyles are not parallel with the horizontal plane, making them parallel will inevitably lead to inaccuracy in reading the condylar axis, even if, as Dawson[117] maintains, this imprecision has an insignificant effect on the closing arc of the two arches. The repercussions from the occlusal point of view are minimal, provided that the intermaxillary registration has been correctly taken at the specified VDO. Though these small inaccuracies are clinically of little significance, the alignment of the facebow with the horizontal plane is a determining factor for ideal esthetic-functional integration of the rehabilitation because it allows the technician to preserve or create the ideal orientation of the occlusal plane and the correct verticality of the interincisal line.

FIG 14 *(a)* For correct transfer of information to the laboratory, the arms of the facebow must be parallel to the horizon. On the articulator, in fact, the condyles are aligned on a horizontal plane. *(b)* Even if the patient has a misalignment of acoustic meatuses and/or asymmetry of the intercondylar axis, the clinician must nonetheless take care to align the arms of the facebow with the horizontal plane so that the technician can reproduce the true clinical situation in the articulator *(c and d)*.

CORRECT REGISTRATION

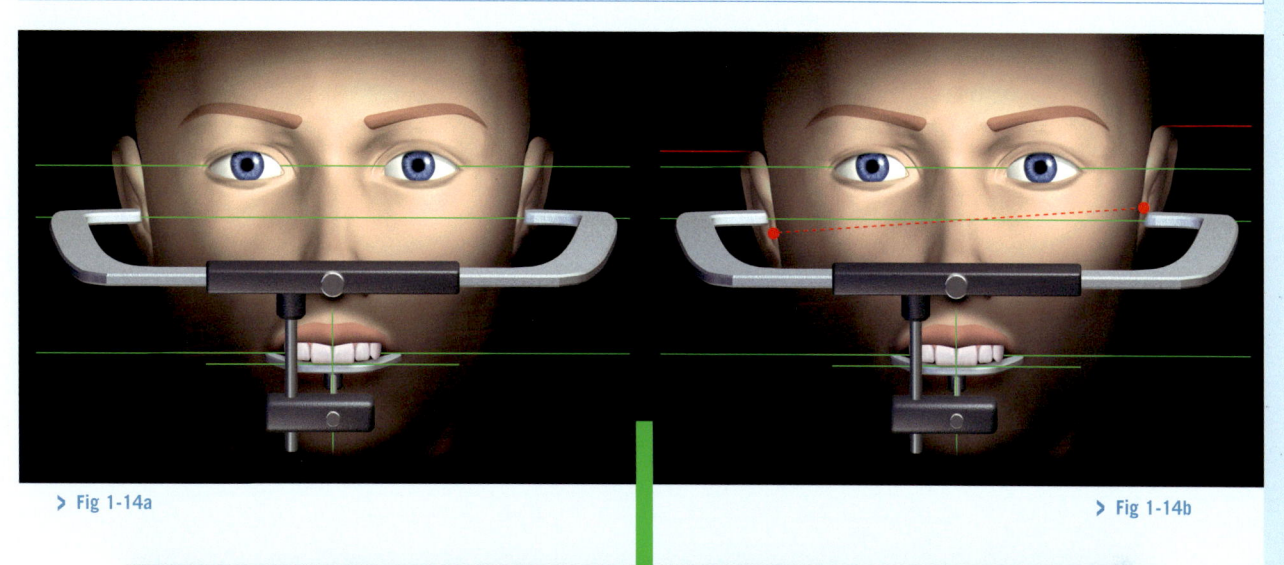

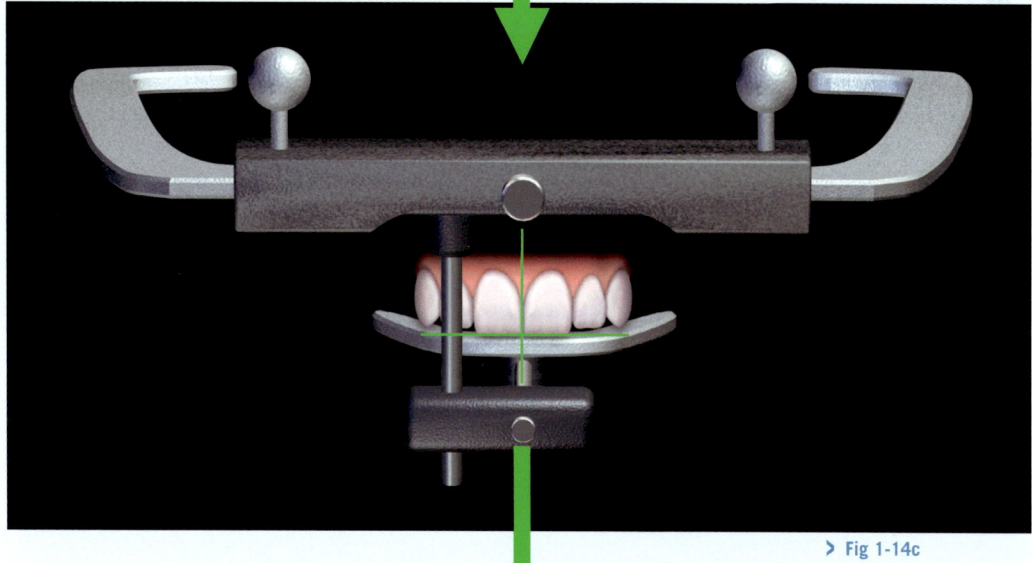

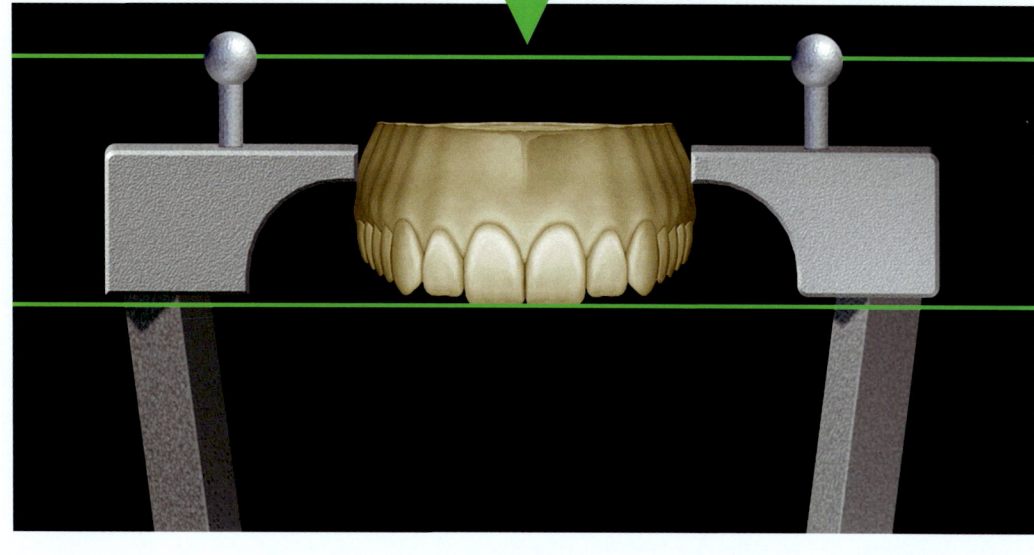

> Fig 1-14a

> Fig 1-14b

> Fig 1-14c

> Fig 1-14d

HORIZONTAL INCISAL PLANE

INCORRECT REGISTRATION

If bad positioning of the ear inserts on a facebow (Fig 1-15a) or a true condylar misalignment (Fig 1-15b) results in incorrect registration with an oblique axis, the maxillary cast will be mounted on the articulator at the wrong angle. For this reason, the intercondylar axis registered on the patient with an oblique orientation automatically becomes a horizontal intercondylar axis in the articulator (Figs 1-15c and 1-15d).

In the laboratory, the condyles are forcibly aligned with the horizon. If the incisal plane is parallel with the horizontal plane, this case is incorrectly reproduced in the articulator and results in incorrect inclination of the anterior teeth (Fig 1-15d). In turn, the technician will correct the outline of a seemingly oblique occlusal plane by realigning the restorations with the horizontal reference dictated by the working plane (Figs 1-15e and Fig 1-15f). The inevitable consequence is restorations that, once positioned in the oral cavity, show an unexpectedly inclined outline in the context of the patient's face, with an undoubtedly negative impact on the final esthetic outcome (Fig 1-15g).

If, when standing in front of the patient, a lack of parallelism is apparent between the arms of the facebow and the horizon, the clinician can accurately reproduce the initial clinical situation in the articulator with just a slight correction. This correction can be made by moving the ear inserts of the facebow to re-establish the parallelism between the arms of the facebow and the horizontal plane (Figs 1-16a to 1-16f).[115,117]

FIG 15 *(a and b)* The arms of the facebow may be inclined either because of incorrect positioning or because of an actual misalignment of acoustic meatuses and/or inclination of the intercondylar axis. *(c and d)* Although the patient's incisal plane may be parallel to the horizon, if the facebow has been recorded with the arms inclined, the cast mounted on the articulator is tilted toward the side opposite that of the facebow. *(e to g)* If the technician tries to change the angle, making the occlusal plane parallel to the horizontal plane in the prosthetic rehabilitation, the incisal plane will be oblique once the restorations have been positioned in the mouth, with the same incorrect inclination at which the facebow was recorded.

INCORRECT REGISTRATION

malpositioning misalignment of meati

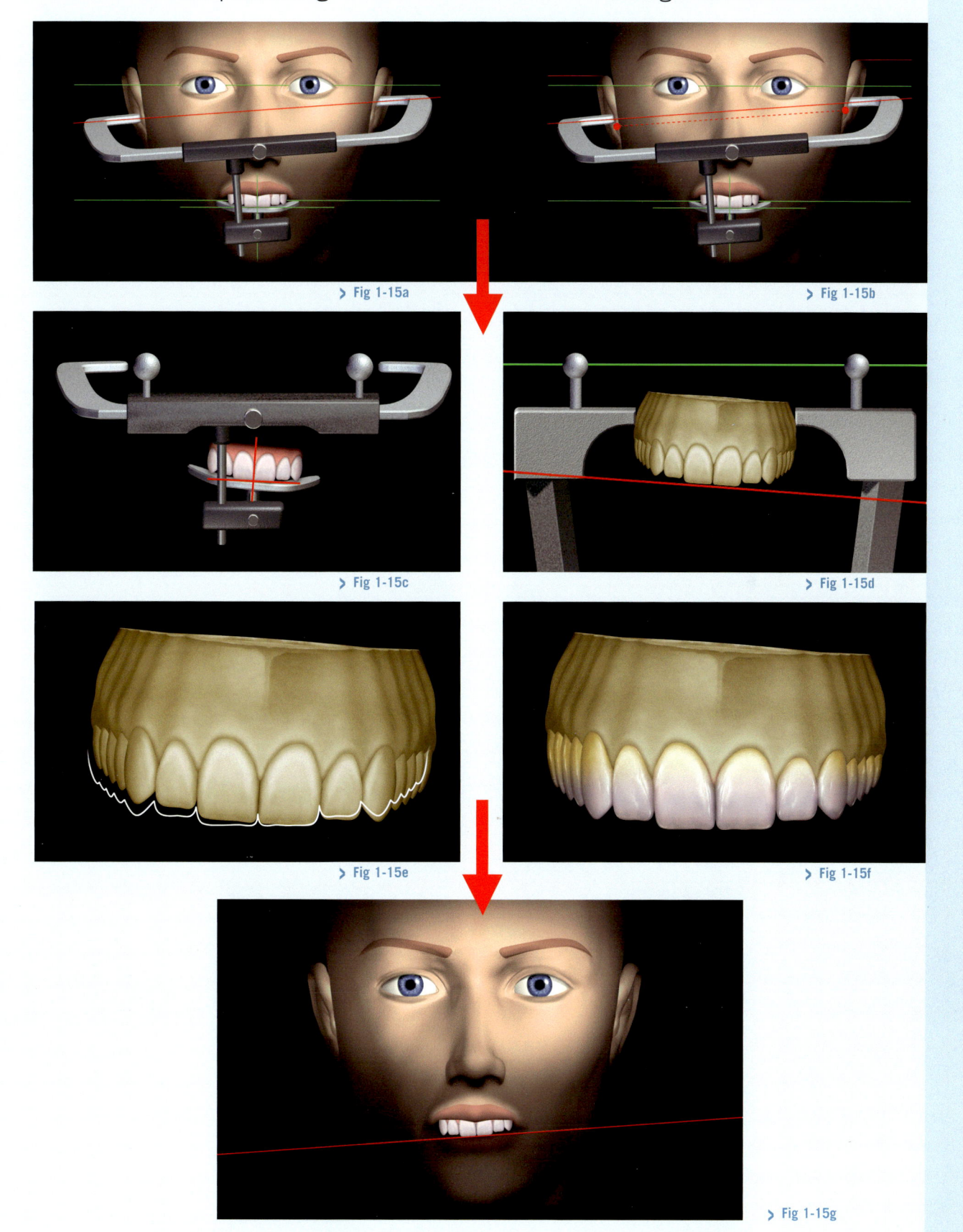

> Fig 1-15a

> Fig 1-15b

> Fig 1-15c

> Fig 1-15d

> Fig 1-15e

> Fig 1-15f

> Fig 1-15g

INCORRECT REGISTRATION—malpositioning

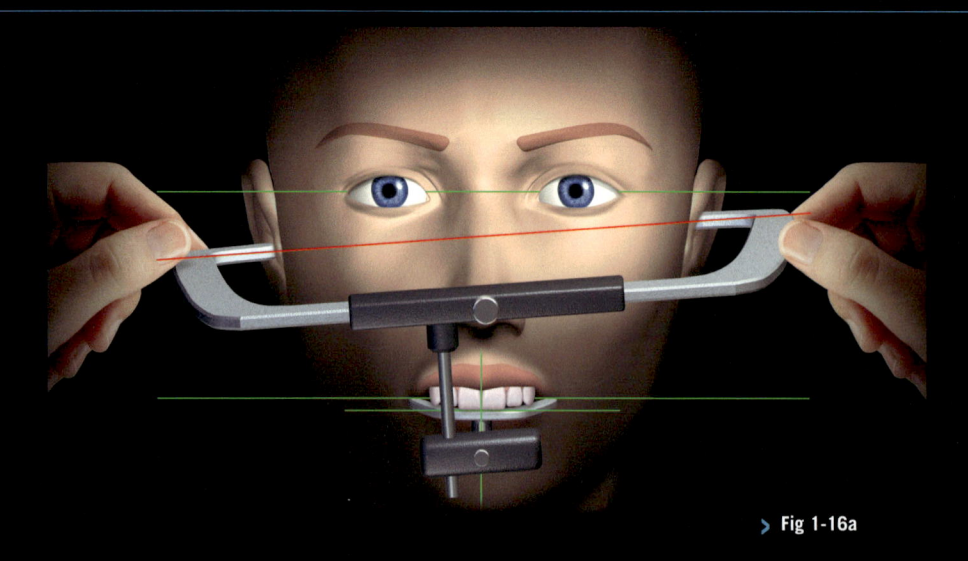

> Fig 1-16a

CORRECTION

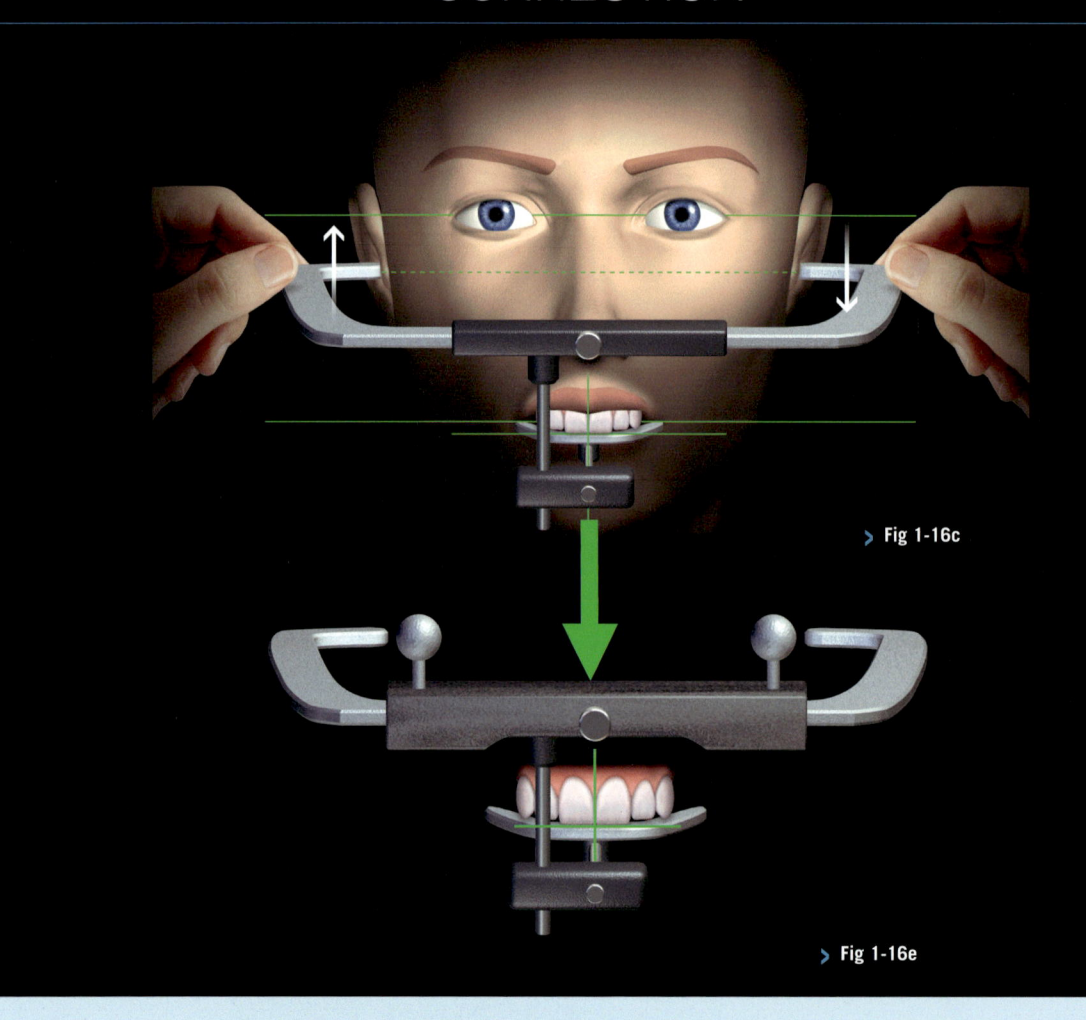

> Fig 1-16c

> Fig 1-16e

FIG 16 *(a to d)* In cases of incorrect facebow positioning, misalignment of the meatus, and/or true inclination of the intercondylar axis, the oblique position of the facebow can easily be corrected by hand because of the elasticity of the acoustic meatuses, orienting

INCORRECT REGISTRATION—misalignment of meati

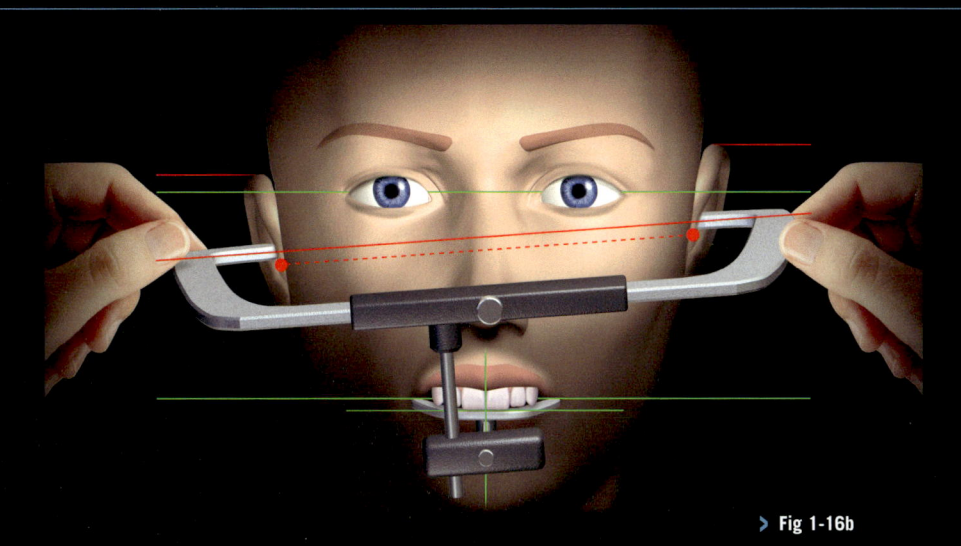

> Fig 1-16b

CORRECTION

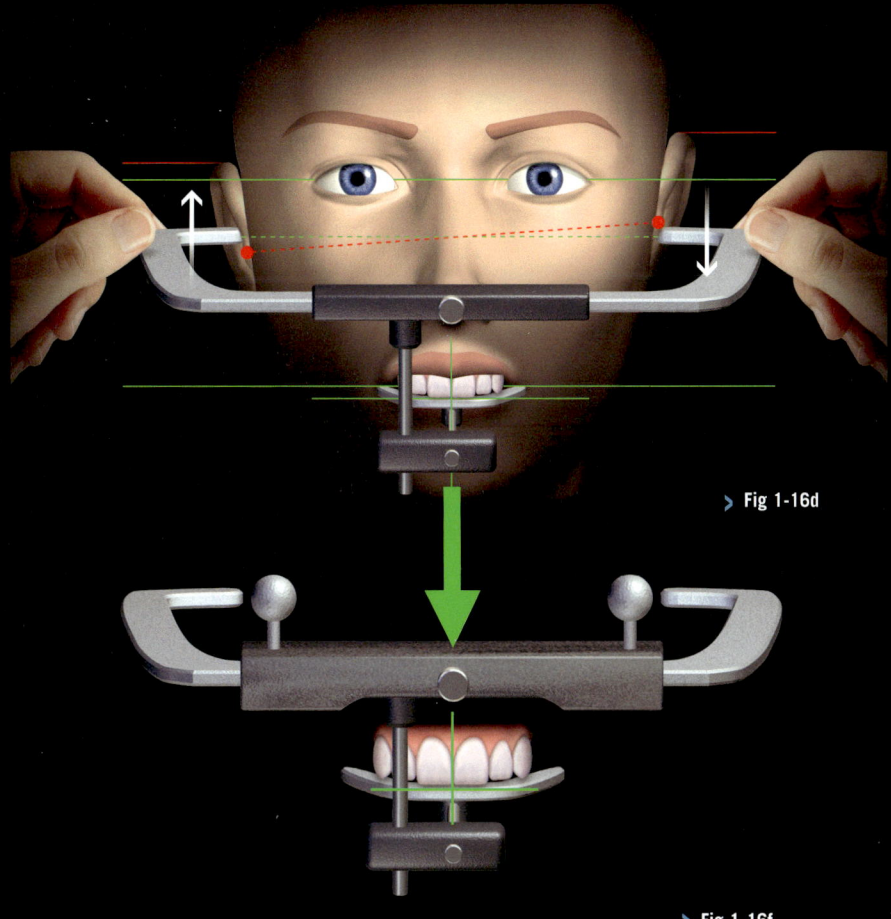

> Fig 1-16d

> Fig 1-16f

the facebow parallel to the horizon. *(e and f)* This allows a faithful reproduction of the orientation of the patient's incisal plane in the articulator.

FACEBOW   REFERENCE: HORIZON

INCLINED INCISAL PLANE

CORRECT REGISTRATION

In cases where the patient's incisal plane is inclined, whether or not it is associated with an inclination of the commissural line (Figs 1-17a and 1-17b), the facebow needs to be oriented parallel with the horizon (Fig 1-17c) for the technician to correctly reproduce its inclination on the workbench (Figs 1-17d and 1-17e).

It is the clinician's task, after checking for the possibility of clinical intervention, to note in the appropriate section of the laboratory checklist the method for correcting the occlusal plane inclination. If this obliquity corresponds to the same inclination of gingival contour, the correction can highlight a difference in level in the cervical margins. If the patient has a medium to high smile line, this lack of parallelism can be corrected with surgical-periodontal, maxillofacial, and/or orthodontic therapy (Fig 1-17f). If the smile line is low, gingival misalignment is not an esthetic limitation, and the clinician's intervention can be aimed purely at ensuring adequate parallelism between the occlusal plane and the horizon (Fig 1-17g). To transfer the patient's actual clinical situation to the technician and clarify any modifications requested, the facebow must be oriented parallel with the horizon regardless of the angle of the incisal plane.

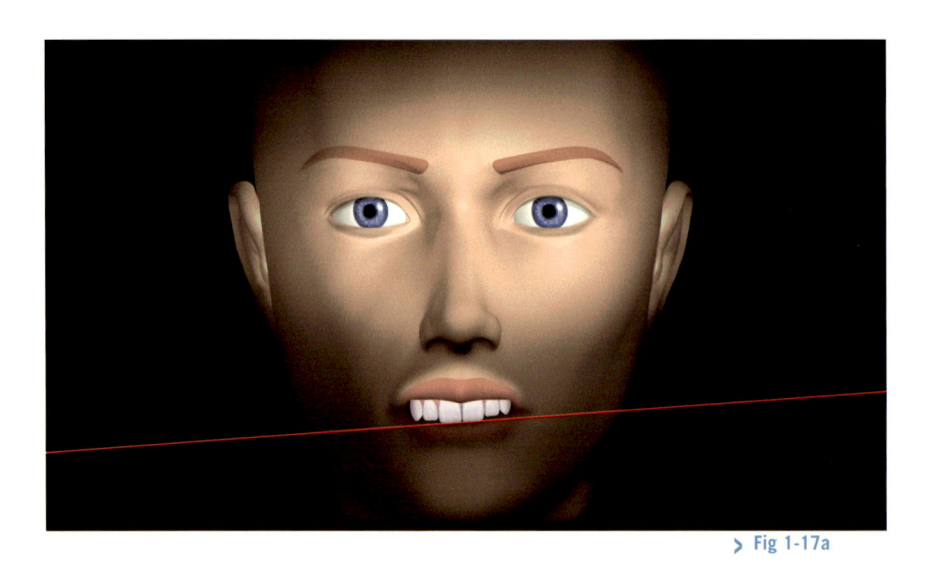

> Fig 1-17a

FIG 17 *(a to d)* If the incisal plane results in a significantly tilted but correct facebow recording, placing the arms parallel to the horizon allows the obliquity of the incisal plane to be replicated in the articulator. *(e and f)* The technician is therefore able to mark the inclination of the incisal plane and correct it according to the indications specified by the clinician on the laboratory checklist. This substantial modification of the occlusal plane is generally only possible if a multidisciplinary clinical approach is adopted. *(g)* At the end of treatment, the discrepancy between the interpupillary line and the incisal plane is corrected, resulting in a realignment of the incisal plane with the horizontal plane.

CORRECT REGISTRATION

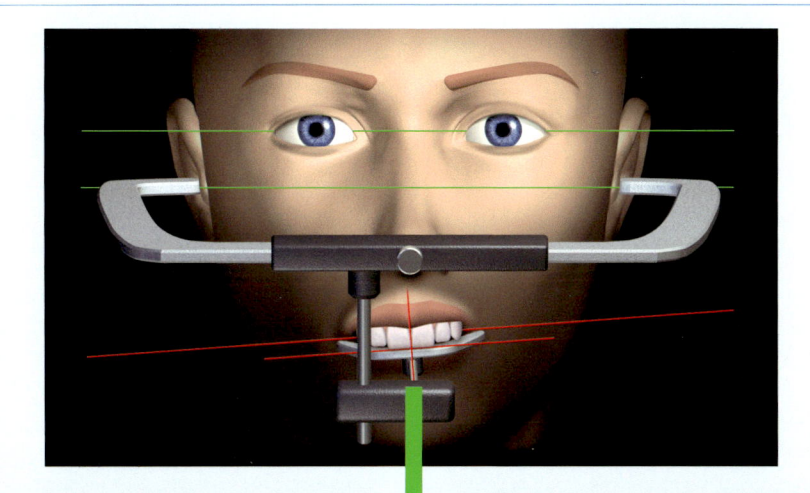

› Fig 1-17b

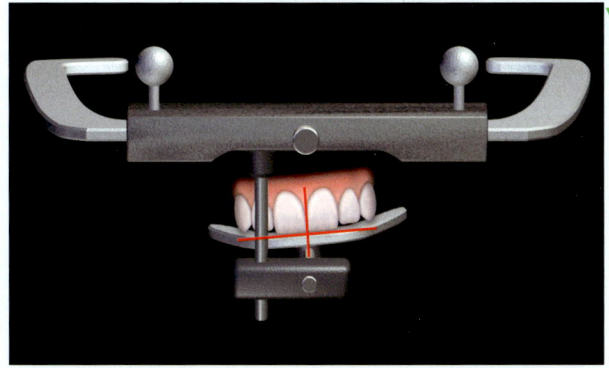

› Fig 1-17c

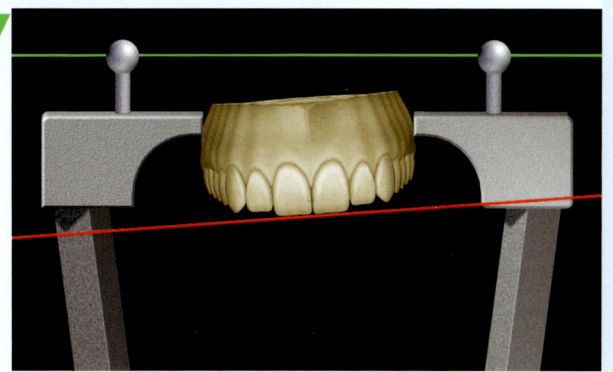

› Fig 1-17d

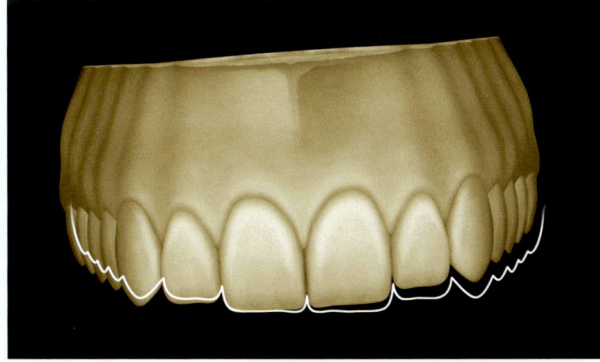

› Fig 1-17e

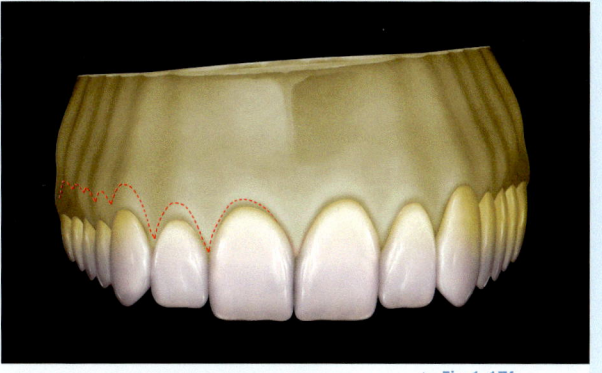

› Fig 1-17f

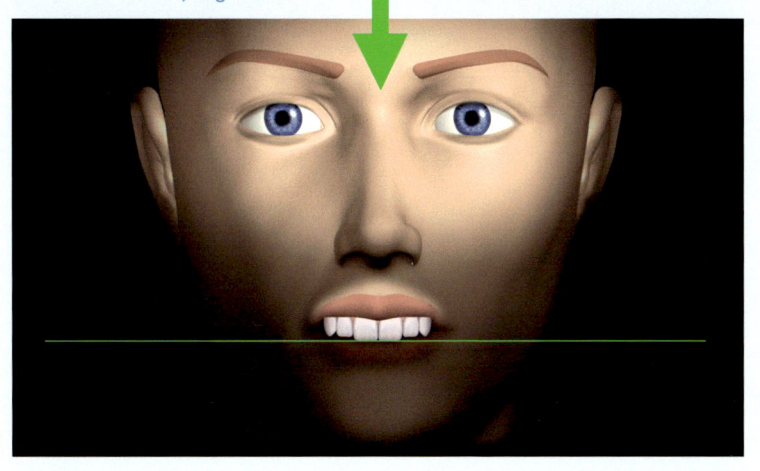

› Fig 1-17g

FACEBOW REFERENCE: HORIZON

INCLINED INCISAL PLANE

INCORRECT REGISTRATION

In the case of an inclination of the incisal plane accompanied by a misalignment of condyles and/or acoustic meatuses, the clinician could fall into the trap of taking the facebow recording while orienting the arms parallel with the inclined occlusal plane (Fig 1-18a). An inclined recording of the facebow that is parallel with the inclined occlusal plane could also occur simply due to bad positioning. In both cases, the technician will find a parallelism between the occlusal plane and the working plane (Figs 1-18b and 1-18c). In the absence of specific requests to modify the plane inclination, the technician will then proceed with the fabrication of the restorations without making any corrections. Once positioned in the mouth, the restorations will reproduce the inclination of the occlusal plane that was initially recorded erroneously (Fig 1-18d). If, on the other hand, after taking an incorrect facebow recording, the clinician specifies on the laboratory checklist the modifications necessary to correct the inclinations in the occlusal plane and dental axes, the technician will find it impossible to check the noted discrepancies against the horizontal plane on the casts mounted on the articulator. Effective communication with the laboratory will allow the clinician, in such a case, to promptly identify a procedural error, which can easily be resolved with a new, correct facebow recording.

In nature, as noted earlier, a lack of parallelism between occlusal plane, interpupillary line, commissural line, and horizontal plane is found frequently upon close analysis of the face. This common occurrence can often lead to an incorrect orientation of the facebow. Regardless of inclination in one or more of the reference lines, the goal of the clinician is to ensure, by correction if necessary, that the arms of the facebow are oriented parallel to the horizontal plane, allowing the technician to correctly reproduce the clinical situation in the articulator (Fig 1-19).

FIG 18 *(a and b)* When faced with a tilted incisal plane, if the facebow is recorded without the arms parallel to the horizon but inclined the same way as the occlusal plane, the latter is perfectly horizontal in the articulator. *(c and d)* In the absence of specific indications, the technician therefore maintains the orientation that seems horizontal but that, once the work is complete, is once again tilted when positioned inside the patient's mouth.

Chapter 1 COMMUNICATING TO THE LABORATORY—DIAGNOSTIC WAX-UP

INCORRECT REGISTRATION

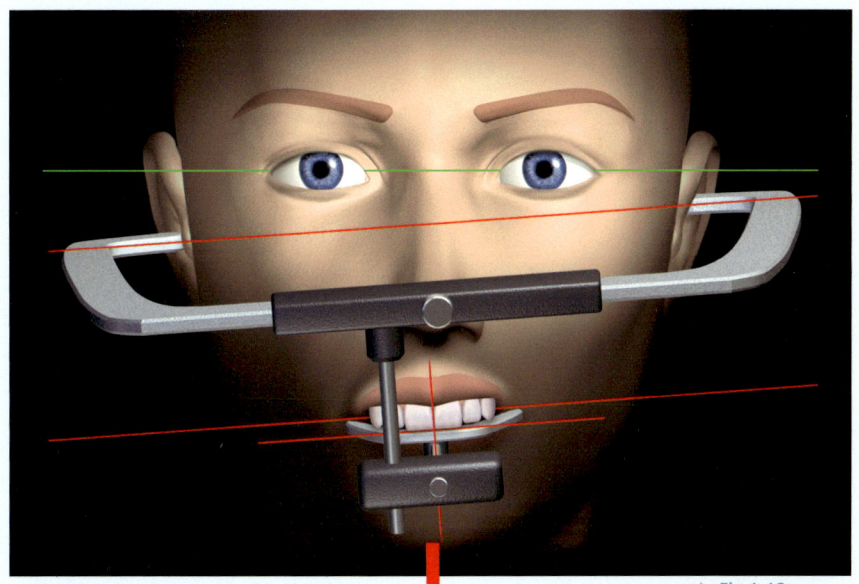

> Fig 1-18a

> Fig 1-18b

> Fig 1-18c

> Fig 1-18d

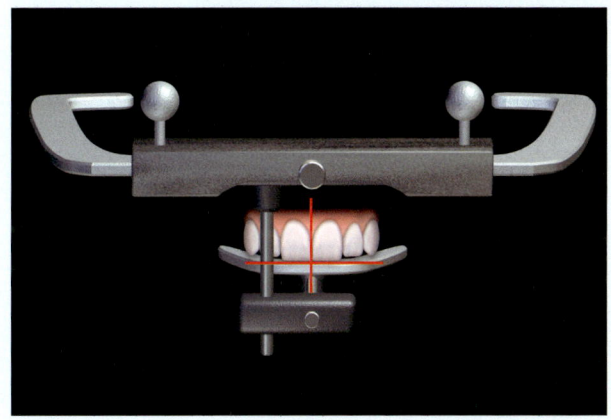

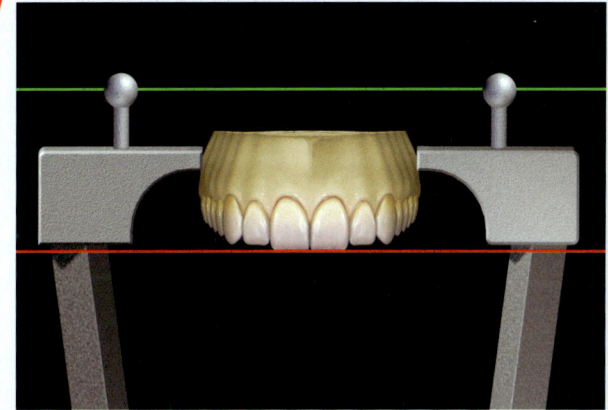

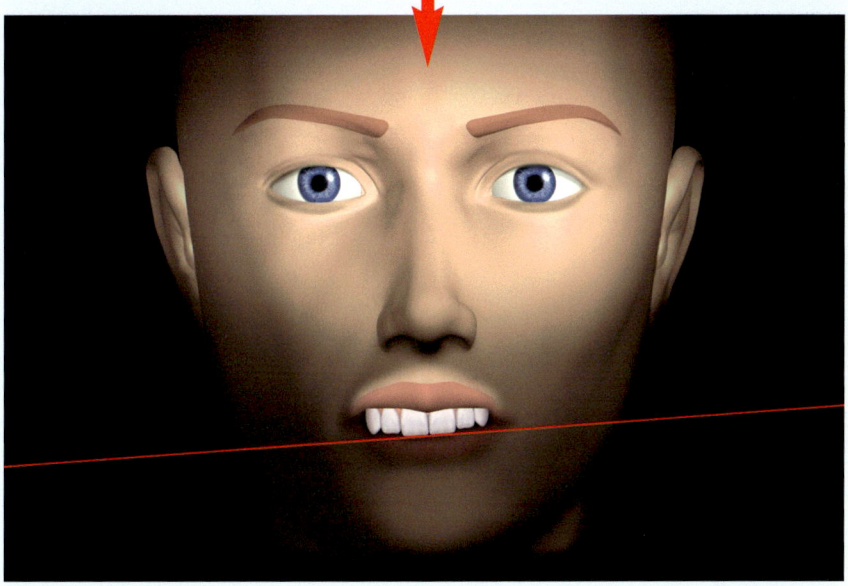

CORRECT REGISTRATION

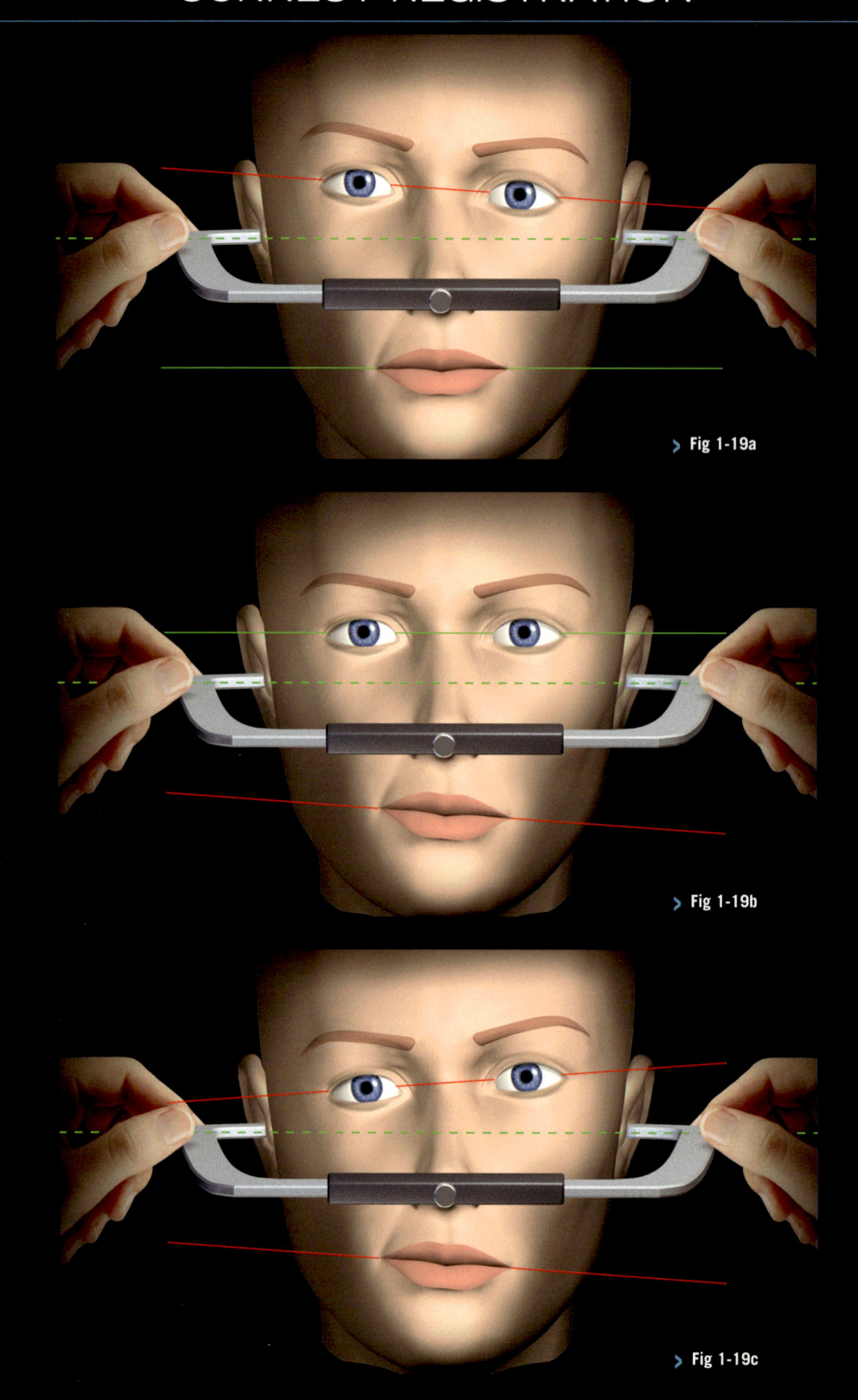

> Fig 1-19a

> Fig 1-19b

> Fig 1-19c

FIG 19 *(a to f)* The occlusal plane, interpupillary line, commissural line, and horizon are not always parallel but may deviate in various ways. In these cases, the horizontal plane is the ideal reference most commonly used to orient the arms of the facebow correctly.

CORRECT REGISTRATION

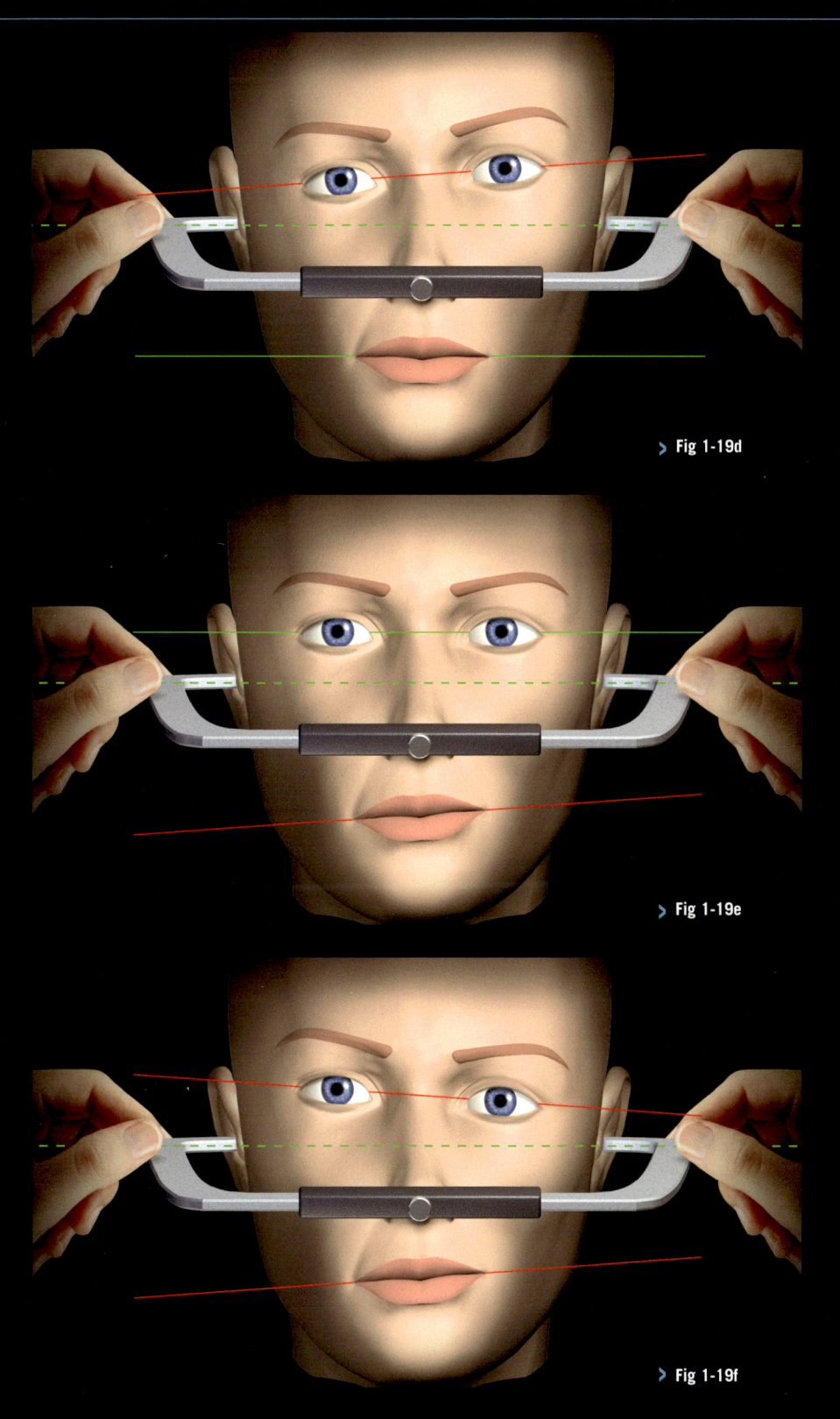

> Fig 1-19d

> Fig 1-19e

> Fig 1-19f

It is therefore necessary for the clinician to check the parallelism of the facebow to the horizon while standing in front of the patient. In case of any misalignment, the arms of the facebow can be adjusted.

FACEBOW REFERENCE: INCLINED

OBLIQUE FACIAL INCLINATION

CORRECT REGISTRATION

It is possible that in some patients the reference lines, like the occlusal plane, are oblique relative to the horizontal plane but parallel to each other (Fig 1-20). This is found especially when there are asymmetries between the right and left sides that give the face a general oblique inclination (see volume 1, chapter 2). In these cases it can be clinically impossible, even with recourse to interdisciplinary treatment, to realign the occlusal plane with the horizon.

Therefore, to integrate the prosthetic rehabilitation into the context of the patient's face so that it fits in with the general oblique inclination, the arms of the facebow must be oriented following the angle of the aforementioned reference lines.

In this way the casts, once mounted on the articulator, will seem to the technician to be perfectly aligned with the horizontal plane (Fig 1-21). Sending photographs of these patients to the laboratory is, as a rule, a major reason to give precise indications to the technician. Highlighting the discrepancy between the obliquity of the occlusal plane seen from the photos and the casts that are instead perfectly aligned with the horizon, the technician could be tempted to modify the inclination of the occlusal plane, ignoring the choice made by the clinician and approved by the patient.

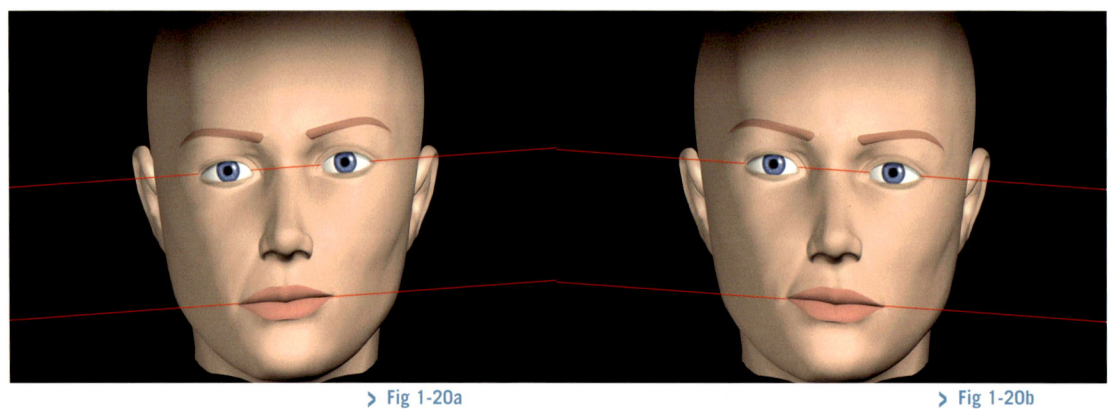

> Fig 1-20a   > Fig 1-20b

FIG 20 *(a and b)* Sometimes a general oblique inclination of the face is found, with the horizontal reference lines and incisal plane oblique in relation to the horizon but parallel to each other, which produces a kind of harmonic asymmetry.

FIG 21 *(a and c)* To integrate the prosthetic rehabilitation into the general oblique inclination of the patient's face, it is useful in these cases to confirm the inclination of the incisal plane, recording the facebow with the arms inclined but parallel to the oblique reference lines. *(b)* The technician, duly informed by the clinician of this specific operational choice, will find perfect alignment of the occlusal plane with the horizon in the articulator and will therefore not have to make any alterations to the orientation of the rehabilitation.

Chapter 1 COMMUNICATING TO THE LABORATORY—DIAGNOSTIC WAX-UP

CORRECT REGISTRATION

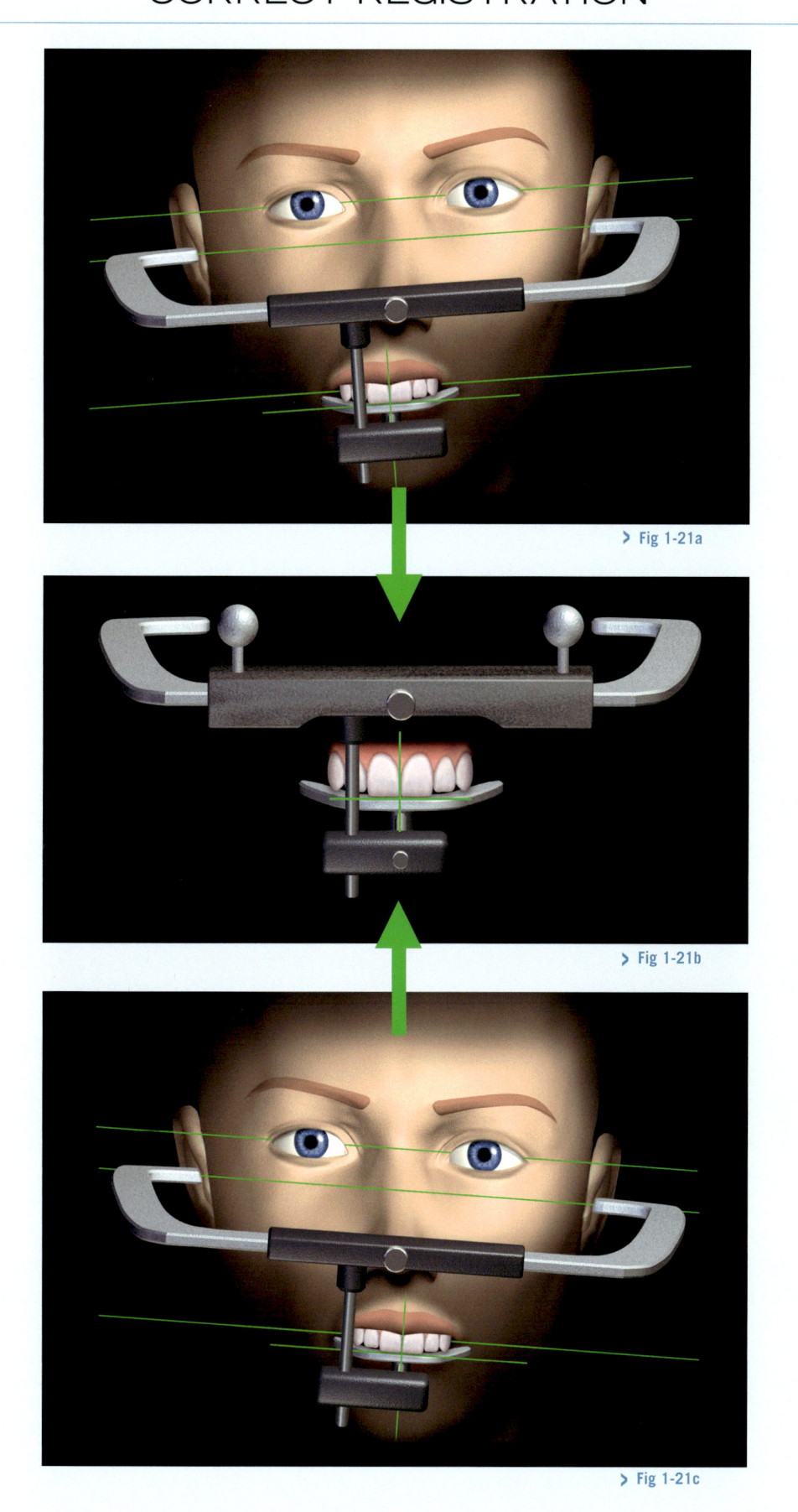

> Fig 1-21a

> Fig 1-21b

> Fig 1-21c

CLINICAL-PRACTICAL SUGGESTIONS

If the interpupillary line is parallel with the horizon and is the chosen reference plane, the clinician can easily orient the arms of the facebow by standing in front of the patient and looking at the eyes. Where there is any doubt as to the parallelism of the facebow in relation to the horizontal plane, a level can be used (Fig 1-22).

Arbitrary versus kinematic facebow All of the suggestions offered until now for reproducing the patient's true occlusal plane do not apply if using a kinematic facebow. In cases where, on the frontal plane, the two condyles are asymmetric (one higher than the other), the clinician must accept the inclination of the kinematic facebow in relation to the horizontal plane without being able to make any correction, because this would negate the purpose of an instrument that depends on the supposition of registering the individual intercondylar axis[120] (Fig 1-23a). In these cases the technician, unable to show the inclination of the intercondylar axis (since even on the fully adjustable articulator the condyles are set on a horizontal plane and are not normally adjustable in height), finds that the maxillary cast has a different occlusal plane inclination from that of the patient (Figs 1-23b and 1-23c). In the absence of specific instructions, this could lead the technician to correct the inclination found in the articulator by shortening and/or lengthening the teeth (Figs 1-23d and 1-23e). Once the restorations are positioned in the mouth, the incorrect orientation of the prosthetic rehabilitation in the context of the patient's face would result in a significant esthetic-functional deficit[124] (Fig 1-23f).

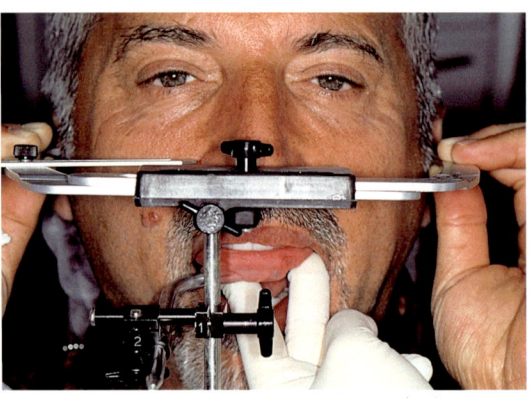

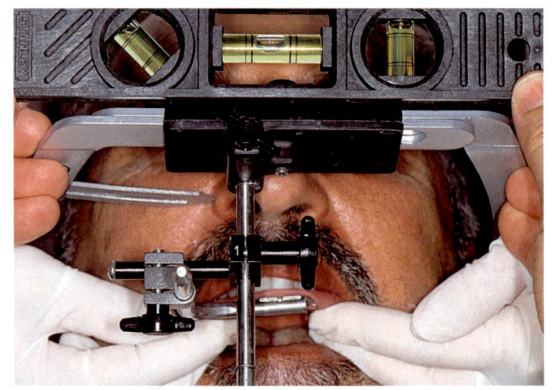

> Fig 1-22a

> Fig 1-22b

FIG 22 (a and b) A level can be used to make sure the arms of the facebow are correctly positioned in relation to the horizon.

FIG 23 (a to c) The premise for using the kinematic facebow is identification of the terminal hinge axis (intercondylar axis) by means of the pantograph or axiograph. If the incisal plane is parallel to the horizon but the intercondylar axis is misaligned, causing the arms to be oblique, the incisal plane will show the opposite angle to that of the facebow once the cast is mounted on the articulator. (d to f) Should the technician, in the absence of specific instructions, decide to realign the incisal plane with the horizon, the prosthetic rehabilitation will show an oblique outline, at the same angle at which the facebow was recorded.

> Fig 1-23a

> Fig 1-23b

> Fig 1-23c

> Fig 1-23d

> Fig 1-23e

> Fig 1-23f

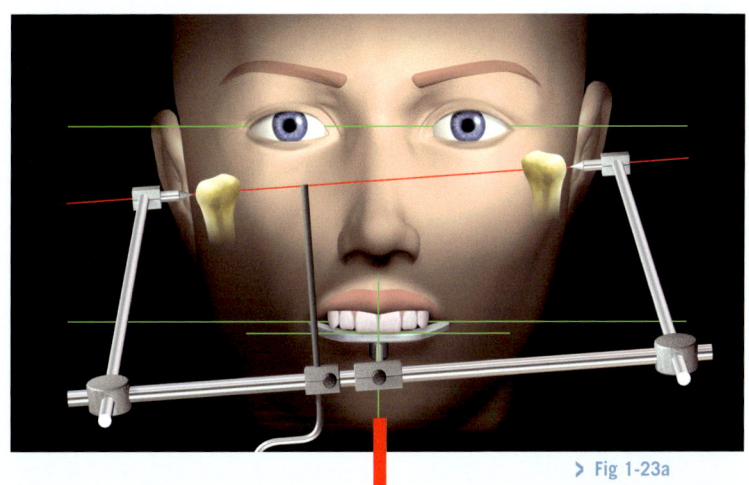

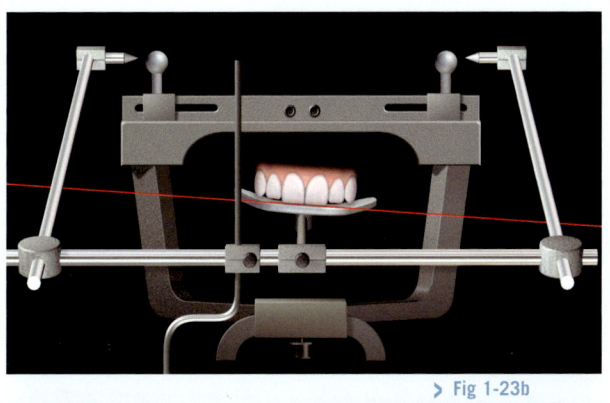

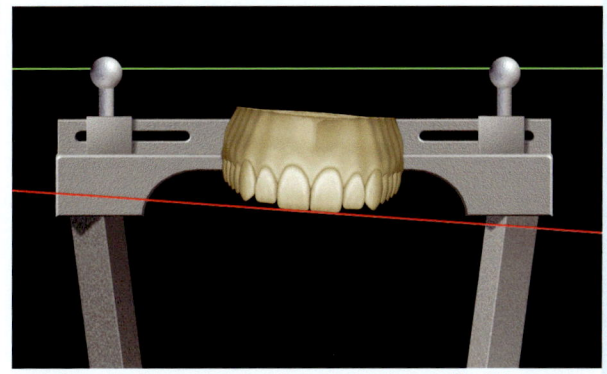

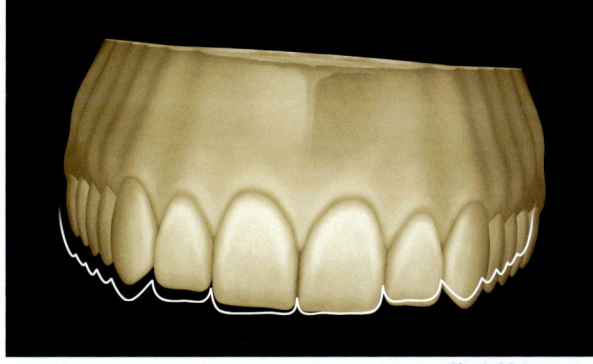

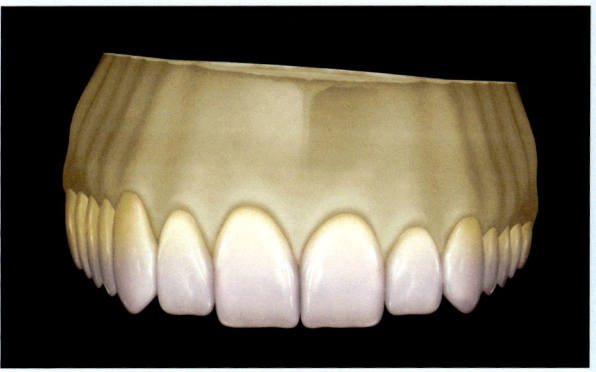

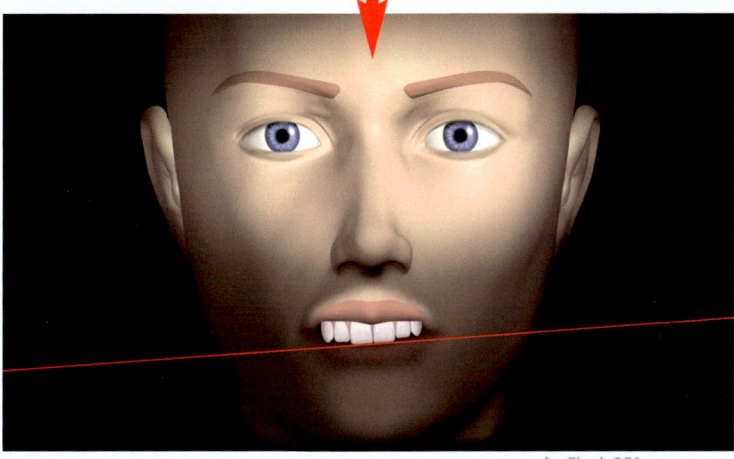

MOUNTING THE CASTS ON THE ARTICULATOR

After receiving the impressions of the two arches, the occlusal registration in CR, the protrusive wax-up, and the facebow recording, the technician has all of the details necessary for mounting the plaster casts on the articulator (Fig 1-24). Articulators are mechanical instruments that make it possible to reproduce both static and dynamic relationships of the maxillary and mandibular arches in the three spatial planes.[105]

FULLY ADJUSTABLE ARTICULATORS

Only after complete muscle relaxation of the stomatognathic system can the border movement of the patient's mandibular dynamics be analyzed using the pantograph, which allows the clinician and the technician to adjust the articulator individually (Fig 1-25a). This will allow adjustment of both the exact inclination of the condylar eminence and the path of the condyle in mandibular translation, since the condylar fossae of the articulator have adjustable walls also equipped with curved inserts (Figs 1-25b and 1-25c). This device is useful in the rehabilitation of especially complex cases, even though it may appear complicated and not without possible errors for those who do not use it regularly.[112–114,116]

SEMI-ADJUSTABLE ARTICULATORS

Semi-adjustable articulators are used more commonly (Fig 1-26a) than fully adjustable articulators. They allow certain adjustments to the condylar fossae (Figs 1-26b and 1-26c) that must be made before embarking upon the prosthetic work, such as the following:
- Inclination of the condylar eminence
- Progressive mandibular lateral translation
- Immediate mandibular lateral translation

The values assigned to these adjustments are at the discretion of the clinician and can either be extrapolated from the occlusal analysis of the patient being treated or established arbitrarily. The articulator (Fig 1-27) is programmed to give the restorations the necessary occlusal stability and to guarantee separation of the posterior teeth during all excursive movements.

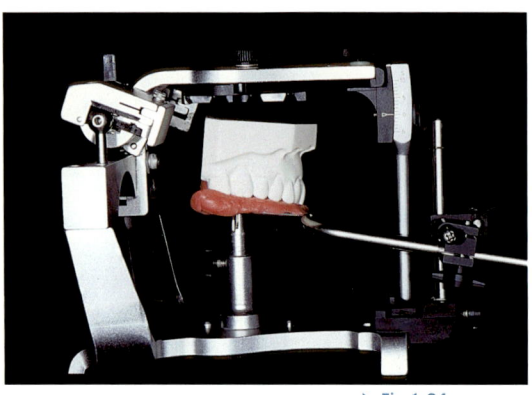

> Fig 1-24a

> Fig 1-24b

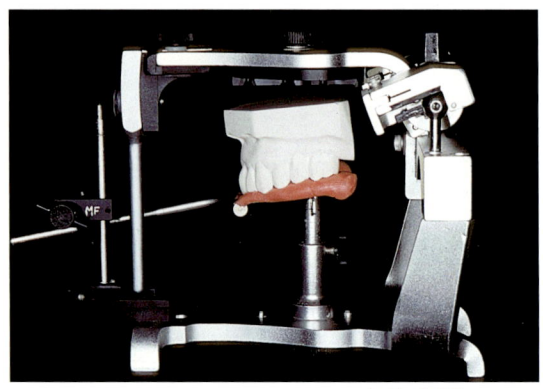

FULLY ADJUSTABLE ARTICULATOR

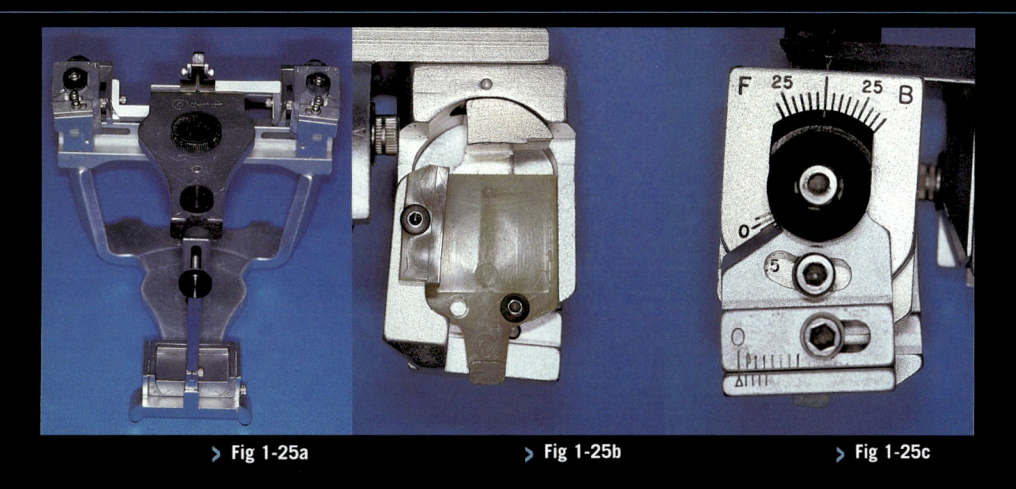

> Fig 1-25a   > Fig 1-25b   > Fig 1-25c

SEMI-ADJUSTABLE ARTICULATOR

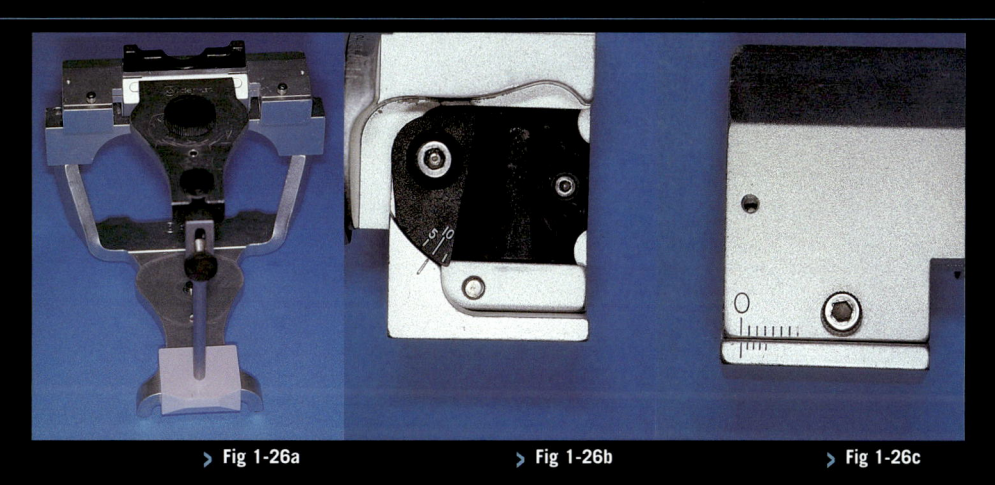

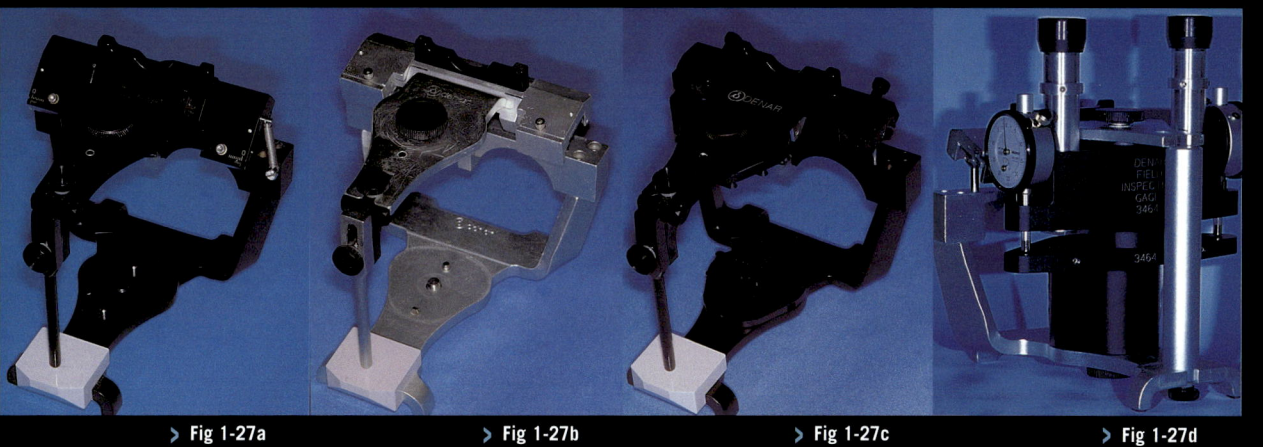

> Fig 1-26a   > Fig 1-26b   > Fig 1-26c

> Fig 1-27a   > Fig 1-27b   > Fig 1-27c   > Fig 1-27d

FIG 24 *(a and b)* The maxillary cast is mounted on the articulator according to the facebow recording.

FIG 25 *(a to c)* The fully adjustable articulator allows ample adjustment of the fossae.

FIG 26 *(a to c)* The semi-adjustable articulator allows less complete adjustments to be made compared with the fully adjustable articulator.

FIG 27 *(a to d)* Semi-adjustable articulators by the same maker, though different models, are interchangeable with the aid of a calibrator, which can make identical adjustments to all of the instruments used.

Adjustment of the condylar path (the posterior setting) along with the route of the anterior guidance (the anterior setting) allows for disocclusion of the posterior sectors. As demonstrated by Slavicek[138] through axiographic studies on more than 3,000 patients, the profile of the anterior guidance is not the same as that of the condylar path. Arbitrarily making the anterior guidance the same as a distinctly inclined condylar path can in fact cause a functional restriction, with extreme difficulty in the excursive movements. The anterior guidance created based on a flattened condylar path could, instead, create excessive shortening and buccal positioning of the maxillary incisal margins, with inevitable interferences when closing the lips, phonetic difficulty, and esthetic-functional deficits.

ADJUSTMENTS

To safeguard against possible posterior interferences during eccentric movements, the semi-adjustable articulator can be adjusted in the following ways:

Inclination of the condylar eminence This is determined by the inclination of the posterior wall of the articular eminence on which the condyle slides during protrusive and nonworking movements. It is advisable to take a protrusive interocclusal wax-up that will give an articulator adjustment closer to the clinical situation (Fig 1-28), although the need to make small occlusal refinements in the oral cavity is not excluded. Lundeen[139,140] has shown that the average condylar angle is 45 degrees. An arbitrary adjustment much less than this value (eg, 20 degrees) (Fig 1-29) almost always gives greater separation of the posterior teeth in the mouth compared with on the articulator.[141] In addition, semi-adjustable articulators usually have a flat path as opposed to the convex condylar path found naturally; this causes an even greater separation between the posterior teeth, constituting a further safety factor[104] (Fig 1-30a). The occlusal morphology obtained in this way is rather flat, with a possible reduction in masticatory efficiency.[142]

FIG 28 (a to e) Once the protrusive interocclusal registration has been positioned, the condylar fossae can then be adjusted; in this particular case, the inclination is roughly 40 degrees. (f) Once the wax has been removed, this inclination gives a marked separation of the two arches in the posterior sectors.

FIG 29 (a and b) If the clinician does not take a protrusive interocclusal registration, the condylar fossa adjustments can be made at an arbitrary value of 20 degrees. (c) In this case the separation between the arches is clearly less accentuated, conditioning the occlusal morphology of the posterior teeth.

FIG 30 (a and b) In the articulator, adjusting the condylar slant to 20 degrees prevents any contact between the posterior teeth during disocclusive movements, because the convexity of the condylar eminence of the same value (20 degrees) ensures greater disocclusion of the posterior sectors in the mouth.

Chapter 1 COMMUNICATING TO THE LABORATORY—DIAGNOSTIC WAX-UP

Setting: PROTRUSIVE INTEROCCLUSAL RECORD

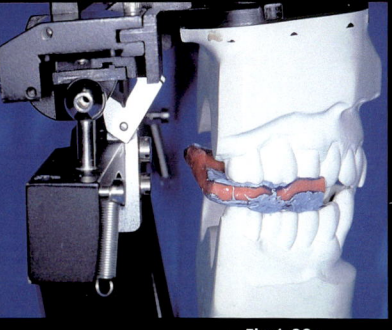

> Fig 1-28a

> Fig 1-28b

> Fig 1-28c

> Fig 1-28d

> Fig 1-28e

> Fig 1-28f

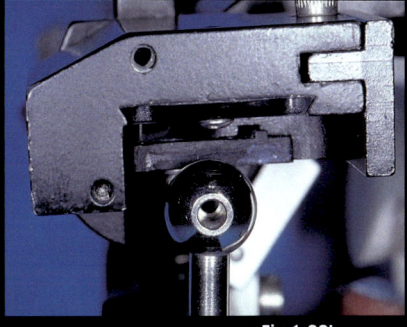

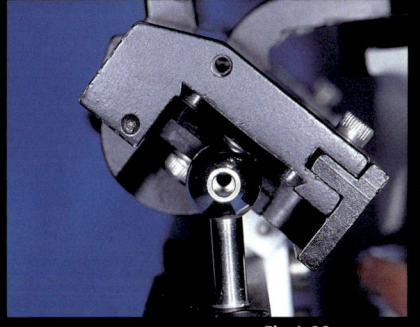

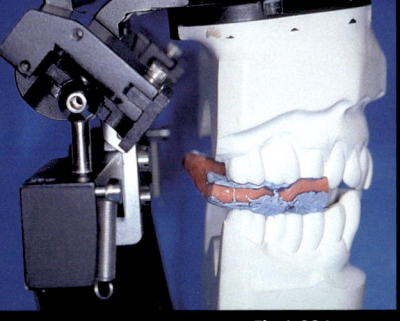

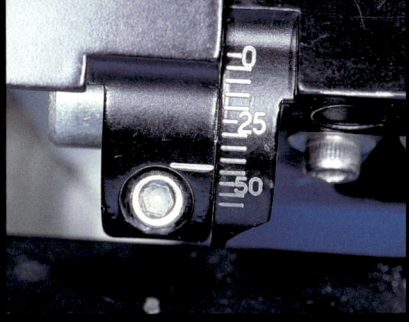

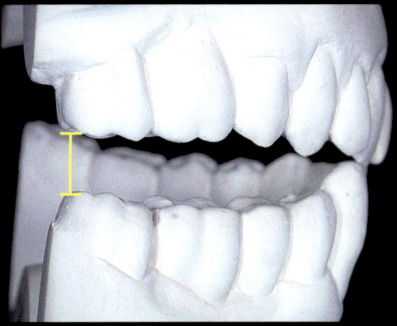

Setting: ARBITRARY 20 DEGREES

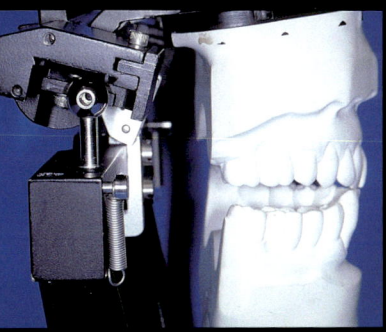

> Fig 1- 29a

> Fig 1-29b

> Fig 1-29c

> Fig 1-30a

> Fig 1-30b

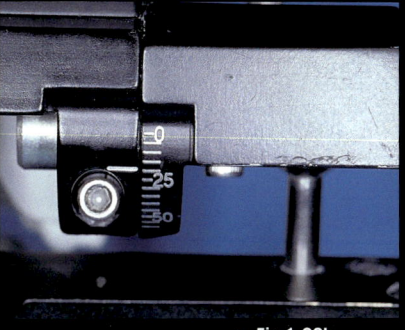

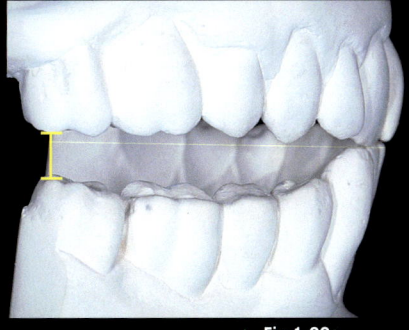

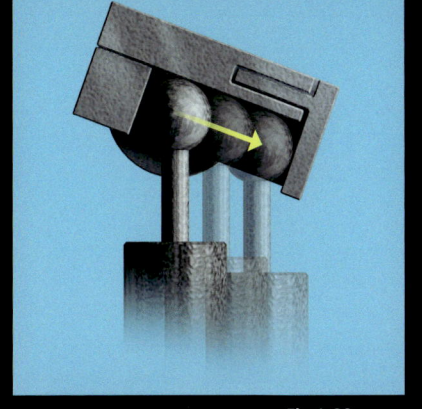

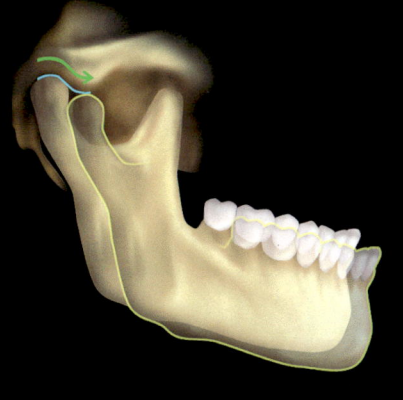

Immediate mandibular lateral translation In the initial phase of lateral mandibular movement, some authors have shown, on a substantial number of subjects, an in toto movement of the mandible in the laterolateral direction (immediate mandibular lateral translation) with values that reach 2.4 mm.[143–147]

Lundeen[139,140] has found a canine guidance in the majority of subjects with immediate mandibular lateral translation, which does make disocclusion of the posterior sectors possible. Asking the technician to make a canine guidance provides enough guarantee of avoiding any occlusal interference without necessarily having to enter into the articulator an immediate mandibular lateral translation, even of a minimum value (Figs 1-31, 1-32a, and 1-32b). When rehabilitating the patient in CR, the condyles should also be positioned against the medial wall of the articular eminence. This makes it virtually impossible for them to move in the laterolateral direction (ie, any immediate mandibular lateral translation is highly improbable).[104,148] Nevertheless, the temporomandibular joint is made up of structures that have a certain degree of elasticity and can, therefore, be subject to anatomic changes over time, leading to an immediate mandibular lateral translation.[149] To provide for this clinical situation, it is quite feasible to enter an immediate mandibular lateral translation value (1.0 mm) into the articulator, which will make it possible to create anatomically suited restorations in this specific case[150] (Figs 1-32c to 1-32f).

Progressive mandibular lateral translation The progressive mandibular lateral translation represents the actual translatory lateral movement of the mandible.[78] To reduce the risk of interferences in the eccentric movements, it is preferable to enter progressive mandibular lateral translation values (eg, 10 degrees) in the articulator that are greater than average values found in nature[139,140] (about 7 degrees) (Fig 1-33). Once the provisional restoration is positioned in the mouth, it is the clinician's task to check that the canine guidance allows adequate disocclusion of the posterior teeth.

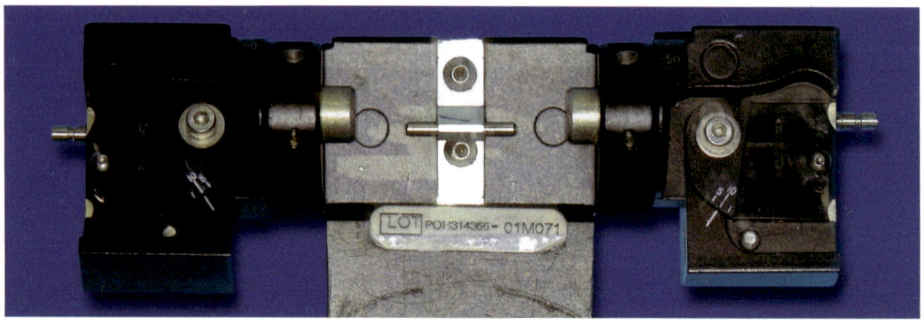

> Fig 1-31

FIG 31 View looking down upon the fossae of the semi-adjustable articulator.

FIG 32 *(a and b)* In setting up the articulator, the immediate value is usually kept at 0 mm. *(c and d)* Alternatively, the clinician can enter a mandibular lateral translation value of 1 mm. In this case, the first part of the lateral pathway has a horizontal movement of the condyles in the articulator. *(e and f)* The condyle on the working side is separated from the wall of the fossa (white line), while the contralateral condyle is, of course, in contact. This adjustment, even where a canine guidance is present, can affect the anatomy of the restorations in the posterior sectors.

FIG 33 *(a and b)* The progressive mandibular lateral translation value is usually set to 10 degrees to minimize the possibility of interference in the posterior sectors during lateral movements.

IMMEDIATE MANDIBULAR LATERAL TRANSLATION

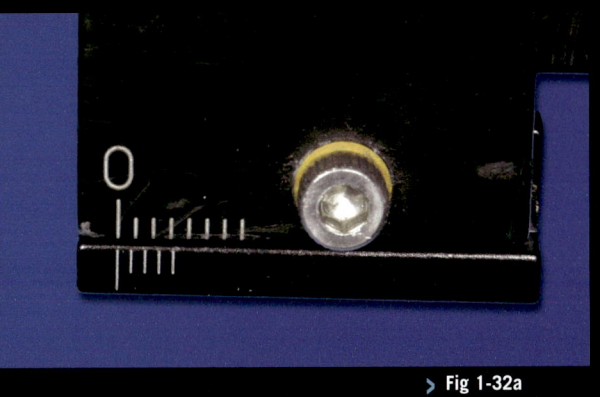

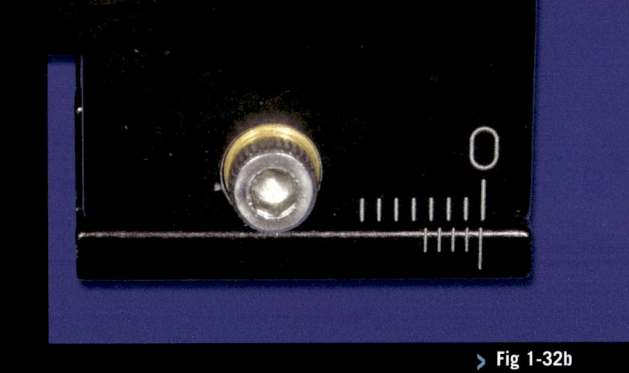

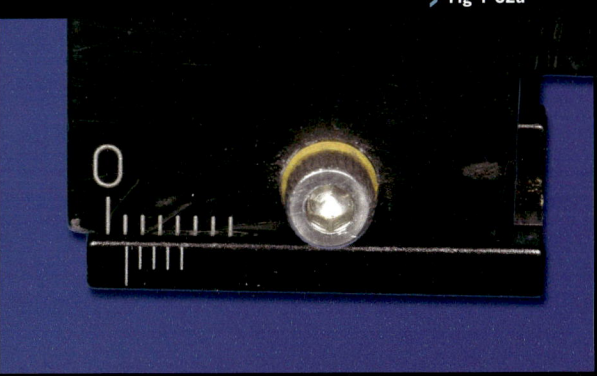

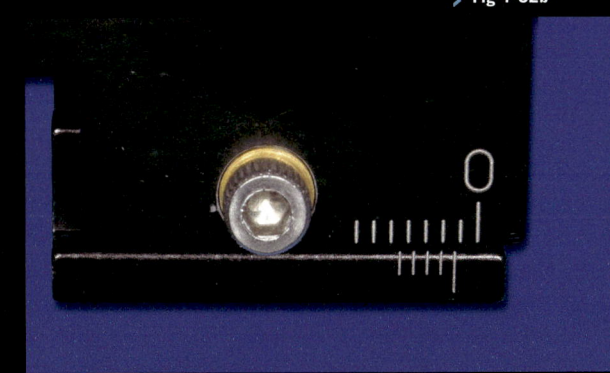

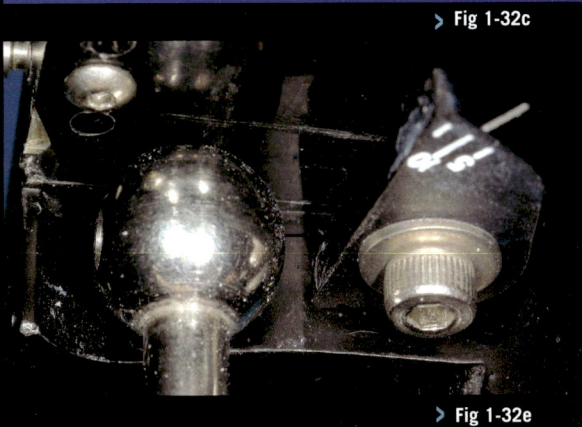

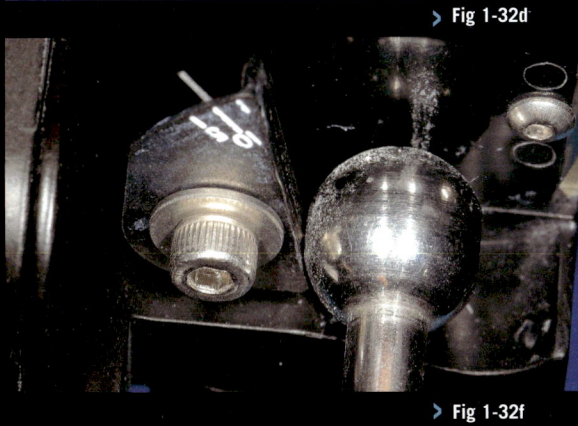

> Fig 1-32a

> Fig 1-32b

> Fig 1-32c

> Fig 1-32d

> Fig 1-32e

> Fig 1-32f

PROGRESSIVE MANDIBULAR LATERAL TRANSLATION

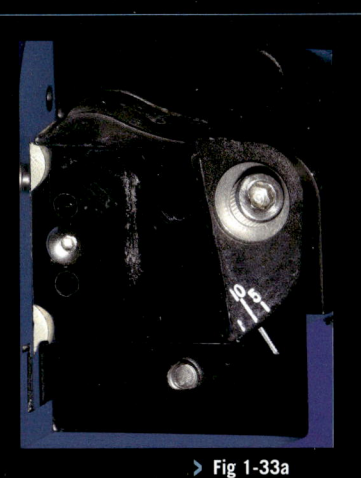

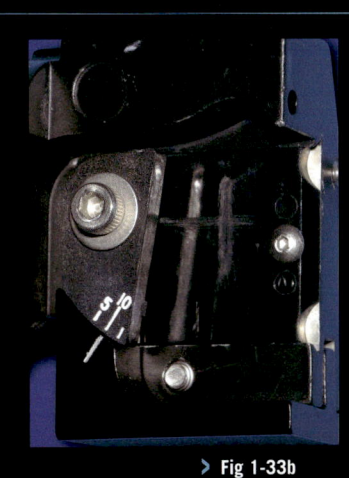

> Fig 1-33a

> Fig 1-33b

DIAGNOSTIC WAX-UP

When the clinician fills in the laboratory checklist correctly, the technician can make the diagnostic wax-up, which represents a preview of the definitive restoration's appearance and should optimize the esthetic-functional modifications (Fig 1-34) established as the treatment objective. After comparing the details noted by the clinician on the laboratory checklist with those observed on the stone casts (which must be large enough to cover the anatomic areas [palate, tuberosities and retromolar trigone, fornices, etc]), the technician mounts the casts on the articulator and adjusts it according to the registration wax-ups (protrusive CR) or preset values (20 degrees for the condylar guide and 10 degrees for the progressive mandibular lateral translation).

If a limited number of teeth are to be reconstructed and there is sufficient stability in the posterior sectors, the diagnostic wax-up can be made in MI. If, however, the prosthetic treatment involves several sextants of the posterior sectors or a whole arch, and a registration in CR is taken, the technician must make sure that the wax has no holes before setting the casts.

→ ...from page 71

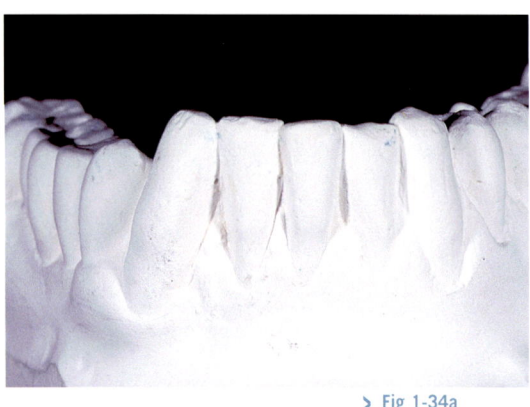

> Fig 1-34a

> Fig 1-34b

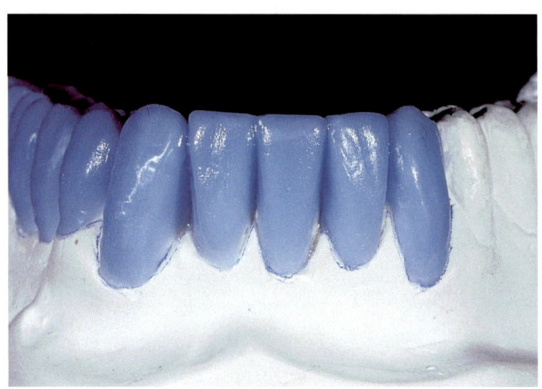

FIG 34 *(a)* The frontal view of the initial plaster cast of the mandibular arch shows the marked occlusal discrepancy between the right and left sides with an intrusion of the right quadrant of about 4 mm in relation to the contralateral quadrant. *(b)* The diagnostic wax-up shows the changes made to the occlusal plane based on the indications given by the clinician on the laboratory checklist.

LABORATORY WORK ORDER

Dr name XXXXX XXXXXXXX	Dental lab name XXXXXXXX
Address XX XXXXXXXXXXXXXX XXX	Address XX XXXXXXXXXXXXXX XXX
City XXXXX State XX	City XXXXX State XX
Telephone XXXXXXXXXX	Telephone XXXXXXXXXX

Date XX/XX/XX Work order no. XX
Patient/Code ___ Age XX [X] Male [ ] Female

■ TYPE OF WORK

[X] Diagnostic waxing [ ] Indirect mock-up [X] Provisional [ ] Fixed prosthesis [ ] Removable prosthesis

■ Description *Idealize the incisal plane, the occlusal scheme, tooth shape and position as indicated in the first 3 pages*

■ SCHEMA

o = Natural abutment □ = Implant X = Missing tooth

❶ 18 (17) ~~16~~ (15) (14) (13) (12) (11) | (21) (22) (23) [24] [25] [26] 27 28 ❷

❹ 48 (47) [46] [45] (44) (43) (42) (41) | ~~31~~ (32) 33 34 35 36 37 38 ❸

PFM: Porcelain-fused-to-metal **PS1:** Presoldering **PS2:** Postsoldering **MM:** Metal margins
MCM: Metal-ceramic margin **CS:** Ceramic shoulder **PC:** Post and core **ABU:** Abutment
AC: All-ceramic **RB:** Resin-bonded **V:** Veneer **IN:** Inlay **ON:** Onlay

Alloy:
Ceramic:

COLOR

2A *2A*

Shade Guide
[ ] Vitapan
[ ] 3D Master
[ ] Ivoclar
[X] Other SR IVOCRON

Value
High [ ] [X] [ ] [ ] Low [ ]

TRY-INS

Try-in *Provisional*	Date XX/XX/XX Notes:	[ ] Attachment No.
Try-in	Date __/__/__ Notes:	[ ] Attachment No.
Try-in	Date __/__/__ Notes:	[ ] Attachment No.
Delivery	Date __/__/__ Notes:	[ ] Attachment No.

Dentist's signature XXXXXXXXX

Copyright © 2008 by Quintessence Publishing Co. Inc

Only at this point does the technician move on to measure the thickness of the wax in the anterior indentation area to establish how much to raise the incisal pin (Figs 1-35a to 1-35c), which must be at level zero with the two arches in occlusion once the registration is removed.

OCCLUSAL ADJUSTMENT OF STONE CASTS

If, upon closing the articulator, the technician finds some areas of contact between the arches that prevent the incisal pin from being positioned at level zero (Figs 1-35d to 1-35f), occlusal reshaping must be performed on the casts until this position is reached (Figs 1-35g to 1-35l).

These modifications on the stone casts are done to achieve stability in centric occlusion (CO) with punctiform, synchronous, and well-distributed contacts[151–154] (see volume 1, chapter 5). However, the opening movement in the articulator could follow the arc of a circle that is not necessarily coincident with the movement made by the patient's condyles. Once the provisional restoration is positioned in the oral cavity, any occlusal inaccuracies would be noticeable and would require further, though slight, occlusal reshaping by the clinician.[109,116,126,155,156]

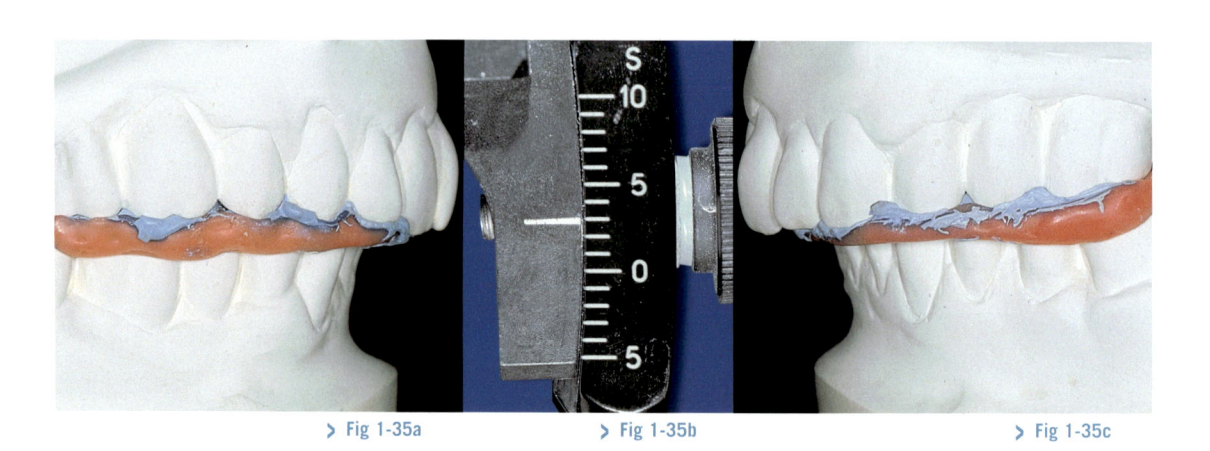

> Fig 1-35a   > Fig 1-35b   > Fig 1-35c

FIG 35 *(a to c)* The CR registration used to mount the casts on the articulator must not contain any holes. Such holes cause an inevitable, though minimal, occlusal rise on the incisal pin. *(d to f)* With the wax removed, the casts are put into occlusion but, because of the interferences, do not reach their MI, preventing the incisal pin from resting on the incisal plane. *(g to i)* In such cases the technician must carry out occlusal reshaping in the articulator until the maxillary and mandibular arches reach CO. *(j to l)* After the occlusal reshaping, the incisal pin should return to zero.

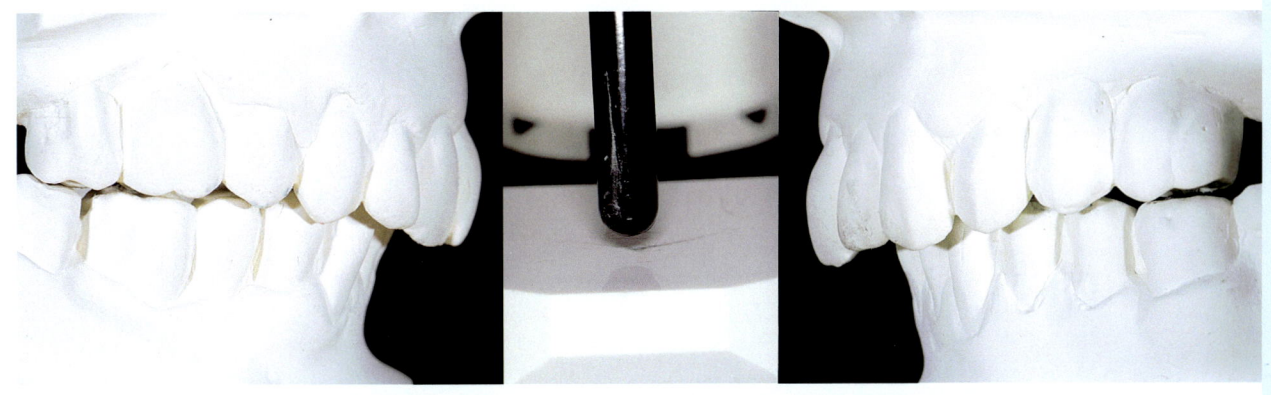

> Fig 1-35d   > Fig 1-35e   > Fig 1-35f

> Fig 1-35g   > Fig 1-35h   > Fig 1-35i

> Fig 1-35j   > Fig 1-35k   > Fig 1-35l

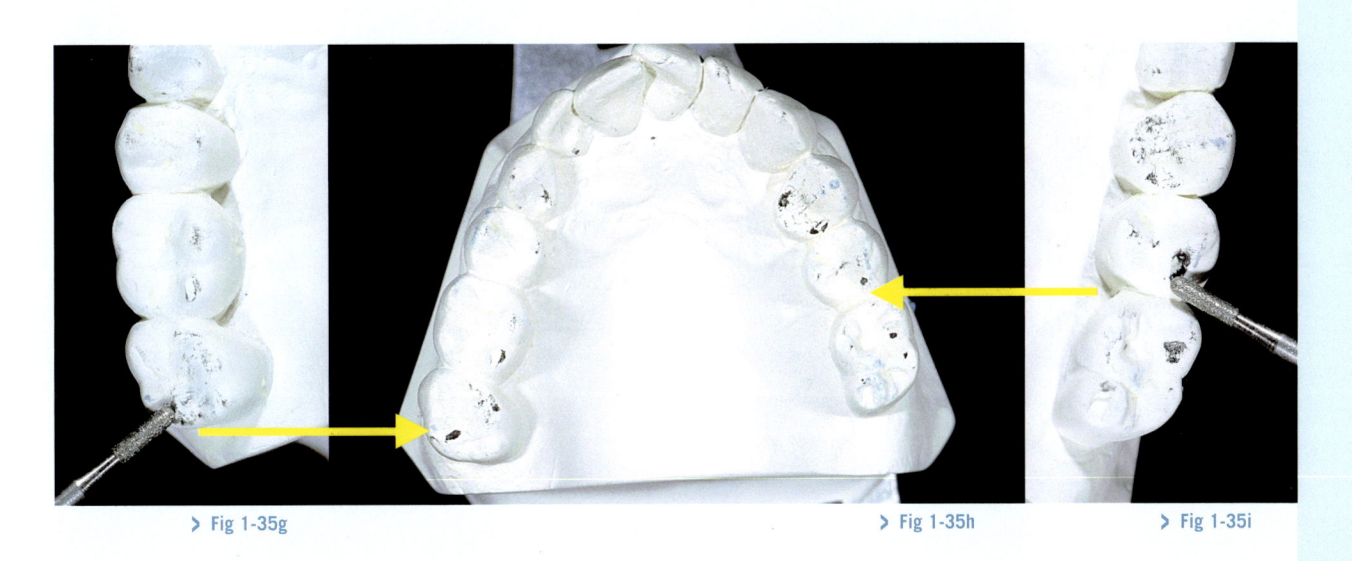

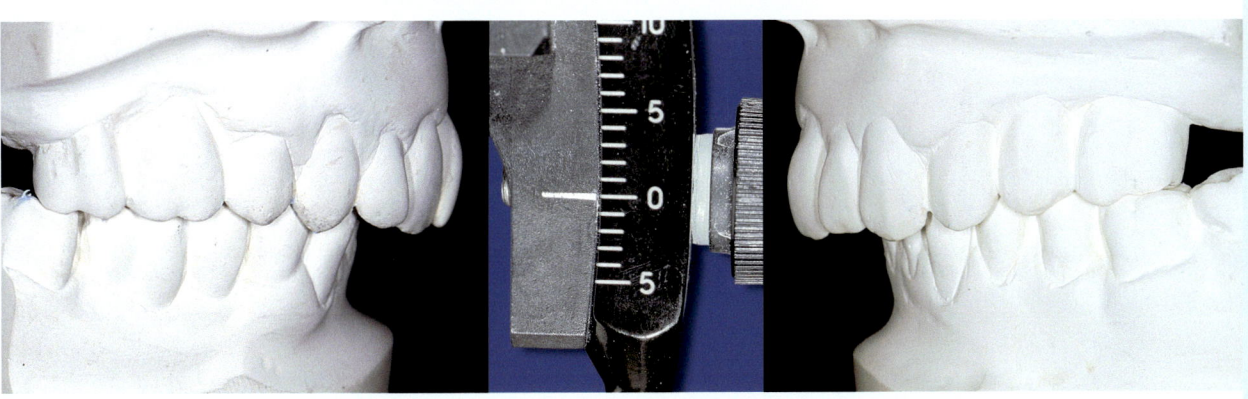

107

The technician also checks the appropriateness of overjet and overbite levels (Figs 1-35m and 1-35n) to optimize the anterior guidance (Figs 1-35o and 1-35p) and to allow adequate disocclusion of the posterior sectors, thereby avoiding occlusal interferences in these areas.

Based on the information received from the clinician, the technician arranges the wax-up on the casts mounted on the articulator as he or she starts to design the anterior teeth to optimize both esthetic and functional aspects. It is therefore possible to determine, by means of correct use of the facebow, the inferior and superior incisal planes, which are the starting point for determining the occlusal plane.[90]

Correct inclination of the incisal edge of the mandibular incisors also allows the technician to guarantee stability of the contacts between the anterior teeth. To adapt itself correctly to the morphology of the palatal concavity of the maxillary incisors and combine both esthetic and functional aspects, the lingual side of the incisal edge of the mandibular incisors must be slightly higher than the buccal edge (see volume 1, chapter 5). Moving the lower incisal margins in the articulator maps out the morphology of the lingual concavity of the anterosuperior teeth, allowing development of an appropriate anterior guidance[138] (Figs 1-35q to 1-35t). The incisal edge of the mandibular incisors in MI should ideally come into contact with the lingual concavity of the maxillary incisors at the top of the cingulum. This provides optimal axial distribution of the forces on the tooth, an appropriate occlusal stop, and progressivity of the disocclusive path angle, which minimizes stress in the excursive movements[138] (see volume 1, chapter 5).

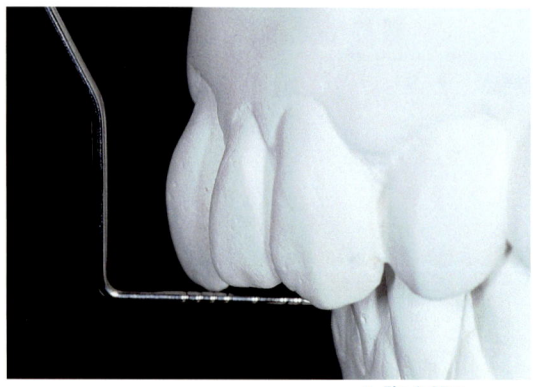

> Fig 1-35m

> Fig 1-35n

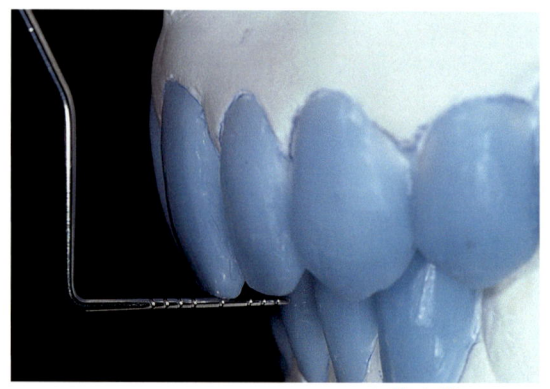

FIG 35 *(m and n)* The prominent initial overjet (8 mm) was reduced significantly (4.5 mm) in the diagnostic wax-up. These substantial modifications, decided upon only after the patient refused to undergo orthodontic treatment, can only be made by performing the prosthetic rehabilitation with full observation of the neutral zone. For this purpose a careful esthetic-functional and phonetic examination are essential to confirm the accuracy of the clinical choice. To optimize the anterior guidance, it is fundamental to draw an adequate palatal concavity of the maxillary anterior teeth. *(o)* If the lingual area is not suitably shaped, the resulting forces are exerted in the transverse direction with an inevitable occlusal overload. *(p)* Correct anatomy allows instead a soft disocclusion and development of a force that is exerted in the axial direction. *(q and r)* Close-up views of the original casts compared with the diagnostic wax-up highlight the reduction in overjet, the achievement of evenly distributed occlusal contacts, and the more congruous tooth arrangement achieved. *(s and t)* A slight contact between the anterior teeth is deemed sufficient and supplies the necessary occlusal stability; this represents the point of departure for a correct disocclusive pattern.

> Fig 1-35o

> Fig 1-35p

> Fig 1-35q

> Fig 1-35r

> Fig 1-35s

> Fig 1-35t

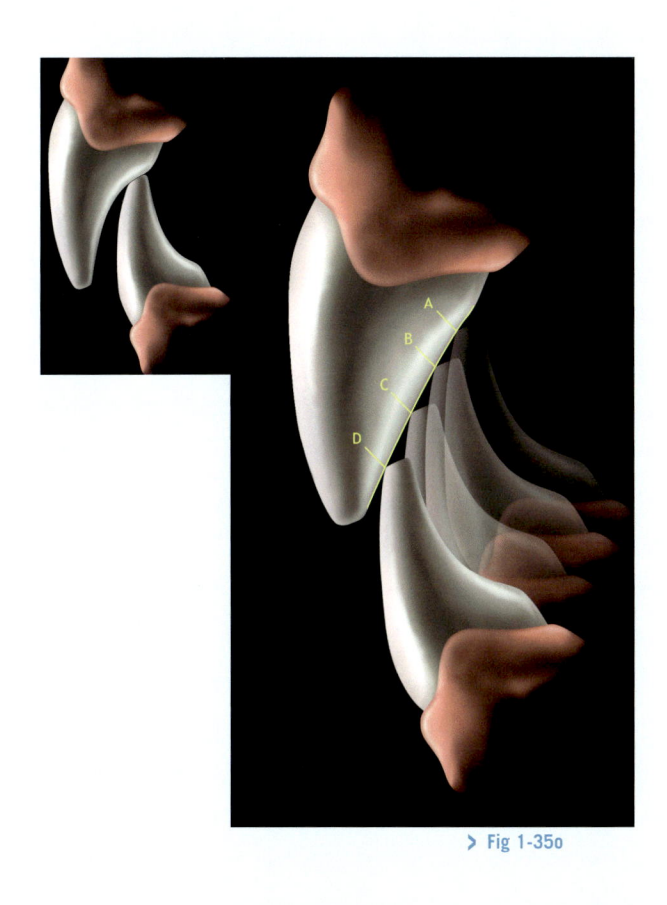

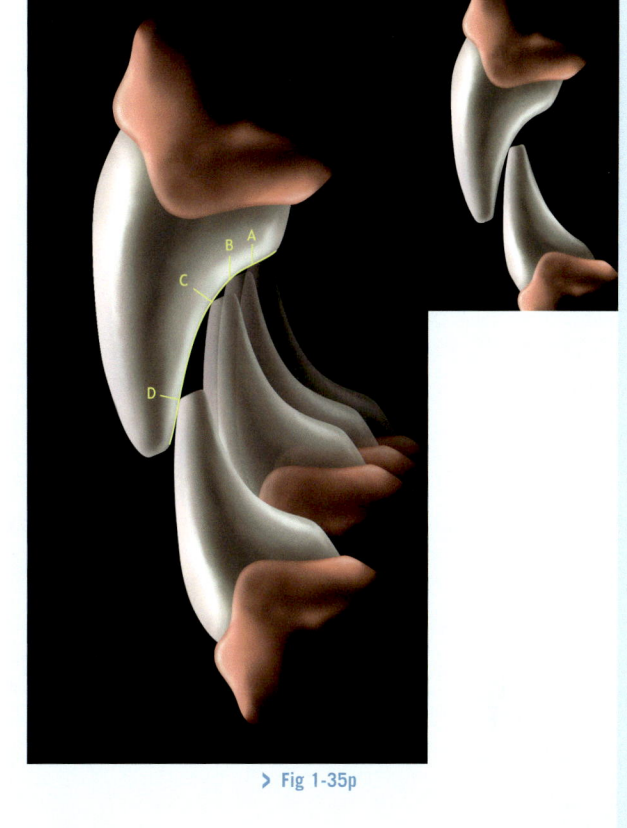

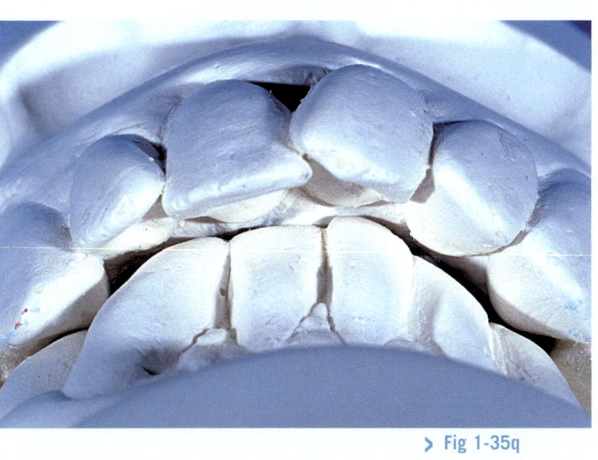

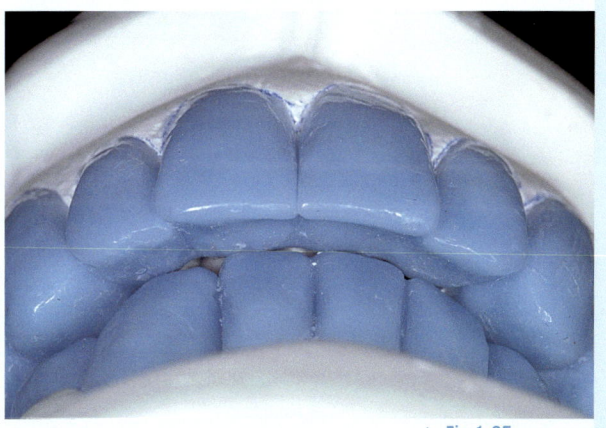

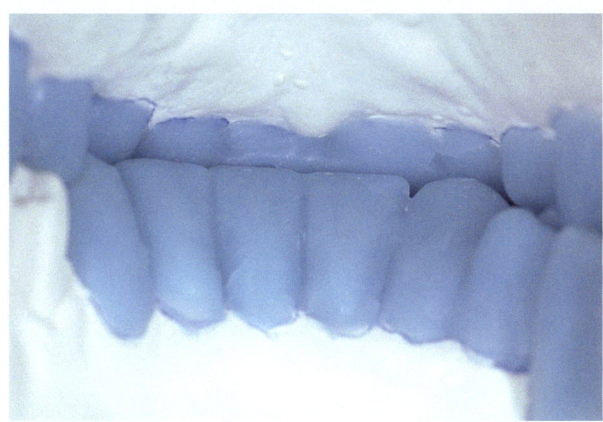

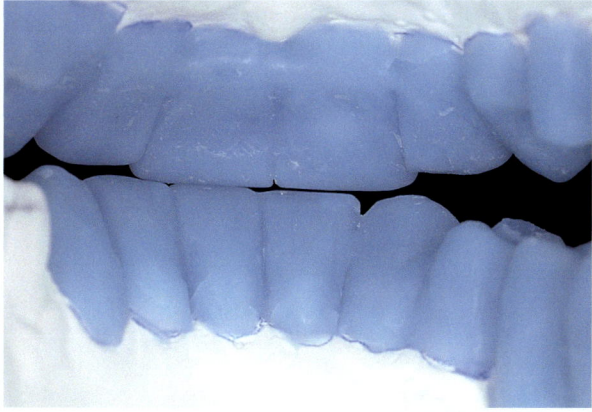

109

The morphology of the posterior teeth is then established. Through punctiform, synchronous, and well-distributed contact, the morphology must ensure the necessary occlusal stability of the posterior sectors.[151-154] The suitability of the anterior guidance ensures that these teeth do not make contact during protrusive and lateral movements, thereby avoiding any working or nonworking interferences and excessive involvement of the neuromuscular complex. Based on available space, the technician anticipates both the final appearance of the restorations and the ideal position of the units (including the pontic areas) in the wax-up, giving the clinician indications as to the necessary parallelism of the tooth preparations. When creating the wax-up, the technician pays special attention to checking the accuracy of the occlusal plane and the curves of Spee and Wilson, especially in cases where there are supraeruptions that can significantly limit the space needed for the prosthetic reconstruction.

Any changes to the occlusal plane, the achievement of correct occlusal stability in the posterior sectors, and the anterior guidance as defined in the articulator (Figs 1-35u to 1-35bb) are then carefully tested in the patient's mouth by means of the provisional restorations. By observing these elements during function, it is possible to confirm the accuracy of changes made to the morphology of the anterior teeth.[138]

DIAGNOSTIC WAX-UP

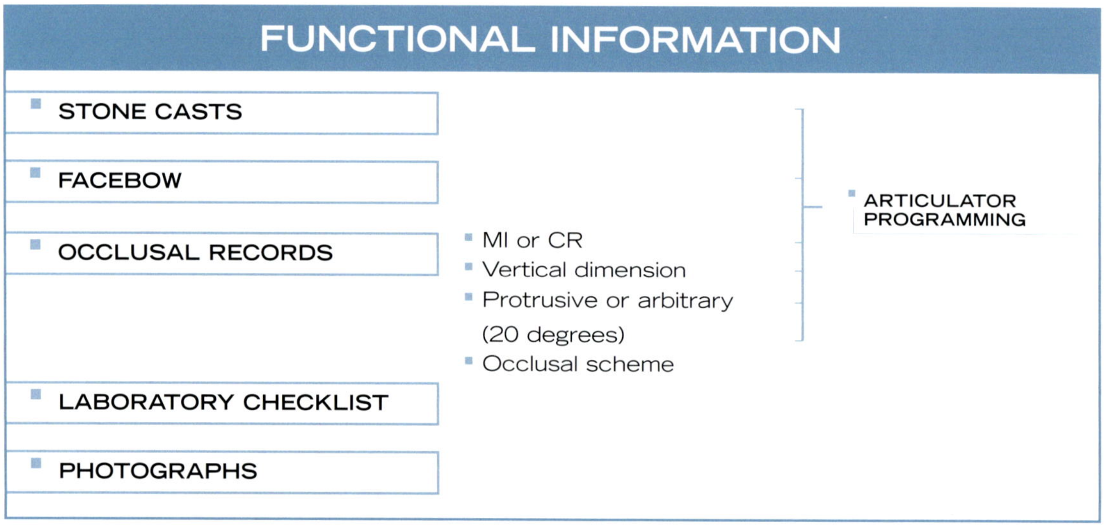

FUNCTIONAL INFORMATION

- STONE CASTS
- FACEBOW
- OCCLUSAL RECORDS
  - MI or CR
  - Vertical dimension
  - Protrusive or arbitrary (20 degrees)
  - Occlusal scheme
- LABORATORY CHECKLIST
- PHOTOGRAPHS

→ ARTICULATOR PROGRAMMING

FIG 35 *(u and v)* Frontal view of the original casts in MI and in the edge-to-edge position. *(w and x)* Frontal view of the diagnostic wax-up in CO and the edge-to-edge position. *(y and z)* From the lateral view of the diagnostic wax-up it is possible to see the good occlusal stability achieved in CO and the reduction in the amount of overjet. *(aa and bb)* The separation between the posterior teeth in the edge-to-edge position now seems much more appropriate.

> Fig 1-35u

> Fig 1-35v

> Fig 1-35w

> Fig 1-35x

> Fig 1-35y

> Fig 1-35z

> Fig 1-35aa

> Fig 1-35bb

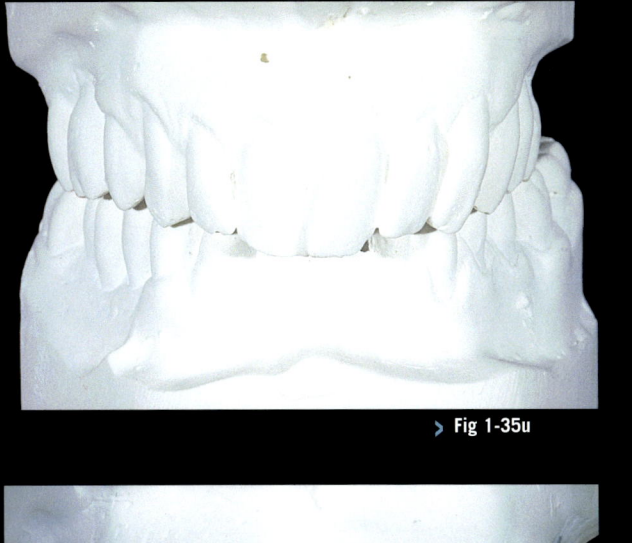

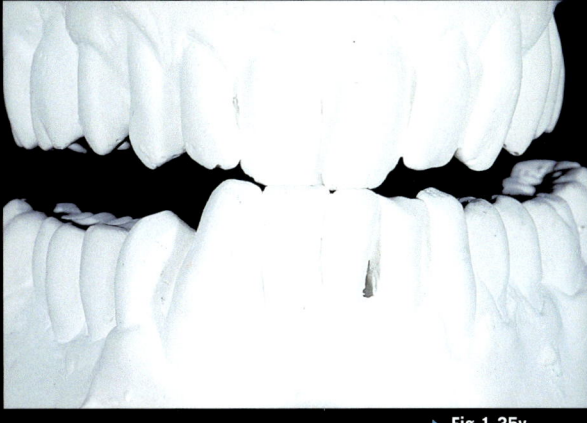

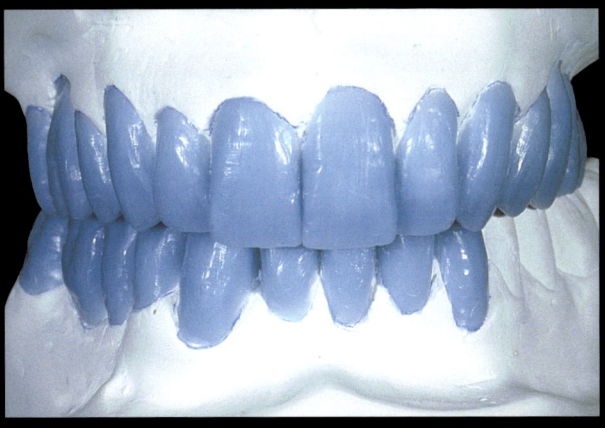

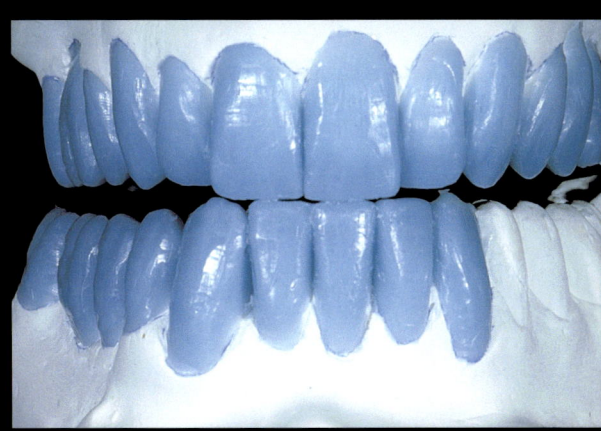

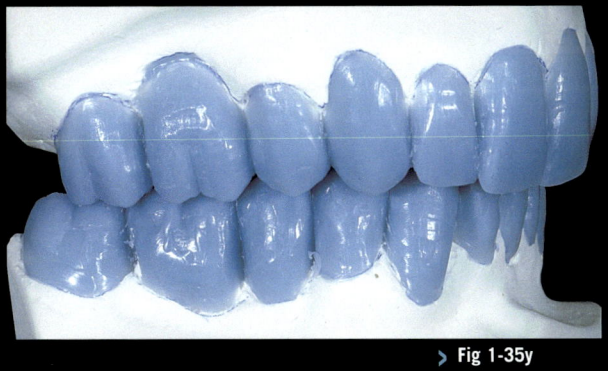

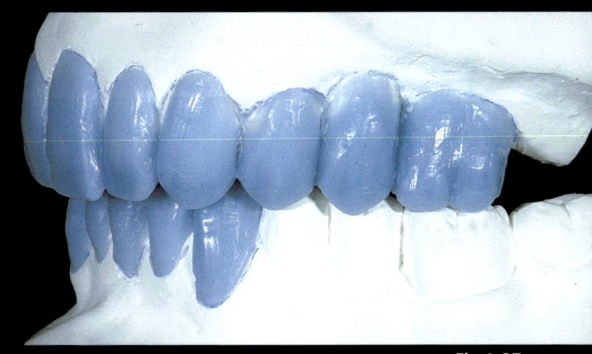

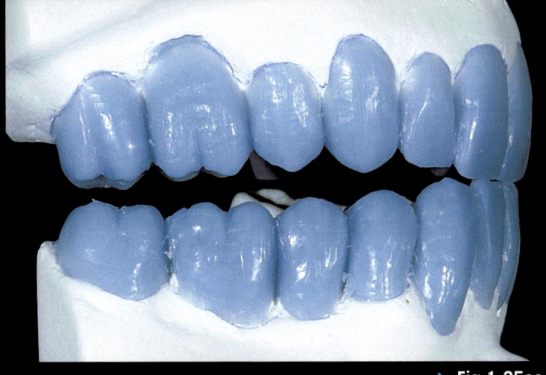

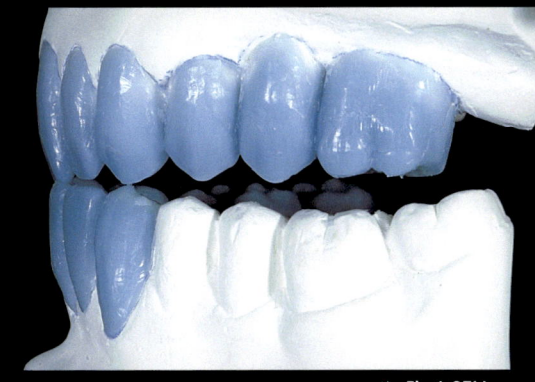

ADDITIVE DIAGNOSTIC WAX-UP

Studying the diagnostic wax-up can easily suggest the most suitable therapeutic course. Although in the majority of cases it confirms the accuracy of the intended treatment plan, it can sometimes reveal the need to modify the work sequence instead by introducing additional therapies of an endodontic, orthodontic, or surgical nature. The wax-up should be created on the stone casts without preparing the teeth on the plaster, as is usually done. The exception to this rule is removing the overcontours of old prostheses or modifying the contours of teeth that, based on the indications on the laboratory checklist, have to change position (Figs 1-35cc to 1-35hh and 1-35ii to 1-35ll). In addition to being a useful point of reference, the preservation of original integral teeth prevents the technician from having to excessively constrict the occlusal table following an overly conical preparation on the plaster casts, often the cause of a problematic insertion of the provisional restoration in the mouth (see chapter 2, page 140).

A silicone mockup and an acetate mockup can be produced from an alginate impression of the diagnostic wax-up. Once in the patient's mouth, these mockups give the clinician the opportunity to check the tooth position and arrangement during the clinical phases and to evaluate the suitability of the thickness of the tooth preparation.

FIG 35 *(cc and dd)* The substantial modification of the occlusal plane made in the diagnostic wax-up can be evaluated using a caliper. *(ee to hh)* After the diagnostic wax-up of the two arches is finalized, the mandibular and maxillary provisional restorations are fabricated.

FIG 35 *(ii to ll)* A comparison between the diagnostic wax-up and provisional restorations of the maxillary and mandibular arches confirms the accuracy of the choices made from the initial phase and the thorough replication from the wax-up to the acrylic restorations. Before finalizing the prosthetic rehabilitation, all of the modifications set out in the treatment plan should be tested in the provisional restoration to ascertain their clinical validity.

> Fig 1-35cc

> Fig 1-35dd

> Fig 1-35ee

> Fig 1-35ff

> Fig 1-35gg

> Fig 1-35hh

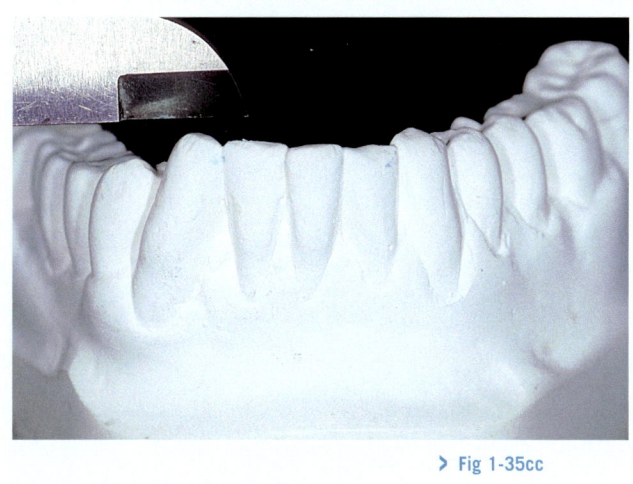

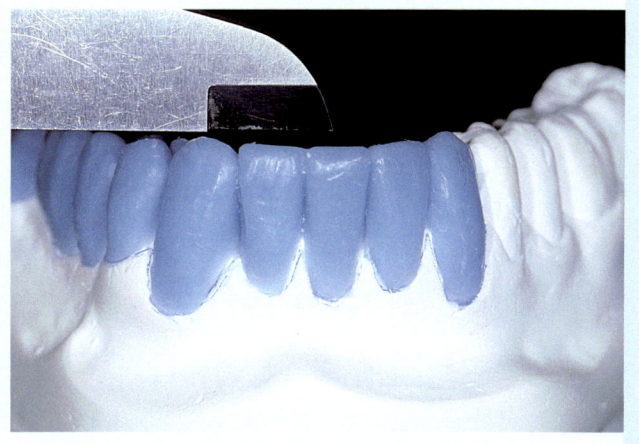

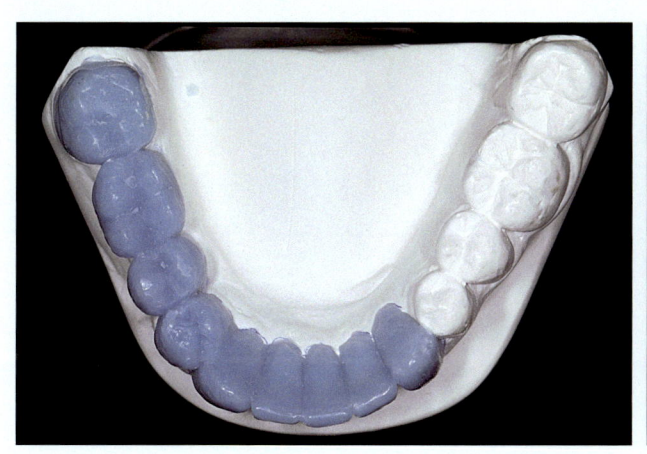

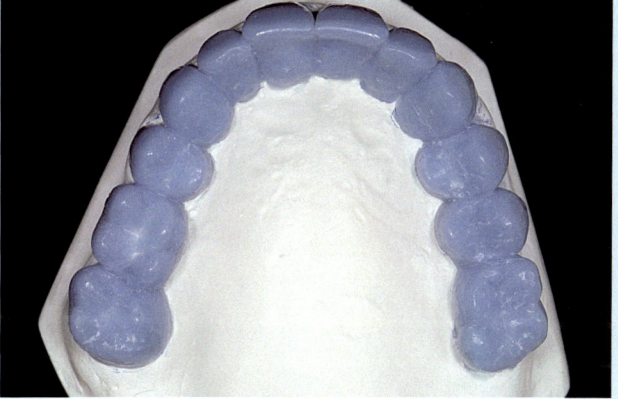

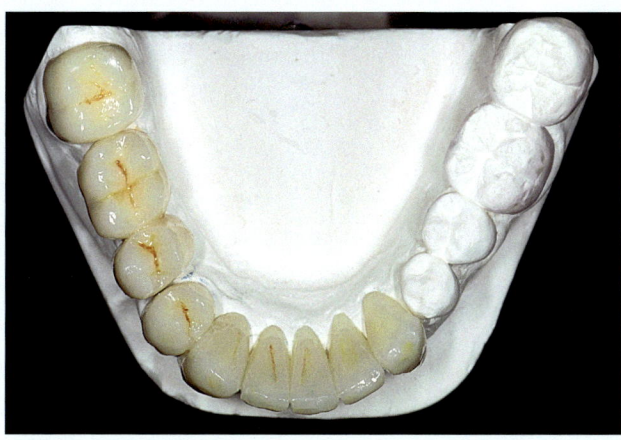

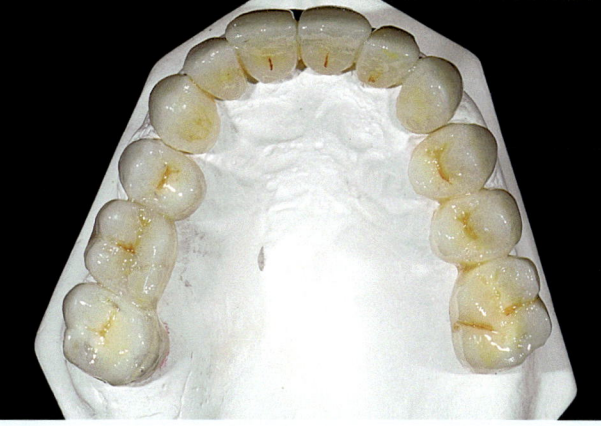

113

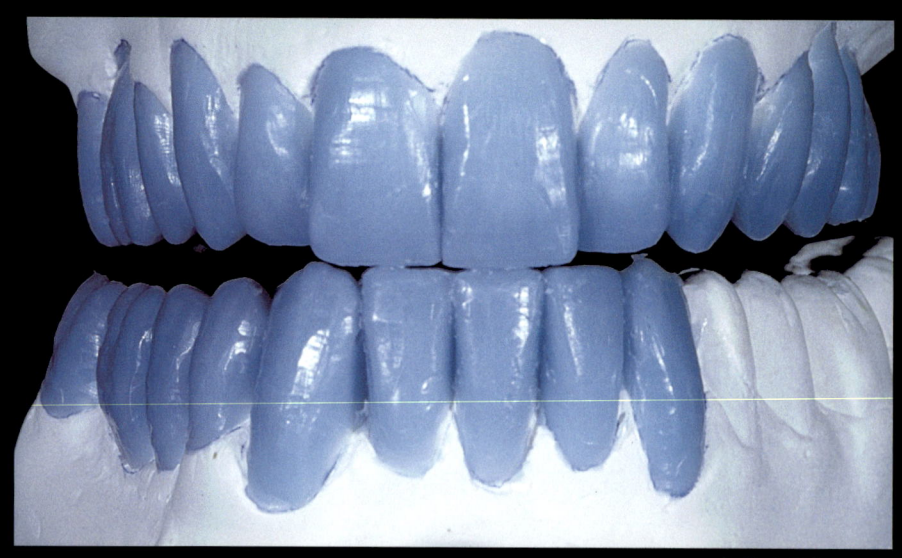

> Fig 1-35ii

DIAGNOSTIC WAX-UP

OBJECTIVE

FUNCTIONAL	ESTHETIC
Curves of Spee and Wilson	Tooth shape and size
Occlusal plane	Tooth-to-tooth proportion
Occlusal stability	Tooth position and arrangement
Overjet – overbite	Tooth axes
Anterior guidance	Interproximal areas
Posterior sector disocclusion	Interincisal embrasures

PROTOTYPE FOR THE PROVISIONAL

> Fig 1-35jj

> Fig 1-35kk

> Fig 1-35ll

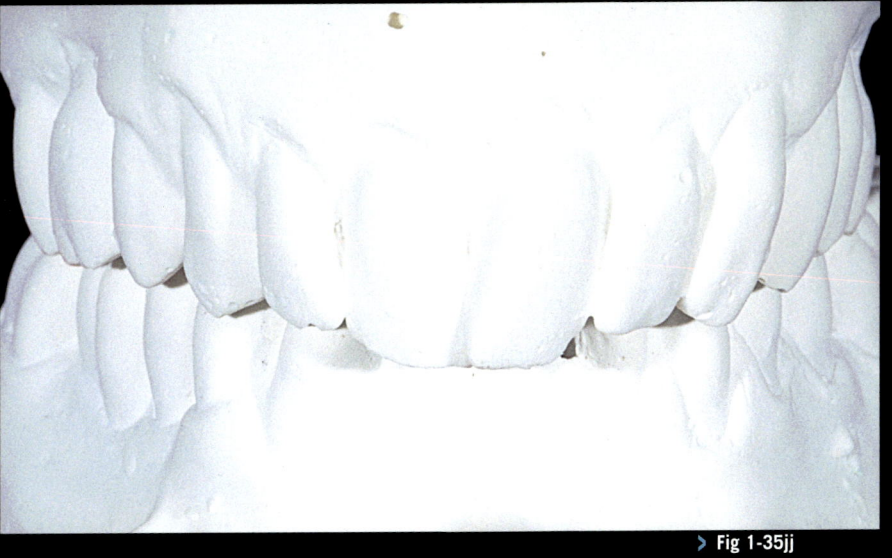

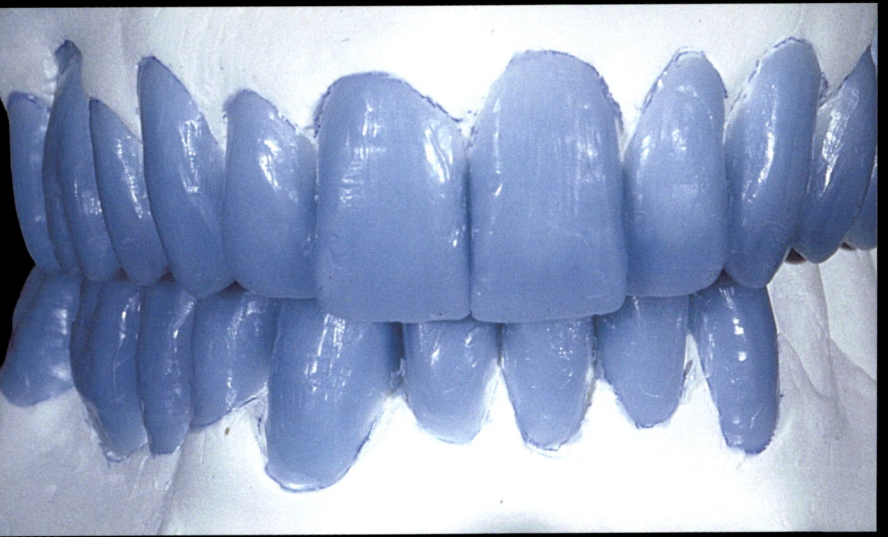

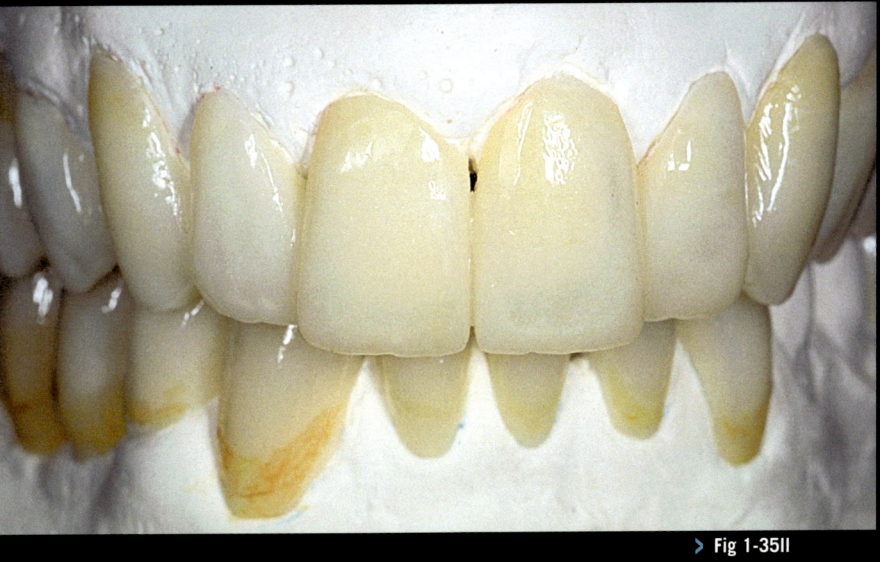

→ continues on page 125

REFERENCES

1. Epstein O et al. Clinical Examination, ed 2. St Louis: Mosby, 1997.

2. Little JW et al. Dental Management of the Medically Compromised Patient, ed 5. St Louis: Mosby, 1997.

3. Calandriello M, Carnevale G, Ricci G. Semeiologia, diagnosi, prognosi e piano di trattamento delle malattie parodontali. In: Calandriello M, Carnevale G, Ricci G (eds). Parodontologia. Torino, Italy: Editrice Cides Odonto Edizioni Internazionali, 1986:138–152.

4. Nyman S, Lindhe J. Examination of patients with periodontal disease. In: Lindhe J, Karring T, Lang NP (eds). Clinical Periodontology and Implant Dentistry, ed 4. Oxford: Blackwell Munksgaard, 2003:403–413.

5. Van Sickels JE, Bianco HJ Jr, Pifer RG. Transcranial radiographs in the evaluation of craniomandibular (TMJ) disorders. J Prosthet Dent 1983;49:244–249.

6. Blaschke DD, Solberg WK, Sanders B. Arthrography of the temporomandibular joint: review of current status. J Am Dent Assoc 1980;100:388–395.

7. Laurell KA, Tootle R, Cunningham R, Beltran J, Simon D. Magnetic resonance imaging of the temporomandibular joint. Part I: literature review. J Prosthet Dent 1987;58:83–89.

8. Laurell KA, Tootle R, Cunningham R, Beltran J, Simon D. Magnetic resonance imaging of the temporomandibular joint. Part II: comparison with laminographic, autopsy, and histologic findigs. J Prosthet Dent 1987;58:211–218.

9. Laurell KA, Tootle R, Cunningham R, Beltran J, Simon D. Magnetic resonance imaging of the temporomandibular joint. Part III: use of a cephalostat for clinical imaging. J Prosthet Dent 1987;58:355–359.

10. Rufenacht CR. Fundamentals of Esthetics. Chicago: Quintessence, 1990.

11. Chiche GJ, Pinault A. Esthetics of Anterior Fixed Prosthodontics. Chicago: Quintessence, 1994.

12. Krogh-Poulsen WG, Olsson A. Occlusal disharmonies and dysfunction of the stomatognathic system. Dent Clin North Am 1966;10:627–635.

13. Solberg WK. Occlusion-related pathosis and its clinical evaluation. In: Clark JW (ed). Clinical Dentistry, vol 2. Hagerstown, MD: Harper & Row, 1976:ch 35.

14. Pullinger AG, Liu SP, Low G, Tay D. Differences between sexes in maximum jaw opening when corrected to body size. J Oral Rehabil 1987;14:291–299.

15. Baelum U, Feyerskov O, Karring T. Oral hygiene, gingivitis and periodontal breakdown in adult tanzanians. J Periodontal Res 1986;21:221–232.

16. Hugoson A, Laurell L, Lundgreen D. Frequency distribution of individuals aged 20–70 years according to severity of periodontal disease experience in 1973 and 1983. J Clin Periodontol 1992;19:227–232.

17. Loe H, Anerud A, Boysen H. The natural history of periodontal disease in man: prevalence, severity and extent of gingival recession. J Periodontol 1992;63:489–495.

18. Goodson JM. Selection of suitable indicators of periodontitis. In: Bader JD (ed). Risk Assessment in Dentistry. Chapel Hill, NC: Univ of North Carolina Dental Ecology, 1989.

19. The American Academy of Periodontology: Epidemiology of periodontal diseases. J Periodontol 1996;67:935.

20. Rosen H. Operative procedures on mutilated endodontically treated teeth. J Prosthet Dent 1961;11:973–986.

21. Eissman HF, Radke RA. Postendodontic restoration. In: Cohen S, Burns RC (eds). Pathways of the Pulp, ed 4. St Louis: CV Mosby, 1987:640–643.

22. Sorensen JA, Engelman MJ. Ferrule design and fracture resistance of endodontically treated teeth. J Prosthet Dent 1990;63:529–536.

23. Ingle JI, Teel S, Wands DH. Restoration of endodontically treated teeth and preparation for overdenture. In: Ingle JI, Bakland LK (eds). Endodontics, ed 4. Philadelphia: Lea and Febiger, 1994:897.

24. Morgano SM, Brackett SE. Foundation restorations in fixed prosthodontics: current knowledge and future needs. J Prosthet Dent 1999;82:643–657.

25. Zhi-yue L, Yu-xing Z. Effect of post-core design and ferrule on fracture resistance of endodontically treated maxillary central incisors. J Prosthet Dent 2003;89:368–373.

26. Ante IH. The fundamental principles of abutments. Mich State Dent Soc Bull 8:14 July 1926.

27. Tylman SD, Malone WFP. Tylman's Theory and Practice of Fixed Prosthodontics, ed 7. St Louis: Mosby,1978:15.

28. Dykema RW et al. Johnston's Modern Practice in Fixed Prosthodontics, ed 4. Philadelphia: WB Saunders, 1986:4.

29. Shillingburg HT Jr, Hobo S, Whitsett LD, Jacobi R, Brackett SE. Fundamentals of Fixed Prosthodontics, ed 3. Chicago: Quintessence, 1997:11–24.

30. Nyman S, Ericsson I. The capacity of reduced periodontal tissues to support fixed bridgework. J Clin Periodontol 1982;9:409–414.

31. Freilich MA, Breeding LC, Keagle JG, Garnick JJ. Fixed partial dentures supported by periodontally compromised teeth. J Prosthet Dent 1991;65:607–611.

32. Decock V, De Nayer K, De Boever JA, Dent M. 18-year longitudinal study of cantilevered fixed restorations. Int J Prosthodont 1996;9:331–340.

33. Nyman S, Lindhe J, Lundgren D. The role of occlusion for the stability of fixed bridges in patients with reduced periodontal tissue support. J Clin Periodontol 1975;2:53–66.

34. Laurell L, Lundgren D, Falk H, Hugoson A. Long-term prognosis of extensive polyunit cantilevered fixed partial dentures. J Prosthet Dent 1991;66:545–552.

35. Smith RA, Berger R, Dodson TB. Risk factors associated with dental implants in healthy and medically compromised patients. Int J Oral Maxillofac Implants 1992;7:367–372.

36. Bain CA, Moy PK. The association between the failure of dental implants and cigarette smoking. Int J Oral Maxillofac Implants 1993;8:609–615.

37. Haber J, Wattles J, Crowley M, Mandell R, Joshipura K, Kent RL. Evidence for cigarette smoking as a major risk factor for periodontitis. J Periodontol 1993;64:16–23.

38. De Bruyn H, Collaert B. The effect of smoking on early implant failure. Clin Oral Implants Res 1994;5:206–264.

39. Bain CA. Smoking and implant failure-benefits of a smoking cessation protocol. Int J Oral Maxillofac Implants 1996;11:756–759.

40. Lindquist LW, Carlsson GE, Jemt T. Association between marginal bone loss around osseointegrated mandibular implants and smoking habits: a 10-year follow-up study. J Dent Res 1997;76:1667–1674.

41. Wilson TG Jr, Nunn M. The relationship between the interleukin-1 periodontal genotype and implant loss. Initial data. J Periodontol 1999;70:724–729.

42. Penarrocha M, Palomar M, Sanchis JM, Guarinos J, Balaguer J. Radiologic study of marginal bone loss around 108 dental implants and its relationship to smoking, implant location, and morphology. Int J Oral Maxillofac Implants 2004;19:861–867.

43. Quirynen M, Listgarten MA. Distribution of bacterial morphotypes around natural teeth and titanium implants ad modum Branemark. Clin Oral Implants Res 1990;1:8–12.

44. Jemt T, Lekholm U. Oral implants treatment in posterior partially edentulous jaws: A 5-year follow-up report. Int J Oral Maxillofac Implants 1993;8:635–640.

45. Lekholm U, Van Steenberghe D, Hermann I, Bolender C, Folmer T, Gunne J, Higuchi K, Laney W, Linden U. Osseointegrated implants in the treatment of partially edentulous jaws. A prospective 5-year multicenter study. Int J Oral Maxillofac Implants 1994;9:627–635.

46. Lazzara R, Siddiqui AA, Binon P, Feldman S, Weiner R, Phillips R, Gonshor A. Retrospective multicenter analysis of 3i endosseous dental implants placed over a 5-year period. Clin Oral Implants Res 1996;7:73–83.

47. Bragger U, Burgin WB, Hammerle CH, Lang NP. Associations between clinical parameters assessed around implants and teeth. Clin Oral Implants Res 1997;8:412–421.

48. Gouvoussis J, Sindhusake D, Yeung S. Cross-infection from periodontitis sites to failing implant sites in the same mouth. Int J Oral Maxillofac Implants 1997;12:666–673.

49. Holmgren K, Sheikholeslam A, Riise C, Kopp S. The effects of an occlusal splint on the electromyographic activities of the temporal and masseter muscles during maximal clenching in patients with a habit of nocturnal bruxism and signs and symptoms of craniomandibular disorders. J Oral Rehabil 1990;17:447–459.

50. Okeson JP. Management of Temporomandibular Disorders and Occlusion, ed 4. St Louis: Mosby, 1998:ch 15.

51. Wright KW, Yettram AL. Reactive force distributions for teeth when loaded singly and when used as fixed partial denture abutments. J Prosthet Dent 1979;42:411–416.

52. Cheung GS, Dimmer A, Mellor R, Gale M. A clinical evaluation of conventional bridgework. J Oral Rehabil 1990;17:131–136.

53. Yang HS, Chung HJ, Park YJ. Stress analysis of a cantilevered fixed partial denture with normal and reduced bone support. J Prosthet Dent 1996;76:424–430.

54. Rosenstiel SF, Land MF, Fujimoto J. Contemporary Fixed Prosthodontics, ed 3. St Louis: Mosby, 2001:63–88.

55. Carnevale G, Pontoriero R, di Febo G. Long-term effects of root-resective therapy in furcation-involved molars. A 10-year longitudinal study. J Clin Periodontol 1998;25:209–214.

56. Hardt CR, Grondahl K, Lekholm U, Wennstrom JL. Outcome of implant therapy in relation to experienced loss of periodontal bone support: a retrospective 5-year study. Clin Oral Implants Res 2002;13:488–494.

57. Wennstrom JL, Ekestubbe A, Grondahl K, Karlsson S, Lindhe J. Oral rehabilitation with implant-supported fixed partial dentures in periodontitis-susceptible subjects. A 5-year prospective study. J Clin Periodontol 2004;31:713–724.

58. Truhlar RS, Farish SE, Scheitler LE, Morris HF, Ochi S. Bone quality and implant design-related outcomes through stage II surgical uncovering of Spectra-System root form implants. J Oral Maxillofac Surg 1997;55:46–54.

59. Kayser AF. Shortened dental arches and oral function. J Oral Rehabil 1981;8:457–462.

60. Aukes JN, Kayser AF, Felling AJ. The subjective experience of mastication in subjects with shortened dental arches. J Oral Rehabil 1988;15:321–324.

61. Sarita PT, Witter DJ, Kreulen CM, Van't Hof MA, Creugers NH. Chewing ability of subjects with shortened dental arches. Community Dent Oral Epidemiol 2003;31:328–334.

62. Witter DJ, van Elteren P, Kayser AF. Migration of teeth in shortened dental arches. J Oral Rehabil 1987;14:321–329.

63. Kuboki T, Okamoto S, Suzuki H, et al. Quality of life assessment of bone-anchored fixed partial denture patients with unilateral mandibular distal-extension edentulism. J Prosthet Dent 1999;82:182–187.

64. Sarita PT, Kreulen CM, Witter D, Creugers NH. Signs and symptoms associated with TMD in adults with shortened dental arches. Int J Prosthodont 2003;16:265–270.

65. Armellini D, von Fraunhofer JA. The shortened dental arch: A review of the literature. J Prosthet Dent 2004;92:531–535.

66. Spear FM. Occlusion in the new millennium: the controversy continues. Part 1. Tonawanda, Great Lakes Orthodontics, Spear Perspective newsletter;3(1).

67. Witter DJ, van Elteren P, Kayser AF, van Rossum MJ. The effect of removable partial dentures on the oral function in shortened dental arches. J Oral Rehabil 1989;16:27–33.

68. Witter DJ, Van Elteren P, Kayser AF, Van Rossum GM. Oral comfort in shortened dental arches. J Oral Rehabil 1990;17:137–143.

69. Allen PF, Witter DF, Wilson NH, Kayser AF. Shortened dental arch therapy: Views of consultants in restorative dentistry in the United Kingdom. J Oral Rehabil 1996;23:481–485.

70. Marzola R, Derbabian K, Donovan TE, Arcidiacono A. The science of communicating the art of esthetic dentistry. Part I: patient-dentist-patient communication. J Esthet Dent 2000;12:131–138.

71. Magne P, Belser U. Bonded Porcelain Restorations in the Anterior Dentition. A Biomimetic Approach. Chicago: Quintessence, 2002:179–236.

72. Duchenne GB. The Mechanism of Human Facial Expression. New York: Cambridge Univ Press, 1990.

73. Shillingburg HT Jr, Hobo S, Whitsett LD, Jacobi R, Brackett SE. Fundamentals of Fixed Prosthodontics, ed 3. Chicago: Quintessence, 1997:35–45.

74. Gross M, Nemcovsky C, Tabibian Y, Gazit E. The effect of three different recording materials on the reproducibility of condylar guidance registrations in three semi-adjustable articulators. J Oral Rehabil 1998;25:204–208.

75. Breeding LC, Dixon D. Compression resistance of four interocclusal recording materials. J Prosthet Dent 1992;68:876–878.

76. Chiche GJ, Pinault A. Communication with the dental laboratory: Try-in procedures and shade selection. In: Chiche GJ, Pinault A (eds). Esthetics of Anterior Fixed Prosthodontics. Chicago: Quintessence, 1994:115–142.

77. Peregrina A, Reisbick MH. Occlusal accuracy of casts made and articulated differently. J Prosthet Dent 1990;63:422–425.

78. Academy of Prosthodontics. The Glossary of Prosthodontic Terms, ed 7. St Louis: Mosby, 1999.

79. Weinberg LA. The role of muscle deconditioning for occlusal corrective procedures. J Prosthet Dent 1991;66:250–255.

80. Tripodakis AP, Smulow JB, Mehta NR, Clark RE. Clinical study of location and reproducibility of three mandibular positions in relation to body posture and muscle function. J Prosthet Dent 1995;73:190–198.

81. Dawson PE. Temporomandibular joint pain-dysfunction problems can be solved. J Prosthet Dent 1973;29:100–112.

82. McKee JR. Comparing condylar position repeatability for standardized versus nonstandardized methods of achieving centric relation. J Prosthet Dent 1997;77:280–284.

83. Tarantola GJ, Becker IM, Gremillion H. The reproducibility of centric relation: A clinical approach. J Am Dent Assoc 1997;128:1245–1251.

84. Dawson PE. A classification system for occlusions that relates maximal intercuspation to the position and condition of the temporomandibular joints. J Prosthet Dent 1996;75:60–66.

85. Hansson T, Nordstrom B. Thickness of the soft tissue layers and articular disk in temporomandibular joints with deviations in form. Acta Odontol Scand 1977;35:281–288.

86. Rosenstiel SF, Land MF, Fujimoto J. Contemporary Fixed Prosthodontics, ed 3. St Louis: Mosby, 2001:27–62.

87. Dawson PE. Evaluation, Diagnosis, and Treatment of Occlusal Problems, ed 2. St Louis: Mosby, 1989:56–71.

88. Spear FM. Occlusion in the new millennium: the controversy continues. Part 2. Tonawanda, Great Lakes Orthodontics, Spear Perspective newsletter;3(2).

89. Dahl BL, Krogstad O. Long-term observations of an increased occlusal face height obtained by a combined orthodontic/prosthetic approach. J Oral Rehabil 1985;12:173–176.

90. Dawson PE. Evaluation, Diagnosis, and Treatment of Occlusal Problems, ed 2. St Louis: Mosby, 1989:298–319.

91. Landa JS. The free-way space and its significance in the rehabilitation of the masticatory apparatus. J Prosthet Dent 1952;2:756–779.

92. Mehringer EJ. The use of speech patterns as an aid in prosthodontic reconstruction. J Prosthet Dent 1963;13:825–836.

93. Gibbs CH, Messerman T, Reswick JB, Derda HJ. Functional movements of the mandible. J Prosthet Dent 1971;26:604–620.

94. MacGregor AR. Fenn, Liddelow and Gimson's Clinical Dental Prosthetics. London: Wright, 1989:89.

95. Chiche GJ, Pinault A. Artistic and scientific principles applied to esthetic dentistry. In: Chiche GJ, Pinault A (eds). Esthetics of Anterior Fixed Prosthodontics. Chicago: Quintessence, 1994:13–32.

96. Pound E. The mandibular movements of speech and their seven related values. J Prosthet Dent 1966;16:835–843.

97. Pound E. Let /S/ be your guide. J Prosthet Dent 1977;38:482–489.

98. Manns A, Miralles R, Palazzi C. EMG, bite force, and elongation of the masseter muscle under isometric voluntary contractions and variations of vertical dimension. J Prosthet Dent 1979;42:674–682.

99. Silverman ET. Speech rehabilitation: Habits and myofunctional therapy. In: Seide L (ed). Restorative Procedures in Dynamic Approach to Restorative Dentistry. Philadelphia: Saunders, 1980.

100. Rivera-Morales WC, Mohl ND. Variability of closest speaking space compared with interocclusal distance in dentulous subjects. J Prosthet Dent 1991;65:228–232.

101. D'Amico A. The canine teeth-normal functional relation of the natural teeth of man. J South Calif Dent Assoc 1958;26:6–23,49–60,127–142,175–182,194–208, 239–241.

102. D'Amico A. Functional occlusion of the natural teeth of man. J Prosthet Dent 1961;11:899–915.

103. Thornton LJ. Anterior guidance: Group function/canine guidance. A literature review. J Prosthet Dent 1990;64:479–482.

104. Dawson PE. Evaluation, Diagnosis, and Treatment of Occlusal Problems, ed 2. St Louis: Mosby, 1989:206–237.

105 ■ Weinberg LA. An evaluation of basic articulators and their concepts. Part I: basic concepts. J Prosthet Dent 1963;13:622–644.

106 ■ Schallhorn RG. A study of the arbitrary center and the kinematic center of rotation for face-bow mountings. J Prosthet Dent 1957;7:162–169.

107 ■ Lauritzen AG, Bodner GH. Variations in location of arbitrary and true hinge axis points. J Prosthet Dent 1961;11:224–229.

108 ■ Teteruck WR, Lundeen HC. The accuracy of an ear face-bow. J Prosthet Dent 1966;16:1039–1046.

109 ■ Walker PM. Discrepancies between arbitrary and true hinge axes. J Prosthet Dent 1980;43:279–285.

110 ■ Simpson JW, Hesby RA, Pfeifer DL, Pelleu GB Jr. Arbitrary mandibular hinge axis locations. J Prosthet Dent 1984;51:819–822.

111 ■ Palik JF, Nelson DR, White JT. Accuracy of an earpiece face-bow. J Prosthet Dent 1985;53:800–804.

112 ■ Kurth L, Feinstein IK. The hinge axis of the mandible. J Prosthet Dent 1951;1:327–332.

113 ■ Borgh O, Posselt U. Hinge axis registration: Experiments on the articulator. J Prosthet Dent 1958;8:35–40.

114 ■ Lauritzen AG, Wolford LW. Hinge axis location on an experimental basis. J Prosthet Dent 1961;11:1059–1067.

115 ■ Preston JD. A reassessment of the mandibular transverse horizontal axis theory. J Prosthet Dent 1979; 41:605–613.

116 ■ Bowley JF, Michaels GC, Lai TW, Lin PP. Reliability of a facebow transfer procedure. J Prosthet Dent 1992; 67:491–498.

117 ■ Dawson PE. Evaluation, Diagnosis, and Treatment of Occlusal Problems, ed 2. St Louis: Mosby, 1989: 238–260.

118 ■ Wilkie ND. The anterior point of reference. J Prosthet Dent 1979;41:488–496.

119 ■ Pitchford JH. A reevaluation of the axis-orbital plane and the use of orbitale in a facebow transfer record. J Prosthet Dent 1991;66:349–355.

120 ■ Gracis S. Clinical considerations and rationale for the use of simplified instrumentation in occlusal rehabilitation. Part 1: Mounting of the models on the articulator. Int J Periodontics Restorative Dent 2003;23:57–67.

121 ■ Lee RL. Standardized head position and reference planes for dento-facial aesthetics. Dent Today 2000 Feb:19(2).

122 ■ Gonzales JB, Kingery RH. Evaluation of planes of reference for orienting maxillary casts on articulators. J Am Dent Assoc 1968;76:329–336.

123 ■ Bailey JO, Nowlin TP. Evaluation of the third point of reference for mounting maxillary casts on the Hanau articulator. J Prosthet Dent 1984;51:199–201.

124 ■ Stade EH, Hanson JG, Baker CL. Esthetic considerations in the use of face-bows. J Prosthet Dent 1982; 48:253–256.

125 ■ Castellani D. Elements of Occlusion. Bologna, Italy: Edizioni Martina, 2000:103–126.

126 ■ Weinberg LA. An evaluation of the face-bow mounting. J Prosthet Dent 1961;11:32–42.

127 ■ Rufenacht CR. Fundamentals of Esthetics. Chicago: Quintessence, 1990:33–58.

128 ■ Lombardi RE. The principles of visual perception and their clinical application to denture esthetics. J Prosthet Dent 1973;29:358–382.

129 ■ Roach RR, Muia PJ. Communication between dentist and technician: An esthetic checklist. In: Preston JD (ed). Perspectives in Dental Ceramics: Proceedings of the Fourth International Symposium on Ceramics. Chicago: Quintessence, 1998:445–455.

130 ■ Fradeani M. Esthetic Rehabilitation in Fixed Prosthodontics, Vol 1. Esthetic Analysis: A Systematic Approach to Prosthetic Treatment. Chicago: Quintessence, 2004:35–61.

131 ■ Viazis AD. A cephalometric analysis based on natural head position. J Clin Orthod 1991;25:172–181.

132 ■ Arnett GW, Bergman RT. Facial keys to orthodontic diagnosis and treatment planning. Part I. Am J Orthod Dentofacial Orthop 1993;103:299–312.

133 ■ Rifkin R. Facial analysis: A comprehensive approach to treatment planning in aesthetic dentistry. Pract Periodontics Aesthet Dent 2000;12:865–871.

134 ■ Paul SJ. Smile analysis and face-bow transfer: Enhancing aesthetic restorative treatment. Pract Proced Aesthet Dent 2001;13:217–222.

135 ■ Padwa BL, Kaiser MO, Kaban LB. Occlusal cant in the frontal plane as a reflection of facial asymmetry. J Oral Maxillofac Surg 1997;55:811–816.

136 ■ Chiche GJ, Aoshima H. Functional versus aesthetic articulation of maxillary anterior restorations. Pract Periodontics Aesthet Dent 1997;9:335–342.

137 ■ Chiche GJ, Kokich VG, Caudill R. Diagnosis and treatment planning of esthetic problems. In: Chiche GJ, Pinault A (eds). Esthetics of Anterior Fixed Prosthodontics. Chicago: Quintessence, 1994: 33–52.

138 ■ Dawson PE. Evaluation, Diagnosis, and Treatment of Occlusal Problems, ed 2. St Louis: Mosby, 1989: 274–297.

139 ■ Lundeen HC, Wirth CG. Condylar movement patterns engraved in plastic blocks. J Prosthet Dent 1973; 30:866–875.

140 ■ Lundeen HC, Shryock EF, Gibbs CH. An evaluation of mandibular border movements: their character and significance. J Prosthet Dent 1978;40:442–452.

141 ■ Weiner S. Biomechanics of occlusion and the articulator. Dent Clin North Am 1995;39:257–284.

142 ■ Molina M. Concetti Fondamentali di Gnatologia Moderna. Milano, Italia: Riccardo Ilic Editrice, 1988:199–241.

143 ■ Preiskel HW. Ultrasonic measurements of movements of the working condyle. J Prosthed Dent 1972;27: 607–615.

144 ■ Bellanti ND, Martin KR. The significance of articulator capability. Part II: The prevalence of immediate side shift. J Prosthet Dent 1979;42:255–256.

145 ■ Hart JK, Sakamura JS. Mandibular lateral side-shift and the need of gnathologic instrumentation. J Prosthet Dent 1985;54:415–420.

146 ■ Hobo S. Formula for adjusting the horizontal condylar path of semi-adjustable articulator with interocclusal records. Part 1: correlation between the immediate side shift, the progressive side shift and the Bennet angle. J Prosthet Dent 1986;55:422–426.

147 ■ Hobo S. Formula for adjusting the horizontal condylar path of semiadjustable articulator with interocclusal records. Part 2: practical evaluations. J Prosthet Dent 1986;55:582–588.

148 ■ Levinson E. The nature of the side-shift in lateral mandibular movement and its implications in clinical practice. J Prosthet Dent 1984;52:91–98.

149 ■ Gracis S. Clinical considerations and rationale for the use of simplified instrumentation in occlusal rehabilitation. Part 2: setting of the articulator and occlusal optimization. Int J Periodontics Restorative Dent 2003;23:139–145.

150 ■ Wiskott HW, Belser UC. A rationale for a simplified occlusal design in restorative dentistry: historical review and clinical guidelines. J Prosthet Dent 1995; 73:169–183.

151 ■ Krogh-Poulsen WG, Olsson A. Management of the occlusion of the teeth: background, definitions, rationale. In: Schwartz L, Chayes C (eds). Facial Pain and Mandibular Dysfunction. Philadelphia: WB Saunders, 1968.

152 ■ Dawson PE, Arcan M. Attaining harmonic occlusion through visualized strain analysis. J Prosthet Dent 1981;46:615–622.

153 ■ Ramfjord S, Ash MM. Occlusion, ed 3. Philadelphia: WB Saunders, 1983.

154 ■ Dawson PE. Evaluation, Diagnosis, and Treatment of Occlusal Problems, ed 2. St Louis: Mosby, 1989:14–17.

155 ■ Piehslinger E, Bauer W, Schmiedmayer HB. Computer simulation of occlusal discrepancies resulting from different mounting techniques. J Prosthet Dent 1995; 74:279–283.

156 ■ Adrien P, Schouver J. Methods for minimizing the errors in mandibular model mounting on an articulator. J Oral Rehabil 1997;24;929–935.

VOLUME 2 PROSTHETIC TREATMENT

Chapter 1 COMMUNICATING TO THE LABORATORY—DIAGNOSTIC WAX-UP

VOLUME 2 PROSTHETIC TREATMENT

ESTHETIC REHABILITATION IN FIXED PROSTHODONTICS

Chapter 2

CREATING AND INTEGRATING THE PROVISIONAL RESTORATION

The provisional restoration is derived from the diagnostic wax-up and must faithfully reproduce the changes that were made in it. The use of a specific technique to create the provisional restoration allows it to be fitted correctly and thus to verify the clinical suitability of the revision choices. Formerly just one procedure in the prosthetic treatment plan, the provisional restoration has taken on a fundamental role to such an extent that it can be considered a testing ground for evaluating and verifying function, esthetics, phonetics, and biologic integration before proceeding with the preparations and the final impressions.

OBJECTIVE _ To create and properly fit a provisional restoration that, once suitably integrated, will serve as the prototype for the definitive rehabilitation.

CREATING AND INTEGRATING THE PROVISIONAL RESTORATION

To achieve optimal integration and to accommodate the associated therapies frequently included in the treatment plan of a prosthetic rehabilitation, it is often necessary to leave the provisional restoration in the oral cavity for some time. In such cases, it is sufficient to make only the preliminary preparations for fitting the provisional restoration, leaving the final preparations and impressions for a later phase.

Especially in cases where tooth position and restorative contour have been modified, extended wear of the provisional restoration allows the validity of the changes made to it to be tested clinically with regard to their biologic, esthetic, and functional integrity. Only after this objective has been met is it possible to proceed with finalizing the work. For these reasons, the chapter on the methods of making and integrating the provisional restoration (chapter 2) chronologically precedes the chapters discussing final preparations (chapter 3) and final impressions (chapter 4).

OBJECTIVE

The main objective in creating a provisional restoration is to produce a faithful reproduction of the diagnostic wax-up (Fig 2-1a) that can be correctly fitted into the oral cavity (Figs 2-1b and 2-1c).

PROVISIONALS

OBJECTIVES

- Replace missing teeth
- Replace incorrect prostheses
- Correct tooth malposition
- Verify and stabilize tooth mobility
- Restore ideal occlusal stability (in MI or CR)
- Restore suitable vertical dimension (VD)
- Keep occlusal trauma under control
- Protect tooth tissue after preparing abutments
- Check parallelism of abutments
- Facilitate associated therapies
- Suggest other possible operating needs (ortho, perio, implants, etc)
- Restore optimal function
- Improve esthetics
- Check and improve phonetics
- Maintain adequate patient hygiene
- Facilitate examination for surgery
- Preserve and condition marginal periodontium
- Serve as a prototype for the definitive restorations

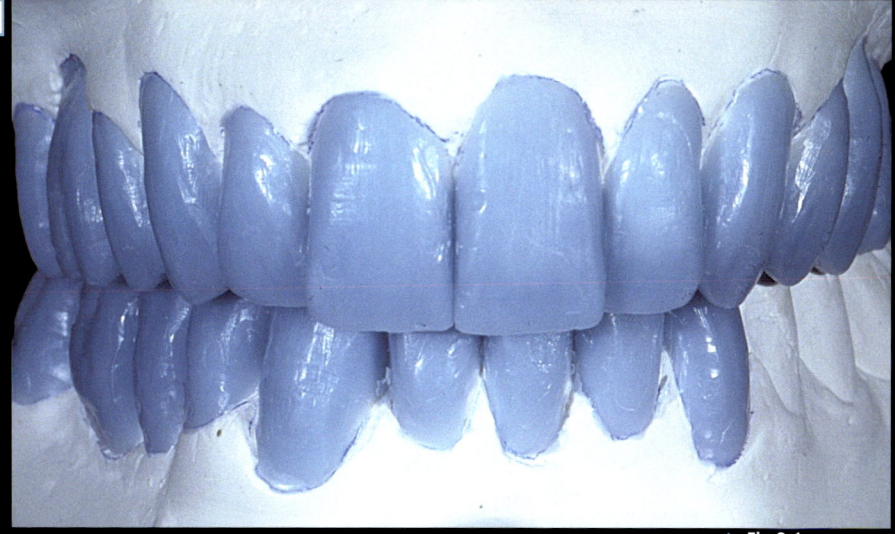

> Fig 2-1a

> Fig 2-1b

> Fig 2-1c

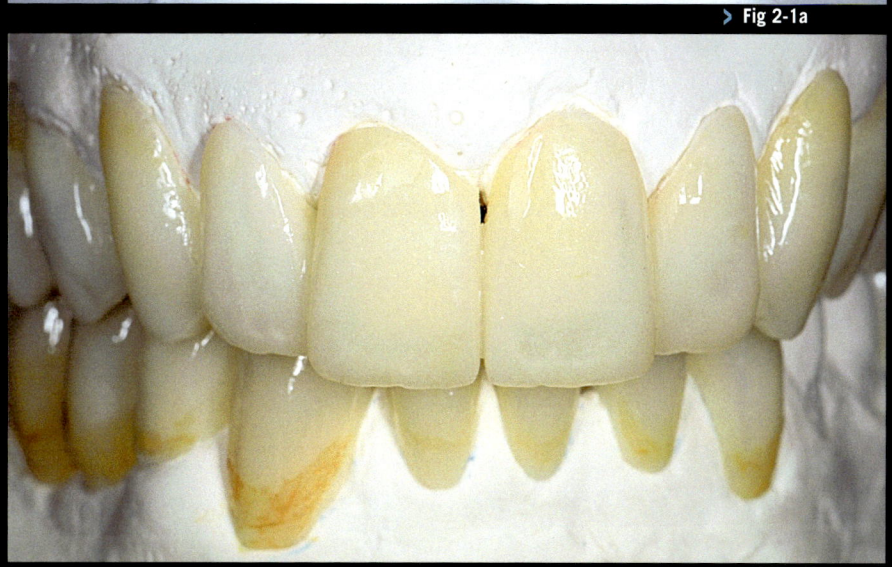

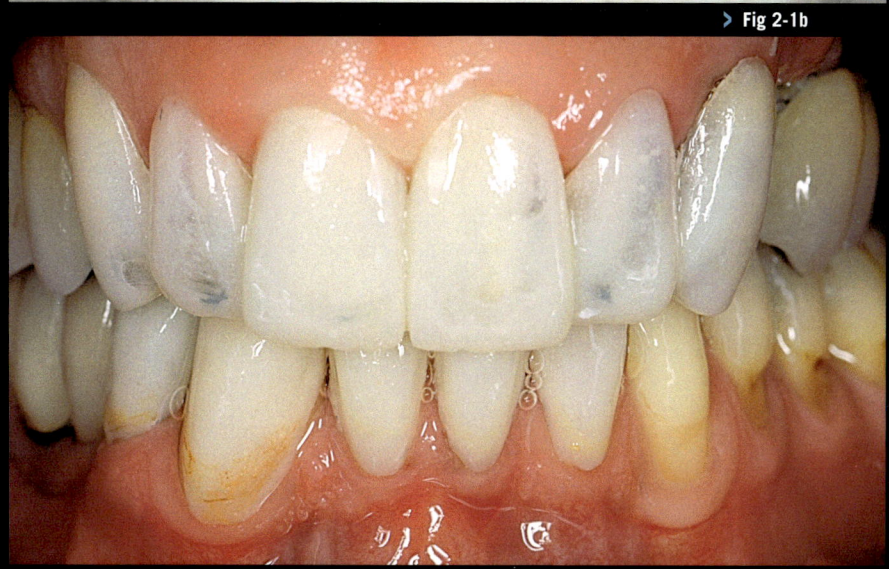

FIG 1 *(a to c)* All of the variations requested by the clinician and executed by the technician in the diagnostic wax-up must be faithfully reproduced in the provisional restoration.

Once the provisional restoration is in the mouth, it must be possible to clinically assess the accuracy of the changes made as a result of the esthetic and functional analysis of the patient. Scrupulous preliminary planning and the correct completion of all stages during fabrication, fitting, and relining of the provisional restoration simplify the work of the clinician and the technician and reduce the working time considerably. The skill, precision, and maximum care applied by the clinician in this initial phase of the treatment affect much more than the choice of materials to be used, which is a crucial factor in the success of the case.[1]

The provisional restoration must guarantee the patient a suitable esthetic appearance as well as comfort if he or she is to have confidence and faith in the treatment undertaken.[2,3] It is therefore necessary to minimize the risk of decementation or fracture, which are almost always the result of an inappropriate occlusal situation, inadequate preparations, or incorrect relining. Once optimal esthetic, functional, and biologic integration has been achieved (Figs 2-1d to 2-1f),[4-10] the provisional restoration must, above all, serve as an essential reference or prototype for the prosthetic rehabilitation. All of the information contained in the impression can be transferred to the laboratory, so that every detail is reproduced in the definitive work (see chapter 4).

REQUIREMENTS

The provisional restoration must have the right characteristics to allow it to remain in the oral cavity for long periods. It must be resistant to abrasion and of sufficient strength to minimize the risk of fracture during function. It must also allow gingival health to be main tained through careful design of the contours, suitable marginal fit, and an appropriately polished surface. If these requirements are not met, then tissue inflammation will inevitably ensue. This condition is often incorrectly and arbitrarily ascribed to the presumed intolerance of the patient to the acrylic material used.

PROVISIONALS

IDEAL REQUISITES

- Easy removal during sessions in the office
- Resistance to fracture and decementation during normal masticatory function
- Resistance to abrasion
- Maintenance of tooth position and occlusal stability
- Optimal marginal adaptation
- Maintenance of gingival health
- Good working and polishing capabilities
- Color stability

> Fig 2-1d

> Fig 2-1e

> Fig 2-1f

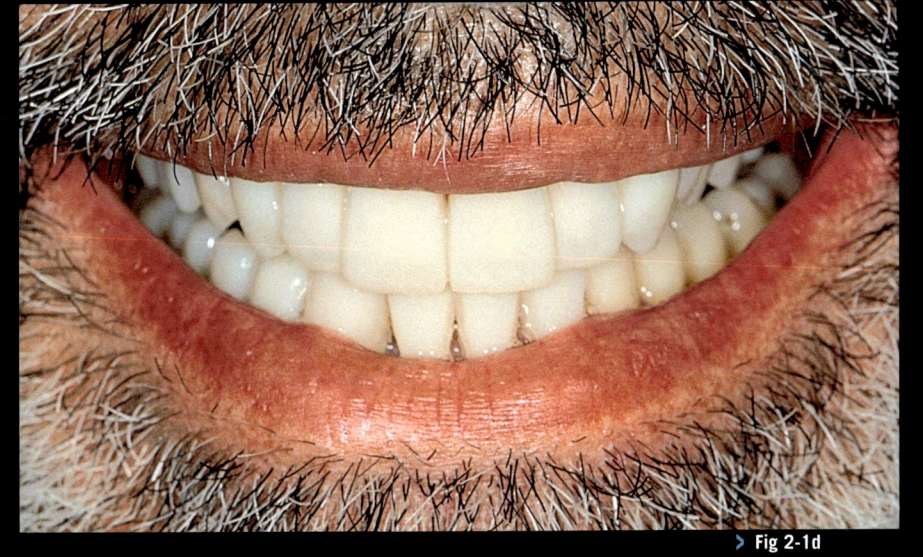

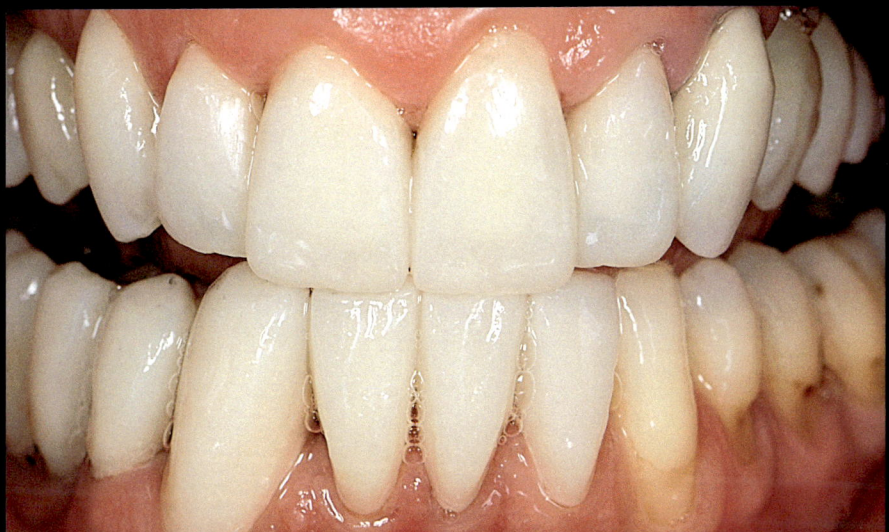

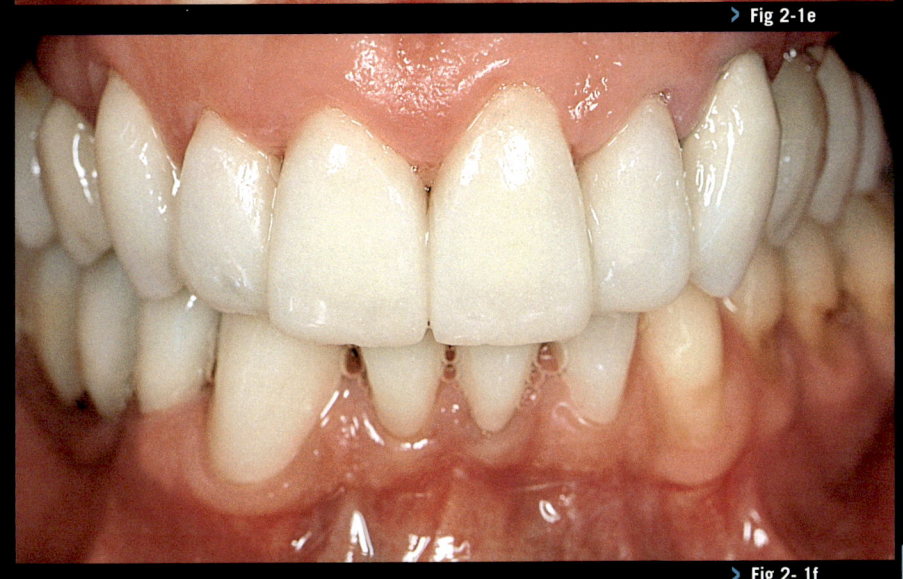

→ continues on page 145

FIG 1 *(d to f)* After relining and finishing, the provisional restoration must appear adequately integrated from the esthetic, functional, and biologic viewpoints.

PROVISIONAL RESTORATIONS

MATERIALS

Acrylic and composite materials, which are both easily modified by subtraction as well as addition, are preferred for constructing and relining provisional restorations using various polymerization methods.[11–15]

ACRYLIC RESINS - Methyl methacrylate

The most widely used material is methyl methacrylate,[15–18] especially for the indirect fabrication technique. It has several good characteristics, most notably adequate marginal fit and satisfactory chromatic stability. Because of its high resistance to fracture, it is usually recommended for creating provisional restorations that will stay in the mouth for a long time.

ACRYLIC RESINS – Ethyl methacrylate

Ethyl methacrylate is considered more suitable for provisional restorations that will have a shorter life.[19,20] The advantage offered by this type of material is its lower exothermic reaction[12,21–23] and a less marked contraction of the acrylic resin than methyl methacrylate.[12,21,22]

Polymerization method Acrylic resins can be divided into two categories: heat-activated and self-curing. *Heat-activated acrylic* resins are ideal for making provisional restorations, by the indirect technique, for medium- to long-term use. The acrylic material that is polymerized by heat is particularly compact and resistant to abrasion and fracture and is chromatically stable[11,16,24] (Fig 2-2a). *Self-curing acrylic* resin is the type most widely used for making provisional restorations by the direct method as well as for relining those made using the indirect technique[15,25] (Fig 2-2b).

RESIN COMPOSITES

Resin composites usually come in self-mixing syringes typical of impression materials (Fig 2-2c). Although the initial surface hardness level of resin composites appears to be high, a notable reduction occurs over time.[26–28] Despite their limited exothermic reaction[22,29,30] and minimal polymerization contraction,[22] these materials have not reached the wide level of use initially expected because many clinicians believe that they are difficult to manipulate[16,25,31–33] and that they significantly compromise the marginal closure due to the presence of air bubbles.[34]

Polymerization method Though usually self-curing, resin composites can also be light curing and dual curing (Fig 2-2d).

FIG 2 *(a and b)* Methacrylate is used in fabricating the provisional restoration through the direct technique as well as for relining the acrylic resin shell. *(c and d)* The resin composites, supplied in convenient self-mixing syringes, are both self-curing and light-curing.

Chapter 2 CREATING AND INTEGRATING THE PROVISIONAL RESTORATION

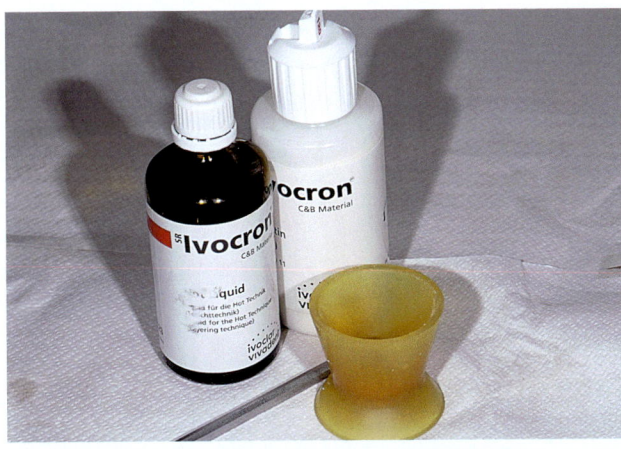

> Fig 2-2a

> Fig 2-2b

> Fig 2-2c

> Fig 2-2d

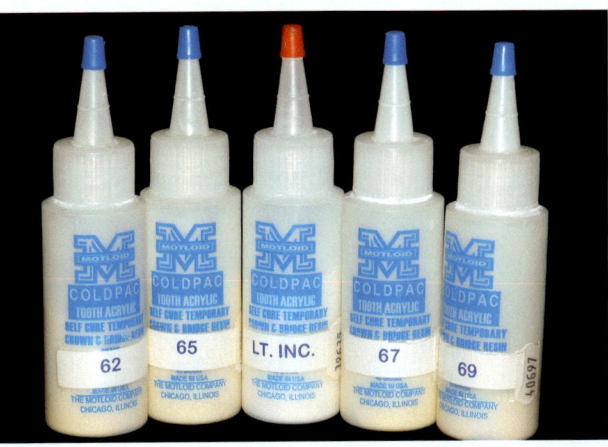

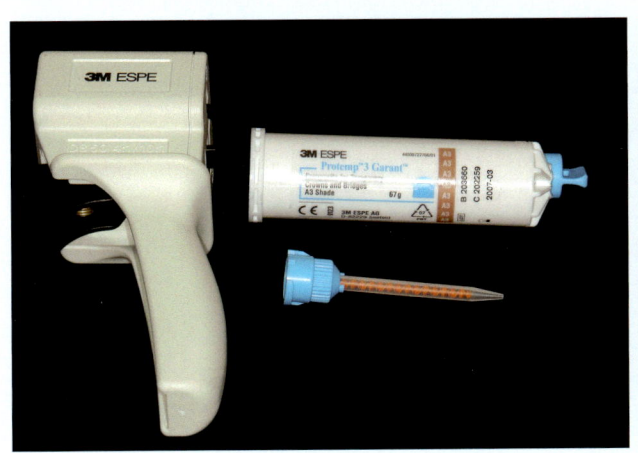

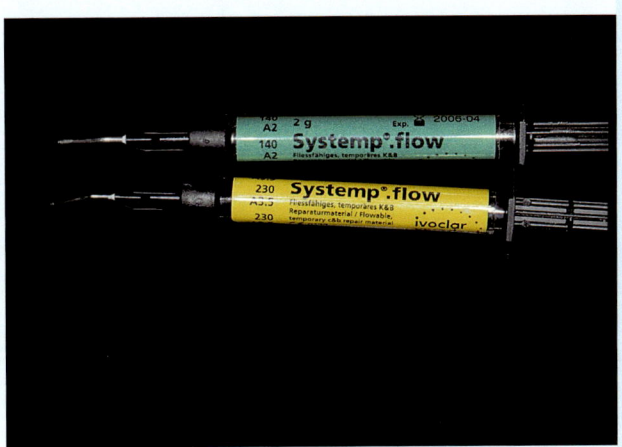

ACRYLIC RESINS—METHYL METHACRYLATE

ADVANTAGES	DISADVANTAGES
■ High resistance to fracture ■ Acceptable marginal precision ■ Satisfactory color stability ■ Good longevity ■ Wide chromatic range	■ Marked exothermia ■ Significant shrinkage

ACRYLIC RESINS—ETHYL METHACRYLATE

ADVANTAGES	DISADVANTAGES
■ Ideal working time ■ Low shrinkage ■ Low exothermic reaction ■ Wide chromatic range	■ Low resistance to abrasion ■ Limited longevity ■ Poor chromatic stability

RESIN COMPOSITES

ADVANTAGES	DISADVANTAGES
■ Low shrinkage ■ Good resistance to adhesion ■ Low exothermic reaction ■ Ease of repair	■ Problematic marginal closure ■ Low strength over time ■ Limited chromatic range ■ Expensive

TOOTH PREPARATION

PLANNING THE PROSTHETIC ABUTMENT

Tooth preparation is a fundamental and irreversible clinical stage of prosthetic rehabilitation and therefore requires maximum care to guarantee easy insertion and adequate retention and resistance of the provisional restoration.

Tooth preparation must be carried out only after the technician has made the diagnostic wax-up based on the esthetic-functional needs of the patient (Figs 2-3a and 2-3b). Abutment reduction is done in accordance with the final three-dimensional volume of the wax-up, which often differs from the dimensions, axes, and inclination that the teeth originally presented. The wax-up therefore serves as a guide to tooth preparation, allowing the clinician to accomplish accurate removal of existing dental tissue.

Transparent acetate matrices and silicone matrices pressed on a stone duplicate of the wax-up itself are used to reach the esthetic and functional objectives and to ensure congruous preparations (Figs 2-3c to 2-3f). These matrices make it possible to immediately check the adequacy of both the axial inclination of the abutments and the thickness of the preparations, helping the clinician identify any modifications. Use of these matrices allows prosthetically guided preparation of the abutments to make it easier to insert the provisional restoration.

PRELIMINARY PREPARATION

Preliminary preparations are generally vertical (knife edge or slight chamfer). The main goals are to remove the undercuts between the teeth and to obtain parallelism of the abutments. Preparing the definitive abutments (see chapter 3, pages 324–351) and taking accurate impressions (see chapter 4, pages 384–409) can be deferred to a later stage. This minimally invasive approach proves especially useful in complex rehabilitation cases. If the treatment plan involves extractions, periodontal procedures, and/or implant-surgical procedures, these preparations will then require apicalization of the gingival levels, with consequent lengthening of the clinical crown after the provisional restorations are fitted. In the final preparation stage, modification of the axial inclination may therefore be necessary; such modifications will be more conservative where only preliminary preparations have been carried out, eliminating the need to make any excessive reduction of the tooth structure.

> Fig 2-3a

> Fig 2-3b

> Fig 2-3c

> Fig 2-3d

> Fig 2-3e

> Fig 2-3f

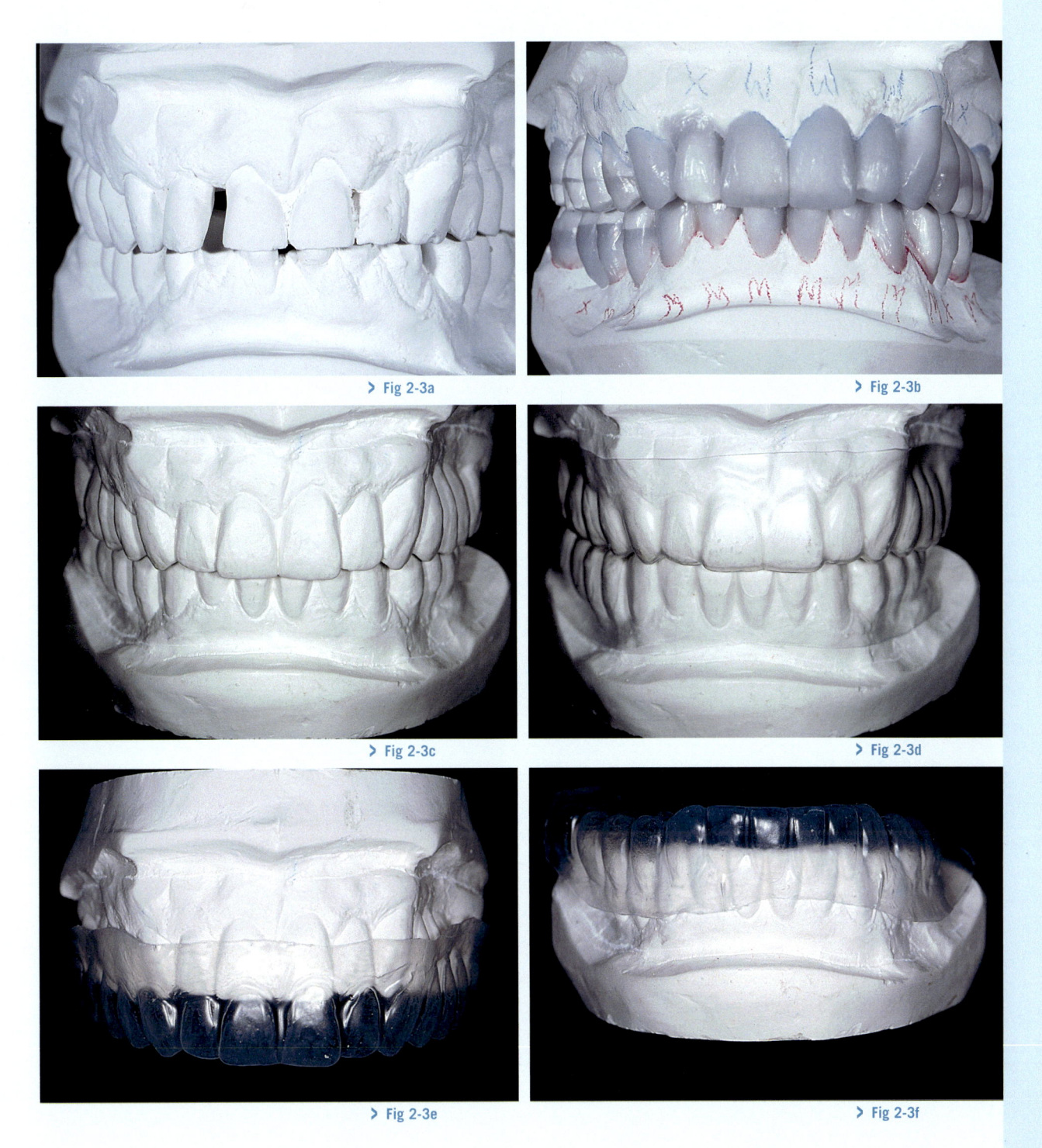

FIG 3 *(a and b)* Stone casts of the preoperative situation and diagnostic wax-up. *(c to f)* On both arches of the stone duplicate of the wax-up, the transparent acetate stents are pressed; these are used by the clinician as a guide to tooth preparation.

Correct insertion of a provisional restoration that secures the abutments of an entire arch can sometimes be impaired by the original inclination of the natural teeth (curves of Spee and Wilson).

In the maxillary arch, for example, the curve of Spee causes a natural divergence between the axial orientation of the anterior teeth, which tend to be buccally positioned, and that of the last molars. Being unable to significantly modify the axis of the anterior teeth, the clinician is sometimes forced to mesialize the distal walls of the molars to avoid excessively reducing the already limited tooth structure and involuntarily varying the overjet to achieve the correct insertion of a fixed provisional restoration on the entire maxillary arch. In the mandibular arch, on the other hand, a complete fit of the provisional rehabilitation may require slight distalization of the mesial walls of the molars.

To counteract a lack of parallelism of the axial inclination often found between the maxillary and mandibular posterior teeth of the two sides, which is caused by the curve of Wilson, the clinician must slightly lingualize the buccal walls of the posterior teeth in the maxillary arch, while in the mandibular arch the lingual walls should be slightly buccally positioned. Even with these measures, perfect parallelism between the teeth of an entire arch is not always easy to achieve, especially in the presence of numerous abutments. If the teeth are only minimally nonparallel, fitting the provisional restoration is sometimes possible by resorting to "special" insertion axes that take advantage of the physiologic tooth mobility, especially in the buccolingual direction. The difficulties of inserting a complete provisional restoration can also be accentuated in the mandibular arch by changes in the width of the mandible at various phases of opening the mouth. Previewing the final sizes of the restorations, provided by the acetate matrix, undoubtedly makes the clinician's task easier (Figs 2-3g to 2-3l). Nonetheless, the final check of the axes should be completed with the aid of large occlusal mirrors that, by reflecting the entire arch, make it possible to compare the opposing surfaces of the abutments prepared according to the established insertion axis.

> Fig 2-3g

> Fig 2-3h

> Fig 2-3i

> Fig 2-3j

> Fig 2-3k

> Fig 2-3l

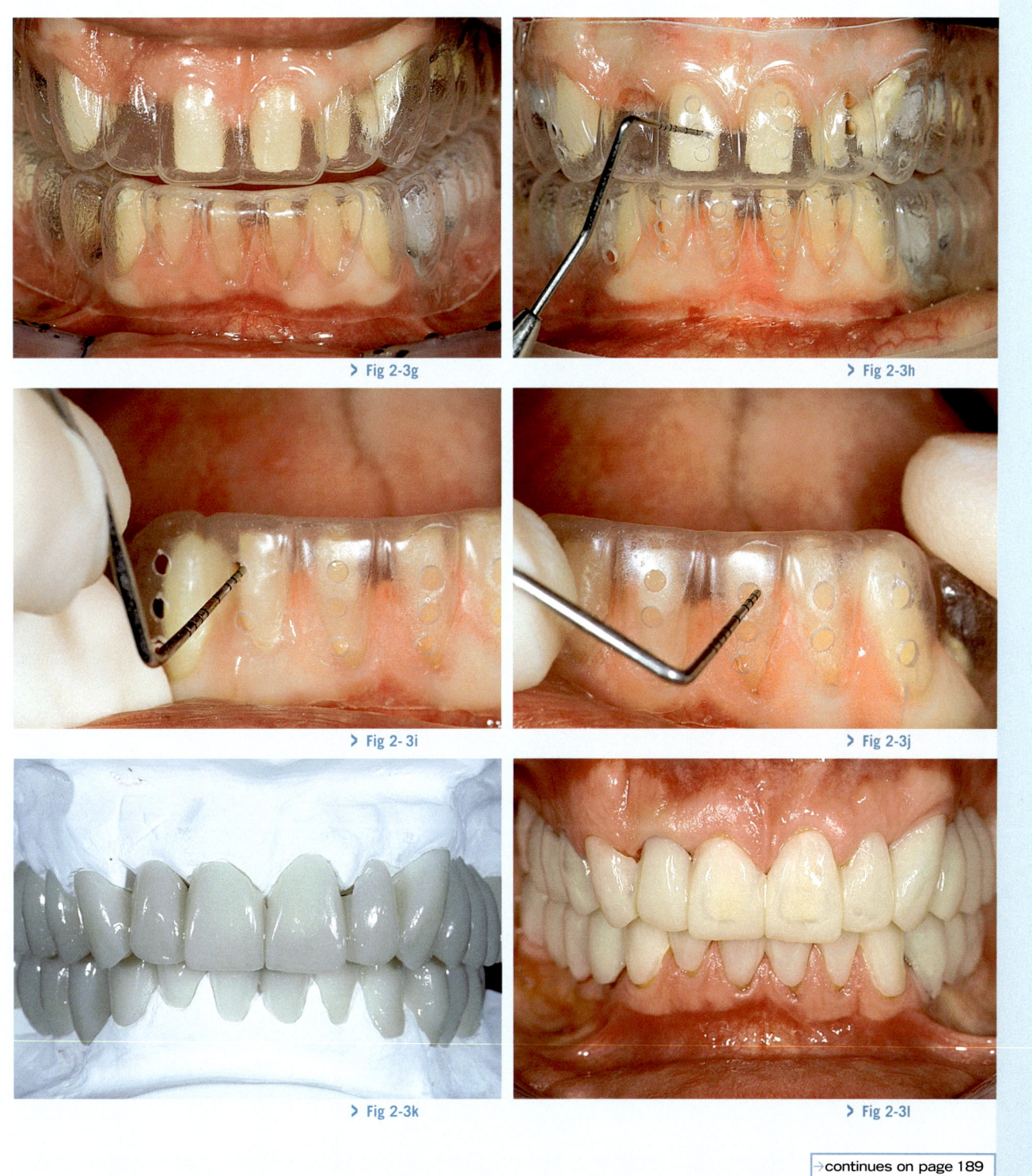

→continues on page 189

FIG 3 *(g to j)* The indices provide valuable indications as to the axial inclination and the preparation thicknesses, which the clinician can check using a millimetric periodontal probe. *(k and l)* The provisional restoration received from the laboratory can at this point be easily fitted, without encountering any resistance to its insertion.

FABRICATING THE PROVISIONAL RESTORATION

DIRECT TECHNIQUE

CHAIRSIDE FABRICATION

With this technique, the provisional restoration is fabricated directly with the patient in the chair[35] by pouring self-curing resin into an acetate matrix[11] or into an impression in silicone or alginate.[36] With each option, the temperature of the acrylic rises considerably during polymerization because of the significant amounts of resin used. The resulting heat is higher when using the silicone or acetate matrix (a difference of up to 7°C), with substantial risks to the pulp vitality.[37] Because of the large quantity of water contained in it, the alginate impression is able to significantly reduce the exothermic reaction.

ACETATE MATRIX

Although it impedes heat dispersion, the acetate matrix has an important advantage: Its transparency allows the clinician to check, throughout the various stages of constructing the provisional restoration, for correct insertion and removal, formation of any air bubbles, and, in complex cases, the correct orientation of the occlusal plane. For this reason, the acetate matrix can be recommended,[22,38-44] but only with the use of abundant water irrigation to minimize the rise in temperature.

While ideal for simple cases, the direct technique can also be used in more complex cases that require modifications to tooth position and shape (Figs 2-4a to 2-4d). In these cases, the acetate matrix must be derived from the stone cast of the diagnostic wax-up made in the laboratory (Figs 2-4e to 2-4g).

The matrix can also serve as a guide for the tooth preparations[31] (Figs 2-4h and 2-4i), becoming an integral part of the patient's clinical documentation, since it allows a new provisional restoration to be made at any time (Figs 2-4j to 2-4t).[39] In complex cases, however, the use of a large amount of acrylic resin, with its high exothermic reaction mitigated only partially by an abundant flow of water, means the matrix undergoes significant polymerization shrinkage, with inevitable repercussions on the marginal precision.[29,45-49] In these cases it is always advisable to reline the provisional restoration after emptying and sandblasting it to ensure good bonding of the relining material.[35,41,50]

For all of the reasons stated above, using the direct technique in complex cases, as opposed to fabricating a provisional restoration with heat-curing resins in the laboratory, must be considered a compromise to be adopted only in certain situations.

> Fig 2-4a

> Fig 2-4b

> Fig 2-4c

> Fig 2-4d

> Fig 2-4e

> Fig 2-4f

> Fig 2-4g

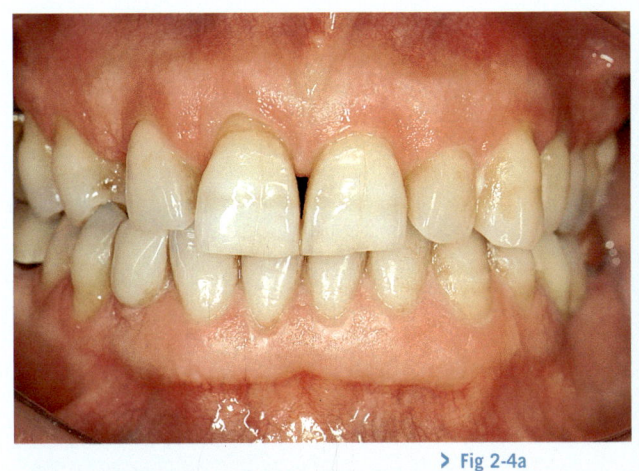

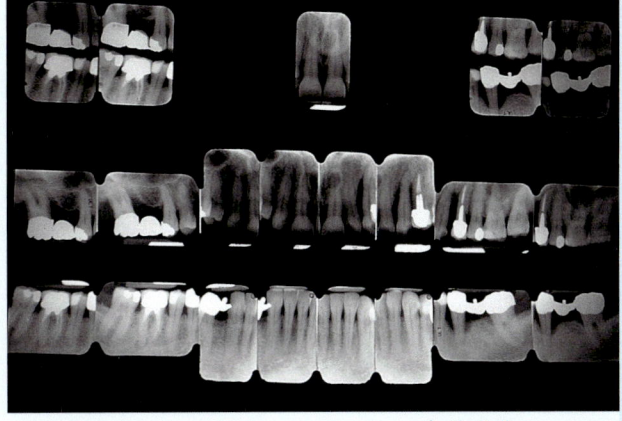

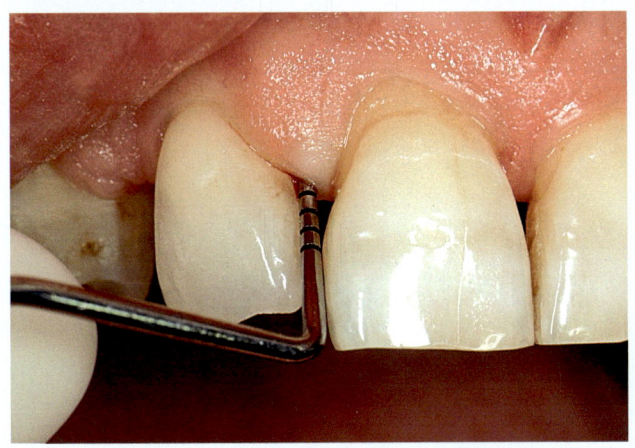

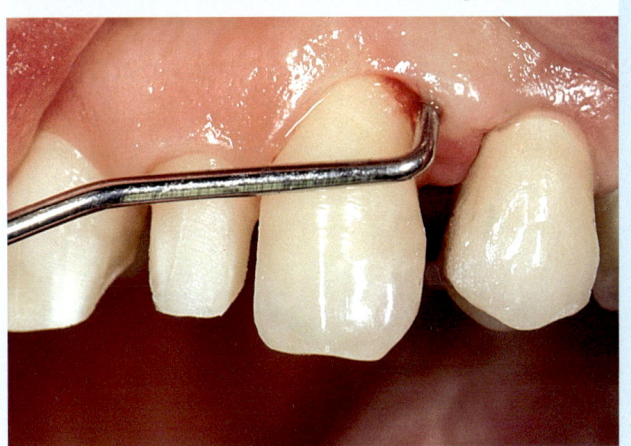

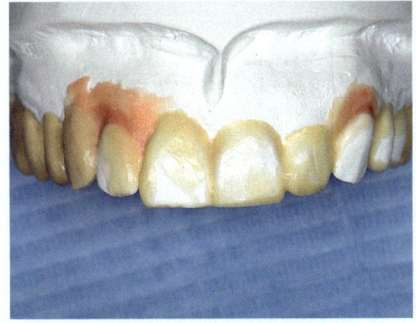

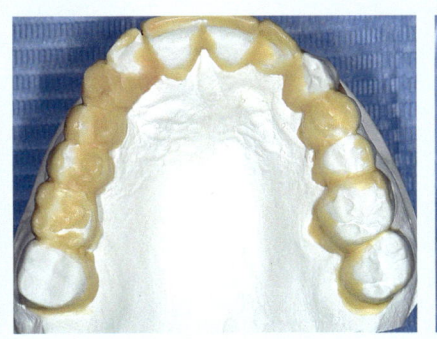

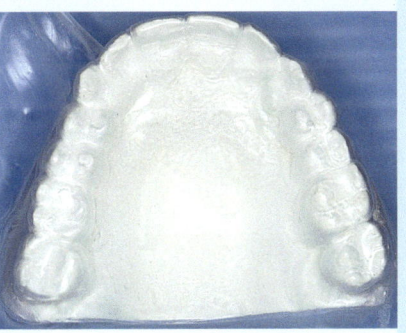

DIRECT TECHNIQUE

ADVANTAGES	DISADVANTAGES
- Practical fabrication - Quick procedure - Low cost	- Difficult fabrication in complex cases - Marked exothermic reaction - Problematic marginal closure

FIG 4 *(a to d)* The patient has a significant loss of periodontal support around some teeth, demonstrated by the complete full-mouth radiographic series and probing values. *(e to g)* After the preliminary diagnostic wax-up, a stone cast is made and subsequently used for pressing an acetate matrix.

> Fig 2-4h

> Fig 2-4i

> Fig 2-4j

> Fig 2-4k

> Fig 2-4l

> Fig 2-4m

> Fig 2-4n

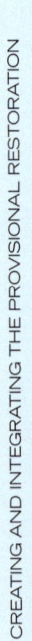

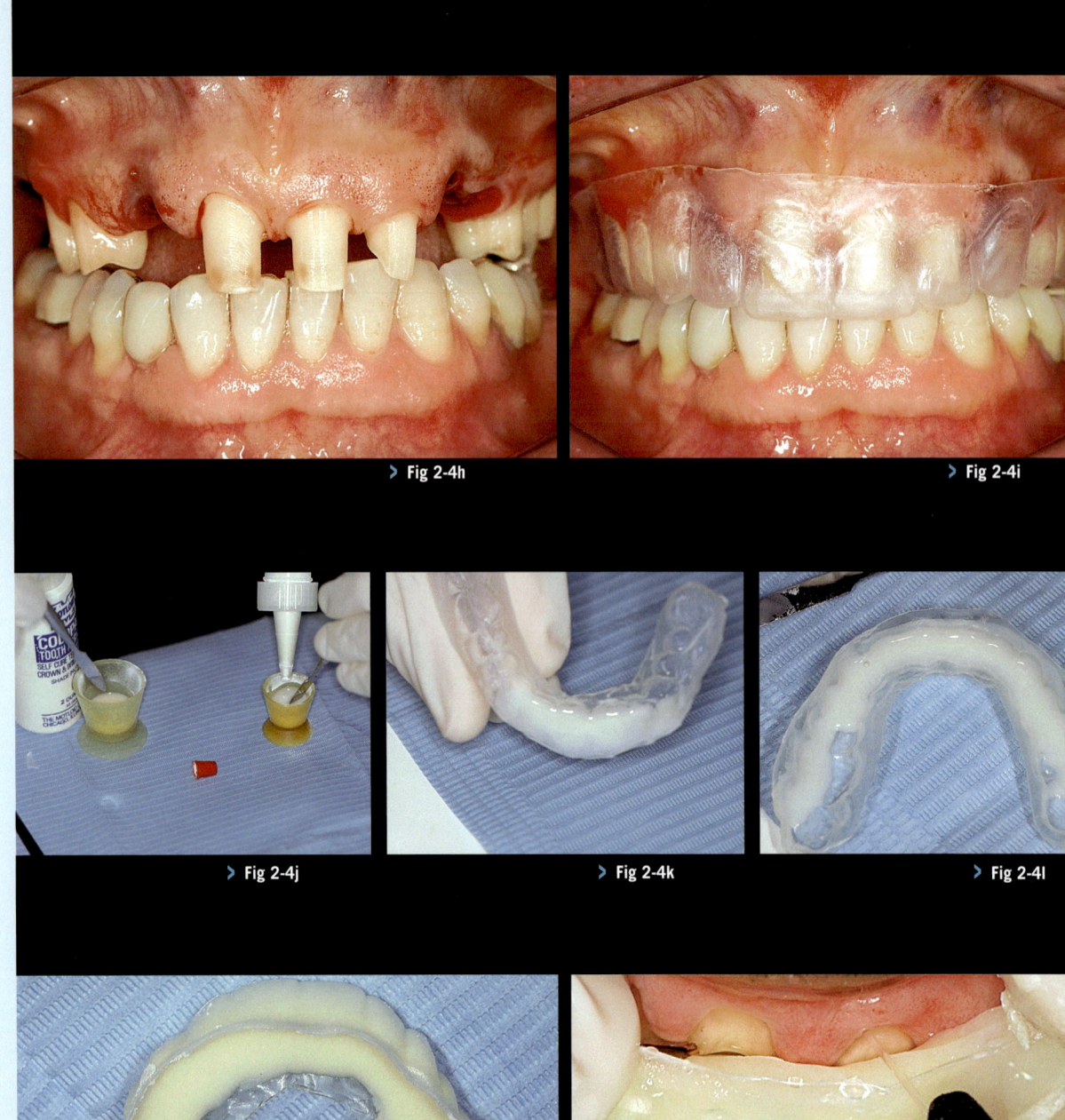

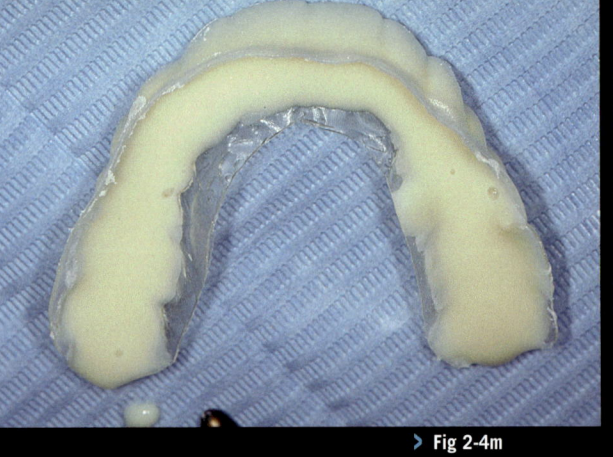

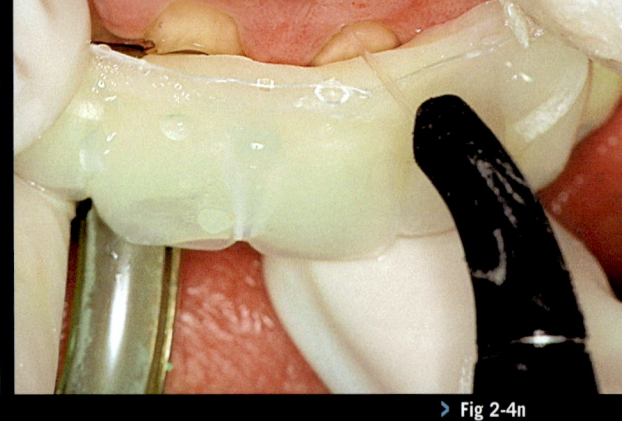

FIG 4 *(h and i)* After the preliminary tooth preparations and the necessary extractions are completed, the transparent matrix is tried in the mouth. *(j and k)* The acrylic resin is then mixed. First a layer of "enamel" is positioned inside the matrix, starting from the anterior sector, to give adequate translucency to the buccal portion of the provisional restoration, which is the most esthetically important part. *(l and m)* At this stage, the clinician should check that no air bubbles have been created before spreading the remaining enamel portion around the rest of the matrix and applying the layer of "dentin." *(n)* During polymerization in the mouth, the marked exothermic reaction resulting from the large amount of acrylic resin is attenuated by irrigation of the abutments, a procedure that further reduces the risk of the acrylic resin adhering to the prepared teeth.

> Fig 2-4o

> Fig 2-4p

> Fig 2-4q

> Fig 2-4r

> Fig 2-4s

> Fig 2-4t

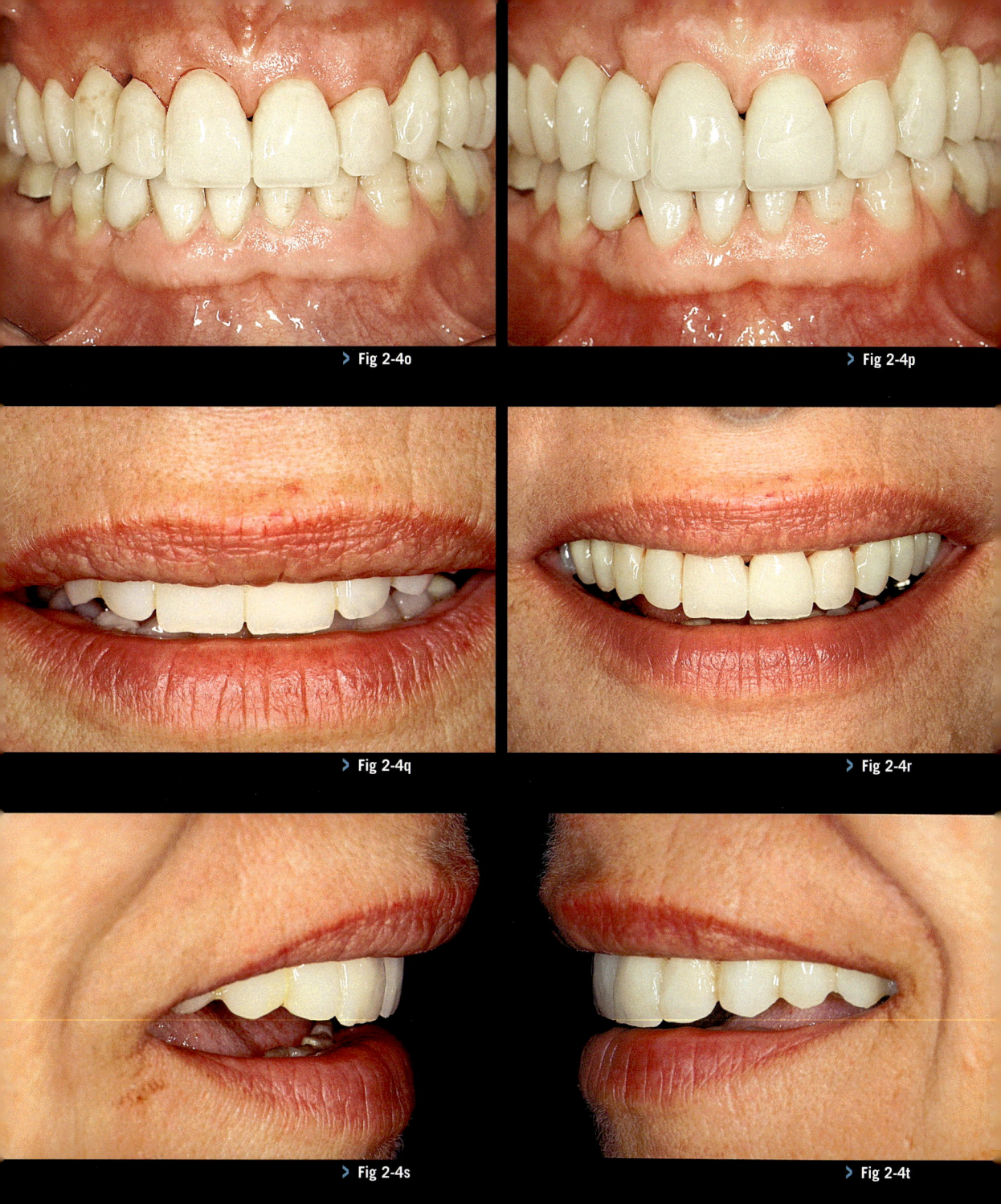

FIG 4 *(o)* Once polymerization is complete, the provisional restoration, removed from the matrix, is adequately finished and polished before being again positioned in the mouth and cemented into place. *(p)* A few weeks later, before it is removed for the supporting therapies (eg, endodontic treatments and periodontal surgery), the provisional restoration appears to be suitably integrated from both the biologic and esthetic viewpoints. *(q to t)* During the various phases of speech and smile it is possible to appreciate the satisfactory esthetic aspect achieved by suitable layering of the thickness of the enamel and dentin.

FABRICATING THE PROVISIONAL RESTORATION
INDIRECT TECHNIQUE

FABRICATION IN THE LABORATORY

In cases that require significant esthetic and/or occlusal alterations, creating the provisional restoration is usually left to the laboratory (indirect technique).[8,25,51–62] A heat-activated acrylic resin or a self-curing resin is normally used in these cases. The provisional restoration can be created either on intact casts (prepared teeth) or on casts on which the tooth preparations have already been carried out. In both cases the clinician receives an acrylic resin shell from the technician that is then relined in the mouth. Compared with the direct technique, fabrication of the shell in the laboratory reduces the amount of acrylic material needed for relining, thus generating less heat and less adhesive contraction and exposing the patient to less of the free monomer. These factors significantly increase overall patient comfort.[63,64]

PROVISIONAL RESTORATIONS FOR UNPREPARED TEETH

A provisional restoration created before the abutment teeth are prepared is made in the laboratory using a stone cast on which the technician prepares the teeth, with the aid of silicone indices derived from the diagnostic wax-up (Fig 2-5). Once the abutments on the patient have undergone a preliminary reduction, the shell is fitted into the mouth and necessarily relined. A certain amount of difficulty in fitting the provisional restoration can arise from inadequate communication between the clinician and the technician, or from problems with the acrylic resin or the technique used to construct the restoration. These problems are augmented if the technician cannot accurately identify the outline of the edentulous areas under old restorations. The design of the provisional restoration in these specific areas must be defined arbitrarily in the laboratory and later checked carefully and modified by the clinician if it prevents the provisional restoration from fitting perfectly.

PROVISIONAL RESTORATIONS FOR PREPARED TEETH

If the clinician has already prepared the teeth, the provisional restoration is made on a cast obtained from impressions of these preparations. This technique can be adopted when replacing old incongruous restorations (Fig 2-6a) or when, having positioned a first provisional restoration in the mouth, the decision is made to make a second one. Compared with cases where the provisional restoration is created before teeth are prepared, having a cast with the prepared teeth available (Fig 2-6b) gives the technician more precise references on which to base the provisional restoration (Figs 2-6c and 2-6d). This ensures that it fits more easily into the patient's mouth, even if it does not prevent the need for relining.

FIG 5 *(a to d)* To construct the provisional restoration before tooth preparation, the technician must perform the diagnostic wax-up on the original cast. From this, a stone cast is made on which the teeth are prepared. *(e)* The preparations are created under the guidance of a silicone index, which is also derived from the wax-up. *(f)* The technician then fabricates the acrylic resin shell on this cast.

UNPREDPARED TEETH

> Fig 2-5a

> Fig 2-5b

> Fig 2-5c

> Fig 2-5d

> Fig 2-5e

> Fig 2-5f

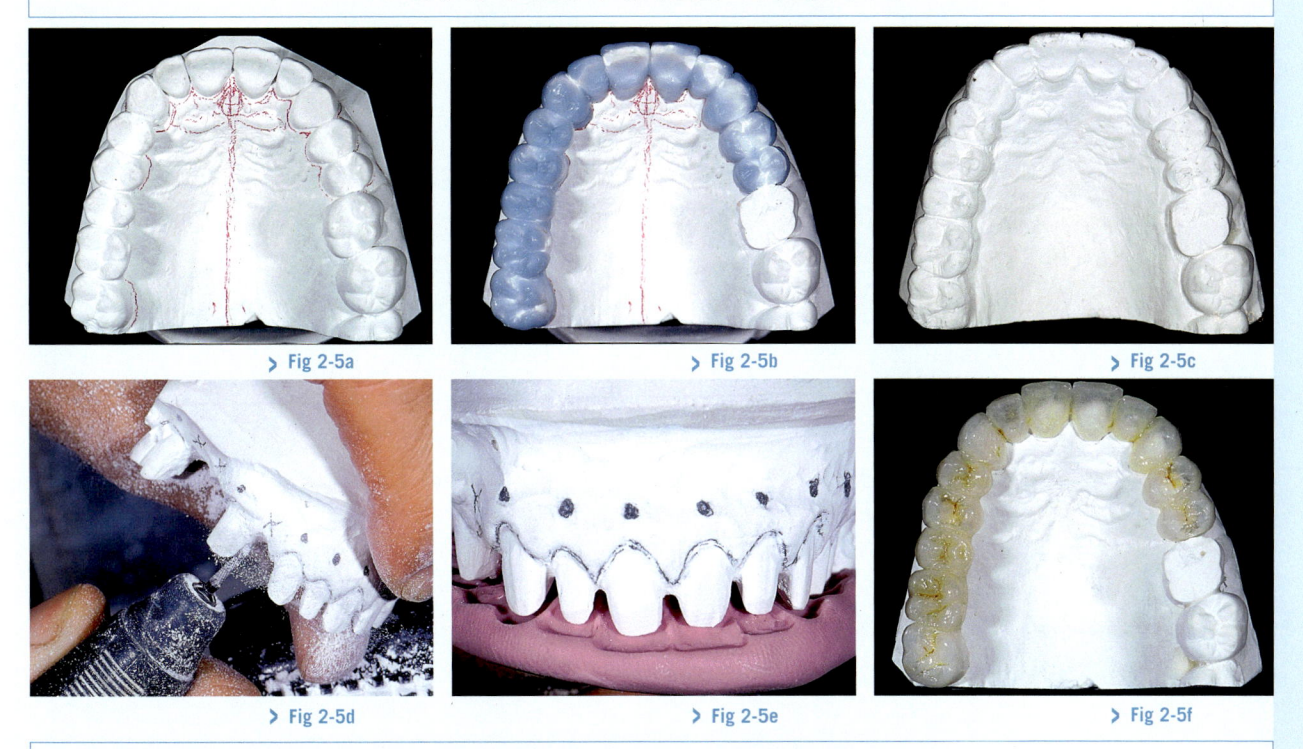

PREPARED TEETH

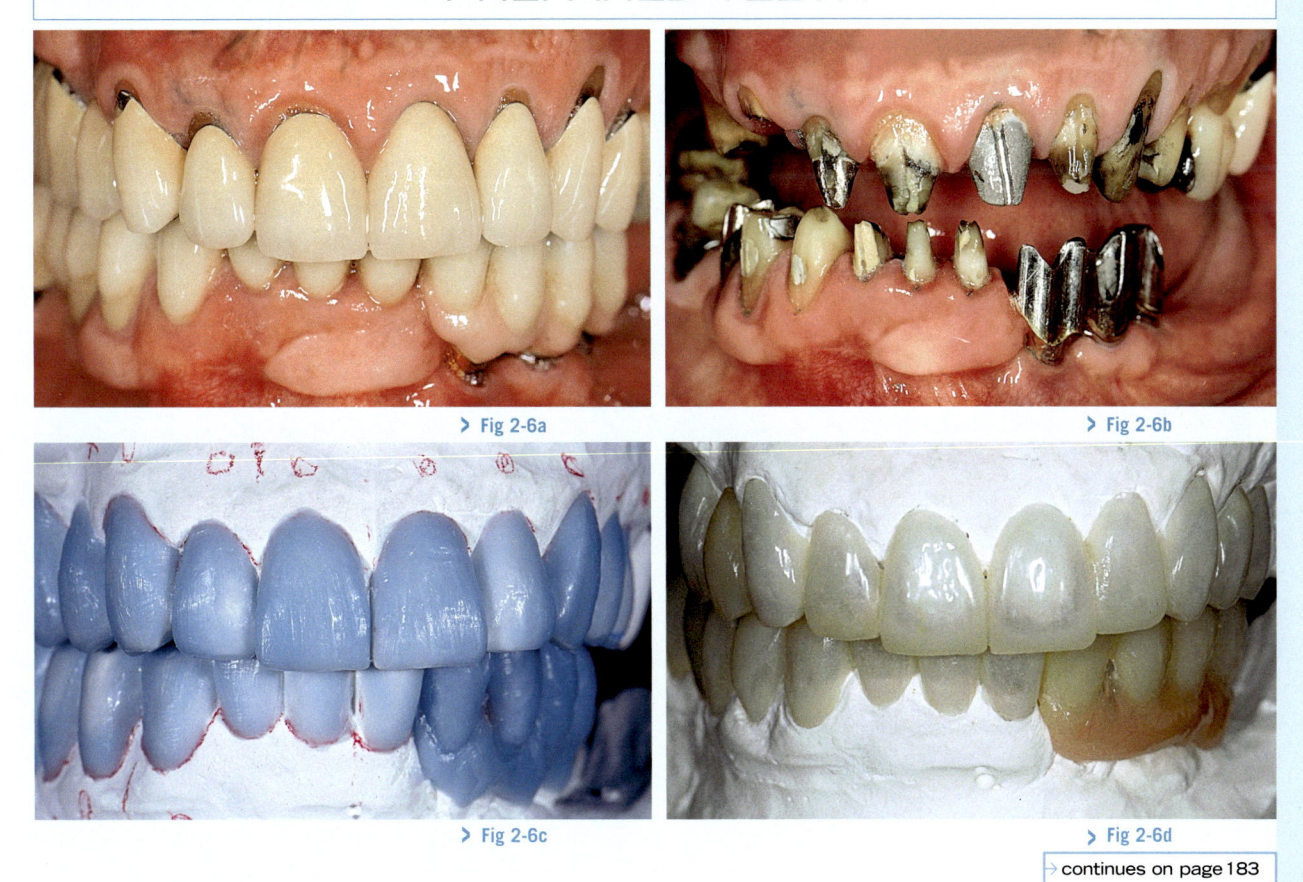

> Fig 2-6a

> Fig 2-6b

> Fig 2-6c

> Fig 2-6d

→ continues on page 183

FIG 6 *(a and b)* After removing the old incongruous prostheses from both arches, the clinician takes the impressions of the abutments. *(c and d)* The technician makes a cast of these, on which the diagnostic wax-up is made. This is used to create the provisional restoration for prepared teeth.

INDIRECT TECHNIQUE

■ FAILED INSERTION ■
UNPREPARED TEETH - CAUSES

In the technique used for unprepared teeth, the clinician very often finds it impossible to fit the provisional restoration received from the laboratory fully into the mouth. This handicap means that the suitability of the esthetic-functional modifications made in the diagnostic wax-up cannot be assessed.

Reduction of occlusal table Inadequate communication between clinician and technician is often the cause of difficulty in fitting the provisional restoration. It is normal to find a narrowing of the occlusal table in a shell that was created before the teeth are prepared, which prevents the provisional restoration from fitting properly into the patient's mouth because of friction on the abutments. This error can be attributed to the relatively common laboratory practice of carrying out the tooth preparations on the stone casts (Figs 2-7a and 2-7b) before the diagnostic wax-up (Fig 2-7c) is made. The result is a loss of all references for correct tooth axis orientation and the information necessary to maintain an adequate occlusal surface (Fig 2-7d) (see chapter 1, page 112). After making the preliminary preparations, the clinician will find it extremely difficult to fit the provisional restoration when positioning it into the oral cavity (Fig 2-7e). There may follow an attempt to intervene in a destructive manner on the tooth preparations, making them more conical and often causing not only irreversible damage to the pulp but also a drastic reduction in the mechanical retention of the restoration. In an attempt to make the restoration fit, the temptation may also arise to dig deeper and deeper into the shell, often leading to the only outcome: perforating it in various points (Fig 2-7f). Despite these various attempts, the clinician may find it impossible to fit the provisional restoration into the oral cavity. Forced to position it to protect the prepared abutments, the clinician nevertheless proceeds with relining the provisional restoration, even though, because of the difficulty in fitting it, there may be an inclined occlusal plane. Apart from giving an unsatisfactory esthetic appearance, this forces the clinician to destroy the occlusal anatomy of the restoration so that the patient can close the mouth completely. In this way all of the care taken by the clinician and technician to identify the modifications to be made, first in the wax-up and then on the cast of the provisional restoration in the articulator, will have been in vain.

FIG 7 *(a and b)* When an entire arch is being rehabilitated, one rather common error that is made during the phase of creating the provisional restoration in the laboratory is to carry out the tooth preparations on the cast before the wax-up is made. *(c and d, dotted red lines)* This often leads to the abutments being too conical and results in an unwanted narrowing of the occlusal table, present in both the diagnostic wax-up and in the provisional restoration derived from it. *(e)* If the reduction in the occlusal table made by the technician is overlooked, when the clinician positions the provisional restoration in the mouth after completing the tooth preparations with appropriate axial tapers (6 to 10 degrees) on the patient, the provisional restoration will prove very difficult to fit due to resistance against the abutments. *(f)* The clinician in turn is forced to make the abutments overly conical and to continually modify the inside of the provisional restoration in order to fit it, which often creates perforations that inevitably weaken it.

Chapter 2 CREATING AND INTEGRATING THE PROVISIONAL RESTORATION

FAILED INSERTION DUE TO REDUCTION OF OCCLUSAL TABLE

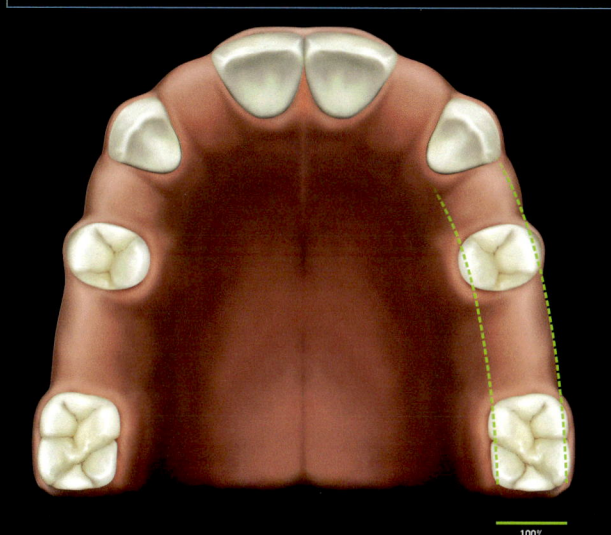

> Fig 2-7a

> Fig 2-7b

> Fig 2-7c

> Fig 2-7d

> Fig 2-7e

> Fig 2-7f

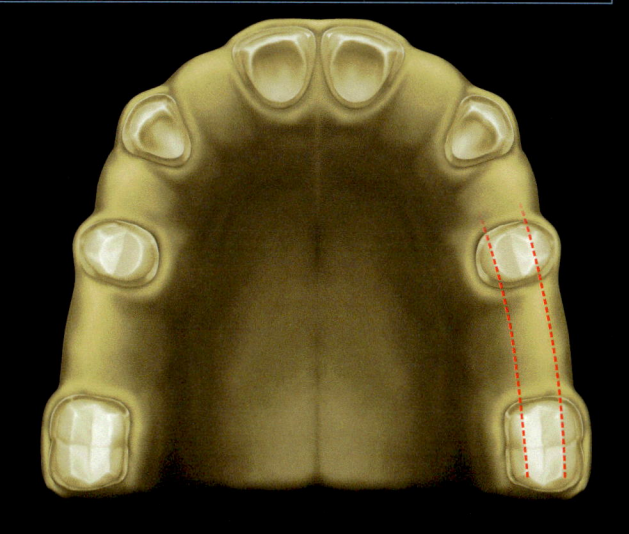

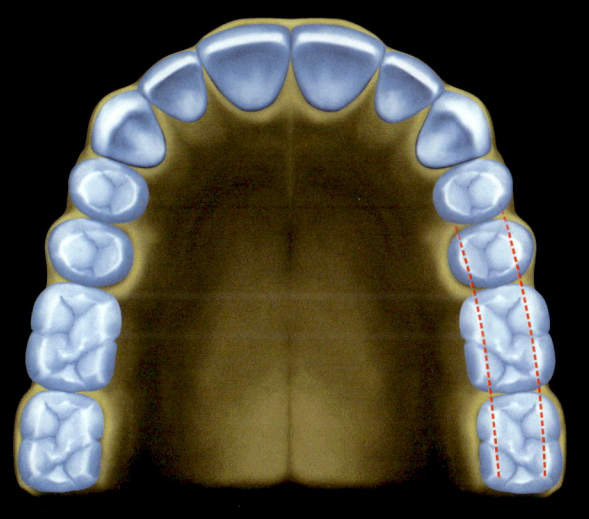

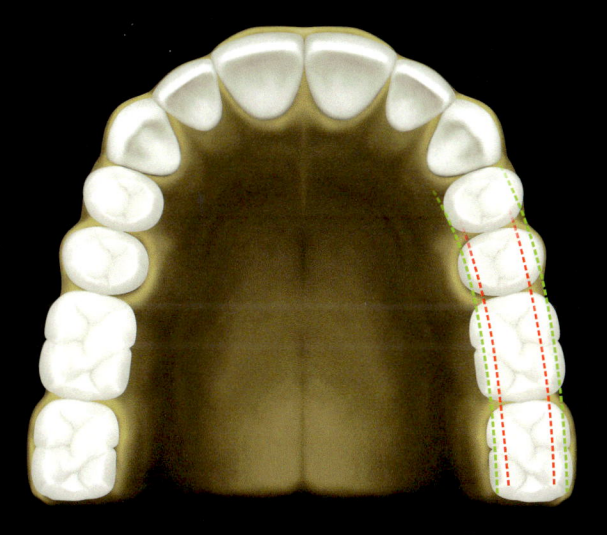

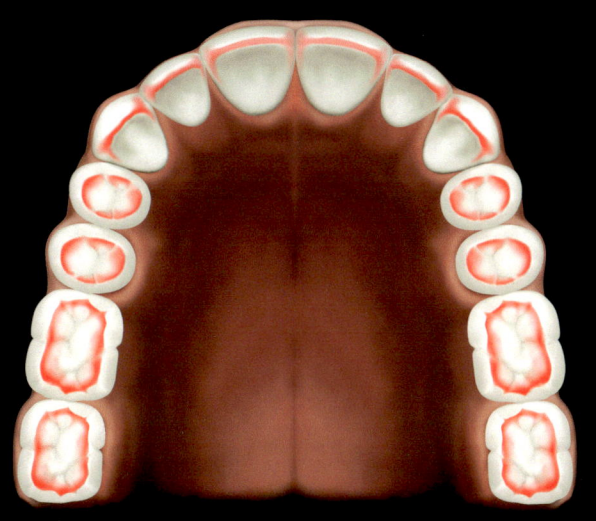

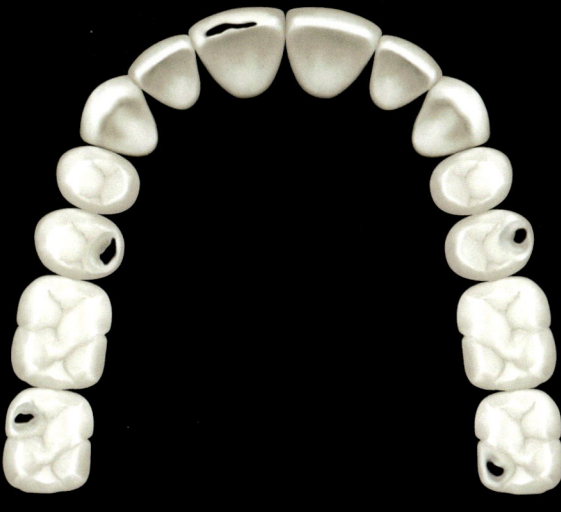

Arbitrary realignment and inadequate tooth preparation It may happen that the technician, in the absence of precise indications for creating the diagnostic wax-up, tries to realign the teeth and/or to optimize the dental composition by making changes to the inclination of the tooth axes (Figs 2-8a and 2-8b). Although most of the time these are minor, the variations made to the tooth arrangement in the provisional restoration must be followed in the abutment preparation phase.

Otherwise, it may become extremely difficult, if not impossible, to fit the provisional restoration (Figs 2-8c to 2-8f). In an attempt to seat the shell completely, the clinician can be tempted to file the abutments excessively, without realizing the need to alter the axial inclination. These actions will, more often than not, only weaken the tooth structure unnecessarily, risking the pulp vitality without allowing a chance to fit the provisional restoration in the correct position.

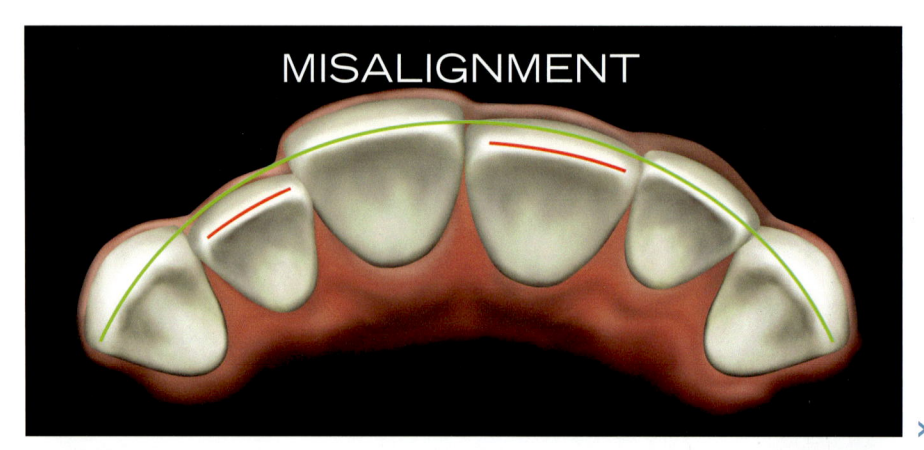

> Fig 2-8a

> Fig 2-8b

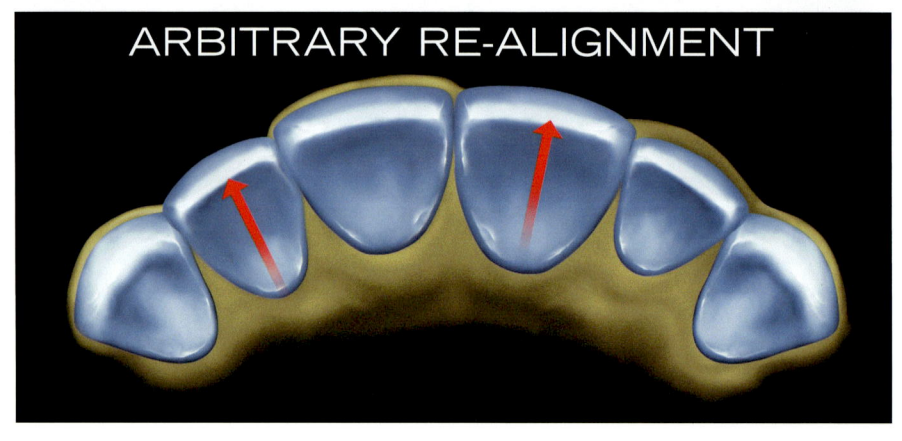

FIG 8 *(a and b)* When slight misalignments are found, the technician may sometimes arbitrarily decide to align the teeth in the diagnostic wax-up in an attempt to optimize the tooth composition, even though not specifically requested to do so. *(c)* In the absence of effective communication between the clinic and the laboratory, the clinician may not notice this immediately and may make the preparations on the patient according to the original tooth axes. When the time comes to insert the provisional restoration, it will be impossible to fit. *(d)* The resistance is a result of the discrepancy between the tooth preparations carried out by the clinician and the axes of the provisional restorations fabricated by the technician. *(e and f)* Only if the clinician notices this change before making the preparations and gives them adequate axial inclination in relation to the realignment carried out by the technician can he or she proceed with correct fitting of the provisional restoration.

FAILED INSERTION DUE TO INADEQUATE TOOTH PREPARATION

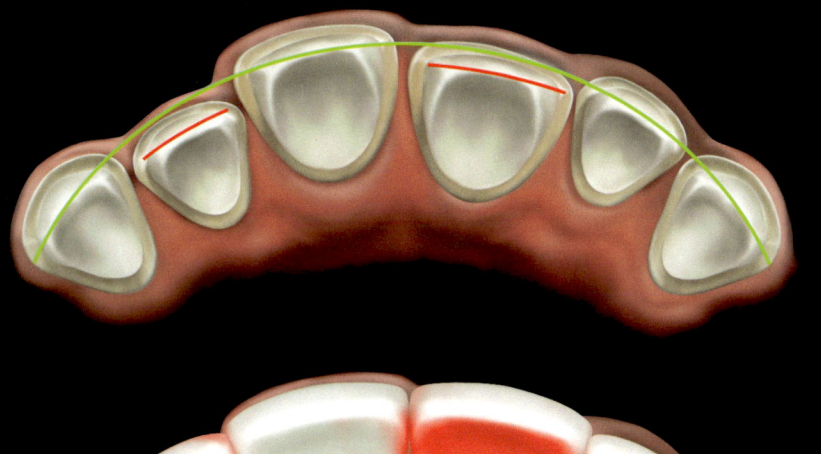

> Fig 2-8c

> Fig 2-8d

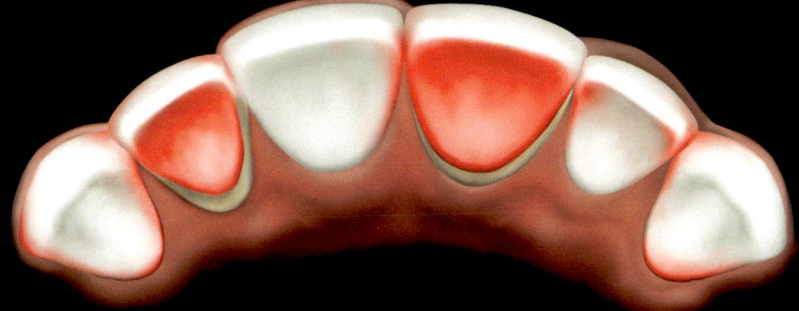

ADEQUATE PREPARATION FOR RE-ALIGNMENT

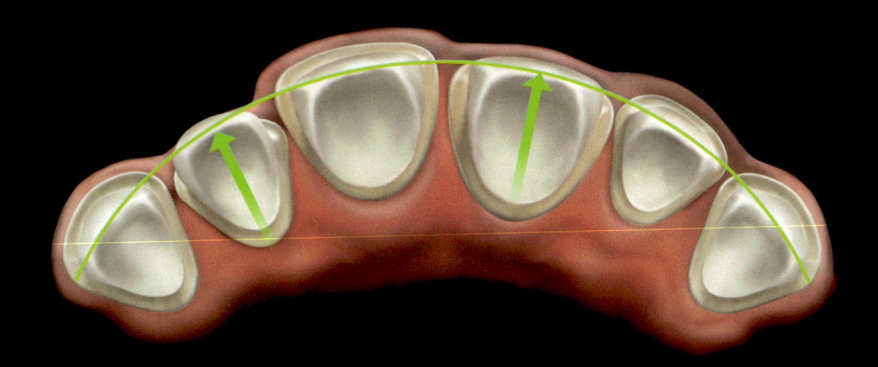

> Fig 2-8e

> Fig 2-8f

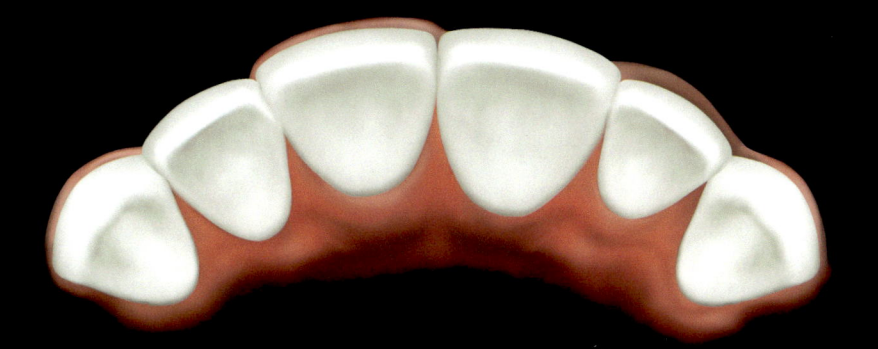

INDIRECT TECHNIQUE

■ FAILED INSERTION ■
PREPARED TEETH - SOLUTIONS

If failure to fit the provisional restoration due to a reduced occlusal table can be avoided simply by making the diagnostic wax-up before undertaking any tooth preparation on the stone casts, it is more complex to create a shell that fits correctly in cases where changes are necessary to the original tooth position, and even more so when these changes are substantial (Fig 2-9).

The necessary variations, copiously detailed on the laboratory checklist, are made by the technician on a duplicate of the original cast mounted on the articulator, correcting the axes with a bur until the required tooth position is achieved only in this initial phase (Figs 2-10a to 2-10d).

Tooth preparation index The diagnostic wax-up is created on the modified cast (Fig 2-10e), and two stone casts are made from it by means of an impression. A silicone index is made on the first of these casts (Fig 2-10f), to be used later for making the provisional restoration, and an acetate index is made as well, which is useful to the clinician for correctly positioning the provisional restoration and assessing the tooth preparations. The second stone cast is used by the technician, at this point only, to make the tooth preparations according to the newly defined axes (Fig 2-10g).

To help the clinician identify the new orientation of the tooth axes, an acrylic resin index or a silicone matrix that extends only to the occlusal/incisal area is created on the cast with the prepared teeth (Figs 2-10h and 2-10i). Use of one of these makes correct positioning of the provisional restoration much easier (Figs 2-10j to 2-10n).

FIG 9 *(a and b)* The patient has a pronounced overjet, which is already greatly reduced in the diagnostic wax-up by means of a simultaneous slight shifting of both the maxillary and mandibular axes. *(c)* Each adjustment made in the diagnostic wax-up has been duly replicated in the provisional restorations. *(d and e)* On the stone cast taken from this provisional restoration, the teeth are prepared, and an acrylic stent created to reproduce the indentation of the occlusal/incisal areas of the preparations made. *(f to i)* Once positioned in the mouth, the index made in this way acts as a fundamental guide that helps the clinician considerably in achieving the correct axial inclination of the tooth preparations, making both fitting and correct relining of the provisional restoration much easier.

Chapter 2 CREATING AND INTEGRATING THE PROVISIONAL RESTORATION

→ ...from page 127

> Fig 2-9a

> Fig 2-9b

> Fig 2-9c

> Fig 2-9d

> Fig 2-9e

> Fig 2-9f

> Fig 2-9g

> Fig 2-9h

> Fig 2-9i

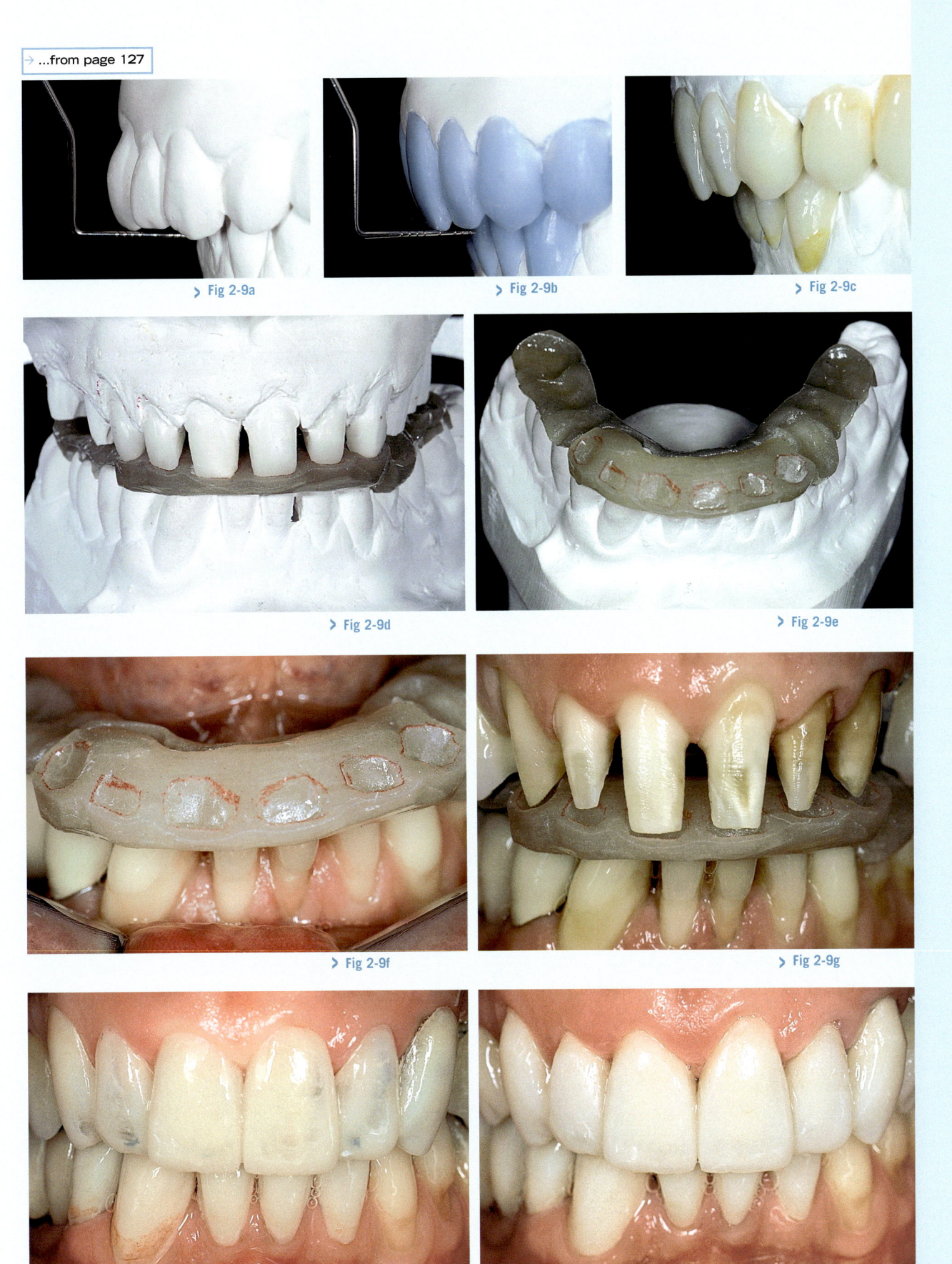

→ continues on page 267

> Fig 2-10a

> Fig 2-10b

> Fig 2-10c

> Fig 2-10d

> Fig 2-10e

> Fig 2-10f

> Fig 2-10g

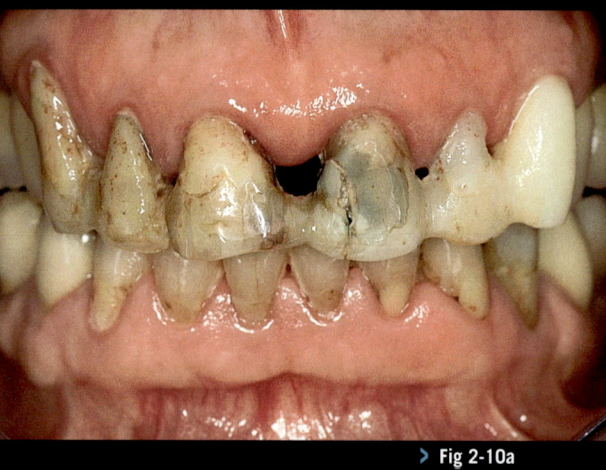

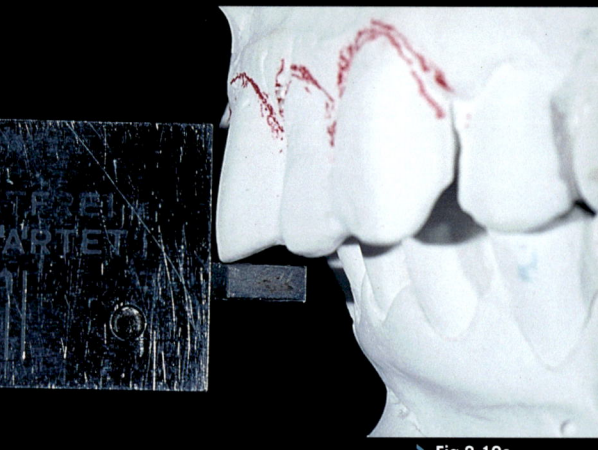

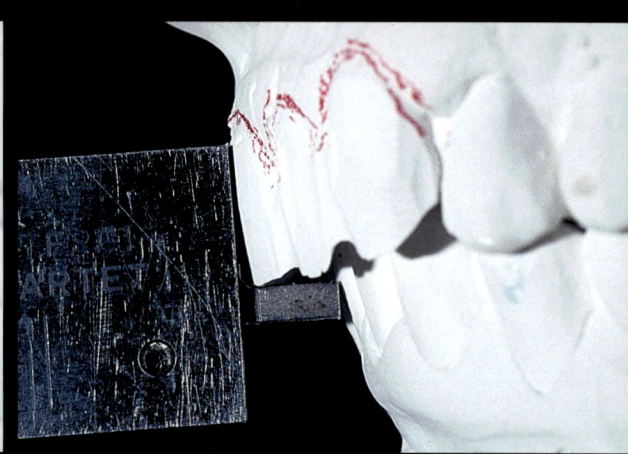

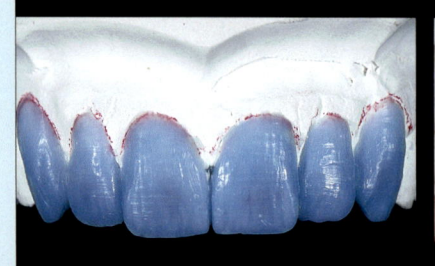

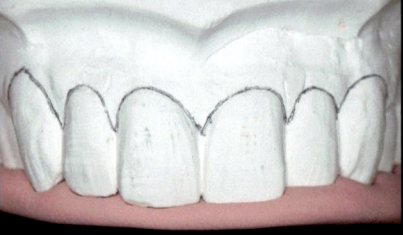

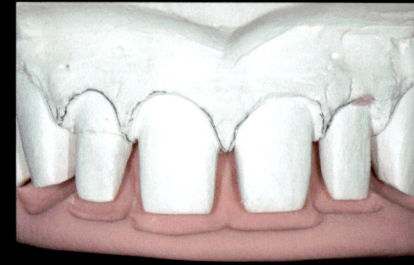

FIG 10 *(a and b)* The patient's dentition shows a considerable lack of periodontal support that, through time, has caused a noticeable degree of overjet and gaps between the anterior teeth. *(c to e)* After modifying the axes of the preparations on the stone cast duplicate of the original cast according to the information received from the clinician, the technician completes the diagnostic wax-up. The corrections made in this specific case on the cast before the wax-up are not intended as tooth preparations, but rather as adjustments of the axial orientations, required in order to design the new incisal profile. *(f and g)* The technician creates a silicone index from the stone cast of the wax-up, which will serve as a guide in the tooth preparations.

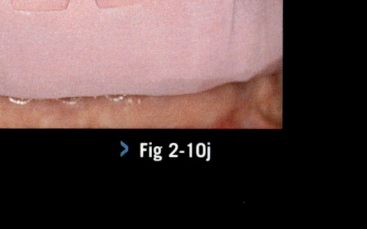

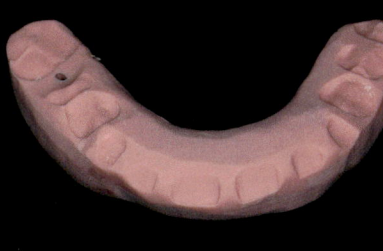

> Fig 2-10h

> Fig 2-10i

> Fig 2-10j

> Fig 2-10k

> Fig 2-10l

> Fig 2-10m

> Fig 2-10n

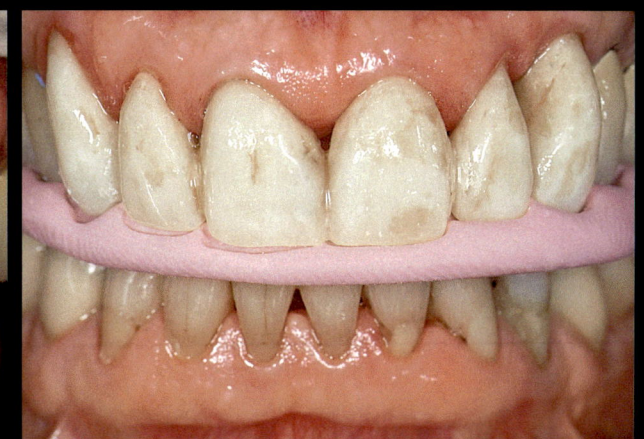

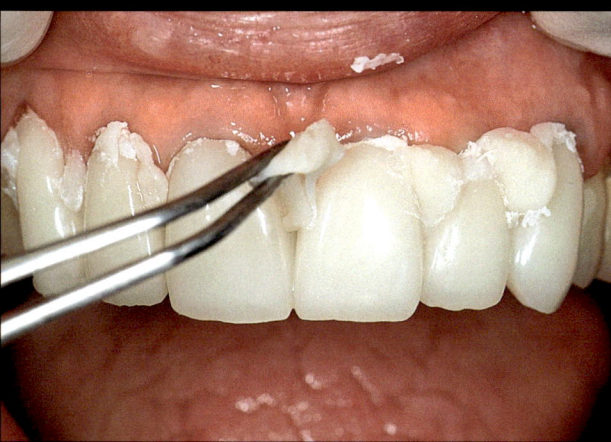

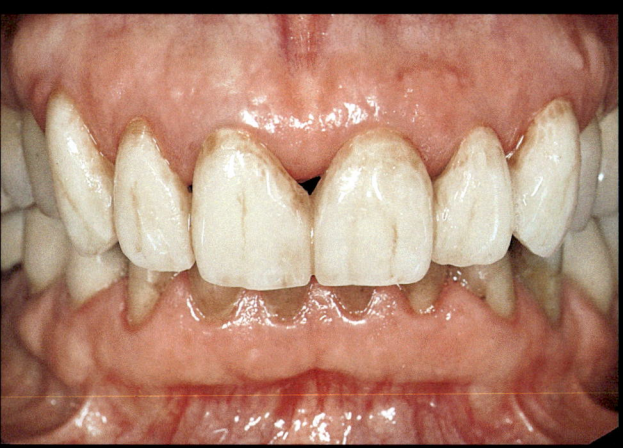

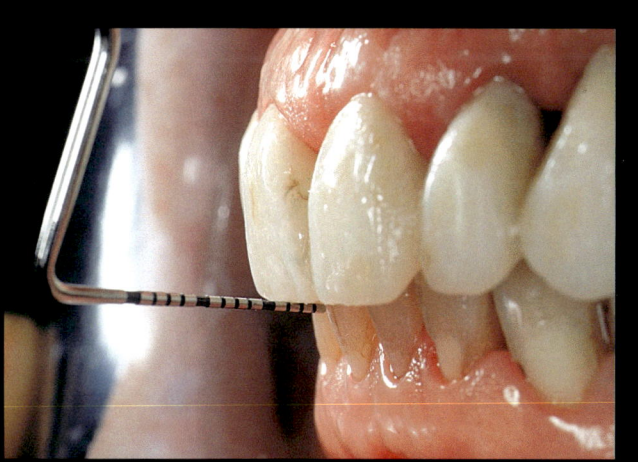

FIG 10 *(h to j)* A new silicone matrix created on the incisal aspect of the abutments prepared with this technique aids the clinician in finding the correct axial inclination of the preparations to be made. *(k)* This procedure allows the shell to be fitted and relined correctly. *(l)* The suitability of the position achieved by the provisional restoration is validated if it matches the silicone index derived from the cast of the wax-up on the provisional restoration. *(m)* Once it has been polished and colored, the provisional restoration demonstrates a satisfactory overall integration. *(n)* From the lateral view, the noticeable reduction in overjet can be appreciated.

INDIRECT TECHNIQUE

■ DIFFICULT INSERTION ■
PREPARED AND UNPREPARED TEETH - CAUSES

Friction Whether the provisional restoration is created before or after tooth preparation, another difficulty in fitting it, which results from a limitation inherent in the traditional indirect technique, is the inevitable though minimal shrinking of the acrylic resin material.

The traditional technique involves creating a wax-up that extends to the dentogingival border (Fig 2-11a). The shell derived from this wax-up is often difficult to fit because of excessive friction, especially in the cervical areas. This friction prevents the provisional restoration from being fully inserted, creating a raised bite as well as marginal shortening and undercontour.

Because of the larger shell size (Figs 2-11b to 2-11d), the friction is more evident when an entire arch is being treated. Obviously, the lack of complete insertion prevents the clinician from assessing the suitability of the provisional restoration, which was made by the technician according to the information transferred to the laboratory. Because the proposed esthetic-functional changes cannot be clinically tested, the provisional restoration cannot fulfill its fundamental purpose of representing the prototype for the definitive restoration.

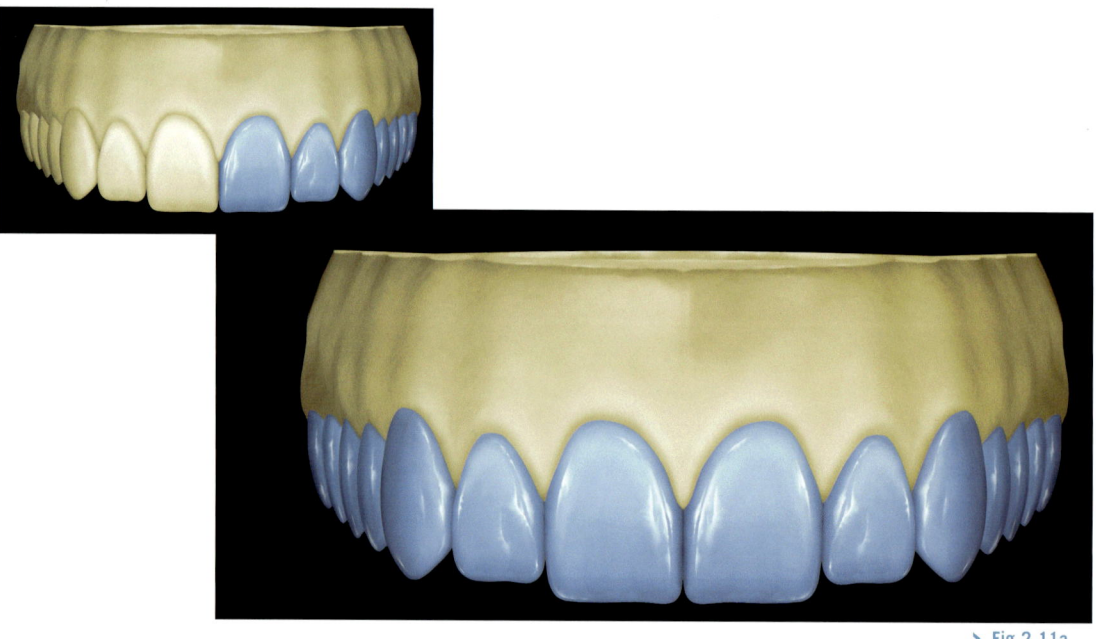

> Fig 2-11a

FIG 11 *(a)* Creating the provisional restoration by the indirect technique involves making an acrylic resin provisional restoration derived from a diagnostic wax-up, the cervical limit of which is drawn exactly at the dentogingival border. *(b)* In the case of a complete rehabilitation of the maxillary arch, the provisional restoration made in this way inevitably proves difficult to fit because of the excessive friction between the shell and the abutments, especially in the cervical areas. *(c)* This resistance prevents the clinician from fitting the provisional restoration completely. *(d)* The occlusal view shows the undercontour caused after the acrylic resin contracted.

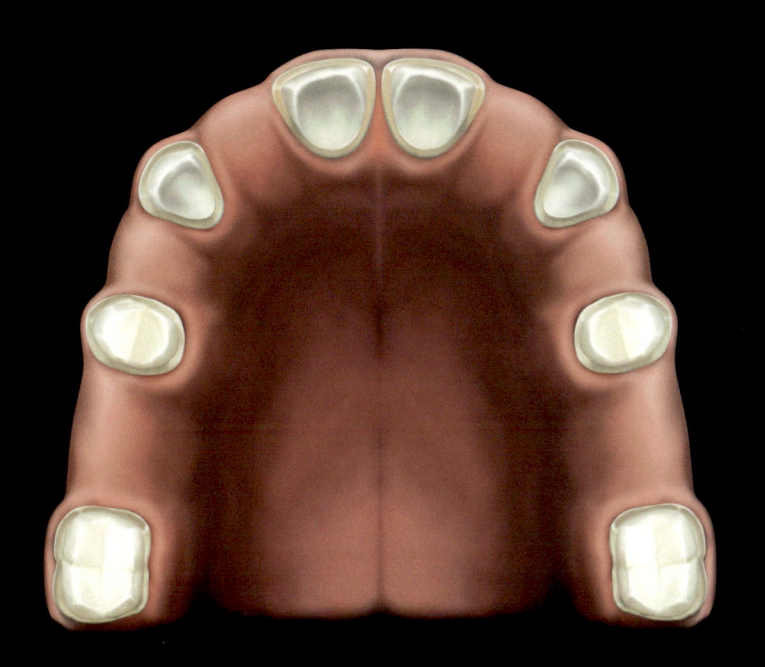

> Fig 2-11b

> Fig 2-11c

> Fig 2-11d

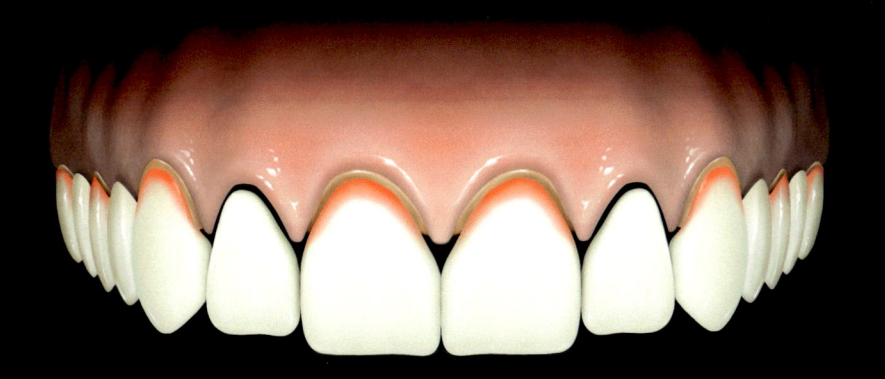

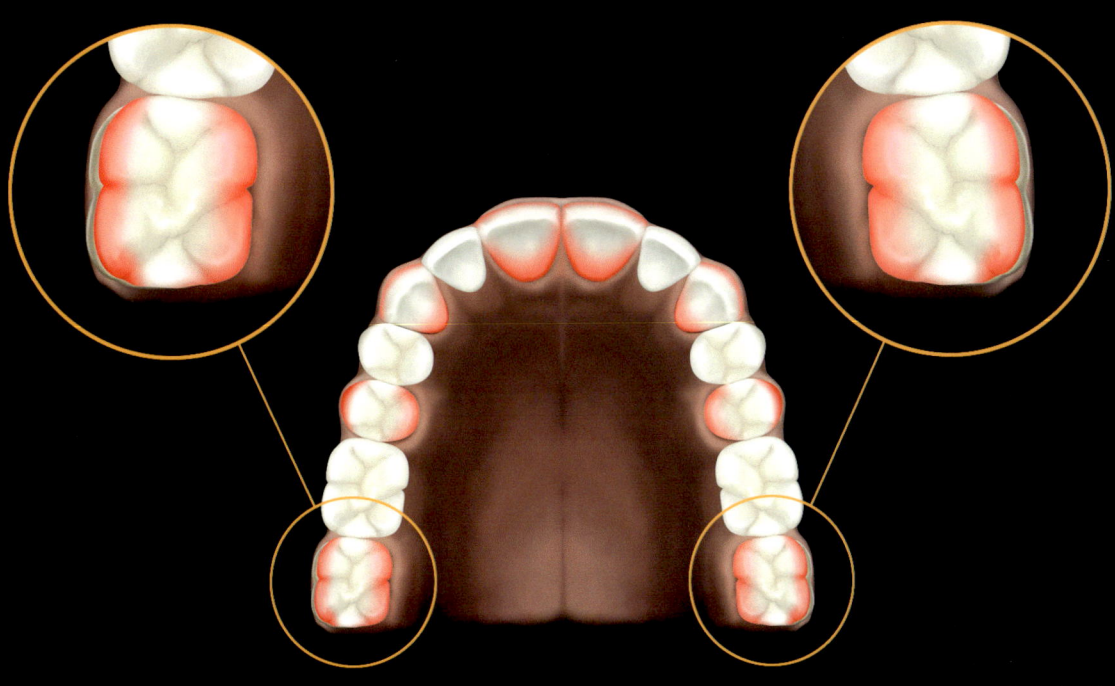

UNSATISFACTORY MARGINAL PRECISION

Another typical problem is the difficulty of achieving adequate marginal precision because of substantial undercontouring and even a small degree of shrinkage in the acrylic shell. This dual imprecision results from improper application of the wax, the extension of which, as can be seen, is limited to the dentogingival border (Figs 2-12a and 2-12b).

Undercontour Especially in cases of extensive rehabilitation, the undercontouring is caused by the slight but unavoidable contraction of the acrylic that occurs during polymerization, which can reduce the volume of the provisional restoration by up to 6%.[65]

If the friction on the axial walls caused by shrinkage can be partly compensated for by emptying the inside of the provisional restoration, the shell will be irremediably undercontoured at the marginal level, remaining inside the thickness of the tooth preparation (Figs 2-12c to 2-12e).

Shortening The slight shortening caused by the acrylic contraction is further accentuated by the processes of finishing and emptying the provisional restoration by the technician. By reducing the thickness of the shell at the marginal level, these necessary modifications can cause unwanted chipping.

The marginal deficit can become even more accentuated if the clinician, when attempting to reduce the friction against the walls of the restoration, tries to widen the shell even further, causing even more shortening.

FIG 12 *(a to e)* The provisional restoration made by the traditionally performed indirect technique almost always shows both an undercontour and a slight shortening at the marginal level, caused by the contraction of the acrylic resin.

> Fig 2-12a

> Fig 2-12b

> Fig 2-12c

> Fig 2-12d

> Fig 2-12e

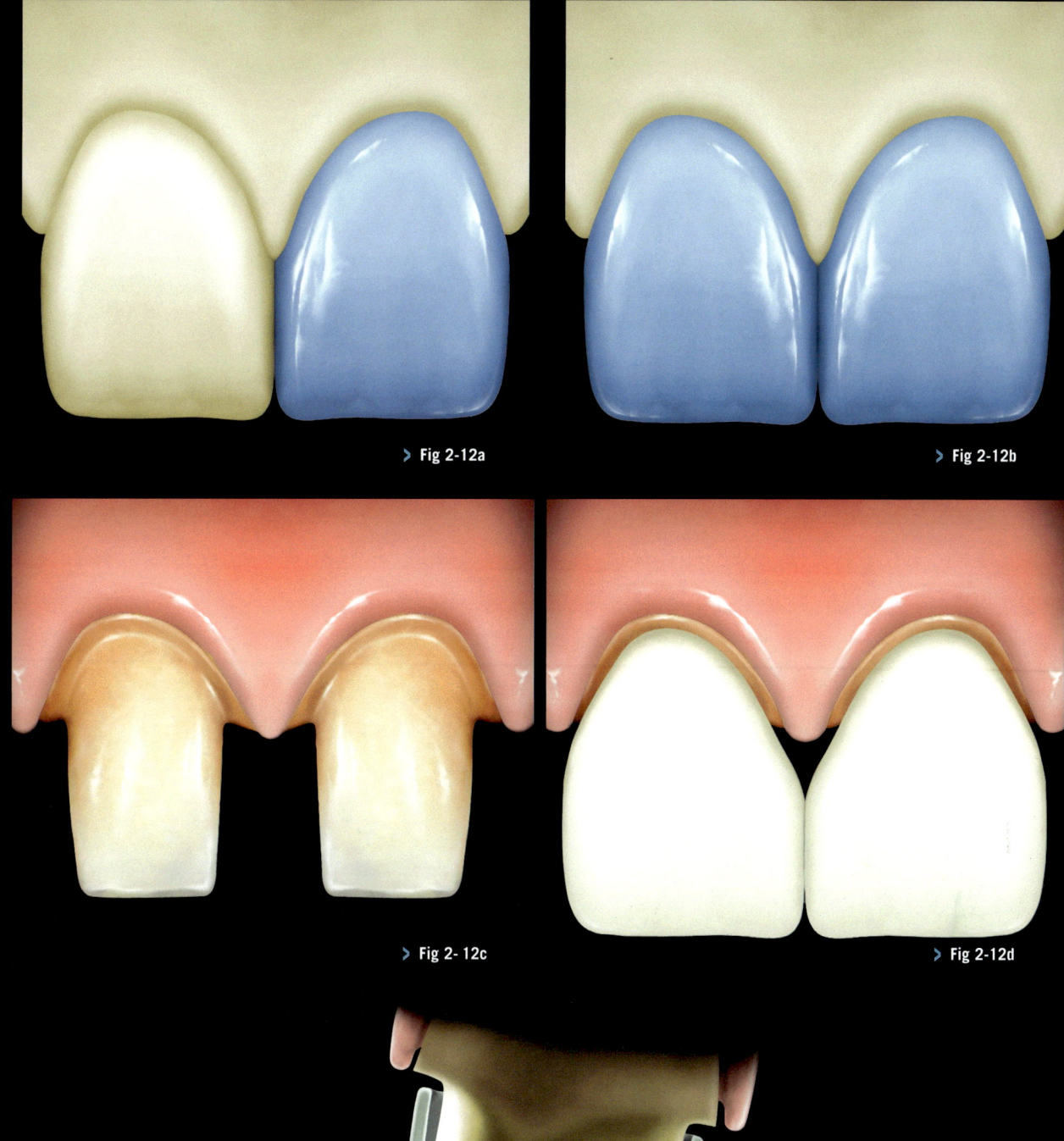

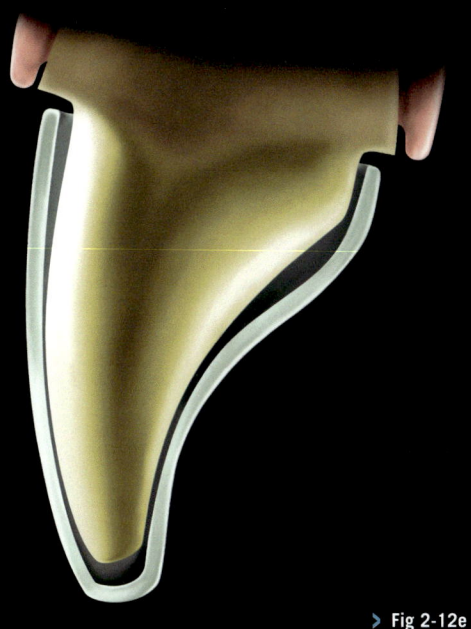

Relining: problems To compensate for the marginal deficit, during relining it is necessary to use the fingers to push a fair amount of acrylic resin material into the cervical area (Figs 2-12f and 2-12g). Only in this way is it possible to see the margin of the preparations and to try to correct the undercontour. It is extremely difficult to distribute the relining material evenly around the perimeter of all units in the provisional restoration so that the margins are covered completely and the acrylic resin material penetrates the sulcus. This requires further relining or re-margining that, on the one hand, allows a satisfactory marginal fit to be achieved but, on the other hand, is not helpful in preventing undercontouring (Fig 2-12h). In addition, an esthetically unattractive demarcation line is visible between the original shell and the relined portion, which can easily become detached during the finishing phase.

Although the provisional restoration is created on the cast with the prepared teeth, too much contraction of the acrylic resin material can prevent the provisional restoration from fitting perfectly. The technician, who should be aware of the possibility of the abutments on the stone cast fracturing while the acrylic resin shell is being pressed, can make a duplicate in advance that can be used to check and if necessary correct both the fit of the provisional restoration and its marginal adaptation. These corrections oblige the clinician to reline the provisional restoration on the patient, which is necessary in any case for adequate retention and a satisfactory marginal closure.

TRADITIONAL INDIRECT TECHNIQUE
CONCERNS

- Difficult to fit
- Poor marginal precision
- Undercontoured emergence profile
- Possible detachment of relining material
- Unsatisfactory esthetics

FIG 12 *(f)* The shortening and the undercontour are further accentuated by the finishing procedures carried out, first by the technician and then by the clinician, to reduce the friction in the marginal area, without completely fitting the shell. *(g)* During the relining phases the clinician is forced to push the excess material with the fingers in an attempt to capture the preparation margin and to achieve a satisfactory marginal closure. *(h)* In any case, this method does not prevent the restoration from being undercontoured or the relining material from detaching, something that often occurs during finishing.

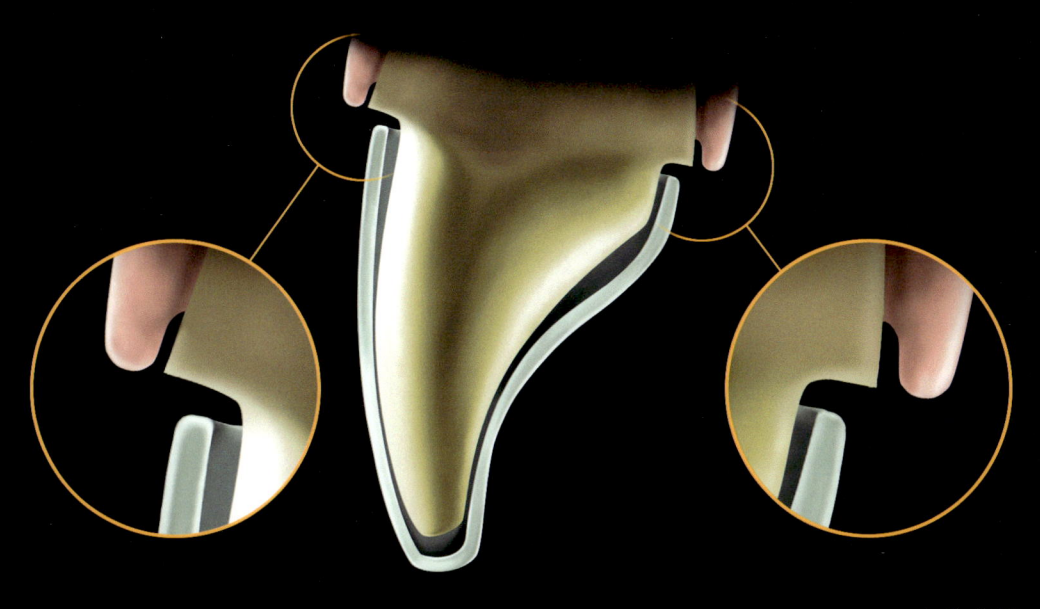

> Fig 2-12f

> Fig 2-12g

> Fig 2-12h

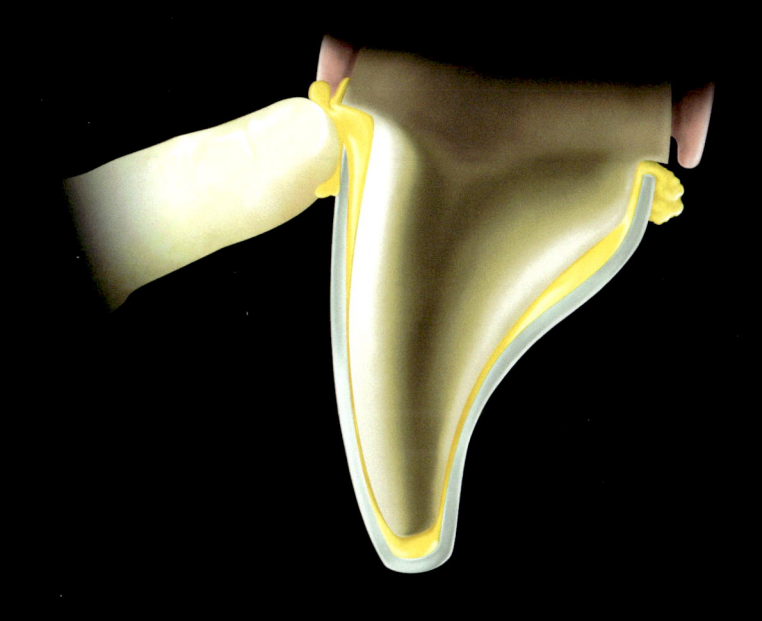

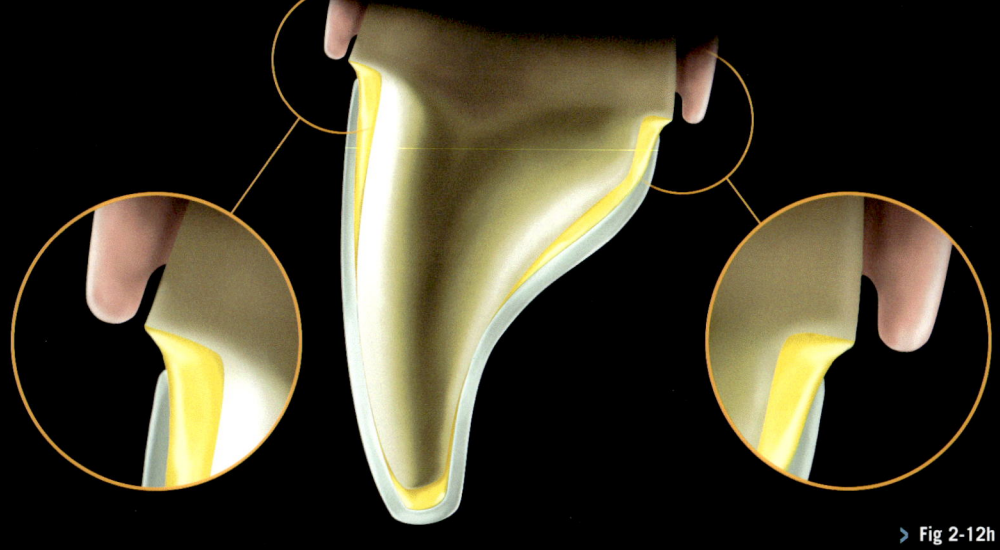

INDIRECT TECHNIQUE

■ DIFFICULT INSERTION ■
PREPARED AND UNPREPARED TEETH—SOLUTIONS
↓

■ MODIFIED INDIRECT TECHNIQUE (MIT) ■

PROVISIONAL RESTORATION WITH FACILITATED INSERTION

To overcome the problems of fitting and precision inherent in the traditional indirect technique described thus far, the authors have been modifying the ways in which provisional restorations are fabricated for over 20 years. The objective from the start was to obtain a shell that, in encountering no hindrances to its insertion, could be guided into the correct position directly by occlusal contact.

Ideal acrylic resin shell insertion is fundamental to relining in the correct position. This can be done by adopting certain measures that prove equally valid whether the provisional restoration is fabricated before or after teeth are prepared.

FITTING

Extending the cervical third This technique involves oversizing the diagnostic wax-up at the cervical level.

Before applying the wax, it is necessary to mark on the cast with a pencil an extension of the margin by about 0.5 to 1.0 mm beyond the tooth limit on both the buccal and the palatal sides (Fig 2-13a). The line marked will be the cervical border of the wax-up (Figs 2-13b and 2-13c), which, being on the gingiva in a position external to the tooth limit, provides not only a lengthening but also a widening of the wax-up at the cervical level.

A groove is then made in the stone with a sharp instrument along the entire section previously marked with the pencil to define the marginal limit of the provisional restoration (Fig 2-13d).

FIG 13 *(a to c)* A pencil line is drawn on the stone cast, extending beyond the dentogingival border by roughly 0.5 to 1.0 mm, representing the limit for spreading the wax. *(d)* A scalpel is then used to make a groove along the entire pencil line, which helps the technician identify the margin of the provisional restoration.

> Fig 2-13a

> Fig 2-13b

> Fig 2-13c

> Fig 2-13d

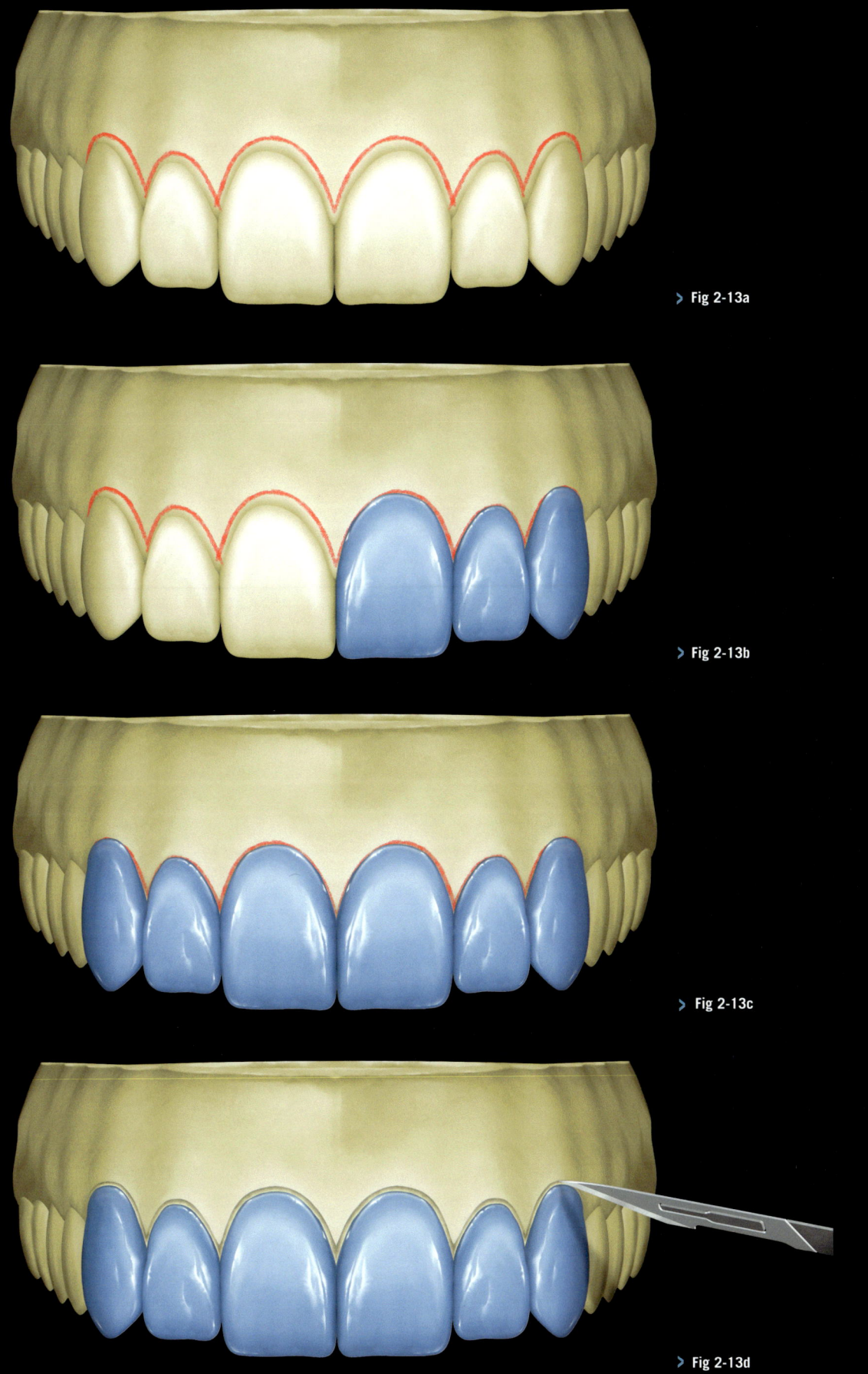

Once the acrylic shell has been made, the oversizing is reduced to roughly 0.2 to 0.4 mm because of the slight shrinkage of the material and the edge finishing. When the shell is inserted into the mouth, a slight extension of the margins remains; since it is beyond the cervical limit of the prepared teeth, this extension will rest on the gingiva.

The result of this procedure is a provisional restoration that is slightly wider in the cervical third yet maintains an ideal anatomy in the middle third as well as in the incisal-occlusal third.

Because of the particular morphologic modification made in the cervical third, the acrylic resin shell must be sufficiently thin to guarantee extreme passivity during fitting, especially for provisional restorations made before tooth preparation, which subsequently proves much easier. With provisional restorations made following tooth preparation, the technician can afford greater acrylic resin thickness when constructing the shell, thus allowing at least a slight layering of the resin.

PRECISION

Container effect The wider shape of the cervical portion contains the marginal limit of the tooth preparation (Fig 2-13e) within the margin of the provisional restoration. Because of this, the clinician can remove all excesses during relining without running the risk of removing relining material from the marginal area (Fig 2-13f).

The widened shell thus acts as a container for the acrylic resin, which, pressed into the cervical area while still in the plastic phase, flows into the sulcus, allowing the margin to be read properly.

Unlike the traditional technique, this method prevents the relining material from detaching during finishing since it is contained inside the shell (Figs 2-13g to 2-13n). One further advantage offered by this technique is the reduction in working time needed for finishing, which is decidedly easier because the excess acrylic resin material will have been removed at an earlier stage.

FIG 13 *(e and f)* After completing the preparations, the clinician relines the provisional restoration directly in the mouth. Use of the MIT technique allows all excess relining material to be removed without the risk of removing acrylic from the marginal area, because the limit of the preparations is confined within the provisional restoration. *(g and h)* Once polymerization is complete, the provisional restoration is modified and finished until adequate marginal precision is achieved, at which point it is fitted into the mouth once more. *(i)* Sectional view of the provisional restoration made using the MIT technique, with a close-up of the widening of the cervical third. *(j and k)* Note how the shell margins are settled on the gingiva. Following relining, the excess acrylic resin is removed with a dental explorer. *(l and m)* Outside the oral cavity, the relined shell has a horizontal step and a vertical overextension of the margin that the clinician must eliminate in the finishing phase. *(n)* After this phase, the provisional restoration, positioned in the mouth, shows adequate precision and a satisfactory marginal closure.

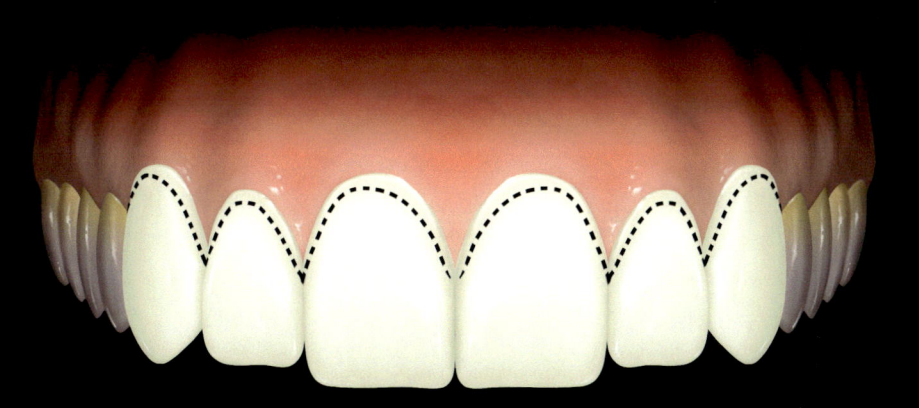

> Fig 2-13e

> Fig 2-13f

> Fig 2-13g

> Fig 2-13h

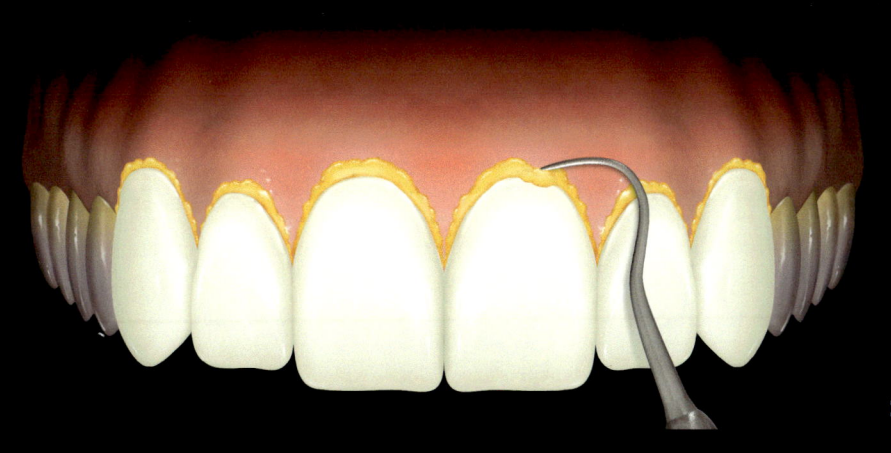

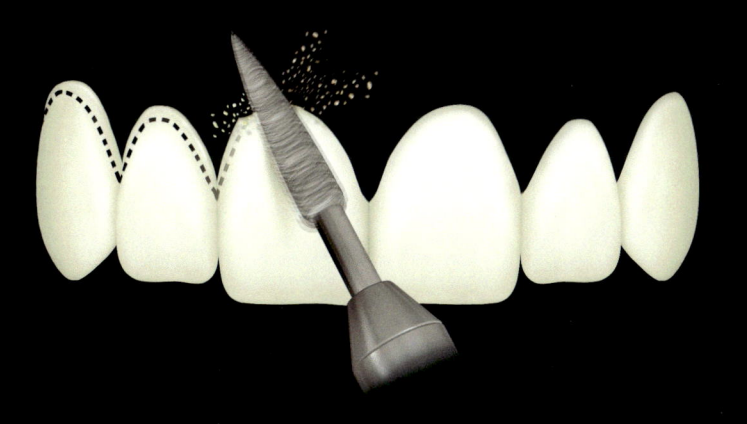

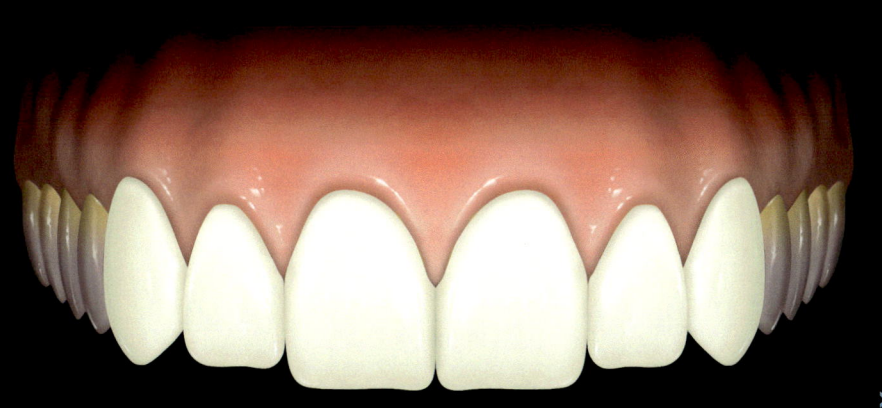

157

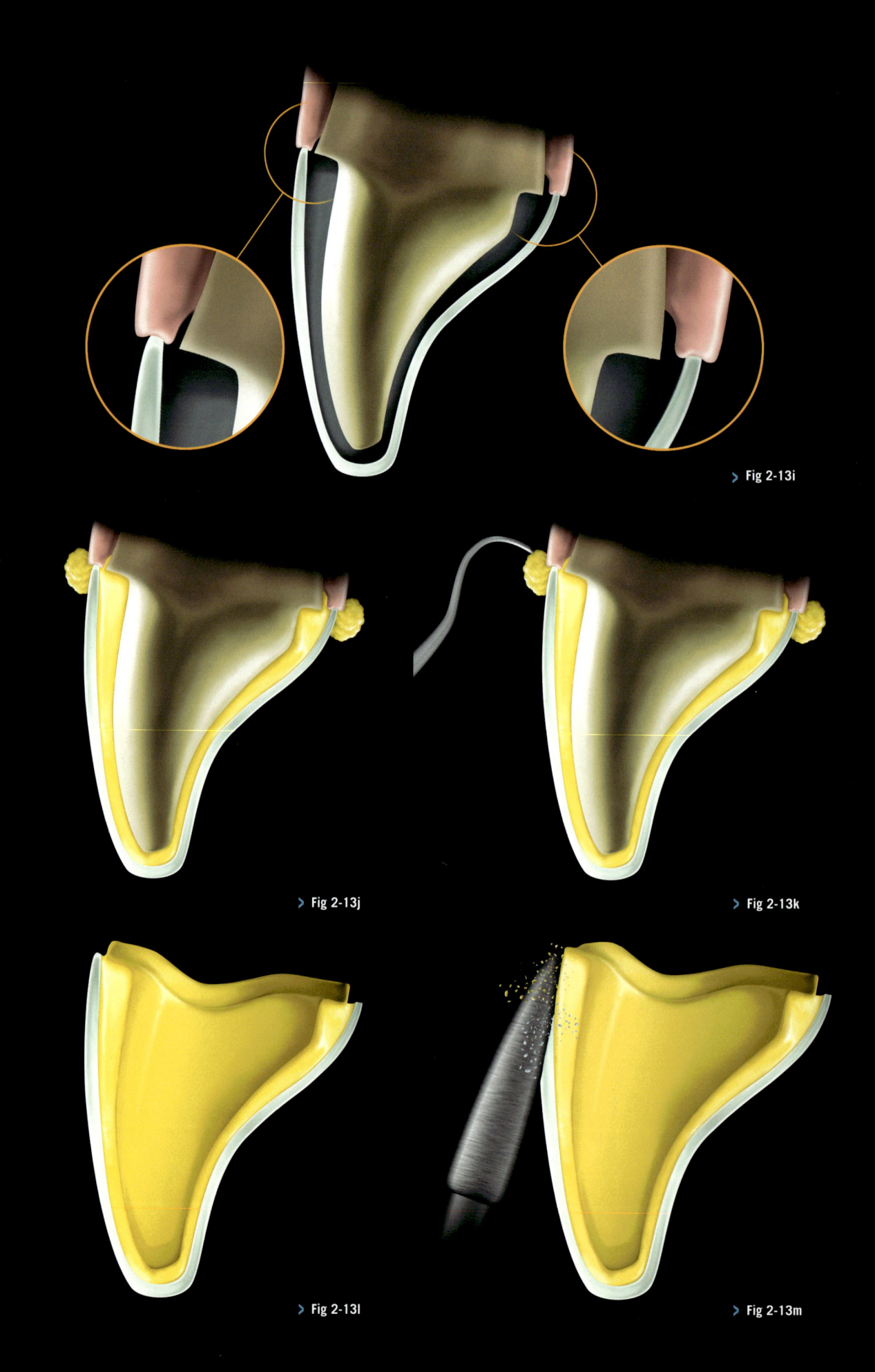

> Fig 2-13i

> Fig 2-13j

> Fig 2-13k

> Fig 2-13l

> Fig 2-13m

> Fig 2-13n

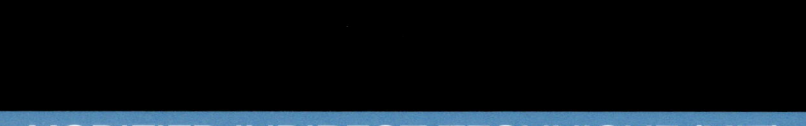

MODIFIED INDIRECT TECHNIQUE (MIT)

PROCEDURE

- With a pencil, mark an overextension of the margin on the stone cast beyond the dentogingival border by roughly 0.5–1.0 mm.
- Perform the diagnostic wax-up, extending it up to the pencil line.
- Make a groove in the stone along the pencil line.
- Fabricate the acrylic shell (overextension: 0.2–0.4 mm).
- Fit and reline the provisional, removing the excess material.
- Refine and polish.

ADVANTAGES

- Passive insertion
- Ideal fit
- Does not raise the bite
- Easy removal of excess material
- Easy penetration of the relining material into the sulcus
- Ideal marginal reading
- Shorter and much easier finishing phases

FABRICATING THE PROVISIONAL RESTORATION—MIT   LABORATORY

■ ANTERIOR REHABILITATION ■
POURING IN THE SILICONE MATRIX (PSM)

This modified technique involves pouring acrylic resin into a silicone matrix (PSM) previously created from the diagnostic wax-up. Because of its ease of application, the technique is mainly used in partial cases in both the anterior and posterior sectors.

TECHNIQUE

An impression of the diagnostic wax-up is taken after the alginate has been spread directly onto the buccal, occlusal, and lingual surfaces with the fingers before an impression tray is applied. This solution faithfully reproduces all of the details of the cast, including the groove previously made at the marginal extension of the wax-up (Figs 2-14a to 2-14d). In addition to being a stable reference, a cast obtained in this way is used to construct an acetate index for the clinician and one in silicone for the laboratory (Figs 2-14e and 2-14f). The technician pours the "acrylic colored dentin" (Figs 2-14g and 2-14h) into the silicone matrix and then places it in the hydropneumatic machine to polymerize the acrylic resin (Fig 2-14i). If a heat-activated acrylic resin is used (Ivocron, Ivoclar Vivadent), it is left in the machine for at least 25 minutes at 100°C and 6 atm. If the decision is made to use a self-curing resin to speed up the process, a polymerization time of 10 minutes at 40°C and 6 atm is sufficient. After it has been fired, the dentin core of the provisional restoration is taken out of the matrix (Fig 2-14j), and the incisal areas are then reduced to allow room for the enamel. Care must be taken during finishing not to remove the resin completely from the gingival area, because it acts as a stop point for reinserting the shell into the matrix while pressing the acrylic. If necessary, the dentin can be colored in this phase, so that the coloring remains inside the provisional restoration, between the layer of dentin already fired and the layer of enamel to be spread over the top of it *(sandwich technique)*.

FIG 14 *(a and b)* Upon receiving the stone cast, the technician draws the overextended margin with a pencil and then proceeds to make the diagnostic wax-up. *(c and d)* A groove is drawn along the cervical limit of the wax-up and, after the technician takes a reliable impression of it in alginate, a stone cast is made on which the previously inscribed groove is evident. *(e to h)* A silicone matrix is taken from this cast, into which the acrylic resin is poured. *(i)* Everything is then put into a hydropneumatic machine to polymerize the acrylic resin. *(j)* When this process is finished, the provisional restoration in dentin is removed from the silicone matrix.

CASE 1

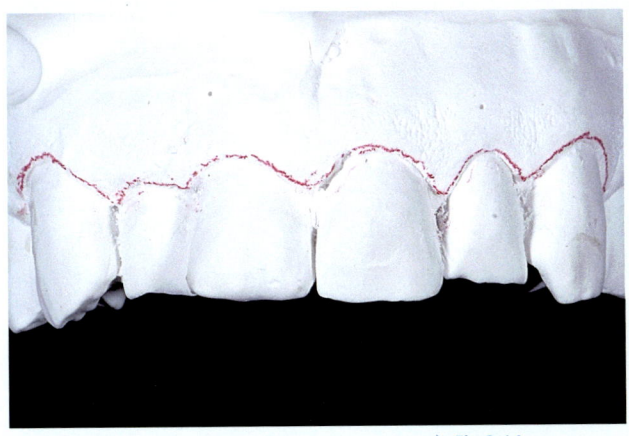

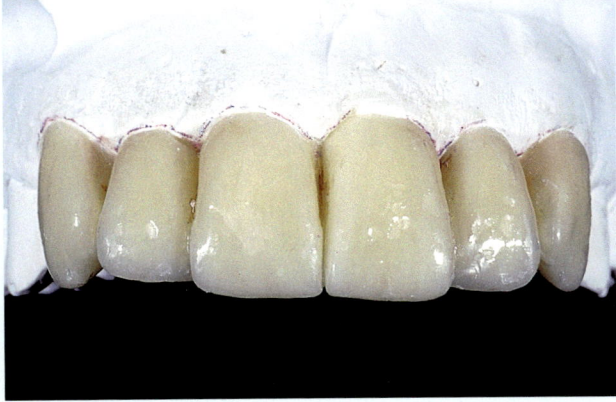

> Fig 2-14a

> Fig 2-14b

> Fig 2-14c

> Fig 2-14d

> Fig 2-14e

> Fig 2-14f

> Fig 2-14g

> Fig 2-14h

> Fig 2-14i

> Fig 2-14j

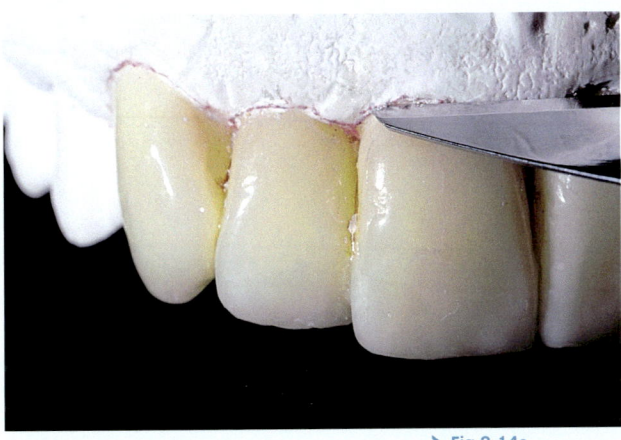

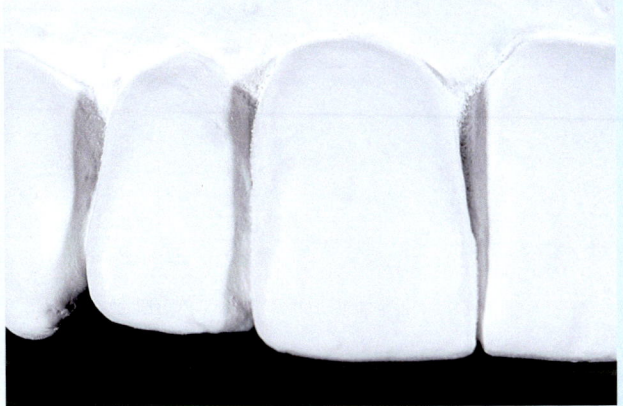

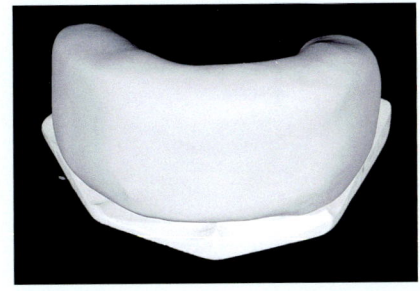

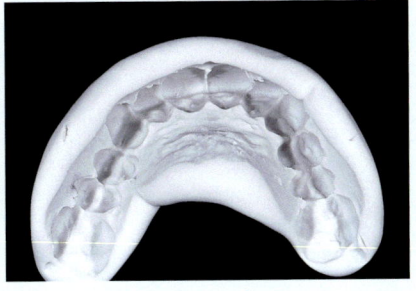

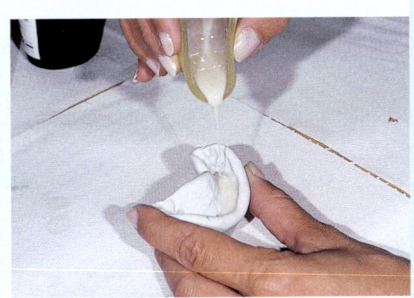

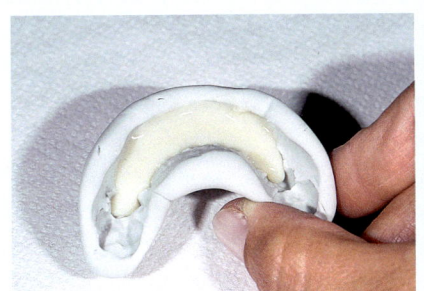

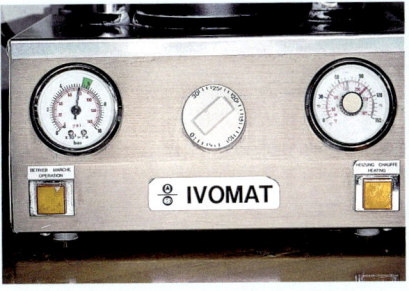

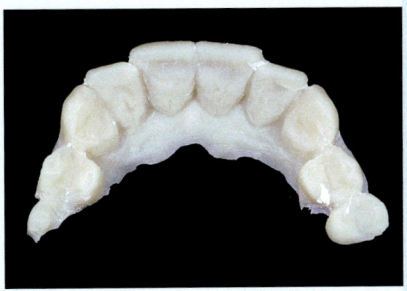

After ensuring the presence of suitable stop points (Fig 2-14k) and cutting the incisal areas (Fig 2-14l), the next phase to be carried out is packing. This is done by pouring "enamel" into the matrix (Figs 2-14m and 2-14n) and replacing the previously fired "dentin" within as well. Only light pressure should be applied to avoid pushing the "dentin" too much and touching the base of the matrix itself, at the risk of reducing the amount of "enamel" in the provisional restoration and obtaining a shell lacking in the necessary incisal translucency. The stop points previously described are helpful in this maneuver. A shallow insertion means more "enamel" but no change to the shape of the actual provisional restoration, which is dictated by the matrix. Once the layer of "enamel" is also polymerized (Fig 2-14o), the cast is again removed from the matrix (Fig 2-14p), and the extended cervical margins, which are immediately recognizable owing to the groove previously inscribed into the wax-up (Figs 2-14q and 2-14r), are once again highlighted with a pencil. The purpose of defining these margins is to allow excess acrylic resin to be removed without touching the specially created margin overcontour (Figs 2-14s and 2-14t). The provisional restoration is then brushed and polished with pumice paste (Figs 2-14u and 2-14v) and, if necessary, the surface is colored more, adding light-hardening glaze that is useful for fixing the pigments correctly and for reinforcing the margins (Figs 2-14w and 2-14x). The next step is hollowing out the space corresponding to the abutment teeth (Figs 2-14y and 2-14z) to achieve passive insertion into the oral cavity, thereby making positioning and relining of the provisional restoration much easier.

TECHNICAL CONSIDERATIONS

This technique is quick and economical since it requires only one duplicate of the wax-up and one silicone matrix to be made. Furthermore, there is no need to mount a cast on the articulator or, consequently, to carry out checks or occlusal alterations in the laboratory.

This method does not allow creation of a well-defined interproximal cervical design, however. The technician must therefore thin and shorten this area arbitrarily to prevent the clinician, when positioning the provisional restoration in the patient's mouth, from experiencing any interference with the tissues that could compromise correct insertion. Nevertheless, to avoid weakening the shell excessively, the interproximal area, although partially shortened, does not need to be eliminated completely.

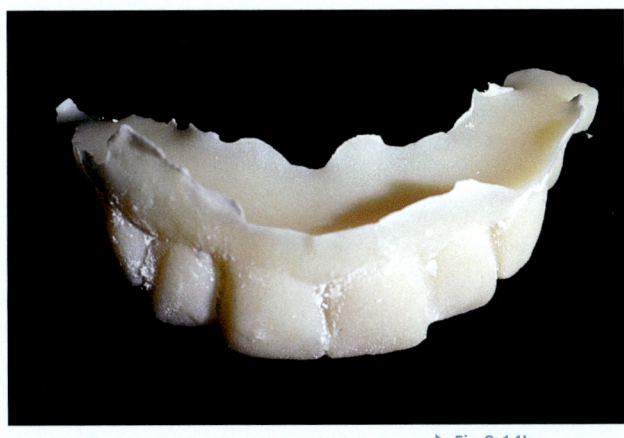

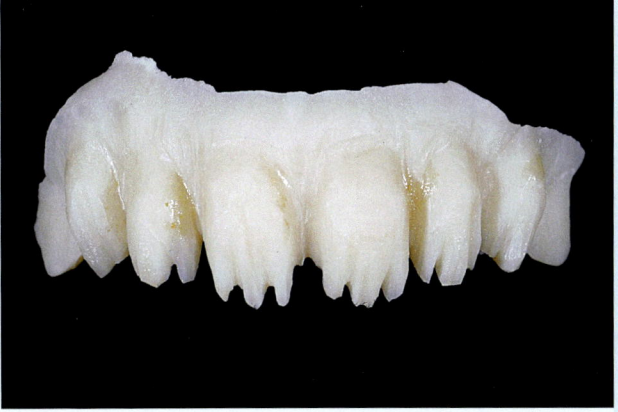

> Fig 2-14k

> Fig 2-14l

> Fig 2-14m

> Fig 2-14n

> Fig 2-14o

> Fig 2-14p

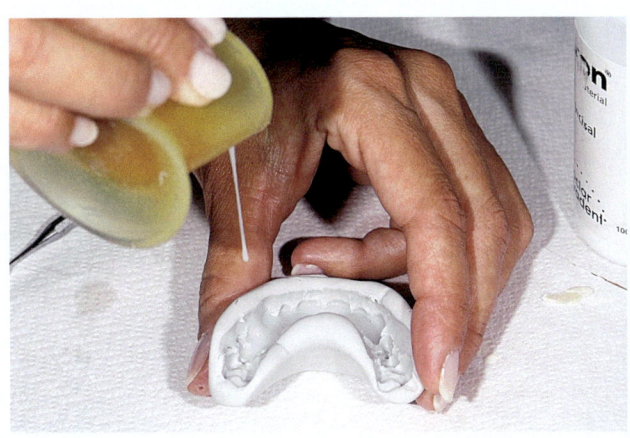

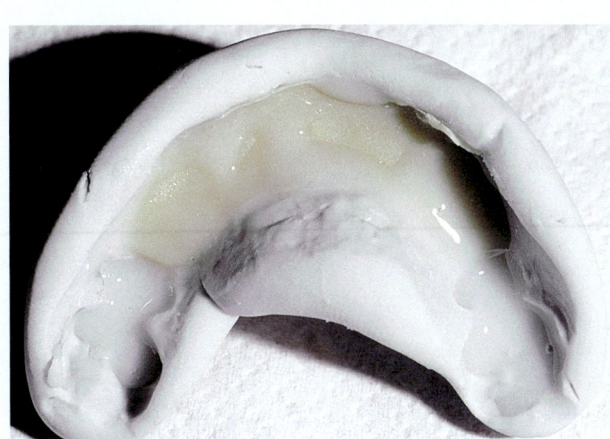

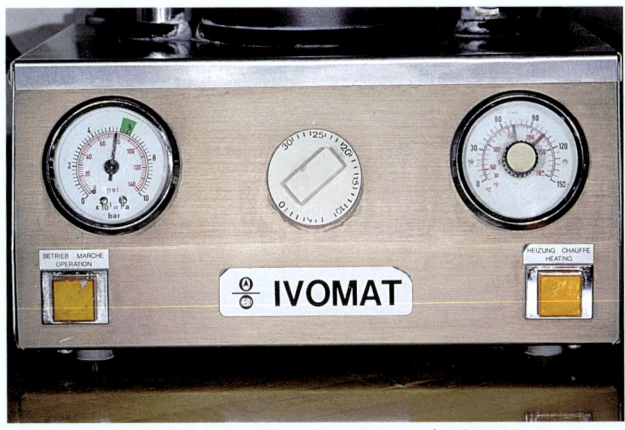

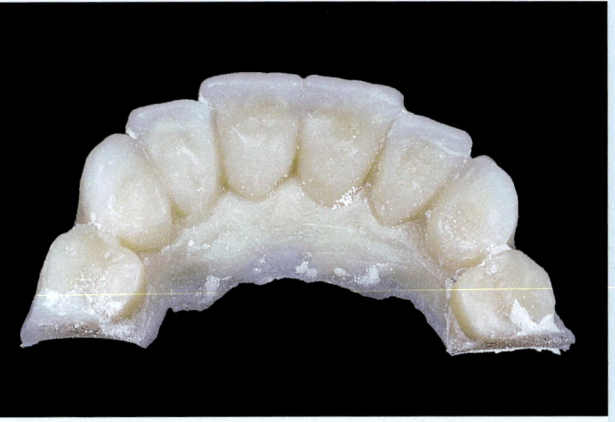

FIG 14 *(k and l)* Before the enamel is packed, cuts restricted to the incisal area are made on the provisional restoration in the dentin layer, which ensures the desired degree of translucency for the provisional restoration. *(m to o)* After the enamel layer is poured into the shell and the provisional restoration is inserted into the dentin layer, it is then polymerized inside the hydropneumatic machine. *(p)* The palatal view of the provisional restoration shows good translucency in the incisal third.

> Fig 2-14q

> Fig 2-14r

> Fig 2-14s

> Fig 2-14t

> Fig 2-14u

> Fig 2-14v

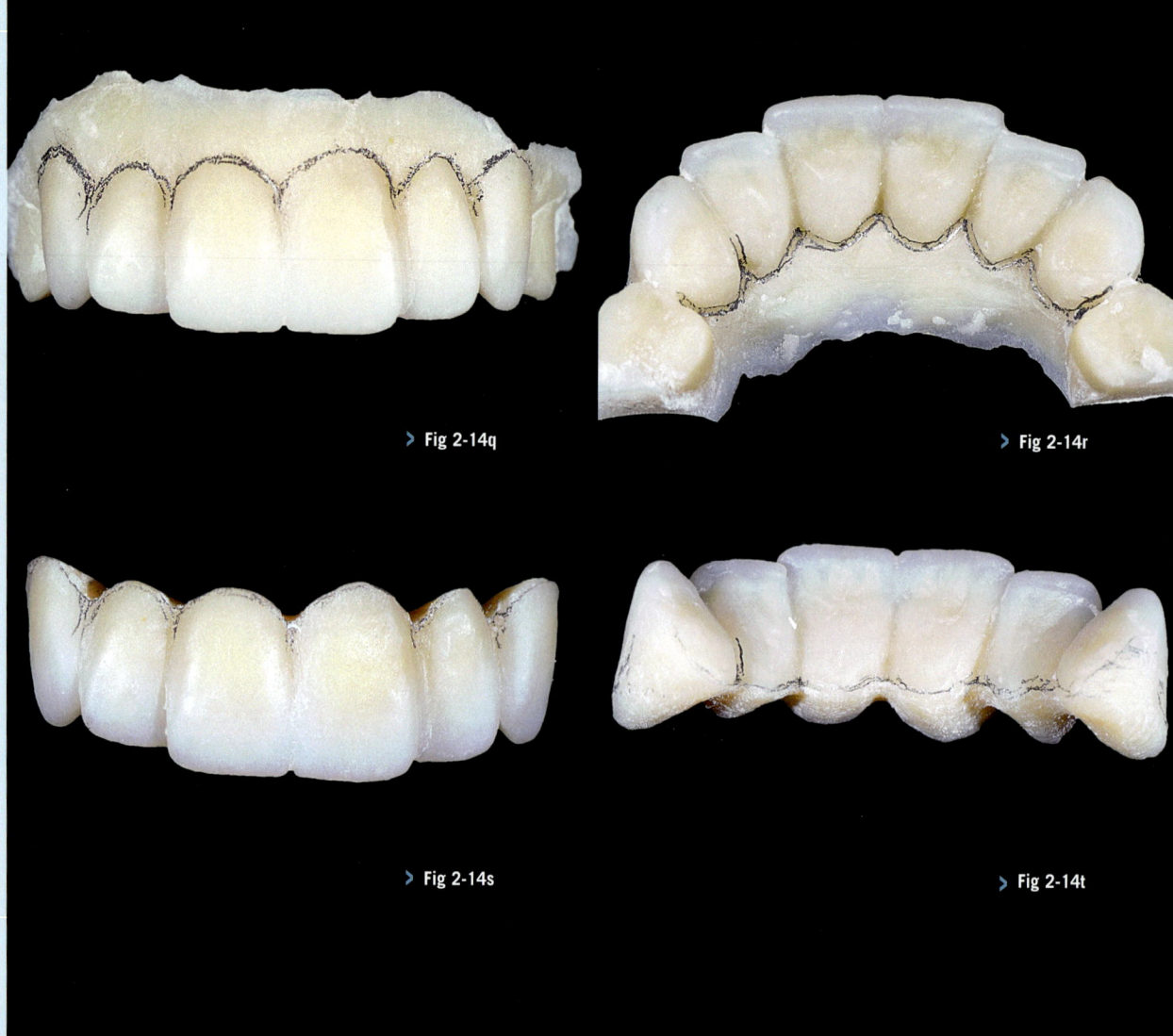

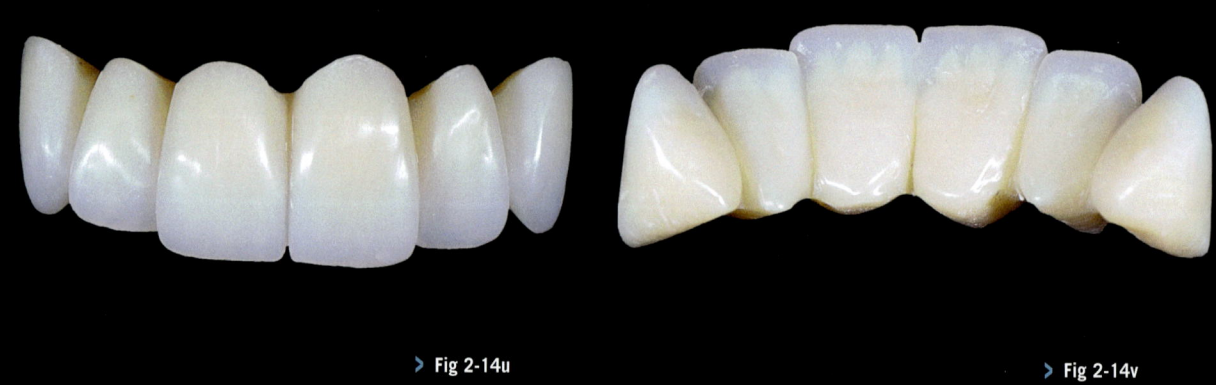

FIG 14 *(q and r)* In both the buccal and palatal areas, the margins of the provisional restoration are easily marked with a pencil thanks to the groove previously inscribed on the stone at the border with the wax. *(s to z)* Once finished and polished, the provisional restoration can be glazed before being completely removed from the shell.

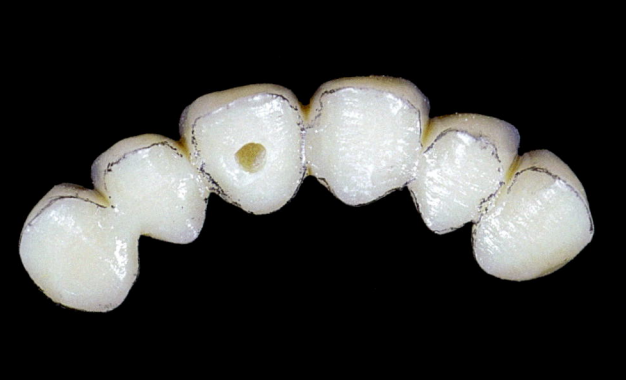

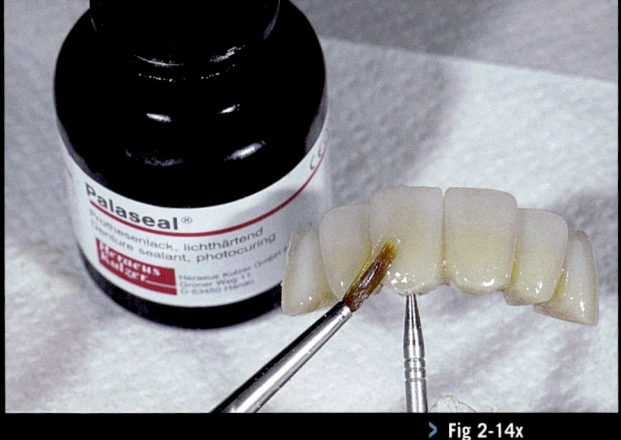

> Fig 2-14w

> Fig 2-14x

> Fig 2-14y

> Fig 2-14z

LABORATORY—MAKING THE PROVISIONAL

POURING IN THE SILICONE MATRIX (PSM)

PROCEDURE

- Make a stone cast of the wax-up, reproducing the overextended cervical groove.
- Make the silicone matrix.
- Pour and polymerize the dentin.
- Remove the provisional from the matrix.
- Proceed with cutting, packing, and polymerizing the enamel.
- Remove the provisional from the matrix once again.
- Highlight the overextended cervical groove.
- Finish and polish the provisional.
- Hollow out the areas where the abutment teeth are located.

ADVANTAGES

- Quick and low-cost technique
- Does not require mounting on articulator and occlusal check

DISADVANTAGES

- Interproximal cervical areas poorly defined
- Cervical design in the edentulous areas impossible to idealize
- Provides very few reference points for correct positioning in the mouth

ANTERIOR REHABILITATION
POSITIONING IN THE ORAL CAVITY

For positioning the provisional restoration in the mouth using the PSM technique, only the occlusal reference is taken, since the one provided by the poorly defined interproximal areas is not reliable.

The patient is asked to close the mouth so that all teeth not being treated make contact. The provisional restoration is thus guided into the correct position by the patient's occlusion.

In the event that insufficient preparations have been made or the shell has not been properly emptied, interference may be found between the shell and the prepared abutments, thereby preventing a correct fit. In these circumstances, despite the friction, the widening of the cervical third specific to the MIT permits a certain adjustment of the shell that allows the patient to bring the adjacent unprepared teeth into contact. The ability to close the mouth completely does not, however, prove that the provisional restoration has reached the correct position. Because of its freedom of movement, the shell could in fact move into a more buccal position in the anterosuperior sextant or a more lingual position in the anterior-inferior sextant, with inevitable esthetic-functional repercussions.

Evaluation and elimination of interferences This error can be avoided by using an acetate index, taken from the cast of the diagnostic wax-up, previously prepared in the laboratory, and extended to one or more teeth adjacent to those being treated. In addition to providing indispensable information on the congruity of the tooth preparations, it can be used to highlight any interference that prevents the provisional restoration, previously positioned inside it, from fitting properly (Figs 2-14aa to 2-14gg).

FIG 14 *(aa)* Taking into consideration the severe abrasions and reduced overjet in the anterior area, an occlusal adjustment was performed in CR to improve the initial overjet before the impression was taken and the stone casts were sent to the laboratory. *(bb)* Under the guidance of the clinician, the technician has modified the patient's misalignment, correcting the original tooth arrangement. *(cc to ee)* An acetate index is made on the cast of the wax-up, into which the acrylic shell made in the laboratory fits perfectly. Extending the transparent stent up to the first premolars, which are not involved in the treatment, acts as a stop for inserting the provisional restoration into the oral cavity. *(ff and gg)* The index proves very useful to the clinician, allowing assessment of the congruity of the completed tooth preparations.

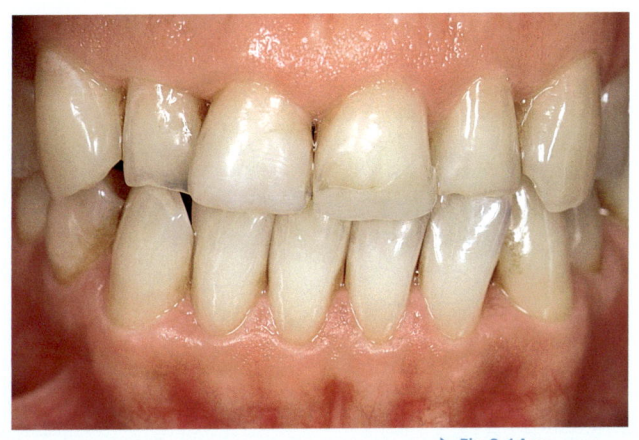

› Fig 2-14aa

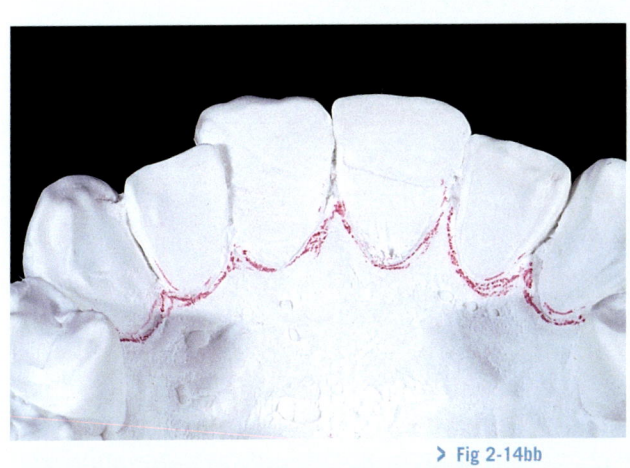

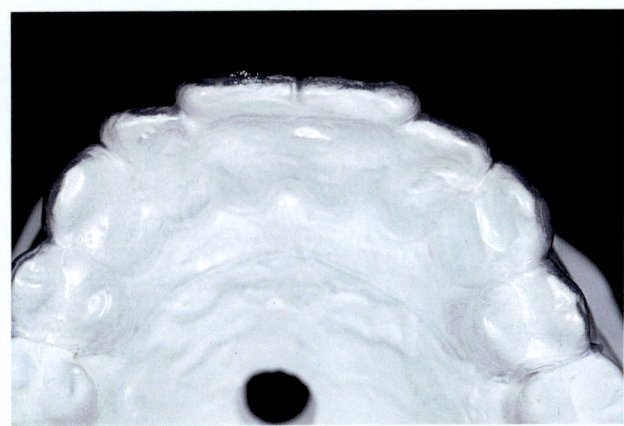

› Fig 2-14bb

› Fig 2-14cc

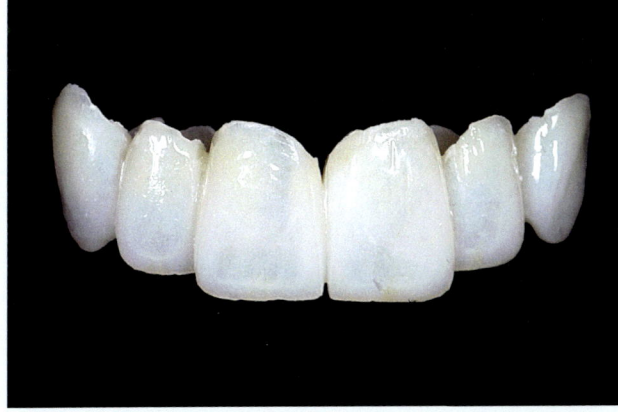

› Fig 2-14dd

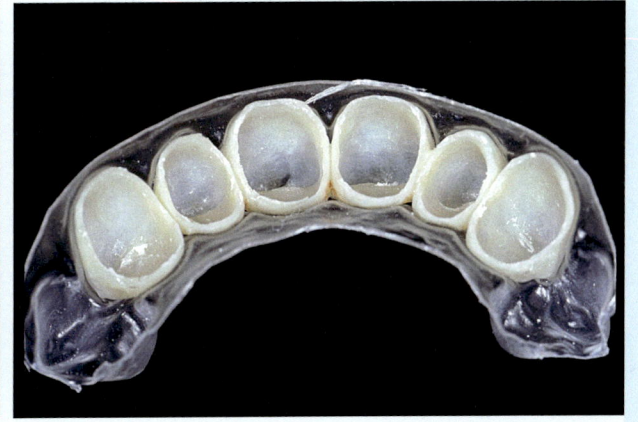

› Fig 2-14ee

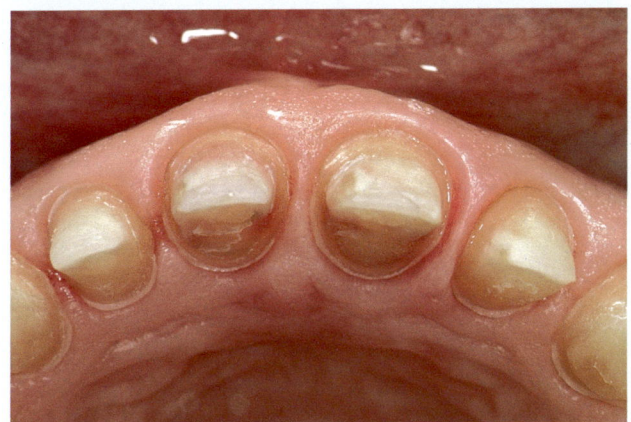

› Fig 2-14ff

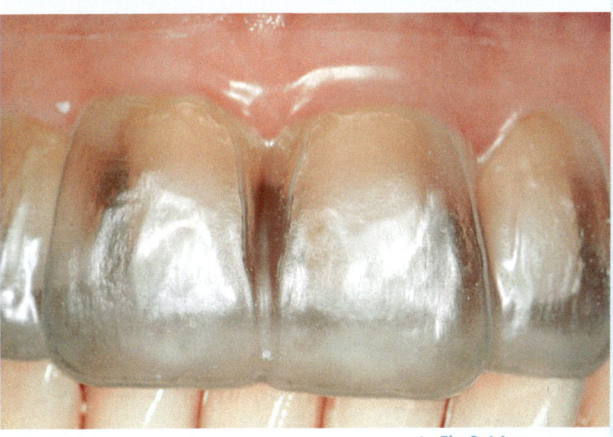

› Fig 2-14gg

167

A perfect fit of the transparent stent is also a good indication for the provisional restoration contained in it and is easily shown by its intimate contact with the unprepared teeth (Fig 2-14hh). The fit is also proven by the cervical overextension of the acrylic shell beyond the dentogingival border. If the index does not position itself perfectly, the interferences that prevent the provisional restoration from fitting properly should be highlighted by means of silicone paste (Fit Checker, GC Dental) and then removed with a bur. In most cases adjustments are necessary in the interproximal areas, where the presence of any tissue ischemia reveals insufficient shortening in the laboratory. These crucial areas must be progressively reduced until the interferences disappear. Once all of the necessary refinements have been made, the index, with the shell inside, is again positioned in the mouth to make sure it fits perfectly.

Fitting guided by occlusion After highlighting any interferences between the provisional restoration and the abutments, thereby serving its purpose, the index is removed (Fig 2-14ii). Its presence during relining would interfere with occlusal verification of the provisional restoration and would furthermore prevent the removal of excess relining material, thus making the finishing work much more difficult. Without any further aid from the acetate index, the provisional restoration is guided into the correct position by the patient's occlusion in MI. Standing in front of the patient, the clinician can now check the accuracy of the occlusal plane inclination, the position of the incisal edge, the level of overjet and overbite, the lengths of the teeth, and the verticality of the interincisal line. It is best to avoid pushing the shell in the apical direction at this stage, which could cause malpositioning of the provisional restoration by putting it into subocclusion.

Only when the clinician is certain that the provisional restoration fits perfectly should relining take place. For that, the patient needs to be asked to gently bring the arches into occlusion until the teeth adjacent to those treated reach MI. All of the excess relining material can then easily be cleaned away (Figs 2-14jj to 2-14mm).

FIG 14 *(hh and ii)* The transparent stent makes it possible to check whether the shell fits into the mouth appropriately. After it is checked for proper fit, the provisional restoration is relined. *(jj and kk)* Because of the extension of the cervical third specific to the MIT, it is possible to eliminate all of the excess relining material without the risk of affecting the marginal area, which is preserved because it is kept within the provisional restoration. After it is finished and polished, the provisional restoration is repositioned and then temporarily cemented. *(ll and mm)* The intraoral photograph and the patient's smile demonstrate overall satisfactory integration.

> Fig 2-14hh

> Fig 2-14ii

> Fig 2-14jj

> Fig 2-14kk

> Fig 2-14ll

> Fig 2-14mm

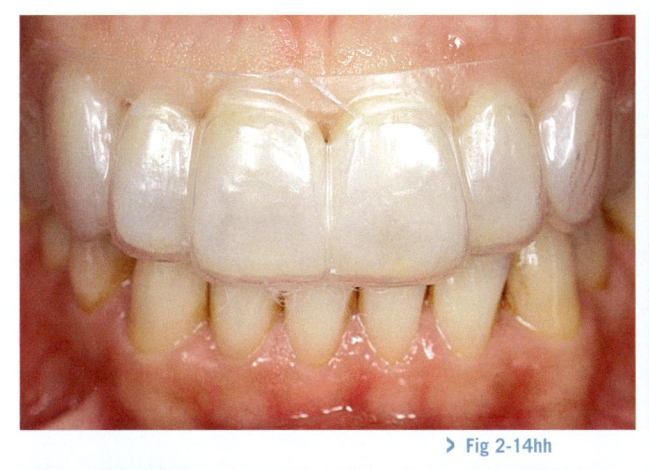

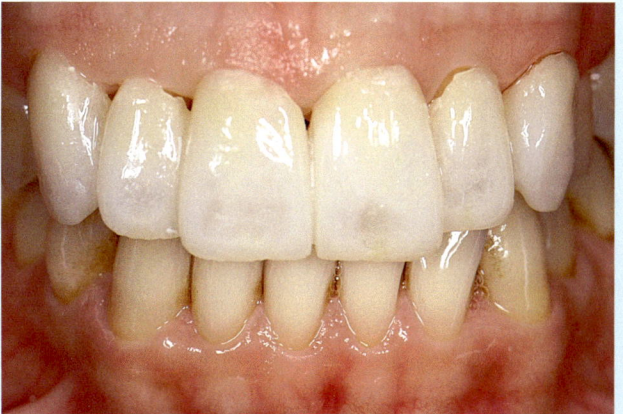

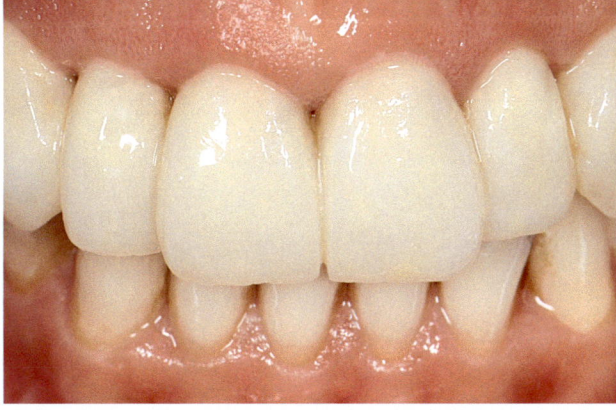

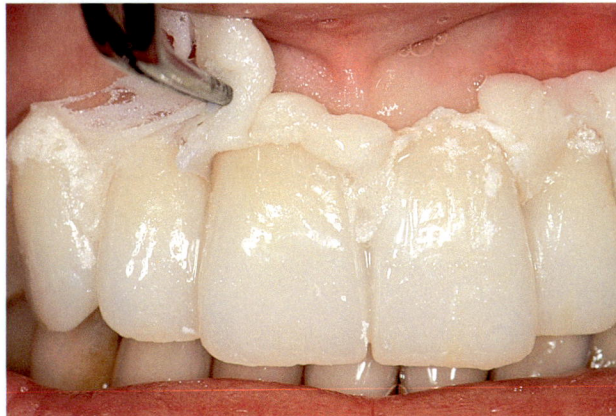

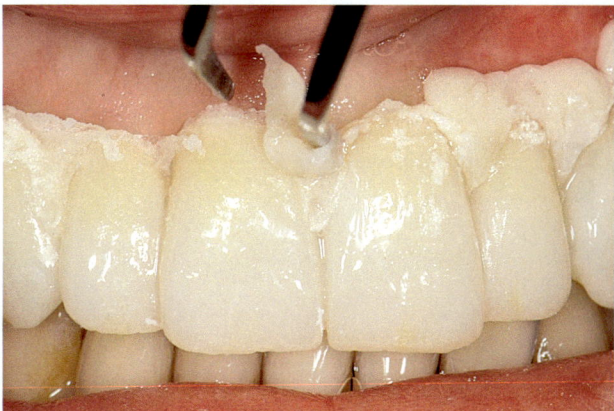

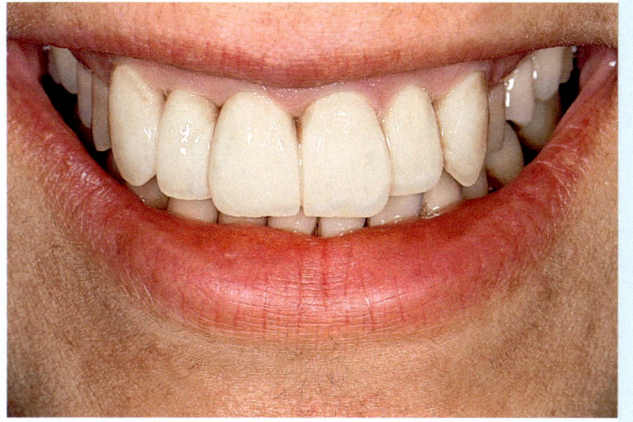

Case 1 →continues on page 345

CLINIC—POSITIONING THE PROVISIONAL

ANTERIOR REHABILITATION

PROCEDURE

- Place the provisional inside the acetate matrix.
- Verify the intimate contact of the acetate matrix with the nonprepared teeth to ensure the complete insertion of the shell.
- Use silicone paste to find interferences, and eliminate them.
- Remove the acetate matrix.
- Guided by occlusion (MI), fit and reline the provisional.
- Check the occlusion, finish, and polish.

FABRICATING THE PROVISIONAL RESTORATION- MIT LABORATORY

■ REHABILITATION OF ONE OR TWO ARCHES ■
PRESSING ON THE STONE CAST (PSC)

This technique involves pressing the provisional restoration directly onto the stone cast (PSC). As we will see, the clinician can prepare both the occlusal and the interproximal references using this method, which makes positioning the provisional restoration in the mouth much easier than the PSM technique, especially in complex rehabilitation cases.

TECHNIQUE

The original cast must be as accurate as possible and must include the anatomic reference points (palate, tuberosities, retromolar trigone, fornices, etc) (Figs 2-15a and 2-15b), so that they also can be reproduced in the stone cast duplicated from the diagnostic wax-up (Figs 2-15c and 2-15d). On the latter, an index in acetate (Fig 2-15e) and four silicone indices (Fig 2-15f) are created. Because they include the anatomic reference points, these can be correctly positioned on any of the patient's casts. The first index is cut to separate the palatal and buccal portions (Figs 2-15g to 2-15i). The technician alternately positions the two portions of the cut index on the original cast (Fig 2-15j). By this means, the palatal and buccal areas can be checked separately and altered with a bur, if necessary, according to how the indices interface with the cast, the tooth positions, and the orientation of the axes (Figs 2-15k and 2-15l). After carrying out these modifications, the technician performs only light preparation (0.8 to 1.0 mm) on all of the teeth involved in the treatment to create the space needed for pressing the provisional restoration. The preparations at marginal level will have to be extended circumferentially up to the pencil line drawn on the cast beyond the dentogingival border (Figs 2-15m and 2-15n) in order for the clinician to be able to count on the container effect of the shell once it is placed in the mouth. After the prepared teeth have been covered with resin-stone insulation (Fig 2-15o), the second silicone index, still in one piece, is filled with "dentin" of the chosen color (Figs 2-15p and 2-15q), taking care to apply it to the area around the preparations and in any edentulous areas (Figs 2-15r to 2-15t) to prevent air bubbles from forming. The index is then placed onto the cast (Fig 2-15u) and, after it is fixed in place with elastic bands (Fig 2-15v), placed into a hydropneumatic machine to polymerize the resin (Fig 2-15w). As described earlier for the PSM technique (see page 160), a firing time of at least 25 minutes at 100°C and 6 atm is required.

CASE 2

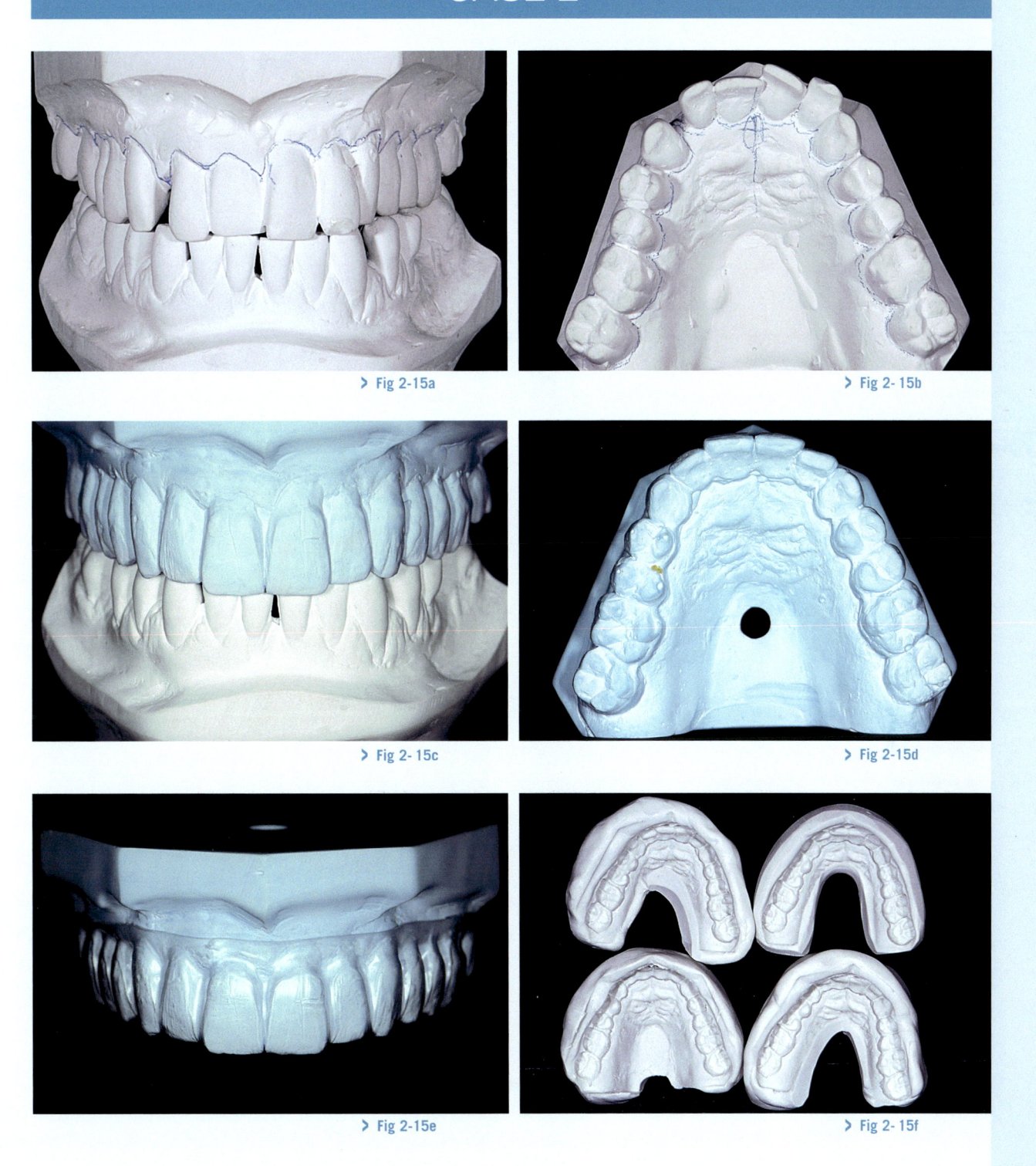

> Fig 2-15a

> Fig 2-15b

> Fig 2-15c

> Fig 2-15d

> Fig 2-15e

> Fig 2-15f

FIG 15 *(a)* The view of the patient's stone cast in MI shows a high degree of occlusal instability. *(b)* On the maxillary arch, the object of the prosthetic rehabilitation to be undertaken, the technician pencils in the cervical extension peculiar to the MIT. *(c and d)* After making the diagnostic wax-up according to the information received on the laboratory checklist, the technician makes a separate stone cast, which, as can be seen from the frontal and occlusal views, makes some important changes to the original tooth position. The occlusal record taken by the clinician guiding the patient in CR does allow the technician to provide the two arches with satisfactory occlusal stability, despite the patient refusing orthodontic-prosthetic treatment of the mandibular arch. *(e and f)* An acetate matrix that will be used by the clinician and four silicone indices that will be used for laboratory purposes are made on this stone cast of the maxillary arch.

> Fig 2-15g

> Fig 2-15h

> Fig 2-15i

> Fig 2-15j

> Fig 2-15k

> Fig 2-15l

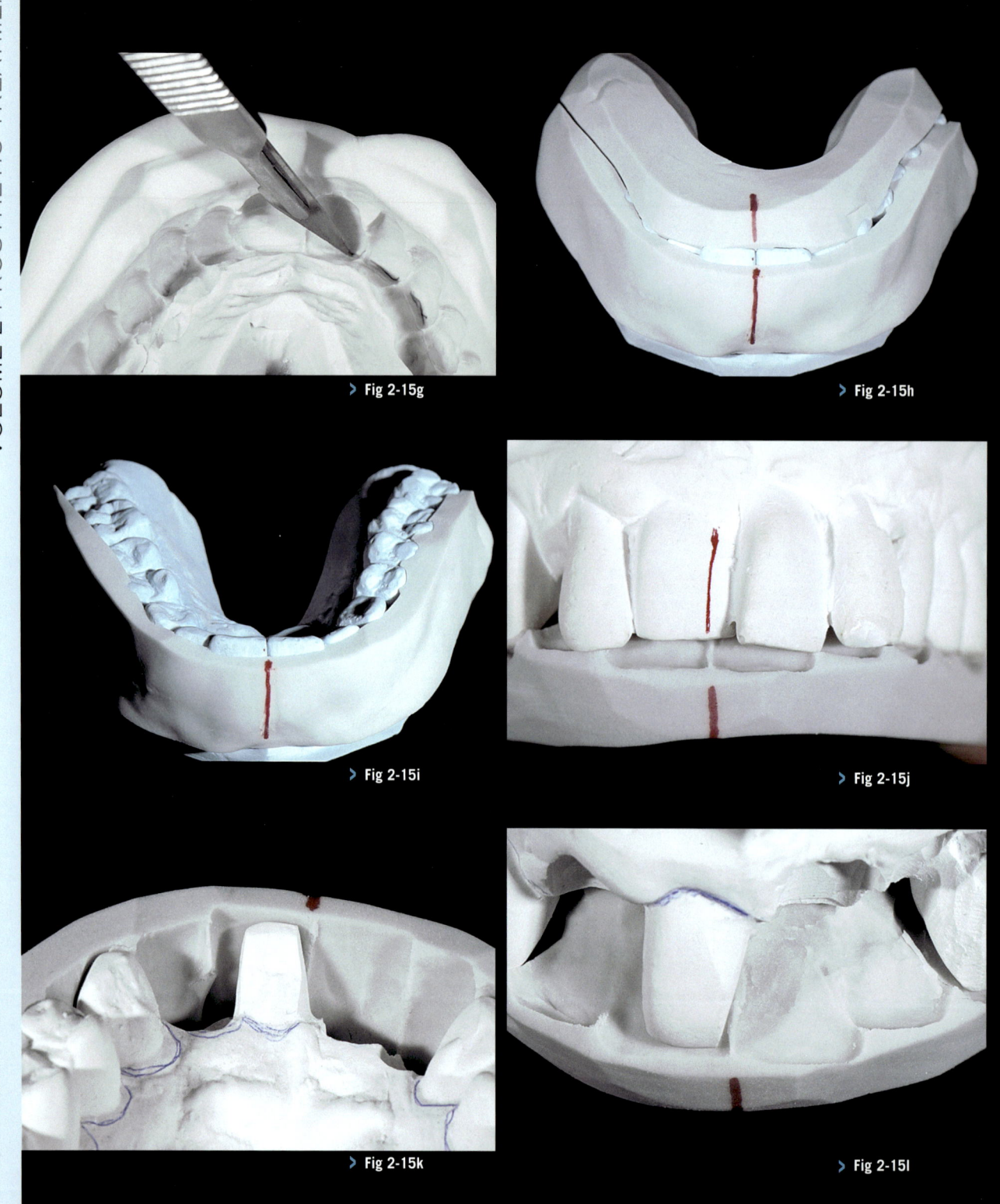

FIG 15 *(g)* The first of the silicone indices made on the diagnostic wax-up is cut with a scalpel to separate the palatal and buccal portions. *(h and i)* A small window is created, and the two parts are positioned on the cast of the wax-up to reveal the interincisal line. *(j)* By positioning the portions of the index on the original cast, the technician can see the incongruities between the initial clinical situation and that previsualized in the wax-up. *(k and l)* This allows the preparation axes for the other teeth to be established, which will be completed on the original cast or on one of its duplicates after the extracted teeth are removed.

> Fig 2-15m

> Fig 2-15n

> Fig 2-15o

> Fig 2-15p

> Fig 2-15q

> Fig 2-15r

> Fig 2-15s

> Fig 2-15t

> Fig 2-15u

> Fig 2-15v

> Fig 2-15w

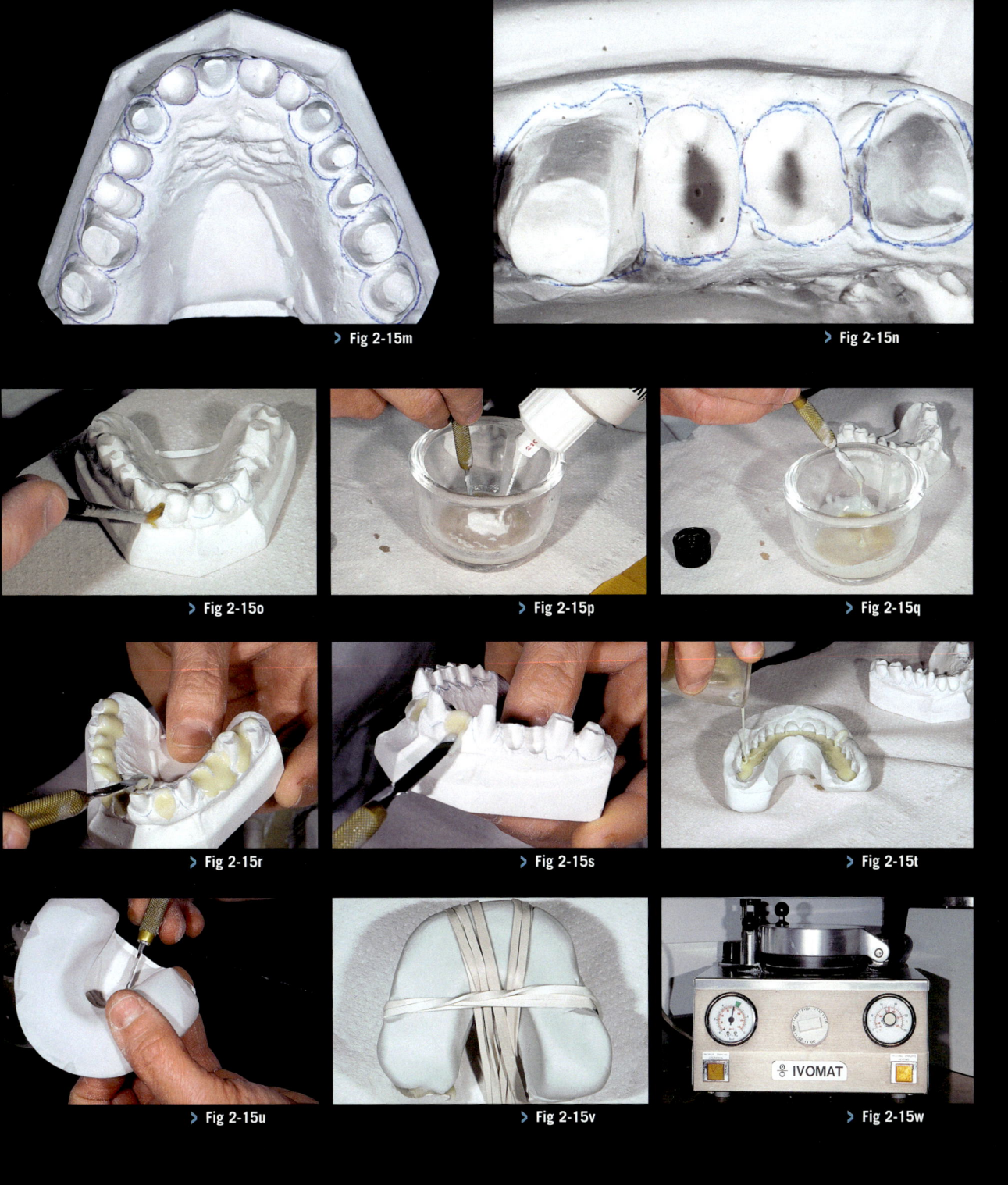

FIG 15 The edentulous areas are created on the cast by hollowing out roughly 3 mm of the root contour. *(m and n)* The resulting concavity must be ovoid and must follow the radicular shape of the extracted tooth to allow adequate cleaning of the area while providing appropriate tissue support, especially on the buccal side. *(o to s)* At this point a resin-stone insulator is applied to the cast, and dentin of the chosen color is prepared, which is distributed evenly around the abutments as well as in the edentulous areas. *(t)* Some of the prepared resin must be poured into the second index. *(u to w)* Once it is positioned on the cast, and the excess resin removed, the cast and the index are firmly fixed together with elastic bands and placed in the hydropneumatic machine for polymerization.

Once polymerization is complete, the index is removed. Leaving the provisional restoration on the cast (Figs 2-15x and 2-15y), the incisal areas are cut to add the "enamel" (Figs 2-15z to 2-15bb). As with the PSM technique, the "dentin" can be colored at this point if necessary so that the colors remain inside the provisional restoration, between the layer of resin already fired and the layer of "enamel" to be placed over it. This procedure is especially useful for provisional restorations created after tooth preparation: The thickness of the layers can be greater because the provisional restoration is not completely emptied out on the inner surface. Then, using the third index, the "enamel" is packed, following the same method as previously described for pressing the "dentin" (Figs 2-15cc to 2-15ee). Once the "enamel" has been polymerized, the provisional restoration must be checked on the articulator. Only in this way is it possible to correct and eliminate the slight raised bite that, despite firmly affixing the index to the cast with elastic bands (Fig 2-15ff), inevitably occurs when the "dentin" and "enamel" are fired. The provisional restoration is then extracted from the cast, and the cervical areas are finished to remove the overruns of resin (Figs 2-15gg and 2-15hh), taking care not to damage the deliberately overextended margin or to reduce even slightly the thickness of the acrylic below 0.4 to 0.5 mm. The provisional restoration is then brushed with a pumice paste and, as with the PSM technique, given further surface coloring. Glaze is added to fix the color (Figs 2-15ii and 2-15jj).

TECHNICAL-CLINICAL CONSIDERATIONS

The need to mount the casts in the articulator to carry out occlusal refinements and tooth preparation means that the PSC technique is more time-intensive than the PSM technique. Nevertheless, unlike the PSM technique, the PSC technique offers the advantage of being able to produce a provisional restoration with well-defined interproximal areas, since the images of the papillae are maintained on the stone. It is thus possible to achieve greater precision in positioning the provisional restoration than with the PSM technique because of the simultaneous presence of both occlusal and interproximal references.

Another advantage over the PSM technique is that, where extractions are necessary, the PSC method allows the technician to draw the exact profile of the provisional restoration in the edentulous areas, tracing the outline of the root trunk. This maneuver is useful for adequately conditioning the tissue. The clinician must in any case scrupulously check the convexity that the technician has given the provisional restoration in the edentulous area (2 to 3 mm) and make alterations if it impairs correct fitting of the restoration by excessively compressing the tissues. Also, given the smaller amount of resin used in the PSC method, there is less volumetric contraction of the acrylic. Finally, the pressing performed on the rigid cast protects the provisional restoration from the risk of distortions that can instead take place with the silicone index used in the PSM technique.

> Fig 2-15x

> Fig 2-15y

> Fig 2-15z

> Fig 2- 15aa

> Fig 2-15bb

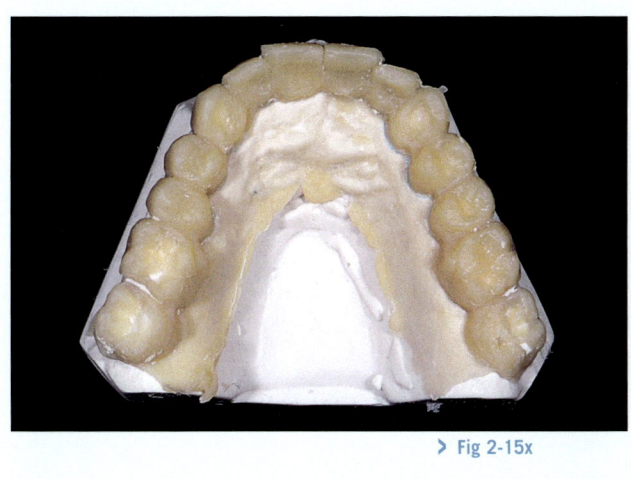

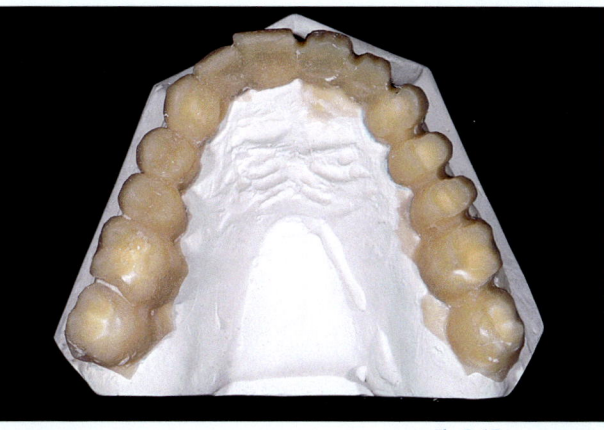

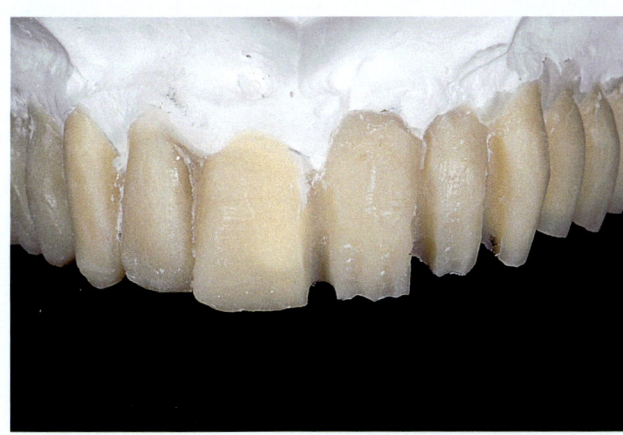

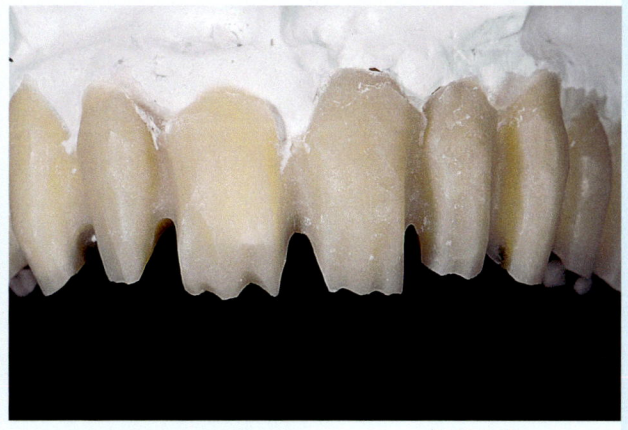

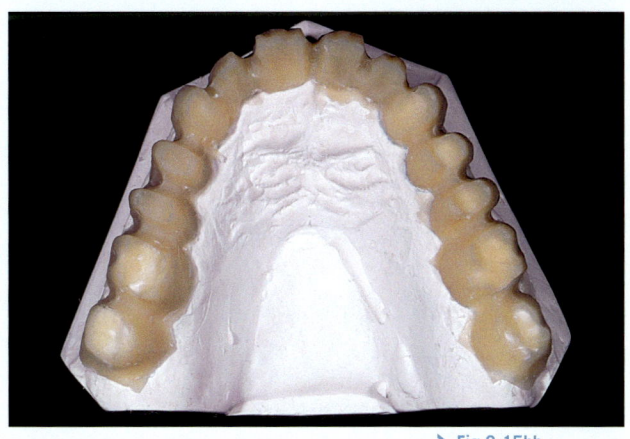

FIG 15 *(x to bb)* When this process is complete, the provisional restoration in dentin is removed from the index and finished. Cuts are made in the incisal areas to help create space for the enamel.

> Fig 2-15cc

> Fig 2-15dd

> Fig 2-15ee

> Fig 2-15ff

> Fig 2-15gg

> Fig 2-15hh

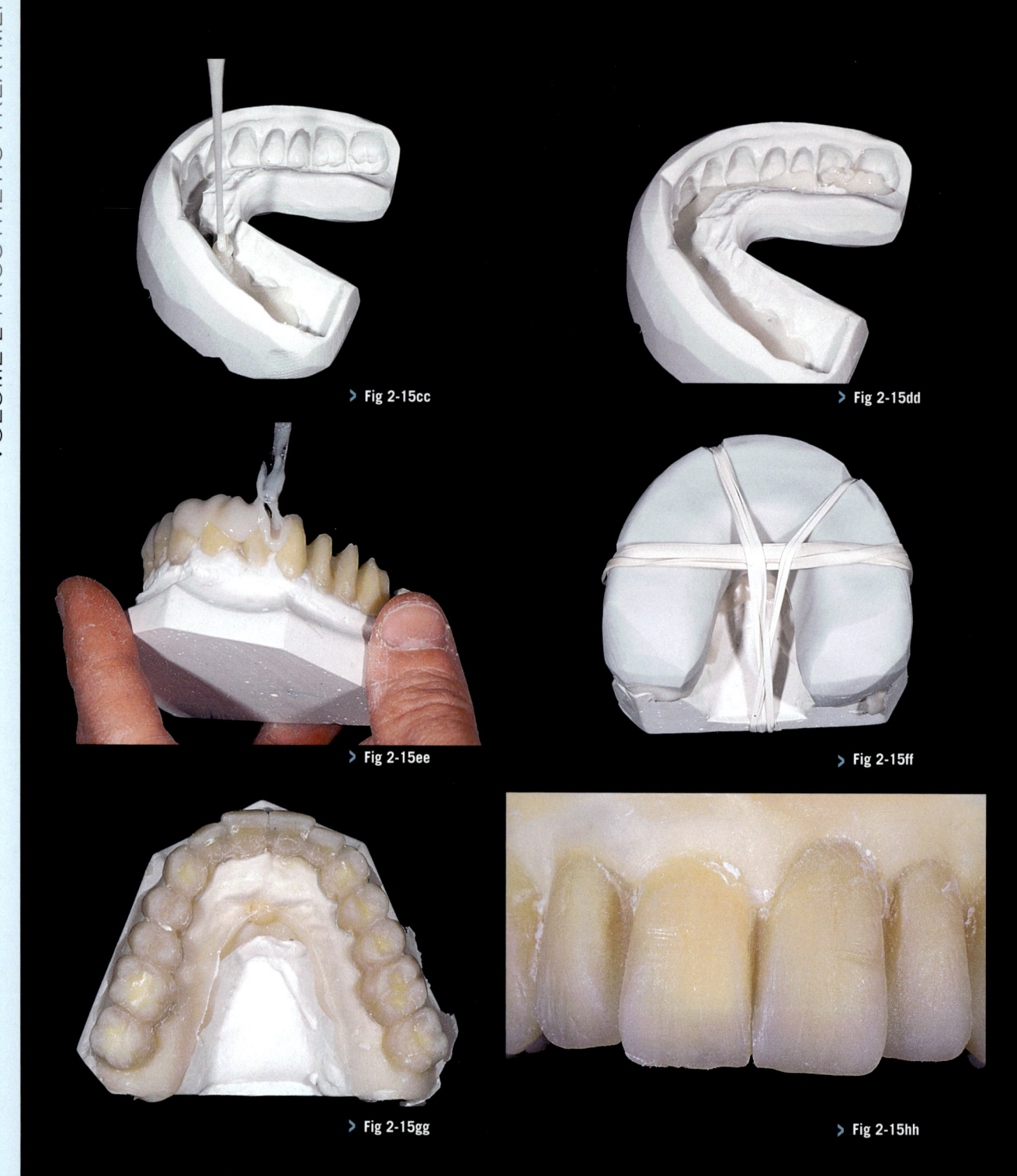

FIG 15 *(cc to ff)* In addition to being poured into the third silicone index, enamel is applied directly to the provisional restoration in dentin still fixed on the stone cast. This is then joined again to the index with elastic bands and put into the hydropneumatic machine. After polymerization, the silicone index is removed. *(gg)* The occlusal view of the provisional restoration shows excess resin, which will be removed before finishing and polishing. *(hh)* A closer view of the provisional restoration shows the good result achieved by layering the enamel over dentin and the adequate translucency that has been given to the incisal third. *(ii and jj)* After the provisional restoration is checked on the articulator to remove the slight but inevitable raised bite, the surface is colored and glazed.

> Fig 2-15ii

> Fig 2-15jj

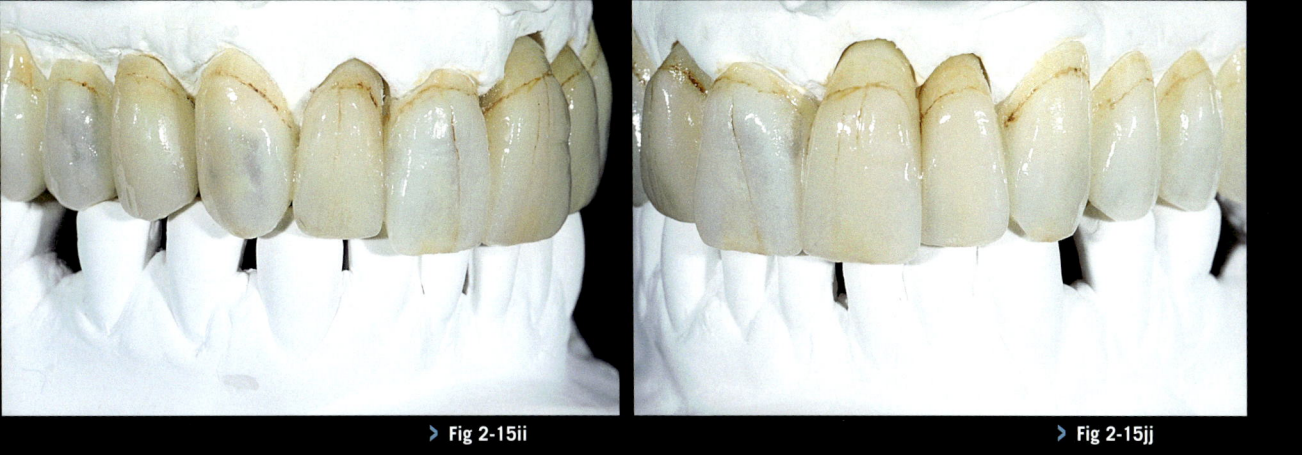

LABORATORY—FABRICATING THE PROVISIONAL

PRESSING ON THE STONE CAST (PSC)

PROCEDURE

- Take an impression extended up to the anatomic reference points.
- Make a stone cast derived from the wax-up reproducing the overextended cervical groove.
- Make four silicone indices and one in acetate:
  - **FIRST SILICONE INDEX** (PALATAL AND BUCCAL PORTIONS):
    – Check insertion on cast
    – Make axial alterations
    – Prepare abutments up to the overextension (pencil mark).
  - **SECOND SILICONE INDEX:** Pour and polymerize the dentin after positioning the index on the cast
  - **THIRD SILICONE INDEX:** Proceed by packing and polymerizing the enamel after positioning the index on the cast
  - **FOURTH SILICONE INDEX AND ACETATE MATRIX:**
    Give to the dentist to check tooth axes and preparations.
- Check occlusion on the articulator.
- Refine and polish.

ADVANTAGES

- Well-defined interproximal areas
- Adequate reference points make positioning in the mouth easier
- Cervical design can be idealized in the edentulous areas

DISADVANTAGES

- Requires occlusal refinements on the articulator with slight alterations to the occlusal anatomy

REHABILITATION OF ONE ARCH
POSITIONING IN THE ORAL CAVITY

If only one of the dental arches requires rehabilitation, it is essential to ensure that the arch not being treated has an adequate occlusal plane and compensation curves compatible with those of the prosthetic treatment to be completed (Figs 2-15kk to 2-15oo).

Evaluating and eliminating interferences The congruity of the tooth preparations is assessed using the acetate index derived from the diagnostic wax-up, which allows the suitability of the new tooth positions, the axial alterations, and the thicknesses of the preparations to be checked (Figs 2-15pp to 2-15tt). It should be pointed out that, when an entire arch is being rehabilitated, the absence of tooth references (intact teeth) makes exact positioning of the transparent stent more complicated. Extending it to the anatomic reference points (palate, retromolar trigone, tuberosities, etc) allows the clinician to achieve adequate insertion of the stent. Once the acrylic resin shell has been put inside the matrix, it is possible, with the aid of silicone paste, to identify any interferences that impair correct positioning of the provisional restoration and hence to eliminate them (Fig 2-15uu).

Fitting guided by occlusion Once the index is removed, the patient is guided in CR (see chapter 1, pages 66–68), until the provisional restoration's intercuspation correctly aligns with the opposing arch. Reaching a correct occlusal relationship is aided by the interproximal walls, adequately designed in the provisional restoration by means of the PSC technique.

At this point the VDO and the levels of overjet and overbite are checked; these should duplicate the situation found with the provisional restoration positioned on the cast. Minimal variations of the preset VDO are not significant from a clinical point of view, especially in this first phase (see chapter 1, page 70). The provisional restoration is now also checked from an esthetic perspective (Figs 2-15vv to 2-15zz). There can be, at times, slight inconsistencies with the orientation of the occlusal plane and the verticality of the interincisal line. Any changes to the setup can be made during relining. The use of an acrylic resin that gives adequate working time allows the clinician the opportunity to check the provisional restoration from both the front and the profile while the resin is still in the plastic phase, allowing any further changes to be made to the final setup of the provisional restoration itself.

Optimizing the orientation of the occlusal plane and the verticality of the interincisal line is imperative even if, in some cases, they do not coincide with the perfect occlusal relationship in CO. When relining is finished, it is still possible to refine any occlusal interference by guiding the patient into CR, easily idealizing the functional aspect of the provisional restoration.

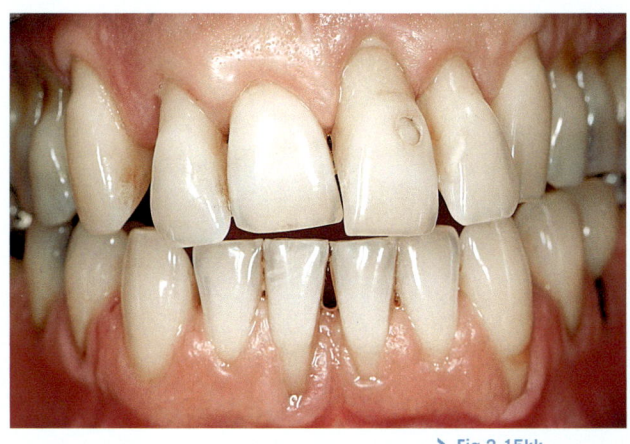

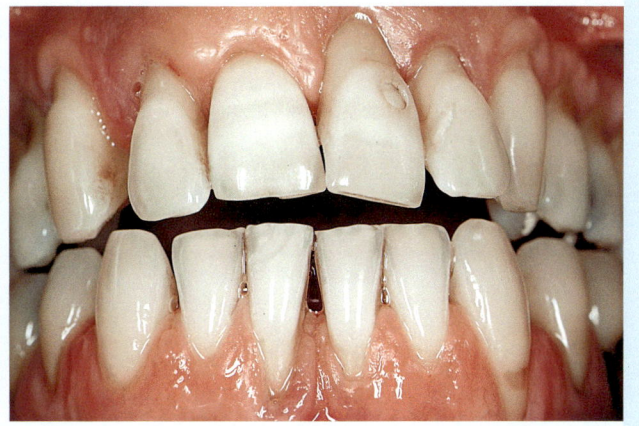

> Fig 2-15kk

> Fig 2-15ll

> Fig 2-15mm

> Fig 2-15nn

> Fig 2-15oo

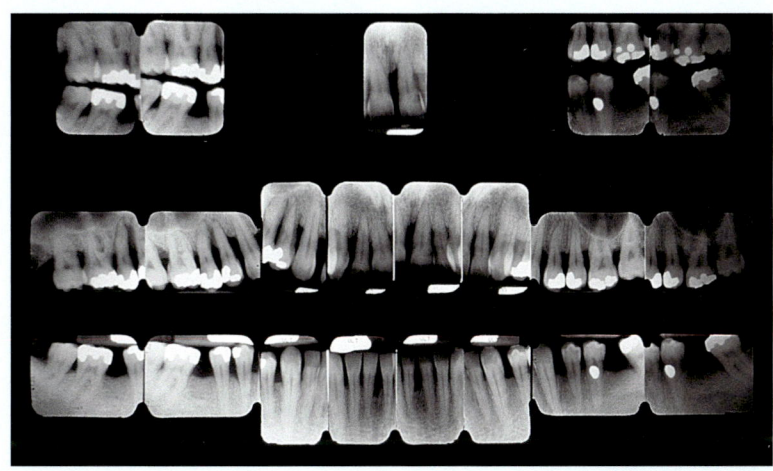

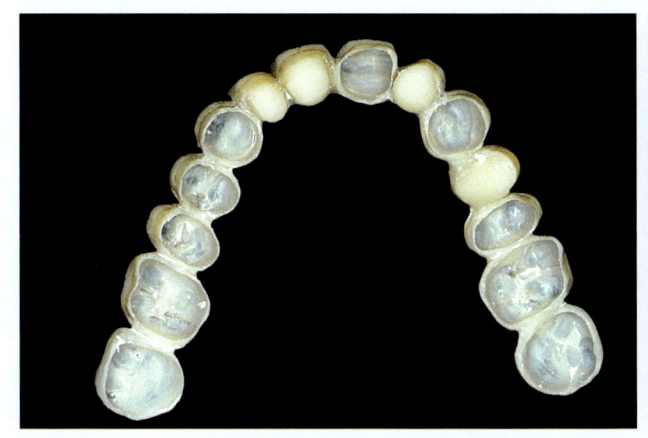

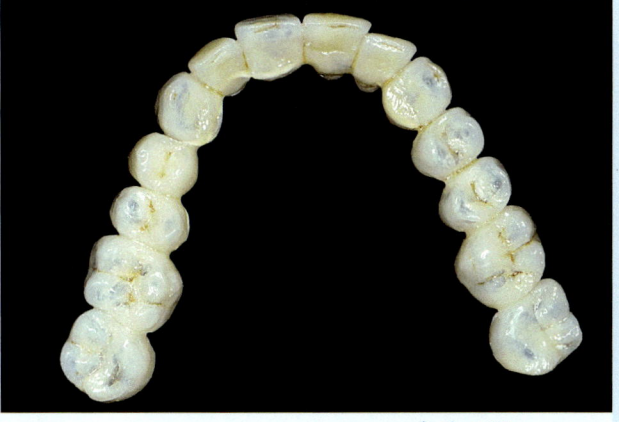

FIG 15 *(kk and ll)* The view of the two arches in MI highlights considerable occlusal instability. The patient shows a significant retrusion of the mandible in CR, with strong occlusal interference in the posterior sectors. *(mm)* The complete full-mouth radiographic series confirms the loss of periodontal support in many maxillary teeth. Orthodontic treatment was recommended in the mandibular arch, but the patient chose not to subscribe to it. However, because the mandibular occlusal plane was judged to be clinically acceptable, it was decided to carry out prosthetic rehabilitation of the maxillary arch alone. *(nn and oo)* The clinician therefore received from the laboratory an acrylic shell with the overextended margins in the cervical third, typical of the MIT.

> Fig 2-15pp

> Fig 2-15qq

> Fig 2-15rr

> Fig 2-15ss

> Fig 2-15tt

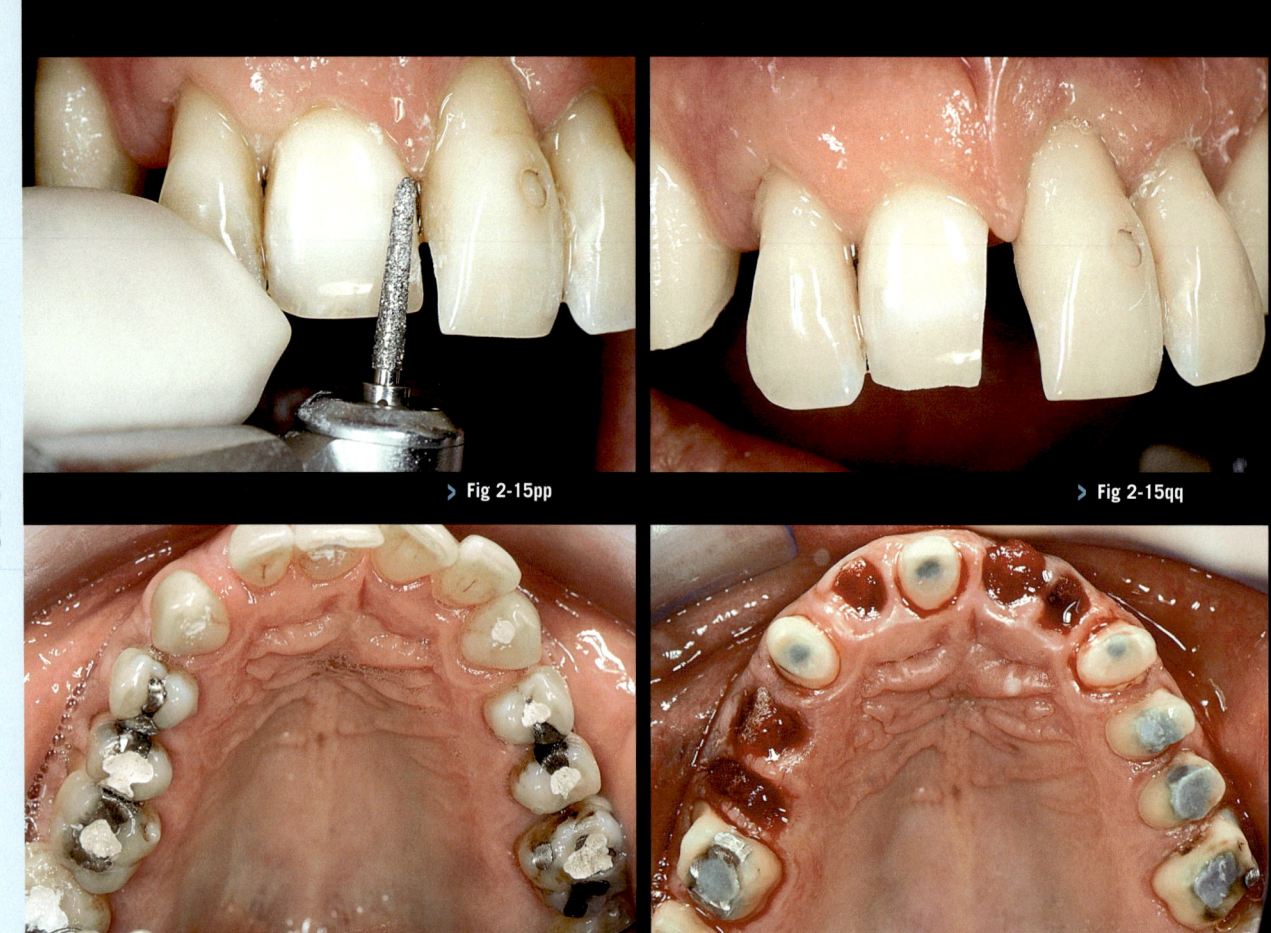

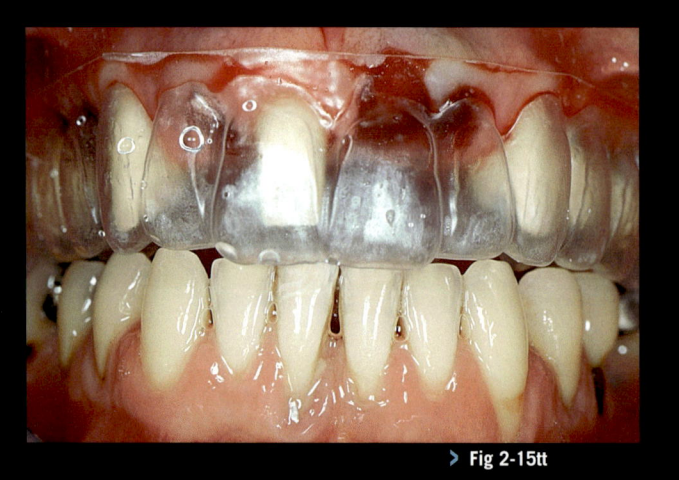

FIG 15 *(pp and qq)* Widening the cervical margin would not be sufficient to fit the shell correctly if the clinician did not follow the newly established axes during the tooth preparations, as requested in the laboratory checklist. *(rr to tt)* Once the periodontally compromised teeth have been extracted and the preparations have been made under the guidance of the acetate index, the provisional restoration inside the transparent stent is positioned in the mouth. *(uu)* Silicone paste is used to assess the accuracy of the positioning and highlight any interferences, which will be eliminated. *(vv and xx)* When the index is removed, the validity of the esthetic-functional alterations made are evaluated. *(yy)* The provisional restoration can then be relined and finished. *(zz)* The photograph of the patient's smile shows the satisfactory esthetic integration.

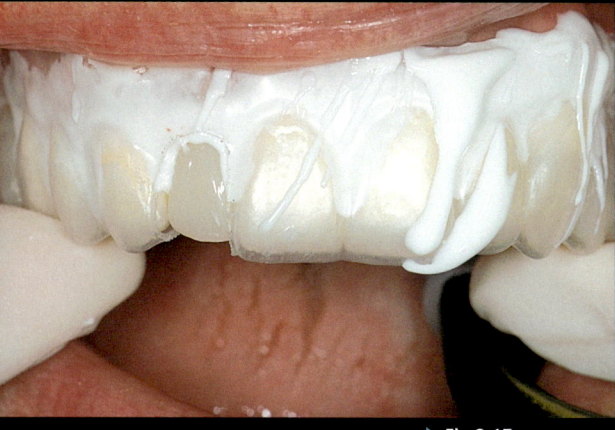

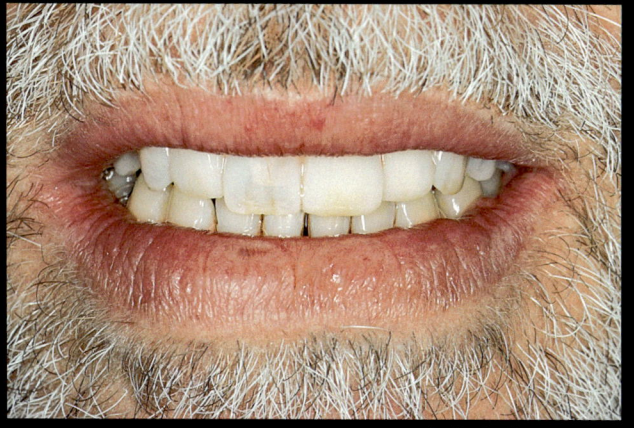

> Fig 2-15uu

> Fig 2-15vv

> Fig 2-15ww

> Fig 2-15xx

> Fig 2-15yy

> Fig 2-15zz

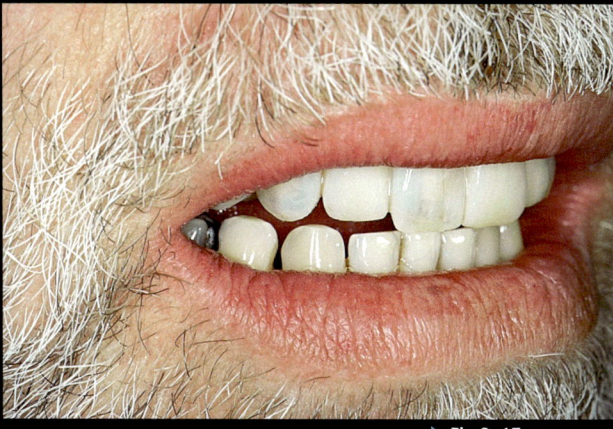

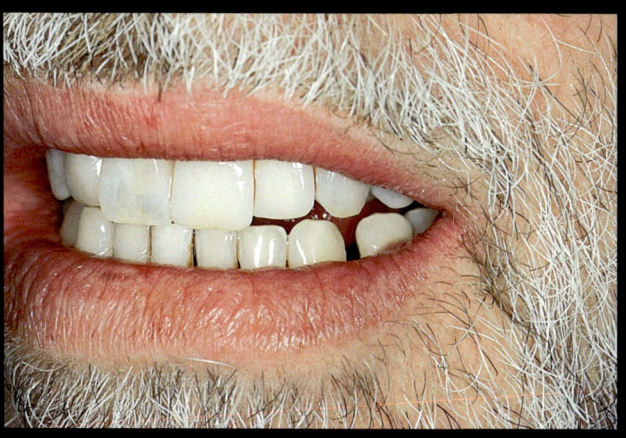

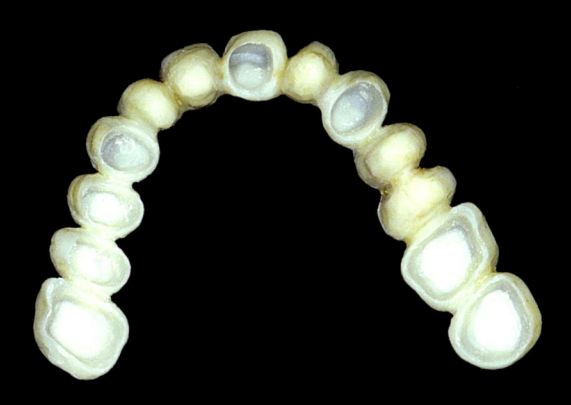

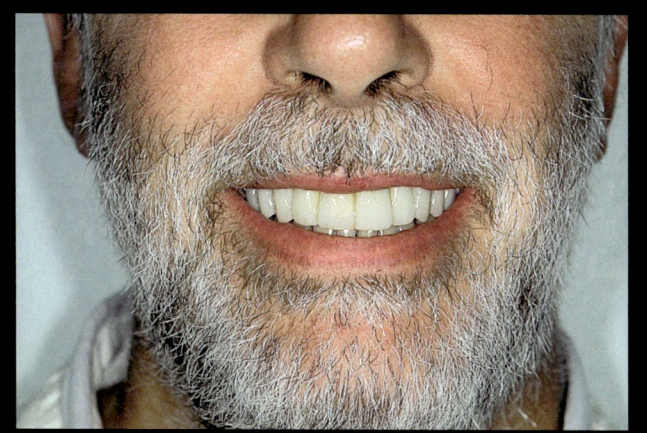

Case 2 → continues on page 317

CLINIC—POSITIONING THE PROVISIONAL

REHABILITATING A SINGLE ARCH

PROCEDURE

- Place the provisional inside the acetate matrix.
- Verify the intimate contact of the acetate matrix with the anatomic reference points to ensure the complete insertion of the shell.
- Use silicone paste to find interferences, and eliminate them.
- Remove the acetate matrix.
- Fit and reline the provisional, guiding the patient in CR.
- Check the occlusion, finish, and polish.

REHABILITATION OF TWO ARCHES
POSITIONING IN THE ORAL CAVITY

If both arches have to be rehabilitated (Figs 2-16a to 2-16c), the clinician can proceed with fitting and relining the provisional restoration in the same way as described for the rehabilitation of just one arch.

Evaluating and eliminating interferences The clinician should check the fit of the two provisional restorations, guided by the acetate indices. Since these are extended up to the anatomic reference points, the transparent stents already used in the tooth preparation phase are useful for checking the correct positioning of the provisional restorations fitted inside them (Figs 2-16d to 2-16g).

Incomplete fit of the index informs the clinician that interferences exist between the provisional restorations and the abutments; these interferences may be attributable to undersizing and/or to the inadequacy of the acrylic resin shell. Such imprecisions can be highlighted and subsequently eliminated using silicone paste. Special attention must be paid to any interferences found in the interproximal areas and in those areas where teeth are to be extracted. Any corrections that are necessary to make shell fitting easier should be made inside the shell to avoid forced modification of the dental preparations. Once the provisional restoration has been relined, the correct shell insertion allows the clinician to minimize the adjustments necessary to guarantee adequate occlusal stability.

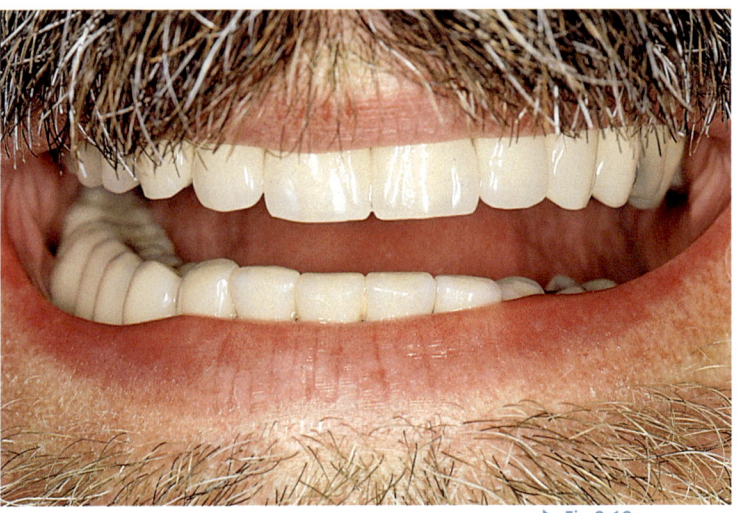

> Fig 2-16a

→ ...from page 139

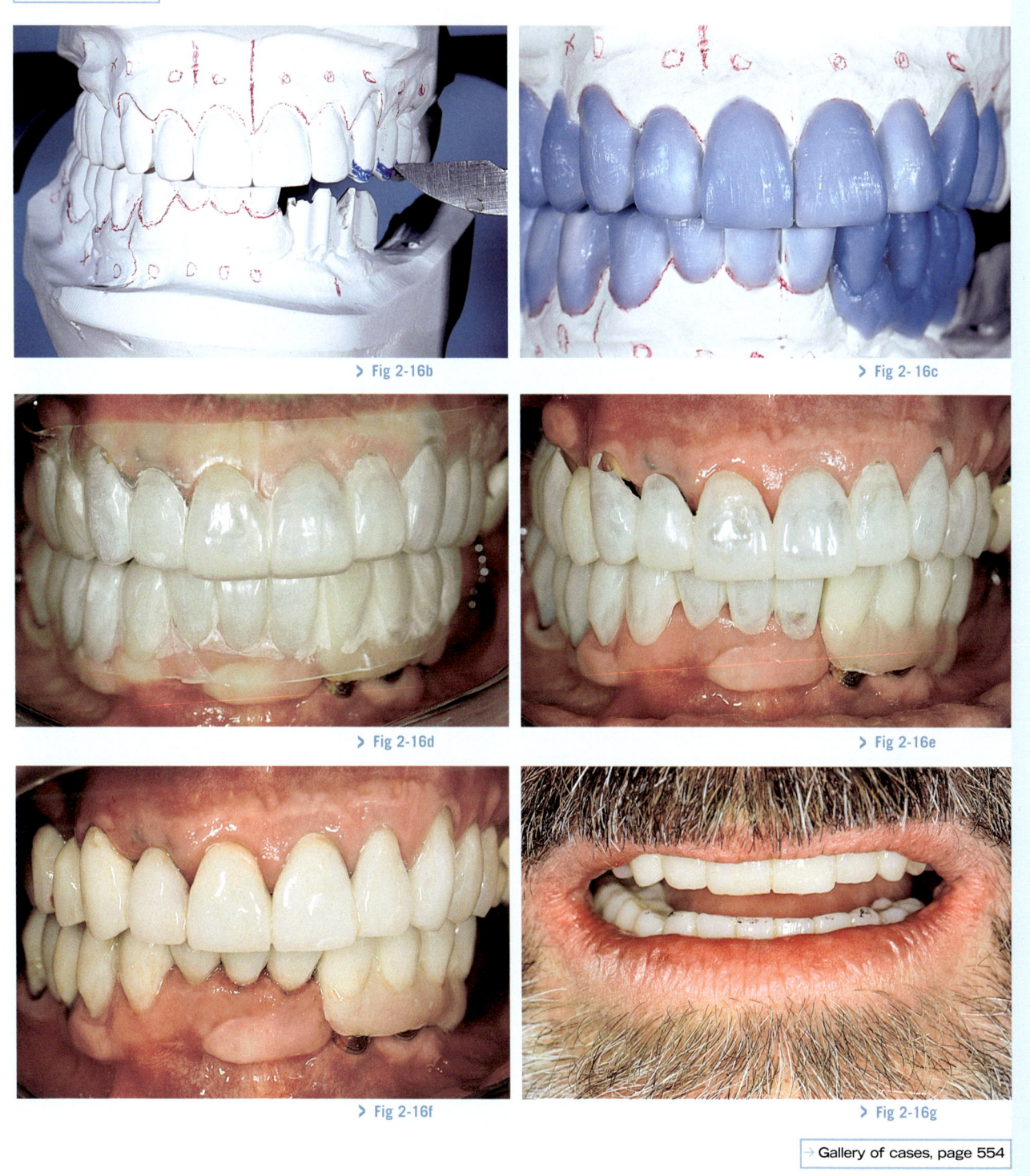

> Fig 2-16b

> Fig 2-16c

> Fig 2-16d

> Fig 2-16e

> Fig 2-16f

> Fig 2-16g

→ Gallery of cases, page 554

FIG 16 The patient complains of a general dissatisfaction with the prosthetic rehabilitation carried out in another office. *(a)* At the visit, and during a deeper examination of the case, the prosthesis reveals a lack of esthetic-functional integration. *(b and c)* After mounting the casts on the articulator using the facebow, the technician first makes the diagnostic wax-up based on the indications received in the laboratory checklist, followed by the provisional restoration, which is a faithful copy of the wax-up. *(d)* Once the two provisional rehabilitations are placed in the mouth, the clinician tests their correct insertion with the aid of the acetate indices. *(e)* When the transparent stents are removed, the shells, which fit passively, are moved into the correct position by guiding the patient in CR. *(f)* If parts of cervical areas are not completely covered by the shell, the excesses can be removed in the relining phase, and this marginal deficit is then filled with the re-margining technique (see page 200). *(g)* The relined and re-margined provisional restoration shows satisfactory esthetic-functional integration and a noticeable improvement in the occlusal plane.

Fitting guided by occlusion Once the indices have been removed, the clinician should verify the correct extension of the cervical limits of the provisional restorations beyond the preparation margin (Figs 2-17a to 2-17o).

When the absence of any interference has been confirmed and the patient has been guided into CR, prior to relining, the arches are temporarily stabilized with silicone paste to allow the clinician to properly check the CO and the suitability of the alterations made from both the esthetic and functional viewpoints.

Normally, the VDO is checked using the dentogingival border as a reference. This can prove difficult with the provisional restorations fitted, because in the MIT technique, the tooth margin is covered by the widened design of the shell. Therefore, the VDO should be measured with the provisional restoration first on the cast and then in the mouth (Fig 2-17p). If the decision is made to leave the VDO unchanged, it should be roughly 1 mm higher than the patient's original VDO. This discrepancy is determined by the marginal overextension of each arch (approximately 0.5 mm) created deliberately using the MIT technique. Maintaining the maxillary provisional restoration in position with silicone paste, the mandibular provisional restoration is relined, again by guiding the patient into CR. Once polymerization has occurred, the mandibular provisional restoration is maintained in position to proceed with relining of the maxillary provisional restoration in the same way. The sequence described above minimizes the alterations that the clinician will have to make to optimize the occlusal contacts in CO and in excursive movements (Figs 2-17q to 2-17s).

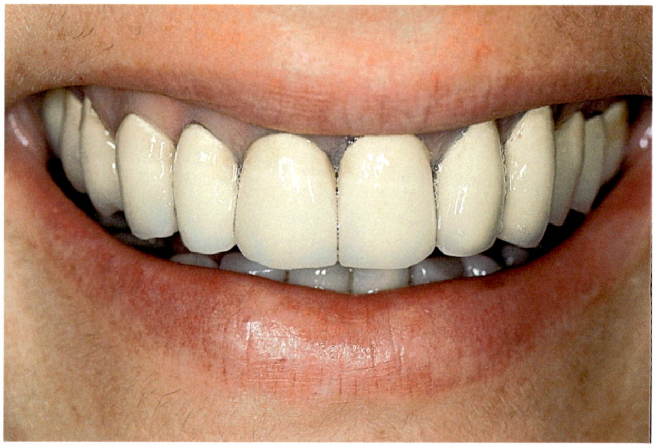

> Fig 2-17a

FIG 17 *(a and b)* About 10 years before this examination the patient underwent orthodontic treatment that preceded the prosthetic rehabilitation of both arches. *(c)* The full-mouth radiographic series shows significant root resorption in many teeth and the presence of excessively sized posts in the anterosuperior sector. *(d and e)* The intraoral lateral views demonstrate an unsatisfactory integration of the restorations, which has driven the patient to seek new treatment. *(f to i)* The same views of the diagnostic wax-up make it possible to see the esthetic-functional alterations planned, then punctually reproduced in the provisional restorations constructed through the MIT.

CASE 3

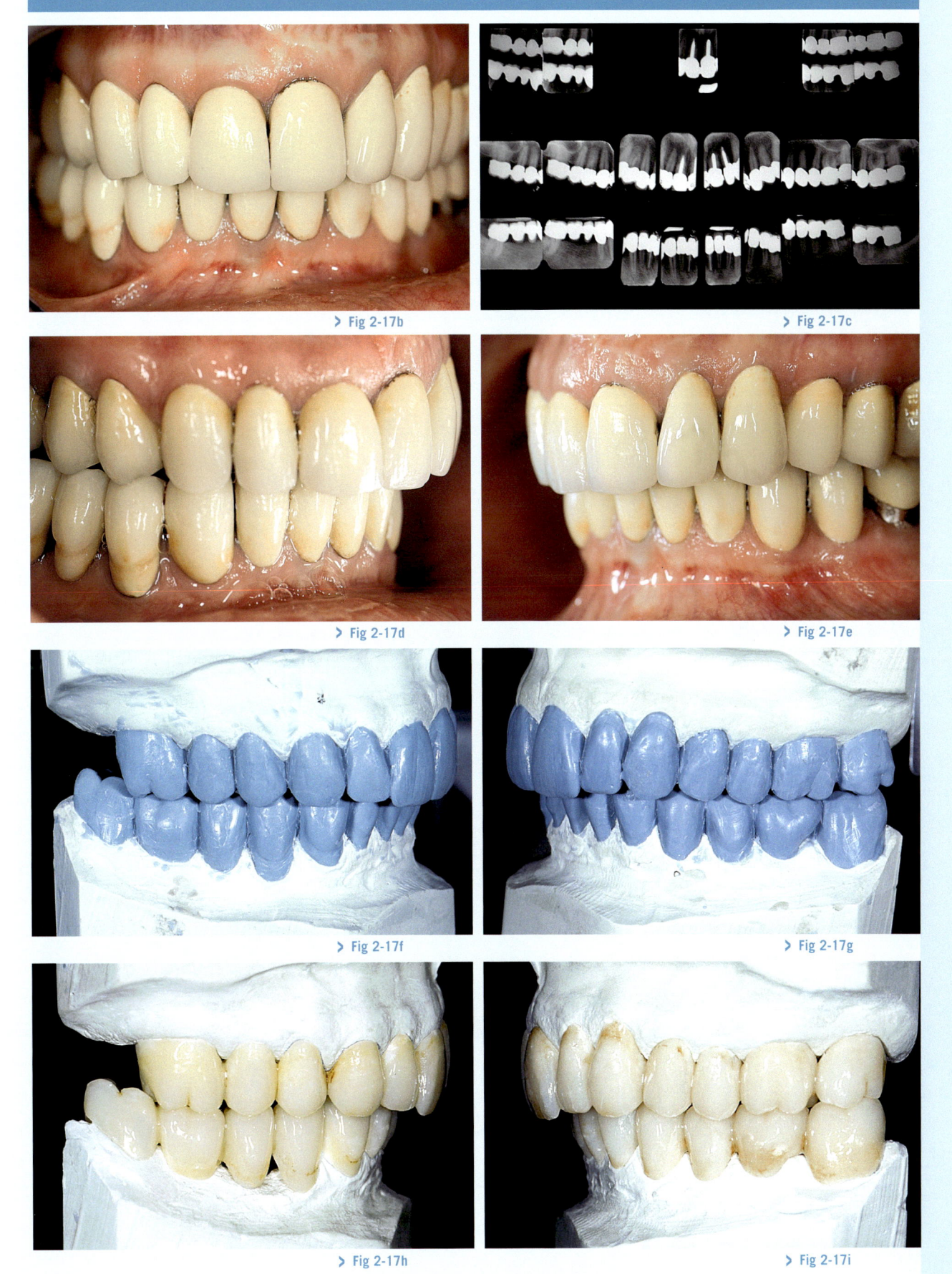

> Fig 2-17b

> Fig 2-17c

> Fig 2-17d

> Fig 2-17e

> Fig 2-17f

> Fig 2-17g

> Fig 2-17h

> Fig 2-17i

185

> Fig 2-17j

> Fig 2-17k

> Fig 2-17l

> Fig 2-17m

> Fig 2-17n

> Fig 2-17o

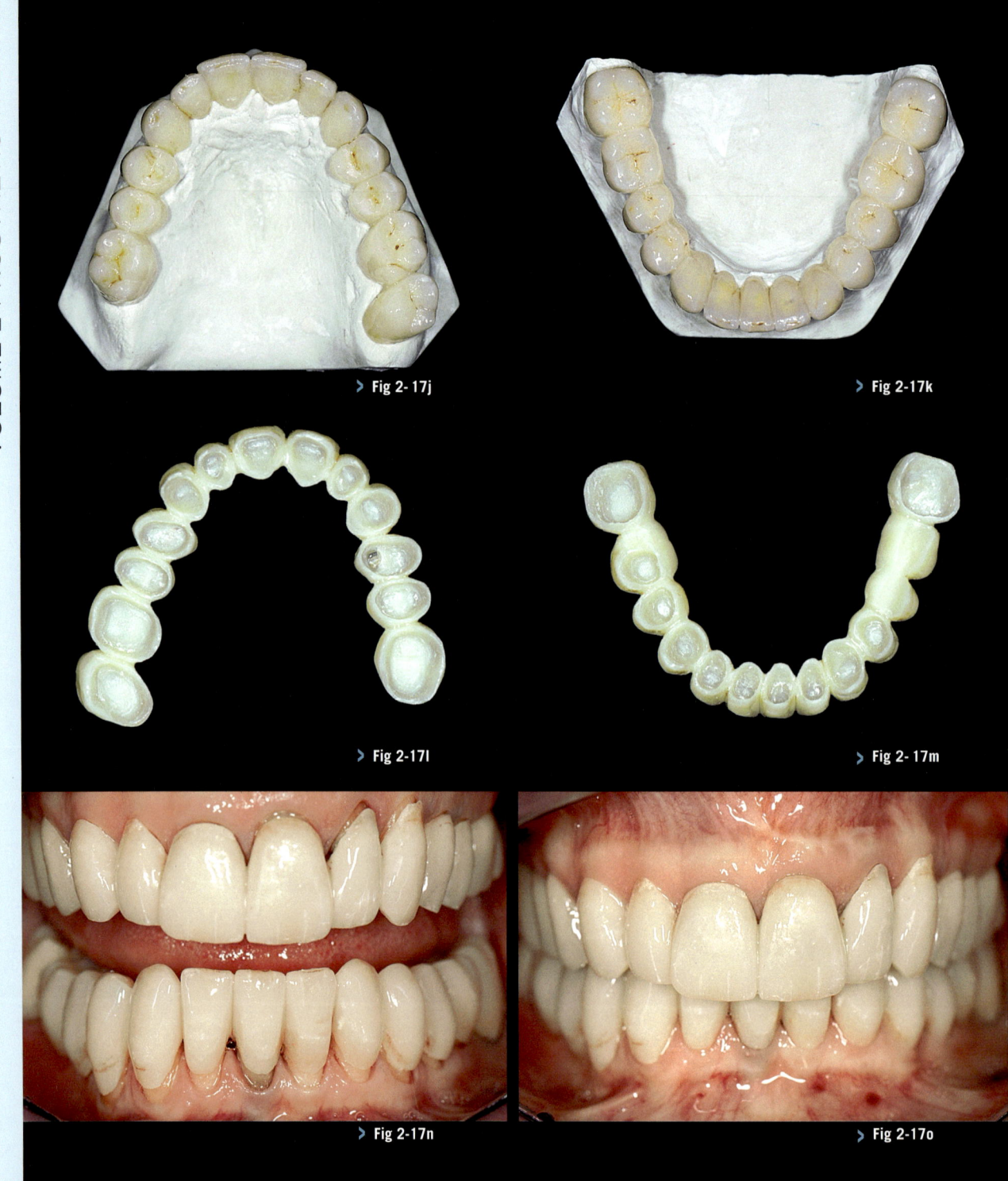

FIG 17 *(j and k)* The occlusal view of the provisional restoration on the stone casts reveals the new occlusal anatomy created. *(l and m)* Upon receipt of the acrylic resin shells, the clinician proceeds to position them in the mouth. *(n and o)* The view of the provisional restorations not yet fully fitted, and the following view in which they are completely inserted by guiding the patient in CR, make it possible to verify complete coverage of the preparation margins due to the cervical overextension and the perfect intercuspation of the two shells in CO. *(p)* After relining, the VDO is checked, which should confirm what was found with the provisional restoration positioned on the stone casts. *(q)* The good occlusal stability and satisfactory overall integration achieved by the provisional restorations can be observed 3 months after fitting, even if there is a height difference in the anterosuperior gingival margins that will later be corrected with surgical-periodontal therapy. *(r and s)* After the provisional restorations are glazed when the associated therapies are carried out, the congruity of the anterior guidance is once more evaluated, which allows adequate disocclusion of the posterior sectors both in the lateral and in the anterior movements.

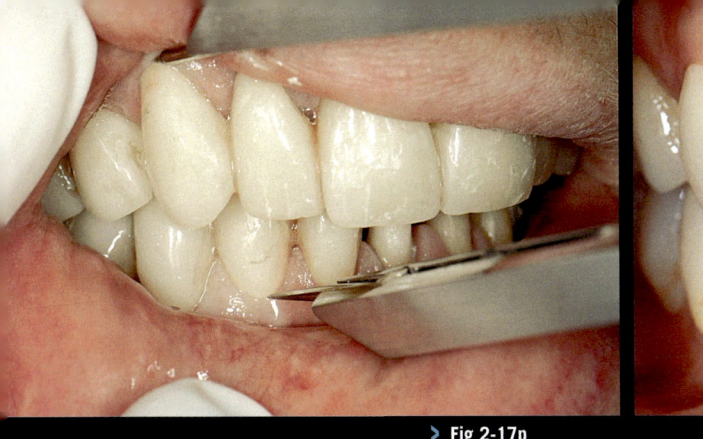

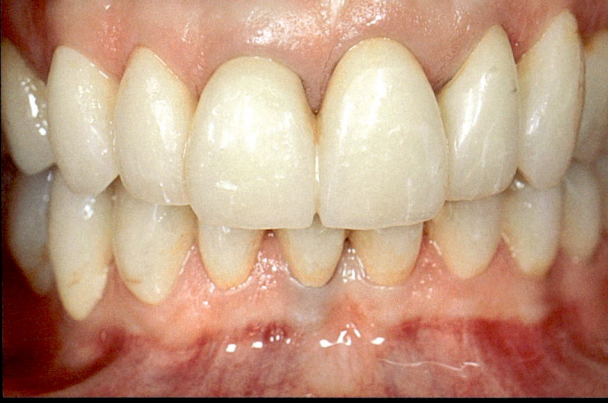

> Fig 2-17p

> Fig 2-17q

> Fig 2-17r

> Fig 2-17s

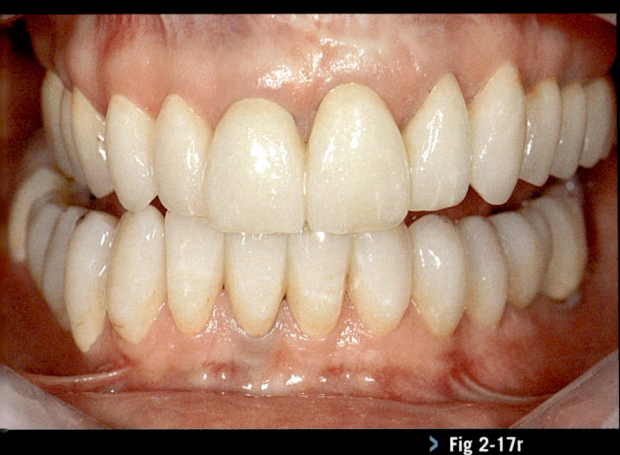

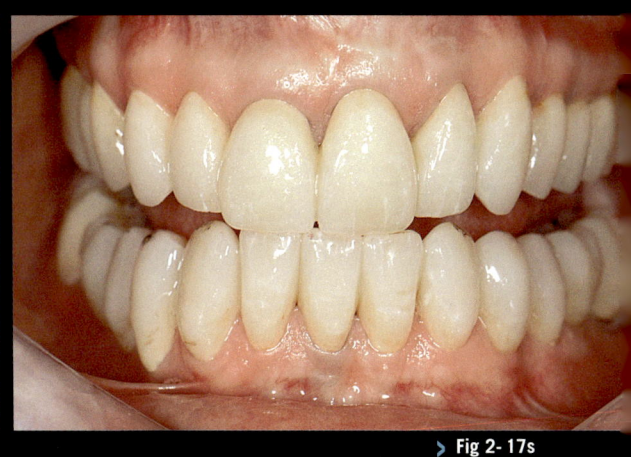

Case 3 →continues on page 295

CLINIC—POSITIONING THE PROVISIONAL

REHABILITATING TWO ARCHES

PROCEDURE

- Place the provisionals inside the acetate matrices.
- Verify the intimate contact of the acetate matrix with the anatomic reference points to ensure the complete insertion of the two shells.
- Use silicone paste to find interferences, and eliminate them.
- Remove the acetate matrices.
- Stabilize the maxillary provisional in CR with silicone paste.
- Reline the mandibular provisional.
- Keep the mandibular provisional relined and proceed with relining of the maxillary provisional.
- Check the occlusion, finish, and polish.

CENTERING DEVICE
FACILITATED INSERTION GUIDE

We have seen how the MIT allows easier fitting of the shell compared with the traditional indirect technique because of the particular overextension of the cervical third that facilitates passive shell insertion. On the one hand, the resulting relatively free movement of the provisional restoration allows the clinician to position it precisely in the mouth, owing to the correct intercuspation created in the shell while the patient is guided into CR. On the other hand, the less experienced clinician may lack confidence in orientating the rehabilitation correctly in the oral cavity and in fitting the acrylic shells at the given VDO. This is especially true in cases involving rehabilitation of both arches. For this reason it can be useful to make use of a special acrylic resin support (centering device) extended to the anatomic areas (palate, retromolar trigone, tuberosities, etc) and joined with the provisional restoration positioned on the cast with a drop of cyanacrylate.

Compared with the acetate index, which could serve the same purpose, the centering device is decidedly more stable because of its greater rigidity, and it ensures excellent precision in positioning the provisional restoration. Unlike the transparent stent, it allows all excess relining material to be easily removed and also makes it possible to check the occlusion by allowing the patient to be brought into CR without causing interference between the occlusal surfaces.

In addition to placing the provisional restorations in the correct position with extreme ease, this technique also makes it possible to see the VDO, as set on the casts in the articulator, replicated in the mouth, which is of great help to many clinicians in more complex rehabilitations (Fig 2-18).

FIG 18 *(a and b)* The patient requires complete rehabilitation of both arches to replace old incongruous prosthetic work, re-establish the correct occlusal planes, and close up the gaps between the teeth. *(c to k)* After mounting the casts in the articulator, the technician makes the diagnostic wax-up and, on a stone cast taken from it, carries out the preparations following the new tooth arrangement set out in the wax-up. *(l to n)* The provisional restorations are then fabricated using the MIT.

...from page 133

> Fig 2-18a

> Fig 2-18b

> Fig 2-18c

> Fig 2- 18d

> Fig 2-18e

> Fig 2-18f

> Fig 2-18g

> Fig 2-18h

> Fig 2-18i

> Fig 2-18j

> Fig 2-18k

> Fig 2-18l

> Fig 2-18m

> Fig 2-18n

189

> Fig 2-18o

> Fig 2-18p

> Fig 2-18q

> Fig 2-18r

> Fig 2-18s

> Fig 2-18t

> Fig 2-18u

> Fig 2-18v

> Fig 2-18w

> Fig 2- 18x

> Fig 2-18y

FIG 18 *(o to t)* To aid the clinician in ideal placement of the provisional restorations, an acrylic support is constructed in the laboratory, extended to the anatomic areas. This, along with the acrylic shell made before the teeth are prepared, allows the same position from the articulator to be found in the mouth. *(u to y)* This centering device and the provisional restoration must be joined together with a drop of cyanoacrylate, preferably at the intermediate teeth, to make removal of the excess relining material easier. *(z)* View of the provisional restoration–centering device union in situ in CO. *(aa)* The stability of the position achieved by the acrylic shells, although not yet relined, is borne out by their lack of mobility even during excursive movements. *(bb and cc)* Relining then takes place, and afterward the provisional restoration is removed from the oral cavity of the relined union. At this point, the provisional restorations are detached from the centering device to proceed with finishing. *(dd and ee)* The intraoral view in CO and in protrusive movement demonstrates the good level of overall integration achieved.

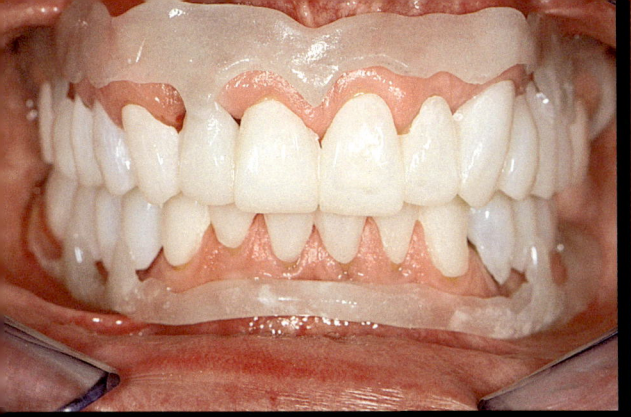

> Fig 2-18z

> Fig 2-18aa

> Fig 2-18bb

> Fig 2-18cc

> Fig 2-18dd

> Fig 2-18ee

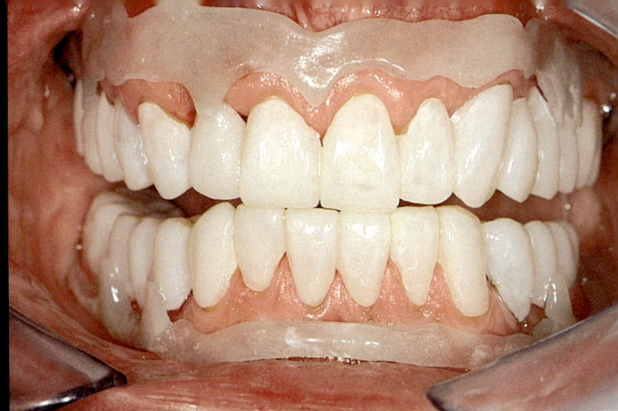

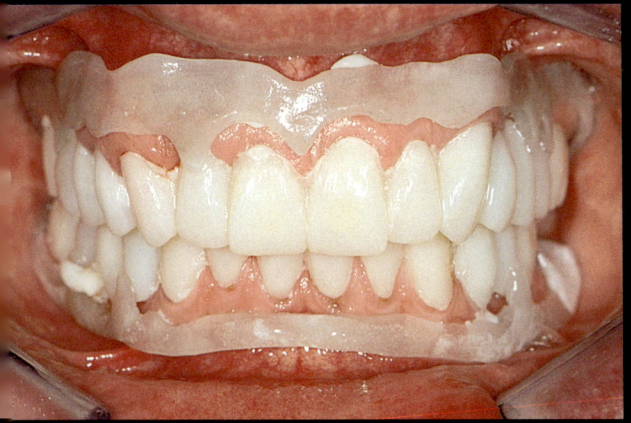

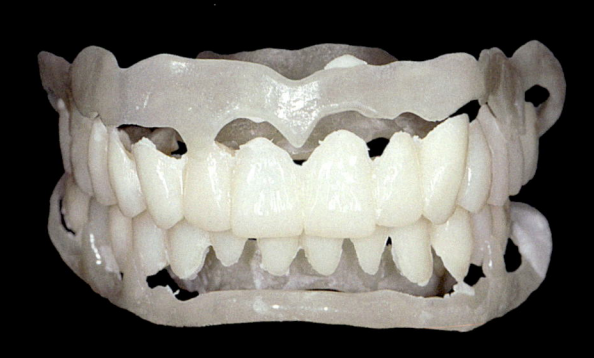

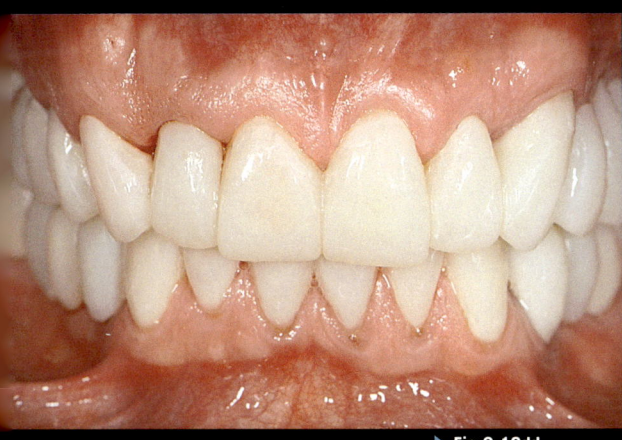

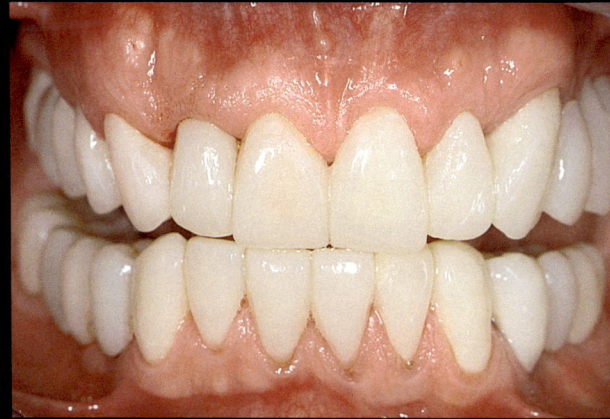

CENTERING DEVICE

PROCEDURE

- Take an extended impression at the anatomic reference points.
- Construct the provisional on the cast.
- Make the centering device on the cast, affixing it to the provisional.
- Fit and reline the provisional under the guidance of the centering device.
- Check the occlusion, finish, and polish.

RELINING

The provisional restoration is normally relined in the mouth one or more times.[66-68] A shell created with the indirect technique, either before or after the teeth are prepared, achieves a much higher marginal precision, once relined, than that of any other non-relined provisional restoration.[69-75] To read the margin correctly, it may be useful to insert retraction cords into the sulcus during relining.[1,31,76,77] After sandblasting and wetting the inside with monomer, the provisional restoration is filled with self-curing resin in a filamentous state (Figs 2-19a to 2-19c). Fitting the shell onto the abutments, which have been wetted with water, must be carried out when the acrylic resin has lost its glossy appearance (ie, in the malleable state) (Fig 2-19d). It is not advisable to cover the abutments with insulating substances (eg, petroleum jelly), which can interfere with the polymerization.

All of the excess resin that overflows the shell margin during relining can easily be removed before polymerization is complete without detachment of any relining material from the marginal area (Figs 2-19e to 2-19j). This is possible only if, as provided for in the MIT, the margins of the preparations remain inside the provisional restoration.

The plasticity of the resin during the initial relining phase allows further slight corrections to be made, if necessary, to the provisional occlusal setup. The provisional restoration is partially slipped out (2 to 3 mm) and then reinserted, while the exposed abutments are carefully and thoroughly irrigated with an air and water spray (Figs 2-19k and 2-19l). This operation, repeated every 15 to 20 seconds, tends to limit the possible repercussions caused by the exothermic reaction and the presence of free monomer to the pulp and gingival tissues.[36,37,68,78-80]

Abundant irrigation with water not only substantially limits the rise in temperature but also prolongs the working time of the relining material and allows any unwanted adhesion to the abutments or retention in undercut areas to be quickly identified, so that they can be corrected before polymerization is complete.[72]

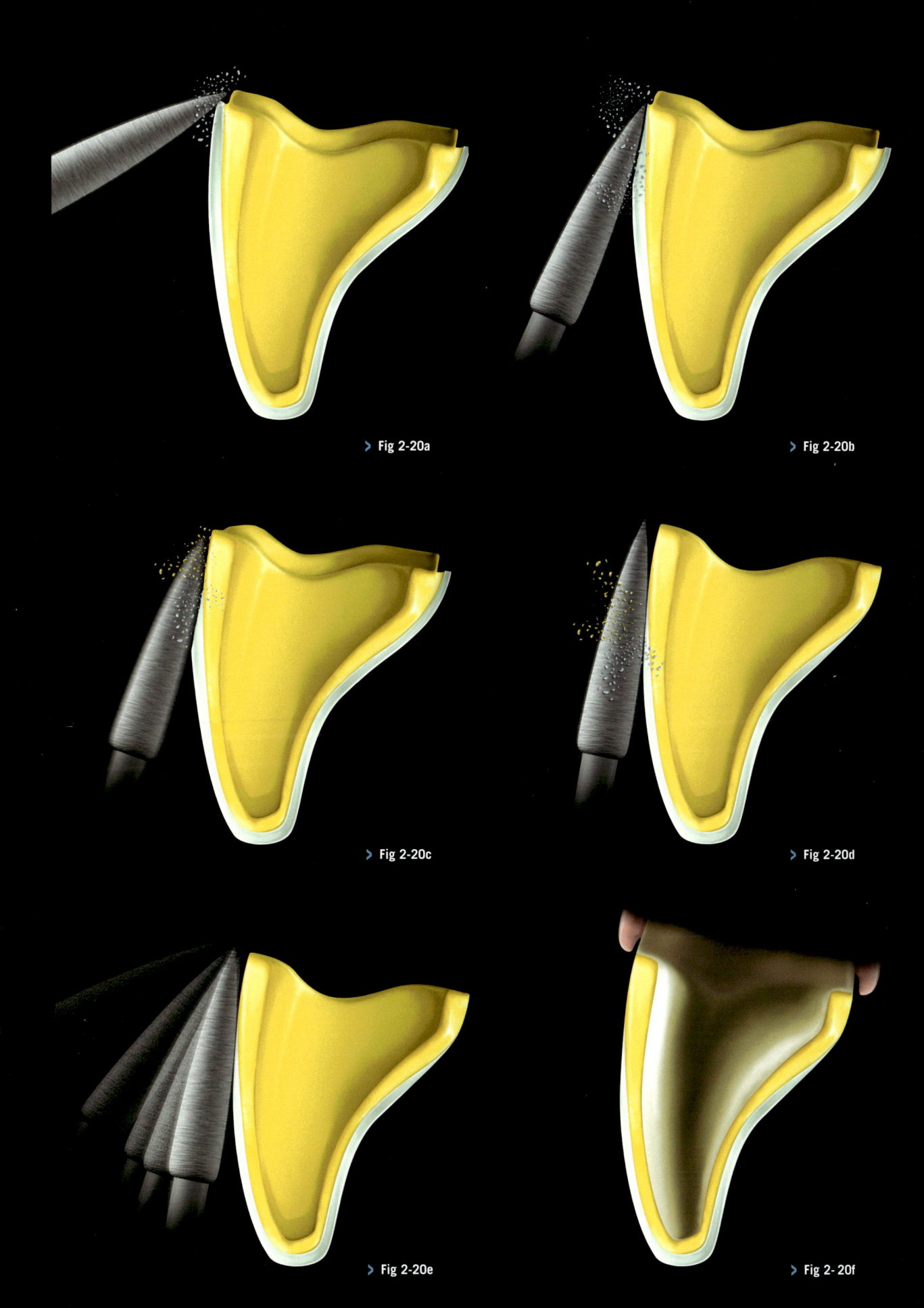

> Fig 2-20a

> Fig 2-20b

> Fig 2-20c

> Fig 2-20d

> Fig 2-20e

> Fig 2-20f

> Fig 2-20g

> Fig 2-20h

> Fig 2-20i

> Fig 2-20j

> Fig 2-20k

> Fig 2-20l

> Fig 2-20m

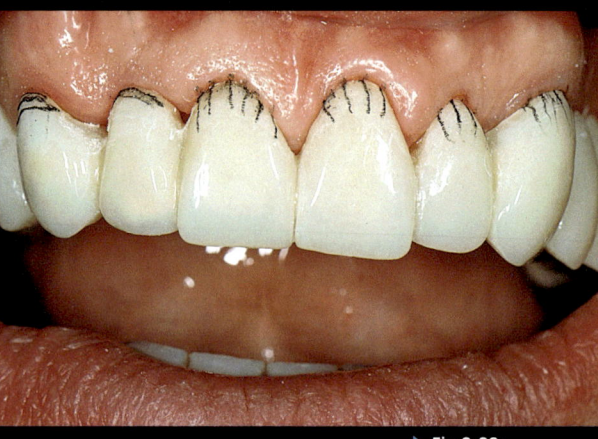

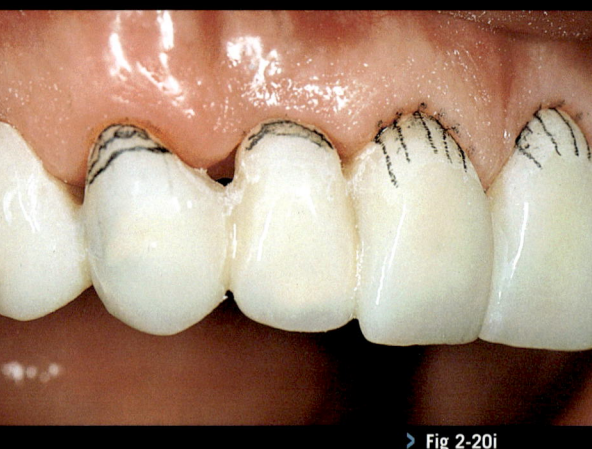

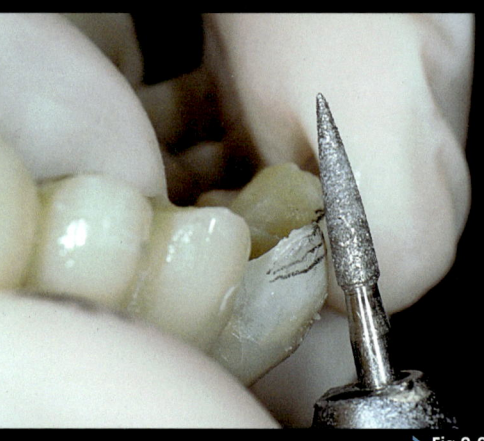

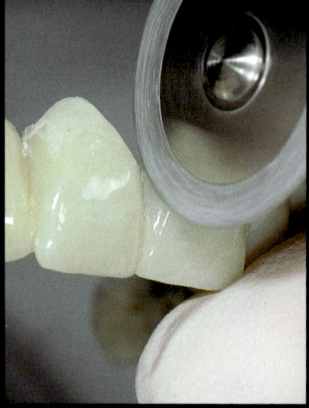

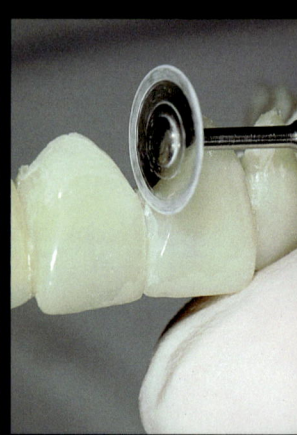

FIG 20 With the provisional restoration positioned in the mouth, any remaining horizontal overcontours are highlighted by horizontal pencil marks. *(g to j)* The emergence profile of the provisional restoration must also be checked, and its excessive convexity marked with vertical pencil lines. *(k)* After the provisional restoration is removed, the necessary corrections are made using a bur mounted on a laboratory handpiece. *(l and m)* To optimize the esthetic appearance of the anterior sector, creating ideal separation between the anterior teeth, diamond disks with a circumference suitable for that area will be used. *(n to p)* Once these corrections have been made with the provisional restoration in hand, the more expert clinician can make further improvements to the cervical contour with a bur directly in the mouth, by slightly removing and reinserting the provisional restoration on the abutments, obviously taking care to avoid creating any interference with the tooth preparations or with the surrounding periodontal structures. *(q to s)* With a sharply pointed explorer, the validity of the marginal closure and the absence of horizontal overcontours, as well as the adequacy of the emergence profile, are then checked.

> Fig 2-20n

> Fig 2-20o

> Fig 2-20p

> Fig 2-20q

> Fig 2-20r

> Fig 2-20s

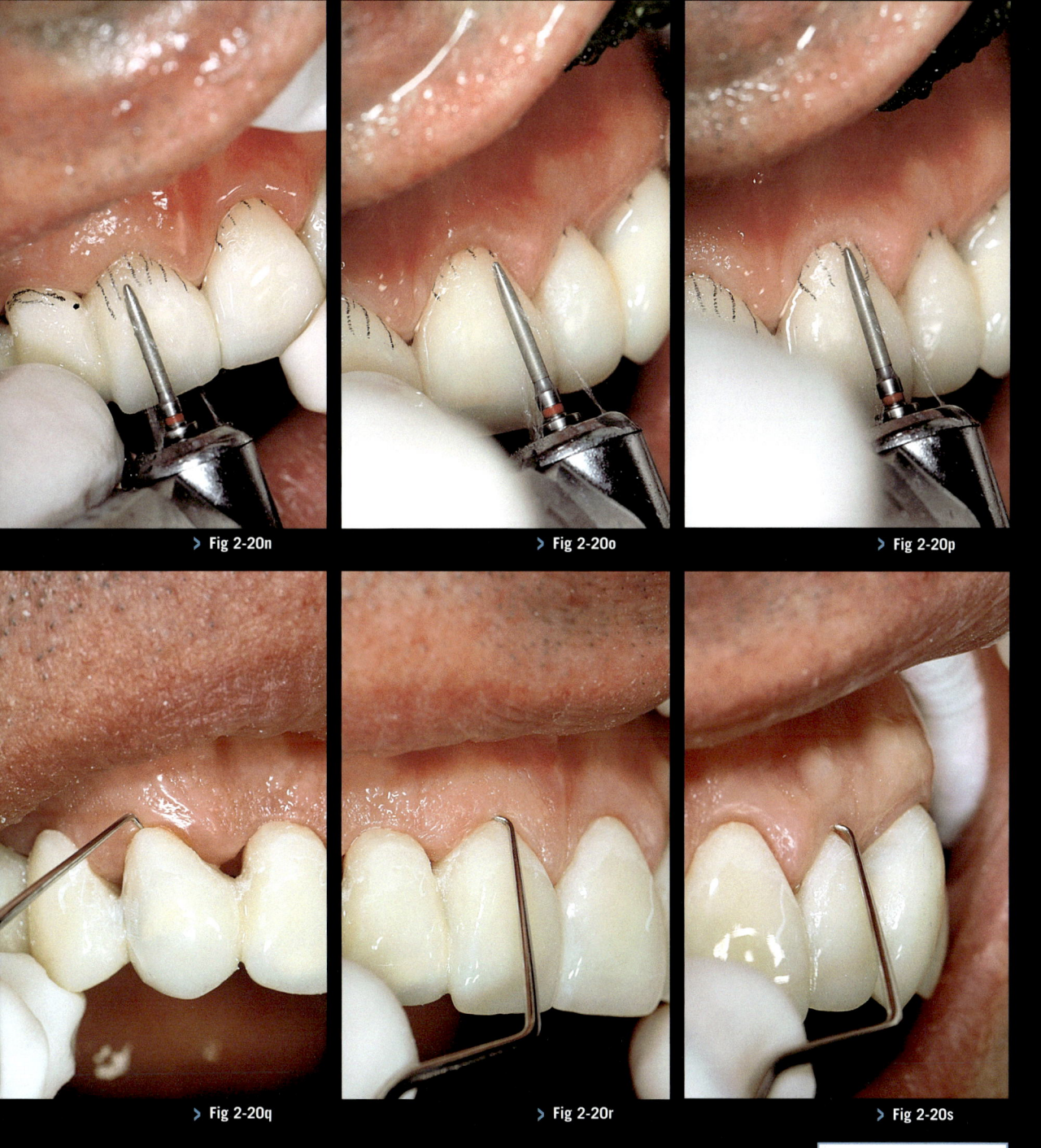

→continues on page 227

FINISHING

PROCEDURE

- Identify the preparation margin.
- Remove the cervical overextension up to the finishing line.
- Check the fit in the mouth and use a pencil to mark any horizontal and vertical.
- Correct the provisional with laboratory burs and rotary handpieces.

RE-MARGINING

SALT AND PEPPER TECHNIQUE

If, after finishing, there are marginal discrepancies limited to certain specific areas, the provisional restoration can be "re-margined" using the *salt and pepper technique* (Fig 2-21a). After the area to be remargined has been sandblasted with the restoration in its exact position, a creamy mixture is applied by dipping a brush in monomer and adding some of the acrylic powder. Given the hydrophobic properties of methacrylate, it is advisable to dry the area to be treated before applying the acrylic resin. Once complete polymerization has taken place, the margin is finished and then polished.

FLOW COMPOSITES

Because of their ease of use, light-curing flow composites are increasingly being used in place of the salt and pepper technique for re-margining (Figs 2-21a and 2-21b). Their use is especially advantageous for multiple imperfections at the marginal level. Thanks to the extremely rapid polymerization of flow composites, the clinician can re-margin the provisional restoration several times within a very short period until perfect closure is achieved. After an initial preliminary polymerization in the mouth (approximately 10 seconds), the provisional restoration is taken out and the process is completed outside the oral cavity. To avoid separation, it is best to choose a flow composite with a level of elasticity similar to that of the acrylic resin used for constructing and relining the provisional restoration. An adhesive may be useful for this as well as for sandblasting the area to be remargined. To finish the areas to be treated, it is critical to use a diamond bur instead of tungsten carbide to minimize the vibrations that could cause the two materials to separate (Figs 2-21c to 2-21e).

FIG 21 *(a and b)* Where a localized marginal deficit (shortening, undercontour, chipping, etc) exists, new relining is not necessary. Instead, a syringe of the light-curing flow composite can be applied to the area in question, while the provisional restoration remains in situ. After a preliminary polymerization (approximately 10 seconds), the provisional restoration is removed from the oral cavity and the light curing completed outside. The clinician must take great care to ensure that the light covers the whole area. *(c to e)* By gradually changing the angle of the bur to eliminate the horizontal step first and then optimize the emergence profile, in a short time it is possible to obtain an optimal coronal contour and marginal fit.

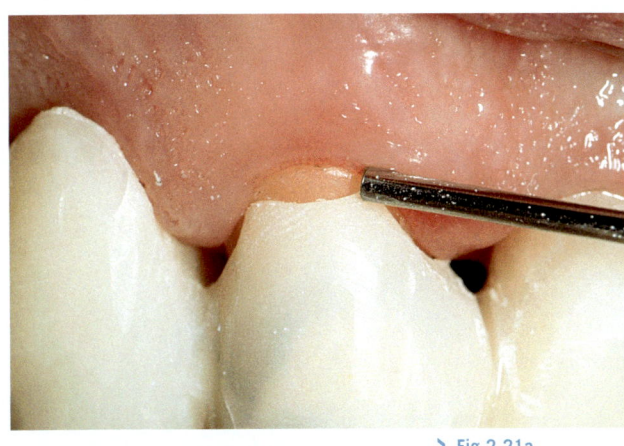

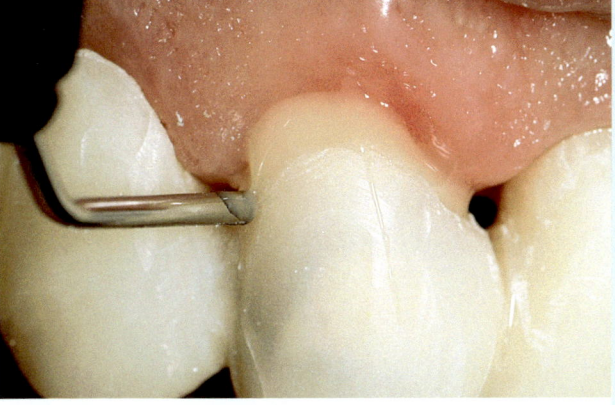

> Fig 2-21a

> Fig 2-21b

> Fig 2-21c

> Fig 2-21d

> Fig 2-21e

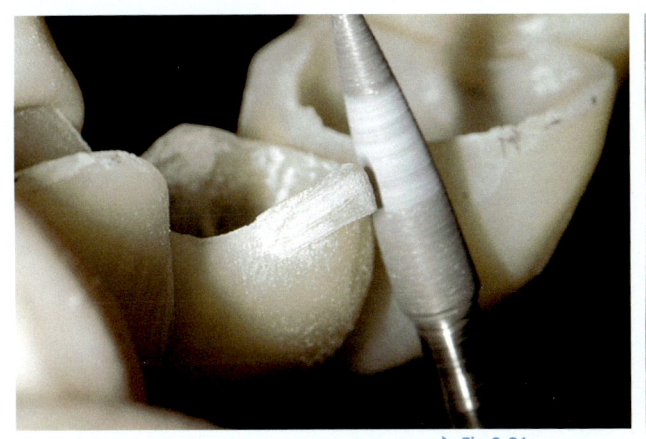

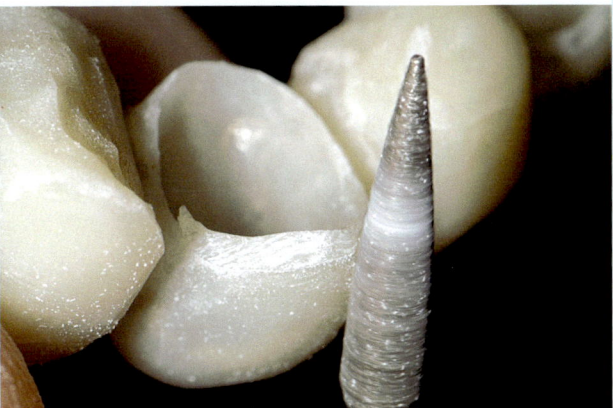

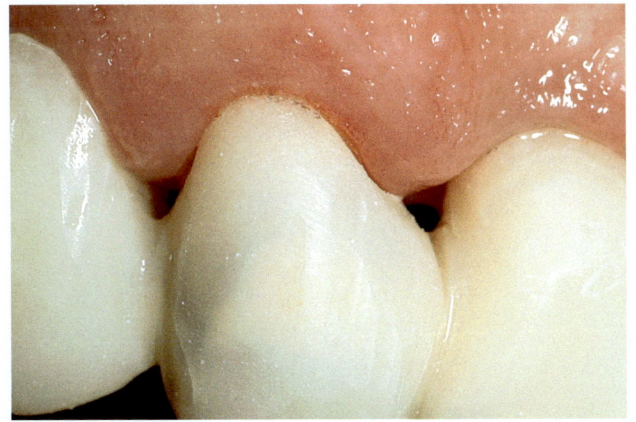

RE-MARGINING

PROCEDURE

- Sandblast the area to be re-margined.
- Position the provisional correctly in situ.
- Cover the area to be re-margined with *flow* composite.
- Complete preliminary light curing in the mouth (approximately 10 seconds).
- Complete final light curing outside the oral cavity (approximately 15–20 seconds).

COLORING AND GLAZING

The stability of the acrylic resin used to construct the shell in the laboratory[84] (Ivocron) and for relining[81] (Coldpac) proves to be an important factor in guaranteeing the patient adequate esthetics, especially in cases where the provisional restoration must remain in the mouth for a prolonged period. Although many acrylic resins now contain stabilizers, contact with pigments derived from the consumption of substances that color (eg, tea and coffee) can nevertheless bring color changes caused by the intrinsic porosity of the material used. In this regard the methyl methacrylates have proved to be the most stable group and the least subject to discoloration.[84,85]

The particular thinness of the shell means that the final color of the provisional restoration is determined not just by the color chosen in the laboratory but also by the color of the resin used in relining, which is therefore chosen by the clinician according to the final chromatic appearance desired. To optimize the esthetic appearance of the provisional restoration (Figs 2-22a to 2-22e) after it has been finished and polished with a polishing rubber and pumice paste, surface colorings can be added and then fixed with a specific acrylic paint (Palaseal, Heraeus-Kulzer)[86]; polymerization requires the use of an ultraviolet oven (Fig 2-22f). The glaze is normally applied to the interproximal areas as well, which are usually difficult to reach with polishing rubbers, while the clinician is very careful not to create an excessive thickness that could affect the ability to cleanse in these spaces. The pleasing esthetic result achieved, although very much appreciated by patients, is not long-lasting (Figs 2-22g and 2-22h). It is therefore advisable to use this solution when the provisional restoration will remain in the mouth for a relatively short time (2 to 4 weeks), or in cases where there is a chance to repeat the application during periodic removals for associated therapies (eg, endodontic treatment, periodontal surgery, implant placement). In provisional restorations where units on prosthetic abutments alternate with pontics, with significant variation in the thickness of the acrylic resin, one method of coloring the basic shade of the provisional restoration consists of adding acrylic pigments to the relining paste during mixing to alter the color (Figs 2-23a to 2-23m). Another useful expedient is that of emptying the intermediate units to unify the crown thicknesses. It is then possible to fill these units with the same amount of relining material, which gives all of the units of the shell the same coloring.

FIG 22 *(a and b)* The patient, who has a low smile line, wishes to replace the old restorations in the anterosuperior sector. *(c and d)* After the provisional restoration is fabricated in the laboratory, it is positioned in the mouth to check the fit. *(e)* Relining takes place by having the patient close in MI and eliminating the excess resin. *(f)* After it is finished, the provisional restoration is given surface coloring, fixed by a thin layer of glaze. *(g and h)* When initially positioned in the mouth the provisional restoration looks especially glossy, but after just 2 months the shiny surface, obtained by using acrylic paint, is noticeably reduced.

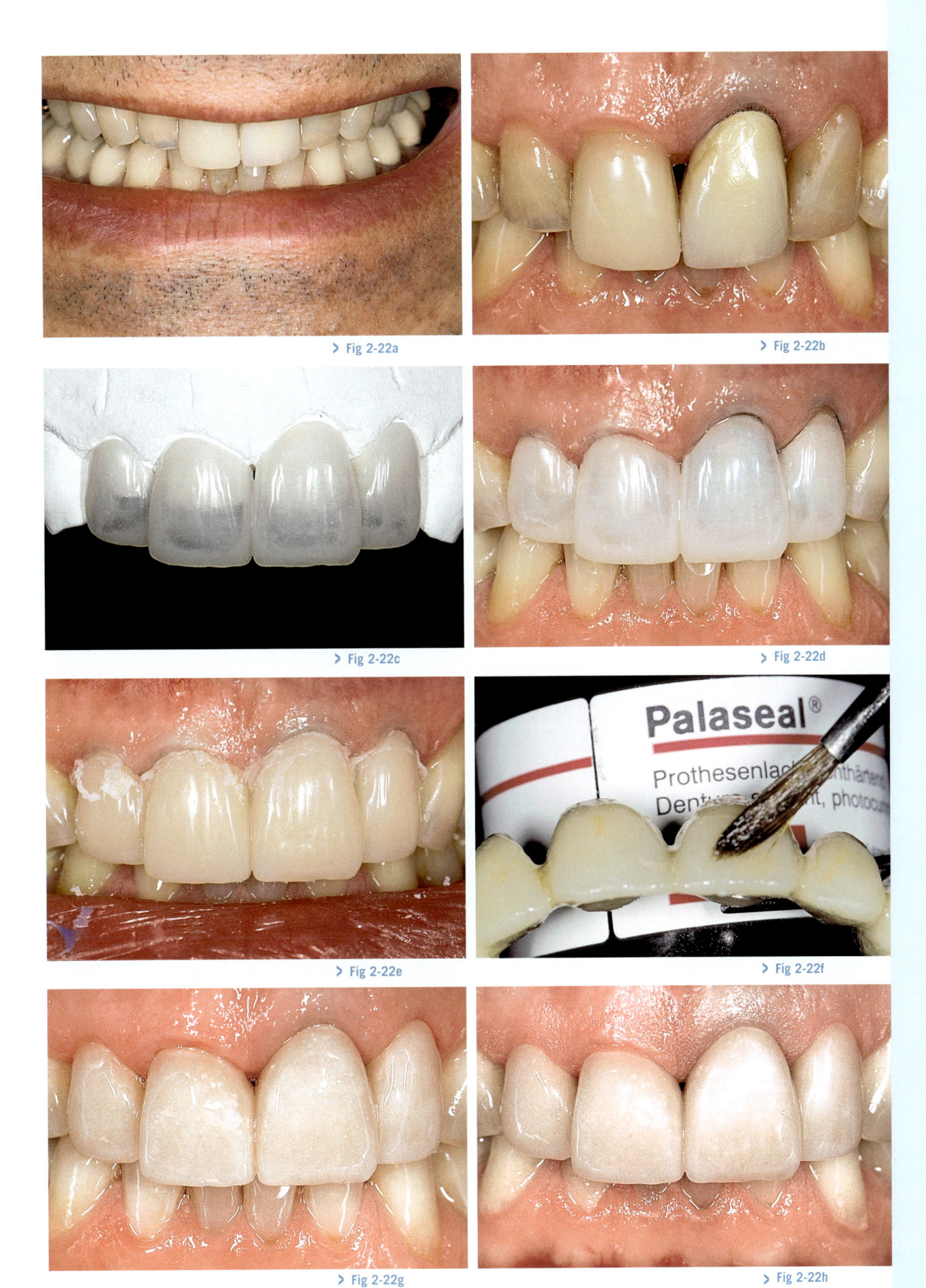

> Fig 2-22a

> Fig 2-22b

> Fig 2-22c

> Fig 2-22d

> Fig 2-22e

> Fig 2-22f

> Fig 2-22g

> Fig 2-22h

> Fig 2-23a

> Fig 2-23b

> Fig 2-23c

> Fig 2-23d

> Fig 2-23e

> Fig 2-23f

> Fig 2-23g

> Fig 2-23h

> Fig 2-23i

> Fig 2-23j

> Fig 2-23k

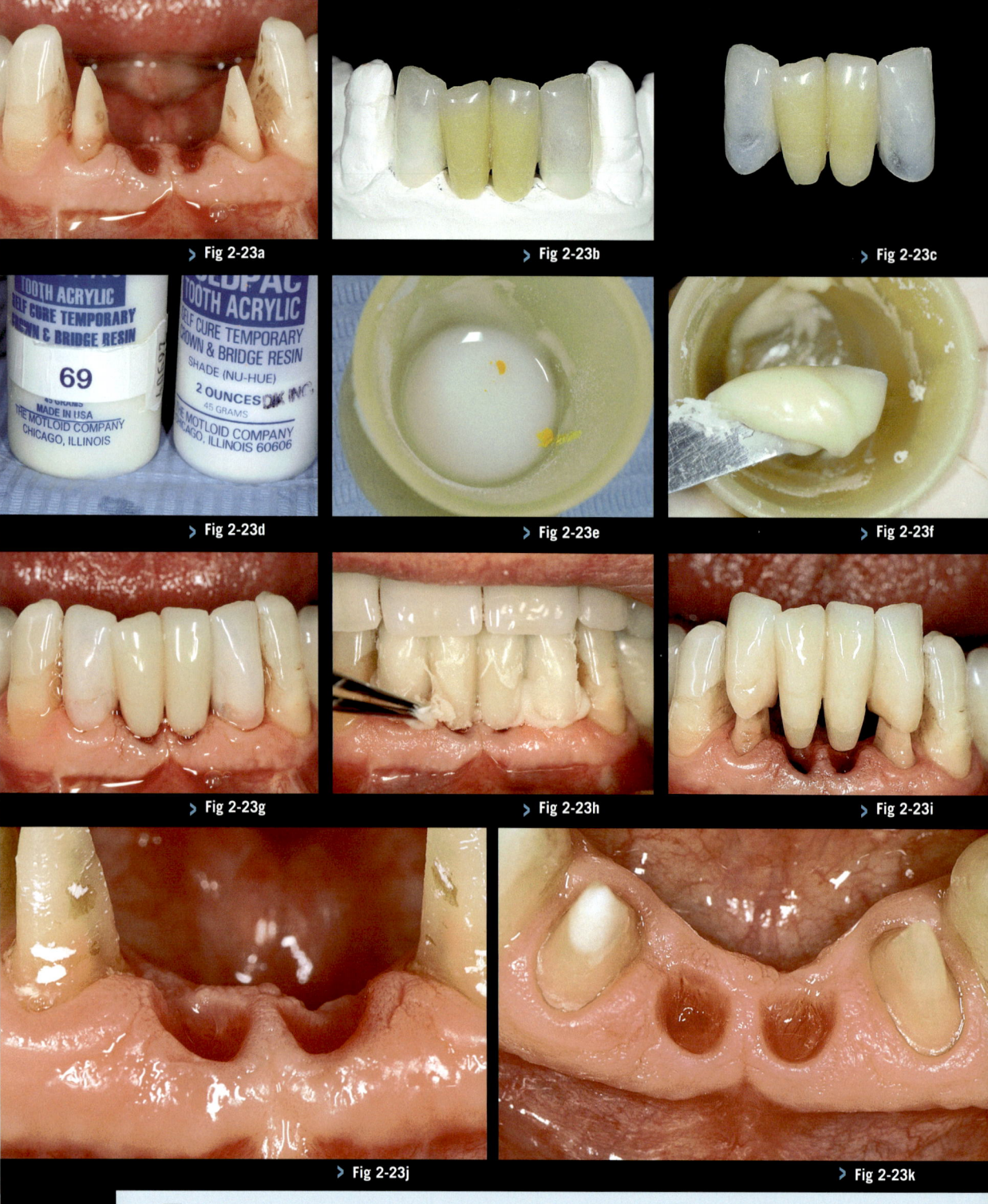

FIG 23 *(a)* The patient needs the mandibular central incisors replaced. *(b and c)* The provisional restoration received from the laboratory shows, both on the cast and when removed, a significant chromatic discrepancy between the central and lateral incisors, which can be attributed to the relative difference in thickness of the acrylic resin between the intermediate teeth and those that will be fitted onto the abutments. *(d to f)* To overcome this chromatic difference, when the relining paste is mixed, superficial colors are added to the dentin and enamel areas to saturate the shading even more. *(g)* Without the relining paste, the provisional restoration in the mouth confirms the color difference between the central incisors and the laterals. *(h)* Relining is then carried out. The patient is asked to close his mouth so that the provisional restoration can reach the correct position guided by MI. *(i)* When the excess relining material has been removed, and finishing and polishing have taken place, the chromatic appearances of the four teeth are more or less identical. *(j to l)* The contour of the provisional restoration has also been appropriately designed at the extraction sites to condition the edentulous ridges and to optimize both the esthetic appearance and the biologic integration. *(m)* The final view of the definitive restorations demonstrates the satisfactory overall integration.

> Fig 2-23l

> Fig 2-23m

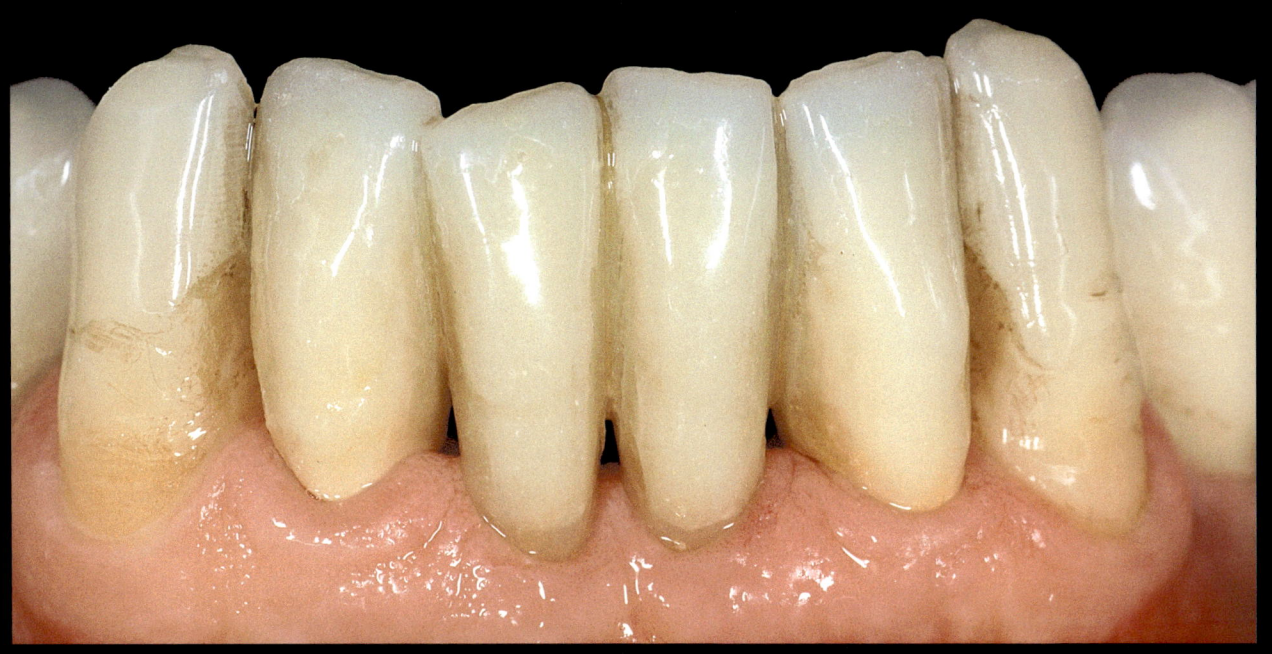

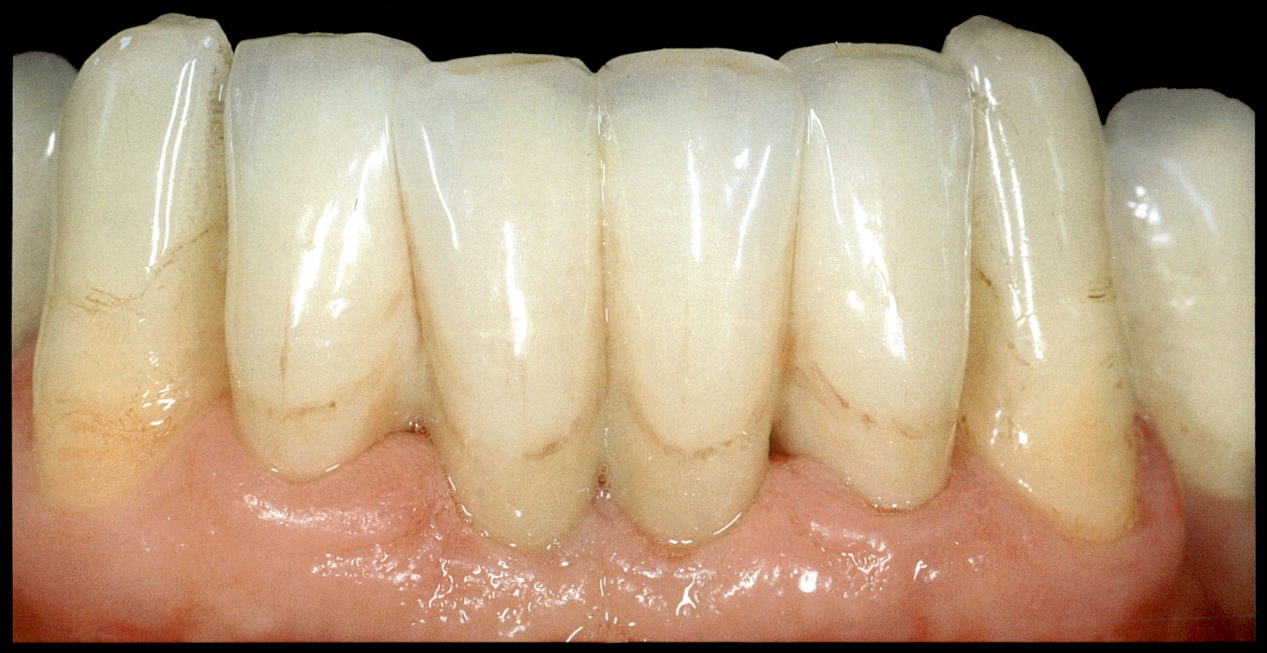

COLORING AND GLAZING

PROCEDURE

- Select the color of the relining paste to achieve the desired shade.
- Polish the exterior surface of the provisional with rubbers and pumice paste.
- Characterize the provisional with pigments and glaze it with acrylic paint.
- Repeat coloring every 2–4 weeks while the associated therapies are being carried out.

CEMENTATION

The cementation of the provisional restoration must allow for an adequate seal between the restoration and the prepared tooth, to prevent phenomena of microleakage and consequent pulp irritation.[65,87] The cements usually used for provisional restorations are based on the following:

- zinc oxide–eugenol
- eugenol-free zinc oxide
- calcium hydroxide
- methacrylate

Nonetheless, all of these cements should allow the clinician to easily remove the provisional restoration when necessary. They should also guarantee adequate stability of the restorations during normal masticatory function. The clinician's need to pursue two contrasting objectives often forces a solution of compromise, wherein a cement is chosen based on individual circumstances.

The zinc oxide–eugenol based cements are undeniably the most commonly used and are especially indicated in the presence of vital teeth because of the antibacterial properties of the eugenol, which can reduce the sensitivity of the abutments[87] (Fig 2-24a). In cases where the provisional restoration has to be relined following cementation, however, the presence of eugenol could interfere with polymerization of the acrylic.[22,88] The most widely used of these cements (TempBond, Kerr) does not seem to manifest this limitation, however.[89] Anyway, if the definitive work is to be fixed with resin-based cements, it is preferable to cement the provisional restoration with products that do not contain eugenol[88] (Fig 2-24b).

Applying colored lubricant such as petroleum jelly to the cervical area inhibits adhesion of the cement to the surface of the provisional restoration, making it easier to completely remove the excesses and reducing the time required to bring this delicate operation to an end (Figs 2-24c to 2-24h). Special care must be taken so that the petroleum jelly does not penetrate and weaken the strength of the cement.

FIG 24 *(a and b)* The most commonly used cements normally have a zinc oxide base, with or without eugenol. *(c to e)* Before proceeding with cementation, it is a good rule to apply some colored lubricant to the outside of the provisional restoration along the entire cervical contour, to make removal of excess material as easy as possible. *(f)* This process minimizes the risk of leaving cement residue inside the gingival sulcus, promoting adequate biologic integration of the provisional restoration, as confirmed by the view of the restorations 2 weeks after temporary cementation. *(g and h)* With the provisional restoration removed, it is possible to see the healthy condition of the gingival tissue, which has been maintained due to ideal margins and contours and accurate removal of excess cement.

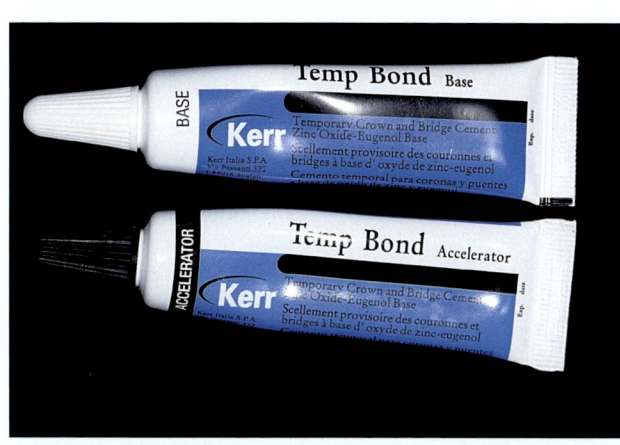

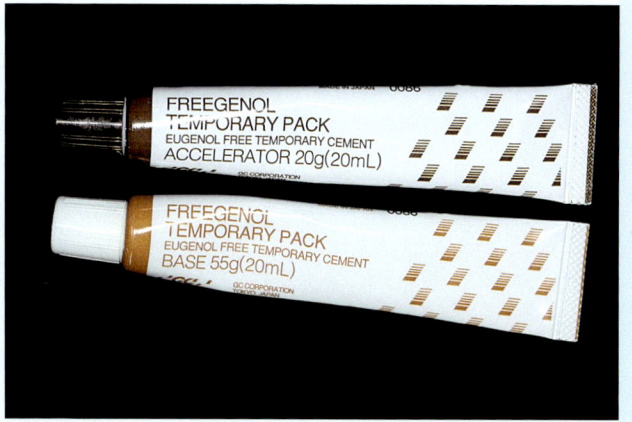

> Fig 2-24a

> Fig 2-24b

> Fig 2-24c

> Fig 2-24d

> Fig 2-24e

> Fig 2-24f

> Fig 2-24g

> Fig 2-24h

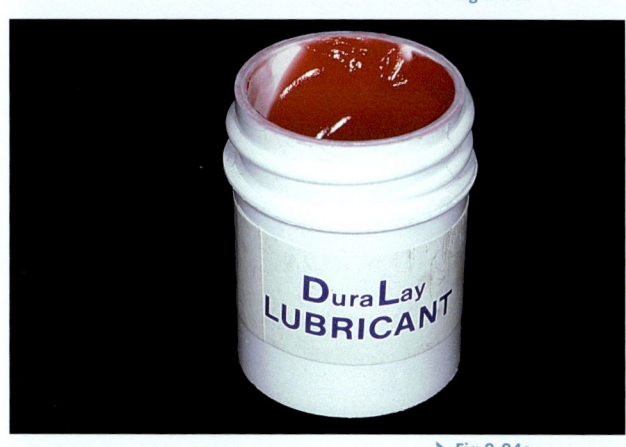

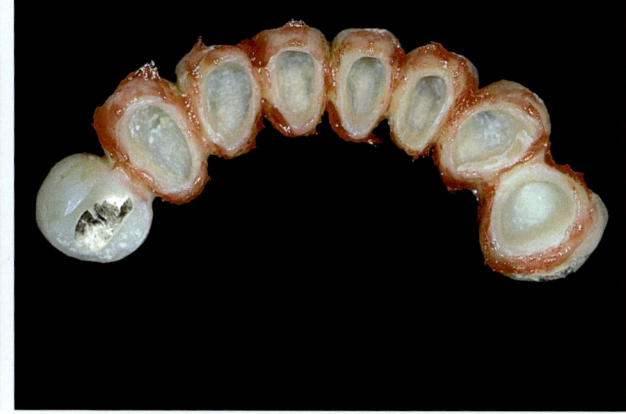

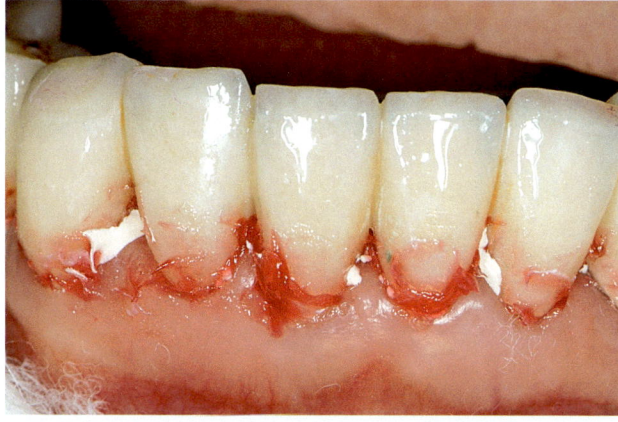

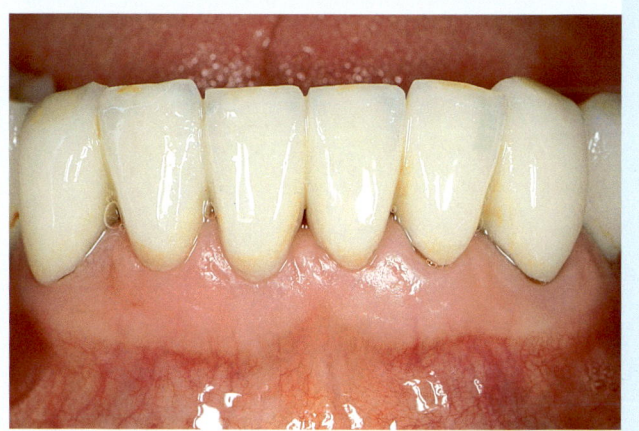

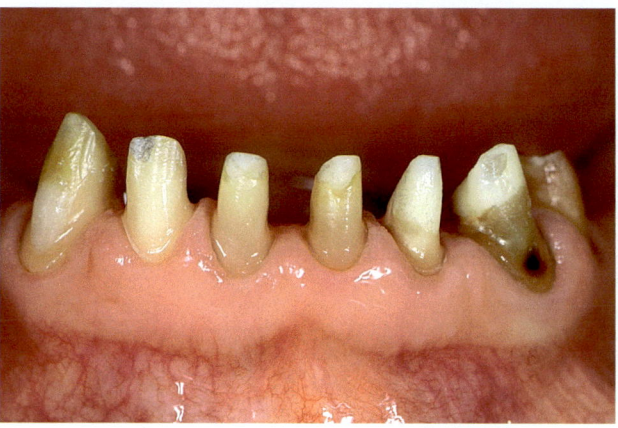

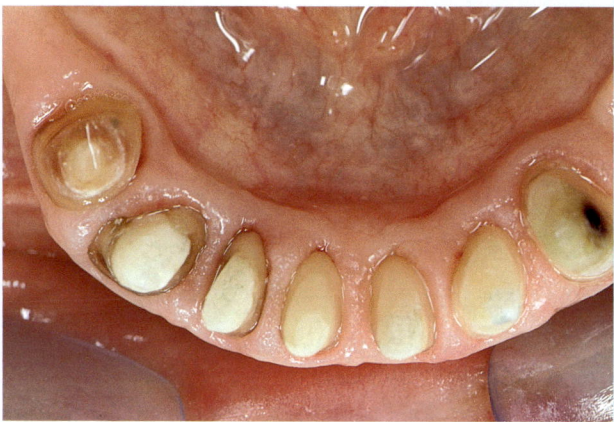

Some authors[87,90] recommend checking and recementing the provisional restoration periodically to avoid any risk of microleakage. The present authors believe this is unnecessary if the provisional restoration has been relined and remargined correctly, leaving the restoration polymerization to complete itself in the oral cavity.

Good retention, achieved through correct relining, combined with adequate marginal precision and meticulous checking of the occlusion makes it possible to avoid both decementation and fracturing of the provisional restoration. Clinical proof of the stability of the provisional restoration in the mouth is provided, on removal, by the presence of evenly distributed cement of normal color (Figs 2-25a and 2-25b). Significant chromatic variations or the absence of cement is, conversely, an unequivocal sign of microleakage. If, despite having taken all precautions, repeated decementation is found, or if the provisional restoration is to remain in the mouth for a long period (> 3 months), it is preferable to use a definitive cement (polycarboxylate or zinc phosphate) mixed with an insulating agent (eg, petroleum jelly). Though it somewhat reduces the high strength of these materials, this method saves the patient excessive discomfort during the removal maneuvers.

For efficacious but delicate removal, the use of tungsten forceps with a knurled or roughened tip and angled about 60 degrees is recommended. This is particularly useful for removing provisional restorations positioned in the mandibular arch and in the posterior sectors of the maxillary arch (Figs 2-25c and 2-25d). Whenever possible, use of the hammer should be avoided; this can be very unpleasant for the patient and could cause the provisional restoration to fracture more easily.

FIG 25 When the provisional restoration is removed from the oral cavity, the temporary cement usually remains adhered to the inside of the acrylic resin shell. *(a and b)* Its coloring should not show any alterations, to verify the absence of any marginal leakages. This is possible only if the provisional restoration has a satisfactory marginal closure and is not destabilized by interference or occlusal overloadings. *(c and d)* To remove the restoration, a pair of forceps with a knurled tip and an angle of approximately 60 degrees proves particularly helpful in the posterior areas.

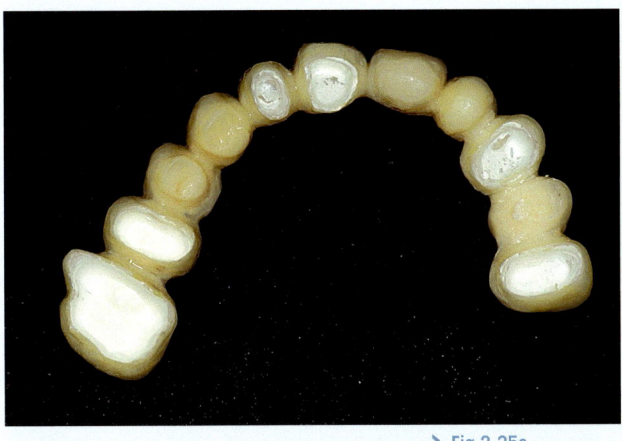

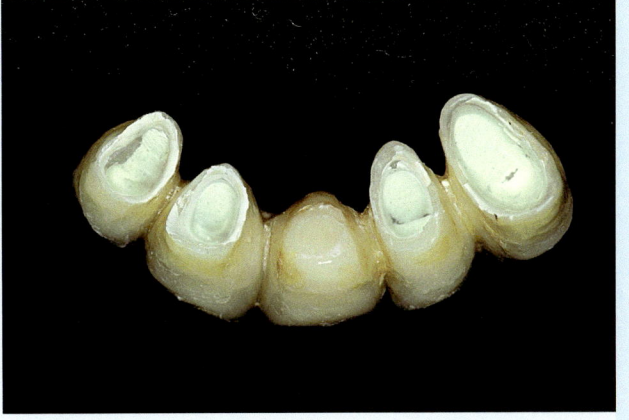

> Fig 2-25a

> Fig 2-25b

> Fig 2-25c

> Fig 2-25d

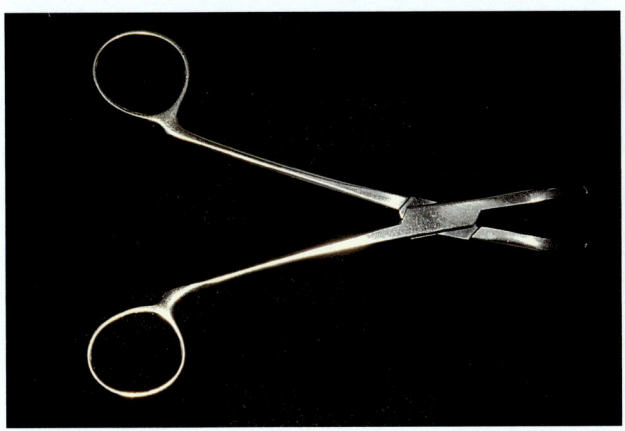

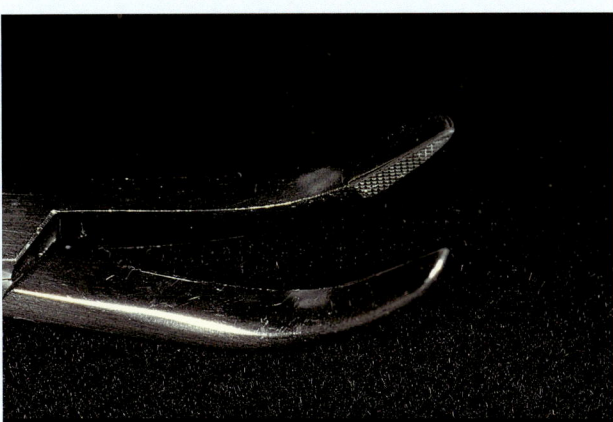

CEMENTATION

REQUISITES

- Stability maintained in the mouth during function
- Easily removed when necessary

SUGGESTIONS

- Achieve satisfactory marginal closure through relining and re-margining of the provisional to prevent decementation.
- Carry out a careful check of the occlusion to avoid fractures and decementations.
- Choose cements on the basis of the time they will remain in the oral cavity and the type of final fixation agent that will be used.
- Spread petroleum jelly (Vaseline) over the exterior of the provisional to facilitate removal of excess.
- If the provisional is removed, check for any leakage before proceeding with a new cementation.

PARTIAL-COVERAGE RESTORATIONS

SHORT-TERM PROVISIONAL RESTORATIONS

Minimally invasive techniques (inlays, onlays, overlays, and veneers)[91,92] possess undeniable clinical advantages, such as preservation of healthy tooth structure, reinforcement of remaining walls,[93] and most of the time, maintenance of pulp vitality. The positioning and stability of the provisional restorations in these cases, however, can be problematic because of the peculiar design of the tooth preparation and because of the mechanical retention, which is decidedly less stable compared with that of the full-coverage crown restorations described up to this point. For this reason, provisional restorations should remain in the mouth only as long as it takes to create and cement the definitive restorations.

POSTERIOR SECTORS

The use of adhesive indirect partial restorations in the posterior sectors, made in either resin composite or ceramic, has become more widespread.

PROVISIONAL INLAYS

If the restoration extension does not involve the cusps, the cavities can be temporarily protected by applying zinc oxide-eugenol–free fillings (Fig 2-26). This was especially done in the past; however, the presence of eugenol on the dentin impairs the adhesion of the restoration during the final cementation phases, consequently reducing its retention.[94] For many years now, provisional fillings in acrylic resin have therefore been used. These are positioned in the cavity in the plastic phase and light polymerized (Fig 2-27). They ensure adequate protection for a very limited period,[95] so their use is recommended only in cases where the definitive restorations will be luted within a period of a few days (maximum 1 week). On the other hand, if the final inlays are to be bonded after a much longer period of time, acrylic provisional inlays are indicated instead, constructed by means of the direct technique (see pages 134–137) using a previously prepared acetate index (Fig 2-28). The finishing of these provisional inlays may be more difficult compared with that traditionally used for complete crowns, since it requires more time and greater attention, especially in defining the occlusal and interproximal areas. Once fixed with a temporary resinous cement, the provisional restorations made in this way guarantee good stability, however, and can therefore remain for a longer period in the oral cavity.

FIG 26 *(a)* In the past, eugenol-free temporary fillings with a zinc base were used to protect the cavities. *(b)* Once the temporary fillings were removed and the cavity surfaces cleaned with a prophy cup and pumice paste, the two definitive inlays were bonded.

FIG 27 *(a)* Today the use of acrylic resin for temporary fillings is particularly widespread. *(b and c)* Thanks to its rubbery consistency, the provisional restoration in acrylic resin can be easily removed from the cavity using a pointed instrument before the definitive restoration is positioned.

FIG 28 *(a)* Before removing the old fillings to be replaced with inlays and carrying out the cavity preparations, an impression of the original situation is taken to make a stone cast, on which an acetate index is made. *(b)* This index is used for constructing the provisional restoration with the direct technique. *(c and d)* When polymerization is complete, the provisional restoration is taken out of the index and accurately finished before being placed into the oral cavity.

> Fig 2-26a

> Fig 2-26b

> Fig 2-27a

> Fig 2-27b

> Fig 2-27c

> Fig 2-28a

> Fig 2-28b

> Fig 2-28c

> Fig 2-28d

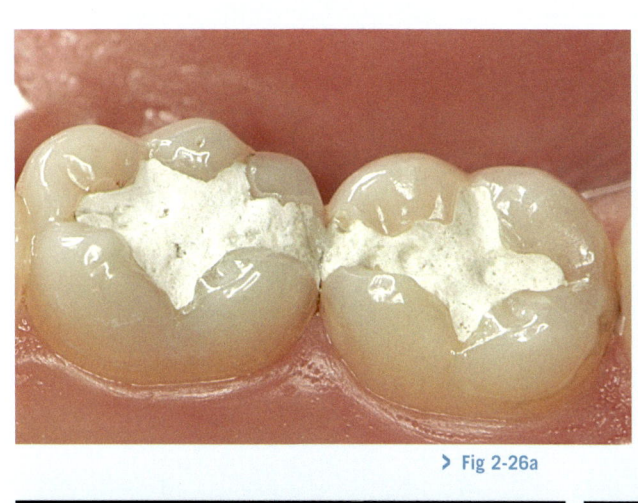

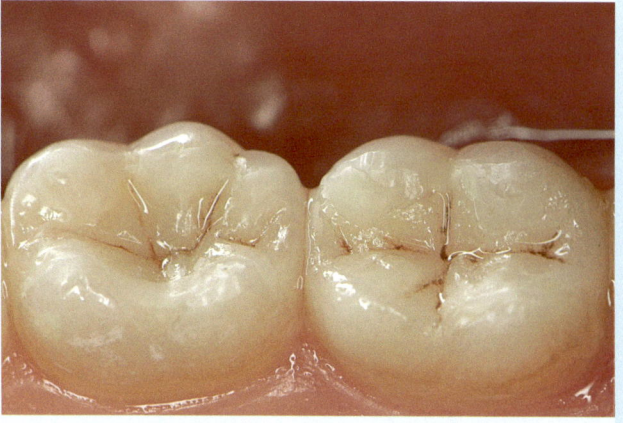

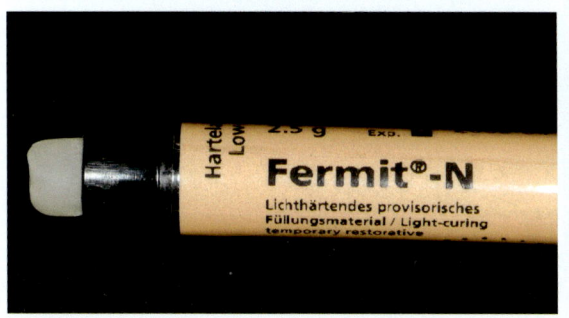

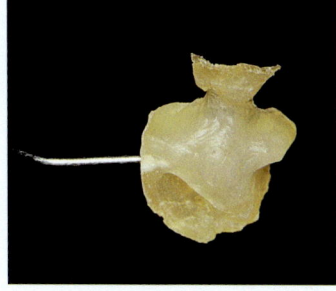

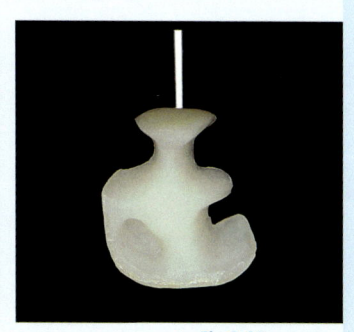

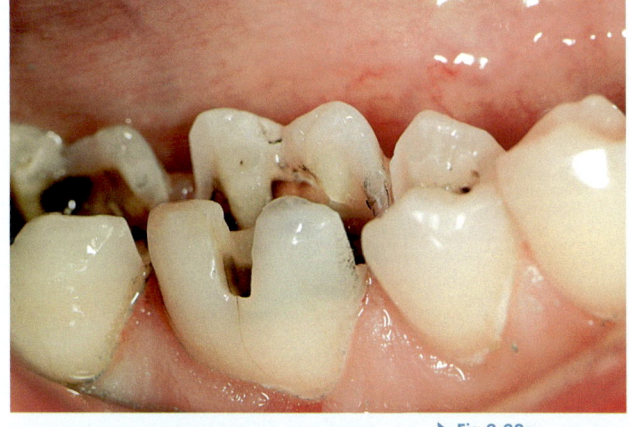

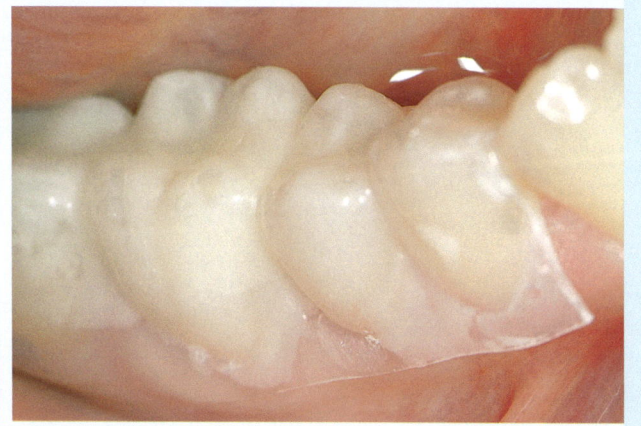

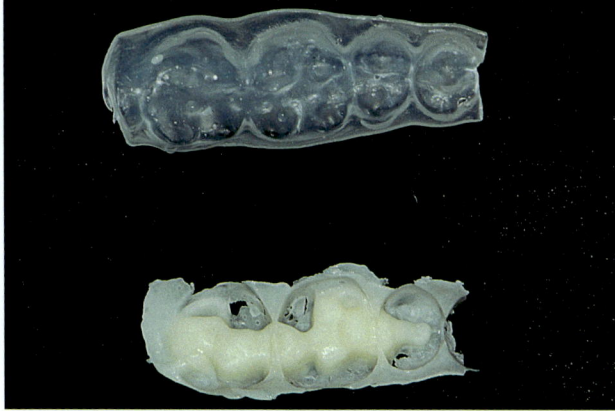

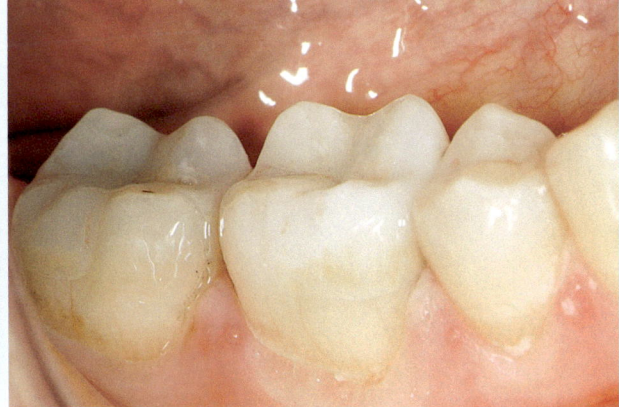

211

PROVISIONAL ONLAYS AND OVERLAYS

Partial posterior restorations with a design requiring one or more cusps to be covered (onlay) or the entire occlusal surface to be covered without extending to the marginal area (overlay) should have provisional restorations that, like complete crowns, are made using both the direct and the indirect technique. Compared with inlays, defining these margins and their finishing is undoubtedly much easier since the greater extension of the restoration, especially at the occlusal level, allows a greater affinity with the techniques for finishing complete crowns. However, on the surface of provisional onlays, alternating areas where the cusps are covered with cavity areas can cause some difficulties for the clinician, who would benefit from the use of magnification loupes during the finishing phases.

With both onlays and overlays, the limited height of the abutment reduces the mechanical retention, thus making decementation of the provisional restoration much more likely. This problem does not arise with the definitive restoration because, despite the absence of any adequate mechanical retention, its cementation by the adhesive technique ensures excellent survival over time.[96–99] The provisional restorations cannot be cemented by adhesive, however, since it would be impossible to remove them to fit the definitive restoration. Therefore, in the absence of sufficient mechanical retention, it may be useful to join the teeth affected by the treatment to exploit the slight inevitable undercuts found between the units. In cases where the dentin has been treated using the "dual bonding" technique before taking the definitive impression,[100] the use of temporary cements with a methacrylate base is not recommended. These cements could create unwanted adhesion of residue of the provisional restoration and/or the cement on the prepared surface that could prove very difficult to remove. It is therefore advisable to perform temporary cementation with eugenol-free zinc oxide cements to prevent the eugenol from reacting with the adhesive procedures of the final cementation. In all cases, whether using zinc oxide–based cements with or without eugenol, or temporary cements with a resinous base, the cavity must be adequately cleaned before proceeding with the final cementation to avoid reducing the adhesive capacity of the definitive restoration (Fig 2-29).[91,101,102]

FIG 29 *(a)* The provisional restorations of three overlays are fixed with eugenol-free cement with a zinc oxide base. *(b)* The marginal finishing line, positioned coronally relative to the gingival margin, is particularly visible due to the opacity of the temporary cement used. *(c and d)* After a few days, the provisional restorations are removed and, with rubber dam in place, the abutments are cleaned so the ceramic overlays can be bonded. *(e and f)* The frontal and occlusal views demonstrate the excellent esthetic integration of the restorations. (Restorations by Dr Riccardo Becciani.)

> Fig 2-29a

> Fig 2-29b

> Fig 2-29c

> Fig 2-29d

> Fig 2-29e

> Fig 2-29f

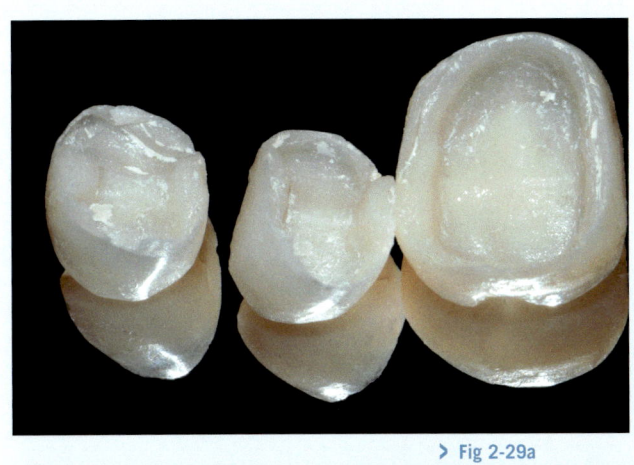

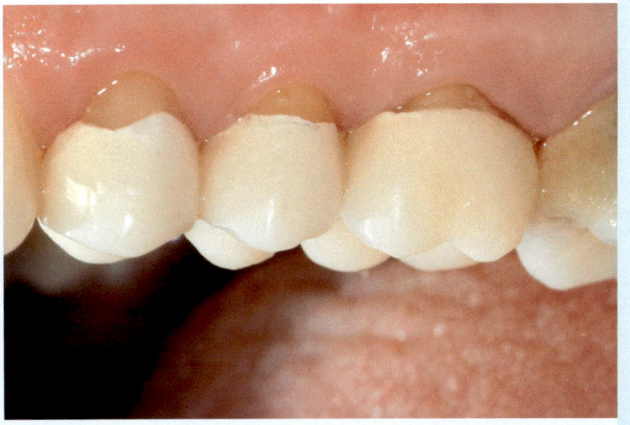

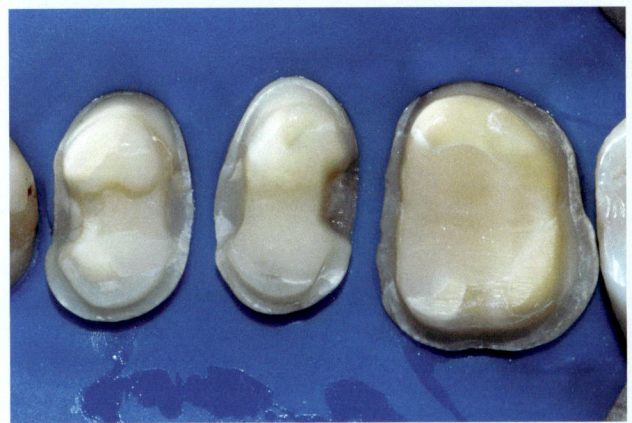

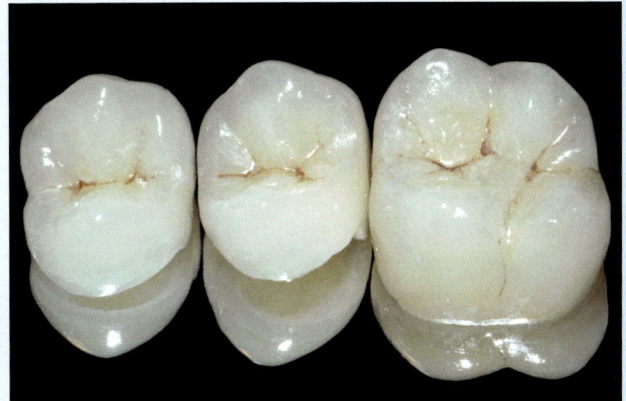

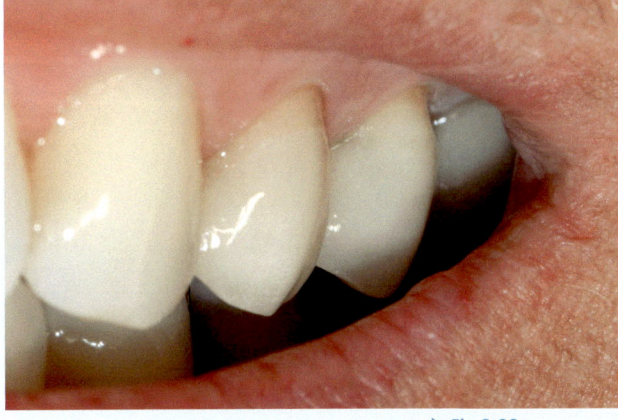

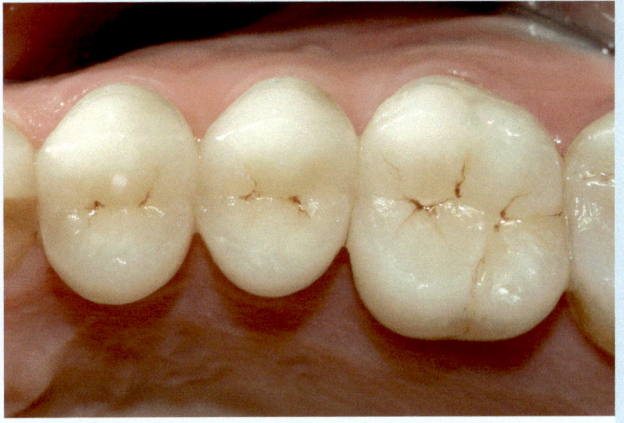

CLINIC—POSITIONING THE PROVISIONAL

INLAYS – ONLAYS

SUGGESTIONS

- Plan to deliver the definitive work within a short period of time.
- INLAYS:
  - Temporarily fill the cavity with light-curing acrylic material.
- ONLAYS:
  - Make an acrylic provisional via the direct or indirect technique.
  - Use eugenol-free cement.

ANTERIOR SECTORS

As with posterior partial restorations, anterior restorations can be made in ceramic or resin composite, even if the former option undoubtedly offers a greater guarantee of esthetic stability over time.[103–107]

PROVISIONAL VENEERS

Originally, the technique for placing ceramic veneers[108] did not involve the use of a provisional phase, since the extension of the tooth preparation was maintained rigorously in enamel and limited to just the buccal side. The encouraging results of clinical follow-ups[109–113] have in time led to a continuous evolution of the indications[114,115] that today involve greater extension of the tooth preparation. This is developed in the interproximal, incisal, and sometimes palatal areas. Provisional veneers, as with onlays and overlays, are constructed with both the direct and the indirect techniques. Self-curing acrylics are normally used for fabrication as well as relining; because of their elasticity, they are more appropriate than resin composites, which are more rigid and therefore more fragile. The greater extension of the tooth preparation allows for fabrication of provisional veneers that possess satisfactory mechanical retention once relined, especially where the restorative therapy involves several adjacent teeth and therefore where the slight undercut action often found between the units can be exploited. It should also be emphasized that keeping the provisional veneers in the mouth is very important if new positions and tooth shapes are to be tested. To ensure maximum stability, the provisional restorations can be cemented using the spot etching technique,[116] which involves etching a small area of the enamel with phosphoric acid and then cementing with fluid resin or composite cement (Fig 2-30). Though this method allows the provisional restoration to be kept in the mouth for long periods, it makes it very difficult to remove the excess cement. Incomplete elimination can mean unsatisfactory adaptation of the ceramic veneers. It is therefore advisable to use a temporary cement while being careful to organize the appointments so as to allow the definitive restorations to be delivered in the space of a few days. Among the temporary luting agents, those with a eugenol-free zinc oxide base are not ideal since the reduced thickness of the provisional veneers easily allows the opacity typical of these cements to show through (Fig 2-31) with inevitable esthetic repercussions. It is therefore best to use a temporary resinous cement (Provilink, Ivoclar Vivadent), which, because of its translucency, allows a satisfactory esthetic result to be achieved. This can be accomplished by coloring and glazing the provisional restorations with a light-curing resin (see pages 202 to 205). This technique is preferable to mechanical polishing because the thickness of the provisional restoration is reduced.

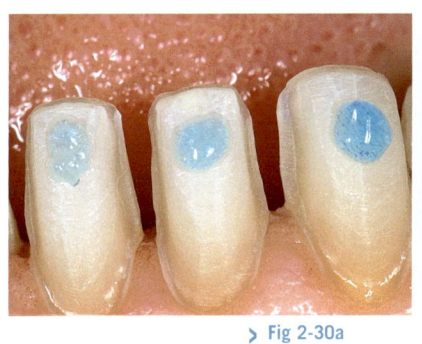

> Fig 2-30a 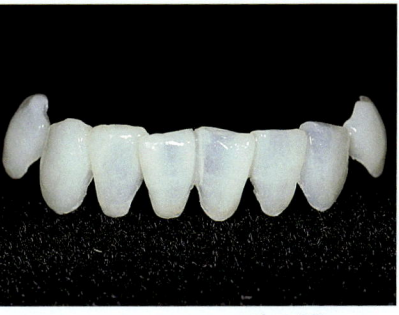 > Fig 2-30b 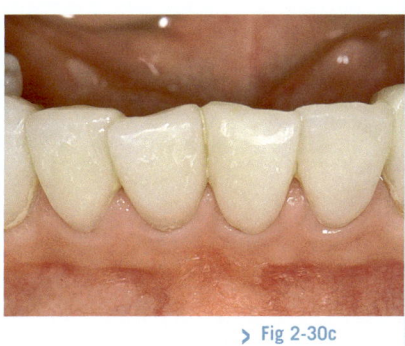 > Fig 2-30c

> Fig 2-31a 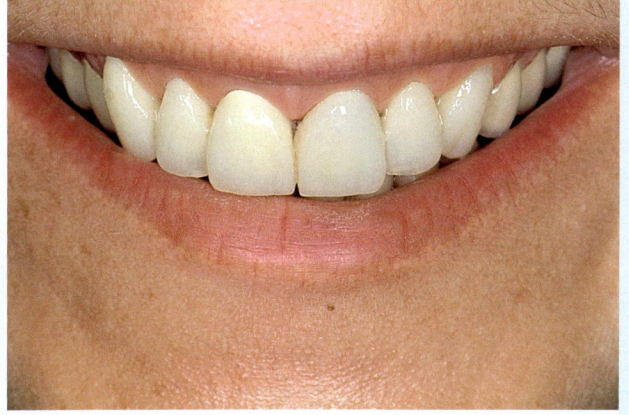 > Fig 2-31b

> Fig 2-31c 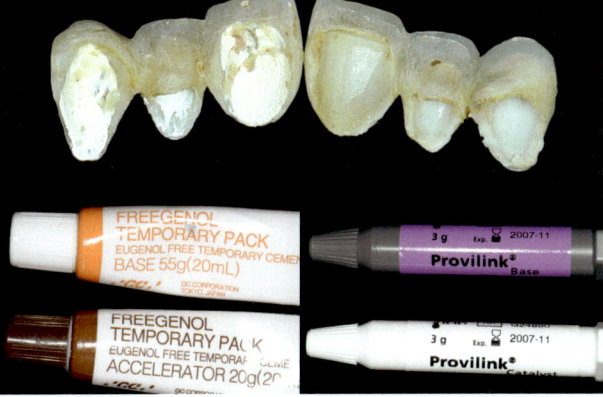 > Fig 2-31d

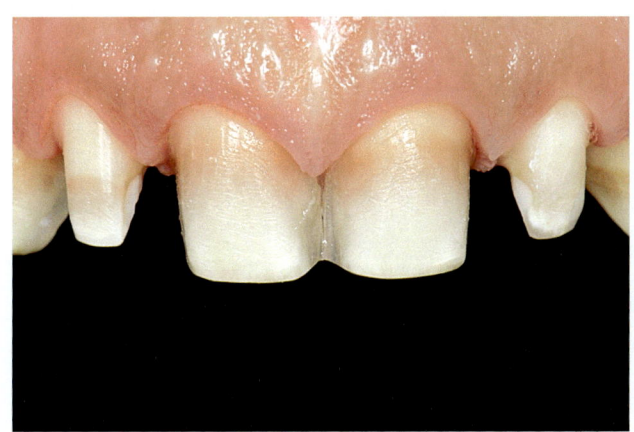

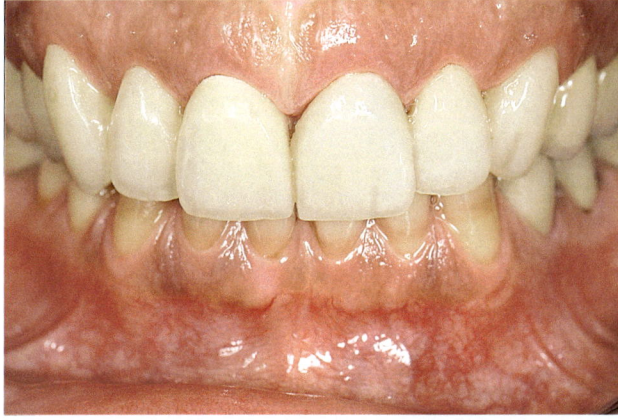

FIG 30 *(a to c)* To ensure maximum retention of the provisional restoration, an area around the enamel of each unit involved in the treatment is etched (spot-etching technique) before the provisional restoration is cemented with fluid resin.

FIG 31 *(a)* Rehabilitation of the anterior sector, as seen from these tooth preparations, involves a combination of ceramic veneers and crowns. Two separate provisional restorations have been made, both extending from the central incisor to the canine, and are fixed with temporary resinous cement. Following the decementation of the right provisional restoration, the patient sought the help of another office, where it was recemented with zinc oxide. *(b to d)* The thinness of the provisional restorations in the buccal area reveals a marked opacity of the right provisional restoration (zinc oxide cement) compared with the left one (temporary resinous cement), which demonstrates the noticeable difference in opacity of the two cements used.

One other factor that undoubtedly plays a decisive role in the stability of provisional veneers is the dynamic occlusal relationships. During protrusive and lateral excursive movements, the restorations are inevitably stressed and in many cases destabilized, with frequent decementations and/or fractures due to unsatisfactory mechanical retention.

Protection matrix One solution to this problem consists of providing the patient with an acetate guard when the provisional restorations are cemented that protects the treated units, especially at night, by redistributing the occlusal loading over all of the teeth in the arch (Figs 2-32 and 2-33). The guard's transparency allows the patient to wear it even during the day without any particular esthetic concern. However, careful arrangement of appointments and close collaboration with the technician, aimed at completing the work as quickly as possible, will be the winning formula for the stability of the provisional restorations, regardless of how they are fabricated and cemented.

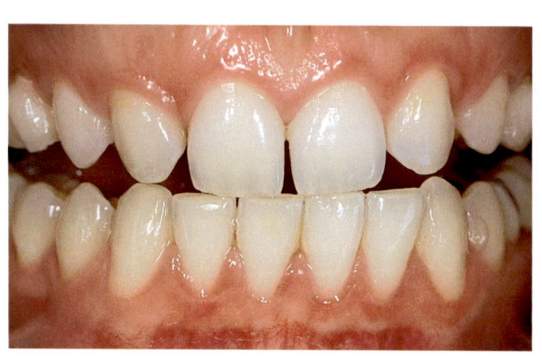

> Fig 2-32a

> Fig 2-32b

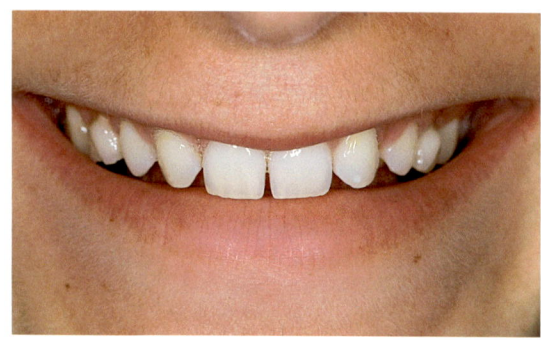

FIG 32 *(a and b)* After undergoing orthodontic treatment in a different office, the patient came to us with a specific request to optimize the esthetic appearance of the anterosuperior sector by closing the diastemata and prosthetically transforming the canines into lateral incisors and the first premolars into canines. *(c to g)* The six acrylic veneers, positioned with a temporary resinous cement, demonstrate correct function during the excursive movements. *(h)* To prevent possible decementation, however, the patient was given an acetate matrix. This device, which guaranteed the stability of the acrylic restorations, made it possible to fulfill the patient's request to postpone delivery of the definitive restorations for a few weeks to allow her to better evaluate the new tooth length. After being in position for 6 weeks, the provisional restorations show a loss of their initial surface brilliance achieved by use of a glaze. *(i)* Nevertheless, a satisfactory functional integration has obviously been maintained.

> Fig 2-32c

> Fig 2-32d

> Fig 2-32e

> Fig 2-32f

> Fig 2-32g

> Fig 2-32h

> Fig 2-32i

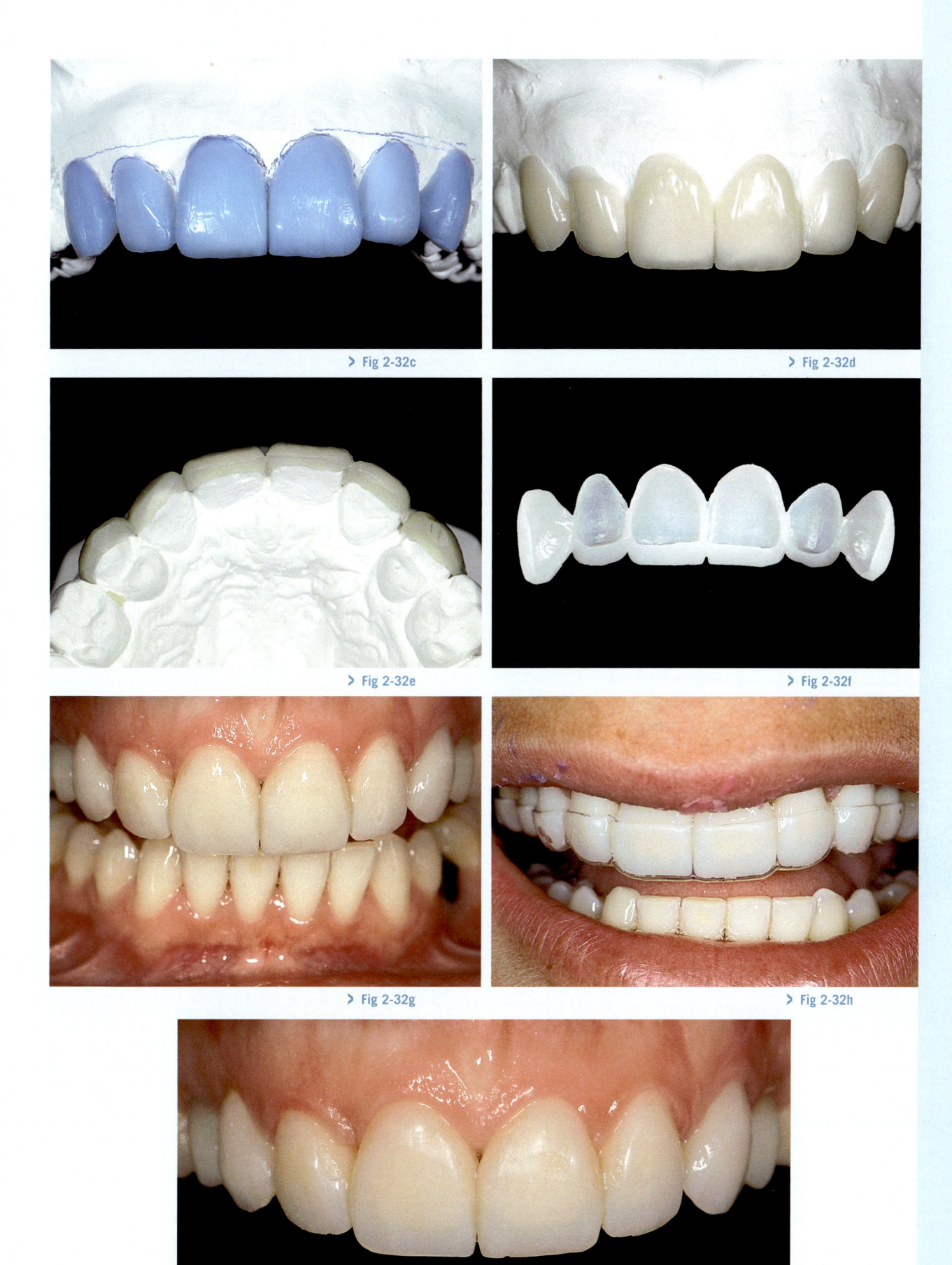

217

> Fig 2-33a

> Fig 2-33b

> Fig 2-33c

> Fig 2-33d

> Fig 2-33e

> Fig 2-33f

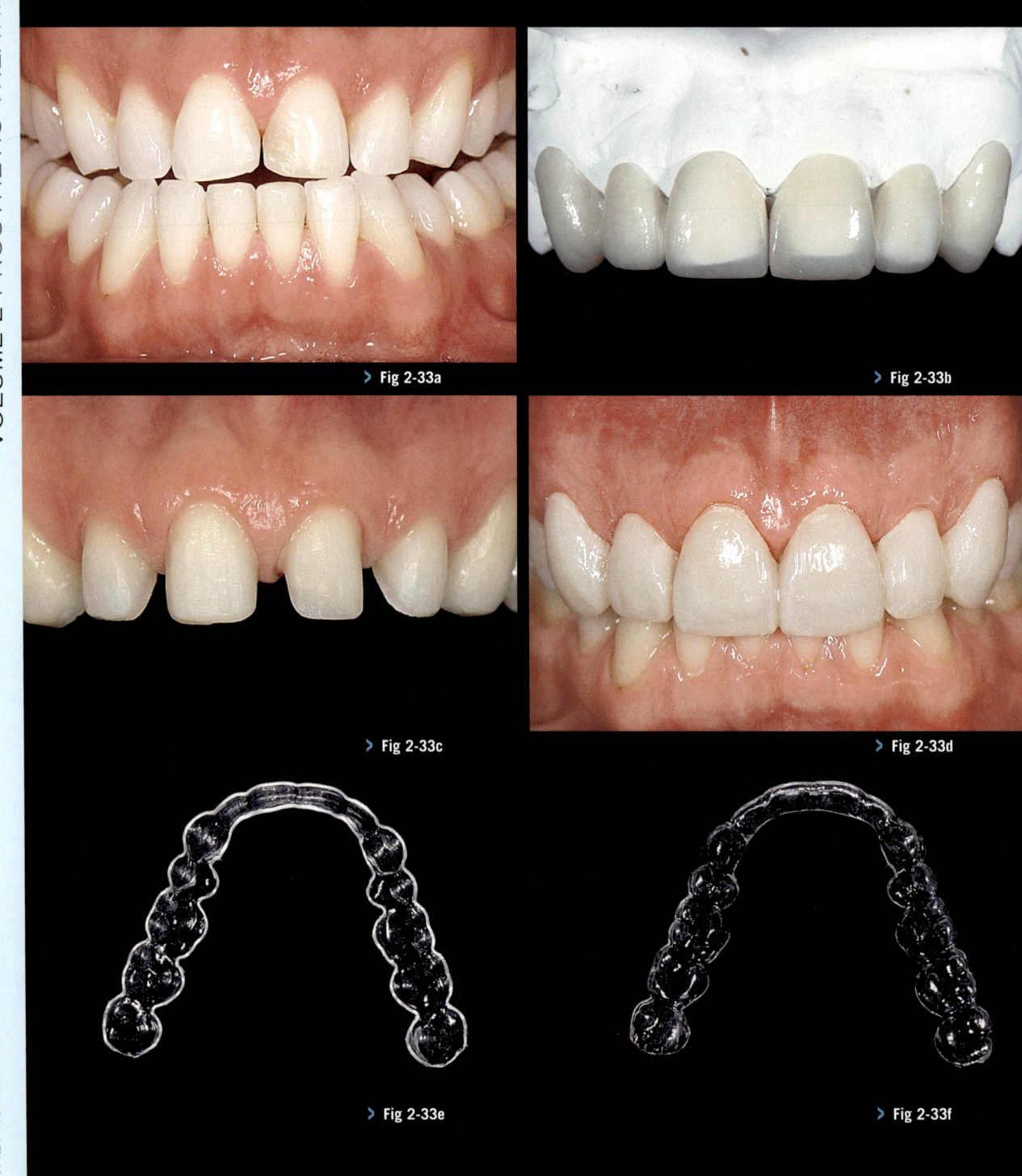

FIG 33 *(a and b)* To prepare for rehabilitation of the anterosuperior sextant, six provisional restorations consisting of a complete crown and five veneers were completed. *(c and d)* Once the tooth preparations were carried out, the provisional restorations were fixed with a temporary resinous cement. *(e and f)* To guarantee greater stability for the provisional restorations, an impression is taken in the oral cavity, from which a stone cast is then made. This is used to create an acetate matrix, which the patient is asked to use until the definitive work is ready. This solution guarantees good stability of the provisional restorations if they are to be kept in the mouth for an extended period. *(g)* Extension of the provisional phase for a long period (8 weeks) because of the patient's health problems is, in this specific case, evidenced by the loss of the glazing applied to the surface of the provisional restorations. *(h)* The matrix protecting the provisional restorations during excursive movements has, however, prevented decementation or fracture. *(i)* View of the six definitive restorations shows the good overall integration.

> Fig 2-33g

> Fig 2-33h

> Fig 2-33i

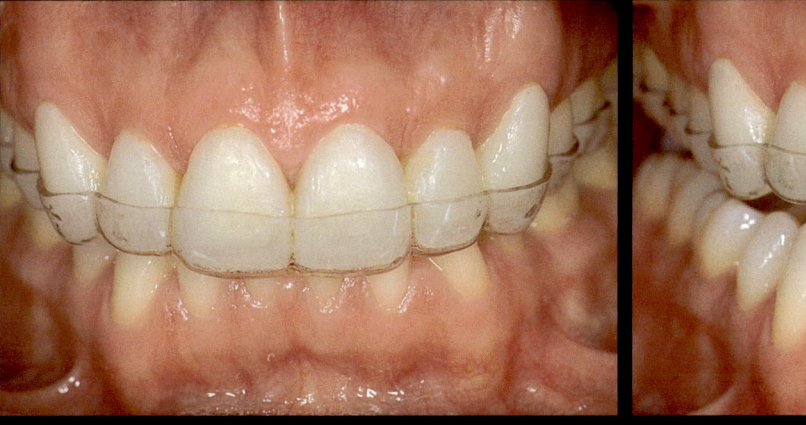

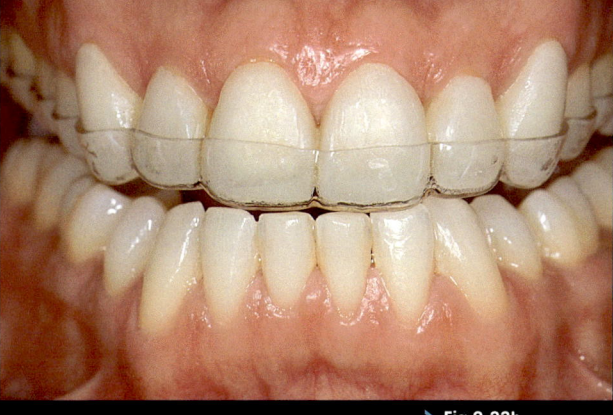

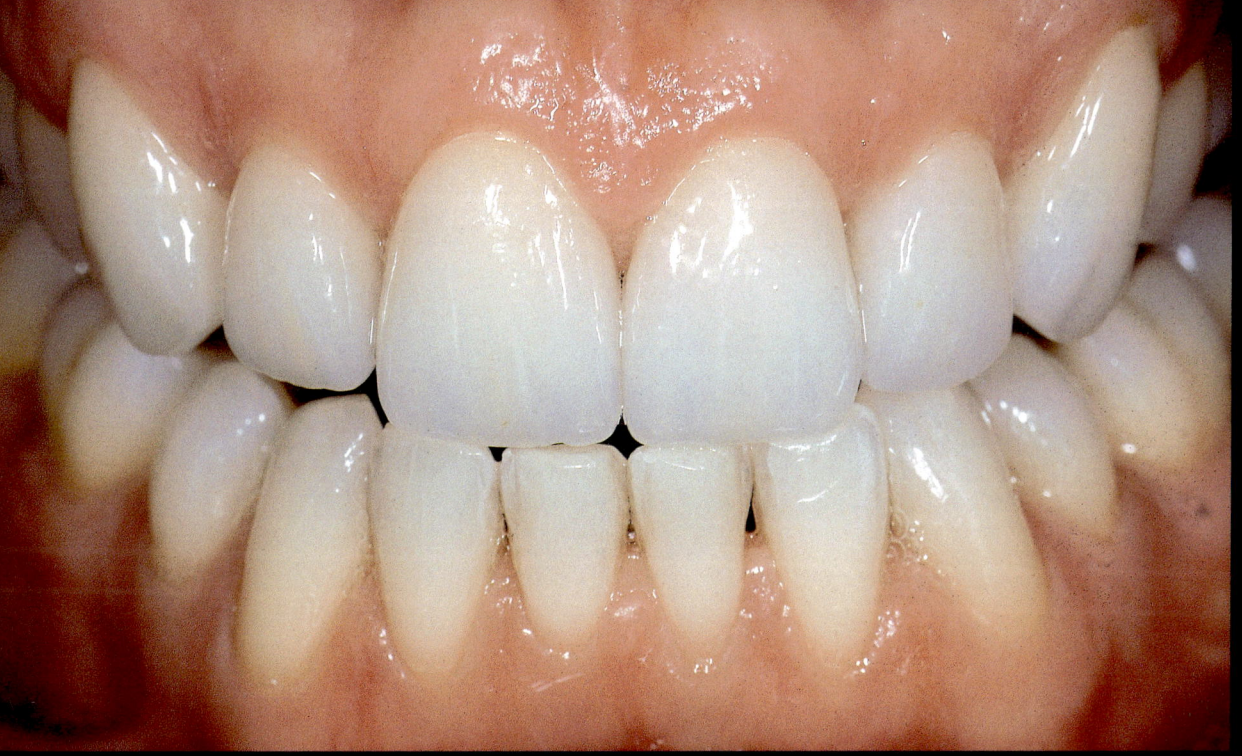

PROVISIONAL

VEENERS

SUGGESTIONS

- Plan to deliver the definitive work within a short period of time.
- Make an acrylic provisional via the direct or indirect technique.
- Take advantage of the undercut between the prepared teeth to increase retention.
    - Good retention: ⟶ Use a temporary resinous cement.
    - Poor retention: ⟶ Use the "spot-etching" technique.
- Have the patient wear a protective acetate occlusal guard.

LONG-TERM PROVISIONAL RESTORATIONS

FIRST PROVISIONAL RESTORATION

Sometimes the provisional restoration must remain in the mouth for long periods, especially in cases requiring associated therapies such as endodontic and orthodontic treatments, preprosthetic reconstructions, and, above all, periodontal and surgical implant treatments (Figs 2-34a to 2-34f).

The need to remove the provisional restoration several times[104,105,107] to carry out these therapies, the potential for spontaneous decementation, and the very real possibility of a fracture can significantly increase the number of appointments necessary. For patients requiring a multidisciplinary approach, the need for repeated interventions to continue the therapies must be considered when drawing up the estimate.

The first provisional restoration is, more often than not, the only one positioned in the mouth, even in cases where it is to remain there for quite some time.

In the authors' experience, recourse to a second provisional restoration is rarely determined by the need to make substantial corrections to the esthetic-functional aspect of the first provisional restoration. In fact, due to the careful analysis made in the planning phase, the extent of the variations in the majority of cases is so limited that only a few further alterations are required. The clinician can easily accomplish these on the first provisional restoration by adding or removing acrylic resin.

SECOND PROVISIONAL RESTORATION

Only in a few specific circumstances is the first provisional restoration replaced by a second one that may or may not be reinforced, depending on the particular clinical needs.

In cases of complex rehabilitations, the particular level of difficulty of the treatment and the extent of the variations to be made can make it impossible to incorporate all of the planned esthetic and functional changes into the first provisional restoration. In these circumstances the clinician may therefore decide to make a second provisional restoration.

FIG 34 *(a and b)* The patient, who has serious periodontal problems, sought our help to resolve the esthetic problem caused by the gaps between the anterosuperior teeth. *(c and d)* The prosthetic rehabilitation of the maxillary arch first involves positioning a provisional restoration before the teeth are prepared. *(e and f)* After preparation of the teeth considered valid for rehabilitation purposes, the right maxillary central incisor is extracted, and the provisional restoration is positioned.

> Fig 2-34a

> Fig 2-34b

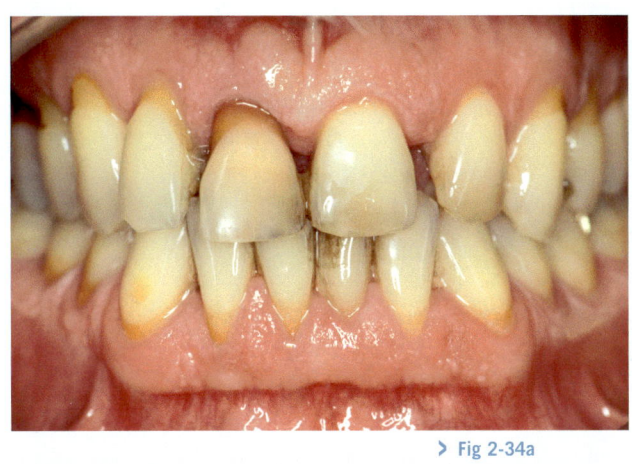

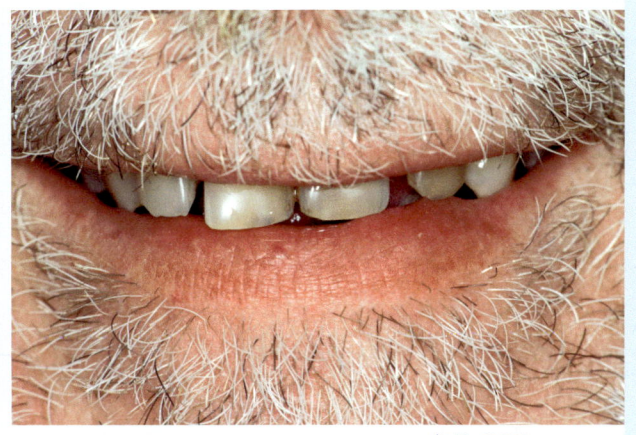

FIRST PROVISIONAL

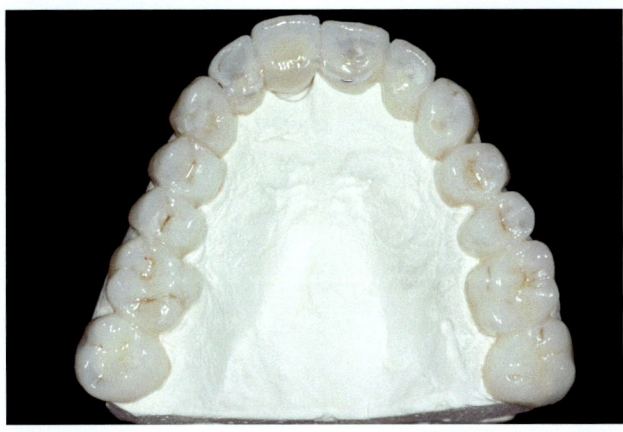

> Fig 2-34c

> Fig 2-34d

> Fig 2-34e

> Fig 2-34f

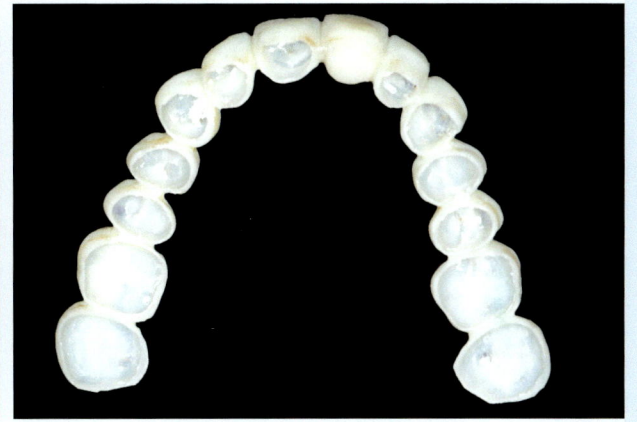

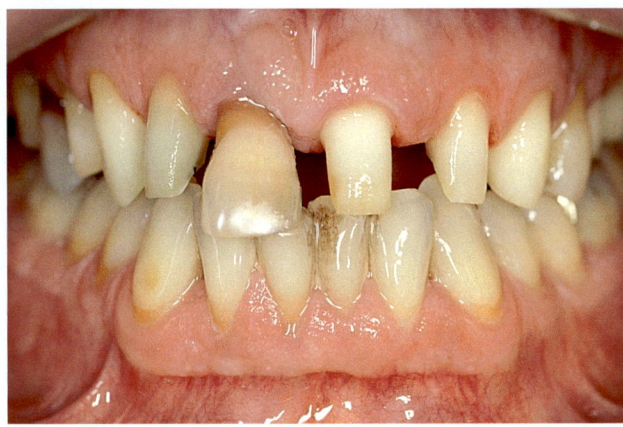

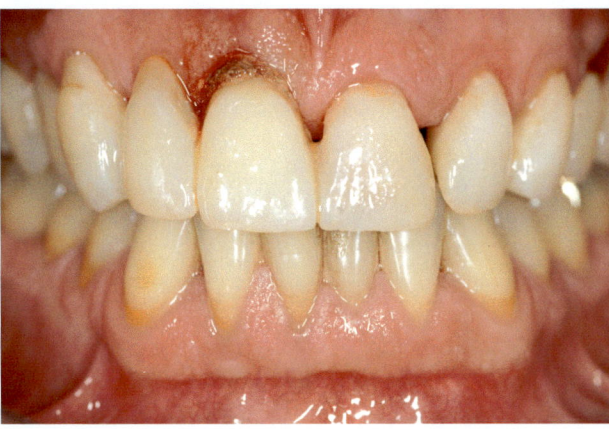

To create the second provisional restoration, the technician is given the cast taken from the impression of the first provisional restoration and the information on the alterations to be made from the laboratory checklist.

The clinician also takes an impression of the prepared teeth, on which the technician will be able to make the new provisional restoration using the methods for prepared teeth described previously (Fig 2-34g) (see page 138). The widened shape of the cervical third and the container effect peculiar to the MIT allow both ideal insertion and the correct relining of the second provisional restoration here as well.

SECOND REINFORCED PROVISIONAL RESTORATION

The creation of a provisional restoration that is reinforced inside is particularly useful in cases where greater structural strength must be guaranteed. In the presence of a restoration with numerous pontic units, or when resective surgical-periodontal therapies are involved with root amputations in the posterior sectors, a second "reinforced" provisional restoration can indeed offer greater support for masticatory forces. Its fabrication may also be necessary in many cases of prosthetic implant therapy. During the osseointegration period (prior to loading) of implants positioned near wide edentulous areas, for example, a reinforced provisional restoration is often made and anchored to the few remaining natural teeth. In addition to guaranteeing the patient adequate resistance and the necessary occlusal stability, the second provisional restoration also satisfies esthetic needs. Various fibers (eg, glass fiber, carbon, Kevlar, polyester, and polyethylene) are used to reinforce the acrylic resin structure of the provisional restoration,[117–119] even if there is some doubt as to their true efficiency.[119] The use of metal reinforcements, made according to different widely documented methods, is therefore preferable (Figs 2-34h to 2-34k).[7,42,44,52,56,60,62,68,120,121]

SECOND REINFORCED PROVISIONAL

INDICATIONS

- Repeated fracture of the first nonreinforced provisional
- Short abutments with inadequate thickness of the provisional in the interproximal area
- Presence of a long span with numerous adjacent pontic elements
- Presence of cantilevers
- Provisional required for long-term wear (6–12 months)
- Presence of excessive occlusal forces

SECOND REINFORCED PROVISIONAL

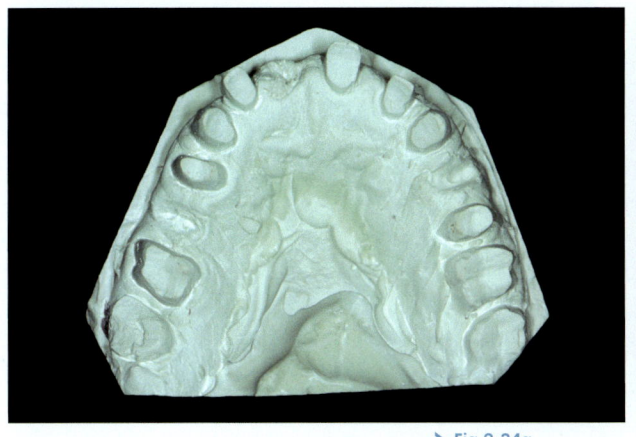

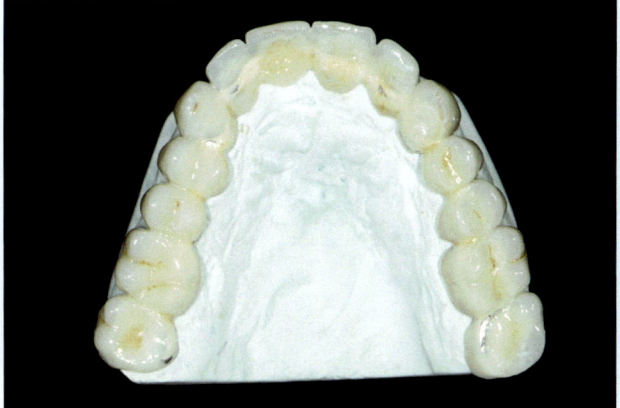

> Fig 2-34g

> Fig 2-34h

> Fig 2-34i

> Fig 2-34j

> Fig 2-34k

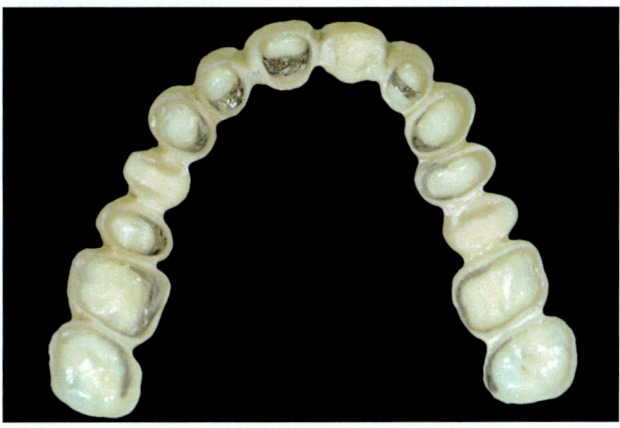

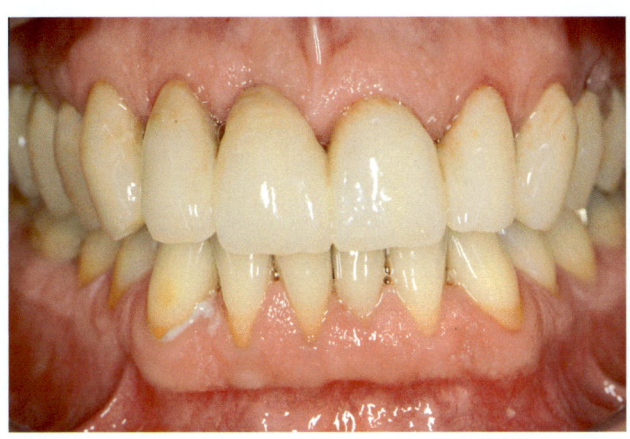

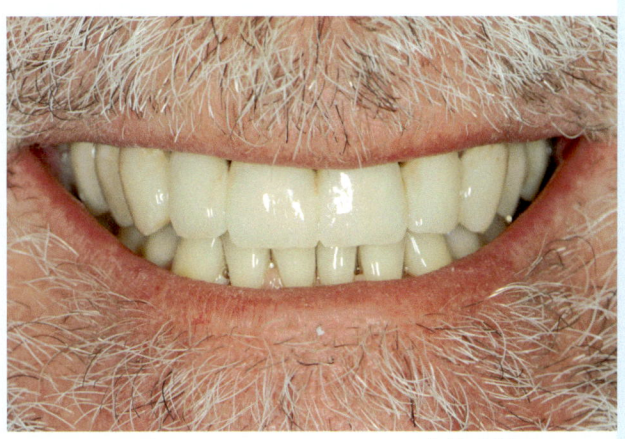

FIG 34 *(g to k)* After taking an impression of the prepared abutments, a second reinforced provisional restoration is created on the stone cast. Because of its metallic structure, the permanence of this provisional restoration in the mouth is guaranteed for as much time as needed to complete the periodontal therapy programmed in the treatment plan.

CAST REINFORCEMENT

For metallic reinforcement, the use of a base metal alloy[14,68,122] is often recommended, even if, in the authors' opinion, the use of a gold alloy has undeniable advantages. One of these is the relative elasticity of the noble metal, which is sufficiently compatible with that of acrylic resin and considerably reduces the risk of fracture. On the contrary, the use of stronger base metal alloys can easily cause the resin to detach from the metal structure due to the substantial difference in the respective degrees of elasticity.

One further advantage offered by gold alloy is its malleability. Where difficulty is encountered in fitting the provisional restoration because of interference between the abutments and the metal reinforcement (highlighted by means of the silicone paste [FitChecker]), the relative softness and malleability of this alloy allow it to be revised so the provisional restoration can be fully inserted.

FABRICATION TECHNIQUE

The framework cast in gold alloy is created on the stone cast with the prepared teeth (Fig 2-35a) under the guidance of a silicone index taken from the stone cast of the first provisional restoration (Fig 2-35b); this allows the correct design to be developed for the reinforcement (Figs 2-35c and 2-35d). In the anterior sector, the reinforcement is normally positioned only on the palatal and interproximal sides of the abutments and not on the buccal side (Figs 2-35e to 2-35h). This is because any changes necessary to the shape on the buccal surface of the provisional restoration that could reduce the thickness of the acrylic could reveal the opacity of the underlying metallic structure, with inevitable esthetic repercussions. In the posterior sectors it is desirable to extend the reinforcement to the buccal area as well, especially near the abutment teeth adjacent to one or more intermediate units. In this way, a ring is established that guarantees the structure more resistance in the area of greatest occlusal loading. Care must be taken, however, to avoid covering the occlusal area with the metal reinforcement and predetermining the height of the abutments in the laboratory, with inevitable obstacles to fitting the provisional restoration in the mouth. To make sure that the metal reinforcement does not lead to oversizing of the overall volume of the individual abutments, the reinforced provisional restorations are created only after the preliminary tooth preparations have been carried out. This avoids both excessive sizing of the provisional restoration and possible interferences with the axis walls.

FIG 35 *(a and b)* Reinforcement of the second provisional restoration is performed on the stone cast of the prepared teeth using a silicone index taken from the cast of the diagnostic wax-up. The index allows the technician to evaluate the final spaces where, once the provisional restoration is finished, both the metallic structure and the acrylic thicknesses are to be included. *(c)* The reinforcement is first created in wax and then cast in gold alloy. After casting, the technician makes the inside of the structure slightly thinner and fixes it on the cast with cyanoacrylate to prevent the reinforcement from coming into contact with the abutments. *(d)* The provisional restoration, made opaque with light-curing opaque shows a slight separation from the prepared teeth, which is essential to allow the clinician to fit the provisional restoration and for correct relining. *(e)* The acrylic resin is then pressed using the PSC technique. *(f to h)* In the close-up one can see how the extension of the metallic structure is limited to just the palatal side in the anterior teeth, while in the molars and in the canines it extends around the perimeter of the abutments to adequately support the occlusal loading that is exerted on the long pontics in the posterior sectors.

Fig 2-35a

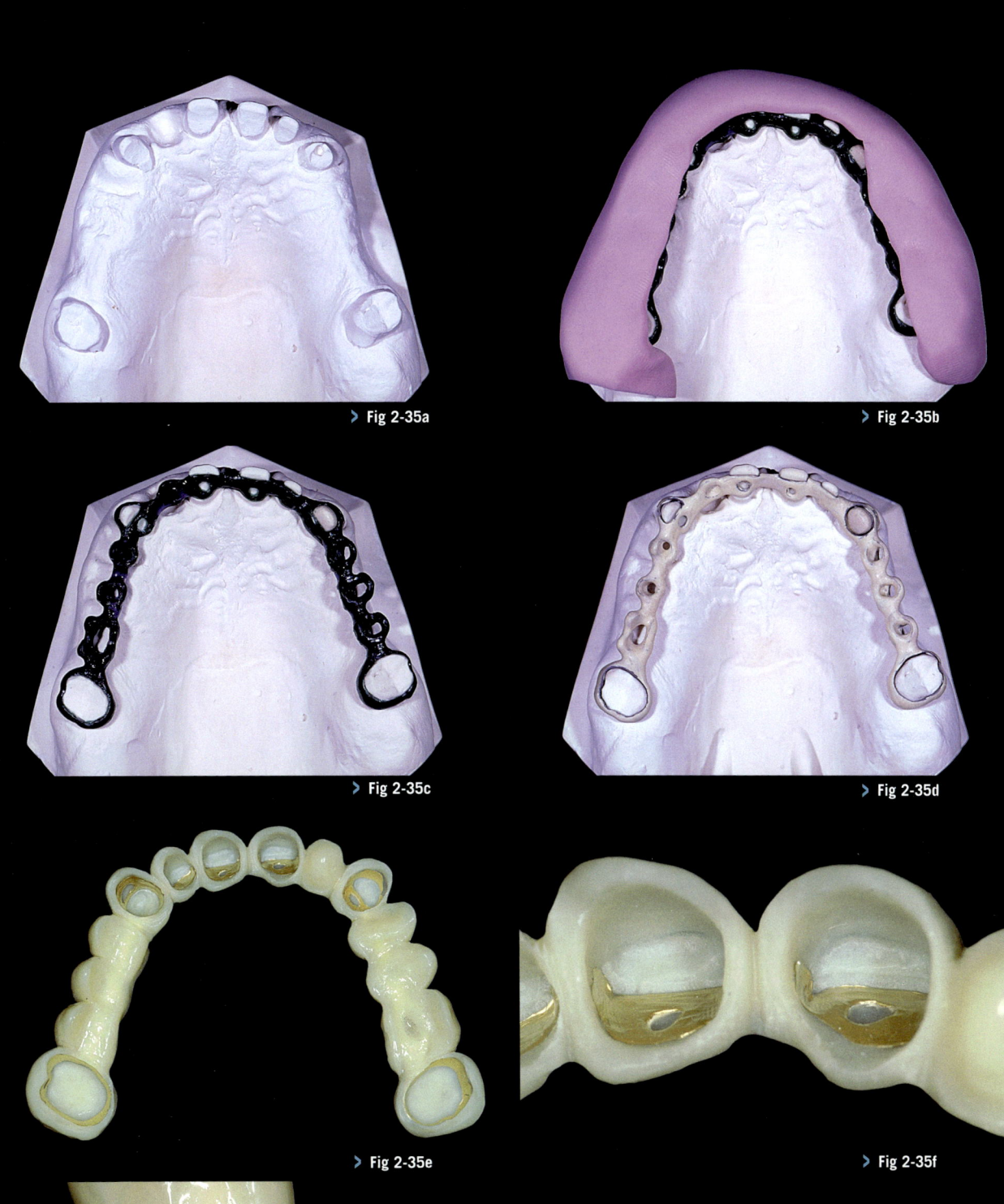

Fig 2-35b

Fig 2-35c

Fig 2-35d

Fig 2-35e

Fig 2-35f

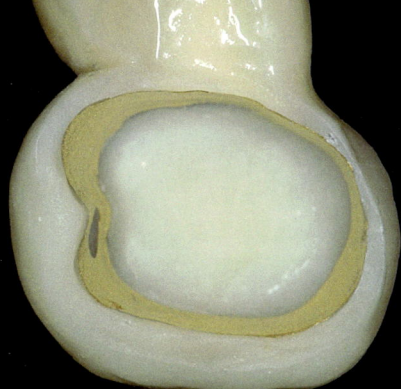

Fig 2-35g

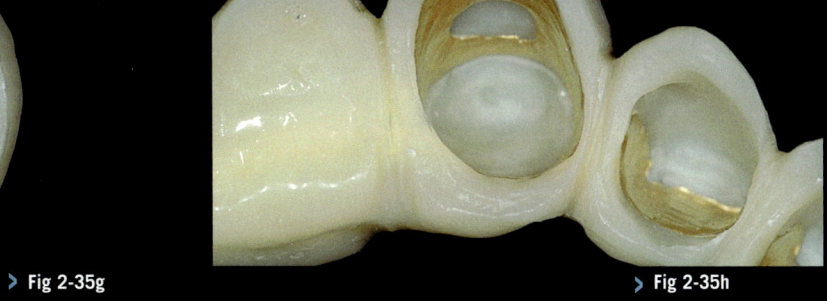

Fig 2-35h

225

LONG-TERM PROVISIONAL RESTORATIONS

THE PROVISIONAL RESTORATION IN PROSTHETIC IMPLANT THERAPY

With increasing frequency, prosthetic implant therapy is the elected treatment for replacing one or more missing teeth. The provisional restoration can be positioned either in the phases that precede implant loading (non–implant-supported) or in those that follow implant placement (implant-supported).

NON–IMPLANT-SUPPORTED PROVISIONAL RESTORATIONS

Non–implant-supported provisional restorations fulfill the need to guarantee the patient good esthetics and masticatory function during the period leading up to the moment when the placed implants can be used to support a provisional or definitive prosthesis. They can be divided into the following categories:
- Removable provisional restorations (with mucosal and/or dental support)
- Fixed provisional restorations (with dental support)

REMOVABLE PROSTHESIS

In partially or fully edentulous patients, wherever a fixed provisional restoration is not possible, a removable acrylic resin prosthesis can be used; once the implants are placed, it must be relined with a particularly resilient material. Despite the stress-relieving service it provides, compression caused by the acrylic resin plates can compromise osseointegration and, in cases where techniques have been carried out to increase the ridge volume, may damage the newly formed tissues. For this reason it is advisable, when possible, to use a removable prosthesis with dental support only.

FIXED PROSTHESIS

The fixed option is the ideal type of provisional restoration because it prevents any unwelcome compressive effect on the soft tissues. The various types are.
- Provisional restoration on natural teeth
- Resin-bonded prosthesis
- Orthodontic provisional restoration

PROVISIONAL RESTORATION ON NATURAL TEETH

A provisional restoration on natural teeth is traditionally used in fixed prosthetics; it is employed when the treatment plan involves prosthetic use of the natural teeth adjacent to the implant sites (Fig 2-36).[123,124] Because of the stability that this type of prosthesis is able to provide, it is an ideal option for the patient, especially from a psychologic point of view. Also important to the clinician is the ease of insertion and removal of the provisional restoration, which in these cases proves to be simple and quick. Should the edentulous area be especially large or if cantilevers are necessary, the prosthesis can be reinforced with a metal structure.[125] While waiting to load the implants with a provisional restoration, in some patients the clinician can use the teeth to be extracted as abutments.[126]

→ ...from page 199

NON-IMPLANT SUPPORTED　　　　　　　　　　　　　　　　　　　　　　　　　　FIXED PROSTHESIS

PROVISIONAL RESTORATION ON NATURAL TEETH

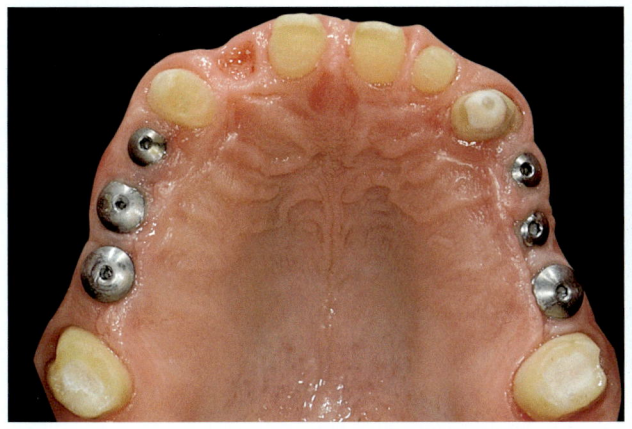

> Fig 2-36a

> Fig 2-36b

> Fig 2-36c

> Fig 2-36d

> Fig 2-36e

> Fig 2-36f

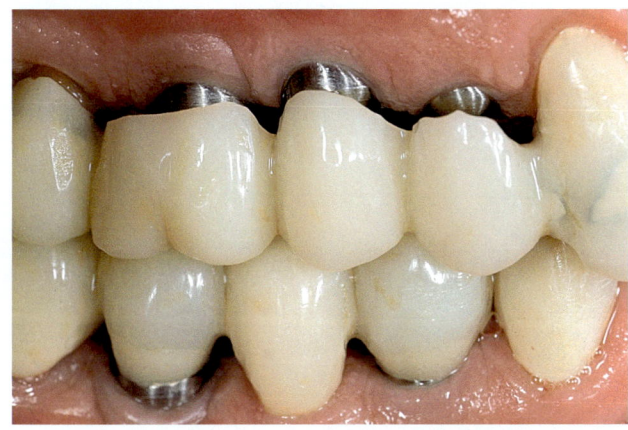

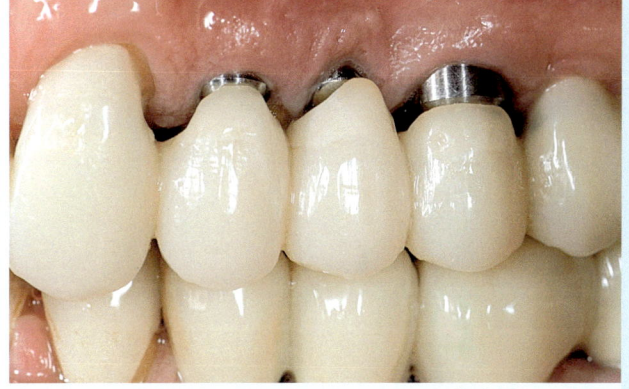

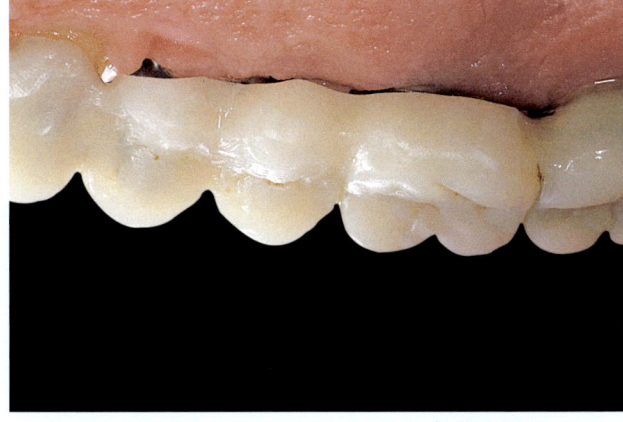

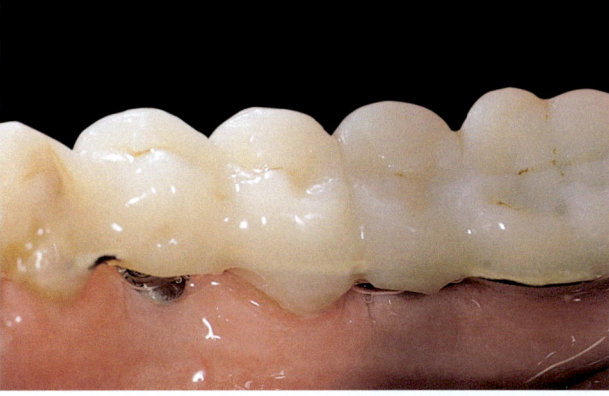

→ continues on page 236

FIG 36 *(a)* As part of the complete rehabilitation of the maxillary arch, implants have been inserted in the posterior sectors and, at the same time, the healing abutments have been positioned (one-stage technique). *(b)* To avoid any repercussions to the osseointegration process, the reinforced provisional restoration is anchored exclusively on the natural abutments, excluding even the slightest contact with the implant abutments. *(c to f)* The lateral and lingual views of the maxillary and mandibular arches reveal how the acrylic index manages to close the gaps quite efficiently, without making any contact with the titanium abutments.

RESIN-BONDED PROSTHESIS

In patients with partial anterior edentulism, it is sometimes useful to employ a resin-bonded prosthesis. This fixed prosthetic solution, which is esthetically viable and particularly comfortable for the patient, is especially indicated where a traditional fixed partial denture would involve the teeth adjacent to the edentulous areas and would therefore be undesirable[127,128] (Figs 2-37a and 2-37b), and/or where it is desirable to avoid compression of the newly formed tissues following a surgical procedure such as bone grafting and/or connective tissue grafting (Figs 2-37c to 2-37f). In addition to the labor-intensive procedures required to remove the prosthesis for the various surgical and prosthetic phases, however, spontaneous decementation can occur, much to the patient's displeasure. In the interest of finding a procedure that is non-invasive to the dental tissues and that is worth carrying out, given the short time for which the resin-bonded prosthesis is used (a few months), it is obviously inadvisable to carry out any tooth preparation on the palatal aspects of the supporting teeth. This is possible only if there is sufficient occlusal space to accommodate the thickness of the bonded proszthesis. If not, at the same time the resin-bonded prosthesis is inserted, an acrylic plate can be fitted that temporarily raises the VDO, thus re-establishing balanced occlusal contact between the two arches and preventing the onset of unwanted tooth extrusions (Figs 2-37g to 2-37j).

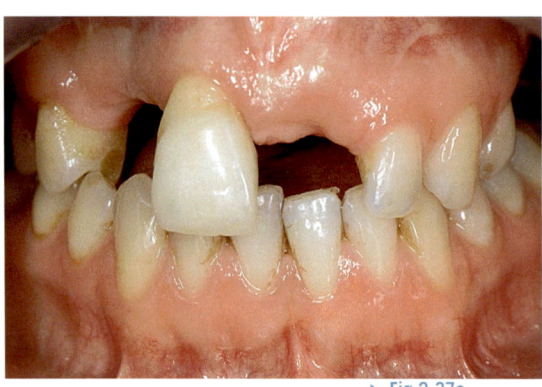

> Fig 2-37a

> Fig 2-37b

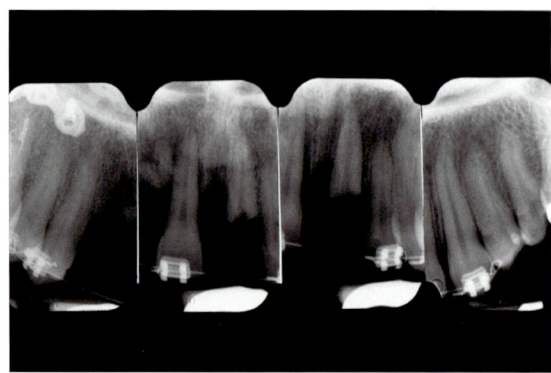

FIG 37 *(a and b)* The young patient has undergone the avulsion of some teeth as the result of an accident. *(c to e)* To rehabilitate the anterosuperior sector, implant positioning is preceded by bone and connective tissue grafting using autologous bone and Bio-Oss (Geistlich Pharma), to augment the ridge volume and optimize the implant position. (Surgery by Prof Massimo Simion.) To prevent any compression of the area involved in the surgical operation while at the same time avoiding the need to make tooth preparations on the adjacent natural teeth, the decision is made to fit a resin-bonded prosthesis. *(f to j)* The limited space between the edentulous ridge and the mandibular incisors makes it necessary to create an acrylic resin plate in the mandibular arch at the same time as the bonded partial denture, which, by raising the occlusion evenly, allows enough space for the resin-bonded prosthesis to be created and averts extrusion of the posterior teeth. The resin-bonded prosthesis, like the acrylic resin plate on the mandibular arch, will be worn by the patient until the provisional restorations can be positioned directly on the implants.

NON-IMPLANT SUPPORTED | FIXED PROSTHESIS

RESIN-BONDED PROSTHESIS

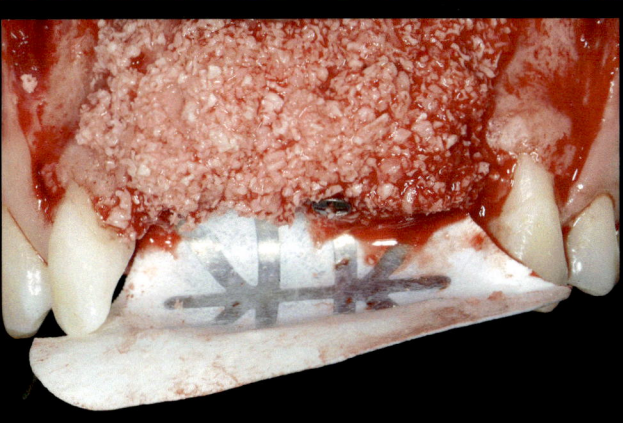

> Fig 2-37c

> Fig 2-37d

> Fig 2-37e

> Fig 2-37f

> Fig 2-37g

> Fig 2-37h

> Fig 2-37i

> Fig 2-37j

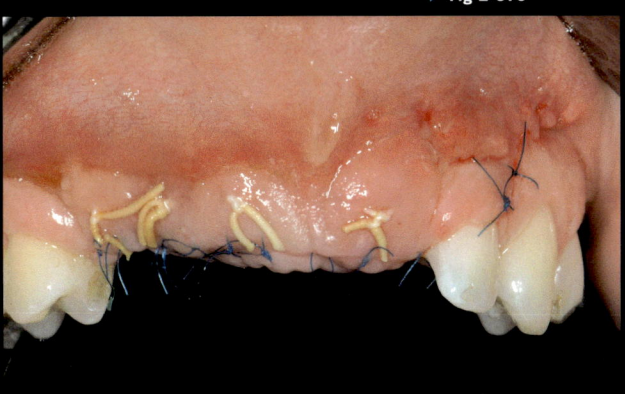

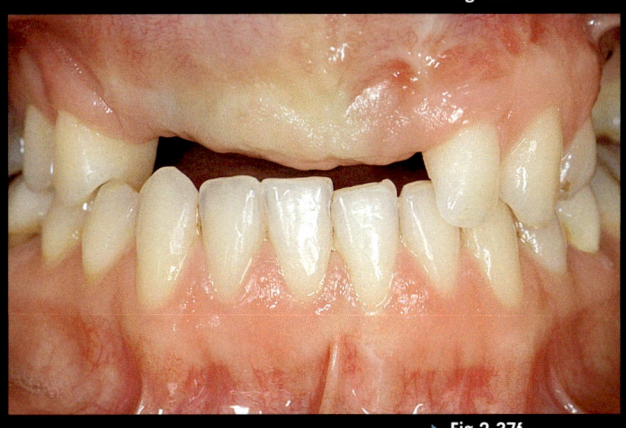

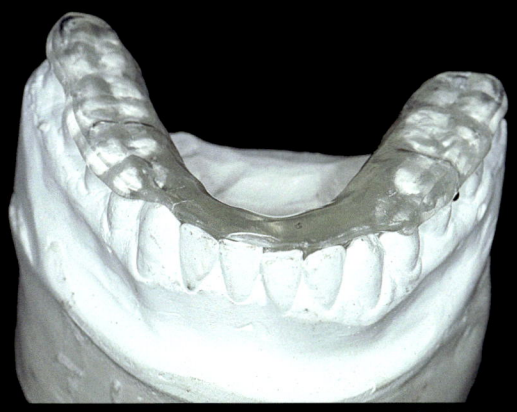

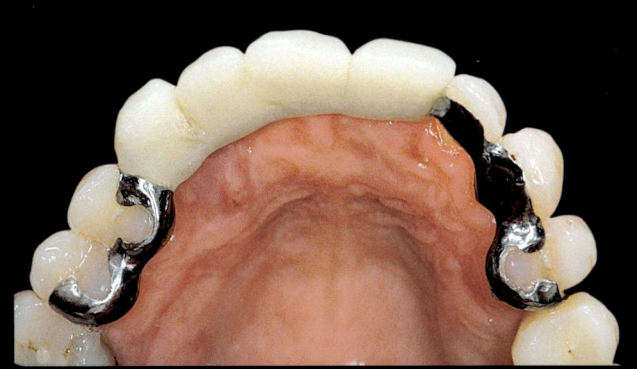

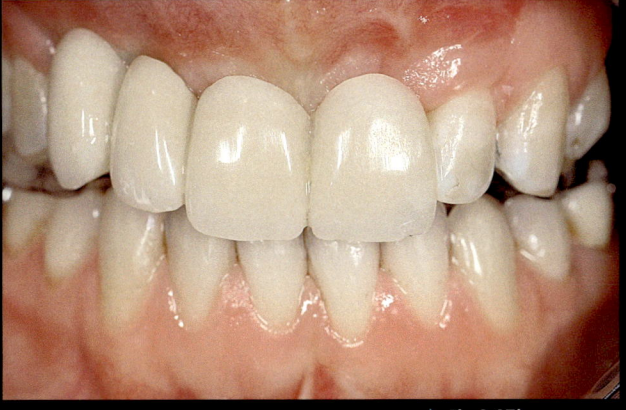

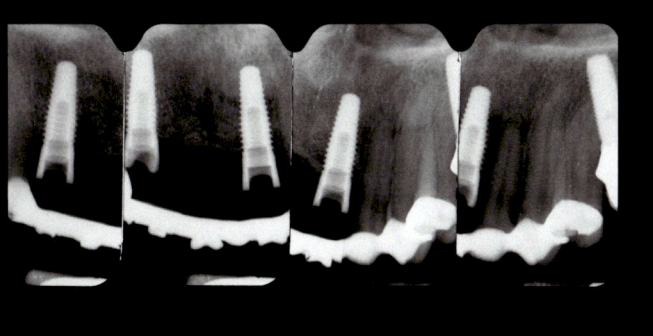

229

ORTHODONTIC PROVISIONAL RESTORATION

For the prosthetic implant treatment of an edentulous area limited to one or two teeth in the anterior sector, before an implant-supported provisional restoration can be used, an orthodontic provisional restoration can be made quickly and used either preoperatively or postoperatively (Figs 2-38a to 2-38l). Using steel wire affixed to brackets bonded to the adjacent teeth, denture teeth can be placed in the edentulous areas for purely esthetic and phonetic functions.[129] The simple and quick application and the low cost of this technique are offset, however, by the limited stability of the resulting provisional restoration.

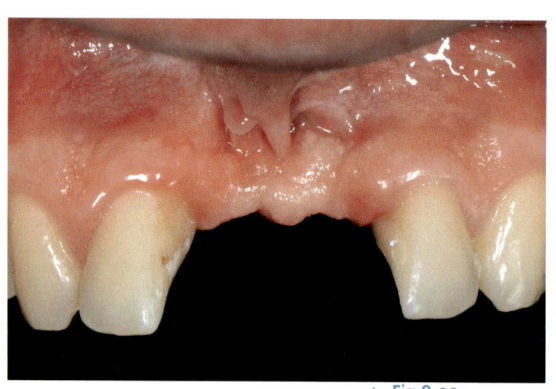

> Fig 2-38a

> Fig 2-38b

> Fig 2-38c

> Fig 2-38d

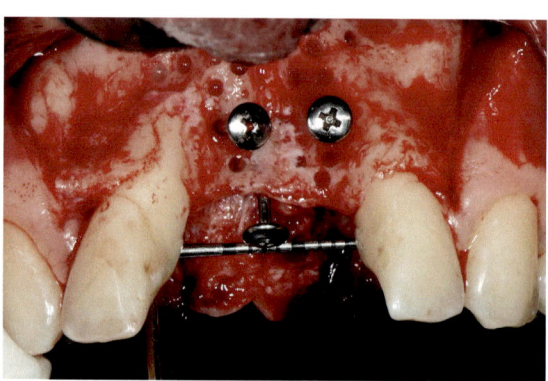

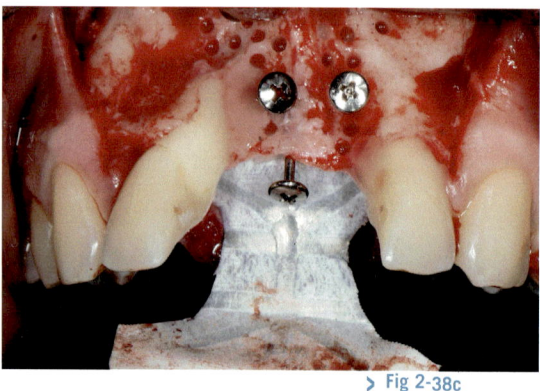

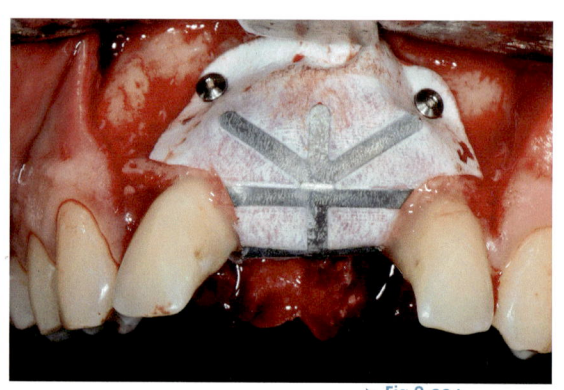

FIG 38 *(a to d)* The traumatic avulsion of the central incisors has made it necessary to carry out a surgical procedure to increase the ridge volume by positioning a reinforced membrane, anchored to specific support screws. (Surgery by Prof Massimo Simion.) *(e and f)* In addition, a periosteal flap has been sutured in a coronal position. *(g and h)* While waiting for complete tissue maturation, an orthodontic provisional restoration was made by anchoring two denture teeth to brackets bonded on the lateral incisors. *(i to k)* Approximately 7 months after the membrane had been positioned, it was removed and, after the adequacy of the osseous volume obtained by the regenerative technique was verified, two implants were placed (NobelPerfect, Nobel Biocare). (Surgery by Prof Massimo Simion.) *(l)* Although implants of reduced diameter (3.5 mm) were selected, the restrictive distance between the lateral incisors, especially with the two teeth emerging from the osseous base, makes it almost impossible to maintain a horizontal biologic space, which ideally should be greater than 1.5 mm between natural tooth and implant and greater than 3.0 mm between implant and implant.

NON-IMPLANT SUPPORTED | FIXED PROSTHESIS

ORTHODONTIC PROVISIONAL

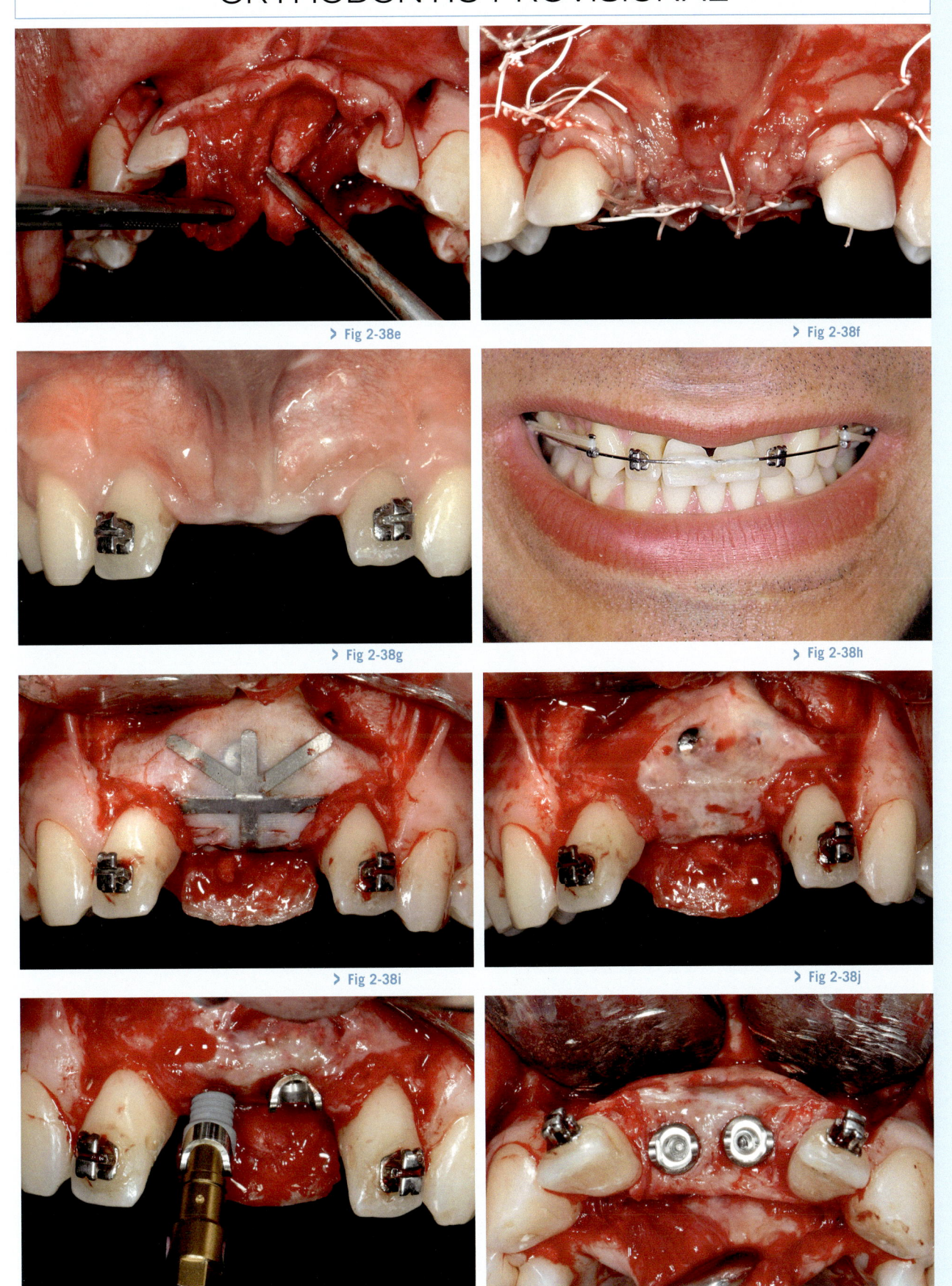

> Fig 2-38e

> Fig 2-38f

> Fig 2-38g

> Fig 2-38h

> Fig 2-38i

> Fig 2-38j

> Fig 2-38k

> Fig 2-38l

231

IMPLANT-SUPPORTED PROVISIONAL RESTORATION

The implant-supported provisional restoration involves anchoring the restoration directly to the implant, with insertion times that vary depending on the difficulty of the individual case. Besides replacing the missing teeth and guaranteeing the patient occlusal, phonetic, and esthetic function, the provisional restoration directly connected to the head of the implant plays an important role by guiding the soft tissues during their healing and maturation process, thus promoting the development of an ideal gingival architecture. Once placed, the implants can be connected to the prosthetic abutments and related restorative, provisional, or definitive prostheses after a defined period based on clinical parameters of a general, surgical, and prosthetic nature (Figs 2-38m to 2-38v). In selected patients, the adoption of appropriate surgical techniques (preparation of the site with a reduced diameter, anchoring the implant bicortically in bone) and the use of implants with a specific design make it possible to achieve primary stability values that allow immediate function and/or prosthetic loading of the implants. The rapid osseointegration, encouraged by the rough surface of the implant, allows a high degree of stability to be maintained even though the initial mechanical integration tends to reduce stability because of the osseous readjustment that takes place after the surgery. To establish a time frame for loading of the implants, the clinician must consider several factors, such as number and position of the implants in the arch, the possibility of joining them together securely, and the adequacy of the occlusal situation in both static and dynamic phases.

Depending on the amount of time that elapses between the placement of the implants and their prosthetic use, the following can be identified:

- *Delayed loading:* Depending on the site, the provisional restoration is fitted between 3 and 6 months after the implants are placed (Figs 2-38w to 2-38ff).
- *Immediate loading:* The provisional restoration is fitted at the same time the implants are placed or, at the most, within 48 hours after.[130–134]
- *Early loading:* The provisional restoration is fitted at some point in the period between immediate loading and delayed loading.

The reliability of delayed loading, a widely tested and practiced technique, and assessment of the risks and benefits of using a provisional restoration immediately, typical of immediate loading, mean that in clinical practice early loading rarely is the chosen option. For this reason, early loading is not specifically addressed in the pages that follow.

FIG 38 *(m and n)* Following the surgical procedure (surgery by Prof Massimo Simion), the flap is sutured into a coronal position to make a greater amount of tissue available during the prosthetic phases. *(o and p)* Roughly 8 months after implant surgery, the implants are exposed and the healing abutments put into position. *(q and r)* With the two abutments removed, the impressions are taken. *(s and t)* By replacing the stone with silicone material in the cast derived from the impressions, the technician will be able to trace the transmucosal path in an ideal way. *(u and v)* After the titanium abutments are positioned on the replica of the head of the implants, the two provisional crowns are fabricated.

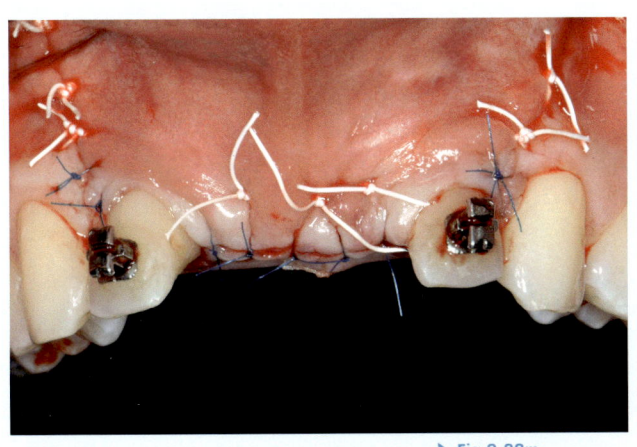

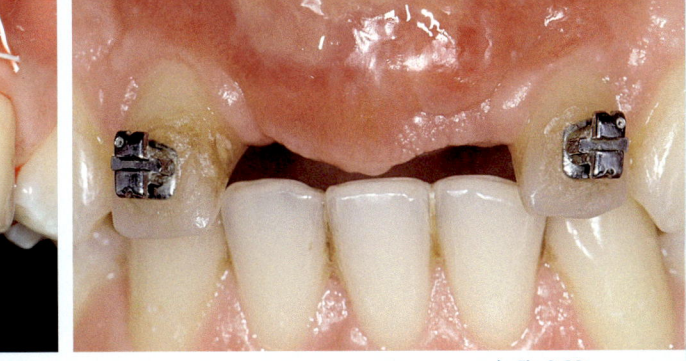

> Fig 2-38m

> Fig 2-38n

> Fig 2-38o

> Fig 2-38p

> Fig 2-38q

> Fig 2-38r

> Fig 2-38s

> Fig 2-38t

> Fig 2-38u

> Fig 2-38v

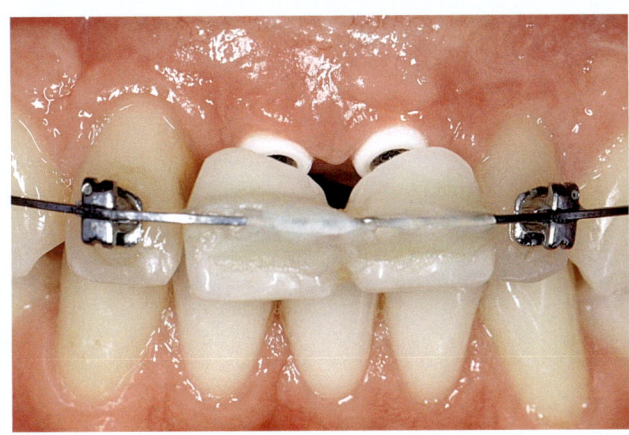

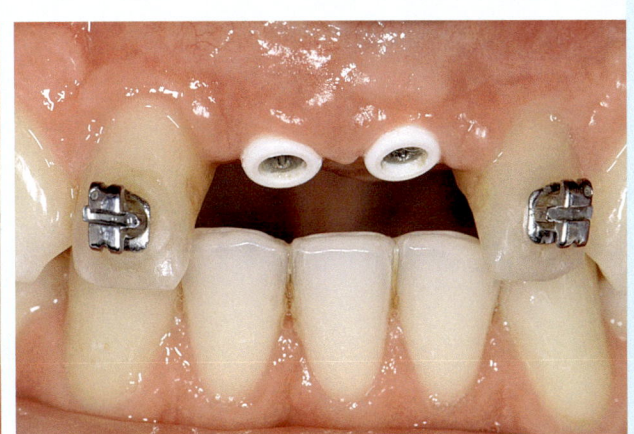

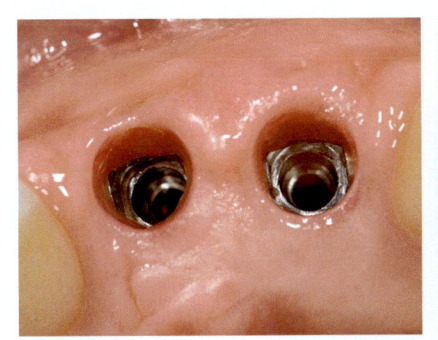

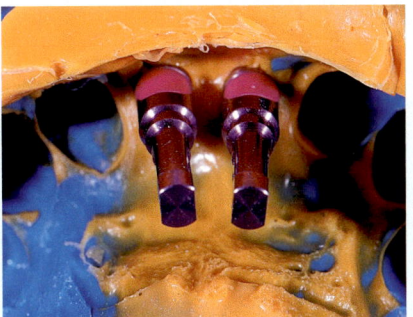

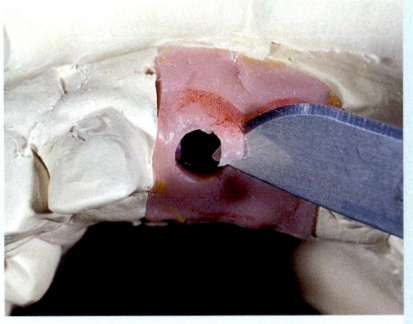

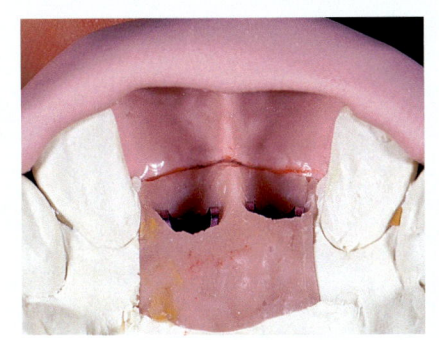

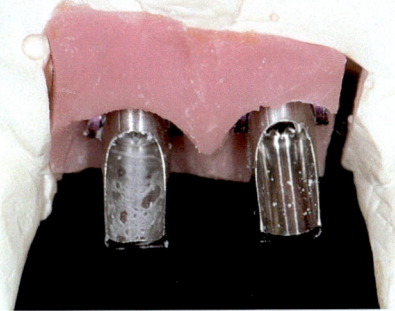

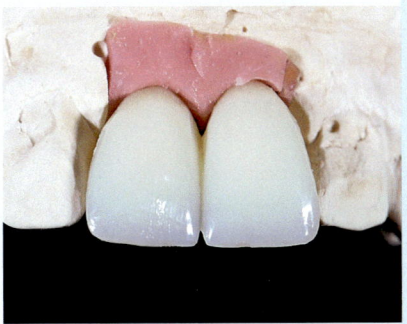

233

> Fig 2-38w

> Fig 2-38x

> Fig 2-38y

> Fig 2-38z

> Fig 2-38aa

> Fig 2-38bb

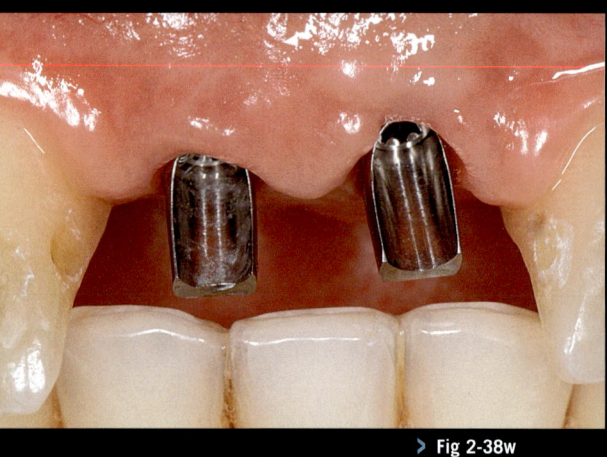

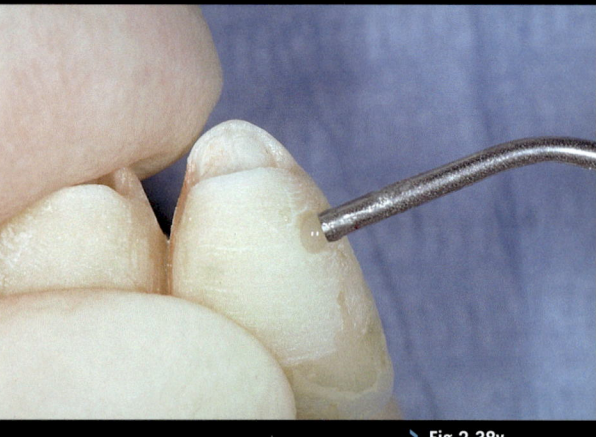

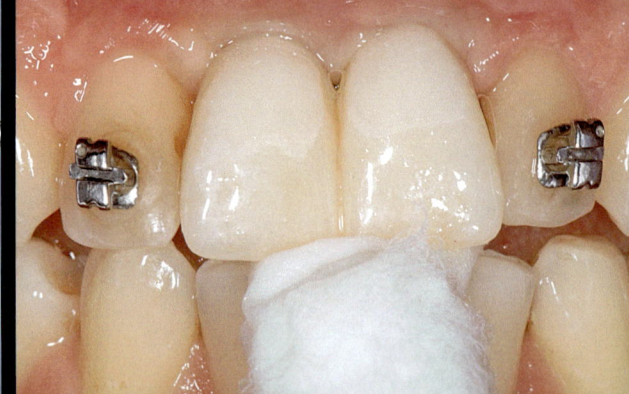

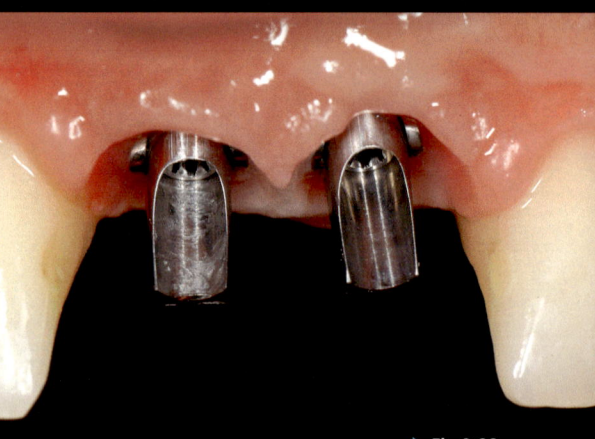

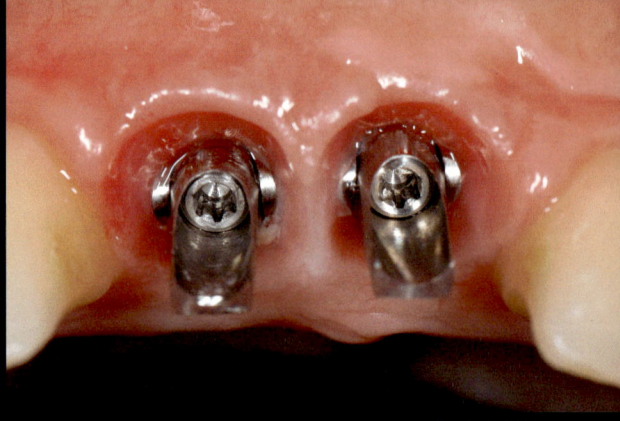

FIG 38 *(w and x)* With the titanium abutments now transferred into the mouth and the provisional restorations in position, one can see that, because of the large amount of soft tissue, the two restorations' margins are in a more coronal position than those of the lateral incisors. *(y and z)* The addition of flowable resin composite in certain specific sites of the cervical area of the provisional restoration, by means of well-applied compression, allows gingival levels and the design of the interproximal spaces to be optimized. *(aa and bb)* One month after positioning, the provisional restorations are removed to inspect the status of the soft tissues, which appear to be healthy and appropriately conditioned. *(cc to ff)* This demonstrates how the problematic preoperative situation has been satisfactorily improved by means of both the surgery and the prosthetic choices. Despite the limited space available, the provisional restorations appear to be pleasingly integrated, also owing to the slight overlap of the central incisors over the laterals, creating an adequately natural look and vitality for the restorations.

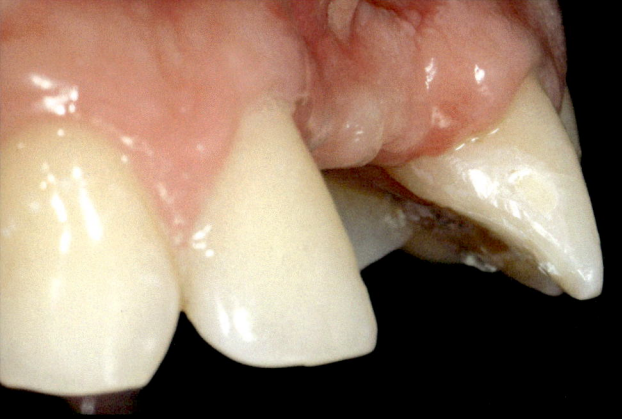

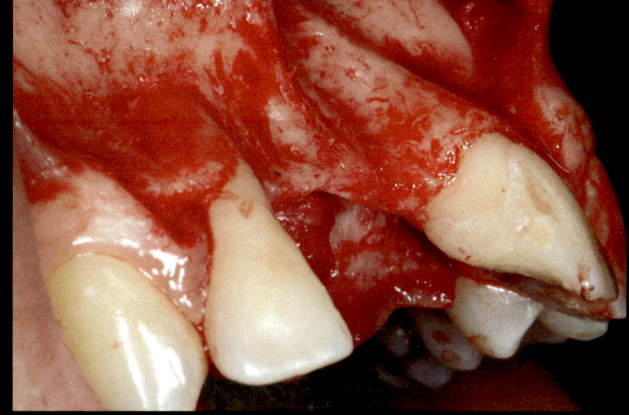

> Fig 2-38cc

> Fig 2-38dd

> Fig 2-38ee

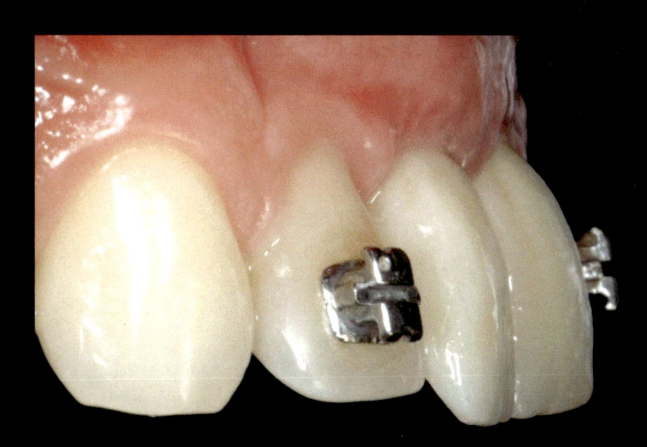

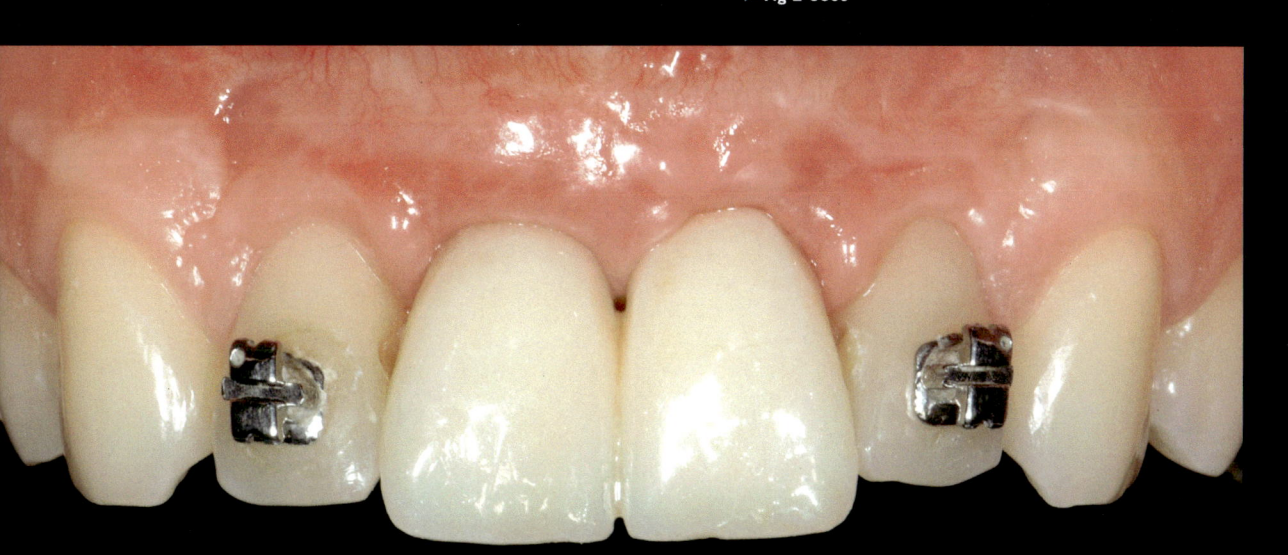

235

IMPLANT-SUPPORTED PROVISIONAL RESTORATIONS

■ DELAYED LOADING ■
PROVISIONAL RESTORATION

From a theoretical point of view, it would always be best to use a provisional abutment before placing the final abutment. In everyday practice, however, patients with partially edentulous areas can have definitive abutments placed directly, especially if it is the posterior sectors to be restored where the esthetic demands are fewer, and/or if the transmucosal path is shallow and therefore the variation in the emergence profile is only slight. This option allows only one provisional phase and offers considerable advantages in both timing and economics, such as avoiding the creation of a second provisional restoration as is necessary in cases of extensive rehabilitation or anterior partial restoration.

PROVISIONAL RESTORATION ON DEFINITIVE ABUTMENTS

The provisional restoration is delivered to the clinician with the definitive abutments and the definitive substructure (Fig 2-39). Once the marginal and occlusal check has been completed, the provisional restoration is fixed, with the clinician carefully and completely removing the excess cement that can remain in the peri-implantar sulcus. This action is usually facilitated by the shallow depth at which the implant platform is generally positioned in the posterior sectors and by the marginal finish limit of the abutment, with the margin specially designated in a juxtagingival or slightly intrasulcular position.

Positioning the provisional restoration directly on definitive abutments while retaining the abutments in the mouth prevents the possible detachment of the junctional epithelium that inevitably occurs every time the definitive abutments are removed and sent to the laboratory to proceed with finalization of the prosthesis. In this way any biologic damage accompanied by possible tissue recession is avoided.

→ ...from page 227

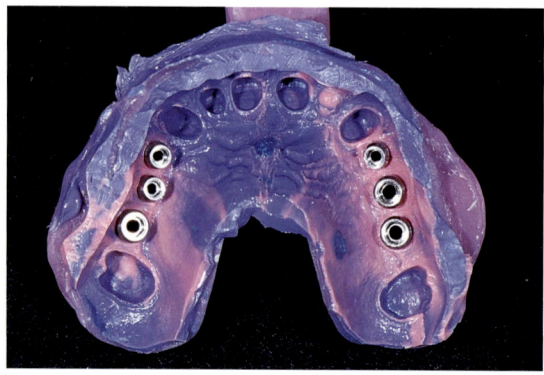

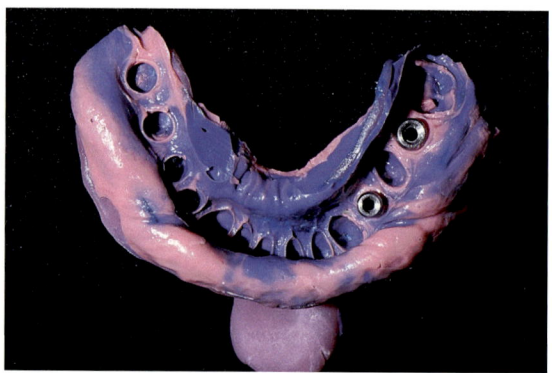

> Fig 2-39a

> Fig 2-39b

> Fig 2-39c

> Fig 2-39d

> Fig 2-39e

> Fig 2-39f

> Fig 2-39g

> Fig 2-39h

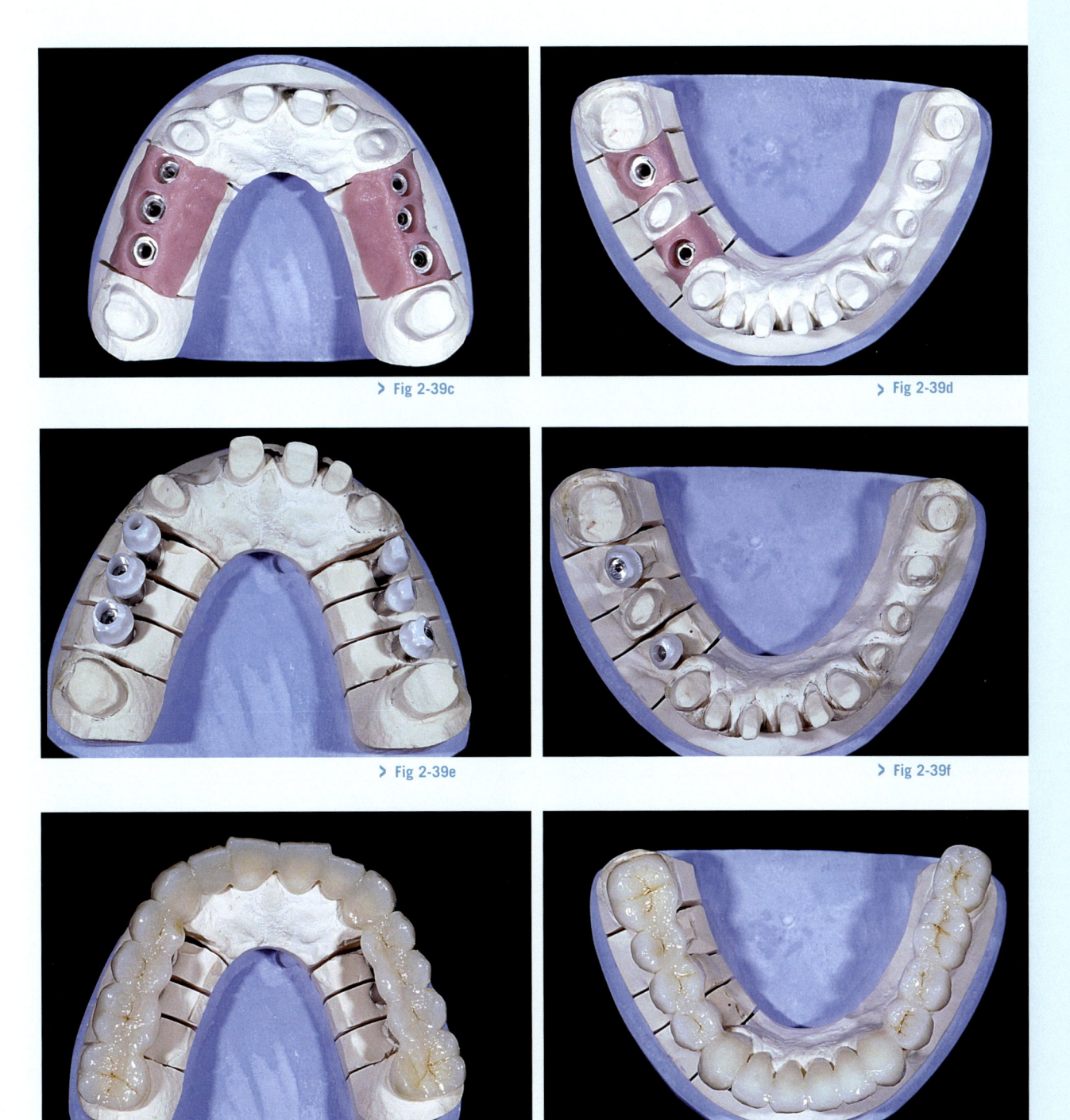

FIG 39 *(a and b)* After waiting an adequate time to achieve osseointegration, impressions are taken both of the implant heads to create the customized abutments in zirconium, and of the abutments of the natural teeth to create the provisional restorations on both complete arches. *(c and d)* On the stone casts, the technician reproduces the gingival soft tissue, using silicone material, in the peri-implant areas. *(e to h)* The zirconium abutments (Procera, Nobel Biocare) are then made and new provisional restorations are fabricated for placement in both arches.

> Fig 2-39i

> Fig 2-39j

> Fig 2-39k

> Fig 2-39l

> Fig 2-39m

> Fig 2-39n

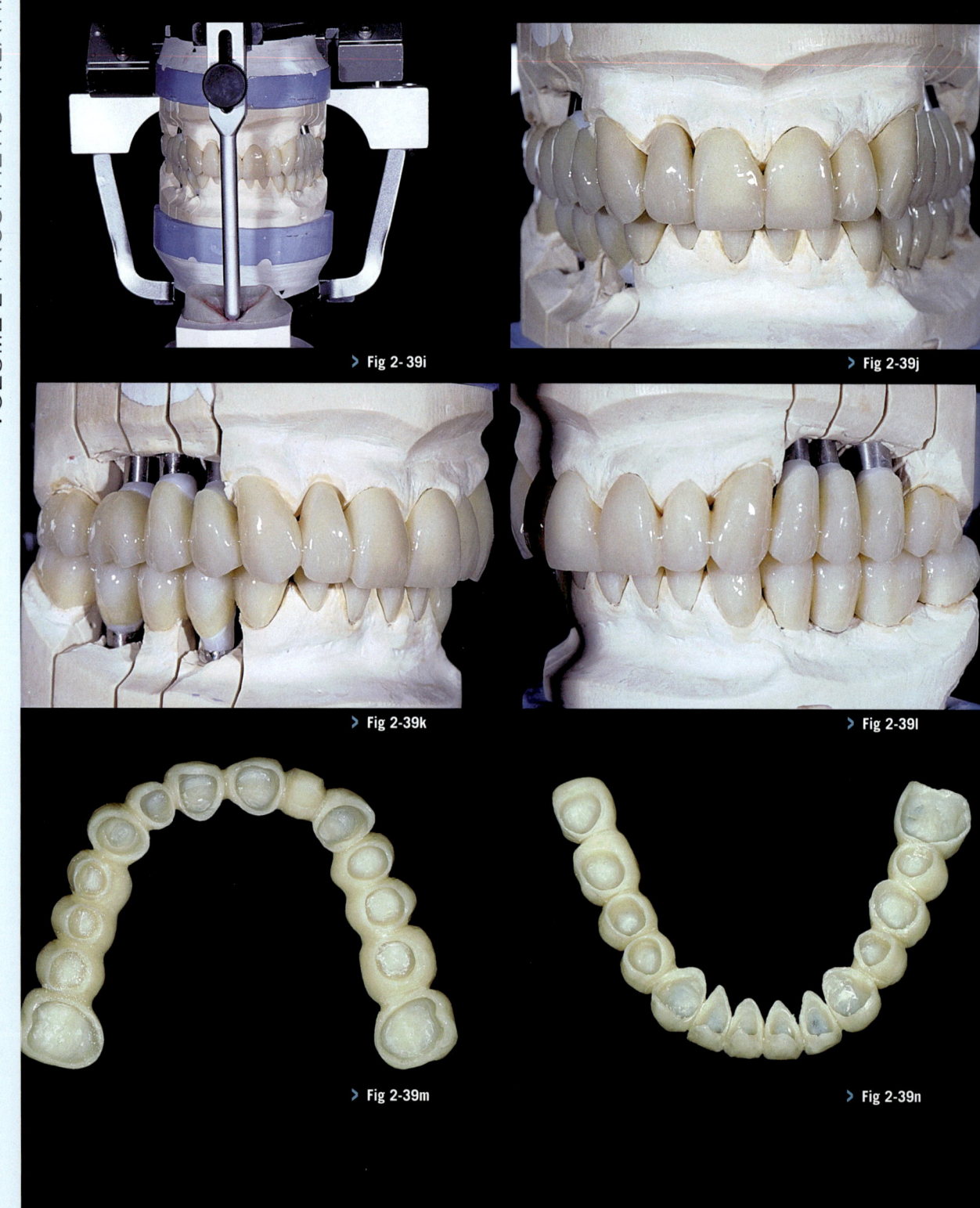

FIG 39 *(i and j)* The provisional restorations mounted on the articulator show the validity of the occlusal relationship. *(k and l)* The lateral view shows the customized zirconium implant abutments. *(m and n)* The provisional restorations, made after tooth preparation with the MIT, are now ready to be relined. *(o to u)* After relining, adequate occlusal stability has been reached, as demonstrated by evenly distributed punctiform contacts on the vertices of the canines, as well as by the presence of the anterior guide with consequent disocclusion of the posterior sectors. *(v)* The patient's smile reveals the satisfactory esthetic integration achieved with the provisional restorations.

> Fig 2-39o

> Fig 2-39p

> Fig 2-39q

> Fig 2-39r

> Fig 2-39s

> Fig 2-39t

> Fig 2-39u

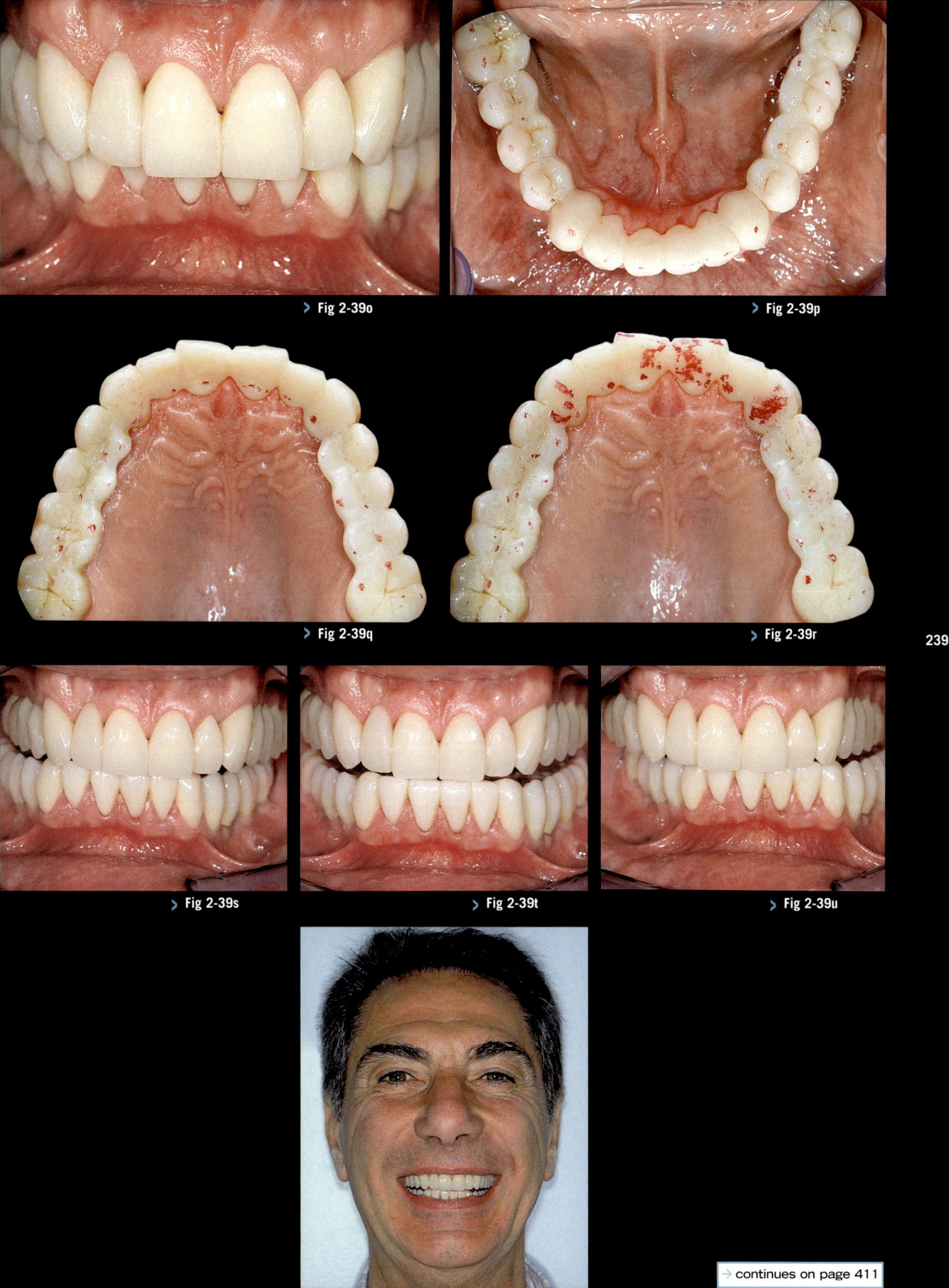

→ continues on page 411

IMPLANT-SUPPORTED PROVISIONAL RESTORATIONS

■ DELAYED LOADING ■
FIRST AND SECOND PROVISIONAL RESTORATIONS

COMPLEX REHABILITATIONS AND ANTERIOR PARTIAL CASES

In many clinical situations, the use of a provisional abutment, preceding construction of the definitive restoration, seems unavoidable.

FIRST PROVISIONAL RESTORATION ON TEMPORARY ABUTMENTS

In fully edentulous arches (Figs 2-40a to 2-40g) and in partial anterior cases, it is an indispensable practice to condition the soft tissues and/or carry out esthetic, phonetic, and/or occlusal checks before the definitive abutments are attached and the case is finalized. In these cases, standard temporary prosthetic abutments in plastic or metal, incorporated into the acrylic resin, are preferred initially because they can be easily modified to suit the specific clinical requirements.[135]

The provisional restoration, with its shape and position perfected in the laboratory, is screw-retained to the implants, and the screw access hole is positioned, if possible, in the occluso-palatal area (Figs 2-40h to 2-40m). The cervical contour should be rather flat, especially if the gingival tissues are not yet completely mature following exposure of the implants. If necessary, the clinician should add or subtract acrylic resin to modify the emergence profile of the intramucosal portion of the provisional restoration.[136]

After all of the necessary esthetic and occlusal checks are completed and the gingival margins and the interimplant papillae are stabilizing, impressions can be taken directly on the head of the implants to construct the definitive abutments on which the second provisional restoration will be anchored.

SECOND PROVISIONAL RESTORATION ON DEFINITIVE ABUTMENTS

Construction of the definitive abutments is accompanied by the fabrication of a second provisional restoration, which may differ from the first based on the need for any esthetic and/or functional modifications requested by the clinician. Retaining the definitive abutments in the mouth prevents the need to remove them again for any tests that could subsequently become indispensable before the work is finalized, thus averting the detachment of the junctional epithelium that inevitably results from this maneuver. Positioning the second provisional restoration on the definitive abutments also makes it possible to evaluate the biologic response of the soft tissues and to confirm, before finalization, the adequacy of the esthetic-functional modifications carried out (Figs 2-40n to 2-40s and 2-41).

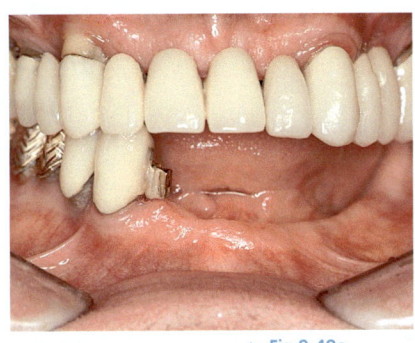

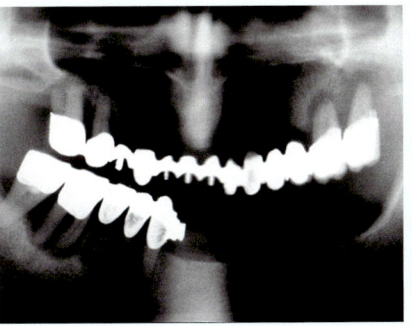

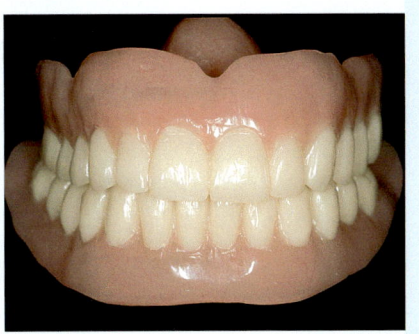

> Fig 2-40a

> Fig 2-40b

> Fig 2-40c

> Fig 2-40d

> Fig 2-40e

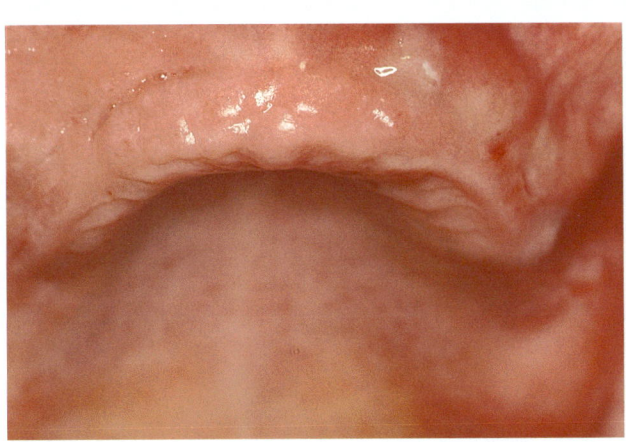

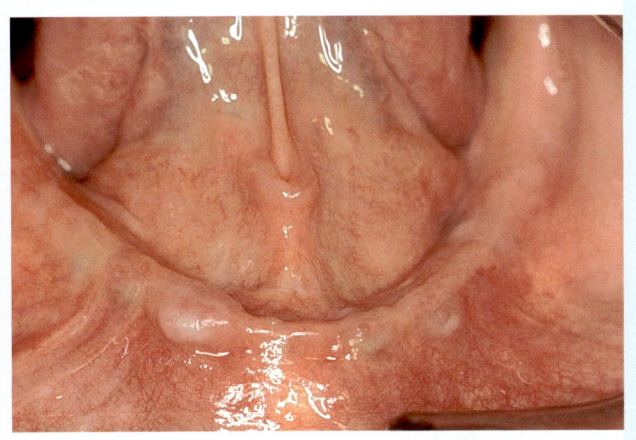

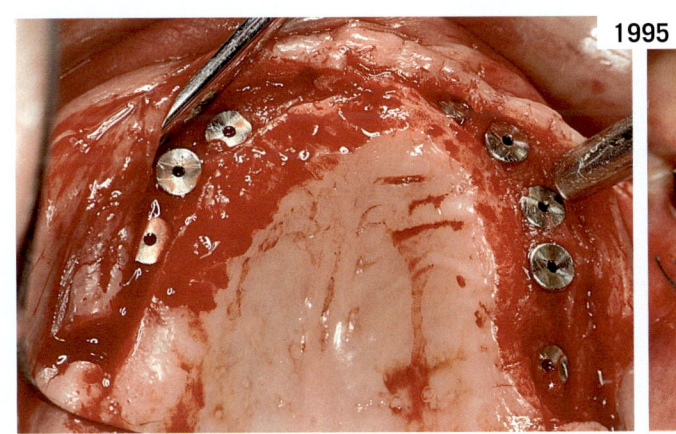

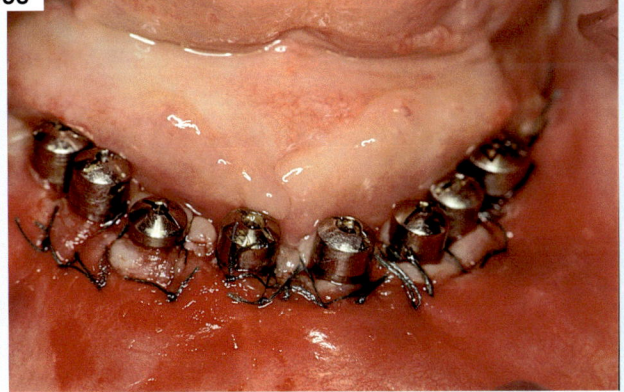

1995

> Fig 2-40f

> Fig 2-40g

FIG 40 *(a to c)* Following extraction of the teeth that supported the old incongruous restorations, the patient is provisionally rehabilitated with two complete dentures. *(d to g)* Roughly 6 months after positioning them and after tissue stability has been achieved, the implants are fitted to the maxillary and mandibular arches.

COMPLEX REHABILITATION

■ FIRST PROVISIONAL ■
REHABILITATION ON TEMPORARY ABUTMENTS

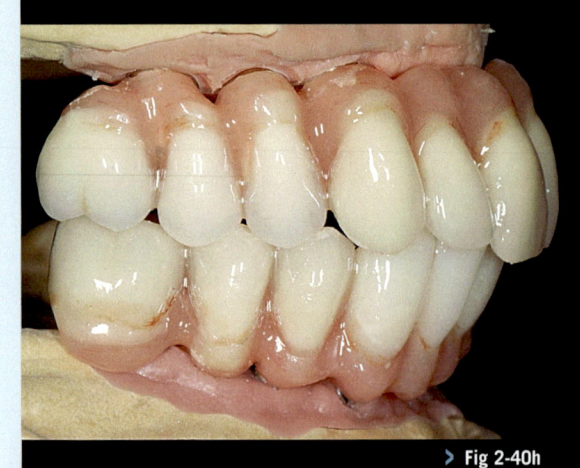

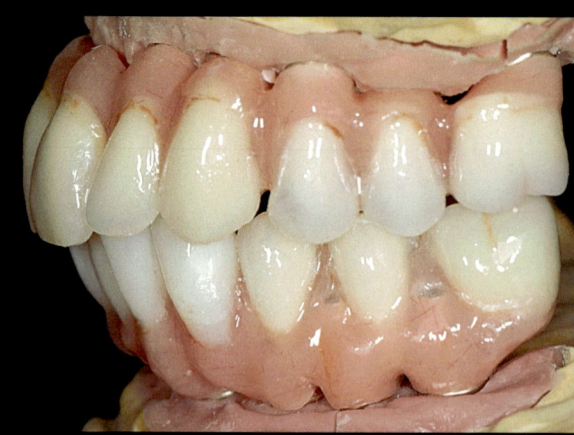

> Fig 2-40h

> Fig 2-40i

> Fig 2-40j

> Fig 2-40k

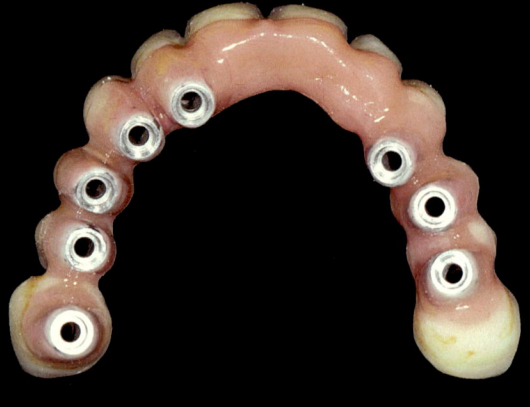

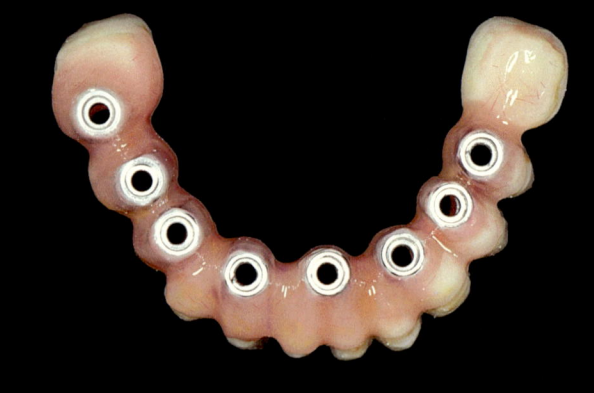

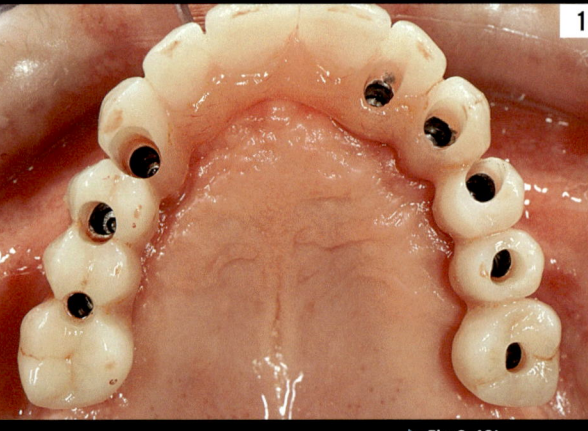

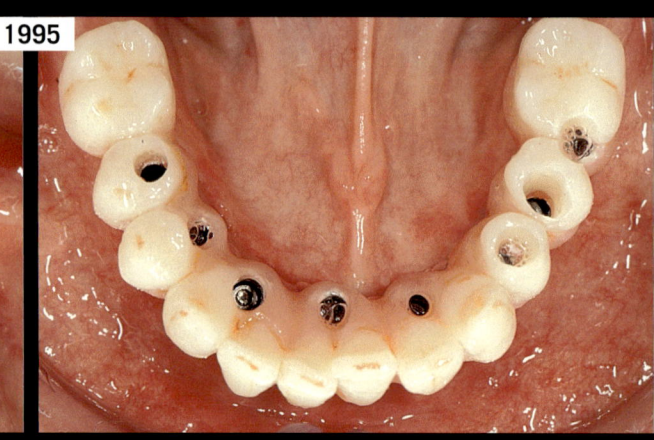

1995

> Fig 2-40l

> Fig 2-40m

FIG 40 *(h to m)* After osseointegration has been achieved, provisional prostheses are constructed and screw-retained directly on the head of the implants, which reflect as closely as possible the esthetic-functional parameters of the removable prostheses. *(n to q)* Once gingival tissue has stabilized, the next step is to fabricate the customized abutments (UCLA) on which a second provisional restoration is made, with slight modifications from the esthetic-functional viewpoint. *(r and s)* This acrylic resin index is bonded in the oral cavity onto the definitive abutments, which will not need to be removed from the oral cavity for subsequent trials of the final restoration.

COMPLEX REHABILITATION

■ SECOND PROVISIONAL ■
REHABILITATION ON DEFINITIVE ABUTMENTS

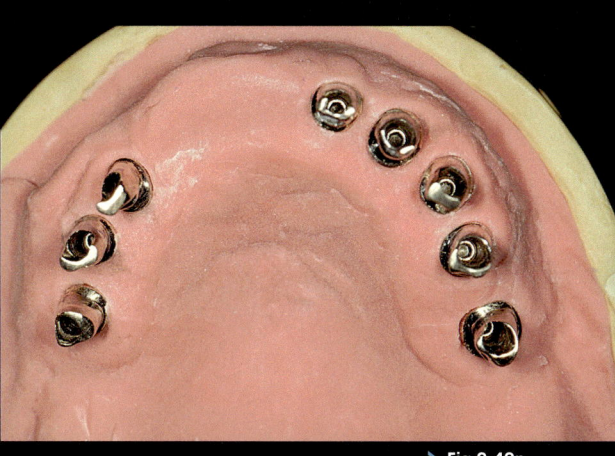

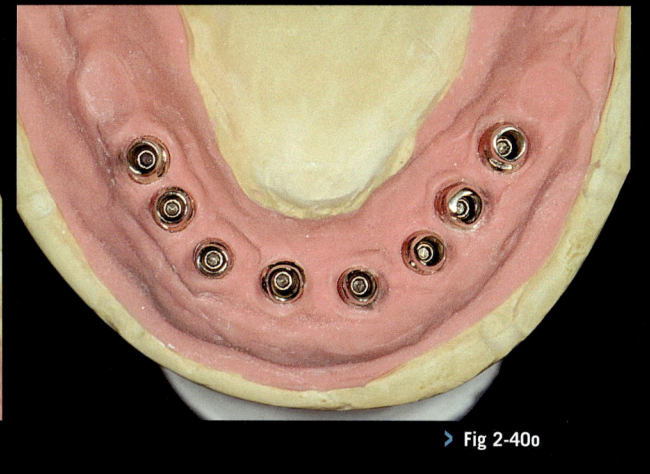

> Fig 2-40n

> Fig 2-40o

> Fig 2-40p

> Fig 2-40q

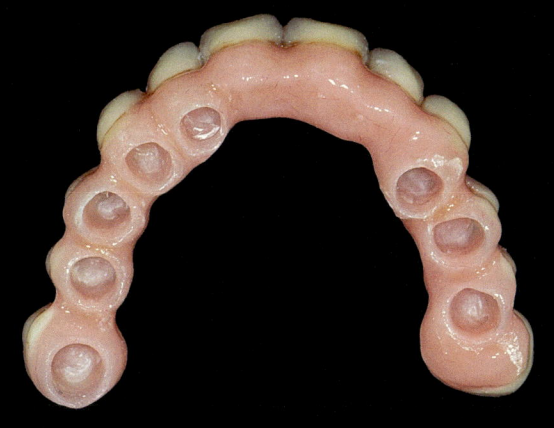

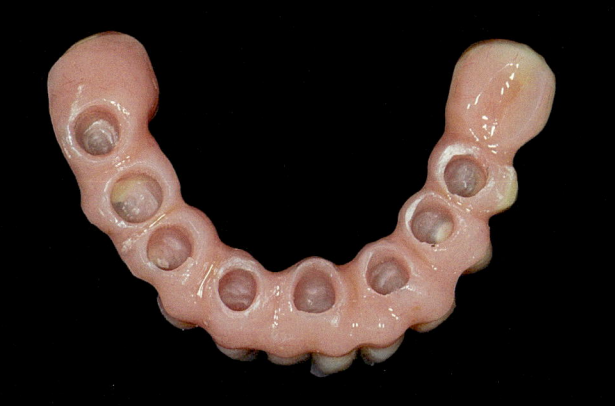

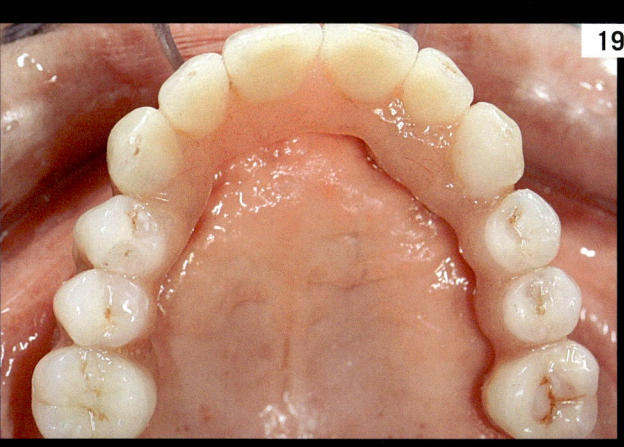

1996

> Fig 2-40r

> Fig 2-40s

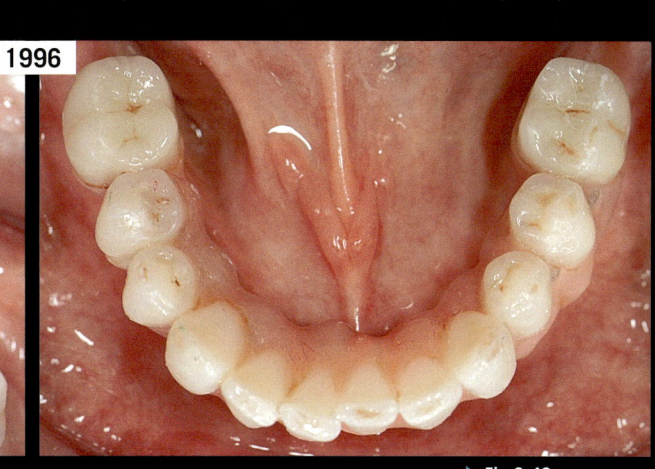

→ Gallery continues on page 526

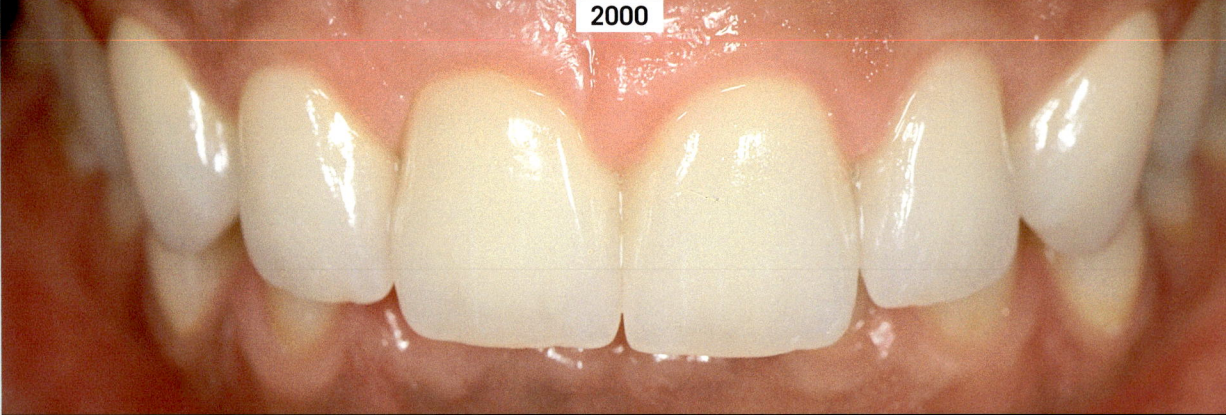

> Fig 2-41a

> Fig 2-41b

> Fig 2-41c

> Fig 2-41d

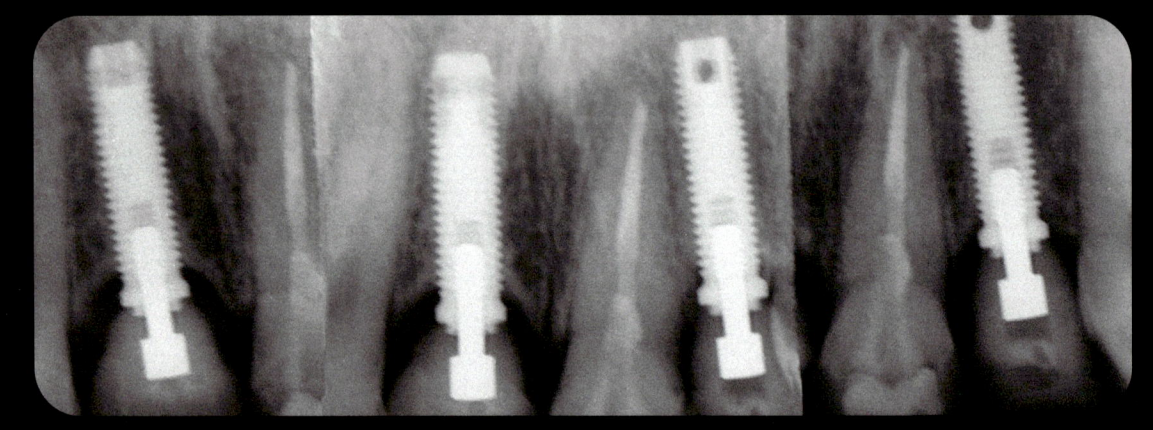

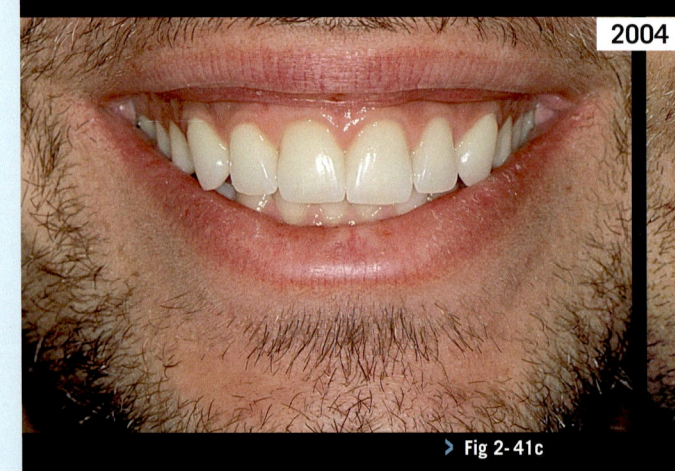

FIG 41 *(a to d)* The patient, rehabilitated some years previously following a road accident and under regular clinical supervision, came to the office after a second damaging accident with a motorcycle. *(e and f)* An intraoral examination of the maxillary arch highlights fractures of 3 restorations and the related prosthetic abutments: 2 on natural teeth (ceramic veneer on the right lateral incisor and an all-ceramic crown on the left central incisor) and 1 on an implant (abutment and all-ceramic crown on the right central incisor). *(g to i)* The occlusal view shows how

> Fig 2-41e

> Fig 2-41f

> Fig 2-41g

> Fig 2-41h

> Fig 2-41i

> Fig 2-41j

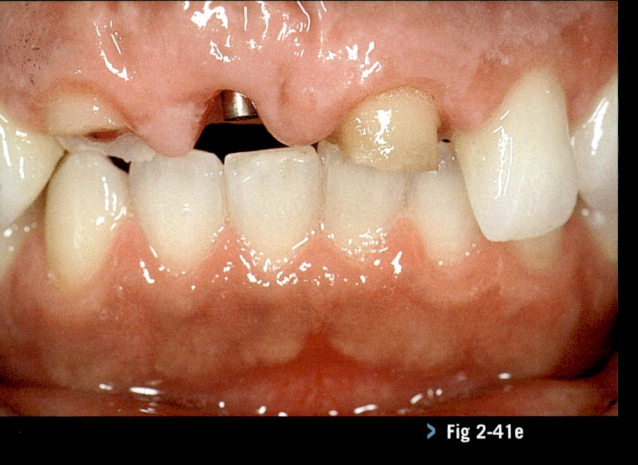

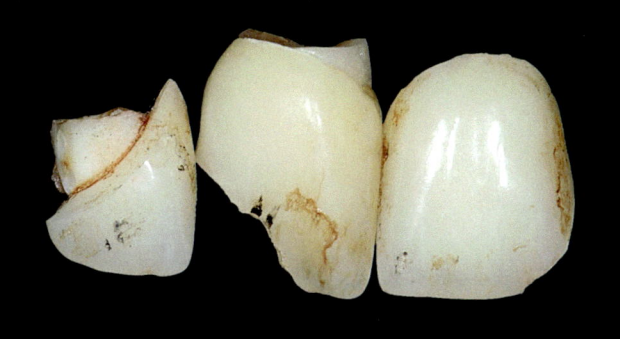

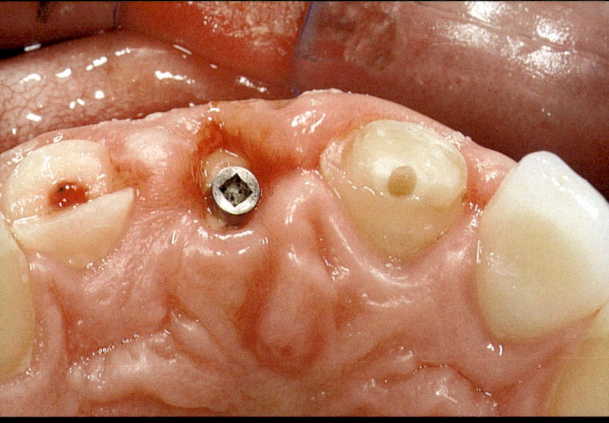

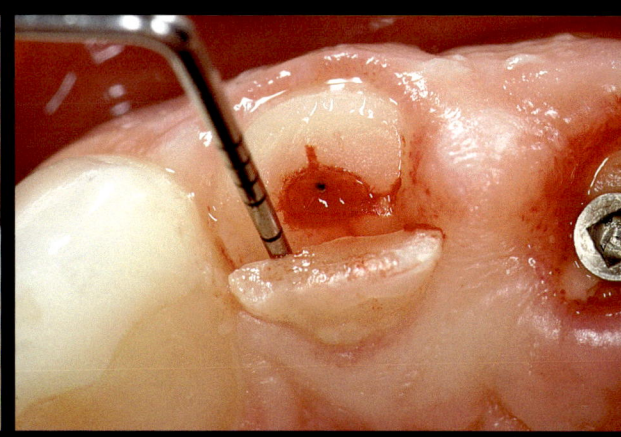

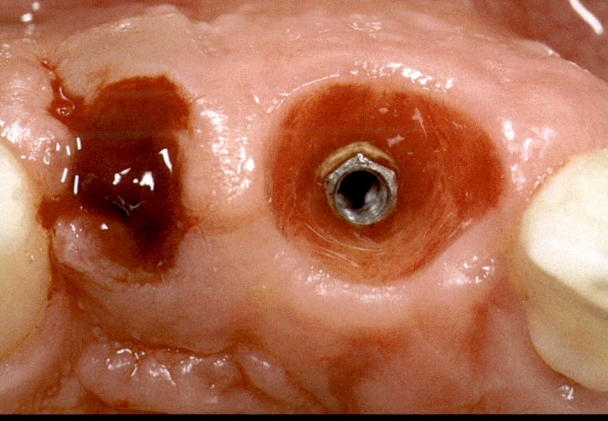

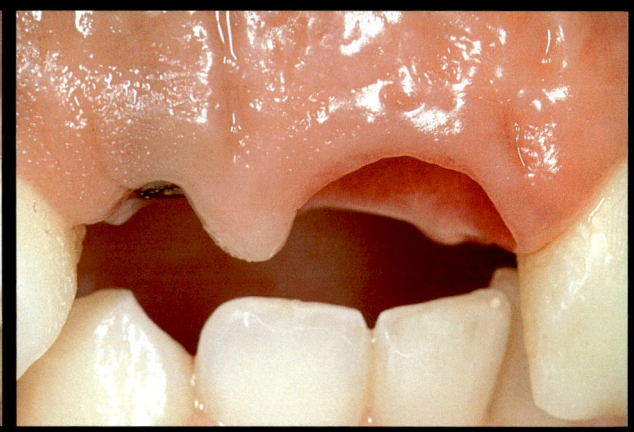

the vertical fracture of the lateral incisor does not allow the tooth to be saved. The tooth is therefore extracted, while at the same time inserting an immediate postextraction implant (one-stage technique) with the placement of a healing abutment 3 mm in height. (Surgery by Dr Sascha A. Jovanovic.) *(j)* It can be seen how, in this phase, the papilla between the right central incisor and the right maxillary lateral still has an ideal height, due to the presence of the connective attachment of the tooth just extracted.

ANTERIOR PARTIAL CASES

■ FIRST PROVISIONAL ■
REHABILITATION ON TEMPORARY ABUTMENTS

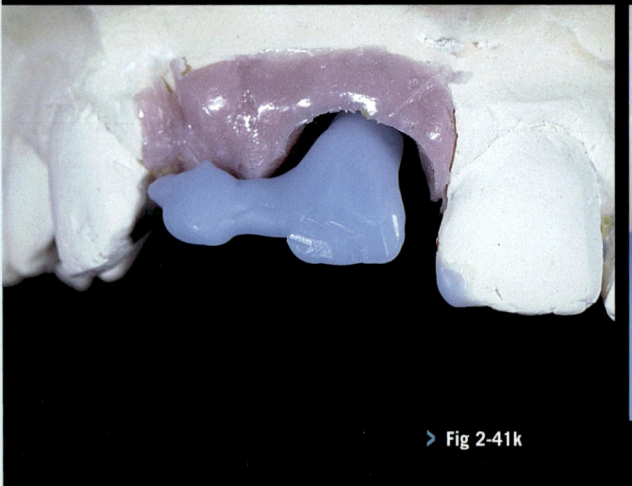

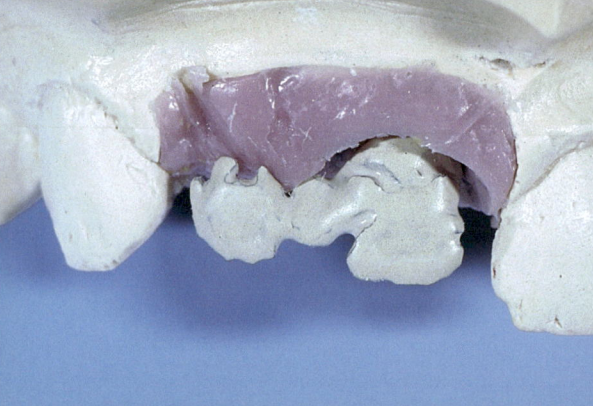

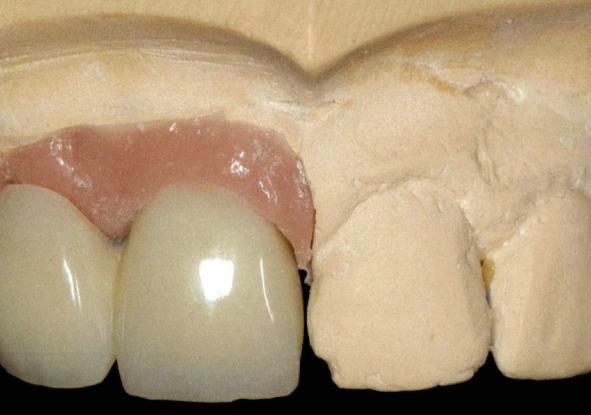

> Fig 2-41k

> Fig 2-41l

> Fig 2-41m

> Fig 2-41n

> Fig 2-41o

> Fig 2-41p

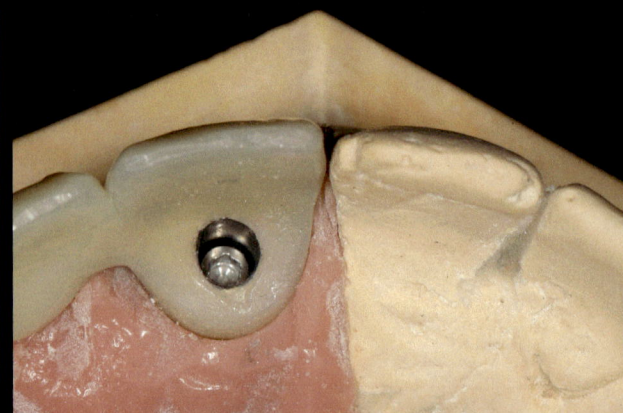

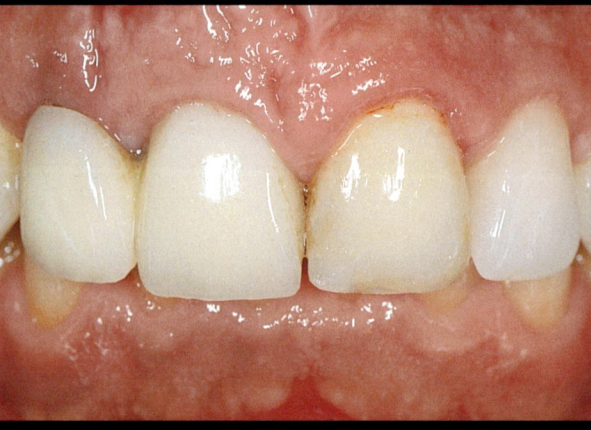

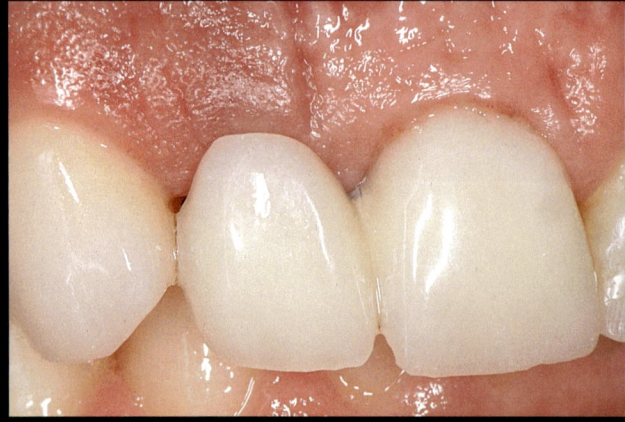

FIG 41 After positioning a provisional tooth on the left central incisor so as not to exert any loading on the implant just inserted on the right lateral, the decision is made to construct a provisional restoration of two teeth anchored to the implant of the right central incisor through a provisional abutment in titanium. *(k)* The provisional restoration, which includes a cantilever unit in the right lateral incisor, is strengthened with a cast metal reinforcement. *(l to n)* After opaqueness of the metal structure has been attained, the provisional restoration is finalized on the stone cast. *(o and p)* Once the restoration is positioned in the mouth, it is easy to see the satisfactory integration achieved.

ANTERIOR PARTIAL CASES

■ SECOND PROVISIONAL ■
REHABILITATION ON DEFINITIVE ABUTMENTS

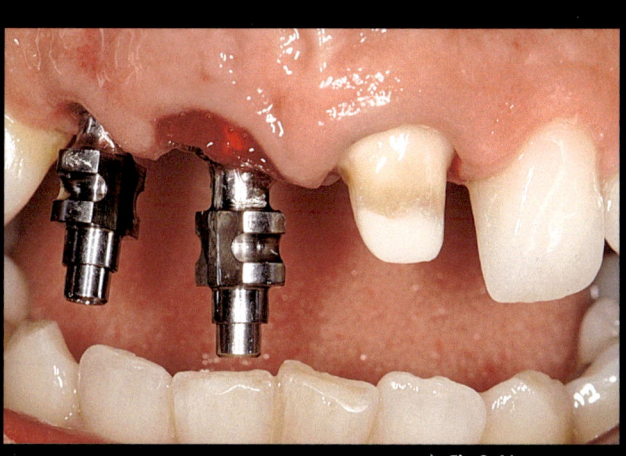

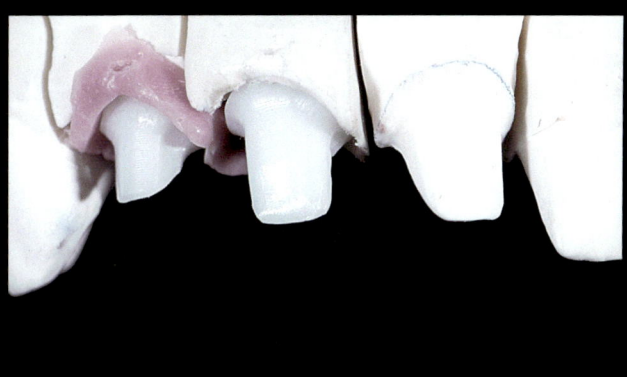

> Fig 2-41q

> Fig 2-41r

> Fig 2-41s

> Fig 2-41t

> Fig 2-41u

> Fig 2-41v

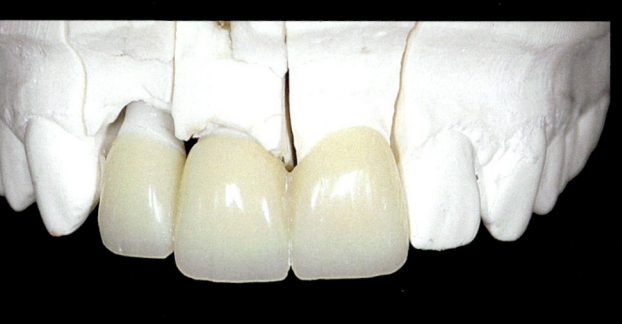

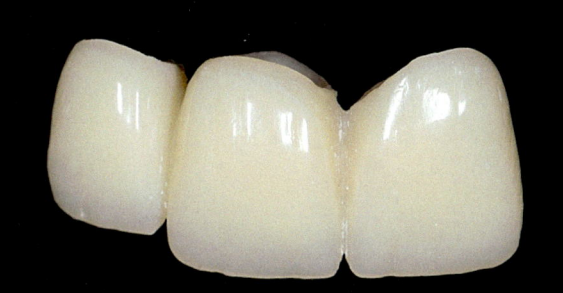

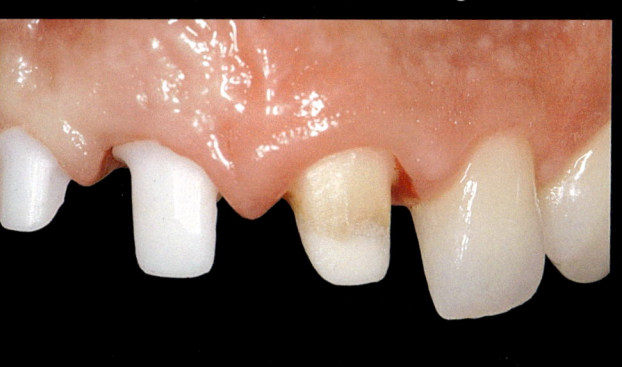

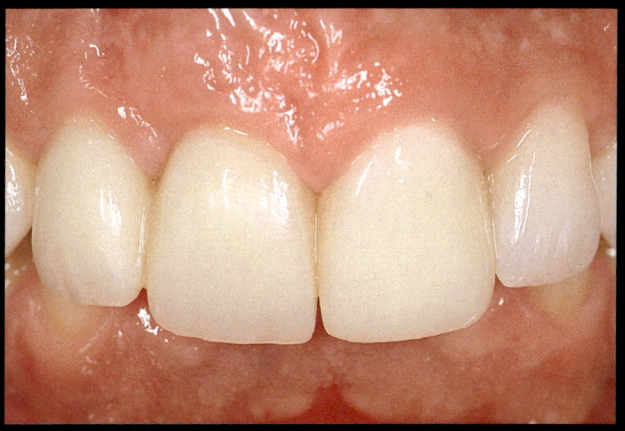

→continues on page 355

A closer view reveals how the healing screw and the provisional restoration have contributed to conserving the adjacent papillae. *(q and r)* After taking the impressions on the implants and on the natural tooth, the final zirconium abutments are made. *(s and t)* The extension of the new provisional restoration includes both the natural tooth and the implants. *(u and v)* The intraoral view of the zirconium abutments makes it possible to appreciate the considerable stability of the height of the interdental papillae, while the photograph of the provisional restoration shows its good integration and the ideal preservation of the gingival levels.

IMPLANT-SUPPORTED PROVISIONAL RESTORATIONS

IMMEDIATE LOADING

In immediate implant loading, the provisional restorations can be divided into the following distinct types, each of which has associated esthetic and functional implications:

- Provisional restoration for partial, single, or multiple edentulous areas[137–143]
- Provisional restoration for implant-prosthetic rehabilitation of entire arches[131,144–151]

Immediate loading can be carried out only on carefully selected patients who are aware of its indubitable esthetic advantages as well as its risks, not necessarily those associated with osseointegration but specifically those related to the stability of the gingival margins[137] and the possible flattening of the buccal bone over time.[152,153] Following placement, the implant must demonstrate good primary stability, assessed on the basis of the insertion torque (> 32 Ncm) or analysis of the resonance frequency (implant stability quotient [ISQ] ≥ 60 to 65).

In cases of single implants as well as the rehabilitation of an entire arch, the screw-retained prosthetic solution is normally used for a provisional restoration. An access hole, which ideally emerges in the occlusopalatal area, makes it possible to insert or remove the prosthesis when necessary, without having to resort to luting agents, whose excesses are always difficult to remove completely.[135]

SINGLE IMPLANT – IMMEDIATE FUNCTION

The provisional restoration is inserted at the same time as positioning the implant, especially in the anterior sector, primarily to satisfy the patient's esthetic and phonetic requirements (Figs 2-42a to 2-42d). Owing to the cervical design perfected in the laboratory, the acrylic resin prosthesis also supports the soft tissues around the implants, maintaining the scalloped shape and height of the papillae during the entire healing period (Figs 2-42e and 2-42f).[137,154,155]

The provisional restoration cannot introduce occlusal contact, either in the static or dynamic phases, to ensure that axial loads or tangential dislocating forces do not interfere with the osseointegration process (Figs 2-42g and 2-42h). These cases are termed *immediate implant function*, although it is always possible that, during the time necessary to achieve satisfactory osseointegration, the patient inadvertently exerts veritable loading forces on the treated tooth.

FIG 42 *(a and b)* The fracture of the buccal wall on the right lateral incisor has an apical extension that does not allow it to be retained. *(c and d)* At the same time that it is extracted, an immediate implant is positioned, with the head of the implant inserted 3 mm more apically than the gingival level of the adjacent teeth. (Surgery by Dr Stefano Gori.) *(e and f)* In the postoperative phase a provisional restoration is put in place by attaching it with screws to the head of the implant, which should serve only an esthetic and phonetic function (immediate function). It can be seen how, after 6 months, the interproximal papillae, like the gingival levels, have not undergone any substantial changes compared with the preoperative situation. *(g and h)* To minimize the risks involved in immediate positioning of the provisional restoration, particular care must be taken to avoid any occlusal contact in both the static and dynamic phases.

> Fig 2-42a

> Fig 2-42b

> Fig 2-42c

> Fig 2-42d

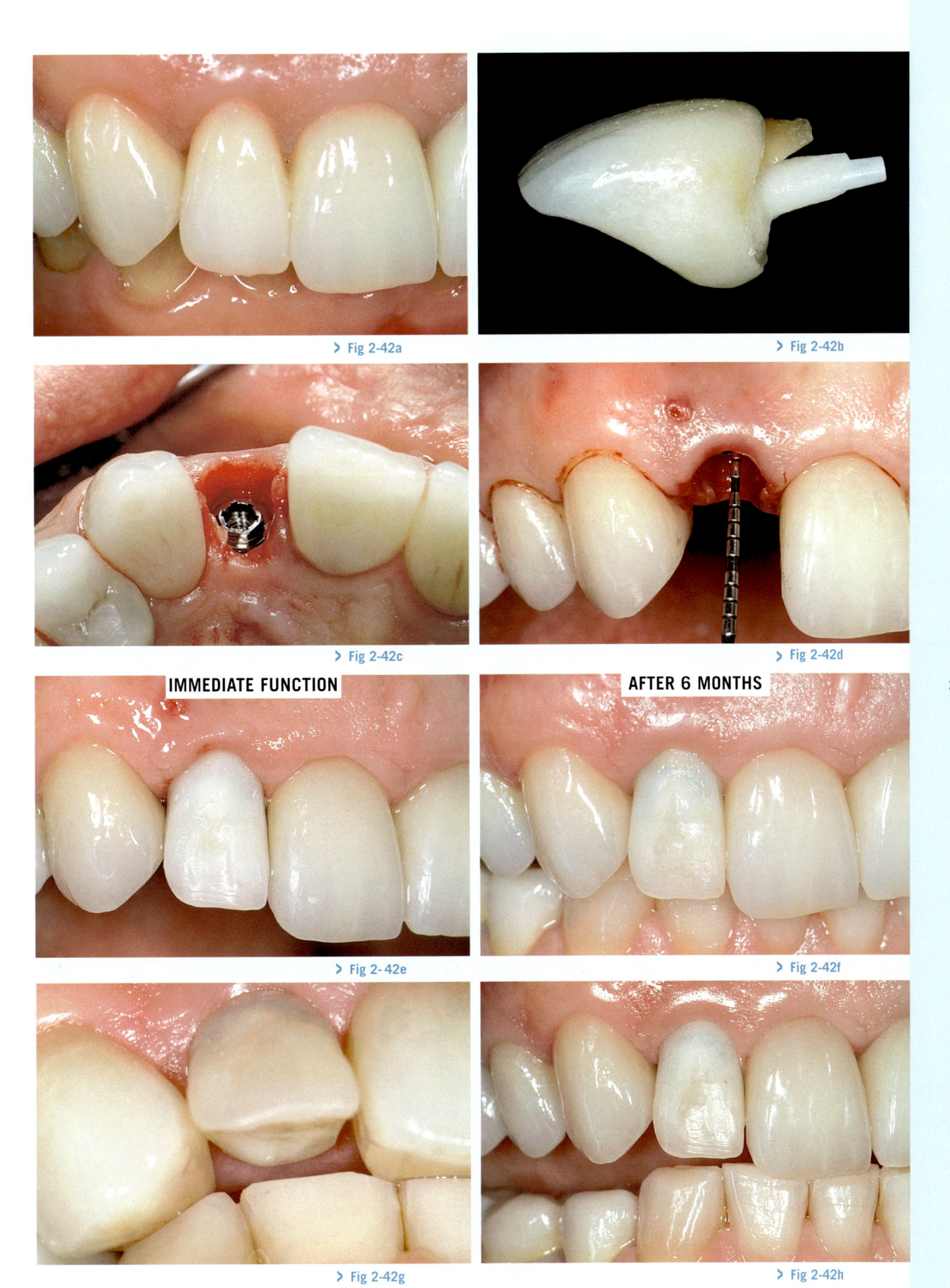

IMMEDIATE FUNCTION

AFTER 6 MONTHS

249

> Fig 2-42e

> Fig 2-42f

> Fig 2-42g

> Fig 2-42h

The provisional restoration for the immediate loading of a single implant is normally fabricated in the laboratory to perfect its shape and contour according to impressions taken before the implant is placed (Fig 2-43). As it is for the natural teeth, relining is carried out directly in the oral cavity after attaching the preformed abutment to the head of the implant. The only precaution in this phase is to ensure that the access allowing the provisional restoration to be screw-retained to the implant is not obstructed by the relining paste. Once relining is completed, the provisional restoration is finished outside the oral cavity and inserted at the end of the surgical session. During the tightening and unscrewing maneuvers for any modifications necessary to the contour, the provisional restoration should be held very still between the fingers so that no twisting forces are transmitted to the implant, at the same time avoiding tightening the screw with excessive torque. As an alternative to the method described above for creating the provisional restoration, the position of the implant can be taken as soon as it is placed, using resin to "block" the transfer coping to the suitably modified surgical stent. The index, made solid with the coping, is fitted onto the same stone cast used to fabricate the surgical stent and then modified to accommodate the coping and the head implant replica, blocked in a position that corresponds with that of the implant. In the laboratory, the technician can then fabricate a provisional restoration that, although not requiring any relining, cannot be inserted into the mouth until 24 to 48 hours after the implant was placed, allowing the time necessary to make the restoration.[156]

The impressions for finalizing the prosthetic work can be taken after a period that varies from 4 to 6 months.

SINGLE IMPLANT—IMMEDIATE FUNCTION

ADVANTAGES

- Single surgical stage
- Increased patient comfort
- Ideal shape and contour
- Easier management of provisionals
- Immediate support for the peri-implant tissues

WARNINGS

- Exclude parafunctional patients and those with deep overbite.
- Achieve adequate primary stability (> 35 N).
- Ascertain the presence of at least 2 mm of buccal bone.
- Check the buccal bone–implant distance (< 2 mm).
- Avoid any occlusal contact in both static and dynamic phases.

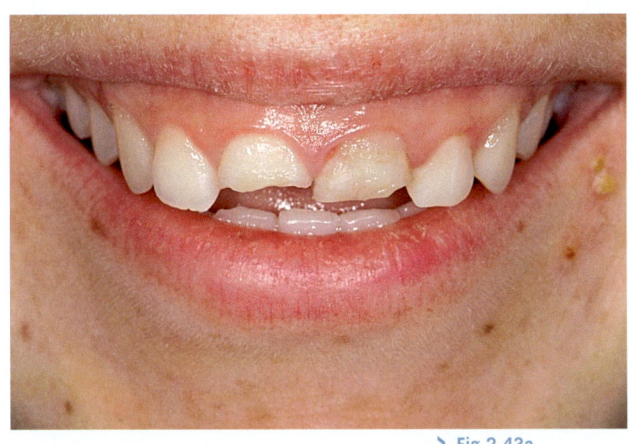

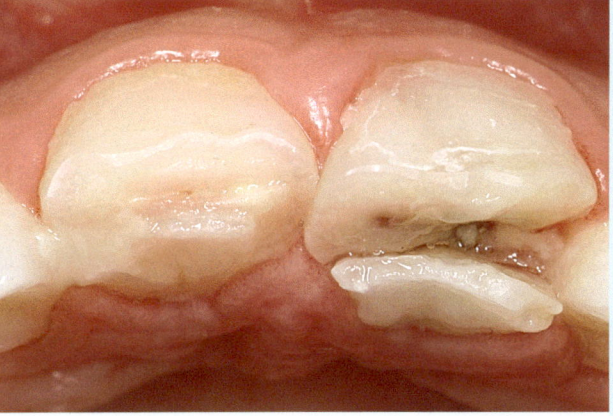

> Fig 2-43a

> Fig 2-43b

> Fig 2-43c

> Fig 2-43d

> Fig 2-43e

> Fig 2-43f

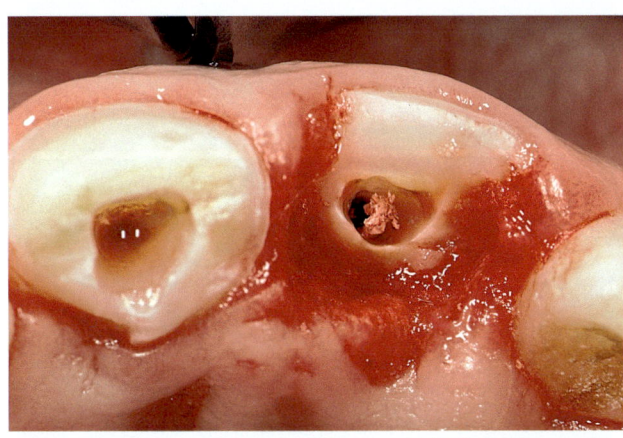

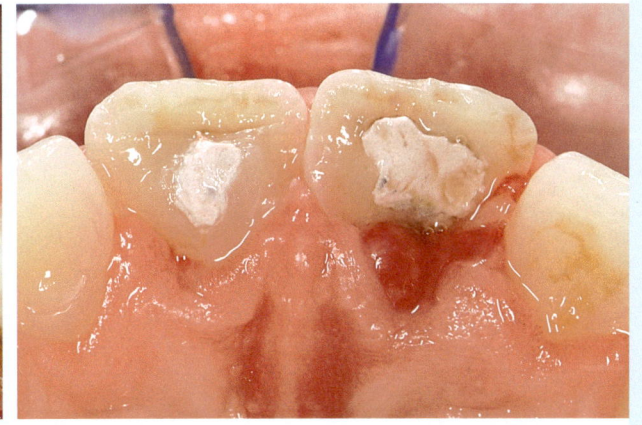

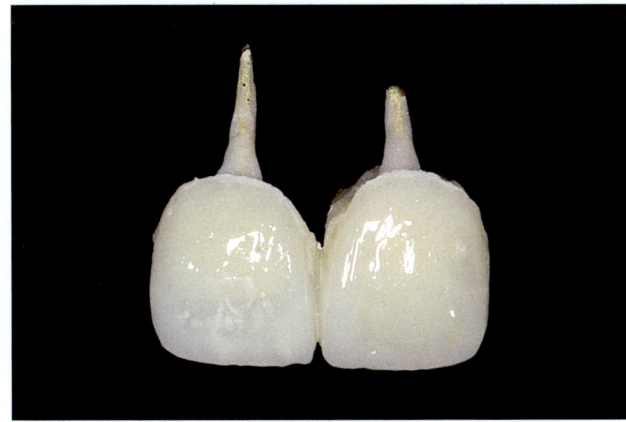

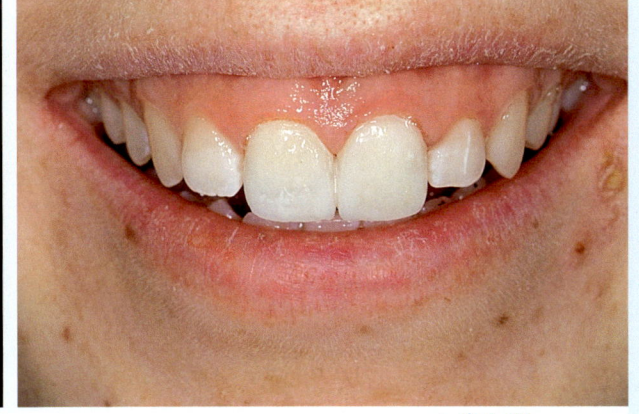

FIG 43 *(a)* The young patient has a fracture of the maxillary central incisors following an accident. *(b)* The occlusal view highlights a vertical fracture of the left central incisor that makes it impossible to save. *(c and d)* Once the fragments have been removed, both teeth are endodontically treated. *(e and f)* This allows two acrylic resin crowns to be temporarily positioned, which achieve adequate stability in the oral cavity after relining due to the presence of two endodontic posts.

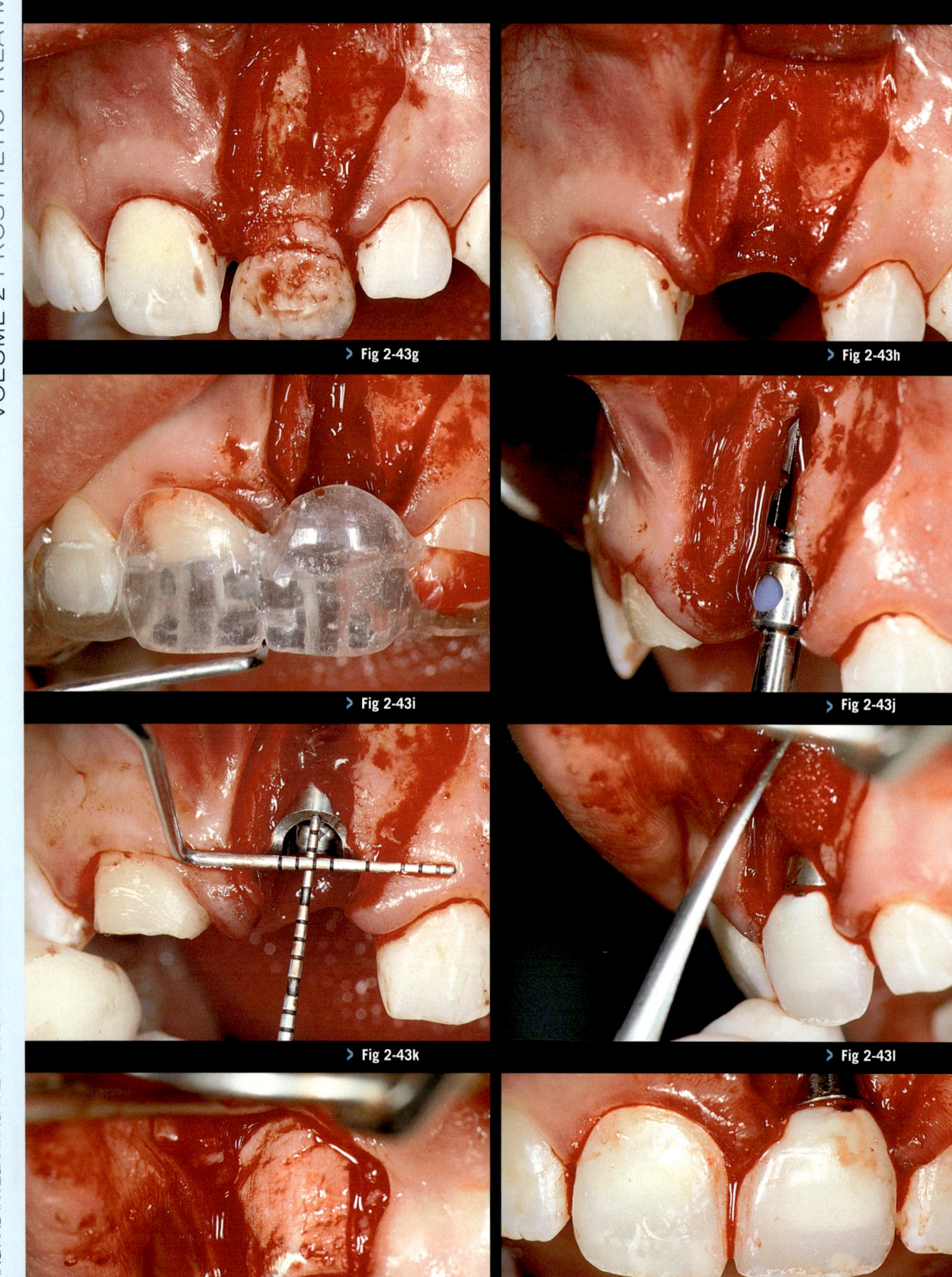

> Fig 2-43g

> Fig 2-43h

> Fig 2-43i

> Fig 2-43j

> Fig 2-43k

> Fig 2-43l

> Fig 2-43m

> Fig 2-43n

> Fig 2-43o

> Fig 2-43p

> Fig 2-43q

> Fig 2-42r

> Fig 2-43s

> Fig 2-43t

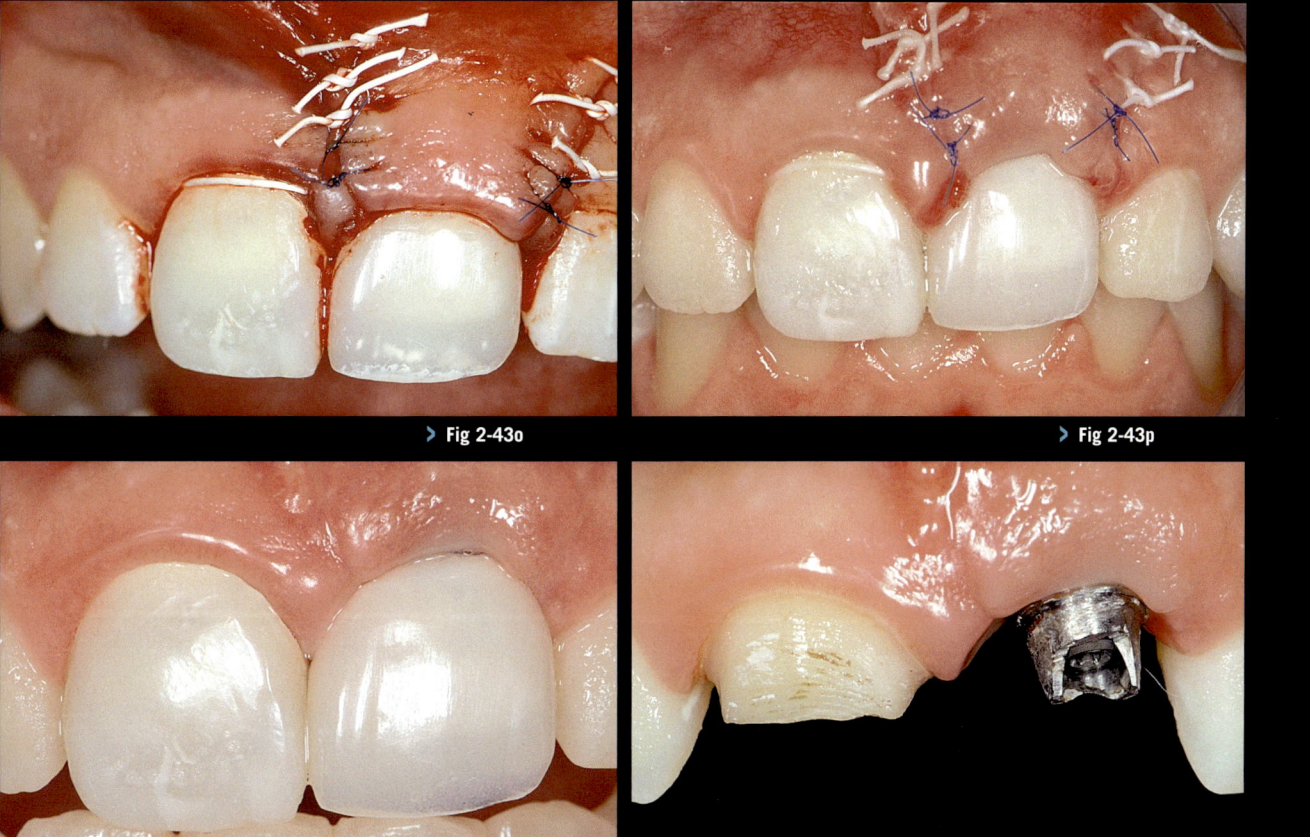

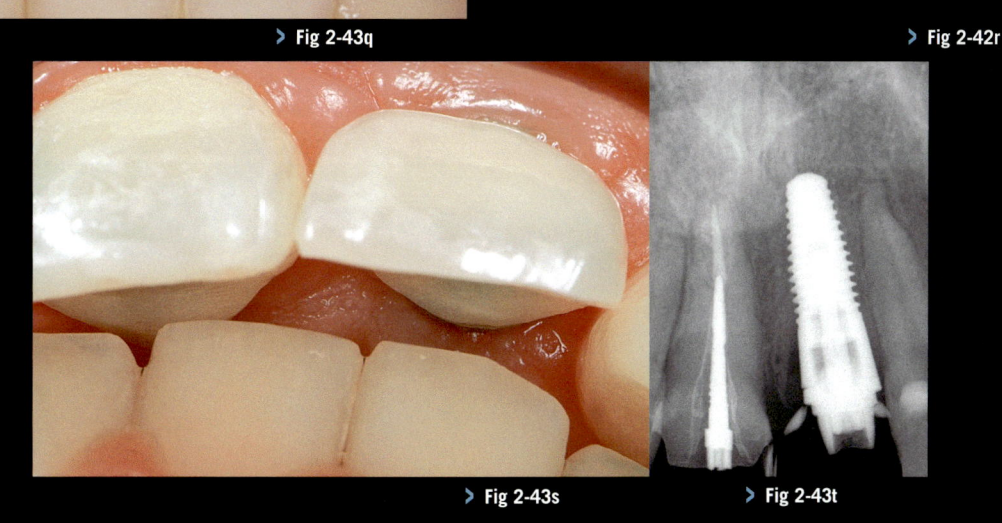

FIG 43 *(g)* With the flap raised, the complete lack of bone is revealed in the buccal wall of the maxilla at the left central incisor. *(h and i)* After the tooth is extracted, a surgical stent is inserted that guides the implant positioning (NobelPerfect). *(j)* The head of the implant is located in the buccal area roughly 2.5 mm from the adjacent gingival levels while, because of the particular shape of the implant, the interproximal peaks remain approximately 1.0 mm subgingivally. (Surgery by Dr Sascha A. Jovanovic.) *(k to m)* At the same time that the implant is inserted, some autologous bone mixed with Bio-Oss is placed to fill the buccal dehiscence, and a resorbable membrane is applied. *(n)* It is at this point that the acrylic resin shell is adapted using a provisional abutment. *(o to r)* With the flap sutured in a coronal position, a slight shrinkage of the soft tissues can be seen after 10 days. This does, however, appear to be contained 6 months postoperatively to allow good alignment of the gingival levels to be maintained. *(s)* The large interocclusal space purposefully left in the palatal aspect of the provisional restoration prevents any contact in both the static and the dynamic phase. *(t)* The radiograph, taken 6 months after positioning, confirms that osseointegration has been achieved.

→ continues on page 362

REHABILITATING ONE OR TWO ARCHES – IMMEDIATE LOADING

The provisional restorations made for rehabilitating entire arches, unlike those for partial ones, must ensure esthetic and phonetic function as well as provide masticatory function (Fig 2-44). This situation describes true "immediate implant loading." It is therefore necessary to give the provisional restoration adequate occlusal stability with punctiform, synchronous, and well-distributed contacts,[157–161] while at the same time creating an anterior guide that, even if not very steep, nevertheless does allow disocclusion of the posterior sectors.[162]

With the aid of a previously fabricated individual impression tray, the impression of the newly placed implants can be taken directly following the surgical procedure. The laboratory can then fabricate a provisional restoration, with possible metal reinforcement,[132,163] that can exist with the solution that has been cemented onto individual abutments. Alternatively, the patient's whole prosthesis can be relined on special abutments, thereby transforming it into a fixed prosthesis screw-retained to implants.[164–166] In this case, too, after waiting a suitable time for osseointegration and for the soft tissues to mature (> 6 months), the definitive impressions can be taken and the case finalized. Software is now available for processing the CT scan, allowing prosthetically and surgically guided implant positioning by means of stereolithographic surgical templates (Figs 2-45a to 2-46).

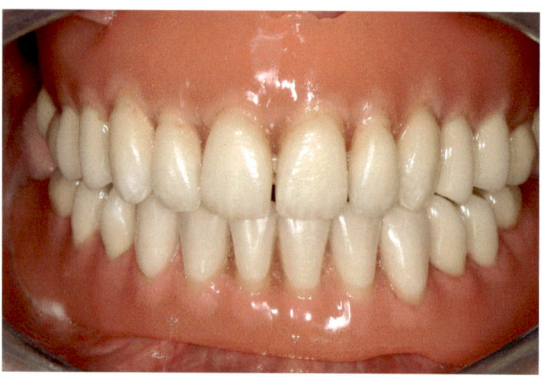

> Fig 2-44a

> Fig 2-44b

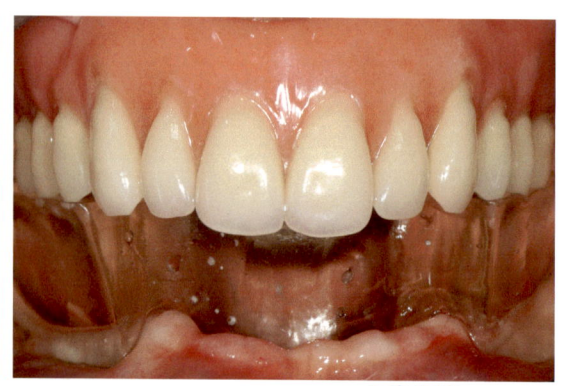

FIG 44 *(a)* The intraoral view of the pre-existing complete removable dentures makes it possible to identify poor stability as well as inadequate esthetics, due to the unsuitable tooth shape and arrangement. *(b)* Try-in of the new maxillary dentures in ideal occlusal relationship, with the transfer matrix positioned at the correct VDO. The ideal identification of the implant sites is marked on the matrix. *(c)* Clinical view of the implant fitting devices, joined to the surgical stent with acrylic resin. *(d)* Assembling the matrix on the master cast makes it possible to check, by means of the impression, the position of the implants and, above all, the accuracy of the occlusal record for mounting on the articulator. *(e)* Just 48 hours after implant surgery the Toronto prosthesis is screw-retained to the mandibular arch. (Treatment by Dr Marco Redemagni and Mr Tom Abbondanza.) *(f)* On both the maxillary and mandibular prostheses, the anterior teeth are ceramic and the posterior ones resin. *(g)* The clinical situation 1 month after inserting the prosthesis. At 6 months postoperatively the prosthesis is removed to reline the cervical areas because of soft tissue shrinkage. *(h)* The healthy condition of the peri-implant tissues is evident. *(i)* A view of the relined mandibular prosthesis, in which the resin teeth have been replaced with ceramic ones in both the maxillary and mandibular posterior sectors. *(j)* The panoramic radiograph carried out 6 months after treatment.

> Fig 2-44c

> Fig 2-44d

> Fig 2-44e

> Fig 2-44f

> Fig 2-44g

> Fig 2-44h

> Fig 2-44i

> Fig 2-44j

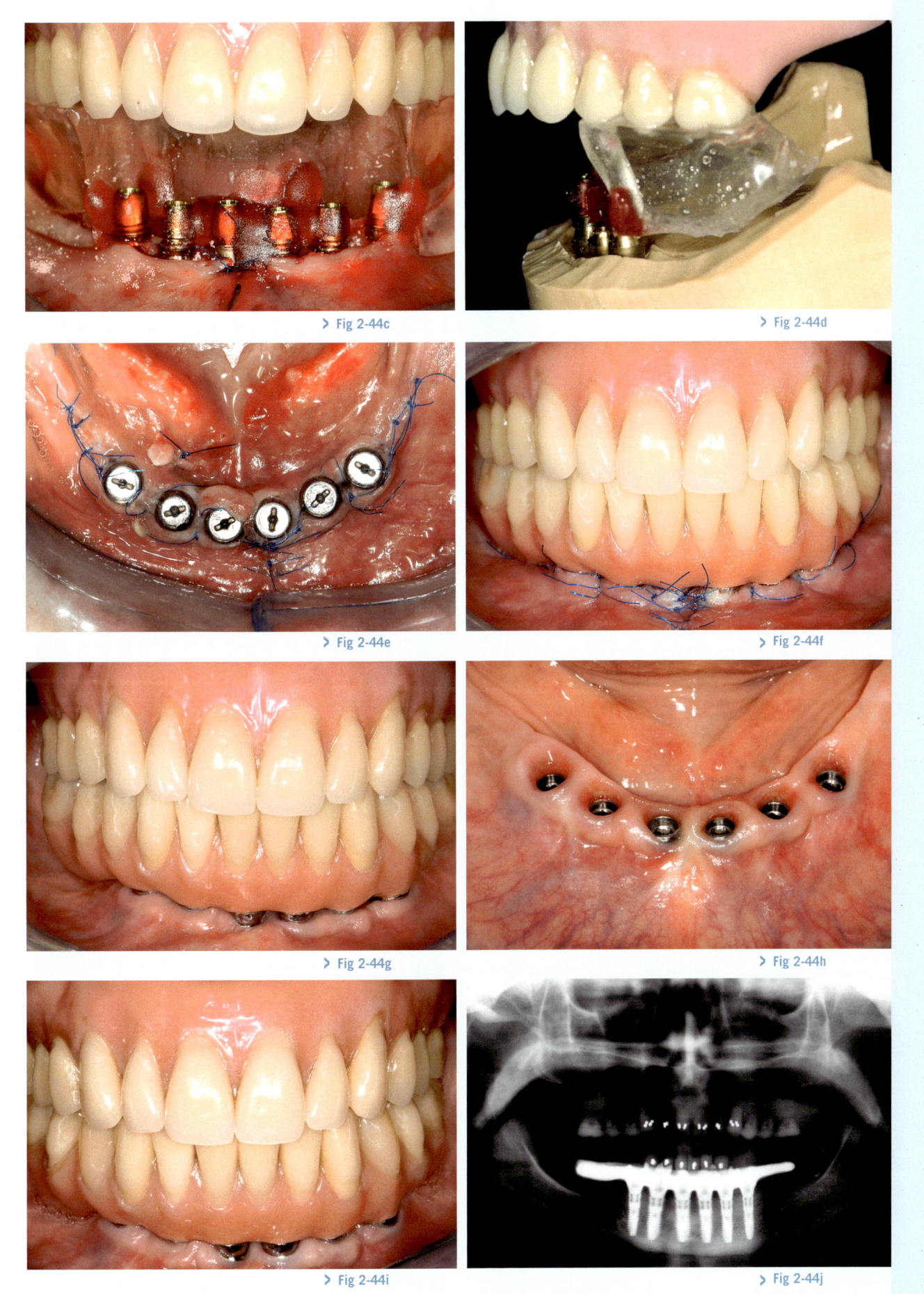

Fig 2-45a

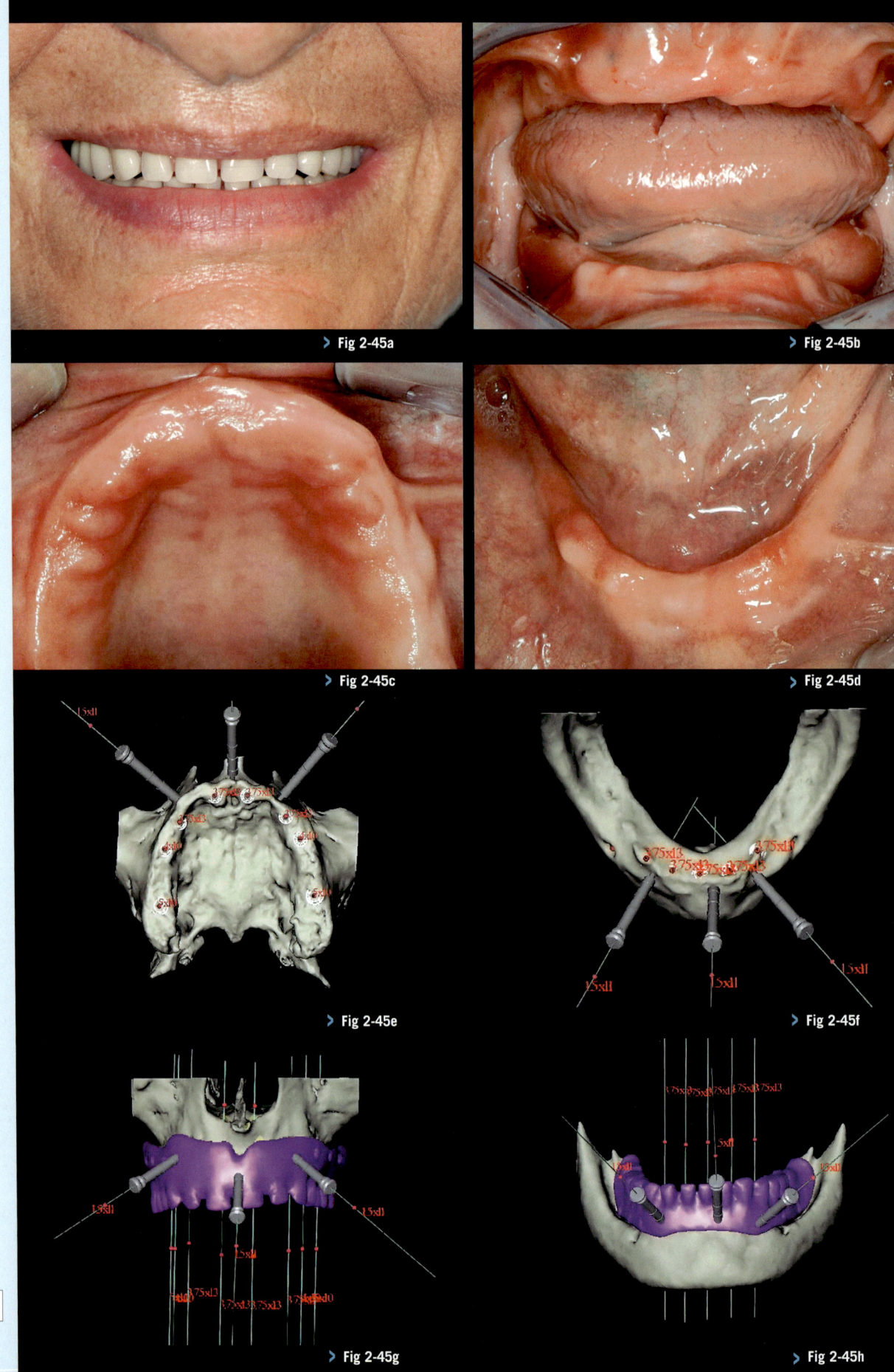

Fig 2-45b

Fig 2-45c

Fig 2-45d

Fig 2-45e

Fig 2-45f

Fig 2-45g

Fig 2-45h

3D PLANNING - CEMENTED PROSTHESIS

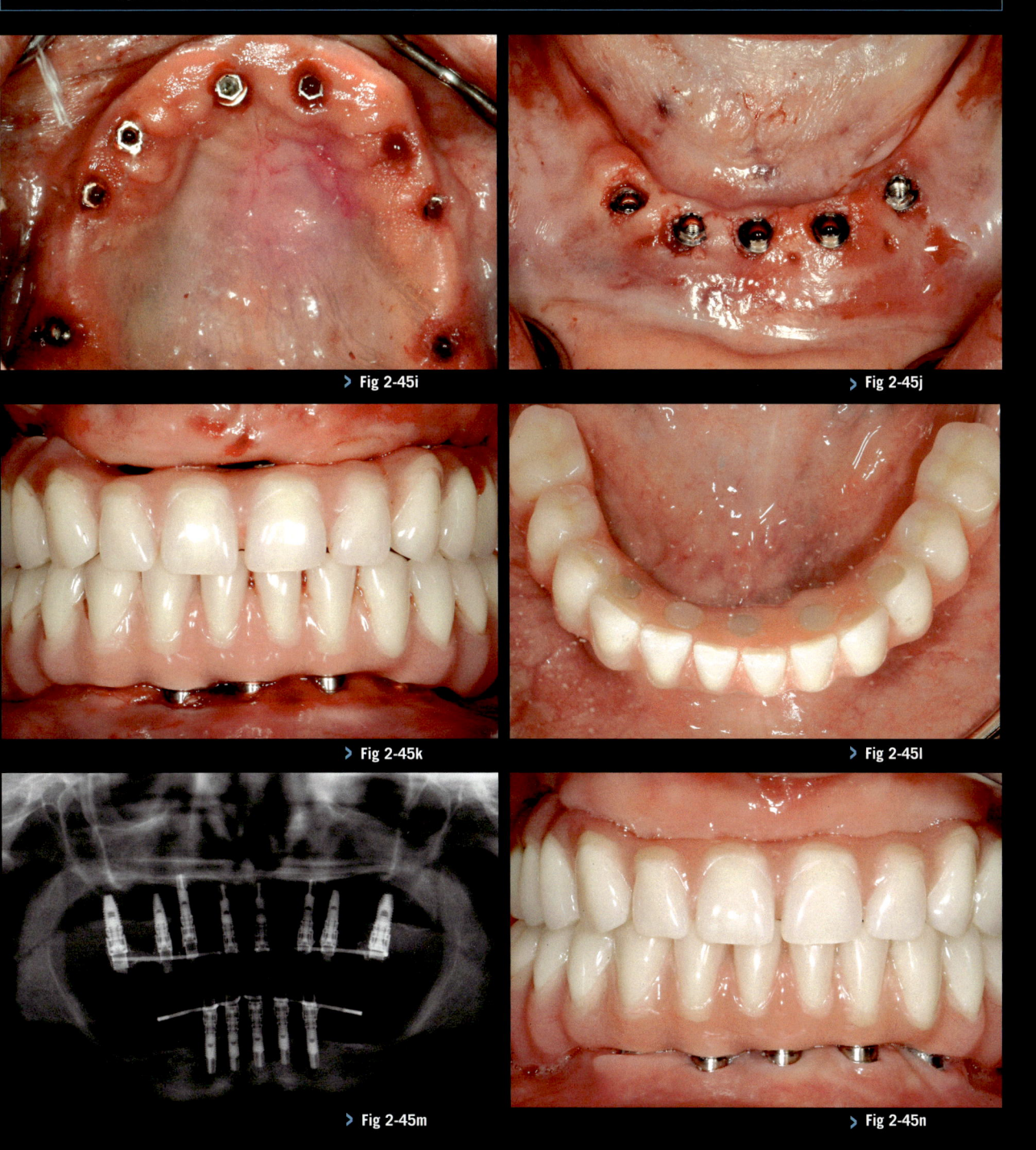

> Fig 2-45i

> Fig 2-45j

> Fig 2-45k

> Fig 2-45l

> Fig 2-45m

> Fig 2-45n

FIG 45 *(a to f)* The patient, who has two complete dentures, requires a fixed rehabilitation. After analyzing both arches using CT, the decision was made to proceed with an implant-prosthetic treatment. Placement of the implants was planned (eight in the maxilla and five in the mandible), paying particular attention to the implant parallelism to guarantee an optimal fit for the prosthetic rehabilitation. *(g and h)* For correct positioning of the implants, two stereolithographic surgical templates were used, derived from the virtual planning for the case (NobelGuide). *(i to l)* After positioning the implants in the oral cavity, the acrylic provisional restorations were screw-retained, supported by a metal structure. *(m and n)* Once the correct positioning, achieved by use of specific expandable abutments, was verified using radiographs, the patient was discharged and subjected to regular checkups during the healing phase. (Treatment by Dr Giampiero Ciabattoni and Mr Valter Neri.)

> Fig 2-46a

> Fig 2-46b

> Fig 2-46c

> Fig 2-46d

> Fig 2-46e

> Fig 2-46f

> Fig 2- 46g

> Fig 2-46h

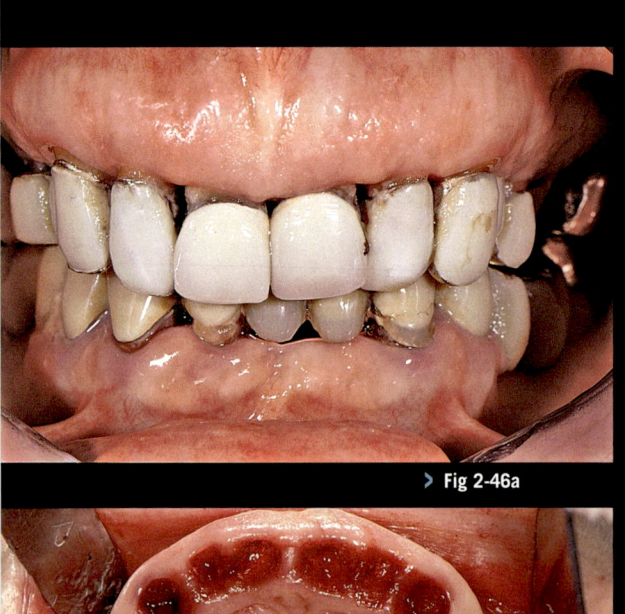

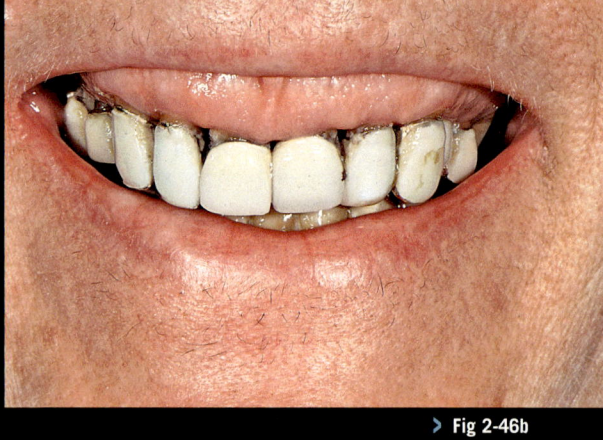

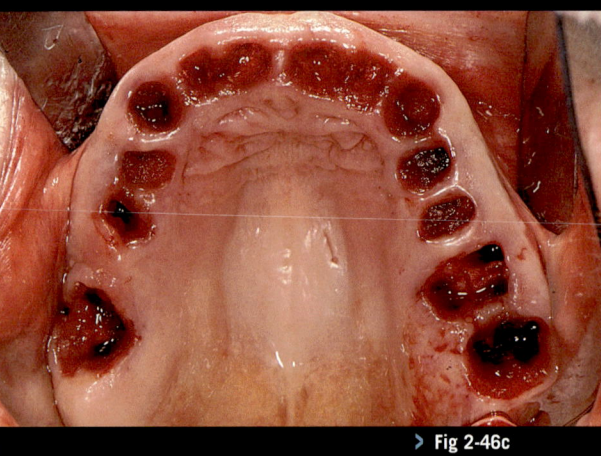

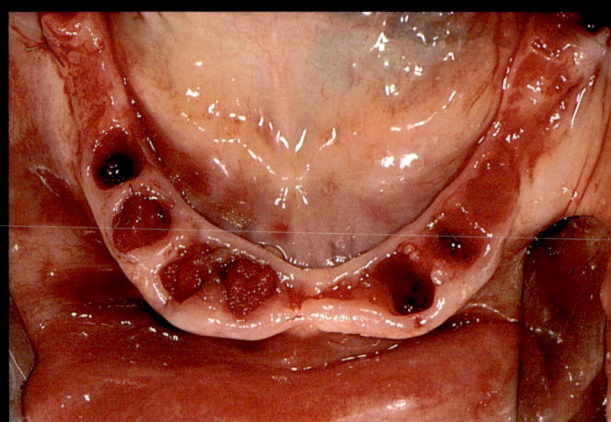

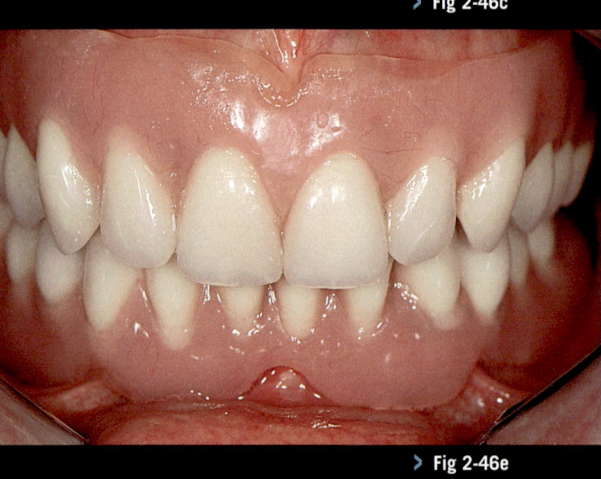

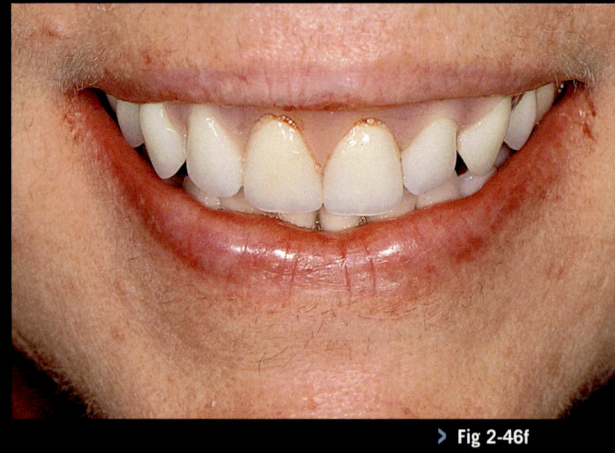

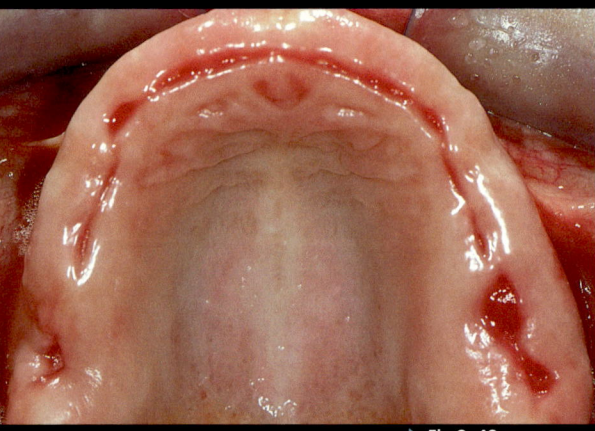

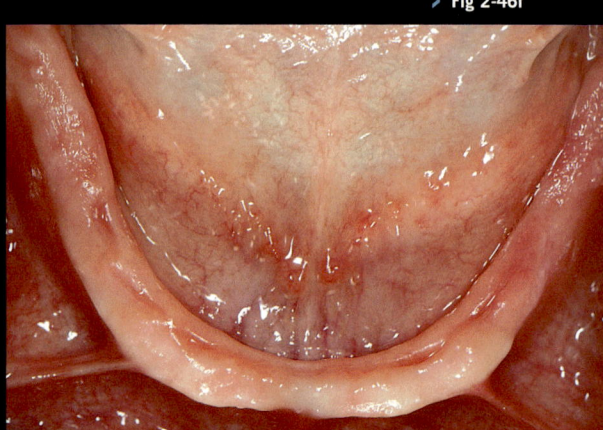

3D PLANNING - CEMENTED PROSTHESIS

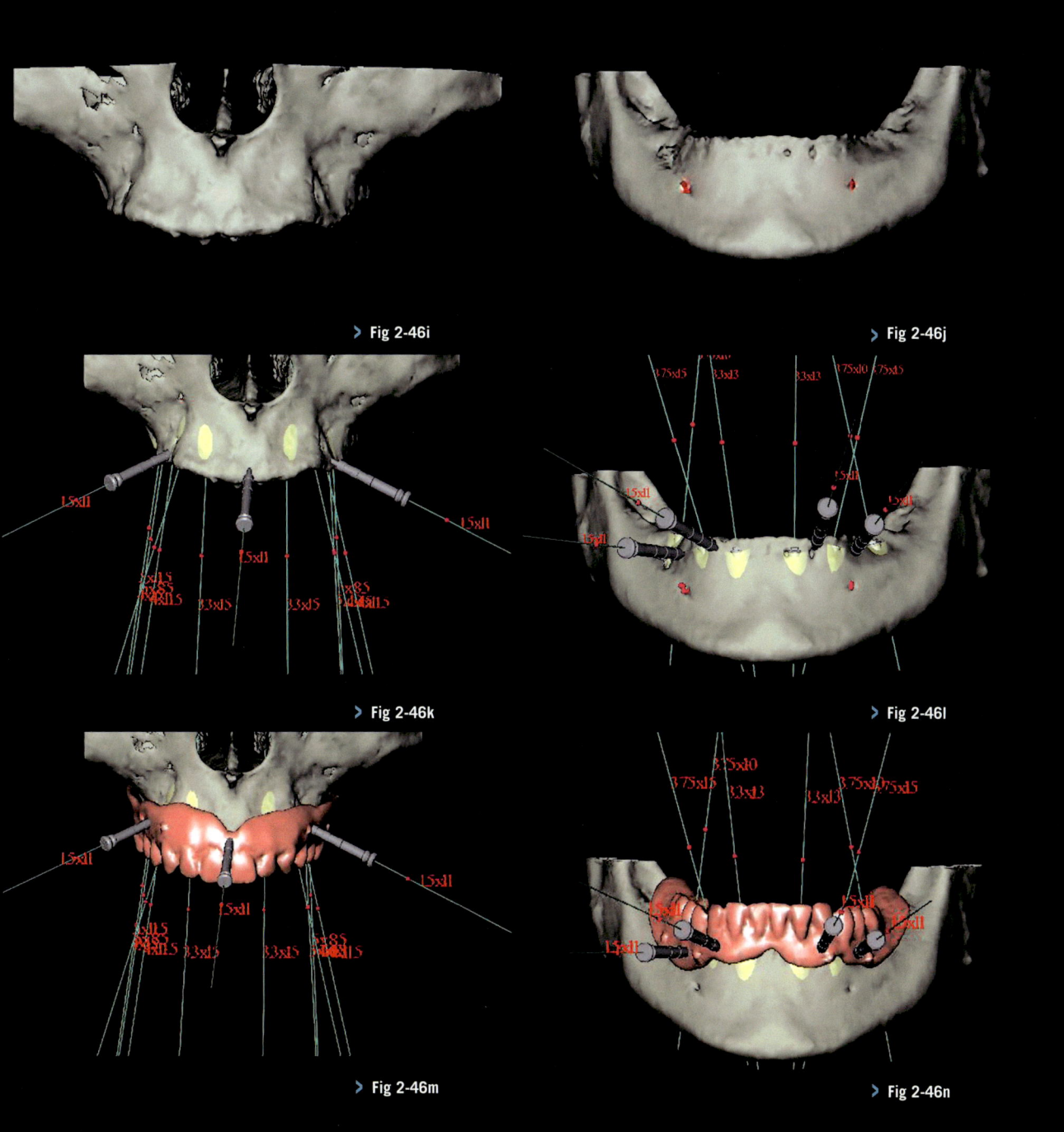

> Fig 2-46i

> Fig 2-46j

> Fig 2-46k

> Fig 2-46l

> Fig 2-46m

> Fig 2-46n

FIG 46 *(a to f)* The serious periodontal compromise of the units in both arches made it necessary to extract them with the consequent positioning of two postextraction complete dentures, in preparation for a subsequent implant prosthetic rehabilitation. *(g and h)* The dentures were then duly relined to ensure perfect adaptation with the soft tissues and adequate stability. *(I and j)* CT of both arches allows an in-depth analysis of the hard and soft tissue anatomy. The next stage is the virtual implant planning. *(k to n)* Given the poor osseous quality and quantity, the decision was made to insert 10 implants into the maxillary arch and 6 into the mandibular arch under the guidance of the stereolithographic surgical templates (NobelGuide).

> Fig 2-46o

> Fig 2-46p

> Fig 2-46q

> Fig 2-46r

> Fig 2-46s

> Fig 2-46t

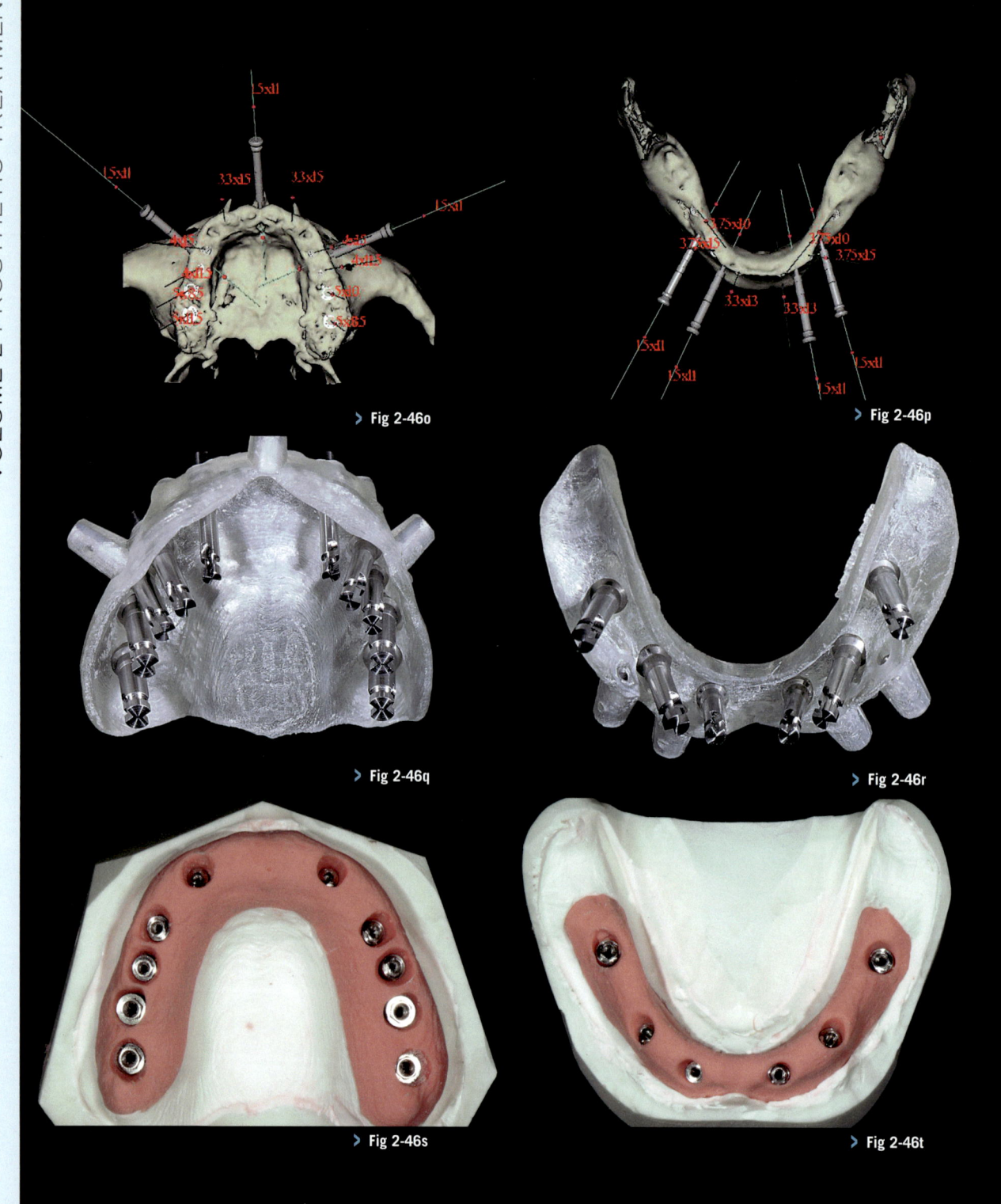

FIG 46 *(o and p)* The insertion of each implant was planned in such a way as to obtain an emergence corresponding to an ideal tooth position. *(q to t)* Positioning the implant replicas on the templates means the master casts can be created before actually inserting the implants into the oral cavity. *(u to x)* The abutments in resin were then molded, idealizing the parallelism and the emergence profile and then, using CAD-CAM technology, the customized zirconium abutments were made (Procera, Nobel Biocare), which are useful for optimizing the esthetics and integrating the restoration at perio-implant tissue level. *(y to bb)* The provisional restorations in resin are positioned on the same day, after the surgical phase, to guarantee the patient adequate comfort and at the same time to achieve a suitable conditioning of the tissues.

Fig 2-46u

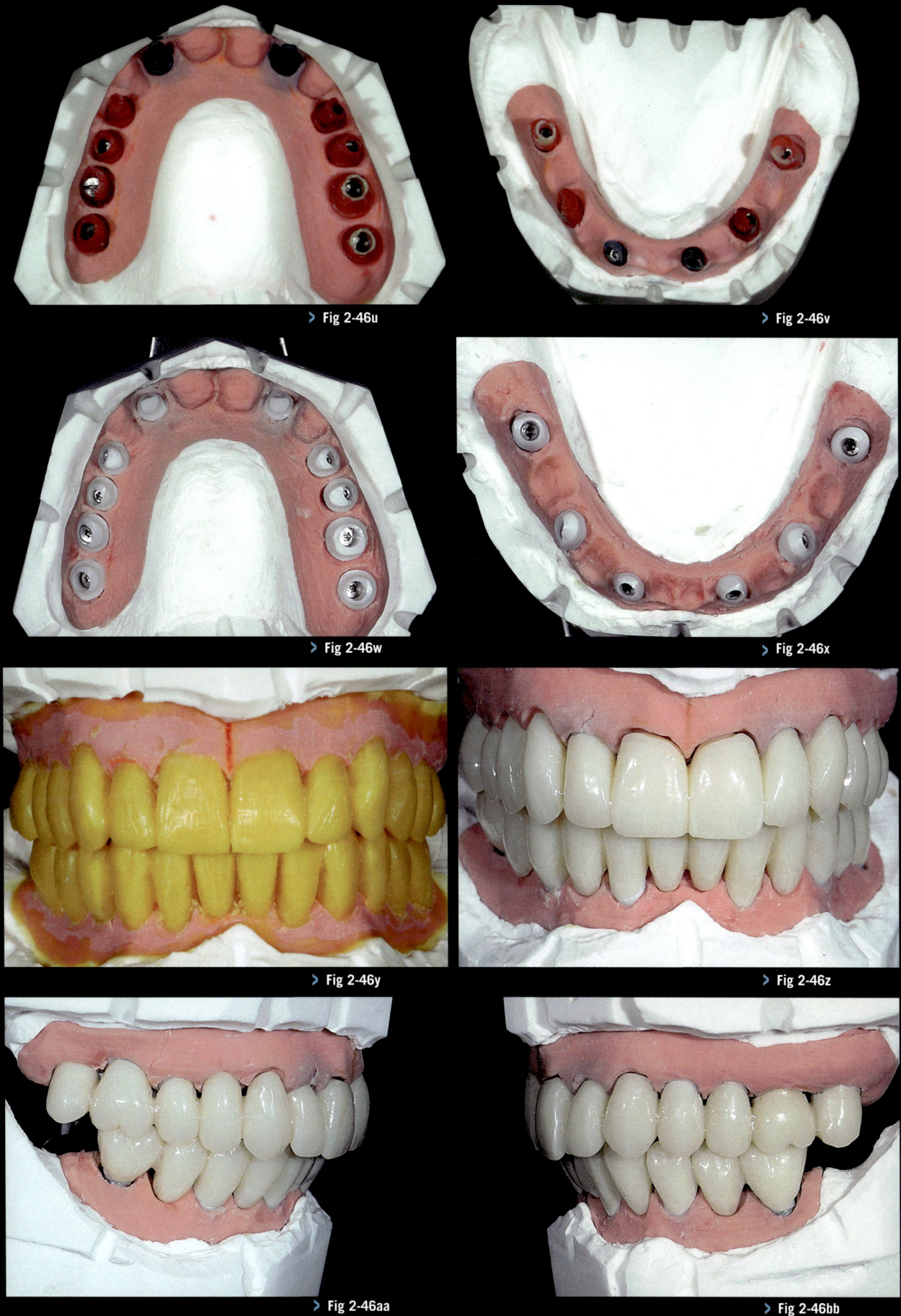

Fig 2-46v

Fig 2-46w

Fig 2-46x

Fig 2-46y

Fig 2-46z

Fig 2-46aa

Fig 2-46bb

> Fig 2-46cc

> Fig 2-46dd

> Fig 2-46ee

> Fig 2-46ff

> Fig 2-46gg

> Fig 2- 46hh

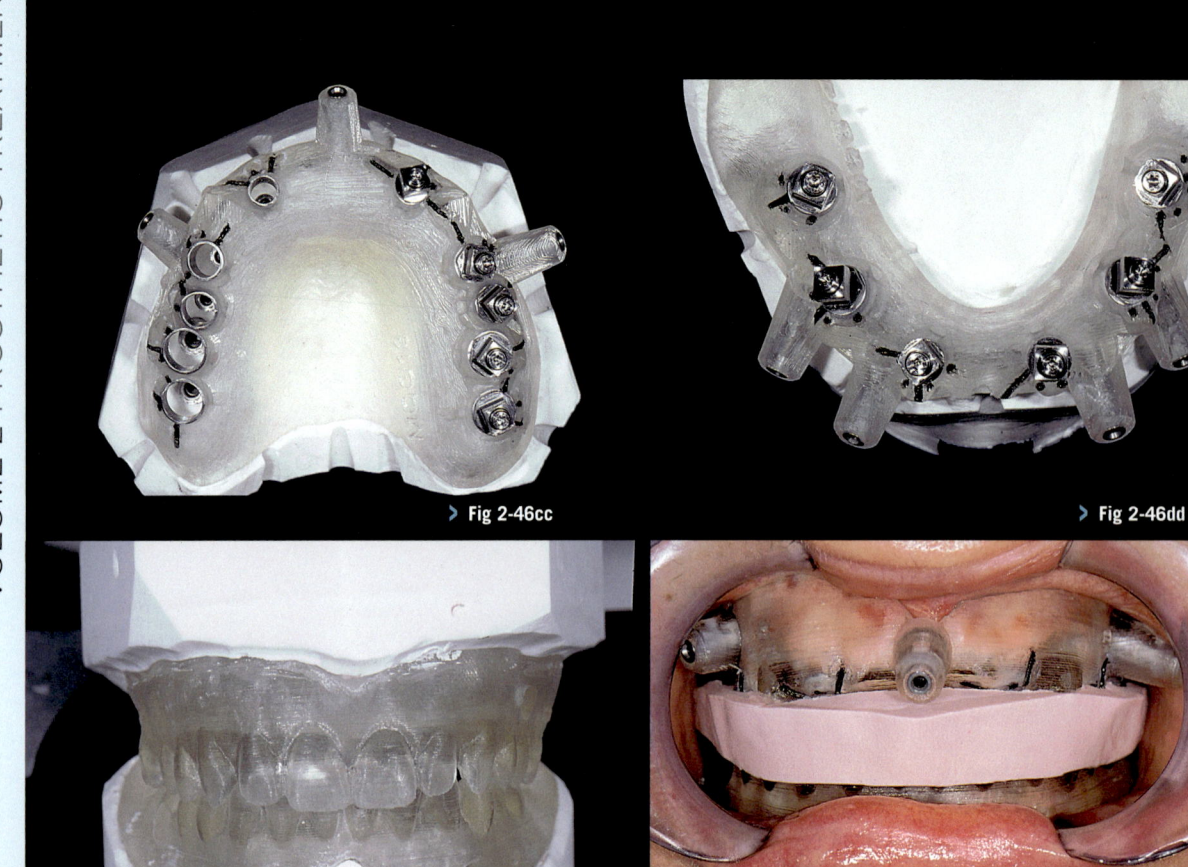

FIG 46 *(cc and dd)* Due to the purposefully drawn specific reference points, the surgical templates allow the implant hexagons to be positioned correctly, thereby ensuring that the abutments are oriented correctly. *(ee)* The stereolithographic copies of the two complete dentures, in CR and at the correct VDO, are mounted on the articulator. By following the cross-mounting technique and by alternating a surgical template and the stereolithographic copy of the opposing denture in the articulator, the silicone indices are made that are needed to correctly position the surgical templates in the oral cavity. *(ff)* View of the maxillary surgical template stabilized in the oral cavity by means of the silicone index positioned on the stereolithographic copy of the mandibular prosthesis. *(gg and hh)* View of the surgical templates with the implants fitted. (Treatment by Drs Stefano Gori and Giampiero Ciabattoni.) *(ii to ll)* A comparison between the preoperative frontal view and the view after positioning the customized zirconium abutments shows the minimal invasiveness of the so-called flapless technique. *(mm and nn)* The occlusal views of the immediate cemented prostheses demonstrate the absence of holes traditionally found in prostheses that are screw-retained, allowing an ideal development of the anatomy of the posterior teeth and, therefore, greater occlusal stability. *(oo)* At the end of the surgical session, the immediate prostheses are relined, refined, and checked in occlusion, ensuring the contacts are punctiform and well distributed in CO. *(pp)* The coincidence between the implant hexagons and abutments is confirmed by the final radiographs. *(qq to tt)* One week later, it is possible to appreciate the overall integration achieved and the clear improvement compared with the preoperative situation.

Fig 2-46ii

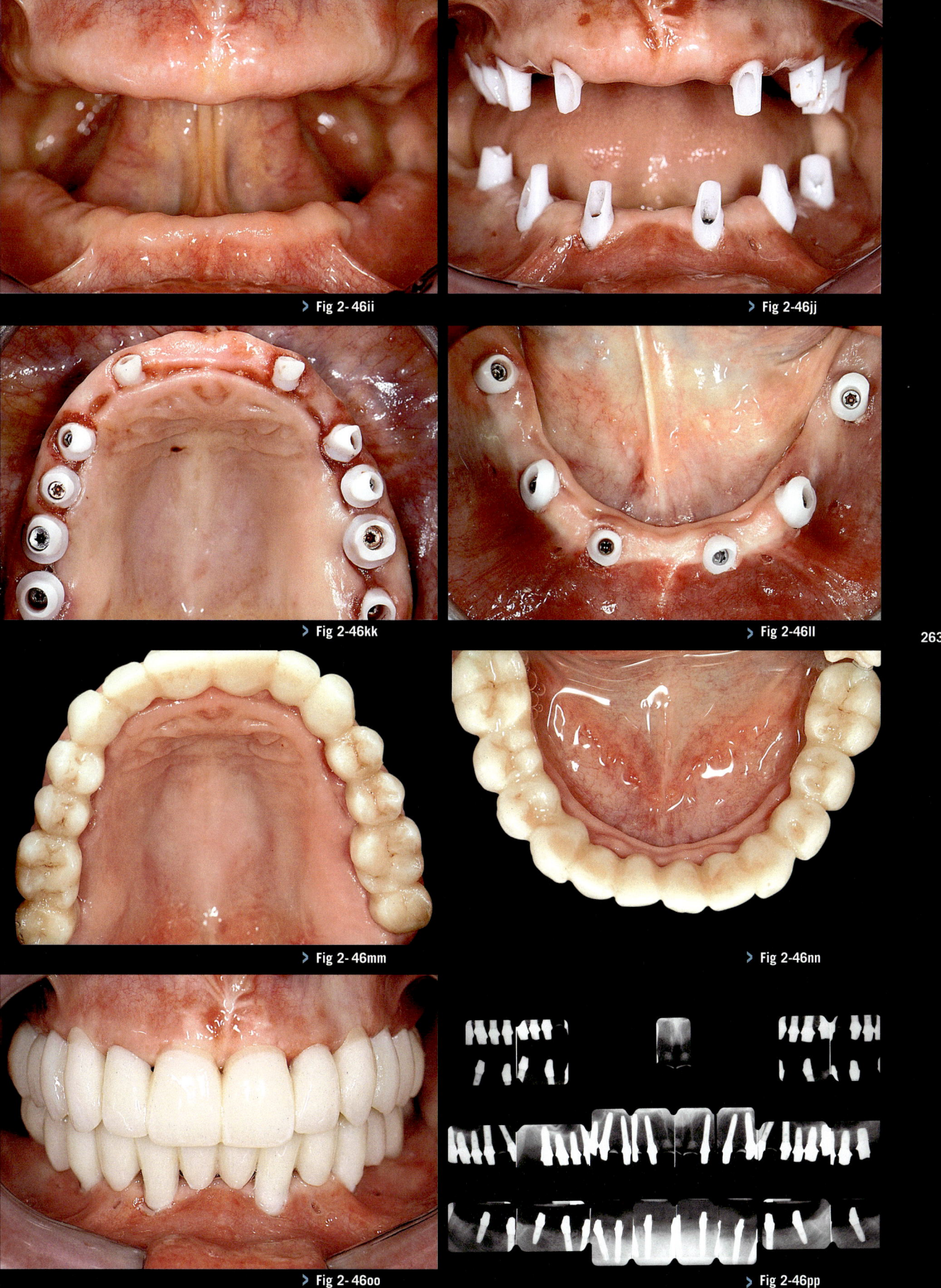

Fig 2-46jj

Fig 2-46kk

Fig 2-46ll

Fig 2-46mm

Fig 2-46nn

Fig 2-46oo

Fig 2-46pp

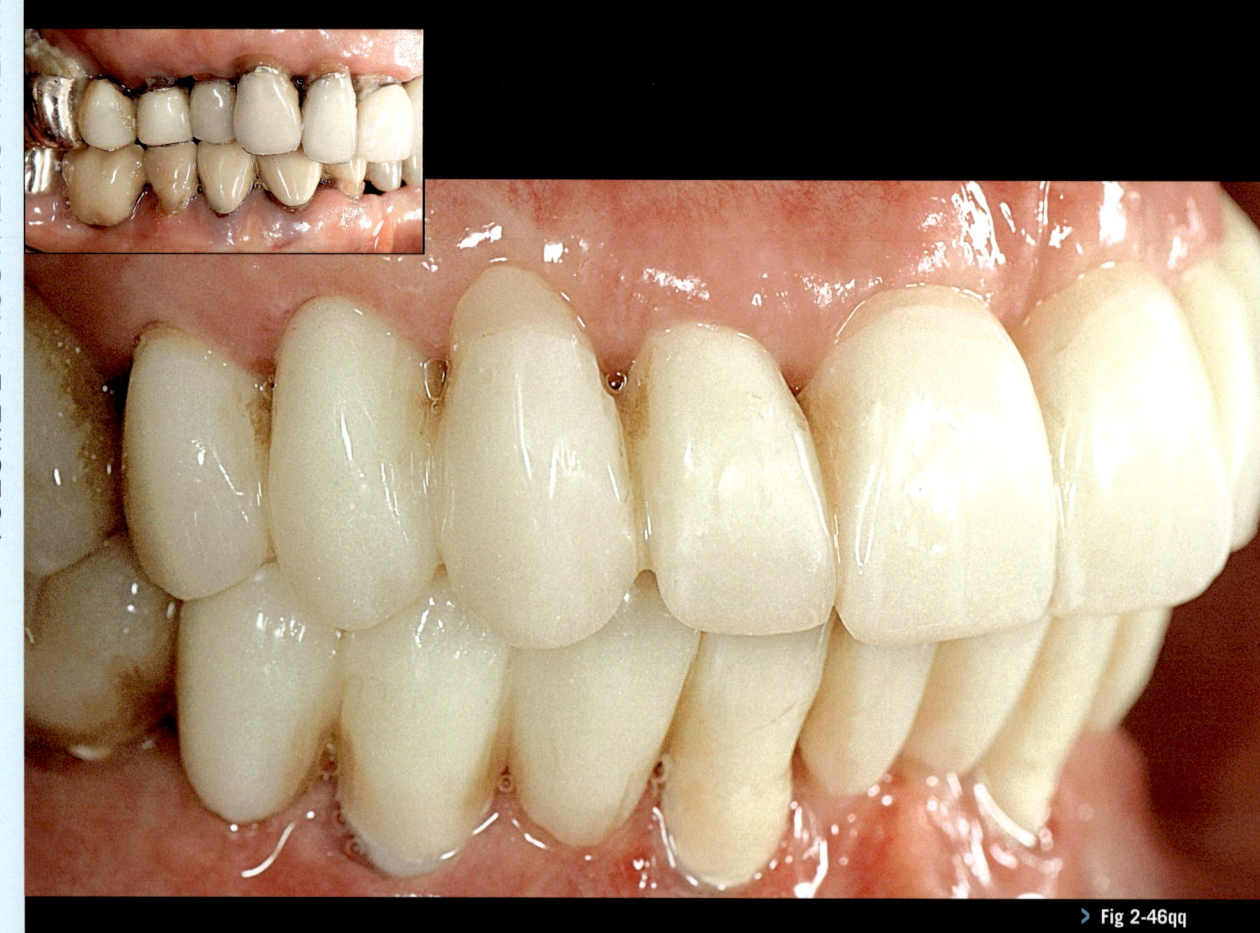

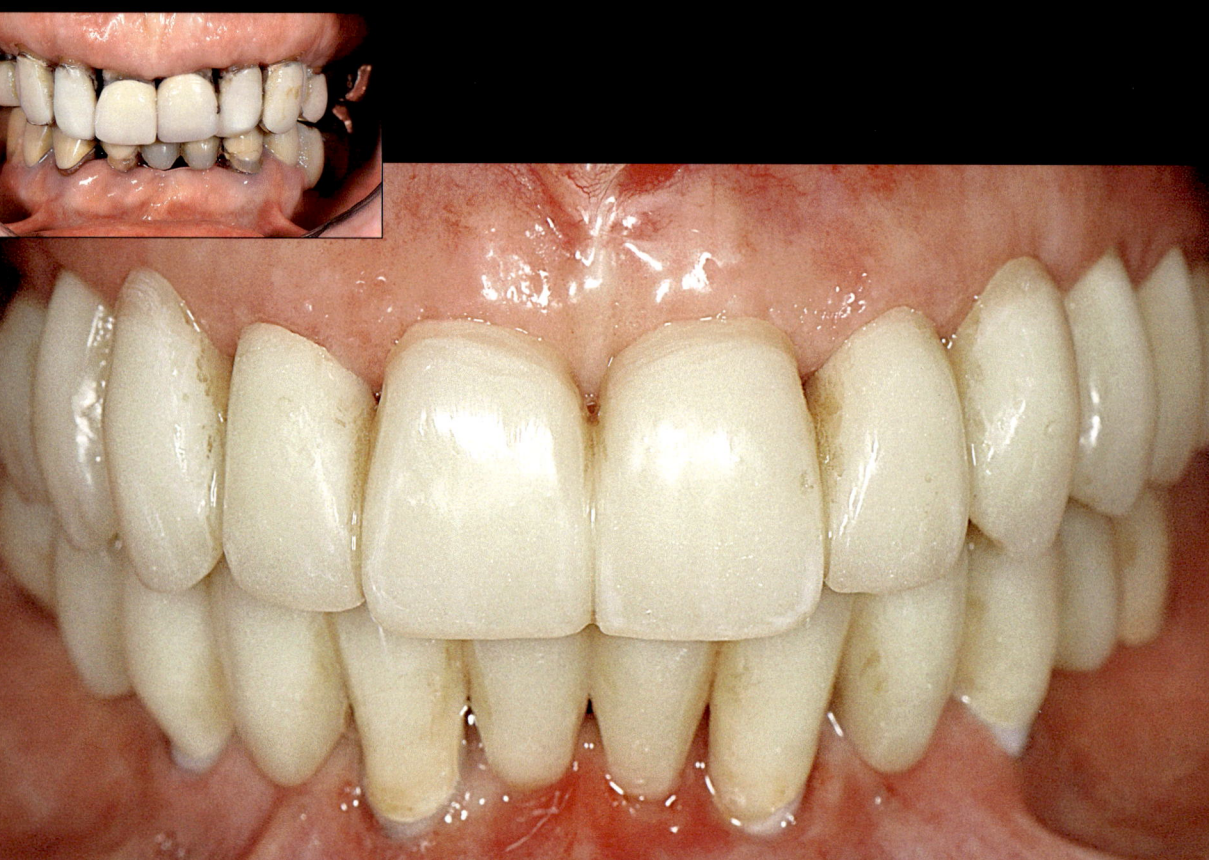

> Fig 2-46qq

> Fig 2-46rr

> Fig 2-46ss

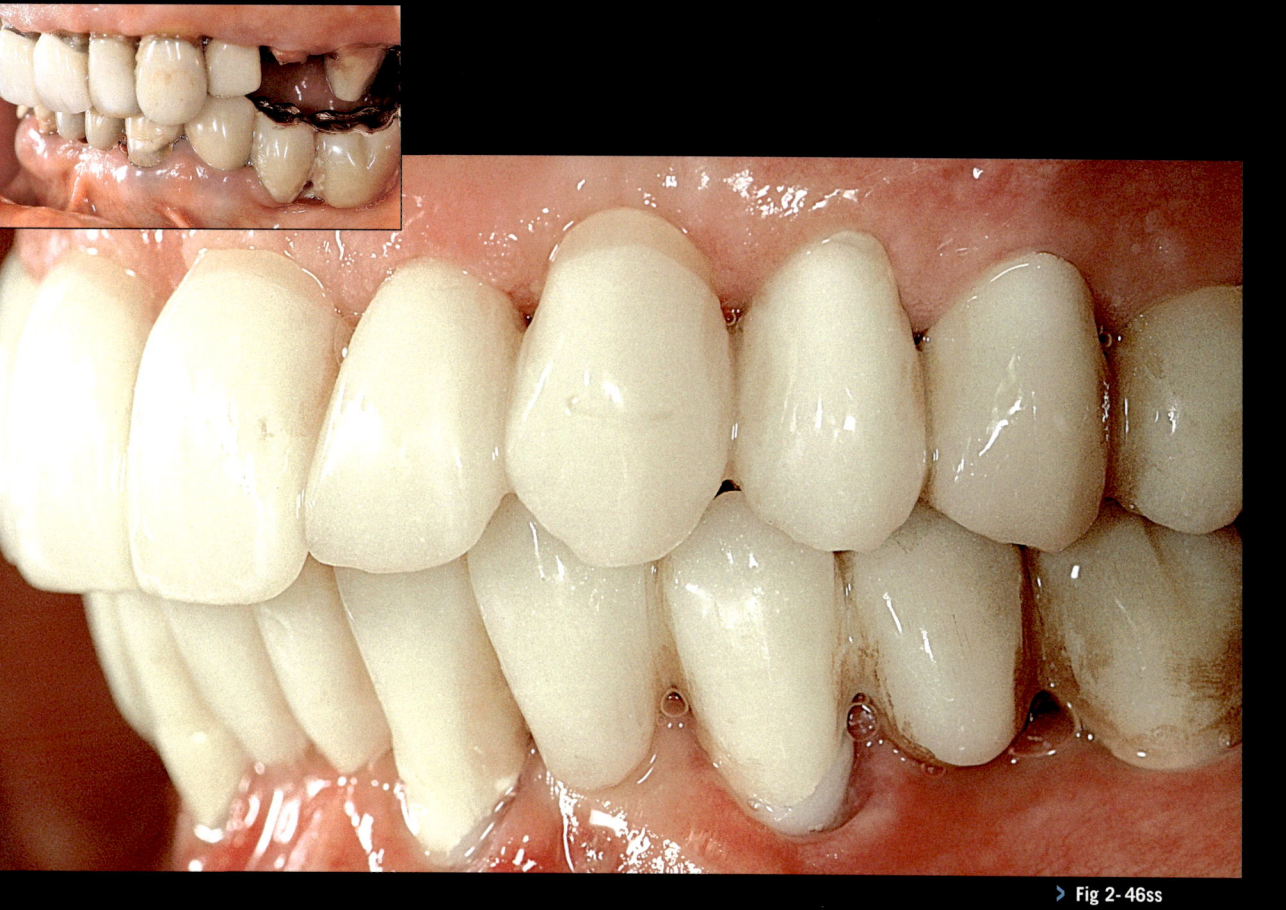

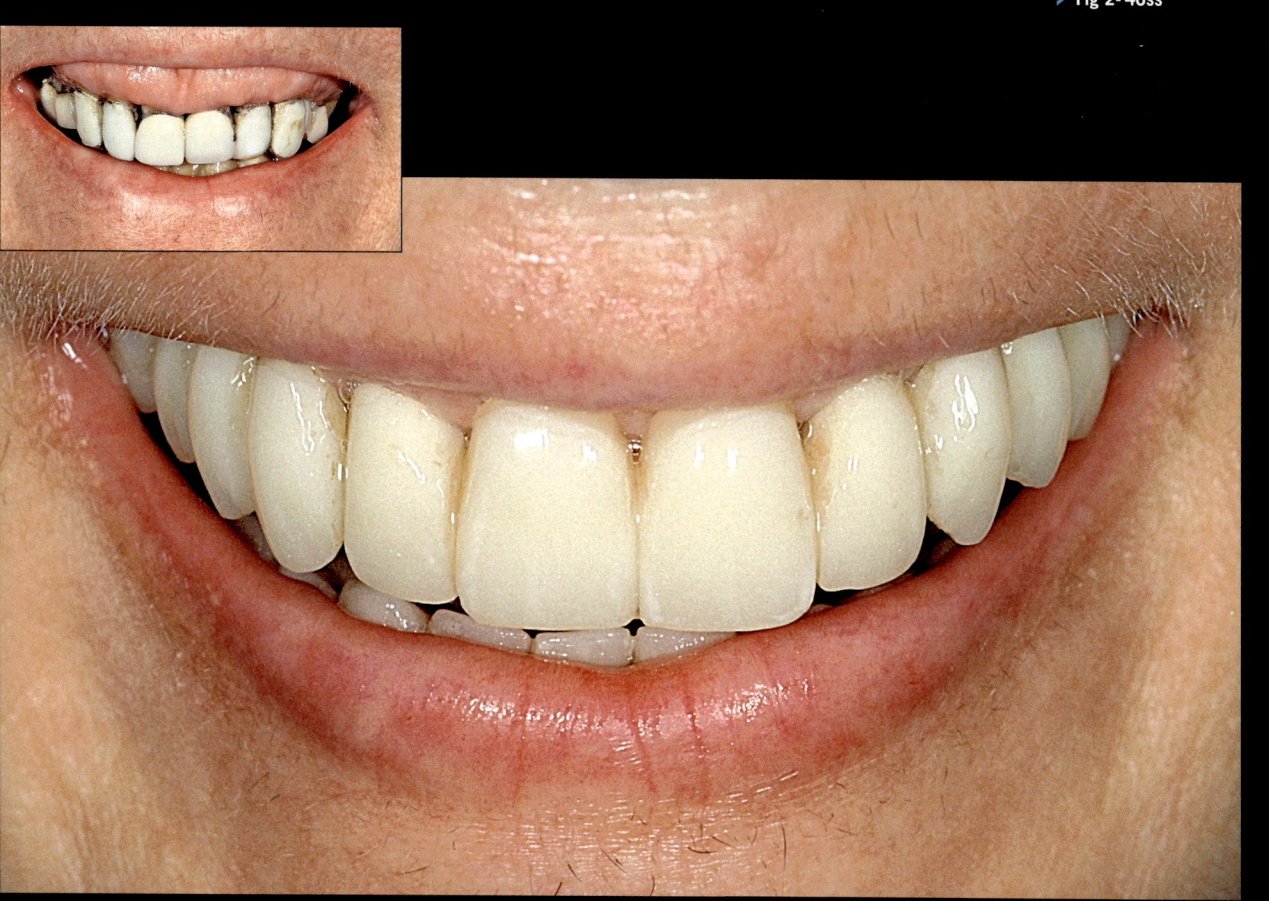

265

> Fig 2-46tt

PROVISIONAL RESTORATIONS — CONCLUSIONS

The techniques of construction, inserting, and relining the provisional restoration described up to this point allow good esthetic, functional, and biologic integration of the prosthesis[7,167–169] and guarantee adequate stability as well in cases where it must remain in the mouth for a long time.

ESTHETIC INTEGRATION

Because of the specific information transmitted from the clinician to the technician by means of the laboratory checklist, the provisional restoration should reflect all of the esthetic modifications requested. Once the provisional restoration is inserted correctly into the mouth, the clinician must ensure that all of the esthetic parameters are optimized through detailed dentolabial and phonetic analysis. During speech and smiling, a check is made to see that the incisal plane and the horizon are once more parallel[170–173] (Fig 2-47a) and that a pleasing harmony has been re-established between the convex outline of the incisal edge and the natural curvature of the lower lip[170–172] (Fig 2-47b). At the same time, a congruous visibility of the anterosuperior teeth at rest, varying between 1 and 5 mm according to the age and sex of the patient, should be present.[174,175] Scrupulous dental and gingival analysis makes it possible to identify any additional incongruities that prevent harmonious development of the tooth composition. On this point, especially in the anterosuperior sector, a check must be made for a suitable dominance of the central incisors over the laterals[176,177] and for the correct progression of the interincisal angles, which gradually widen proceeding from the central incisors toward the canines. The teeth of the provisional restoration must also show such a tooth position and arrangement that the cervical and incisal margins of the laterals are contained within two hypothetical lines traced to join the cervical and incisal margins of the central incisors and canines.

It may be that, despite the completeness of the information supplied to the technician to create the first diagnostic wax-up and then the acrylic resin matrix, the clinician still has to make further corrections to the shape, contour, and tooth arrangement as well. This necessity can especially arise in cases in which a significant number of variations are to be made. Any modifications, easily achieved by adding or subtracting acrylic material, must be perfected in the provisional restoration so that it becomes the prototype to be faithfully replicated in the definitive prosthesis.

ESTHETIC INTEGRATION

REQUIREMENTS

- Parallelism between incisal plane and horizon
- Harmony between convex outline of the incisal edge and lower lip curvature
- Congruity of tooth exposure at rest
- Progression of interincisal angles
- Ideal shape, proportion, contour, and tooth arrangement

> Fig 2-47a

> Fig 2-47b

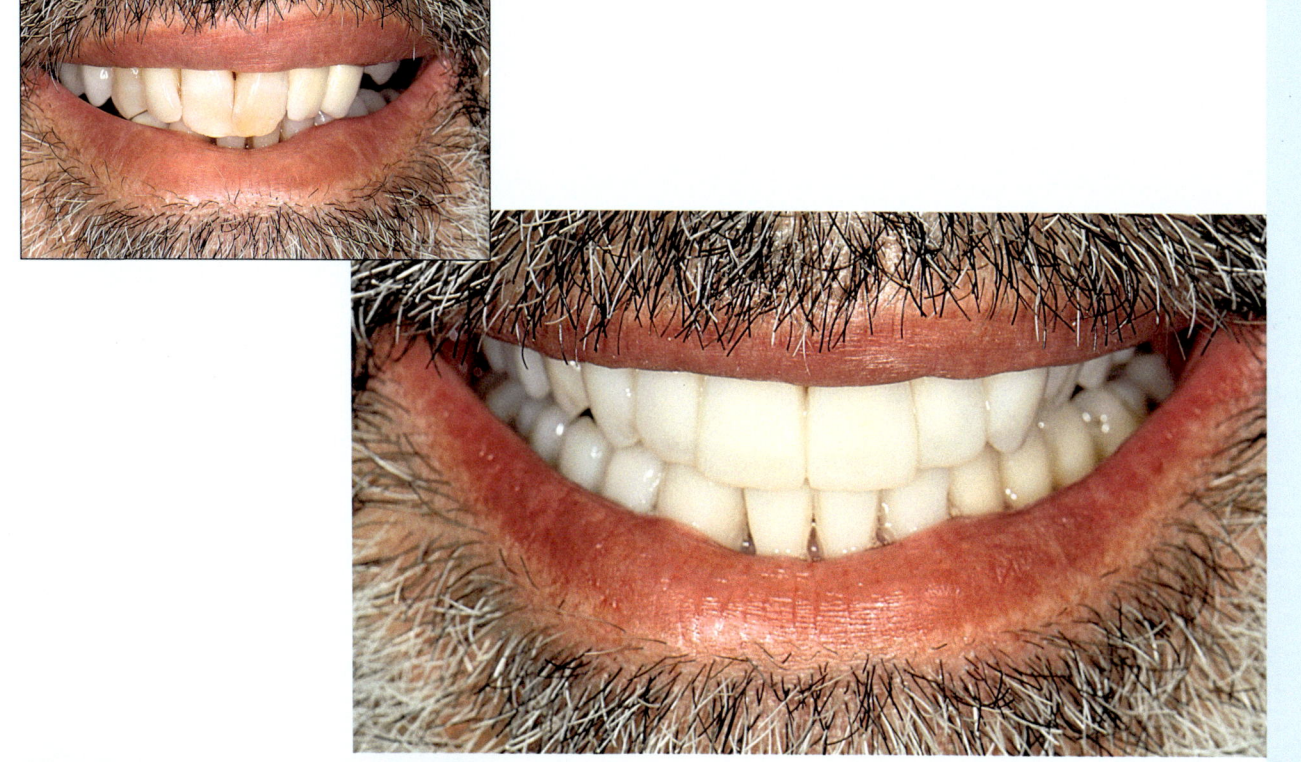

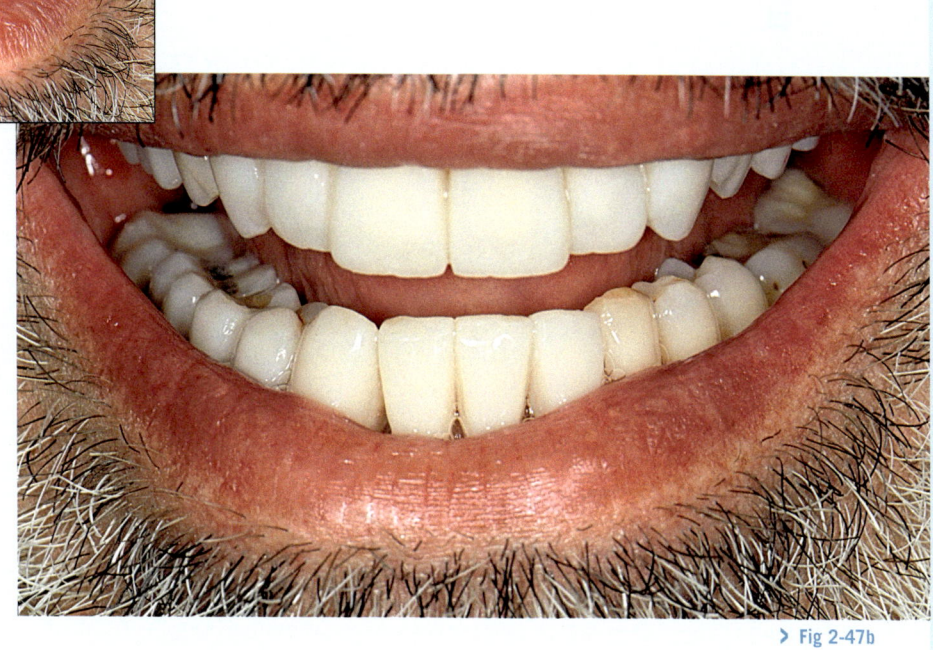

FIG 47 *(a)* The patient was unhappy with the esthetic appearance of his smile and mainly concerned with the overlap of the maxillary central incisors. He is fully satisfied with the overall harmony created with positioning the provisional restoration. *(b)* It is clear that the occlusal plane, previously considerably inclined in the left mandibular sector, has been appropriately compensated by special modifications made first in the wax-up and then replicated in the acrylic shell.

FUNCTIONAL INTEGRATION

Occlusal stability The provisional restoration must demonstrate satisfactory occlusal stability, proven in the posterior sectors by punctiform, synchronous, and evenly distributed contacts[157–161] (Fig 2-47c), unlike in the anterior sector, where light contact that does not cause either mobility or fremitus in the maxillary incisors is sufficient (Fig 2-47d).

Centric relation Positioning the provisional restoration in CR to the correct VDO is of fundamental importance, especially in cases of complete rehabilitation. The methods of reproducing, in the oral cavity, the same position obtained in the articulator have been amply described (see pages 178–191). At this stage, perfect stability of the provisional restoration in CR must be ascertained, making sure there is no occlusal anteroposterior and laterolateral interference in achieving this position.

Vertical dimension of occlusion If changes have been made to the patient's original VDO, the validity of the modifications carried out must be checked as well by having the patient pronounce the sounds M[178–182] and S[183–188] Muscular contraction and soreness indicate the patient's difficulty in adapting to the new height. In these cases it is necessary to explain that this situation could resolve on its own within 2 to 3 days[189–193] thanks to an adaptation mechanism. It is, however, essential to ensure that there is no muscular involvement when the provisional restoration is checked before taking the final impressions.

Anterior guidance It is necessary to assess the level of overjet and overbite and to check the development of an adequate anterior guidance that, by permitting disocclusion of the posterior sectors, allows complete relaxation of the masticatory muscles and applies the smallest load possible to the TMJs (Figs 2-47e to 2-47h).

PROVISIONAL FUNCTIONAL INTEGRATION

REQUIREMENTS

- Occlusal stability:
  - Punctiform, synchronized, and well-distributed contacts
  - No fremitus and/or mobility in the anterior sectors
- Vertical dimension:
  - Adequate pronunciation of letter sounds *M* and *S*
  - Absence of any muscle fatigue
- Anterior guidance:
  - Adequate overbite and overjet
  - No interference in the posterior sectors

> Fig 2-47c

> Fig 2-47d

> Fig 2-47e

> Fig 2-47f

> Fig 2-47g

> Fig 2-47h

→ continues on page 281

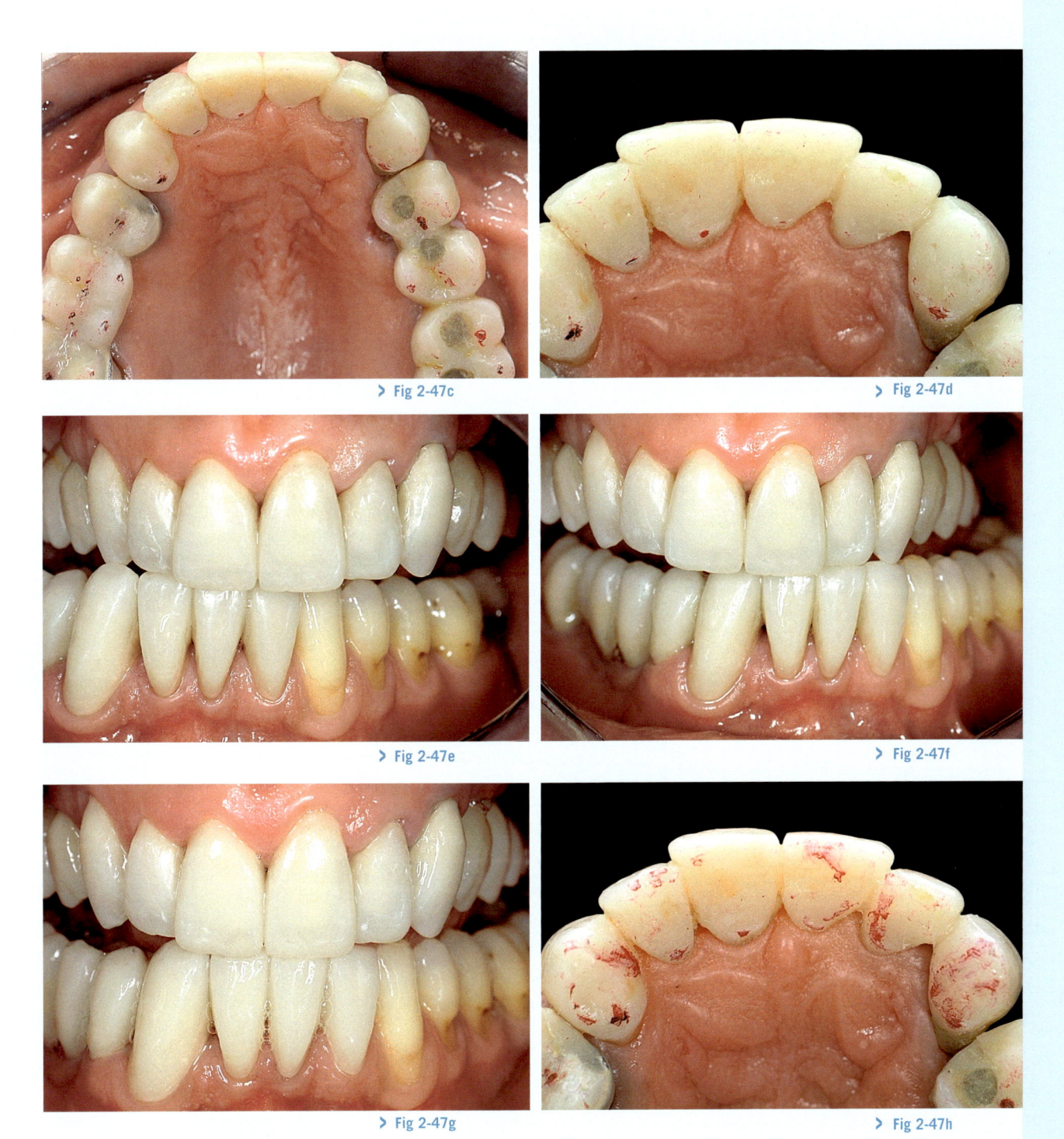

FIG 47 *(c)* On inspection of the maxillary arch, completed only when the provisional restoration was finished, the presence of punctiform, synchronized, and evenly distributed contacts at the centric canines and the fossae bear witness to the appropriate level of occlusal stability achieved. *(d)* The slight contact on the cingulum of the anterior teeth should not generate any fremitus, but instead should constitute the starting point for the development of a correct anterior guidance. *(e to h)* The involvement of the canines and incisors during movements of the mandible, both laterally and protrusively, excludes any contact of the posterior teeth, thereby saving both the stomatognathic muscles and the TMJs from any danger of overloading.

REFERENCES

1. Shavell HM. Mastering the art of tissue management during provisionalization and biologic final impressions. Int J Periodontics Restorative Dent 1988;8:24–43.

2. Conny DJ, Tedesco LA, Brewer JD, Albino JE. Changes of attitude in fixed prosthodontic patients. J Prosthet Dent 1985;53:451–454.

3. Higginbottom FL. Quality provisional restorations: a must for successful restorative dentistry. Compend Contin Educ Dent 1995;16:442,444–447.

4. Preston JD. A systematic approach to the control of esthetic form. J Prosthet Dent 1976;35:393–402.

5. Clements WG. Predictable anterior determinants. J Prosthet Dent 1983;49:40–45.

6. Capp NJ. The diagnostic use of provisional restorations. Restorative Dent 1985;1:92–94–98.

7. Zinner ID, Trachtenberg DI, Miller RD. Provisional restorations in fixed partial prosthodontics. Dent Clin North Am 1989;33:355–377.

8. Kucey BK. Matrices in metal ceramics. J Prosthet Dent 1990;63:32–37.

9. Nemcovsky CE. Transferring the occlusal and esthetic anatomy of the provisional to the final restoration in full-arch oral rehabilitations. Compend Contin Educ Dent 1996;17:72–74 76, 78.

10. Donovan TE, Cho GC. Diagnostic provisional restorations in restorative dentistry: the blueprint for success. J Can Dent Assoc 1999;65:272–275.

11. Burns DR, Beck DA, Nelson SK. A review of selected dental literature on contemporary provisional fixed prosthodontic treatment: report of the Committee on Research in Fixed Prosthodontics of the Academy of Fixed Prosthodontics. J Prosthet Dent 2003;90:474–497.

12. Vahidi F. The provisional restoration. Dent Clin North Am 1987;31:363–381.

13. Skurow HM, Nevins M. The rationale of the preperiodontal provisional biologic trial restoration. Int J Periodontics Restorative Dent 1988;8:8–29.

14. Hazelton LR, Nicholls JI, Brudvik JS, Daly CH. Influence of reinforcement design on the loss of marginal seal of provisional fixed partial dentures. Int J Prosthodont 1995;8:572–579.

15. Christensen GJ. Tooth preparation and pulp degeneration. J Am Dent Assoc 1997;128:353–354.

16. Kaiser DA, Cavazos E Jr. Temporarization techniques in fixed prosthodontics. Dent Clin North Am 1985;29:403–412.

17. Amin AE. The effect of poly-aramide fiber reinforcement on the transverse strength of a provisional crown and bridge resin. Egypt Dent J 1995;41:1299–1304.

18. Duke ES. Provisional restorative materials: a technology update. Compend Contin Educ Dent 1999;20:497–500.

19. Krug RS. Temporary resin crowns and bridges. Dent Clin North Am 1975;19:313–320.

20. Christensen GJ. Provisional restorations for fixed prosthodontics. J Am Dent Assoc 1996;127:249–252.

21. Braden M, Clarke RL, Pearson GJ, Keys WC. A new temporary crown and bridge resin. Br Dent J 1976;141:269–272.

22. Lui JL, Setcos JC, Phillips RW. Temporary restorations: a review. Oper Dent 1986;11:103–110.

23. Driscoll CF, Woolsey G, Ferguson WM. Comparison of exothermic release during polymerization of four materials used to fabricate interim restorations. J Prosthet Dent 1991;65:504–506.

24. Galindo D, Soltys JL, Graser GN. Long-term reinforced fixed provisional restorations. J Prosthet Dent 1998;79:698–701.

25. Boberick KG, Bachstein TK. Use of a flexible cast for the indirect fabrication of provisional restorations. J Prosthet Dent 1999;82:90–93.

26. Koumjian JH, Nimmo A. Evaluation of fracture resistance of resins used for provisional restorations. J Prosthet Dent 1990;64:654–657.

27. Ireland MF, Dixon DL, Breeding LC, Ramp MH. In vitro mechanical property comparison of four resins used for fabrication of provisional fixed restorations. J Prosthet Dent 1998;80:158–162.

28. Diaz-Arnold AM, Dunne JT, Jones AH. Microhardness of provisional fixed prosthodontic materials. J Prosthet Dent 1999;82:525–528.

29. Wang RL, Moore BK, Goodacre CJ, Swartz ML, Andres CJ. A comparison of resins for fabricating provisional fixed restorations. Int J Prosthodont 1989;2:173–184.

30. Moulding MB, Teplitsky PE. Intrapulpar temperature during direct fabrication of provisional restorations. Int J Prosthodont 1990;3:299–304.

31. Passon C, Goldfoge IM. Direct technique for the fabrication of a visible light-curing resin provisional restoration. Quintessence Int 1990;21:699–703.

32. Liebenberg WH. Reducing marginal flash in the fabrication of direct provisional restorations: a new technique using light-cured resin and transparent silicone. J Can Dent Assoc 1995;61:708–713.

33. Luthardt RG, Stossel M, Hinz M, Vollandt R. Clinical performance and periodontal outcome of temporary crowns and fixed partial dentures: a randomized clinical trial. J Prosthet Dent 2000;83:32–39.

34. Tjan AH, Castelnuovo J, Shiotsu G. Marginal fidelity of crowns fabricated from six proprietary provisional materials. J Prosthet Dent 1997;77:482–485.

35. Tjan AHL, Tjan AH, Grant BE. Marginal accuracy of temporary composite crowns. J Prosthet Dent 1987;58:417.

36. Moulding MB, Loney RW. The effect of cooling techniques on intrapulpal temperature during direct fabrication of provisional restorations. Int J Prosthodont 1991;4:332–336.

37. Castelnuovo J, Tjan AH. Temperature rise in pulpal chamber during fabrication of provisional resinous crowns. J Prosthet Dent 1997;78:441–446.

38. Fiasconaro JE, Sherman H. Vacuum-formed prostheses. 1. A temporary fixed bridge or splint. J Am Dent Assoc 1968;76:74–78.

39. Jones EE. Vacuuformed clear resin shells. J Prosthet Dent 1973;29:460–462.

40. Krug RS. Temporary resin crowns and bridges. Dent Clin North Am 1975;19:313–320.

41. Kaiser DA. Accurate acrylic resin temporary restorations. J Prosthet Dent 1978;39:158–161.

42. Fox CW, Abrams BL, Doukoudakis A. Provisional restorations for altered occlusions. J Prosthet Dent 1984; 52:567–572.

43. Chalifoux PR. Temporary crown and fixed partial dentures: new methods to achieve esthetics. J Prosthet Dent 1989;61:411–414.

44. Prestipino V. Visible light-cured resins: a technique for provisional fixed restorations. Quintessence Int 1989;20:241–248.

45. Barghi N, Simmons W. The marginal integrity of the temporary acrylic resin crown. J Prosthet Dent 1976;36:274.

46. Crispin BJ, Watson JF, Caputo AA. The marginal accuracy of treatment restorations: a comparative analysis. J Prosthet Dent 1980;44:283–290.

47. Richards ND, Mitchell RJ. Effects of materials and techniques on accuracy of temporary fixed partial dentures [abstract 1484]. J Dent Res 1984;63:336.

48. Monday JJ, Blais D. Marginal adaptation of provisional acrylic resin crowns. J Prosthet Dent 1985;54:194–197.

49. Koumjian JH, Holmes JB. Marginal accuracy of provisional restorative materials. J Prosthet Dent 1990;63: 639–642.

50. Robinson FB, Hovijitra S. Marginal fit of direct temporary crowns. J Prosthet Dent 1982;47:390.

51. Breeding LC. Indirect temporary acrylic restorations for fixed prosthodontics. J Am Dent Assoc 1982;105:1026–1027.

52. Davidoff SR. Heat processed acrylic resin provisional restorations: an in-office procedure. J Prosthet Dent 1982;48:673–675.

53. Kastenbaum F. Lab processed provisional prosthesis. N Y J Dent 1982;52:39–44.

54. Wood M, Halpern BG, Lamb MF. Visible light-cured composite resins: an alternative for anterior provisional restorations. J Prosthet Dent 1984;51:192–194.

55. Kinsel RP. Fabrication of treatment restorations using acrylic resin denture teeth. J Prosthet Dent 1986;56:142–145.

56. Binkley CJ, Irvin PT. Reinforced heat-processed acrylic resin provisional restorations. J Prosthet Dent 1987;57:689–693.

57. Cho GC, Chee WW. Custom characterization of the provisional restoration. J Prosthet Dent 1993;69:529–532.

58. Moulding MB, Loney RW, Ritsco RG. Marginal accuracy of indirect provisional restorations fabricated on poly(vinyl siloxane) models. Int J Prosthodont 1994;7:554–556.

59. Breeding LC, Dixon DL. Use of light-polymerizing restorative materials in diagnostic cast modification procedures. J Prosthet Dent 1994;72:331–333.

60. Emtiaz S, Tarnow DP. Processed acrylic resin provisional restoration with lingual cast metal framework. J Prosthet Dent 1998;79:484–488.

61. Small BW. Indirect provisional restorations. Gen Dent 1999;47:140–142.

62. Caputi S, Traini T, Paciaffi E, Murmura G. Provisional gold-resin restoration executed through an indirect-direct procedure: a clinical report. J Prosthet Dent 2000;84:125–128.

63. Ferencz JL. Fabrication of provisional crowns and fixed partial dentures utilizing a "shell" technique. N Y J Dent 1981;51:201–206.

64. Chiche GJ, Avila R. Fabrication of a preformed shell for a provisional fixed partial denture. Quintessence Dent Technol 1986;10:579–581.

65. Lepe X, Bales DJ, Johnson GH. Retention of provisional crowns fabricated from two materials with the use of four temporary cements. J Prosthet Dent 1999;81:469–475.

66. Amsterdam M, Fox L. Provisional splinting principles and techniques. Dent Clin North Am 1959;March:73.

67. Schluger S, Yuodelis RA, Page RC. Periodontal Disease. Philadelphia: Lea & Febiger, 1977:638–656.

68. Yuodelis RA, Faucher R. Provisional restorations: an integrated approach to periodontics and restorative dentistry. Dent Clin North Am 1980;285–303.

69. Aviv I, Himmel R, Assif D. A technique for improving the marginal fit of temporary acrylic resin crowns using injection of self-curing acrylic resin. Quintessence Int 1986;17:313–315.

70. Chiche G. Improving marginal adaptation of provisional restorations. Quintessence Int 1990;21:325.

71. Blum J, Weiner S, Berendsen P. Effects of thermocycling on the margins of transitional acrylic resin crowns. J Prosthet Dent 1991;65:642–646.

72. Harrison JD, Chiche GJ, Pinault A. Tissue management for the maxillary anterior region. In: Chiche GJ, Pinault A (eds). Esthetics of Anterior Fixed Prosthodontics. Chicago: Quintessence, 1994:143–159.

73. Liebenberg WH. Improving interproximal access in direct provisional acrylic resin restorations. Quintessence Int 1994;25:697–703.

74. Moulding MB, Loney RW, Ritsco RG. Marginal accuracy of provisional restorations fabricated by different techniques. Int J Prosthodont 1994;7:468–472.

75. Zwetchkenbaum S, Weiner S, Dastane A, Vaidyanathan TK. Effects of relining on long-term marginal stability of provisional crowns. J Prosthet Dent 1995;73:525–529.

76. Lowe RA. The art and science of provisionalization. Int J Periodontics Restorative Dent 1987;7:64–73.

77. Kopp FR. Esthetic principles for full crown restorations. Part II: provisionalization. J Esthet Dent 1993;5:258–264.

78. Zach L, Cohen C. Thermogenesis in operative techniques: comparison of four methods. J Prosthet Dent 1962;12:977–984.

79. Grajower Z, Shaharbani S, Kaufman E. Temperature rise in pulp chamber during fabrication of temporary self-curing resin crowns. J Prosthet Dent 1979;41:535–540.

80. Tjan AH, Grant BE, Godfrey M 3rd. Temperature rise in the pulp chamber during fabrication of provisional crowns. J Prosthet Dent 1989;62:622–626.

81. Scotti R, Mascellani SC, Forniti F. The in vitro color stability of acrylic resins for provisional restorations. Int J Prosthodont 1997;10:164–168.

82. Chee WW, Donovan TE, Daftary F, Siu TM. The effect of vacuum-mixed autopolymerizing acrylic resins on porosity and transverse strength. J Prosthet Dent 1988;60(4):517–519.

83. Ogawa T, Aizawa S, Tanaka M, Matsuya S, Hasegawa A, Koyano K. Effect of water temperature on the fit of provisional crown margins during polymerization. J Prosthet Dent 1999;82:658–661.

84. Yannikakis SA, Zissis AJ, Polyzois GL, Caroni C. Color stability of provisional resin restorative materials. J Prosthet Dent 1998;80:533–539.

85. Crispin BJ, Caputo AA. Color stability of temporary restorative materials. J Prosthet Dent 1979;42:27–33.

86. Borchers L, Tavassol F, Tschernitschek H. Surface quality achieved by polishing and by varnishing of temporary crown and fixed partial denture resins. J Prosthet Dent 1999;82:550–556.

87. Baldissara P, Comin G, Martone F, Scotti R. Comparative study of the marginal microleakage of six cements in fixed provisional crowns. J Prosthet Dent 1998;80:417–422.

88. Rosenstiel SF, Gegauff AG. Effect of provisional cementing agents on provisional resins. J Prosthet Dent 1988;59:23–33.

89. Gegauff AG, Rosenstiel SF. Effect of provisional luting agents on provisional resin addition. Quintessence Int 1987;18:841–845.

90. Sochat T, Schwarz MS. The provisional splint—trouble shooting. J South Calif Dent Assoc 1973;41:92–93.

91. Dietschi D, Spreafico R. Adhesive Metal-Free Restorations. Current Concepts for the Esthetic Treatment of Posterior Teeth. Chicago: Quintessence, 1997.

92. Van Meerbeek B, Vargas M, Inoue S, et al. Adhesive and cements to promote preservation dentistry. Oper Dent (Supplement n°6):119–144, 2001.

93. Douglas WH. Methods to improve fracture resistance of teeth. In: Vanherle G, Smith DC (eds). Posterior Composite Resin Dental Restorative Materials. Utrecht, The Netherlands: Peter Szulc,1985:433–441.

94. Nathanson D. Principles of porcelain use as an inlay/onlay material. In: Garber DA, Goldstein RE (eds). Porcelain and Composite Inlays and Onlays. Esthetic Posterior Restorations. Chicago: Quintessence, 1994:32–37.

95. Burgess JO, Haveman CW, Butzin C. Evaluation for resins for provisional restorations. Am J Dent 1992;5:137–139.

96. Studer S, Lehner C, Brodbeck U, Scharer P. Short-term results of IPS-Empress inlays and onlays. J Prosthodont 1996;5:277–287.

97. Fradeani M, Aquilano A, Bassein L. Longitudinal study of pressed glass-ceramic inlays for four and a half years. J Prosthet Dent 1997;78:346–353.

98. Fuzzi M, Rappelli G. Ceramic inlays: clinical assessment and survival rate. J Adhes Dent 1999;1:71–79.

99. Sjogren G, Lantto R, Granberg A, Sundstrom BO, Tillberg A. Clinical examination of leucite-reinforced glass-ceramic crowns (Empress) in general practice: a retrospective study. Int J Prosthodont 1999;12:122–128.

100. Paul SJ, Scharer P. The dual bonding technique: a modified method to improve adhesive luting procedures. Int J Periodontics Restorative Dent 1997;17:536–545.

101. Woody TL, Davis RD. The effect of eugenol-containing and eugenol-free temporary cements on microleakage in resin bonded restorations. Oper Dent 1992;17:175–180.

102. Terata R, Nakashima K, Obara M, Kubota M. Characterization of enamel and dentin surfaces after removal of temporary cement: effect of temporary cement on tensile bond strength of resin luting cement. Dent Mater 1994;13:148–154.

103. Phillips RW, Avery DR, Mehra R, Swartz ML, McCune RJ. Observations on a composite resin for Class II restorations: three-year report. J Prosthet Dent 1973;30:891–897.

104. Brännström M, Vojinovic O. Response of the dental pulp to invasion of bacteria around three filling materials. ASDC J Dent Child 1976;43:83–89.

105. Powers JM, Fan PL, Raptis CN. Color stablity of new composite restorative materials under accelerated aging. J Dent Res 1980;59:2071–2074.

106. Beham G. IPS Empress: a new ceramic technology. Ivoclar-Vivadent Rep 1990;6:3–15.

107. Dong JK, Luthy H, Wohlwend A, Sharer P. Heat-pressed ceramics: technology and strength. Int J Prosthodont 1992;5:9–16.

108. Rochette A. A ceramic restoration bonded by etched enamel and resin for fractured incisors. J Prosthet Dent 1975;33:287–293.

109. Friedman MJ. A 15-year review of porcelain veneer failure: a clinician's observations. Compend Contin Educ Dent 1998;19:625–632.

110. Peumans M, Van Meerbeek B, Yoshida Y, Lambrechts P, Vanherle G. Five-year clinical performance of porcelain veneers. Quintessence Int 1998;29:211–221.

111. Dumfahrt H, Schaffer H. Porcelain laminate veneers. A retrospective evaluation after 1 to 10 years of service: Part II. Clinical results. Int J Prosthodont 2000; 13:9–18.

112. Magne P, Perroud R, Hodges JS, Belser U. Clinical performance of novel-design porcelain veneers for the recovery of coronal volume and length. Int J Periodontics Restorative Dent 2000;20:441–457.

113. Fradeani M, Redemagni M, Corrado M. Porcelain laminate veneers: 6- to 12-year clinical evaluation. A retrospective study. Int J Periodontics Restorative Dent 2005;25:9–17.

114. Magne P, Belser U. Bonded Porcelain Restorations in the Anterior Dentition. A Biomimetic Approach. Chicago: Quintessence, 2002.

115. Gürel G. The Science and Art of Porcelain Laminate Veneers. Chicago: Quintessence, 2003.

116. Magne P, Belser U. Bonded Porcelain Restorations in the Anterior Dentition. A Biomimetic Approach. Chicago: Quintessence, 2002:239–291.

117. Schreiber CK. The clinical application of carbon fibre/polymer denture bases. Br Dent J 1974;137:21–22.

118. Mullarky RH. Aramid fiber reinforcement of acrylic appliances. J Clin Orthod 1985;19:655–658.

119. Larson WR, Dixon DL, Aquilino SA, Clancy JM. The effect of carbon graphite fiber reinforcement on the strength of provisional crown and fixed partial denture resin. J Prosthet Dent 1991;66:816–820.

120. Amet Em, Phinney TL. Fixed provisional restorations for extended prosthodontic treatment. J Oral Implantol 1995;21:201–206.

121. Hazelton LR, Brudvik JS. A new procedure to reinforce fixed provisional restorations. J Prosthet Dent 1995;74:110–113.

122. Greenberg JR. The metal band-acrylic provisional restoration featuring ultra thin stainless steel bands. Compend Contin Educ Dent 1981;2:7–11.

123. Winkelman RD. Provisionalization of a combination implant/natural abutment restoration. J Dent Technol 1996;13:19–22.

124. Tung FF, Coleman AJ, Lu TN, Marotta L. A multifunctional, provisional, implant-retained fixed partial denture. J Prosthet Dent 2001;85:34–39.

125. Zinner ID, Small SA, Panno FV, Pines MS. Provisional and definitive prostheses following sinus lift and augmentation procedures. Implant Dent 1994;3:24–28.

126. Perel ML. Progressive prosthetic transference for root form implants. Implant Dent 1994;3:42–46.

127. Zinner ID, Panno FV, Pines MS, Small SA. First-stage fixed provisional restorations for implant prosthodontics. J Prosthodont 1993;2:228–232.

128. Palmer RM, Palmer PJ, Smith BJ. A 5-year prospective study of Astra single tooth implants. Clin Oral Implants Res 2000;11:179–182.

129. Breeding LC, Dixon DL. A bonded provisional fixed prosthesis to be worn after implant surgery. J Prosthet Dent 1995;74:114–116.

130. Balshi TJ, Wolfinger GJ. Immediate loading of Brånemark implants in edentulous mandibles. A preliminary report. Implant Dent 1997;6:83–88.

131. Tarnow DP, Emtiaz S, Classi A. Immediate loading of threaded implants at stage 1 surgery in edentulous arches: ten consecutive case reports with 1- to 5-year data. Int J Oral Maxillofac Implants 1997;12:319–324.

132. Horiuchi K, Uchida H, Yamamoto K, Sugimura M. Immediate loading of Brånemark system implants following placement in edentulous patients: a clinical report. Int J Oral Maxillofac Implants 2000;15:824–830.

133. Jaffin RA, Kumar A, Berman CL. Immediate loading of implants in partially edentulous jaws: a series of 27 case reports. J Periodontol 2000;71:833–888.

134. Colomina LE. Immediate loading of implant-fixed mandibular prostheses: a prospective 18-month follow-up clinical study-preliminary report. Implant Dent 2001;10:23–29.

135. Biggs WF, Litvak AL Jr. Immediate provisional restorations to aid in gingival healing and optimal contours for implant patients. J Prosthet Dent 2001;86:177–180.

136. LeSage BP. Improving implant aesthetics: prosthetically generated papilla through tissue modeling with composite. Pract Proced Aesthet Dent 2006;18:257–263.

137. Wöhrle PS. Single tooth replacement in the aesthetic zone with immediate provisionalization: fourteen consecutive case reports. Pract Periodontics Aesthet Dent 1998;10:1107–1114.

138. Ericsson I, Nilson H, Nilner K. Immediate functional loading of Brånemark single tooth implants. A 5-year clinical follow-up study. Appl Osseointegration Res 2001;2:12–16.

139. Hui E, Chow J, Li D, Liu J, Wat P, Law H. Immediate provisional for single-tooth implant replacement with Brånemark system: preliminary report. Clin Implant Dent Relat Res 2001;3:79–86.

140. Kirketerp P, Andersen JB, Urde G. Replacement of extracted anterior teeth by immediately loaded Replace Select HA-coated implants. A one-year follow-up of 35 patients. Appl Osseointegration Res 2002;3;40–43.

141. Groisman M, Frossard WM, Ferreira HMB, de Menezes Filho LM, Touati B. Single-tooth implants in the maxillary incisor region with immediate provisionalization: 2-year prospective study. Pract Proced Aesthet Dent 2003;15:115–122.

142. Maló P, Friberg B, Polizzi G, Gualini F, Vighagen T, Rangert B. Immediate and early function of Brånemark System implants placed in the esthetic zone: a 1-year prospective clinical multicenter study. Clin Implant Dent Relat Res 2003b;5(Suppl 1):37–46.

143. Rocci A, Martignoni M, Gottlow J. Immediate loading in the maxilla using flapless surgery, implants placed in predetermined positions, and prefabricated provisional restorations. A retrospective 3-year clinical study. Clin Implant Dent Relat Res 2003a;5(Suppl 1):29–36.

144. Vassos D. Single-stage surgery for implant placement: a retrospective study. J Oral Implantol 1997;23:181–185.

145. Ericsson I, Nilson H, Lindh T, Nilner K, Randow K. Immediate functional loading of Brånemark single tooth implants. Clin Oral Implants Res 2000;11:26–33.

146. Payne A, Tawse-Smith A, Kumare R, Thomson M. One-year prospective evaluation of the early loading of unsplinted conical Brånemark fixtures with mandibular overdentures immediately following surgery. Clin Implant Dent Relat Res 2001;3:9–19.

147. Chiapasco M, Gatti C. Implant-retained mandibular overdentures with immediate loading: a 3- to 8-year prospective study on 328 implants. Clin Implant Dent Relat Res 2003;5:29–38.

148. Degidi M, Piattelli A. Immediate functional and non-functional loading of dental implants: a 2- to 60-month follow-up study of 646 titanium implants. J Periodontol 2003:74:225–241.

149. Balshi SF, Wolfinger GJ, Balshi TJ. A prospective study of immediate functional loading following the Teeth in A Day protocol: a case series of 55 consecutive edentulous maxillas. Clin Implant Dent Relat Res 2005;7:24–31.

150. Glauser R, Ruhstaller P, Windisch S, et al. Immediate occlusal loading of Brånemark system TiUnite implants placed predominantly in soft bone: 4-year result of a prospective clinical study. Clin Implant Dent Relat Res 2005;7(Suppl 1):52–59.

151. van Steenberghe D, Glauser R, Blomback U, et al. A computed tomographic scan-derived customized surgical template and fixed prosthesis for flapless surgery and immediate loading of implants in fully edentulous maxillae: a prospective multicenter study. Clin Implant Dent Relat Res 2005;7(Suppl1):111–120.

152. Botticelli D, Berglundh T, Lindhe J. Hard-tissue alterations following immediate placement in extraction sites. J Clin Periodontol 2004;31:820–828.

153. Araujo MG, Sukekava F, Wennstrom JL, Lindhe J. Ridge alterations following implant placement in fresh extraction sockets: an experimental study in the dog. J Clin Periodontol 2005;32:645–652.

154. Cooper L, Felton DA, Kugelberg CF, et al. A multicenter 12-month evaluation of single-tooth implants restored 3 weeks after 1-stage surgery. Int J Oral Maxillofac Implants 2001;16:182–192.

155. Park KB, Han TJ, Kenney B. Immediate implant placement with immediate provisional crown placement: three case reports. Pract Periodontics Aesthet Dent 2002;14:147–154.

156. Hochwald DA. Surgical template impression during stage I surgery for fabrication of a provisional restoration to be placed at stage II surgery. J Prosthet Dent 1991;66:796–798.

157. Krough-Poulson WG, Olsson A. Management of the occlusion of the teeth: background, definitions, rationale. In: Schwartz L, Chayes C (eds). Facial Pain and Mandibular Dysfunction. Philadelphia: WB Saunders, 1968.

158. Dawson PE, Arcan M. Attaining harmonic occlusion through visualized strain analysis. J Prosthet Dent 1981;46:615–622.

159. Ramfjord S, Ash MM. Occlusion, ed 3. Philadelphia: WB Saunders, 1983.

160. Dawson PE. Evaluation, Diagnosis, and Treatment of Occlusal Problems, ed 2. St Louis: Mosby, 1989:14–17.

161. Castellani D. Elements of Occlusion. Bologna, Italy: Edizioni Martina, 2000:37–54.

162. Dawson PE. Evaluation, Diagnosis, and Treatment of Occlusal Problems. St Louis: CV Mosby, 1989:274–297.

163. Kinsel RP, Lamb RE, Moneim A. Development of gingival esthetics in the edentulous patient with immediately loaded, single-stage, implant-supported fixed prostheses: a clinical report. Int J Oral Maxillofac Implants 2000;15:711–721.

164. Berglin GM. A technique for fabricating a fixed provisional prosthesis on osseointegrated fixtures. J Prosthet Dent 1989;61:347–348.

165. Schnitman PA, Wöhrle PS, Rubenstein JE. Immediate fixed interim prostheses supported by two-stage threaded implants: methodology and results. J Oral Implantol 1990;16:96–105.

166. Cibirka Rm, Linebaugh ML. The fixed/detachable implant provisional prosthesis. J Prosthodont 1997;6:149–152.

167. Shavell HM. Mastering the art of provisionalization. J Calif Dent Assoc 1979;7:42–49.

168. Rieder CE. Use of provisional restorations to develop and achieve esthetic expectations. Int J Periodontics Restorative Dent 1989;9:122–139.

169. Sze AJ. Duplication of anterior provisional fixed partial dentures for the final restoration. J Prosthet Dent 1992;68:220–223.

170. Rufenacht CR. Fundamentals of Esthetics. Chicago: Quintessence, 1990:67–134.

171. Chiche GJ, Pinault A. Artistic and scientific principles applied to esthetic dentistry. In: Chiche GJ, Pinault A (eds). Esthetics of Anterior Fixed Prosthodontics. Chicago: Quintessence, 1994:13–32.

172. Roach RR, Muia PJ. Communication between dentist and technician: an esthetic checklist. In: Preston JD (ed). Perspectives in Dental Ceramics: Proceedings of the Fourth International Symposium on Ceramics. Chicago: Quintessence, 1998:445–455.

173. Castellani D. Elements of Occlusion. Bologna, Italy: Edizioni Martina, 2000:122.

174. Vig RG, Brundo GC. The kinetics of anterior tooth display. J Prosthet Dent 1978;39:502–504.

175. Arnett GW, Bergman RT. Facial keys to orthodontic diagnosis and treatment planning. Part I. Am J Orthod Dentofacial Orthop 1993;103:299–312.

176. Mack PJ. Maxillary arch and central incisor dimension in a Nigerian and British population sample. J Dent 1981;9:67–70.

177. Chiche GJ, Pinault A. Replacement of deficient crowns. In: Chiche GJ, Pinault A (eds). Esthetics of Anterior Fixed Prosthodontics. Chicago: Quintessence, 1994:53–73.

178. Landa JS. The free-way space and its significance in the rehabilitation of the masticatory apparatus. J Prosthet Dent 1952;2:756–779.

179. Mehringer EJ. The use of speech patterns as an aid in prosthodontic reconstruction. J Prosthet Dent 1963;13:825–836.

180. Gibbs CH, Messerman T, Reswick JB, Derda HJ. Functional movements of the mandible. J Prosthet Dent 1971;26:604–620.

181. MacGregor AR. Fenn, Liddelow and Gimson's Clinical Dental Prosthetics. London: Wright, 1989:89.

182. Chiche GJ, Pinault A. Artistic and scientific principles applied to esthetic dentistry. In: Chiche GJ, Pinault A (eds). Esthetics of Anterior Fixed Prosthodontics. Chicago: Quintessence, 1994:13–32.

183. Pound E. The mandibular movements of speech and their seven related values. J Prosthet Dent 1966;16:835–843.

184. Pound E. Let /S/ be your guide. J Prosthet Dent 1977;38:482–489.

185. Manns A, Miralles R, Palazzi C. EMG, bite force, and elongation of the masseter muscle under isometric voluntary contractions and variations of vertical dimension. J Prosthet Dent 1979;42:674–682.

186. Silverman ET. Speech rehabilitation: habits and myofunctional therapy. In: Seide L (ed). Restorative Procedures in Dynamic Approach to Restorative Dentistry. Philadelphia: Saunders, 1980.

187. Dawson PE. Evaluation, Diagnosis, and Treatment of Occlusal Problems, ed 2. St Louis: Mosby, 1989:298–319.

188. Rivera-Morales WC, Mohl ND. Variability of closest speaking space compared with interocclusal distance in dentulous subjects. J Prosthet Dent 1991;65:228–232.

189. Christensen J. Effect of occlusion-raising procedures on the chewing system. Dent Pract Dent Rec 1970;20(7):233–238.

190. Carlsson GE, Ingervall B, Kocak G. Effect of increasing vertical dimension on the masticatory system in subjects with natural teeth. J Prosthet Dent 1979;41:284–289.

191. Kohno S, Bando E. Die funktionelle Anpassung der Kaumuskulatur bei starker Beisshebung (Functional adaptation of masticatory muscles as a result of large increases in the vertical dimension). Dtsch Zahnärztl Z 1983;38:759–764.

192. Hammond RJ, Beder OE. Increased vertical dimension and speech articulation errors. J Prosthet Dent 1984;52:401–406.

193. Gross MD, Ormianer Z. A preliminary study on the effect of occlusal vertical dimension increase on mandibular postural rest position. Int J Prosthodont 1994;7:216–226.

VOLUME 2 | PROSTHETIC TREATMENT

ESTHETIC REHABILITATION IN FIXED PROSTHODONTICS

Chapter 3

BIOLOGIC INTEGRATION OF THE PROVISIONAL RESTORATION AND DEFINITIVE PREPARATIONS

Once it has been correctly fabricated and fitted, the provisional restoration must be integrated both from an esthetic-functional and a biologic perspective. Maintaining or restoring good periodontal health in surgical as well as nonsurgical situations is a prerequisite to initiating the definitive preparations. Healthy gingival tissue not only indicates correct integration of the provisional restoration but also allows the esthetic appearance of the dentogingival complex to be optimized in the presence of both natural teeth and osseointegrated implants.

OBJECTIVE _ To re-establish and maintain gingival tissue integrity before proceeding with the definitive preparations.

BIOLOGIC INTEGRATION OF THE PROVISIONAL RESTORATION AND DEFINITIVE PREPARATIONS

SOFT TISSUES

Verifying the health of the periodontium prior to any prosthetic treatment is essential[1,2] to ensure stability of the gingival margins during the prosthetic stages.[3] The gingival tissues must not bleed when probed, thereby proving the absence of inflammation.

PERIODONTAL BIOTYPE

The gingival architecture can be generally characterized as either flat with thick tissues or scalloped with very thin tissues. In patients with the latter biotype, it is essential to operate with extreme delicacy to avoid gingival recession phenomena.[4]

ANATOMIC STRUCTURES

Knowledge of the anatomic structures of the periodontal tissues allows the clinician to minimize biologic damage in this extremely delicate area. Through histologic studies, Gargiulo[5] examined the relationship between the tooth and its supporting tissue (Fig 3-1a) and found that connective tissue attachment and epithelial attachment average 1.07 and 0.97 mm in height, respectively, although variation was shown especially in the epithelial attachment.[6,7] In healthy dentitions, it should be obvious that the structure formed by the connective tissue and epithelial attachments has been maintained.[8]

GINGIVAL SULCUS

In his studies, Gargiulo[5] found an average probing depth of 0.69 mm. Clinically, it is easy to demonstrate that this measurement can vary considerably, even around the same tooth, depending on the site probed. In the anterior sectors, for example, probing a healthy sulcus results in greater depths in the interproximal areas (1.0 to 3.0 mm) compared with the buccal areas[10] (0.5 to 1.0 mm).

PROSTHETIC PROCEDURE AND ASSOCIATED BIOLOGIC RISK

The stages of preparing the teeth, inserting the retraction cords, taking the impression, relining the provisional restoration, and removing the excess cement can cause direct damage to the periodontal tissues. The trauma associated with these procedures constitutes a mechanical insult with a related inflammatory response that is usually reversible if confined to the epithelial attachment area.[11] If, however, the connective tissue attachment is also violated, the damage caused to the periodontal tissues is irreversible.[12] All of this is aggravated by the indirect damage caused by the buildup of plaque, encouraged by incorrect contours and roughness on the surface of the restoration. Accuracy in carrying out all of the operative procedures allows the final stages of the prosthetic work to be approached while maintaining adequate gingival health, which guarantees the restoration's correct biologic integration (Figs 3-1b and 3-1c).

Sulcus

Epithelial attachment

Connective tissue attachment

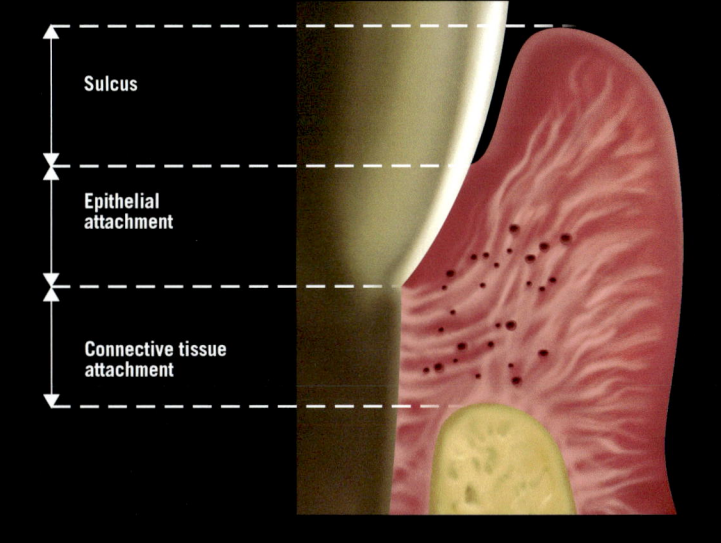

> Fig 3-1a

> Fig 3-1b

> Fig 3-1c

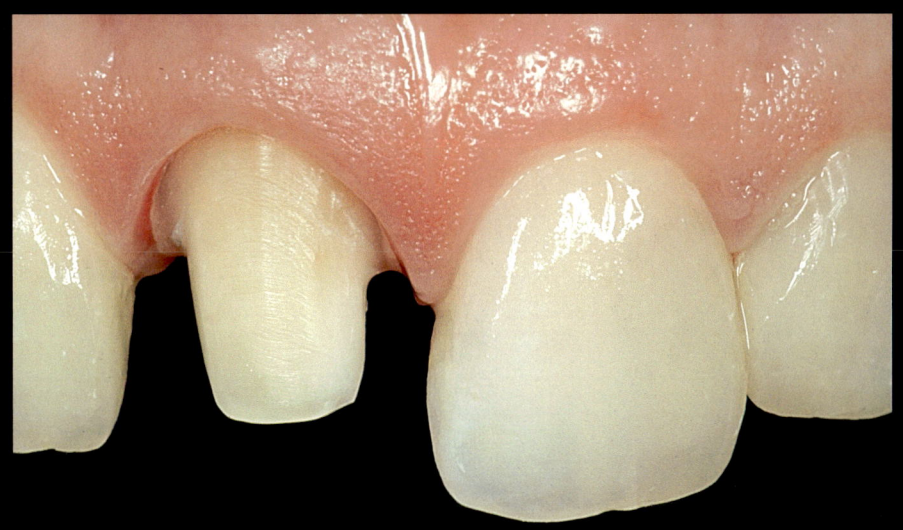

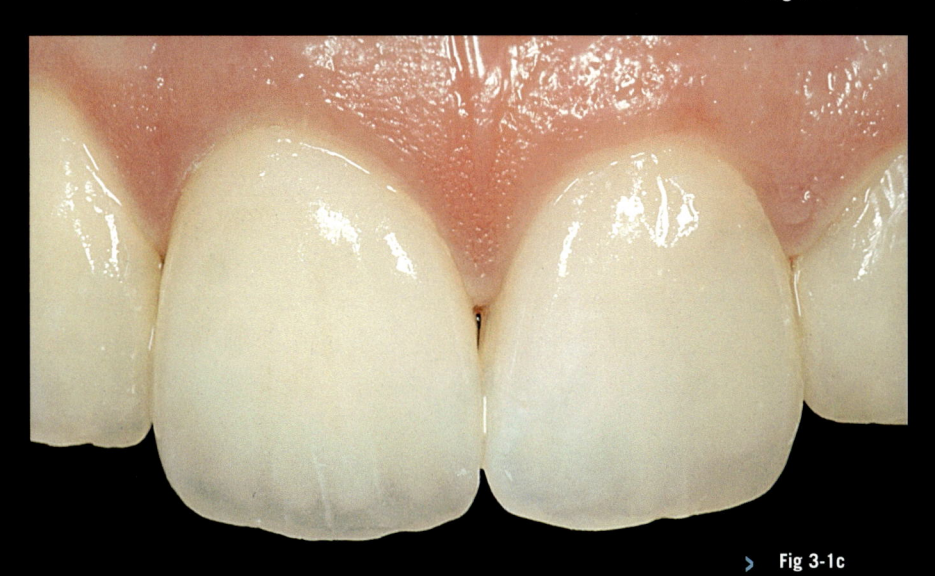

FIG 1 *(a)* Illustration of the periodontal complex, comprising the sulcus, the epithelial attachment, and the connective tissue attachment. *(b and c)* If the clinician has been careful not to violate the epithelial attachment or, more important, the connective tissue attachment during the phases of tooth preparation, final impressions, and relining of the provisional restoration, the gingival tissues will appear to be in a good state of health when the definitive work is delivered.

BIOLOGIC INTEGRATION

PROVISIONAL RESTORATION

RISK FACTORS

The position of the provisional restoration (Figs 3-2a and 3-2b) must in no way affect the optimal state of health of the soft tissues as demonstrated by the absence of bleeding during probing (Fig 3-2c) (see volume 1, chapter 6, pages 244–249), which is a prerequisite for all restorative therapy. The gingival tissues must remain healthy throughout of the period that the provisional restoration stays in the mouth, which can sometimes be quite lengthy (Figs 3-2d to 3-2h). This is especially the case if the treatment involves any associated therapies (endodontic, periodontal, implants, etc) or if true provisional integration following substantial modifications of an esthetic-functional nature is to be tested.

Various authors[13–16] maintain, without adequately specifying the reason, that positioning of the provisional restoration almost inevitably causes inflammation and gingival recession, which diminishes or disappears when the definitive restoration is placed in position. The onset of inflammation around the margins of the provisional restoration cannot, in the majority of cases, be ascribed to the use of acrylic resin. It is almost always the result of inaccurate work by the clinician, who has not satisfactorily checked the contour, marginal fit, and smoothness of the provisional restoration surface.

The acrylic resin used to construct the provisional restoration undoubtedly has less favorable surface characteristics, from a biologic standpoint, than the material used for the definitive restoration. Nevertheless, a correctly made provisional restoration allows good gingival health to be maintained.

A considerable risk factor is the exothermic reaction of the acrylic resin that develops in the resin polymerization phase during relining. As already noted (see chapter 2, page 192), the increase in temperature must be controlled by abundantly irrigating the provisional restoration and abutments with an air-water spray.

Another factor that can jeopardize the biologic integration of the provisional restoration is the amount of free monomer that can remain in contact with the tissues. Though the amount may be minimal and polymerization is complete, this situation can arise during relining if self-curing resin is used,[17] which can occasionally cause sensitization phenomena with allergic stomatitis through contact.[18,19]

FIG 2 *(a and b)* When the shell fits correctly and the relining is complete, the provisional restoration demonstrates satisfactory biologic integration. *(c and d)* The absence of any bleeding on probing indicates a state of good periodontal health even though the tissues still appear to be somewhat irritated after cementation. *(e)* In the mandible, correct insertion of the shell is checked, it is subsequently relined, and then finished. *(f to h)* The slightly supragingival positioning of the marginal limits chosen in this case promotes excellent biologic integration of the restorations.

Chapter 3 BIOLOGIC INTEGRATION OF THE PROVISIONAL RESTORATION AND DEFINITIVE PREPARATIONS

→ ... from page 269

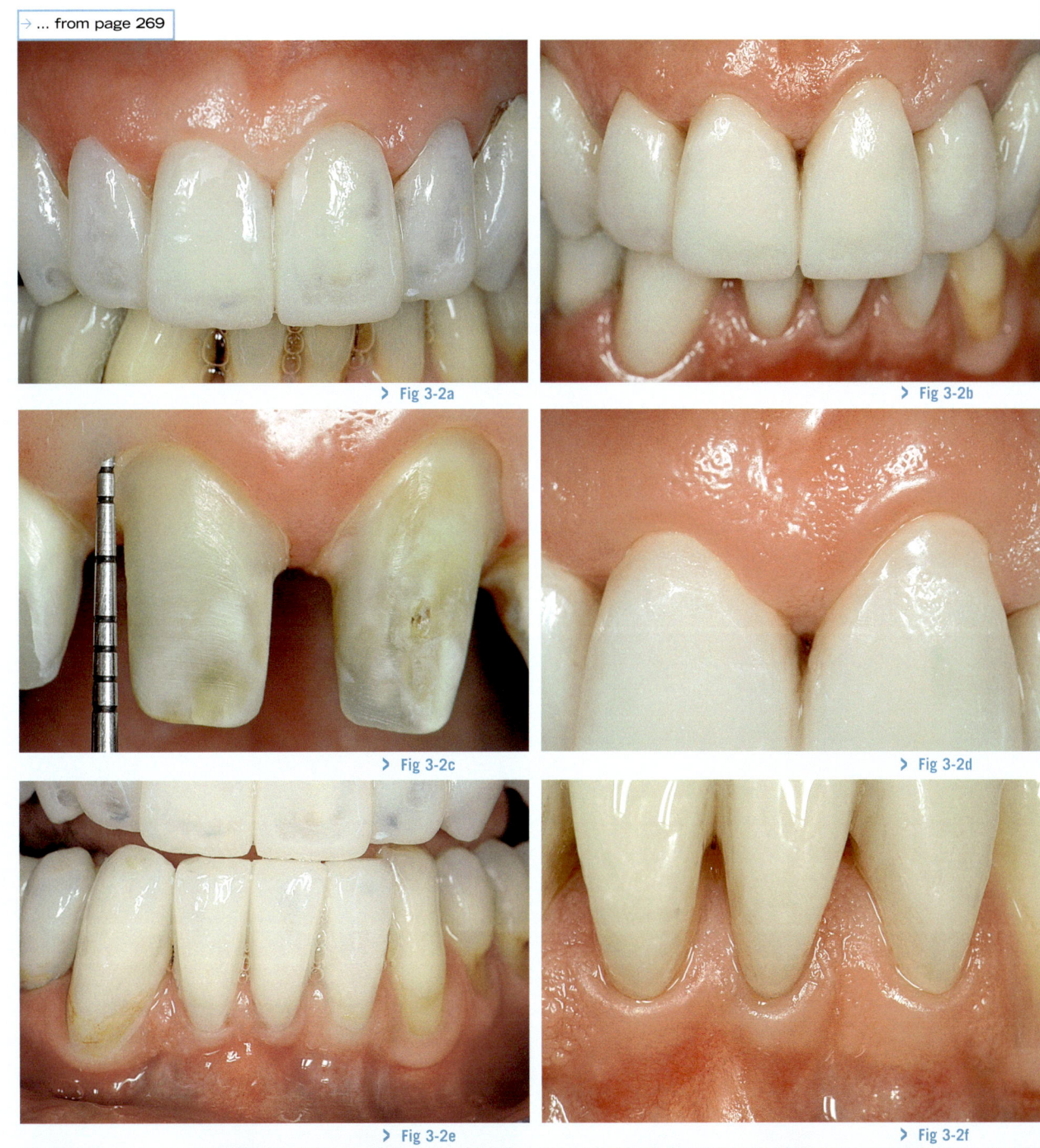

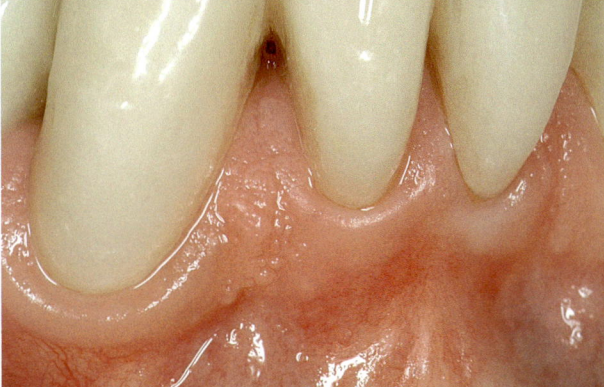

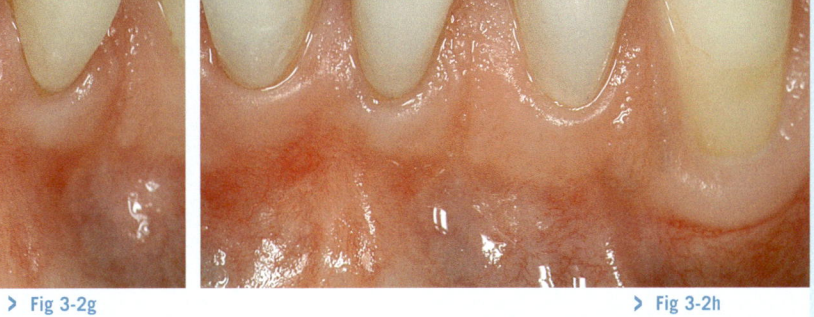

> Fig 3-2a

> Fig 3-2b

> Fig 3-2c

> Fig 3-2d

> Fig 3-2e

> Fig 3-2f

> Fig 3-2g

> Fig 3-2h

→ continues on page 393

The need for prosthetic treatment is often dictated by the need to replace incongruous restorations (Fig 3-3a) that inevitably cause tissue inflammation (Figs 3-3b and 3-3c). Inflammation confined to the surface structures sometimes allows the patient to be treated by just the initial periodontal therapy (Figs 3-3d and 3-3e) and correct positioning of the provisional restoration (Figs 3-3f and 3-3g).

In these cases the provisional restoration must remain in the mouth for some time until a significant improvement is seen in gingival health, promoted by an adequate marginal fit and by the development of an ideal emergence profile. The provisional restoration must be inspected periodically to verify the validity of the coronal contours and to test the patient's ability to prevent plaque buildup through proper oral hygiene. Waiting for the tissues to stabilize (4 to 8 weeks)[20–22] (Figs 3-3h and 3-3i) means the operative stages must be prolonged, directly affecting the time needed to finalize the work. Only after the gingival tissues are stabilized is it possible to proceed with the tooth preparations and take the final impressions. To address subgingival margins presenting with caries lesions or to restore the correct architecture of the hard and soft tissues, it is necessary in some cases to resort to surgical-periodontal treatment before the prosthetic treatment is carried out. This further prolongs the amount of time that the provisional restorations must remain in the mouth.

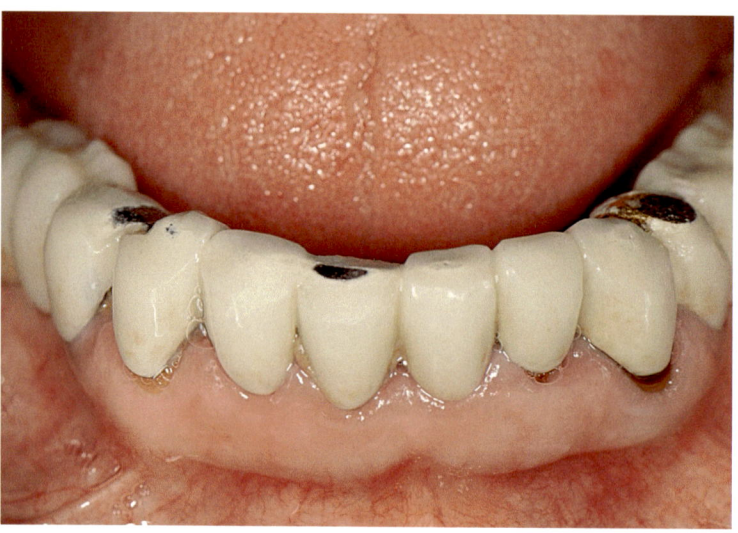

> Fig 3-3a

FIG 3 *(a to c)* Restorations that are poorly integrated under the esthetic-functional profile and have inadequate interdental spaces often cause a substantial inflammatory reaction of the gingival tissues, which is easily identifiable after the original prosthesis is removed. *(d to i)* After the initial periodontal therapy is performed with appropriate instruments, the gingival tissues show a significant improvement approximately 4 weeks after the new provisional restorations have been positioned correctly and relined. Only after complete resolution of the inflammatory condition may the clinician proceed with the prosthetic finalization stages.

Fig 3-3b

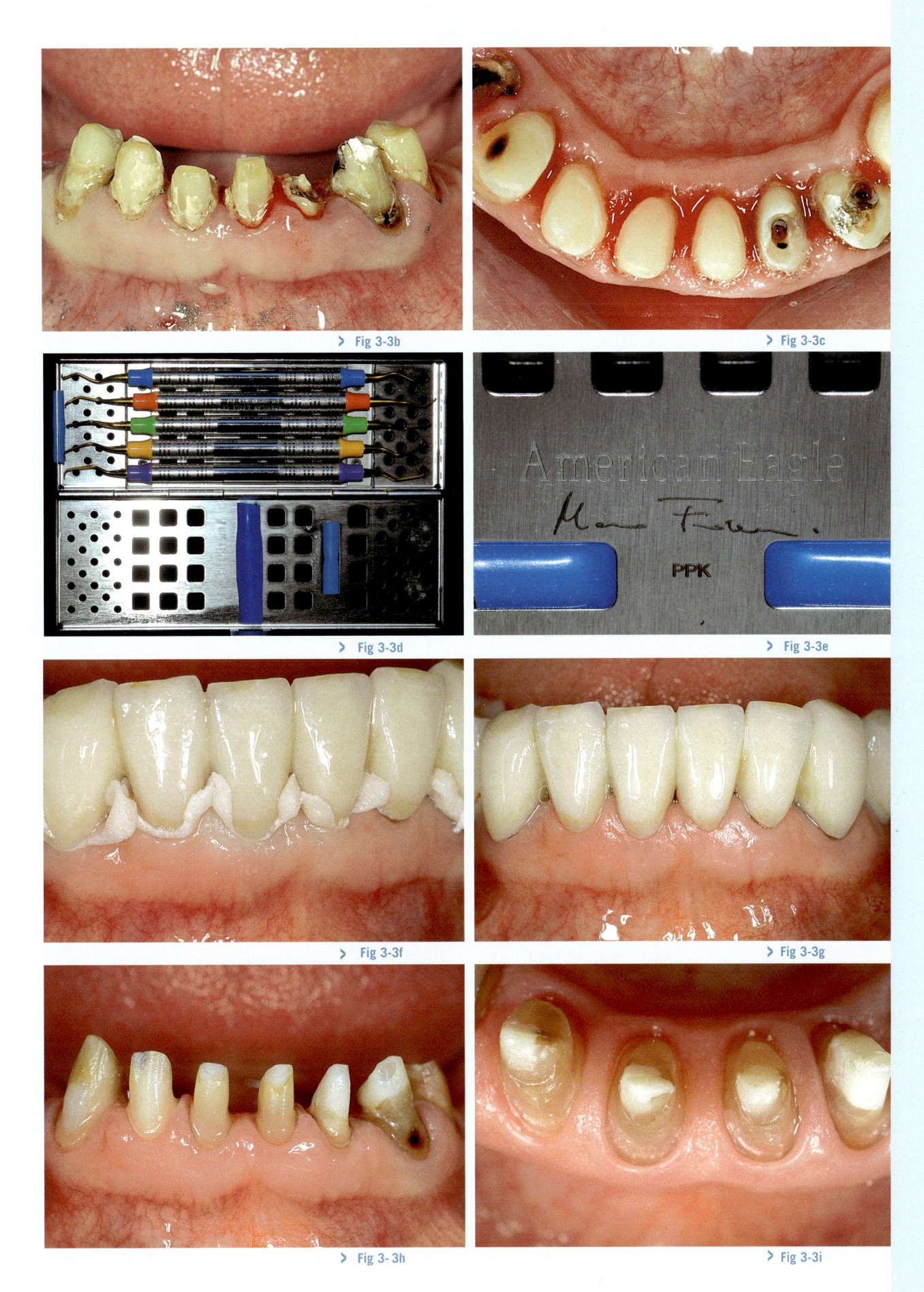

Fig 3-3c

Fig 3-3d

Fig 3-3e

Fig 3-3f

Fig 3-3g

Fig 3-3h

Fig 3-3i

283

GINGIVAL MARGIN STABILITY

To optimize esthetic appearance, the clinician must be able to rely on absolute stability of the gingival margins in all stages of the prosthetic treatment. In addition to the intrinsic properties of the material composing the provisional restoration, other aspects of the prosthetic procedures can directly constitute risk factors that could compromise the health of the soft tissues.

MARGINAL CLOSURE

When existing restorations with pronounced overcontours and inadequate marginal closure (Figs 3-4a to 3-4c) are being replaced, a determining factor in restoring good gingival health is the cervical design of the new provisional restoration (Fig 3-4d). Finishing the provisional restoration in these cases is of fundamental importance. Achieving an optimal marginal fit, despite the less-than-ideal surface of the acrylic resin material, allows the patient to clean the restorations comfortably and thus prevent plaque buildup, which is the main cause of inflammation. Only after observing significant improvement in the tissues (Figs 3-4e and 3-4f) and determining that there is no periodontal damage requiring preprosthetic surgical treatment is it possible to proceed with finalizing the work (Fig 3-4g).

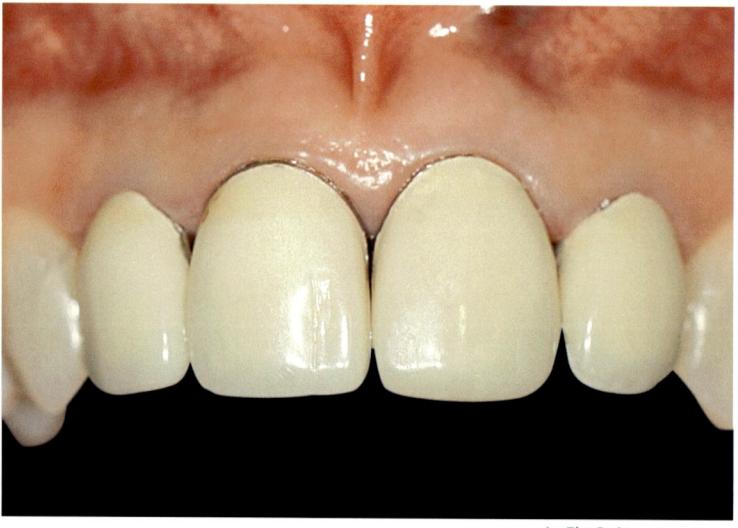

> Fig 3-4a

FIG 4 *(a)* The young patient requests replacement of four anterior restorations, completed some years ago at a different office. *(b and c)* When these are removed, a significant inflammatory tissue response is revealed, especially in the interproximal areas where compromise of the interdental papillae is also evident. *(d to f)* For esthetic reasons, a decision was made to deepen the tooth preparations in the gingival sulcus. Nevertheless, one can see appreciable improvement in the tissues as a result of proper positioning and integration of an adequate provisional restoration. *(g)* The appropriate contours of the provisional restoration contribute significantly to maintaining good gingival health until the definitive work can be delivered, which proves to be adequately integrated under the biologic profile.

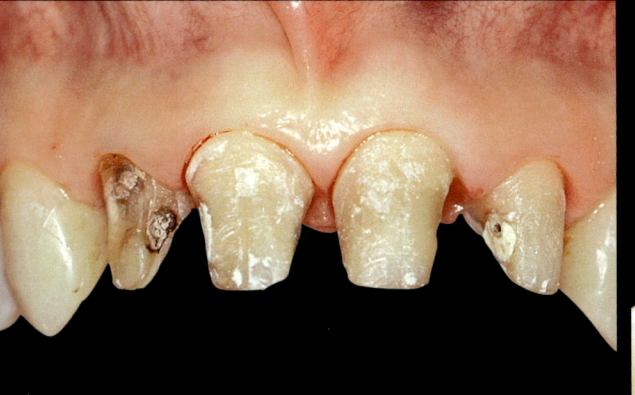

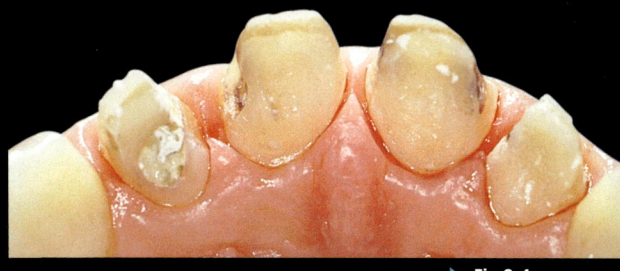

> Fig 3-4b

> Fig 3-4c

> Fig 3-4d

> Fig 3-4e

> Fig 3-4f

> Fig 3-4g

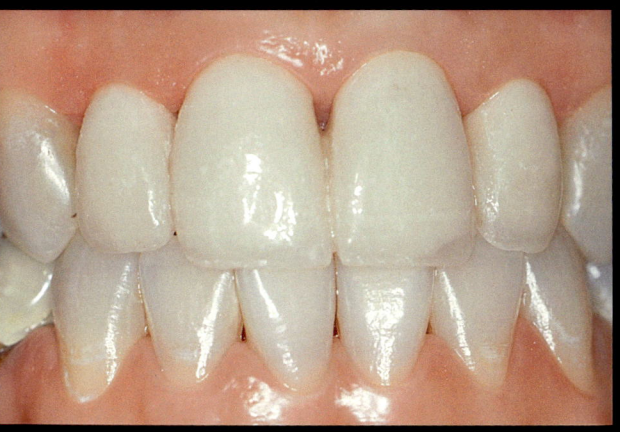

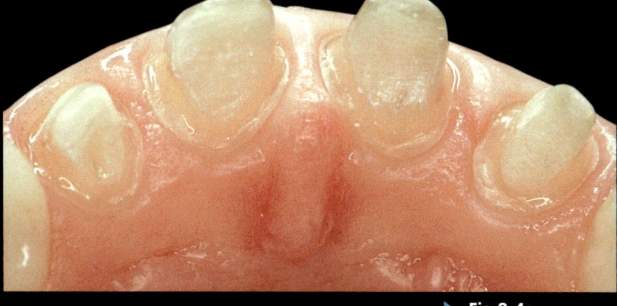

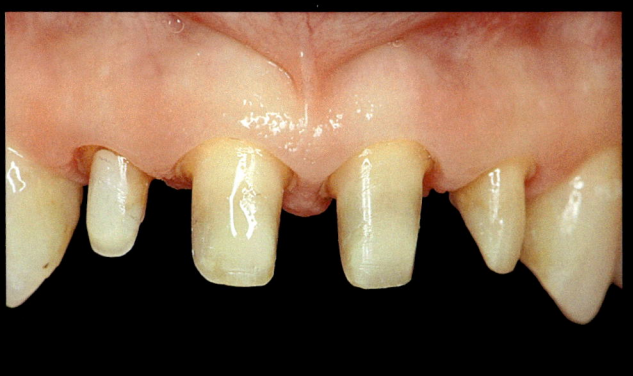

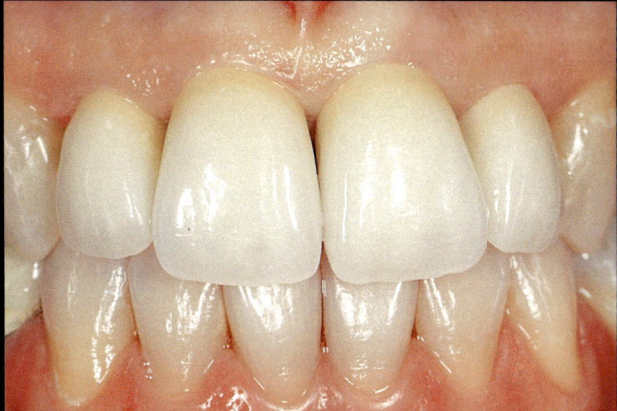

GINGIVAL MARGIN STABILITY

PREREQUISITES

- Optimal marginal fit
- Adequate contour development
- Appropriate polishing of the provisional restoration
- Complete removal of all excess cement

RESTORATION CONTOUR

The restoration contour can play a determining role in the state of health of the periodontium.[23–27] Besides satisfactory marginal closure, the provisional restoration must demonstrate appropriate development of the emergence profiles, both interproximally and at the buccolingual level, to be adequately integrated at a cervical level. This allows the patient to clean the prosthetically involved areas properly, thereby making it easier to maintain gingival health.[28]

INTERPROXIMAL CONTOUR

Where there is excessive space between the teeth (eg, diastemata) (Figs 3-5a and 3-5b), prosthetic modification of the original emergence profile is necessary at the interproximal level (Figs 3-5c and 3-5d). To do this, the preparation must be deepened in the intrasulcular site (Figs 3-5e and 3-5f) (see page 344). Care must be taken to achieve perfect marginal fit without creating any horizontal overcontouring (step). Contour variation appears to be well-tolerated as long as it is restricted to the vertical component (emergence profile) (Fig 3-5g). In the presence of two closely spaced roots, however, even a slight overcontour can compromise the deep periodontium in this very delicate area by encouraging the buildup of plaque, with a consequent inversion of the osseous architecture.[29]

Maintaining oral hygiene While the use of simple dental floss is recommended in the case of single restorations, fixed partial dentures require specific instruments for maintenance of oral hygiene. In the anterior sectors, superfloss effectively prevents the formation of inopportune "black triangles" often caused by the use of interproximal brushes that can traumatize and reduce the height of interdental papillae. The interproximal brush is very useful in the posterior sectors, however, where the patient has fewer esthetic needs. The presence of a significantly less scalloped architecture, and therefore flatter papillae, allows these instruments to be used efficiently in these areas.

FIG 5 *(a)* The patient, who presents with agenesis of the maxillary lateral incisors, complains of the unattractive appearance of the restorations positioned on the central incisors some years previously at a different office. *(b)* When the restorations are removed, the migration of the central incisors due to the missing lateral incisors is even more evident. The patient requests simple replacement of the old restorations to improve the esthetic appearance, declining the proposal to carry out preprosthetic orthodontic correction. *(c and d)* In two separate sessions, the mesial interproximal contour of the provisional restoration was modified on both central incisors in two separate sessions. By this means, the tissues were conditioned in a way that would encourage gradual development of the papilla. *(e and f)* Despite the potential risk involved in the modifications undertaken, the accuracy of the provisional margins allowed an adequate state of gingival health to be preserved. *(g)* Owing to the patient's good home oral hygiene practices, the definitive restorations also show the excellent biologic integration that had been preserved with the provisional restoration.

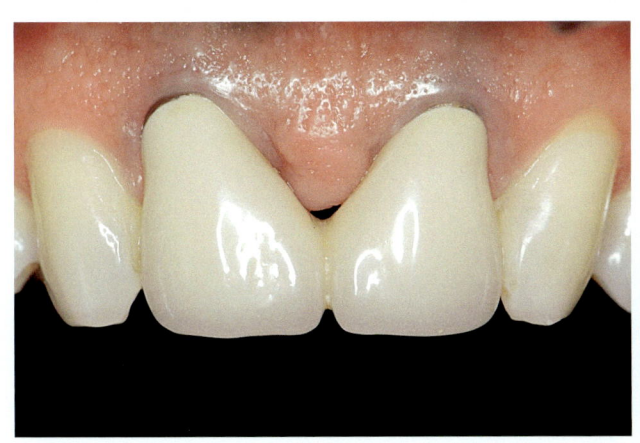

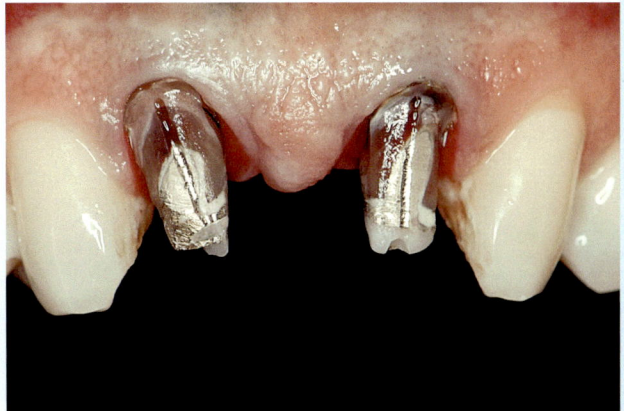

> Fig 3-5a

> Fig 3-5b

> Fig 3-5c

> Fig 3-5d

> Fig 3-5e

> Fig 3-5f

> Fig 3-5g

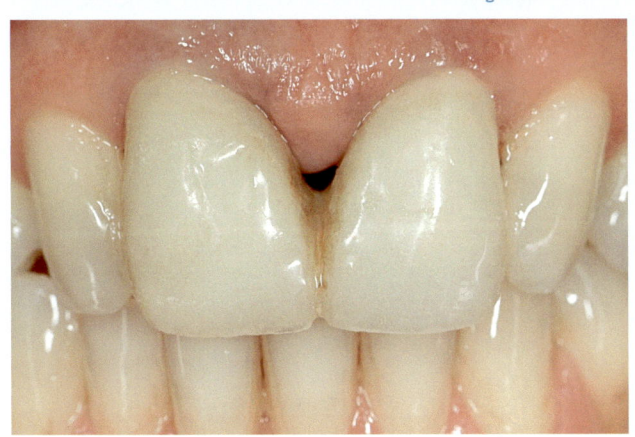

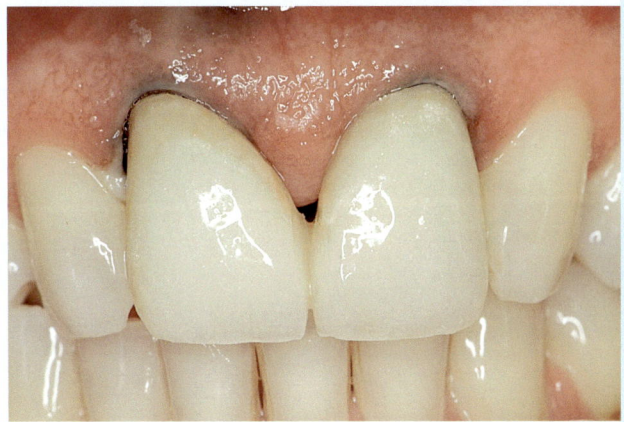

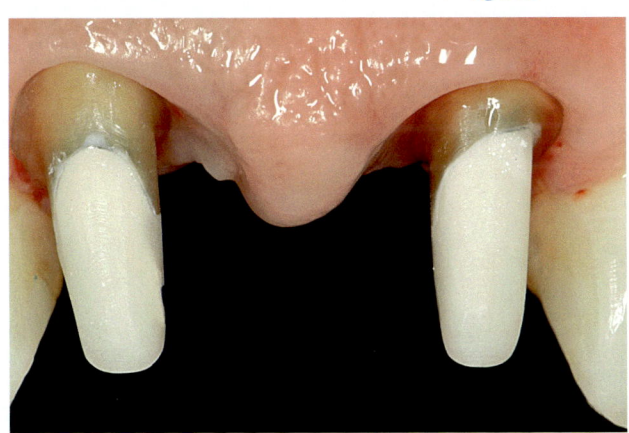

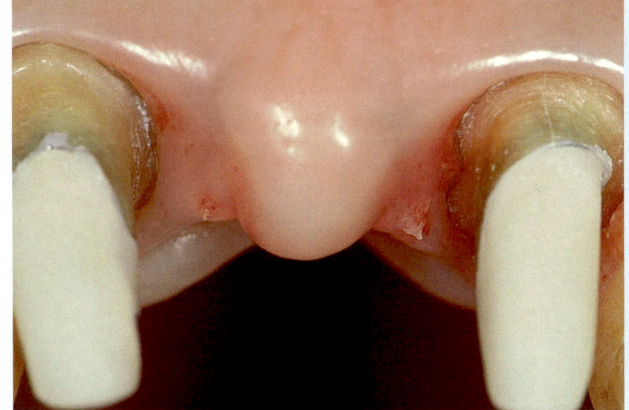

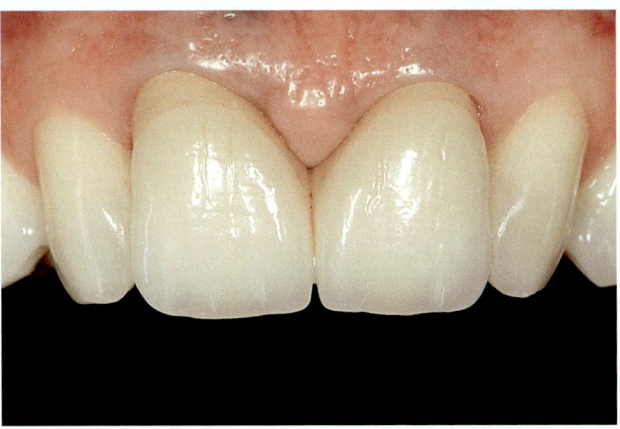

287

BUCCAL CONTOUR

Thin biotype Various studies have examined the relationship between the architecture of the gingival tissues and the cervical contour of the restoration,[4,30] whose buccolingual dimension is frequently found to be greater than that of the original tooth.[31] In the presence of a thin biotype (Fig 3-6a) or in cases where the preparation margin is positioned at the gingival crest, the excessive convexity of the cervical third resulting from insufficient preparations encourages plaque buildup and can lead to inflammation accompanied by gingival recession.[32–34] In such situations it is advisable to develop a provisional contour that is somewhat flattened in the buccal area (Figs 3-6b to 3-6d) to avoid tissue retraction phenomena.[4,35] The choice of a horizontal type of preparation (chamfer or shoulder), which allows the technician to work with adequate thicknesses to create a sufficiently flat restorative profile, is therefore preferable (Figs 3-6e to 3-6h).

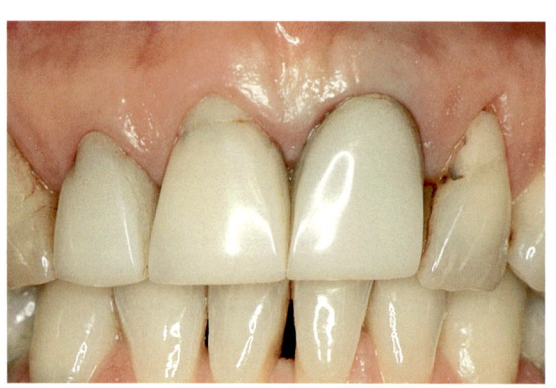

> Fig 3-6a

> Fig 3-6b

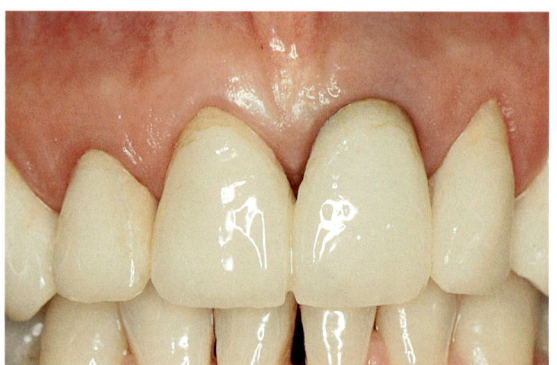

FIG 6 *(a)* Replacement of the old incongruous restorations in the anterosuperior sector requires six complete crowns to be positioned on the canines, lateral incisors, and central incisors. *(b)* After the abutments have been prepared, the provisional restorations are relined, suitably re-margined, and cemented. *(c and d)* Despite the maximum care taken during the operative phases, a slight gingival irritation is visible in this first clinical stage, especially in the presence of a thin biotype. This irritation will regress in the space of a few days if all of the procedures have been properly carried out. *(e to h)* Although a patient with a thin biotype is at greater risk for recession, the appropriate execution of all of the prosthetic phases guarantees, at the time of delivery, satisfactory integration of the definitive restorations, which are well maintained 12 years after they were positioned.

THIN BIOTYPE

Placement of provisional restorations

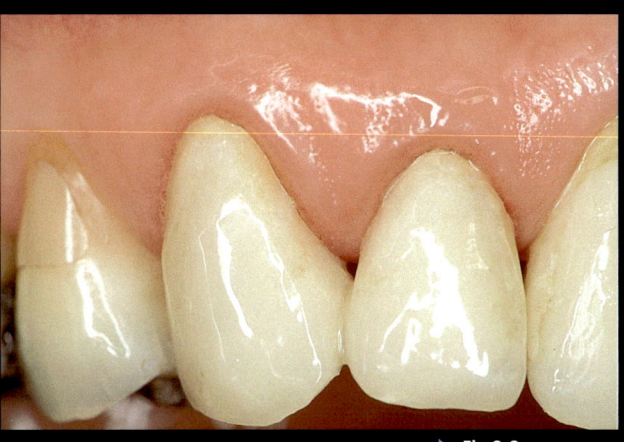

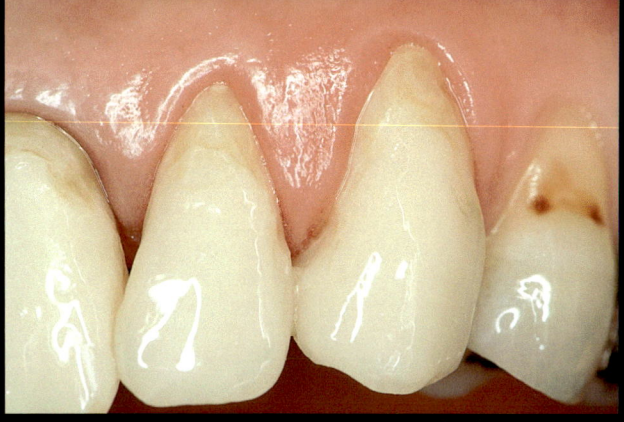

> Fig 3-6c

> Fig 3-6d

Cementation of definitive restorations

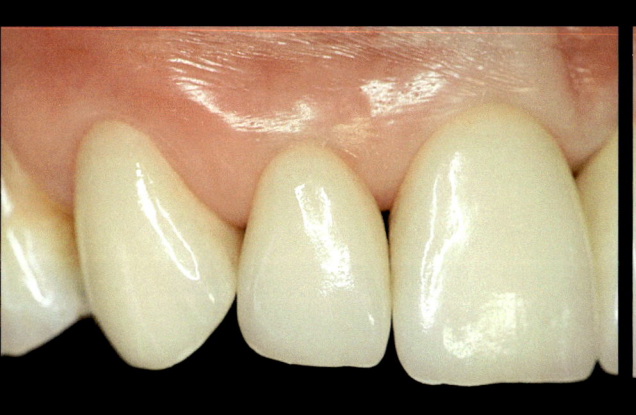

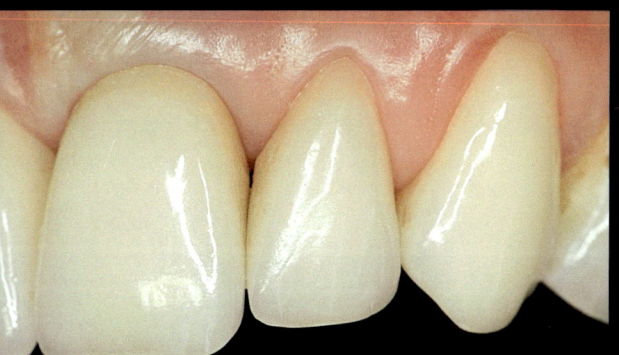

> Fig 3-6e

> Fig 3-6f

Twelve years later

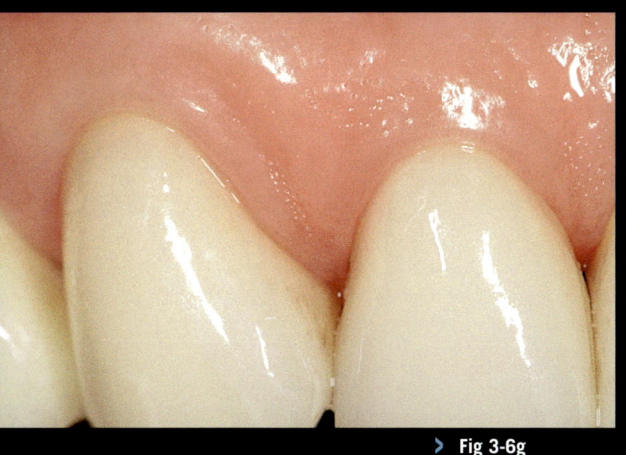

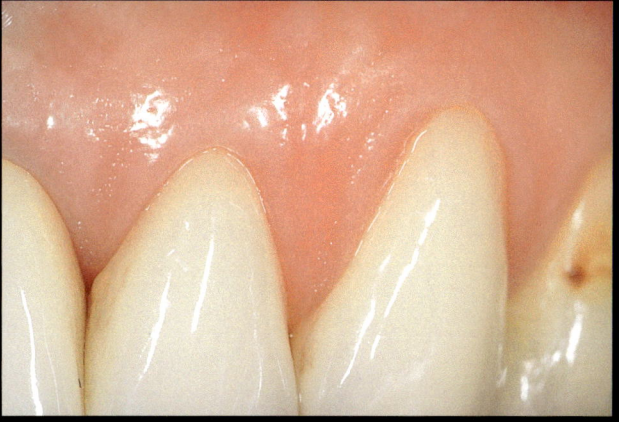

> Fig 3-6g

> Fig 3-6h

Thick biotype In the presence of a thick periodontal biotype (Fig 3-7a), it is preferable to design the emergence profile of the restoration by defining a slight convexity of the cervical third, starting from the intrasulcular area, to better support the gingival tissue[4] (Figs 3-7b to 3-7f). In these patients it has been observed[4,36] that insufficient tissue support from the buccal contour of the restoration can lead to collapse and reddening of the gingival margin.[37] In thick biotypes, however, as with thin tissues, creating a step (horizontal overcontour) causes an inevitable buildup of plaque and gingival inflammation. Instead of gingival recession, periodontal damage is frequently found in these cases in the form of an intraosseous pocket that is revealed by the increased probing depth.

SURFACE CHARACTERISTICS OF THE RESTORATIVE MATERIAL

The surface characteristics of the restorative material can affect the buildup of plaque and its associated gingival inflammation.[38-40] Significant differences have been found in the amount of plaque accumulated based on the materials used to make the prosthetic restoration.[41-45] From a clinical viewpoint, however, this parameter is not always a determining factor in the onset and progression of gingival inflammation. In fact, despite the intrinsic porosity of the acrylic resin used to construct the provisional restoration, a good marginal fit, adequate contour, and correct polishing can result in good integration, even though acrylic resin cannot be rendered as smooth as any other final material[29,46] (Figs 3-8 to 3-13).

EXCESS CEMENT

After cementing the provisional restoration, the clinician should take special care to completely remove all traces of residual cement, which can easily compromise periodontal health.[47] After all excesses have been removed following the suggestions already described (see chapter 2, page 206), it is a good rule to check the patient again 1 week later to make sure that all residue has actually been removed, especially in complex rehabilitation cases. Despite the care taken at this stage, the thinner or thicker line of cement that will inevitably occupy the space in the tooth-restoration interface has an irregular and rough surface appearance that can often contribute to a significant increase in the buildup of plaque.[48-52] The clinician must therefore try to attenuate the surface roughness of the cement by scraping the area delicately with a curette while taking great care not to affect the marginal integrity of the restoration or roughen its surface.

THICK BIOTYPE

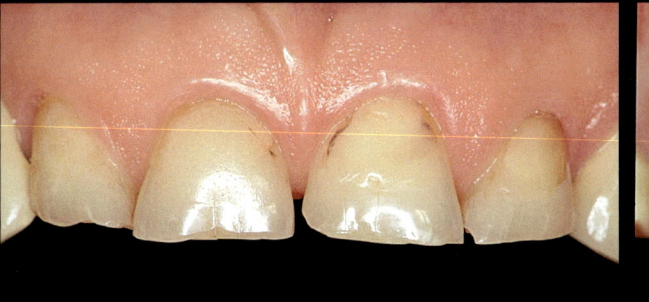

> Fig 3-7a

> Fig 3-7b

> Fig 3-7c

> Fig 3-7d

> Fig 3-7e

> Fig 3-7f

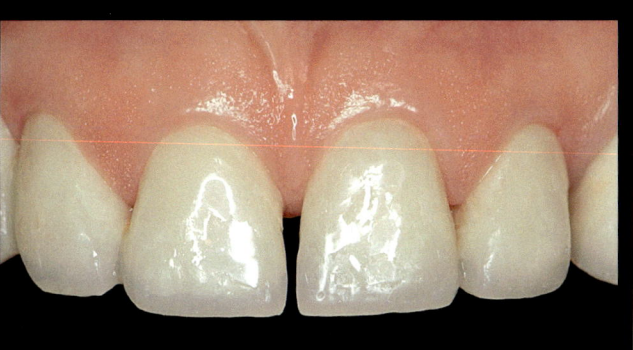

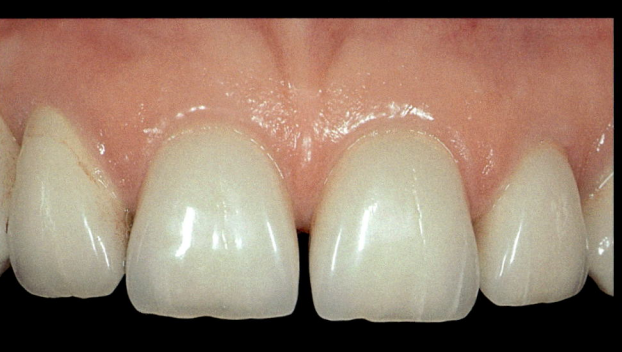

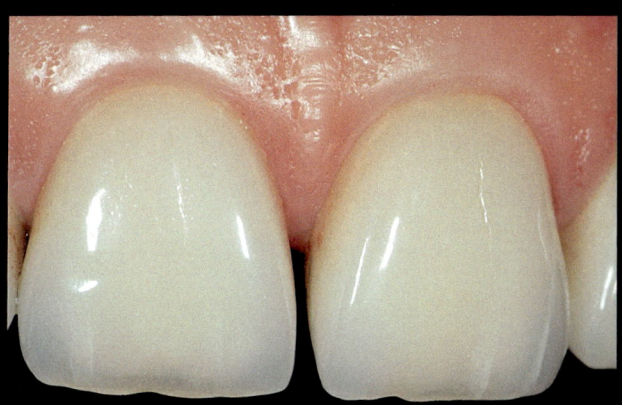

FIG 7 *(a)* The patient, who exhibits a thick periodontal biotype, has significant abrasions of the incisal edges that require complete rehabilitation of the anterosuperior sector. *(b to d)* After the tooth preparations have been carried out and the finish lines positioned in the intrasulcular area, a provisional restoration is inserted that appears to be adequately integrated with the surrounding tissues, even when viewed more closely. *(e and f)* Scrupulous execution of all prosthetic phases guarantees that ideal biologic integration is maintained, even after delivery of the definitive work.

PROVISIONAL RESTORATION

BIOLOGIC INTEGRATION

Placement of provisional restoration **One month later**

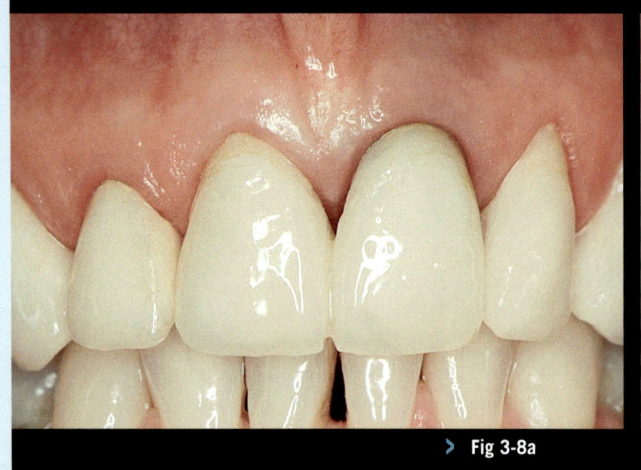

› Fig 3-8a 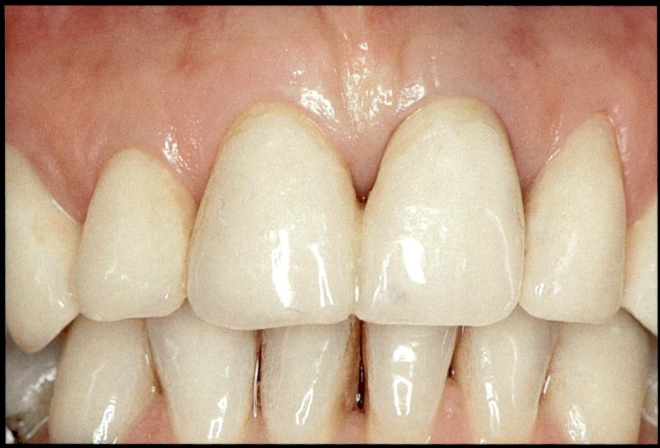 › Fig 3-8b

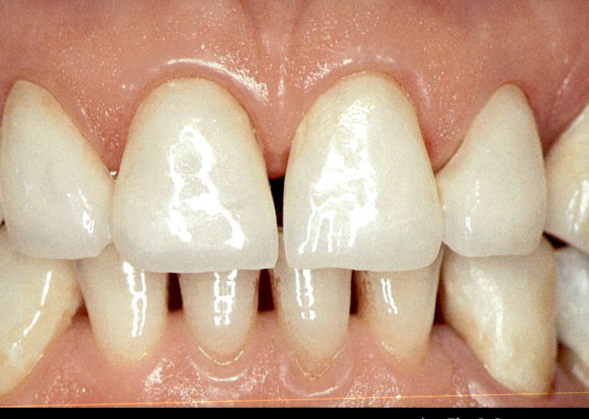

› Fig 3-9a 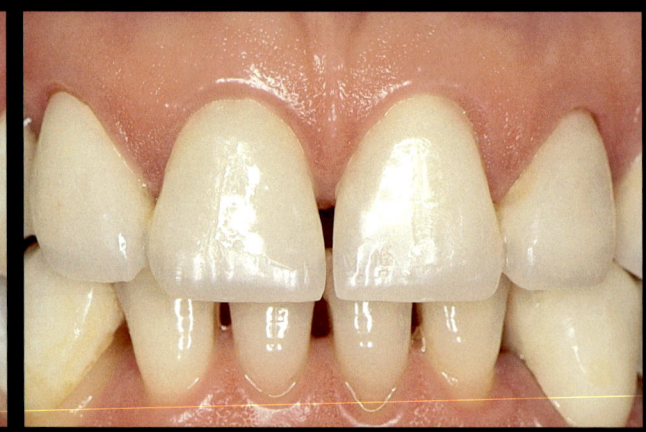 › Fig 3-9b

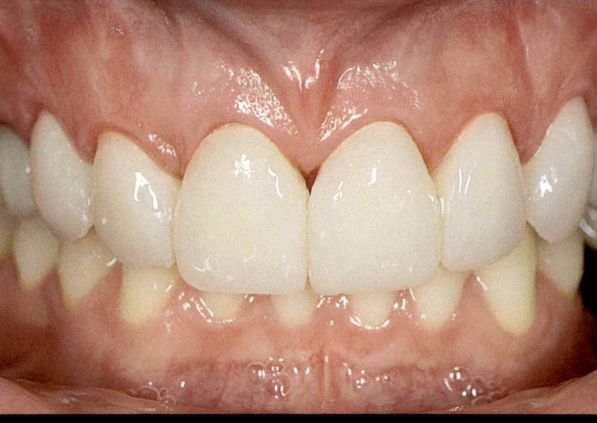

› Fig 3-10a 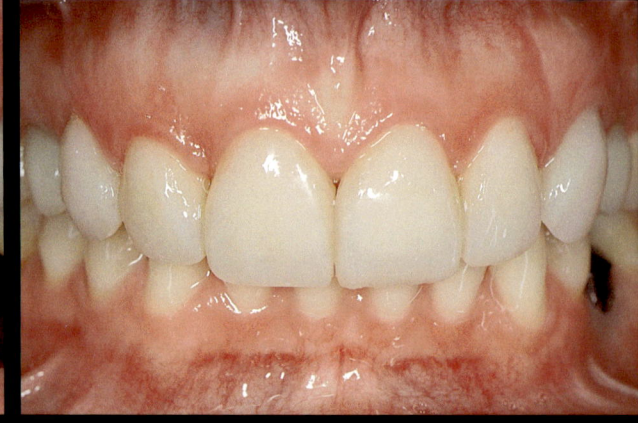 › Fig 3-10b

FIGS 8, 9, 10, 11, 12, 13 *(8a, 9a, 10a, 11a, 12a, 13a)* The operative phases for correct positioning of the provisional restoration can cause slight irritation of the tissues, which is transitory only if a perfect marginal fit and an adequate buccal and interproximal contour are achieved. Of no less importance is the surface smoothness of the provisional restoration, especially in the marginal area, and meticulous removal of all excess cement.

BIOLOGIC INTEGRATION

Placement of provisional restoration

One month later

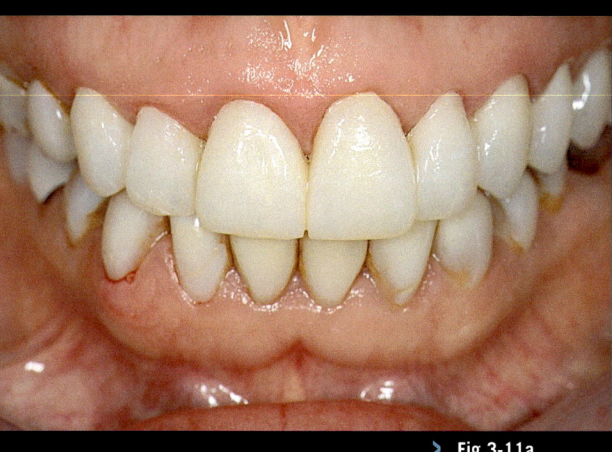

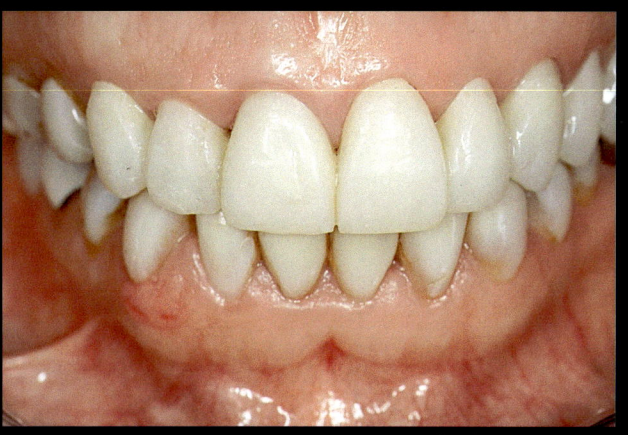

> Fig 3-11a

> Fig 3-11b

> Fig 3-12a

> Fig 3-12b

> Fig 3-13a

> Fig 3-13b

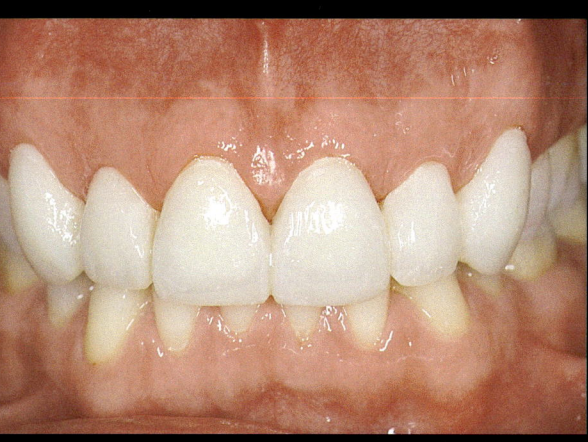

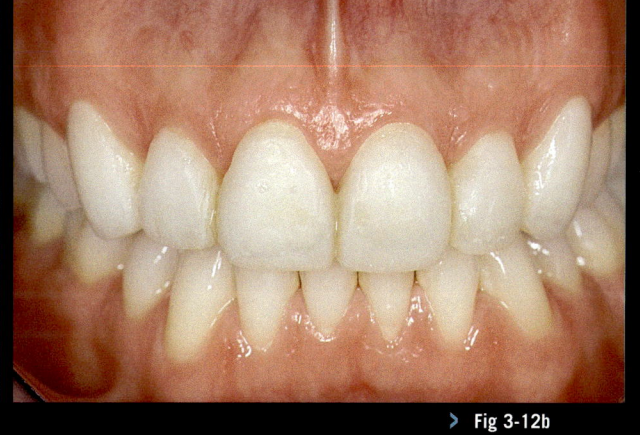

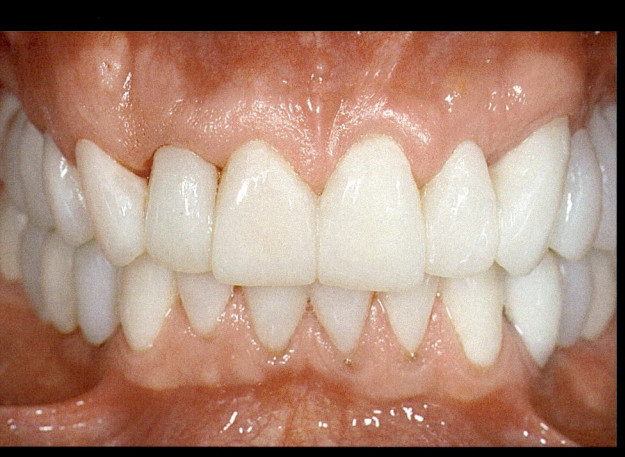

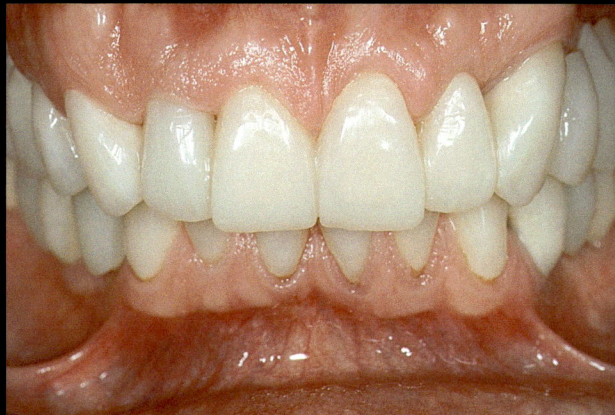

(8b, 9b, 10b, 11b, 12b, 13b) One month after placement, the provisional restorations demonstrate ideal biologic integration, confirming the appropriateness of the prosthetic procedures chosen.

PREPROSTHETIC SURGERY

CLINICAL INDICATIONS

EXPOSURE OF HEALTHY TOOTH STRUCTURE

In finalizing the prosthetic work, surgical treatment may be essential to expose healthy tooth structure.[6,53-55] In some clinical conditions it is impossible to gain adequate visibility and operative access to the gingival margin when dealing with apical lesions (eg, caries lesions or crown-root fractures, root perforations, or root resorptions of the coronal third).

CLINICAL CROWN LENGTHENING

In other cases, preprosthetic surgery is aimed at achieving greater tooth length.[56] Lengthening the clinical crown may be necessary for esthetic reasons (eg, slight asymmetry of the gingival levels) (Fig 3-14) or for biologic purposes, as in the case of removing old restorations with excessive margins extending below the gingival level. Another indication for surgery is the need to guarantee an appropriate ferrule or to improve the retentive capacity of the prosthetic abutments. Having the patient undergo surgical procedures of this nature must, however, be subject to the exclusion of all limiting anatomic factors, such as the following:

- Reduced root length
- Insufficient periodontal support
- Unfavorable crown-root ratio
- Risk of exposing furcations

In the case of combined surgical-prosthetic treatment, positioning of the provisional restoration should precede the surgical phase. The presence of prepared teeth and interdental spaces makes inspection much easier and allows better access during the operative phase.

PREPROSTHETIC SURGERY
INDICATIONS

- Exposure of healthy tooth structure due to:
  - Coronoradicular caries
  - Oblique coronoradicular fractures
  - Radicular perforations (coronal third)
  - External or internal radicular reabsorptions (coronal third)

- Increase in clinical crown length for reasons of:
  - Esthetics: gingival asymmetries
  - Biologic: pre-existing restorations that have violated the connective tissue attachment
  - Retentive: short prosthetic abutments
  - Biomechanical: inadequate ferrule effect
  - Mechanical: limited space in prosthetic connection areas

→ ...from page 187

CASE 3

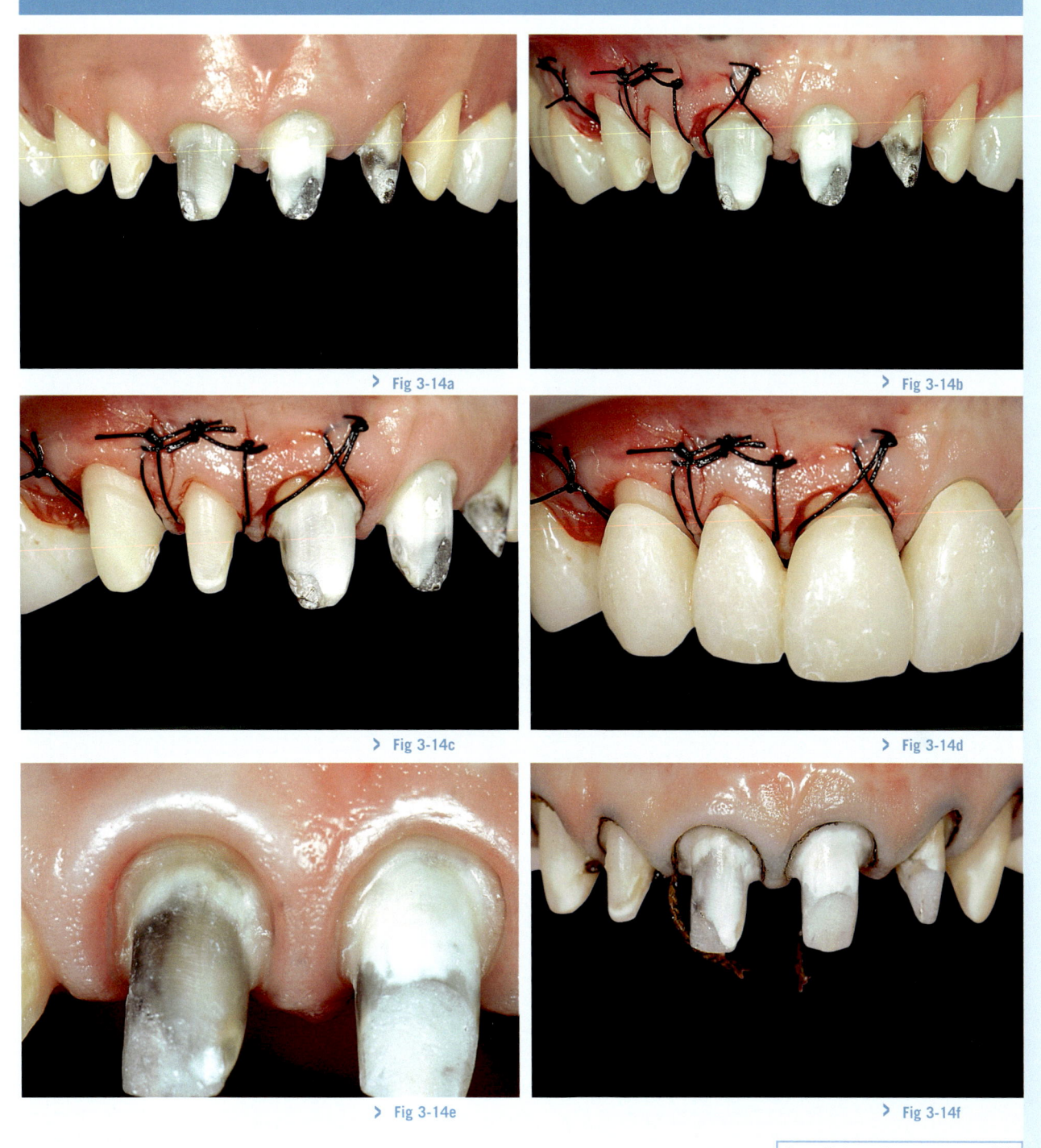

> Fig 3-14a

> Fig 3-14b

> Fig 3-14c

> Fig 3-14d

> Fig 3-14e

> Fig 3-14f

Case 3 → continues on page 377

FIG 14 *(a to c)* The patient has a slight asymmetry of the gingival levels between the right and left sides. This is corrected by means of buccal resective surgery on the right canine and maxillary central incisor combined with a gingivectomy with internal bevel on the right maxillary lateral incisor (periodontal surgery: Dr Roberto Pontoriero). *(d)* Through insertion of the provisional restoration, it is possible to see the amount of clinical crown lengthening achieved in the area where the surgical treatment was undertaken. *(e)* A close-up of the definitive tooth preparations roughly 3 months after they were placed reveals intrasulcular deepening of the finish line. *(f)* After 3 weeks, upon taking the final impressions, the photograph of the abutments with the retraction cords inserted into the sulcus shows the substantial maintenance of tissue apicalization and the harmony of the gingival levels that were achieved surgically.

SURGICAL THERAPY

To expose a sufficient amount of tooth tissue, different surgical procedures are available depending on the treatment objectives and the peculiarities of the clinical case at hand. Caries lesions or fractures located apical to the gingival margin but of limited extension can be treated via subgingival access during minimally invasive surgery. The operative procedure (eg, composite restoration) can be performed at the same time as the surgical phase or immediately afterward to avoid being impaired by the regrowth of tissue in a coronal direction.[56] Even slight asymmetry of the gingival margins deriving from altered passive eruption[57] can sometimes be corrected using minimally invasive surgical techniques, such as gingivectomy with an internal bevel[58] or resective therapy limited to the buccal areas.[58–60] In other cases requiring the exposure of a larger quantity of healthy tooth structure or an increased clinical crown, it is instead necessary to perform resective therapy involving the interproximal areas and apical flap positioning[61–64] (Figs 3-15a to 3-15f). To summarize, depending on the particular needs of the patient, the clinician has a choice of the following surgical options:

- Gingivectomy with internal bevel (with or without removal of the attachment)
- Buccal resective surgery
- Circumferential resective surgery

POSTOPERATIVE MONITORING

This aspect is fundamental in optimizing the results of the surgical therapy.

During the postoperative stage, especially in cases of resective surgery, it is important that the margins and contours of the provisional restoration not be modified to discourage any apicalization of the gingival scallops. The interdental spaces must also be kept unchanged so as not to interfere with the coronal growth of the tissues.

The only modification that is indispensable is confined to the areas where, for example, there are caries lesions. Their removal and the adaptation of the provisional restoration should be completed promptly to "capture" healthy tooth structure before the rise of the soft tissues impedes this procedure. Regular examinations in the office must be scheduled for a length of time that varies from patient to patient depending on the surgical procedure undertaken, to monitor the evolution of the tissue healing and maturation process. The checkups must be scheduled on a weekly basis during the first month, every 2 weeks during the second month, and then, if the surgery undertaken requires a longer maturation time, on a monthly basis.

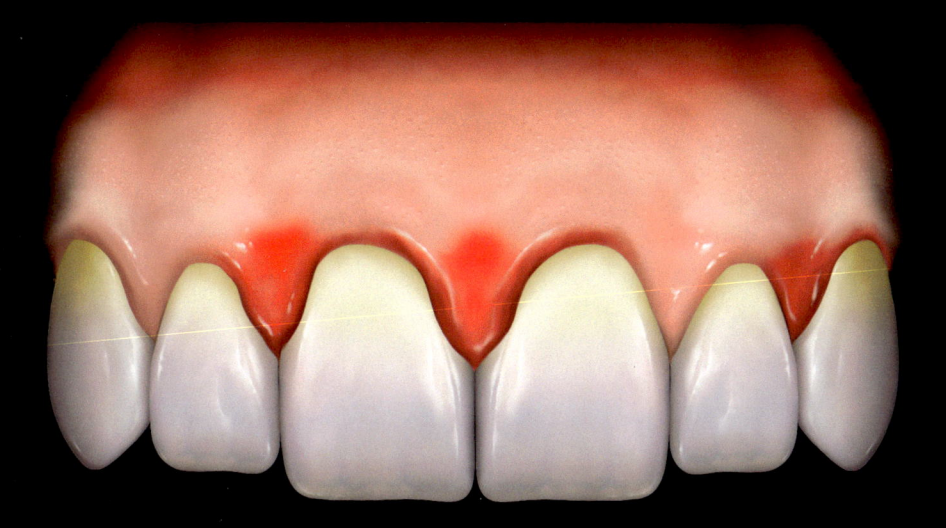

> Fig 3-15a

> Fig 3-15b

> Fig 3-15c

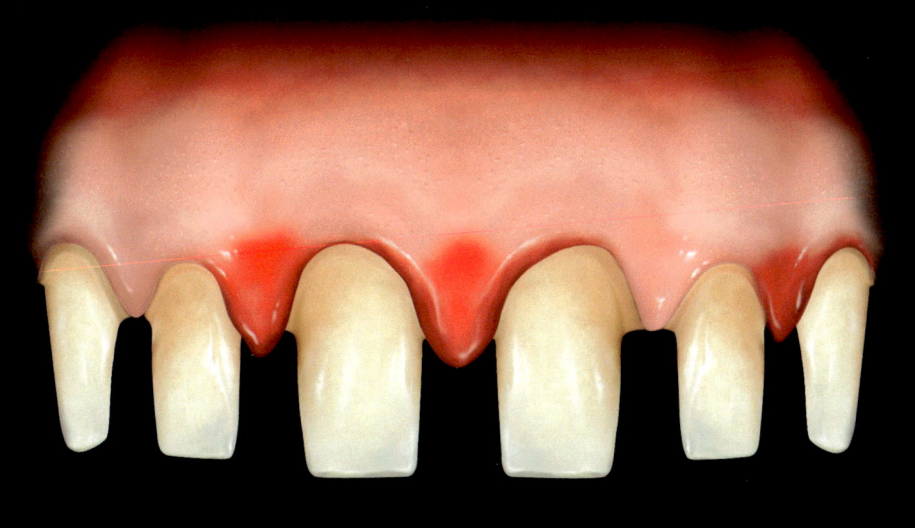

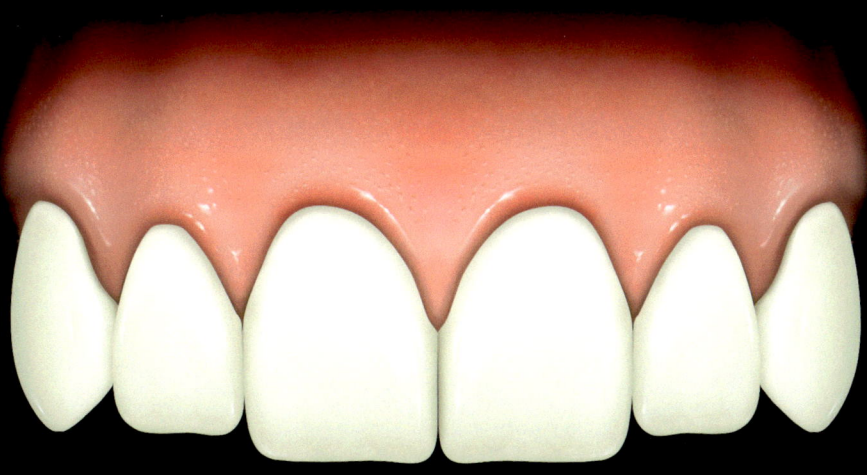

FIG 15 *(a and b)* The examples in the photographs show a considerable inflammatory response in tissues around restorations that have inadequate marginal closure and contours, easily seen with the prosthetic restorations removed. *(c)* Positioning correctly remargined provisional restorations allows satisfactory gingival health to be restored.

The patient, duly informed and made responsible, should ensure maximum compliance regarding the scrupulous daily oral hygiene procedures and observation of the checkup program to be followed in the office. Given the new topography of the gingival levels, the patient must be given specific instructions on how to remove plaque efficiently.

AVERAGE TISSUE MATURATION TIMES

The period needed to achieve tissue healing and maturation, with complete regrowth in the coronal direction, varies according to the type of surgery performed (see volume 1, chapter 6, pages 252–256). In cases where a gingivectomy with internal bevel has been undertaken to correct slight asymmetries of the gingival architecture, a waiting period of 6 weeks will normally suffice, although this period should be increased if the gingival attachment has also been removed. If resective osseous therapy limited to the buccal areas has been performed, a longer monitoring period (> 3 months) is necessary. Finally, if the patient has undergone circumferential resection therapy with an apically positioned flap, the waiting and monitoring time for gingival maturation extends to approximately 6 to 12 months.[56,65-69] Only at the end of this period can regrowth of the tissues in the coronal direction be considered complete.

AVERAGE TISSUE MATURATION TIMES

- Gingivectomy with internal bevel with or without attachment resection → 6–10 weeks
- Buccal resective surgery → > 3 months*
- Resective surgery → > 6 months*

*Monitor the patient and consider individual variability

FIG 15 *(d)* Proper positioning of the provisional restoration has led to an improvement in tissue health, which is a necessary prerequisite for proceeding with the surgical phases. However, when the flap is raised, it is apparent that the pre-existing subgingival collocation of the margin has not allowed the prosthetic margin to be ideally captured. With the flap elevated, minor defects in the periodontal support also are noticeable, with a slight difference in level in the osseous architecture. *(e and f)* After these irregularities have been corrected using a football-shaped bur and suitable surgical instruments to optimize the osseous levels underneath, the flap is positioned apically and sutured at the alveolar ridge level, and care is taken to keep the interproximal areas exposed. Note the large distance between the preparation margin and the new gingival levels achieved following surgery and how the provisional restoration appears correctly contoured following remargining.

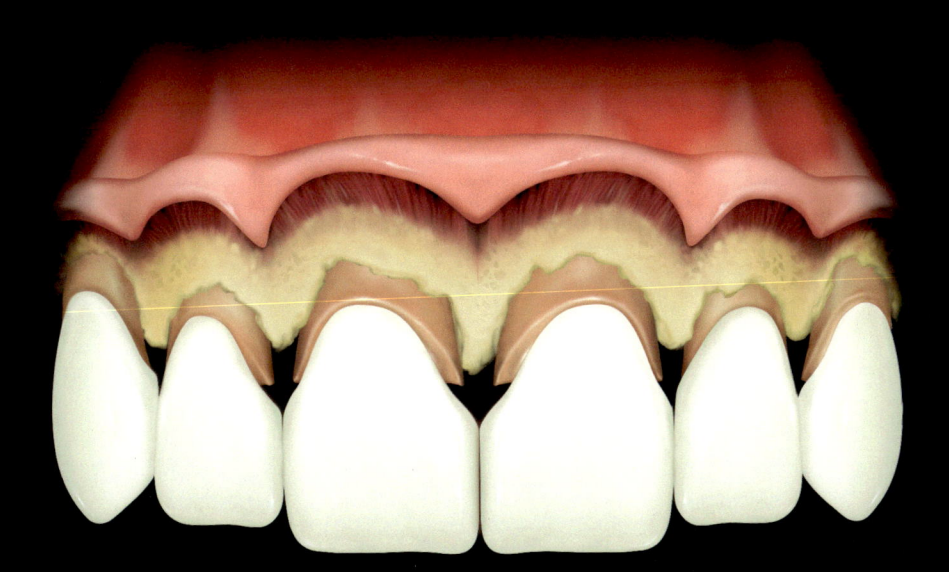

Fig 3-15d

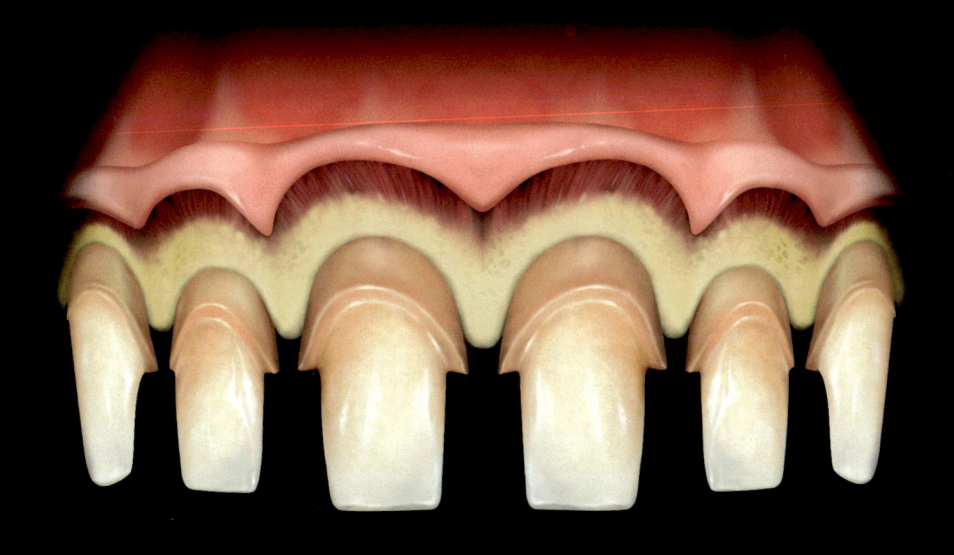

Fig 3-15e

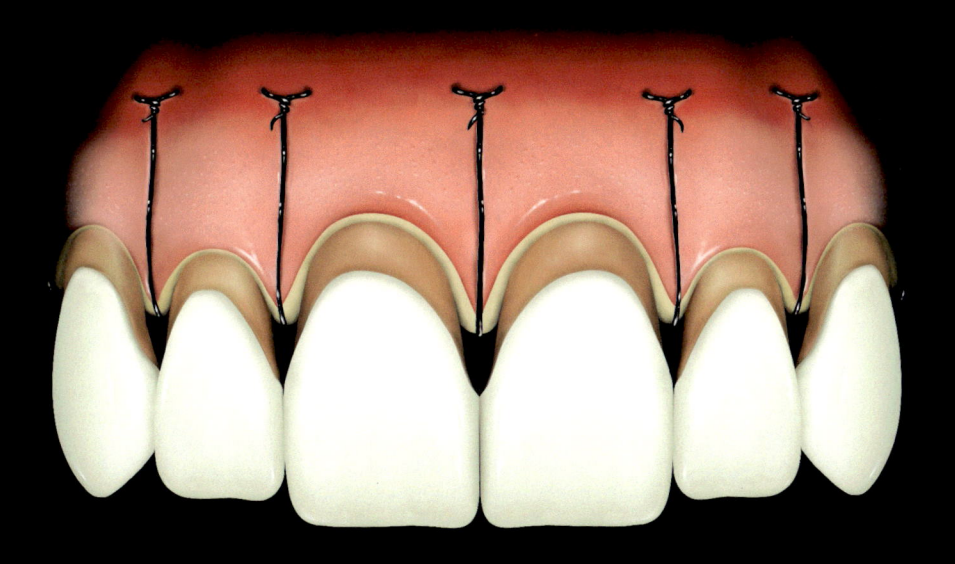

Fig 3-15f

TISSUE REGROWTH VARIABLES

The time ranges stated above obviously refer to average values. Consideration must also be given to variables dependent on the periodontal biotype as well as specific individual variations (Figs 3-15g to 3-15i).

The patient's *periodontal biotype* can play an important role in the amount of tissue regrowth in the coronal direction. Individuals with a thick tissue biotype often show a significantly greater coronal regrowth over a longer period compared with those with a thin tissue biotype.[56]

For the clinician, the biotype is an important factor to take into account before deciding whether to proceed with the tooth preparations, final impressions, and relining of the provisional restoration.

The *individual variations* involve a different rate of tissue regrowth from patient to patient, regardless of periodontal biotype. This individual variability, unlike that associated with periodontal biotype, is impossible to predict. For this reason it is advisable to monitor the patient very carefully during the maturation stages, especially in the interproximal areas, where the coronal growth is greater and takes longer.[69,70]

Standardized parameters have been proposed based on a measurement of the distance between the osseous crest and the interdental point of contact; this should allow a prediction for definitive maturation of the interdental papilla.[71] However, as already stated, the periodontal biotype, the individual variations, the distance between the roots and their more or less conical shape inevitably account for some differences in the coronal regrowth of the tissues. It is therefore preferable to follow each patient clinically to assess the individual level of tissue regrowth, identify definitive maturation accurately, and then proceed with the definitive preparations and relining of the provisional restoration. Observation of the behavior of each patient over time will avoid incorrect predictions. It is important, therefore, to avoid proceeding prematurely with the final stages of completely closing the interdental spaces, which could cause periodontal problems when the restorative contours interfere with the tissues while they are still in the growth phase, as well as the obvious related esthetic repercussions.

Even after observing the maturation times recommended above and considering the tissue regrowth yet to be completed, it is still preferable to leave a space at the interproximal level. It is frequently found that the tissues tend to grow further in the coronal direction even a short time after delivery, remodeling themselves around the restorations and therefore also closing the small remaining black triangles.

FIG 15 *(g)* Ten days after surgery, a slight crestal resorption is evidenced by the thin pinkish margin that surrounds the teeth involved in the treatment at the cervical level. *(h and i)* After roughly 1 month, the tissues show a regrowth in the coronal direction that appears more pronounced 6 months after surgery.

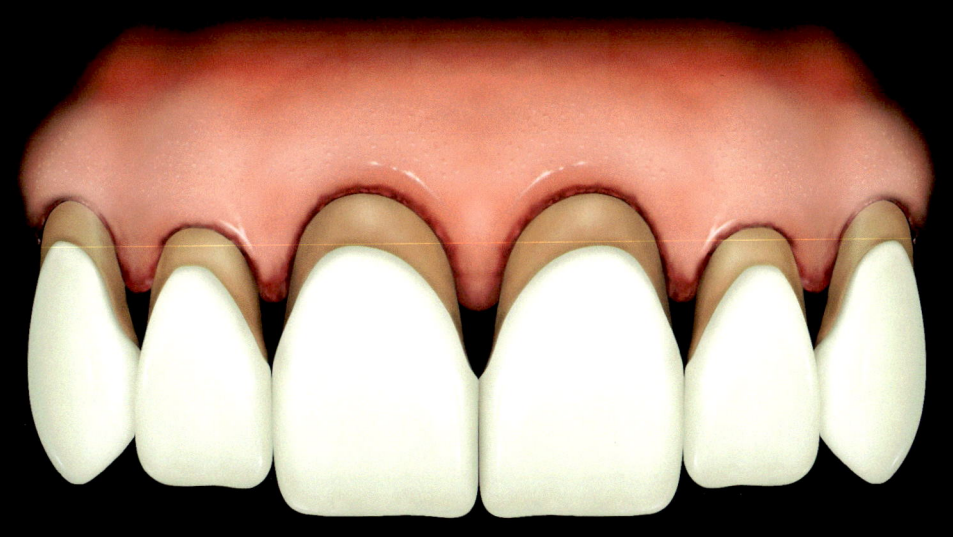

Fig 3-15g

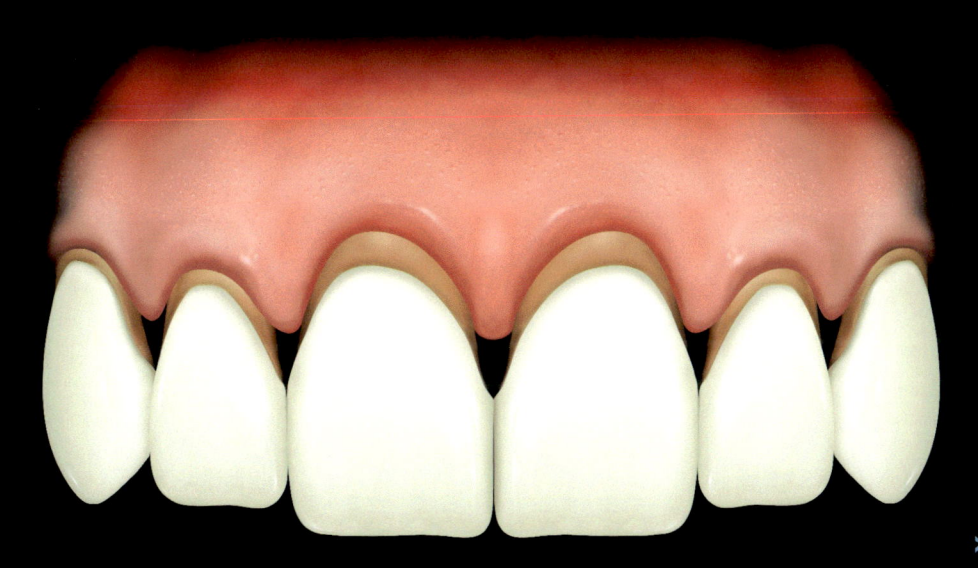

Fig 3-15h

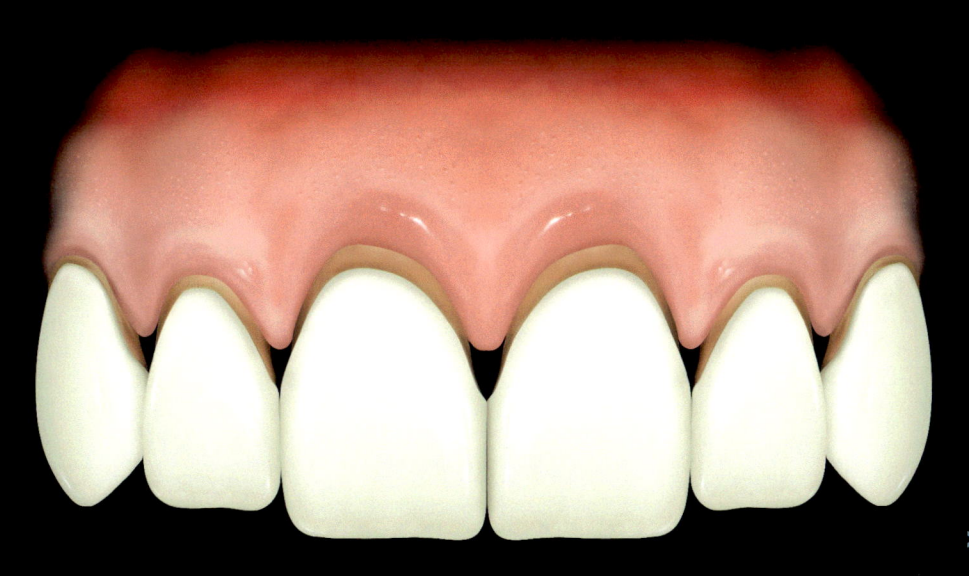

Fig 3-15i

INDICATORS OF TISSUE MATURATION

There are some reference parameters that may provide indications as to the level of tissue maturation. These include:

- Reappearance of typical pink coloring
- Return of surface stippling (in patients/sites where it was previously present)
- Reformation of a well-defined gingival sulcus, detectable on probing
- Stability of the gingival margin

Confirmation that tissue stability has been achieved can be obtained by measuring the distance of previously selected dentogingival reference points over time. Noting the values on the clinical record makes it possible to compare them until they are observed to be stable and constant over time.

This process allows the clinician to identify the moment when final tissue maturation is complete, indicating that it is possible to proceed with the definitive tooth preparations and relining of the provisional restoration (Figs 3-15i to 3-15m).

RELINING AND PROSTHETIC FINALIZATION

Posterior sectors In these areas the patient is less sensitive to esthetic problems because the restorations are less visible. While it is always advisable to observe complete tissue maturation, in these areas it may be possible to reduce the times and move the final restorative stages up in the treatment schedule. A waiting time of 3 to 4 months should be sufficient to achieve soft tissue healing even if they are not completely mature, allowing the clinician to proceed with the prosthetic finalization. In these cases it is necessary to end the margin either at the gingival level or at the supragingival level, leaving interproximal spaces that are large enough to allow for further regrowth of the interdental papillae. Their size should be such as to avoid a buildup of residual food. Because of the rather flat outline of the cementoenamel junction (CEJ) in the posterior sites, the growth of the tissues should prove to be quite limited. To clean the interproximal areas, the use of interdental brushes, decreasing in size over time, is advised to adapt to progressive tissue maturation.

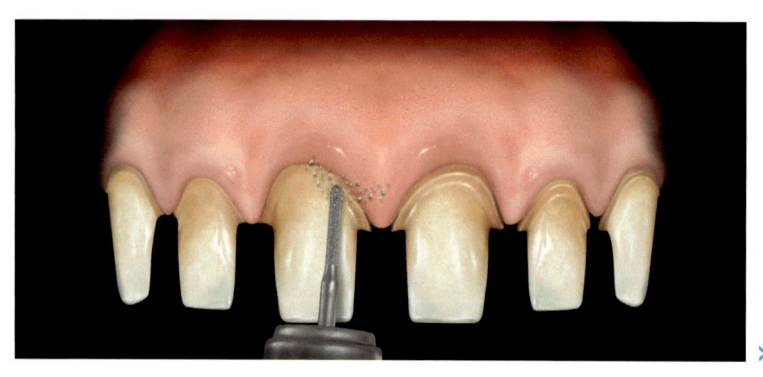

> Fig 3-15j

FIG 15 (j and k) Once the gingival tissues have matured (6 to 12 months), the abutments are prepared to the new gingival level. (l and m) Subsequently, the provisional restorations are relined, and care is taken to leave small spaces in the interproximal areas to allow for any further maturation and adaptation of the tissues in these specific areas over time.

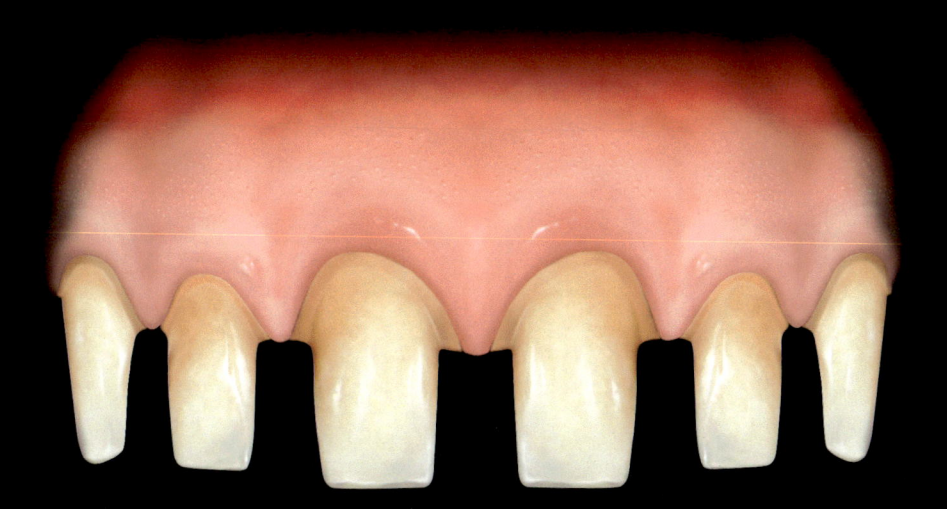

> Fig 3-15k

> Fig 3-15l

> Fig 3-15m

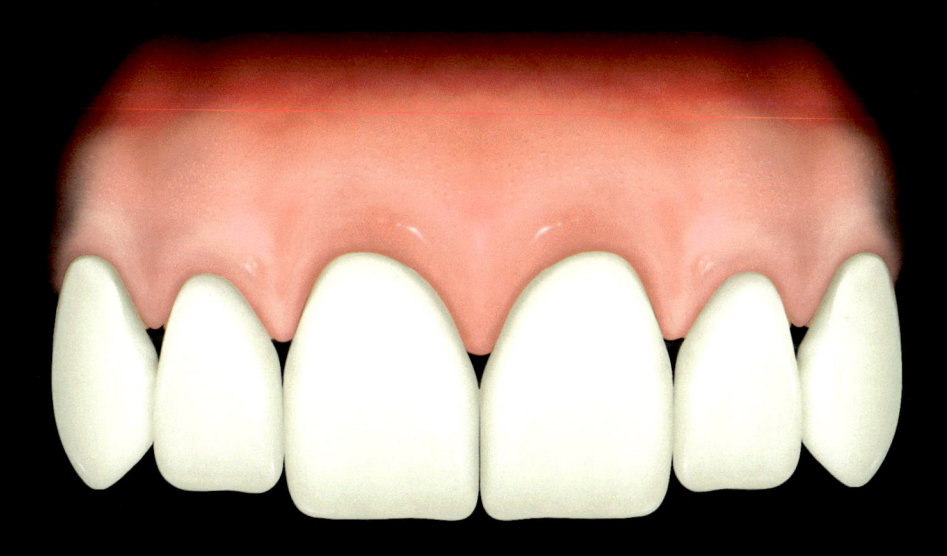

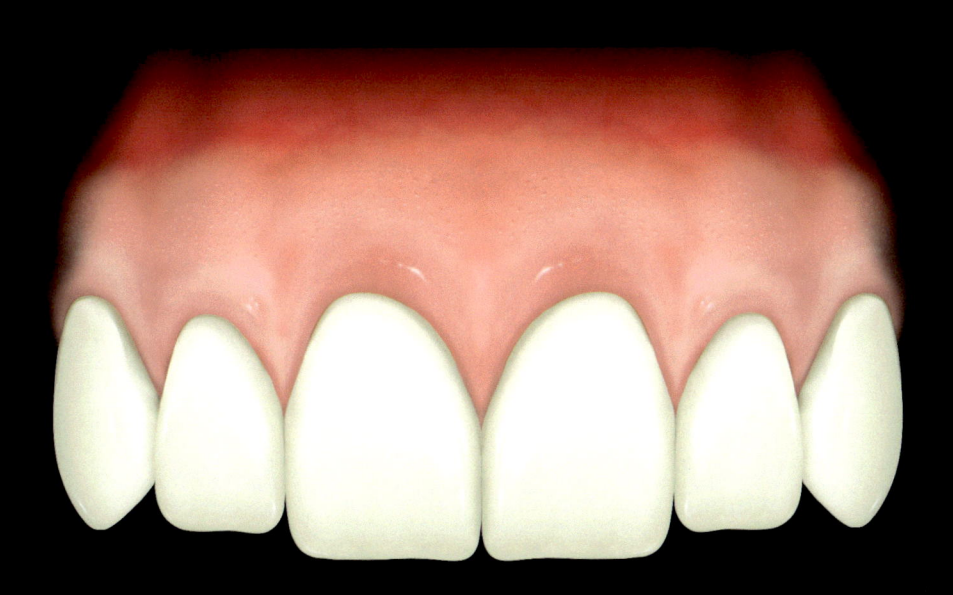

Anterior sector In this area, if esthetic appearance is a priority, it is obligatory to wait until tissue stability has been reached for two fundamental reasons:
- To conceal the prosthetic margins in the intrasulcular site
- To accurately close the gaps between the teeth

Maturation must be monitored very closely. During the healing stage the provisional restorations need to be kept at a distance from the gingival margins, and the interdental black triangles found during this initial period should be kept open so as not to interfere with growth of the tissues. Consequently, especially where a high smile line exists, the patient may complain of esthetic and phonetic problems. Although previously informed of the absolute necessity to observe the rather lengthy waiting times before starting the final stage of the prosthetic therapy, patients may insist on a solution to guarantee greater comfort. The clinician must resist the temptation to apicalize the preparations, remargin the provisional restoration, and close the interdental spaces too early, to avoid the risk of finding, at the end of the tissue regrowth process, excessively subgingival margins with the papillae forced into interdental spaces that are too narrow. The patient should be previously notified that, just 2 weeks after removing the second periodontal pack, a sizeable reduction in the spaces can be seen. Indeed, 1 month after surgery, the coronal regrowth of the tissues will already have developed to 40% buccolingually and to 60% interdentally compared with the final position of the gingival margin.[56]

Considering the average tissue maturation times following resective surgery in the anterior sectors, it is necessary to wait a minimum of 6 to 9 months before finalizing the prosthetic work. Once tissue stability has been ascertained through application of the dentogingival reference points described earlier, the clinician may proceed with definitive preparation of the abutments and relining of the provisional restorations. Reduced spaces retained at the interproximal level are useful for accommodating the gingival tissues as they physiologically adapt to the new coronal contours. The final impressions are delayed by 3 to 4 weeks to test the biologic integration of the restorations. These spaces, although minimized, must also be maintained when the definitive restorations are delivered, to allow for the possibility that the tissues will further adapt as time goes on (Figs 3-16 and 3-17).

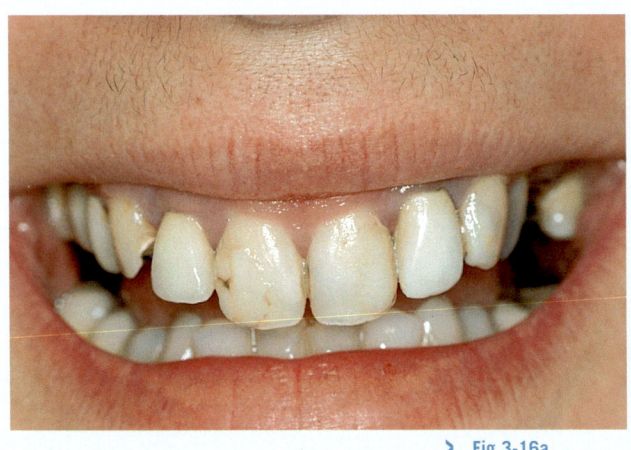

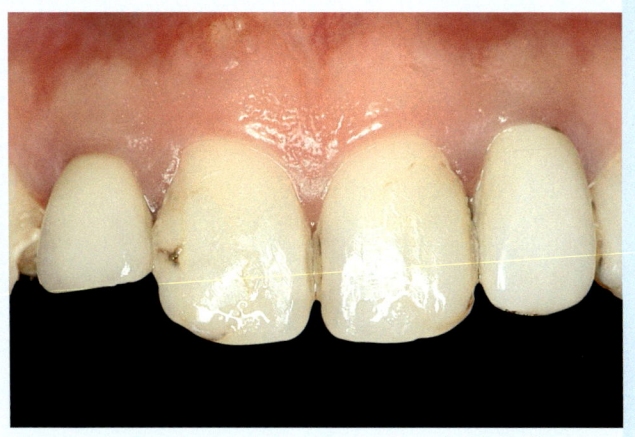

> Fig 3-16a

> Fig 3-16b

> Fig 3-16c

> Fig 3-16d

> Fig 3-16e

> Fig 3-16f

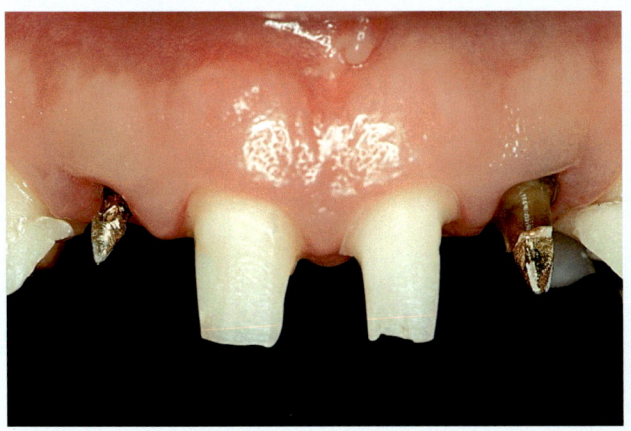

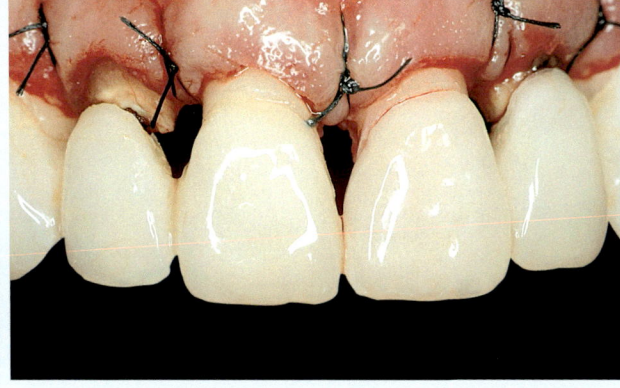

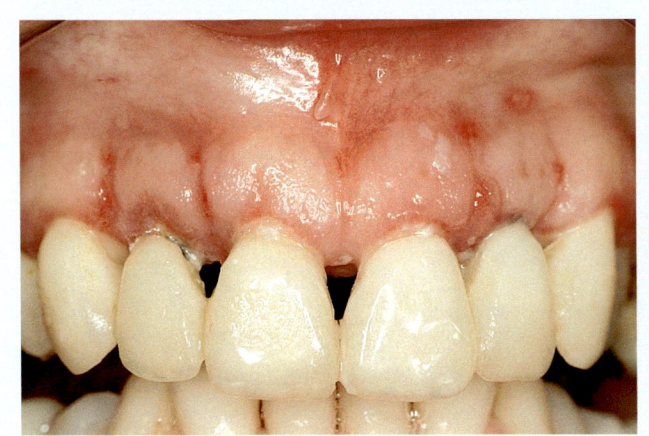

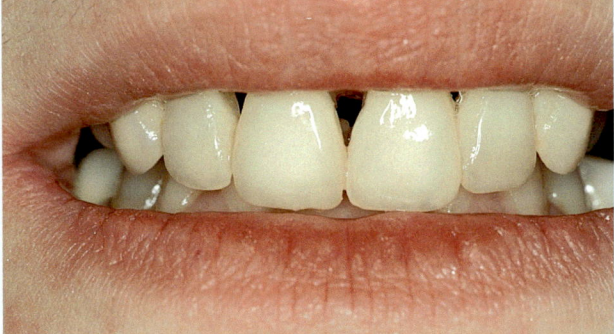

FIG 16 *(a and b)* The patient, who has a high smile line, needs rehabilitation of the anterior sector because of existing incongruous coronal restorations on the maxillary lateral incisors and the presence of microleakage around the composite reconstructions on the maxillary central incisors and canines. *(c)* Once the crowns on the lateral incisors are removed, the impossibility of detecting the prosthetic margin is revealed. *(d)* Resective surgery is carried out with apical repositioning of the flap. (Periodontal surgery by Dr Stefano Parma Benfenati.) By means of this procedure, the gingival margins of the right maxillary side are realigned, and an adequate portion of healthy dentin is exposed. *(e)* At 10 days postsurgery, the periodontal pack and the sutures are both removed. *(f)* The provisional restorations leave wide interdental spaces that undoubtedly constitute an esthetic limitation. However, they could not be modified to allow for tissue regrowth. The patient's discomfort will diminish significantly within the first month, when tissue regrowth takes place.

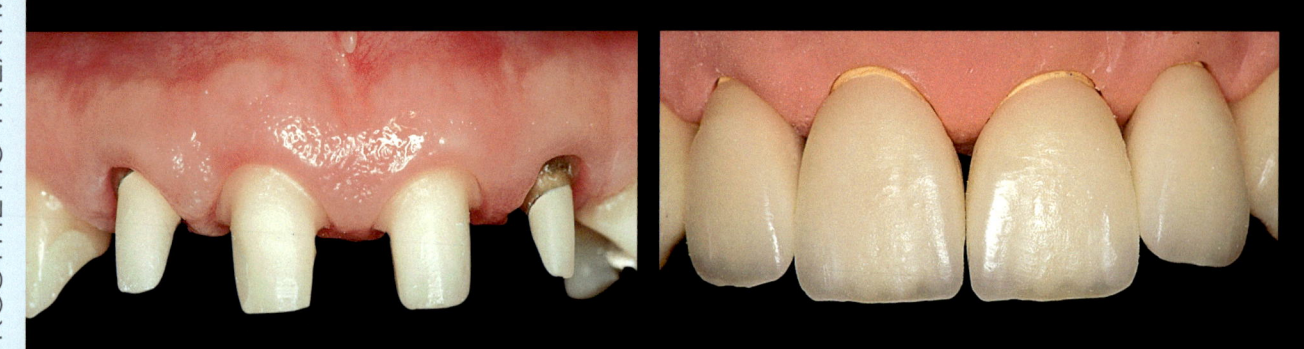

> Fig 3-16g

> Fig 3-16h

3 months

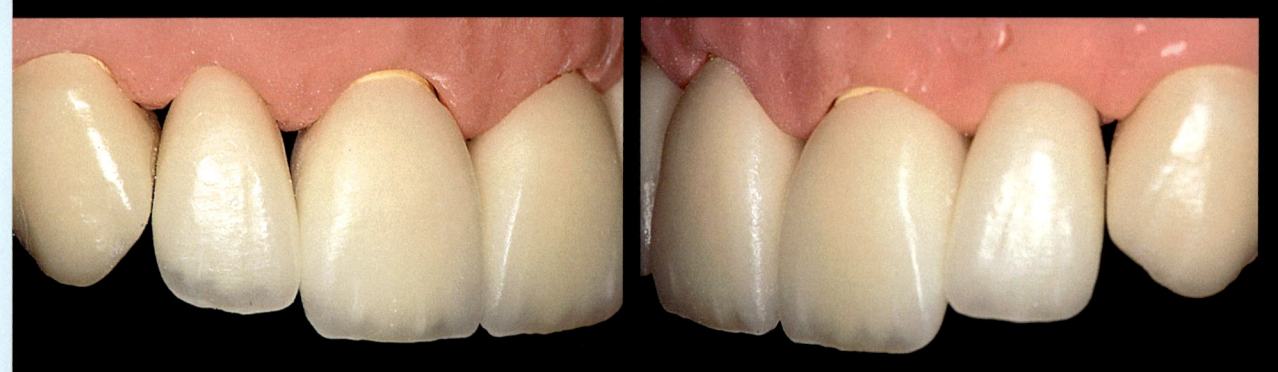

> Fig 3-16i

> Fig 3-16j

4 months

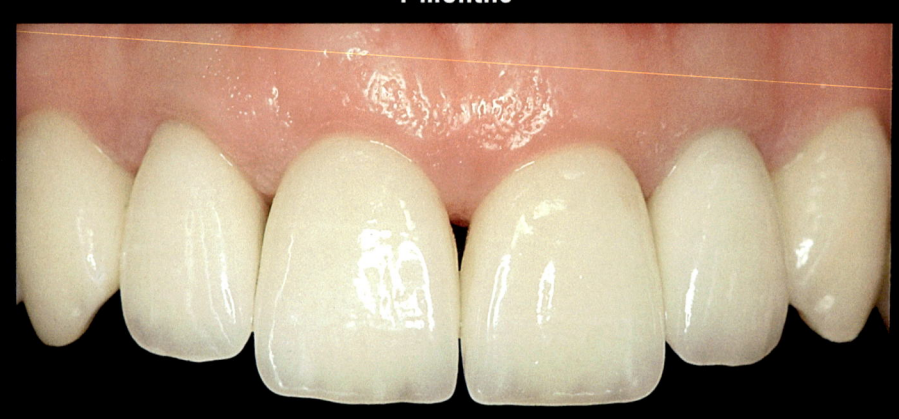

> Fig 3-16k

FIG 16 *(g)* Three months after surgery, the patient had to be absent for a long period. This made it necessary to contract the treatment times by moving up the appointments for the preparations and the final impressions. *(h to j)* Assuming that tissue maturation was not yet complete, specific instructions were given to the technician to maintain the spaces between the anterior teeth so that the tissues could adapt to the anticipated regrowth at the interproximal level. *(k)* The presence of unesthetic interdental spaces in the definitive restorations may initially be met with confusion regarding the esthetic result achieved. *(l)* In a close-up view of the smile, the interdental spaces are particularly evident. *(m)* After 1 year, however, as a demonstration of the successful maturation process, the space between the central incisors has reduced considerably, with significant improvement in the overall esthetic appearance. *(n)* The adaptation of the tissues to the prosthetic restorations is ideal 3 years after delivery of the restorations, fully justifying a clinical choice that was apparently questionable at the beginning of treatment.

4 months

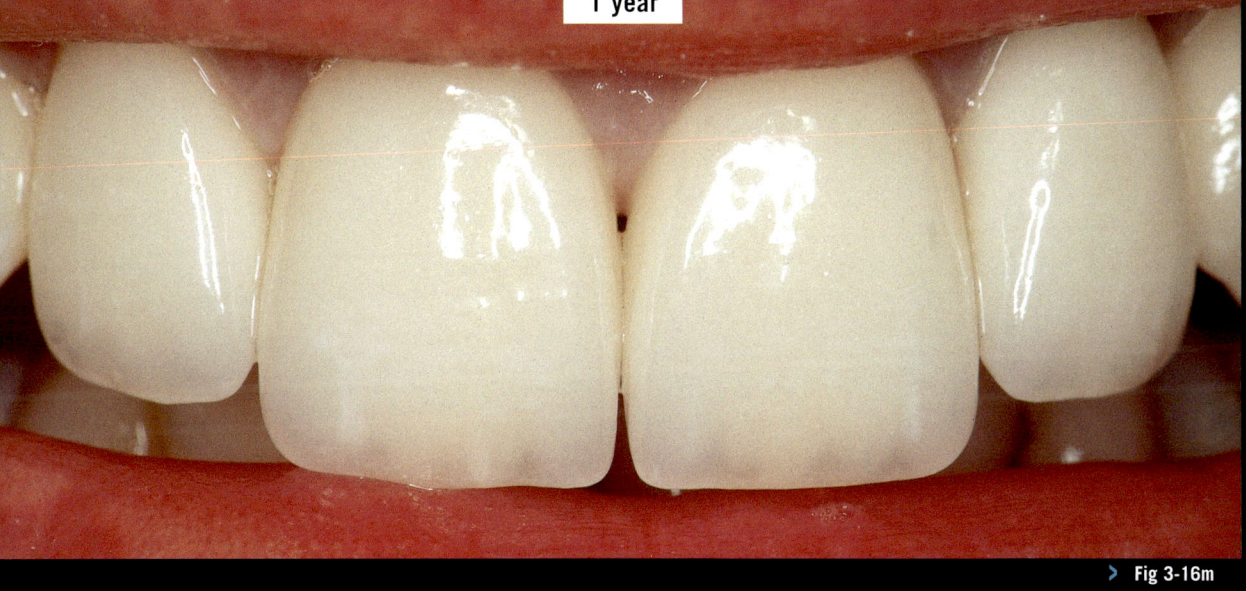

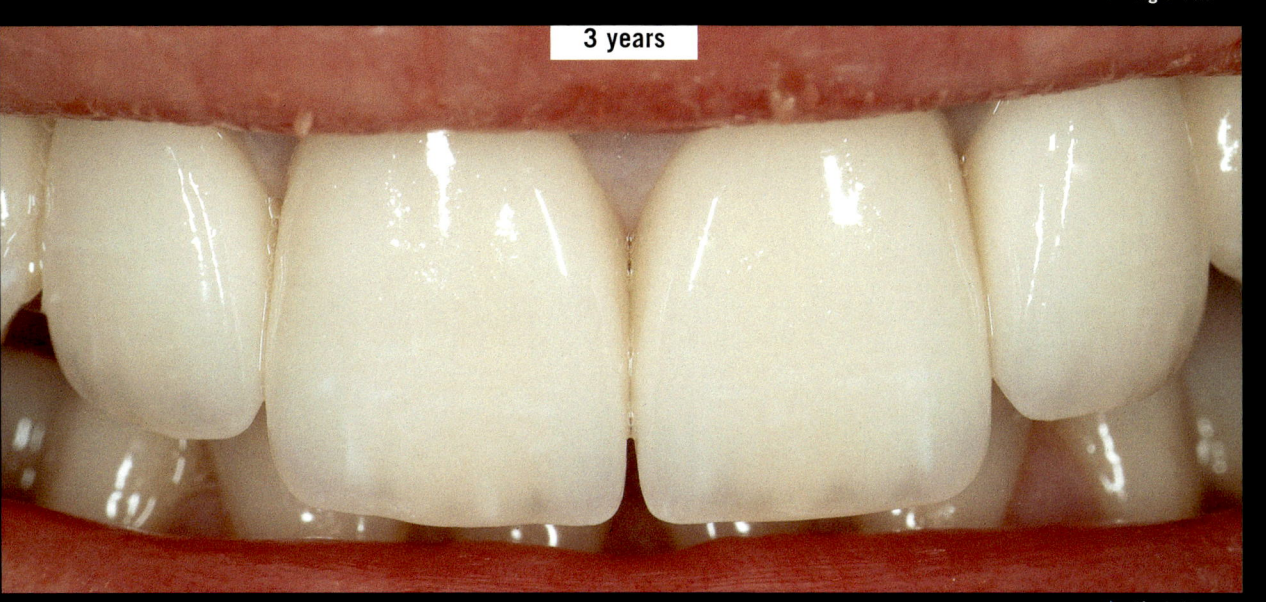

> Fig 3-16l

1 year

> Fig 3-16m

3 years

> Fig 3-16n

> Fig 3-17a

> Fig 3-17b

> Fig 3-17c

> Fig 3-17d

> Fig 3-17e

> Fig 3-17f

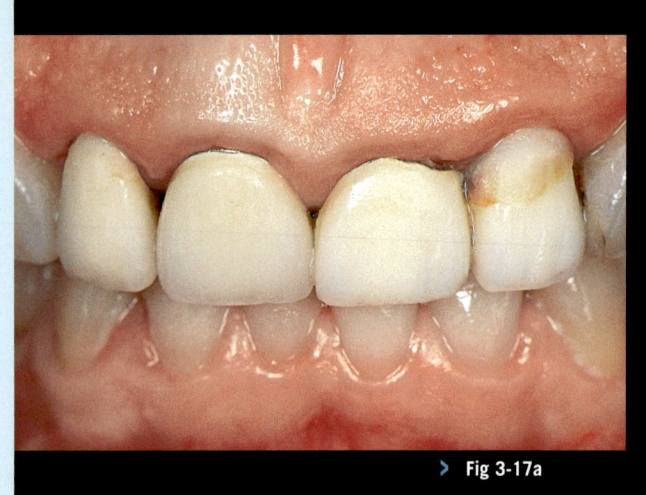

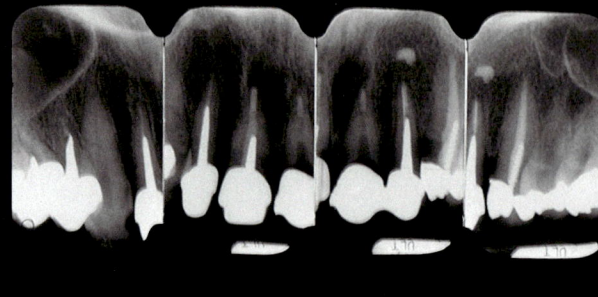

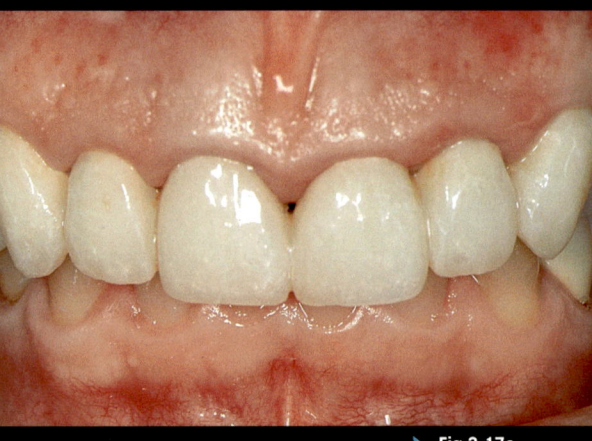

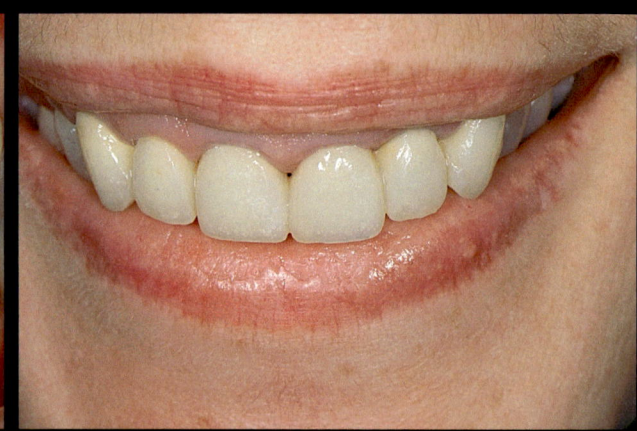

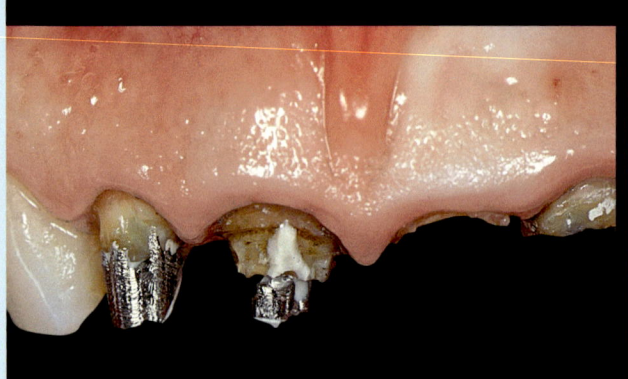

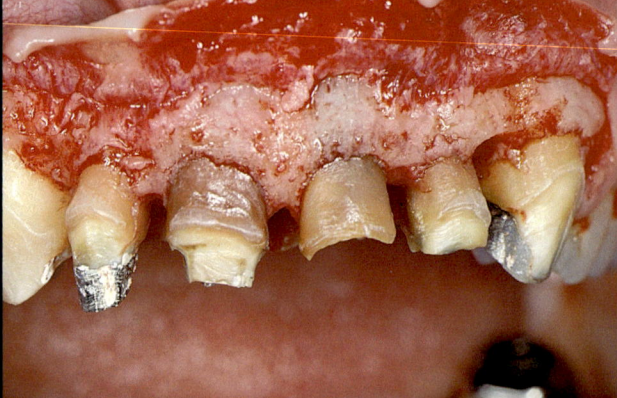

FIG 17 *(a and b)* The patient needs prosthetic treatment of the maxillary teeth between the right second premolar and the left second premolar. *(c to f)* Once the old restorations are removed, the provisional restorations are placed prior to lengthening of the clinical crown, which is essential because of the need to expose healthy tooth tissue. (Periodontal surgery by Dr Roberto Pontoriero.) After surgery, the significant distance between the new gingival levels and the provisional margins, previously in contact with the soft tissues, is evident. *(g to j)* Photographs of the anterosuperior sextant at the time of surgery, after 1 month, 3 months, and 10 months show progressive tissue regrowth, easily referenced by the provisional restoration, which has remained unchanged over time. It is possible to see not only the considerable tissue growth in the coronal direction, but also the progressive closing of the interdental spaces (black triangles).

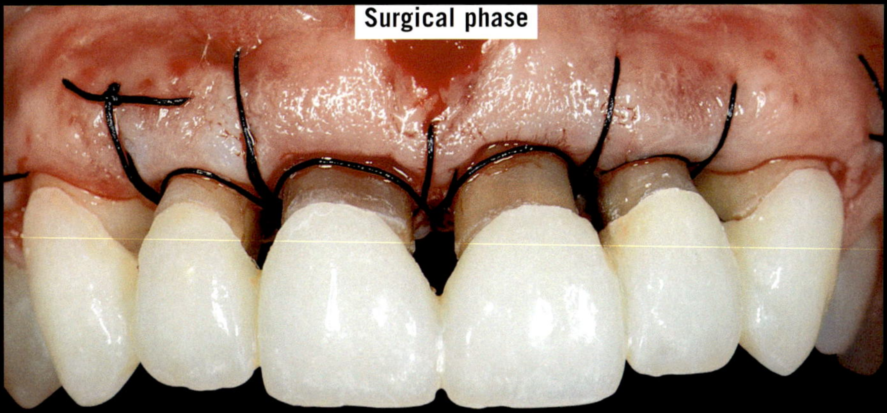

Fig 3-17g — Surgical phase

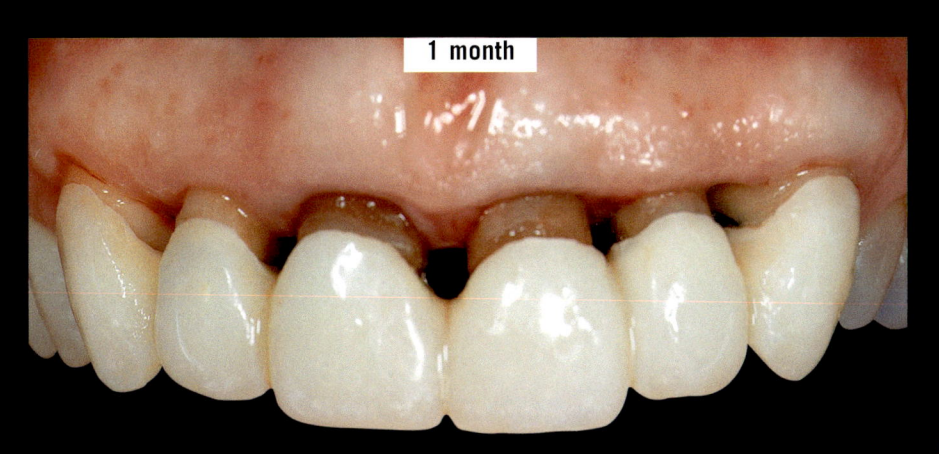

Fig 3-17h — 1 month

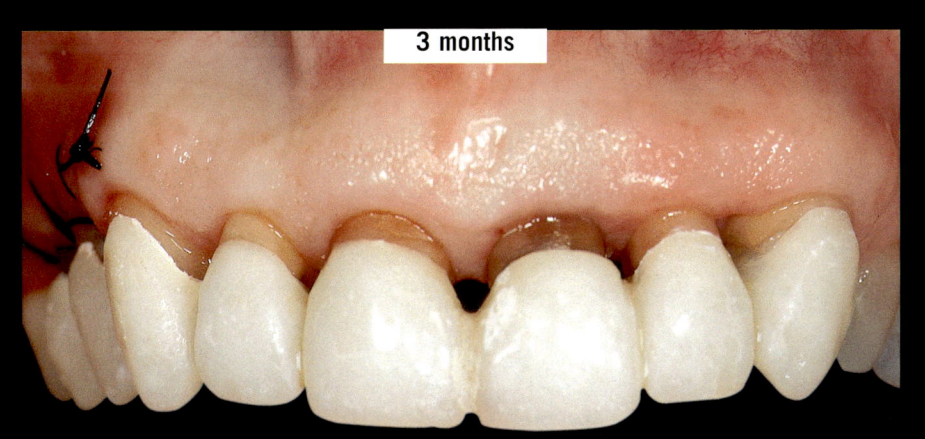

Fig 3-17i — 3 months

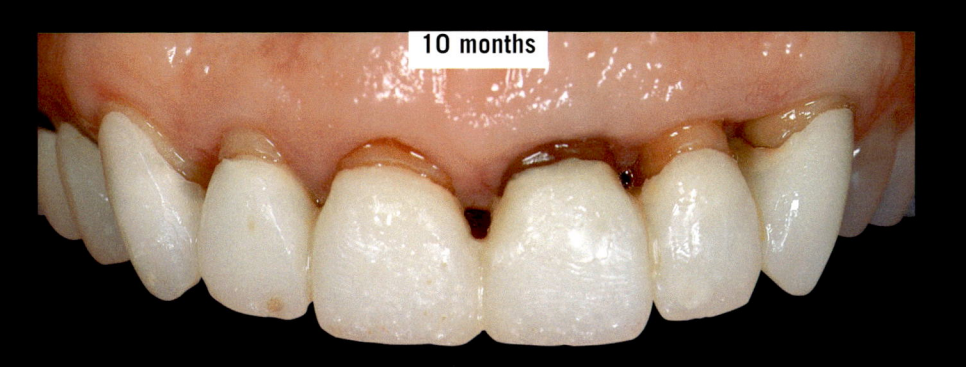

Fig 3-17j — 10 months

> Fig 3-17k

> Fig 3-17l

> Fig 3-17m

> Fig 3-17n

> Fig 3-17o

> Fig 3-17p

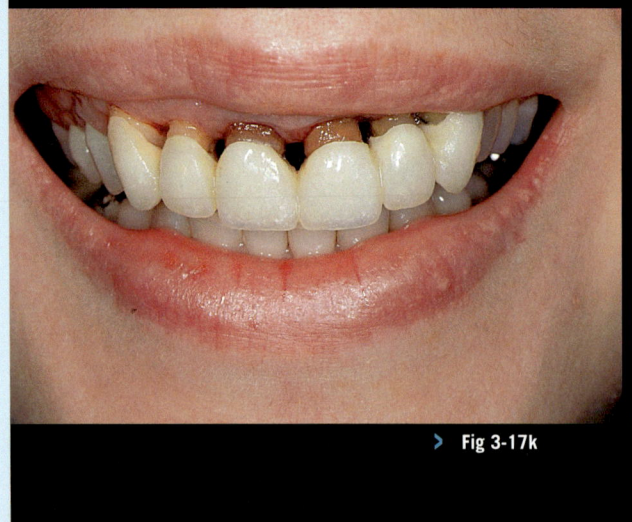

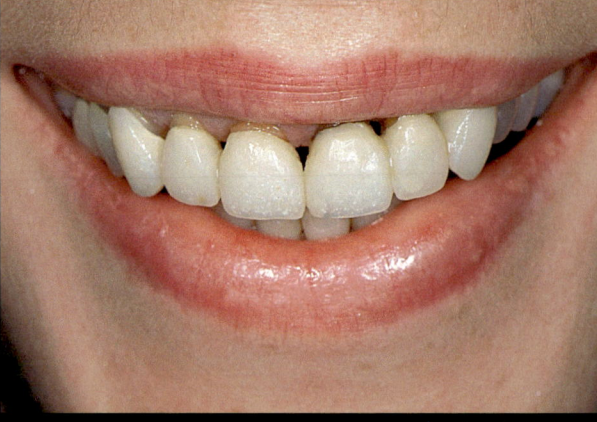

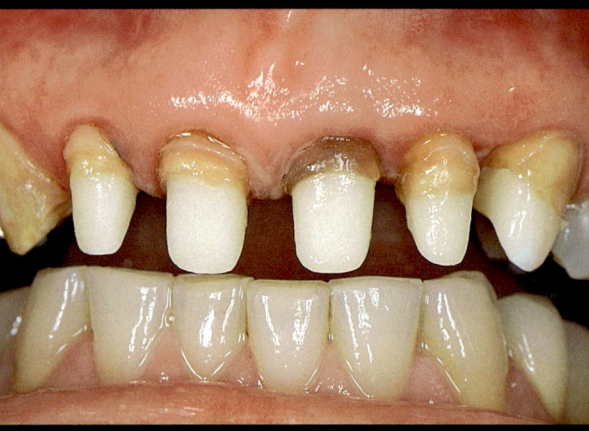

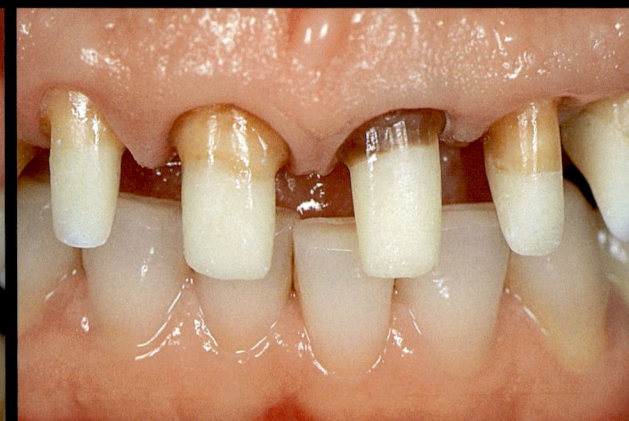

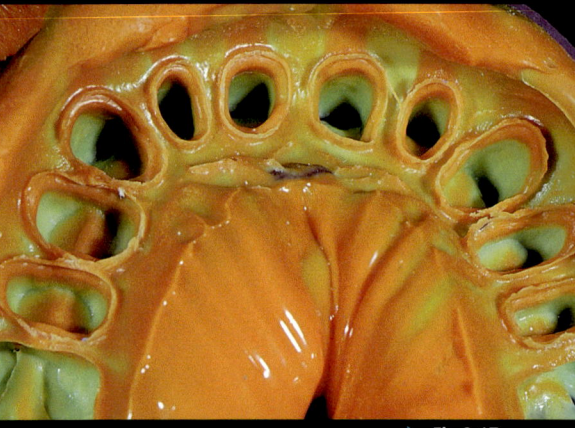

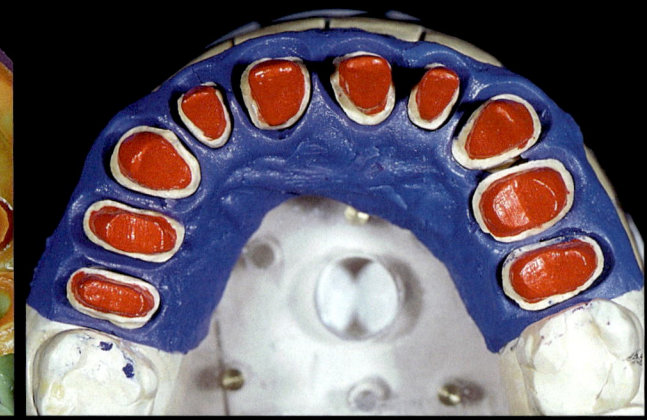

FIG 17 *(k and l)* The postoperative maturation and considerable tissue regrowth in the coronal direction are clearly revealed via comparison of the views of the patient's smile at 1 month and 10 months postoperatively. *(m and n)* Based on the assumption that tissue maturation is complete, the provisional restorations are removed and the abutments definitively prepared. *(o to q)* Once the final impressions are taken and the master cast made, the work is finalized by construction of 10 single all-ceramic restorations. *(r to t)* Although 1 year had passed since surgery at the time the definitive crowns were delivered, it was nevertheless preferred to maintain small interdental spaces, which are completely closed in the photograph taken 1 year after cementation (2 years after surgery), thanks to further maturation and adaptation of the gingival tissues.

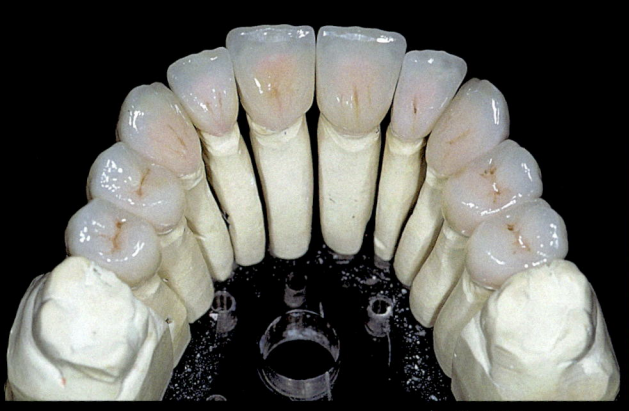

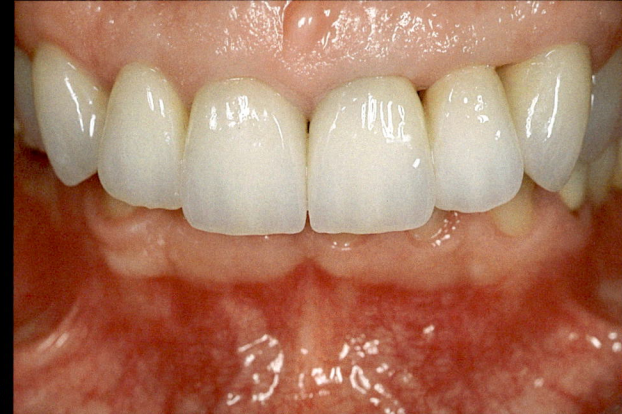

> Fig 3-17q

> Fig 3-17r

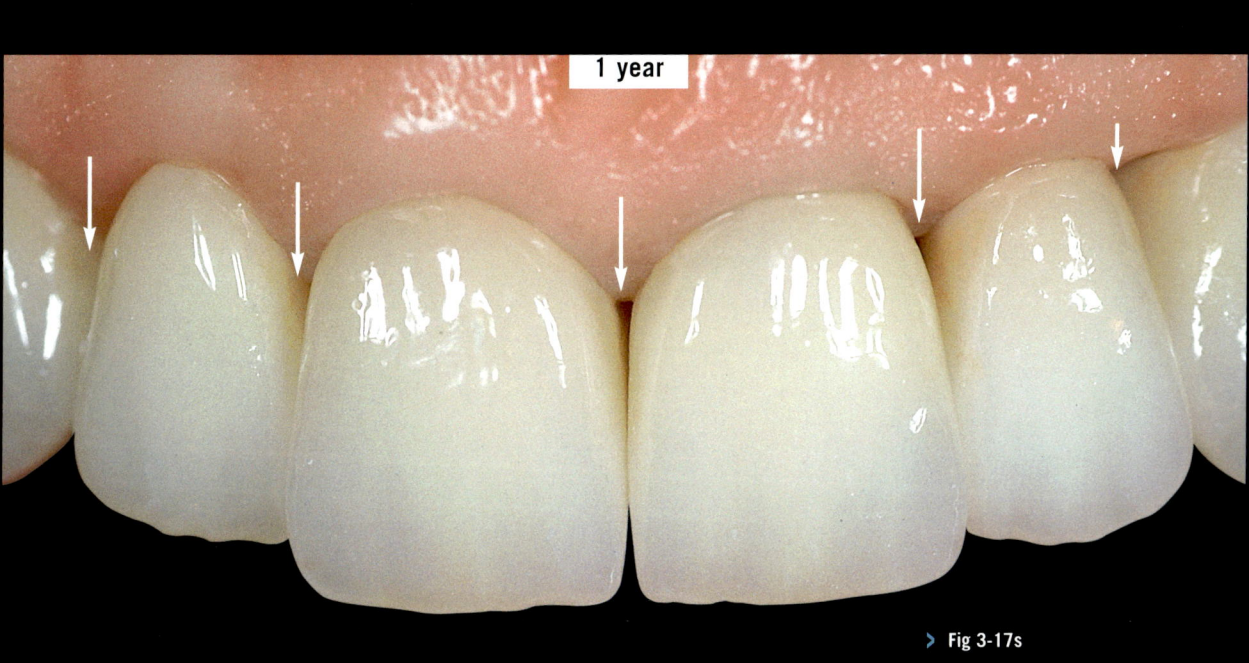

1 year

> Fig 3-17s

2 years

> Fig 3-17t

BIOLOGIC INTEGRATION — PERIODONTALLY COMPROMISED PATIENTS

PROSTHETIC-PERIODONTAL THERAPY

Prosthetic-periodontal therapy is aimed at halting the progression of periodontal disease and eliminating defects through resection that redefines osseous and gingival architecture at a more apical level compared with the preoperative situation.[72] Because of the conical shape of the roots, it results in large interdental spaces that require different treatment between the anterior and posterior sectors.

POSTERIOR SECTORS

Periodontal defects in the posterior sectors frequently involve furcations (Figs 3-18a and 3-18b). Depending on the seriousness and the location of the defects, the clinician will have to decide whether to save or extract each tooth and then proceed with positioning of the implants. However, anatomic limitations commonly found in these areas make implant therapy impossible unless combined with elevation of the maxillary sinus and/or placement of bone grafts, which are not routine procedures for all clinicians. Retaining the teeth through resective root therapy that allows some of the roots of the posterior teeth (ie, molars) to be preserved remains an important therapeutic option.[73] Before the advent of osseointegrated implants, prosthetic-periodontal therapy was sometimes the only method for using a fixed prosthesis in the posterior sectors. To comply with the wishes of some patients, clinicians often resorted to this therapy in the most extreme cases, with very high risks and obvious repercussions to the prognosis. Today, based on experience, certain essential prerequisites can be identified to improve the reliability of this type of therapy, such as minimally invasive root canal treatment, the presence of residual periodontal support of at least 50%, and reduced extension of the edentulous pontic unit.

RELINING AND PROSTHETIC FINALIZATION

Following resective surgery, in the case of root amputations (Fig 3-18c), the provisional restoration is relined immediately and carefully adapted to the new topography while the margins are maintained at a suitable distance from the tissues (Fig 3-18d). If kept at the level of the gingival crest, the definitive preparations can be completed 4 to 6 months after surgery (Figs 3-18e and 3-18f). As noted earlier, the clinician must be careful to leave open interproximal spaces to support the use of interdental brushes (Figs 3-18g to 3-18n). In these cases the topography is extremely different from its original form, which compels the clinician to teach the patient the most efficient ways of cleaning the area (Figs 3-18o to 3-18r).

FIG 18 *(a to c)* The presence of periodontal lesions with compromised molar furcations and reversal of the deep architecture of the entire maxillary right quadrant led to resective surgery with root amputations and hemisections. (Surgery by Dr Roberto Pontoriero.) *(d)* At the time of surgery, the provisional restoration was suitably relined to fill the spaces left after the root amputations; care was taken not to apicalize the margins so as not to interfere with the tissue growth. *(e and f)* The level of maturation appears to be well enough advanced to proceed with the final prosthetic stages 7 months later.

> Fig 3-18a

> Fig 3-18b

> Fig 3-18c

> Fig 3-18d

> Fig 3-18e

> Fig 3-18f

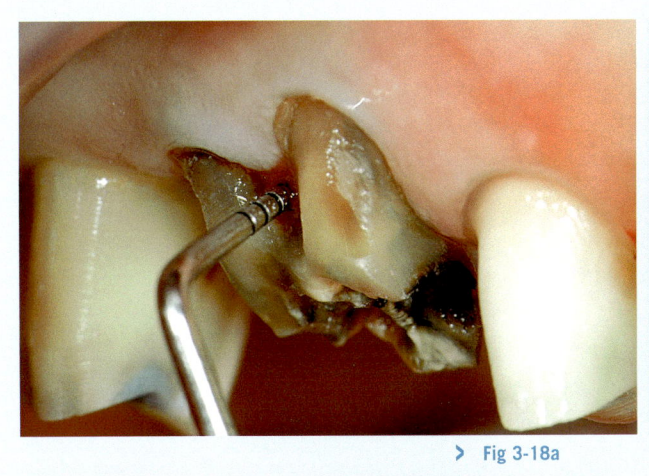

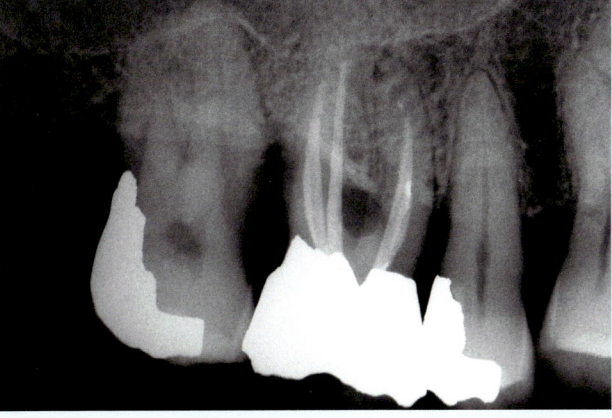

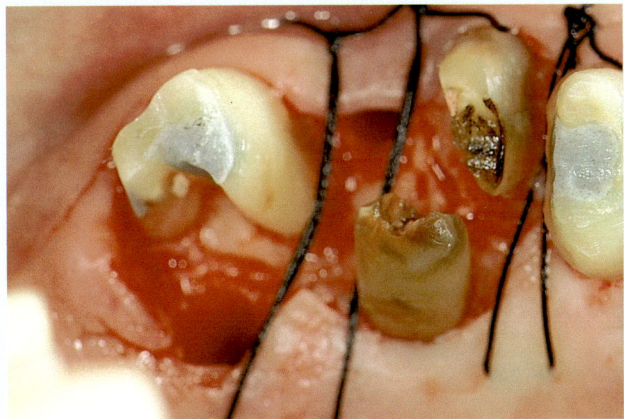

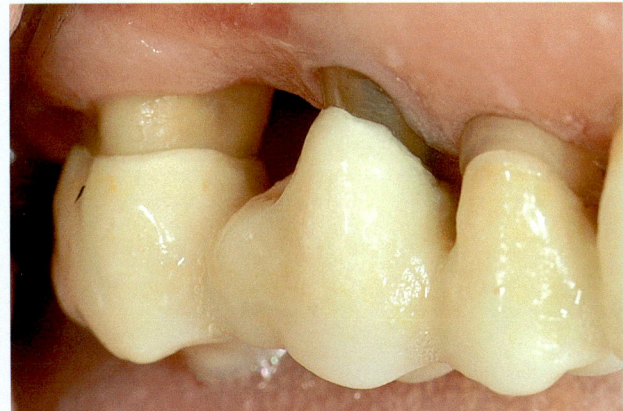

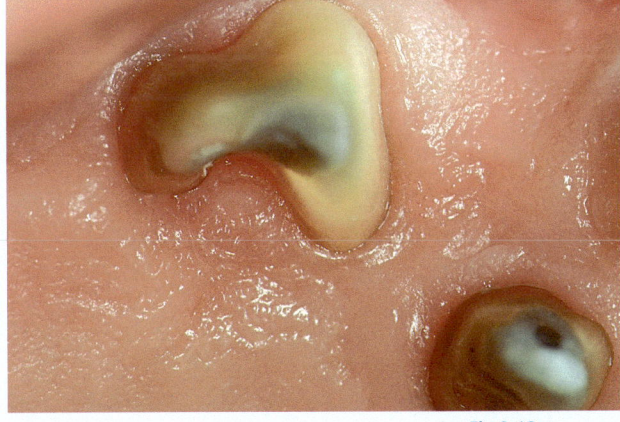

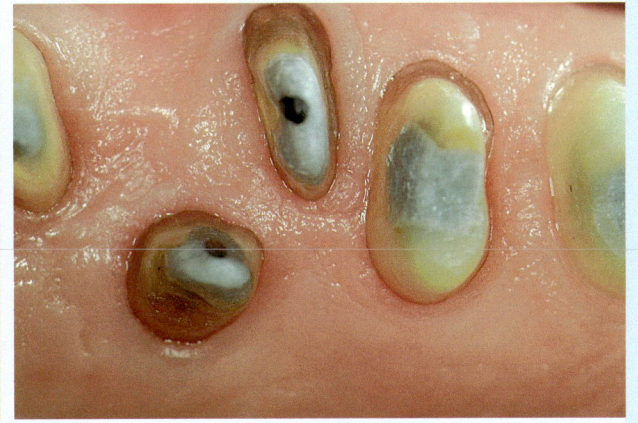

RESECTIVE ROOT SURGERY – POSTERIOR SECTORS

PREREQUISITES

- Patient with low carioreceptivity
- Favorable endodontic conditions
- Appropriate root length and shape
- Periodontal support ≥ 50%
- Limited extension of edentulous span
- Absence of parafunctional activity
- Optimal hygiene maintenance

> Fig 3-18g

> Fig 3-18h

> Fig 3-18i

> Fig 3-18j

> Fig 3-18k

> Fig 3-18l

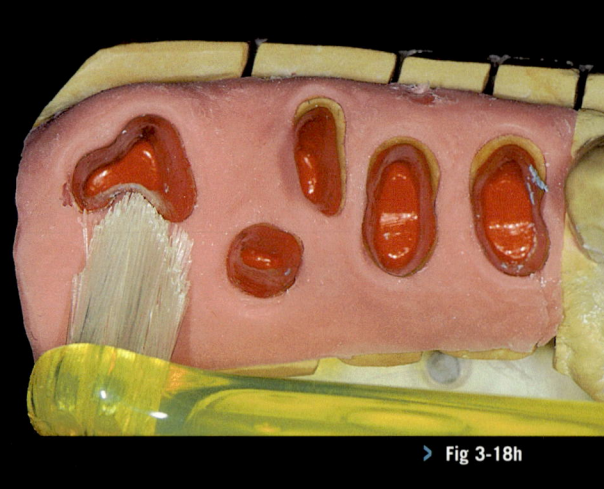

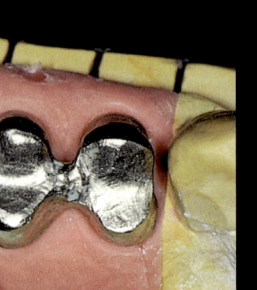

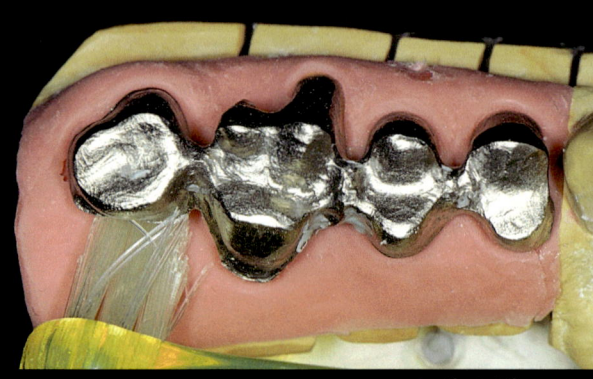

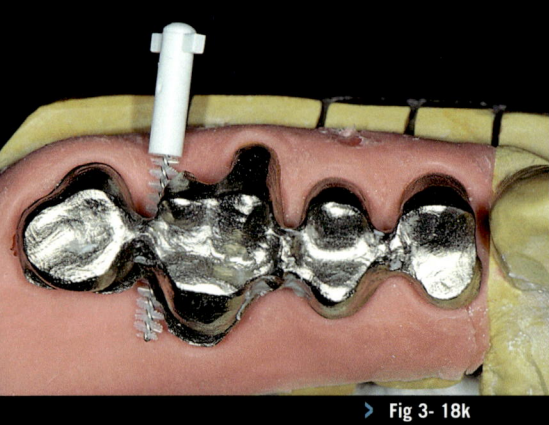

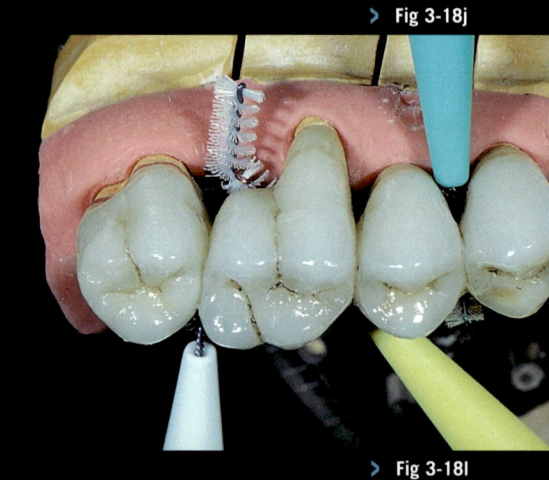

FIG 18 Once the final impressions have been taken, the master cast is made in the laboratory using a technique that makes it possible to replicate the appearance of the soft tissues. *(g to l)* The methods of inserting the interdental brushes, which should trace those that the patient has already been able to test for an adequate period with the provisional restoration in the mouth, will help the technician to correctly design first the metal substructure and then the ceramic-layered fixed partial denture. *(m and n)* It is possible to discern, especially in the cervical aspect, the relationship between the view of the provisional restoration turned upside down and that of the definitive restoration in metal-ceramic. *(o to r)* Over time, the space maintained in the interproximal areas of the definitive restorations to ensure that the patient can practice correct oral hygiene at home allows an excellent state of gingival health to be preserved.

> Fig 3-18m

> Fig 3-18n

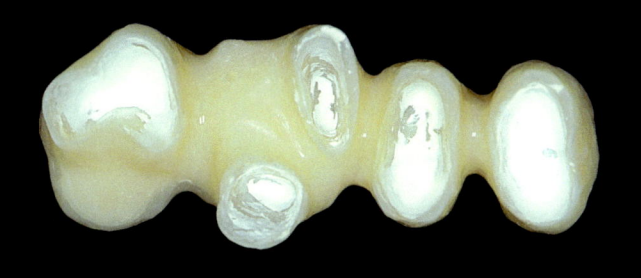

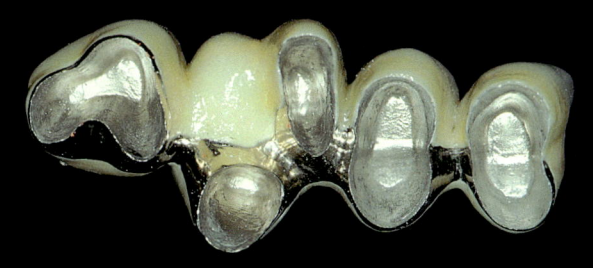

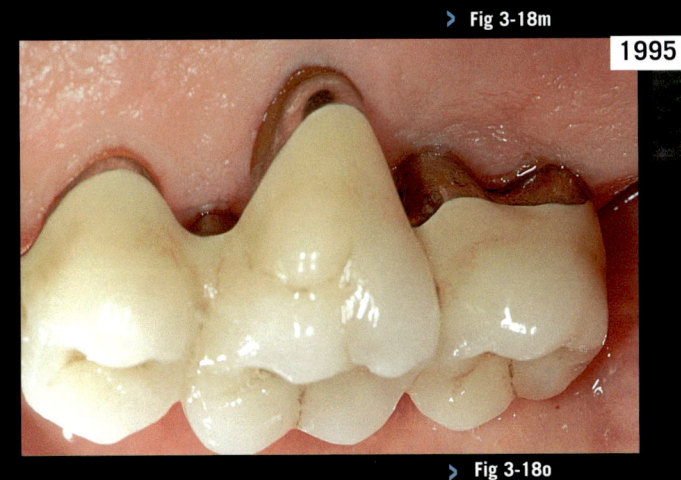

1995

> Fig 3-18o

> Fig 3-18p

2007

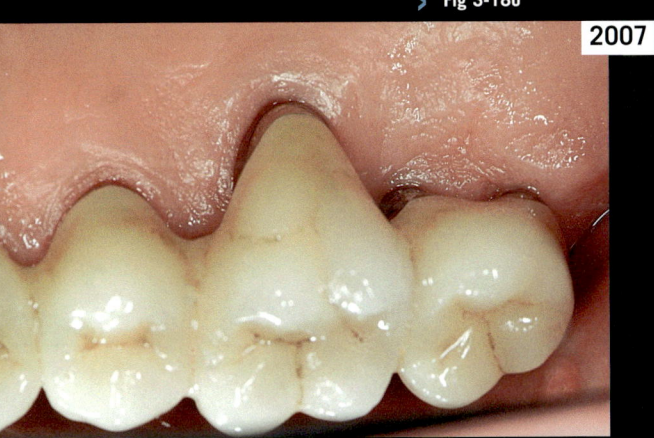

> Fig 3-18q

> Fig 3-18r

RESECTIVE ROOT SURGERY – POSTERIOR SECTORS

RELINING THE PROVISIONAL RESTORATION

- Keep the margins of the provisional restoration 2–3 mm apart in the postoperative healing stages.
- Instruct the patient in hygiene maintenance of the new interradicular spaces.
- Reline the provisional restoration after complete tissue maturation, carrying out preparations at the gingival crest.
- Idealize the interradicular shape of the provisional restoration to assist hygiene maintenance.
- Give the technician all of the information to replicate in the definitive restorations the contours and embrasures of the provisional restoration.

ANTERIOR SECTOR

Depending on the severity of the conical shape of the roots, resective therapy in the anterior sector can cause very large interdental spaces to appear. In periodontal patients, similar to patients requiring preprosthetic surgery, the tissue maturation stage requires a rather long time,[37,74,75] with seemingly less regrowth coronally than is seen in healthy patients.[56,76] The cause can be attributed, at least in part, to the increase in the interradicular distance in a more apical position. If surgical-periodontal therapies are involved in the anterior sector (Figs 3-19a to 3-19c) as well as the posterior sector (Figs 3-19d and 3-19e), the anterior areas are treated first, to allow more time for the maturation stage, if the restorative margins are to be positioned in the intrasulcular position. During this period, the patient must be constantly monitored and instructed in cleaning the surgically treated area properly, paying particular attention to the interproximal spaces (Figs 3-19f and 3-19g).

RELINING AND PROSTHETIC FINALIZATION

The clinician can make sure postoperative tissue maturation is complete by measuring the dentogingival reference points described earlier (see page 302). In the anterior sector it is still necessary to wait a minimum of 6 months before carrying out the definitive preparations, preferably positioning the margin at the level of the gingival crest (Figs 3-19h and 3-19i). Apicalization of the gingival levels following resective surgery and the consequent tooth lengthening mean that the marginal limit of the restorations is often not even visible during maximum smile, so any intracrevicular deepening is unnecessary. Watson[77] has found that many patients, when informed of the potential risks connected with subgingival positioning of the finish line, prefer to safeguard their periodontal health and accept visibility of the prosthetic margin, rather than risk compromise of the restoration's biologic integration.

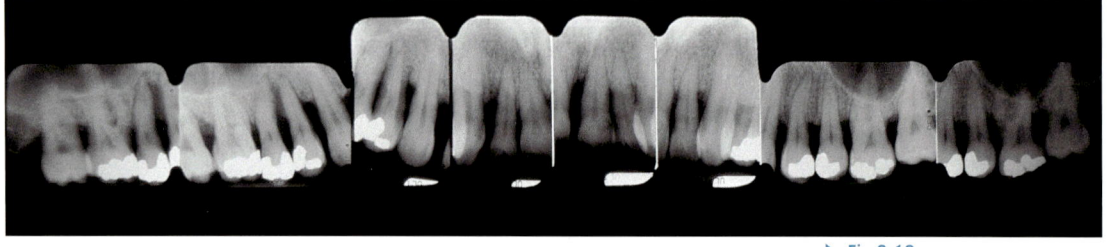

> Fig 3-19a

FIG 19 *(a to c)* The patient, treated for prosthetic-periodontal rehabilitation of the maxillary arch, initially underwent resective therapy in the anterior sector to eliminate periodontal defects. (Periodontal surgery by Dr Roberto Pontoriero.) *(d and e)* In the posterior sectors, the involvement of the buccal furcations of the molars (degree 1) has made intrasurgical tooth preparation of the abutments ("barreling-in" and "barreling-out") necessary to reduce the sinuous shape of the interradicular areas. *(f and g)* During the subsequent relining of the provisional restorations, compensation for the increase in space caused by the intrasurgical tooth preparations was only made horizontally, and care was taken not to extend the cervical margins in the apical direction, thereby avoiding interference with the maturing tissues. *(h and i)* The definitive preparations were completed 8 months after the last surgical procedure.

→ ...from page 181

CASE 2

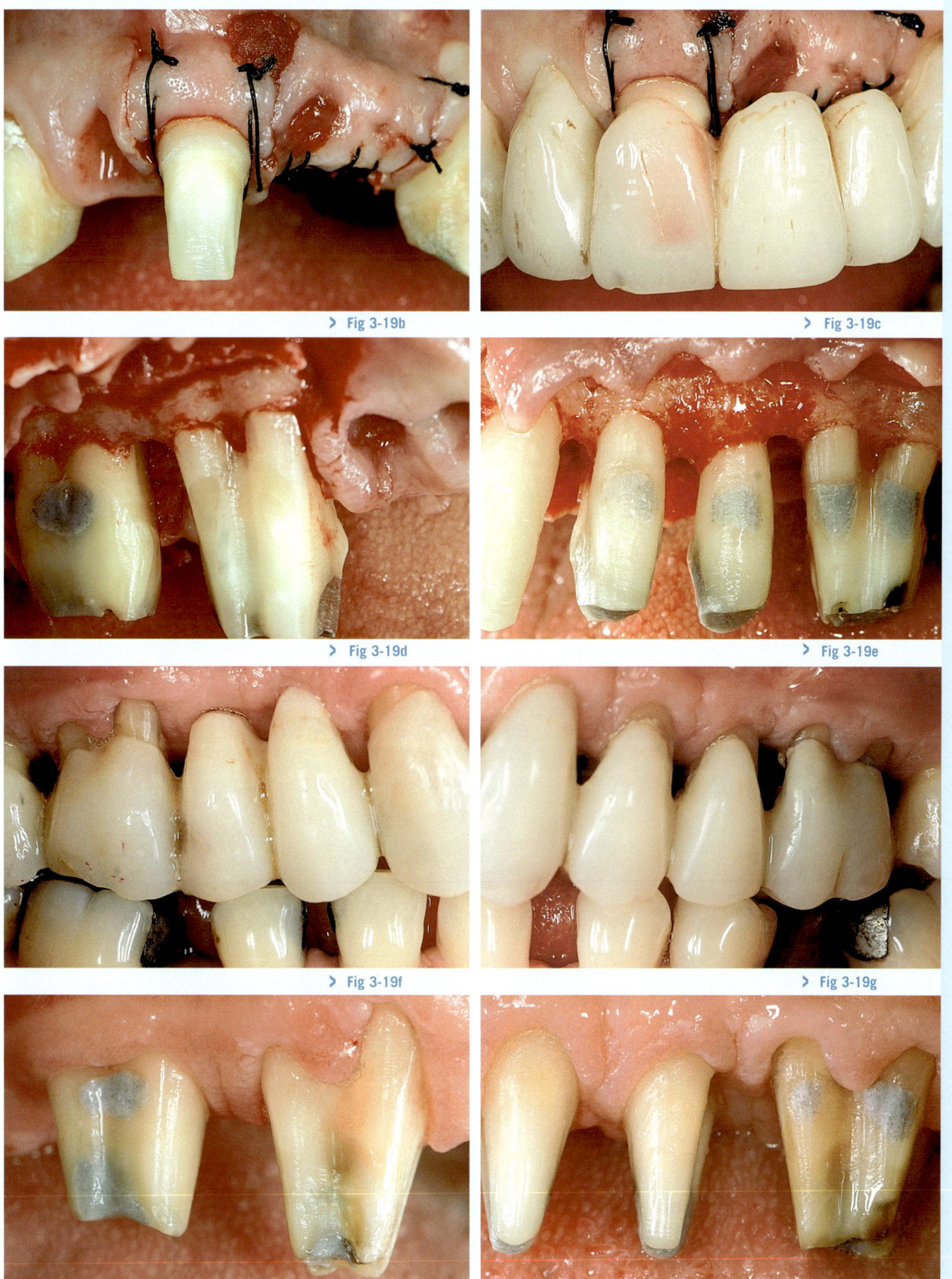

Fig 3-19b

Fig 3-19c

Fig 3-19d

Fig 3-19e

Fig 3-19f

Fig 3-19g

Fig 3-19h

Fig 3-19i

Once the definitive preparations have been made, the clinician can proceed with relining of the provisional restoration, which allows the majority of the interproximal spaces to be closed at the same time that the margins of the prosthesis are adapted to the new finish lines. In cases where the relining method is used, the clinician cannot be supported by the container effect of the MIT. As a result, the relining material should be compressed in the cervical area in order to detect a "reading" of the prosthetic margin and for correct recontouring of the provisional restoration (Figs 3-19j to 3/19o). If, for esthetic and/or phonetic reasons, the patient requests closure of the black triangles between the teeth (Figs 3-20a to 3-20v), the clinician should explain that the presence of a space, even though minimal, is of fundamental importance for the case maintenance, especially considering the possible further tissue maturation that could occur over time at the interproximal level. In cases of periodontal patients, it is not possible to use dental floss because the teeth need to be joined together; instead a superfloss should be used that can only pass through if there is sufficient interdental space. The use of interdental brushes must be discouraged since they can traumatize the papillae and contribute to the formation of unattractive interproximal spaces.

Biologic integration, so fastidiously achieved by means of the surgical therapy and correct postoperative prosthetic management described above, is checked when the final impressions are taken, at a minimum of 3 to 4 weeks after the provisional restoration is relined.

PROSTHETIC FINALIZATION: TIME LINE

"NONSURGICAL" PROSTHETIC CASES

- Absence of inflammation → **STAGE 1:**
  - Final tooth preparations
  - Final impressions
  - Positioning and relining of the provisional restoration

- Presence of inflammation → **STAGE 1:**
  - Removal of old restorations and preliminary preparations
  - Positioning and relining of the provisional restoration

  STAGE 2: (after 4–8 weeks)
  - Final preparations
  - Final impressions and relining of new provisional restoration

"SURGICAL" PROSTHETIC CASES

- **STAGE 1** — Preliminary preparations – positioning and relining of provisional restoration
- **STAGE 2** — Preprosthetic or periodontal surgery
- **STAGE 3** — Wait for tissue maturation (6 weeks to 9 months depending on type of surgery)
  - Final preparations and relining of provisional restorations
- **STAGE 4** — Wait 3–4 weeks → final impressions

> Fig 3-19j

> Fig 3-19k

> Fig 3-19l

> Fig 3-19m

> Fig 3-19n

> Fig 3-19o

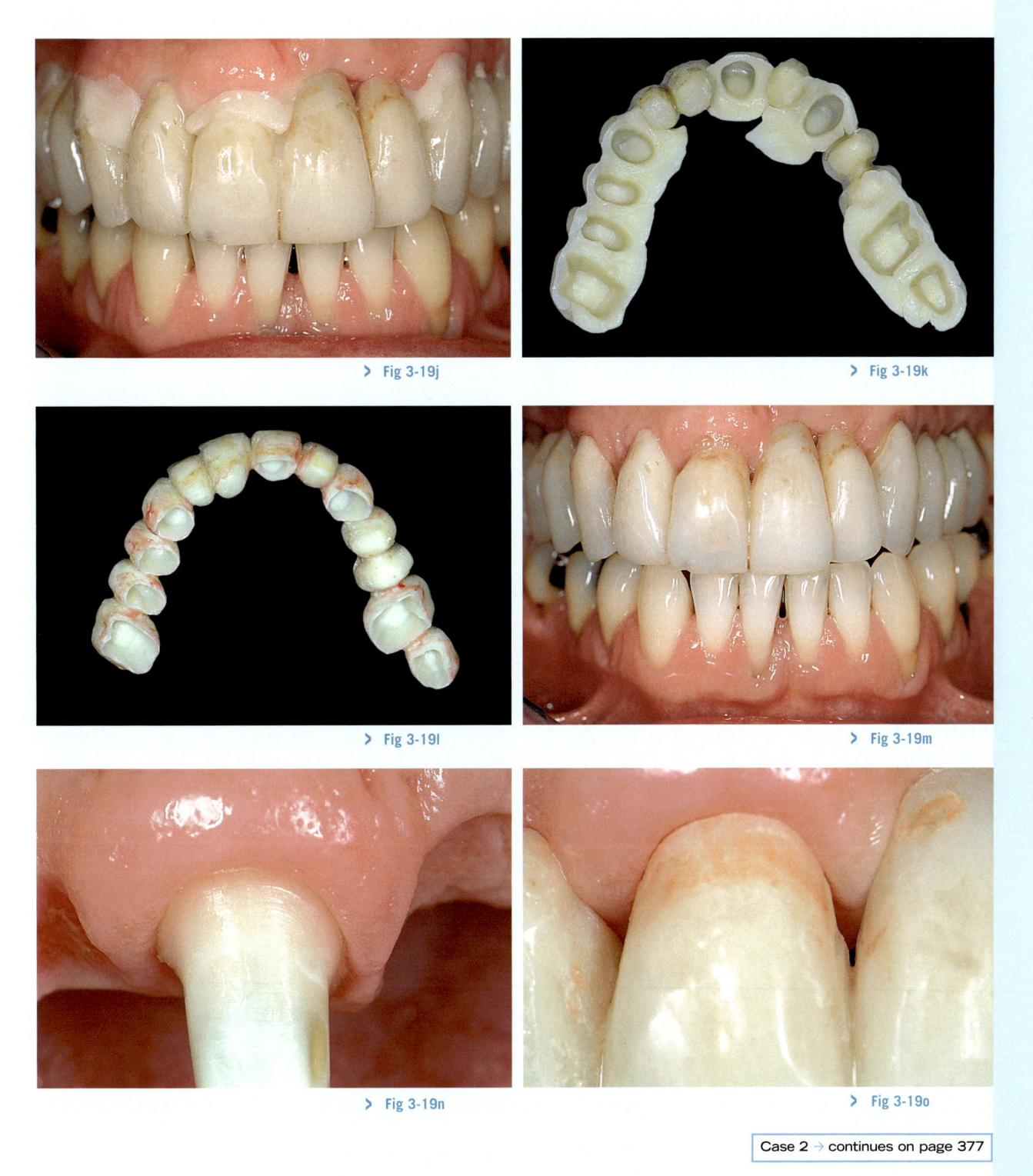

Case 2 → continues on page 377

FIG 19 *(j and k)* Extension of the surgical-periodontal treatment to the entire maxillary arch and the need to allow for complete tissue maturation have meant that the provisional restoration was virtually unchanged for more than 12 months before it was relined using the traditional technique (given the impossibility of using the MIT in this patient). Therefore, to cover the tooth preparation margins adequately, the excess relining material is kept in the cervical area until it is completely polymerized. *(l and m)* After the marginal areas are finished, petroleum jelly is applied to its external surface, and the provisional restoration is cemented and tested from the esthetic and functional viewpoints. *(n and o)* Ensuring that the tooth preparation margin of the right maxillary central incisor is positioned at the gingival crest and that the marginal fit and restorative contour are satisfactory contributes to optimal biologic integration.

→ ...from page 277, Vol 1, Ch 6

1996

> Fig 3-20a

> Fig 3-20b

> Fig 3-20c

> Fig 3-20d

> Fig 3-20e

> Fig 3-20f

> Fig 3- 20g

> Fig 3-20h

> Fig 3-20i

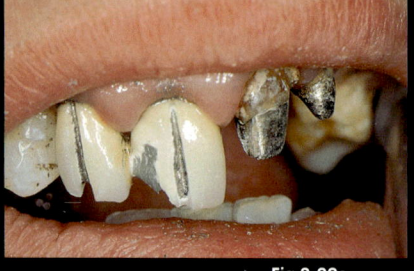

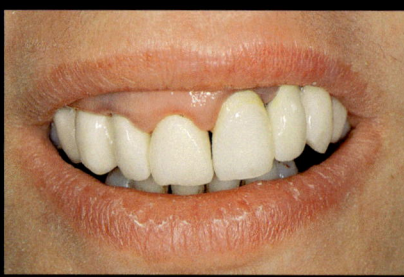

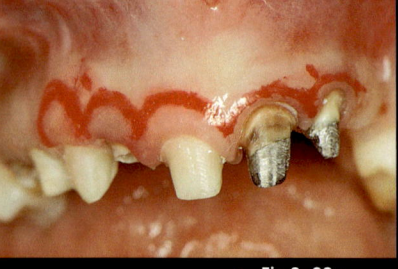

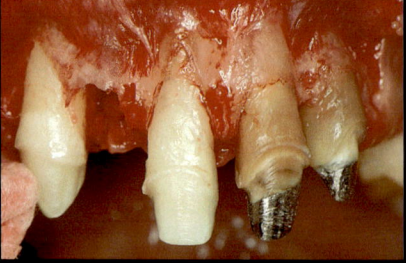

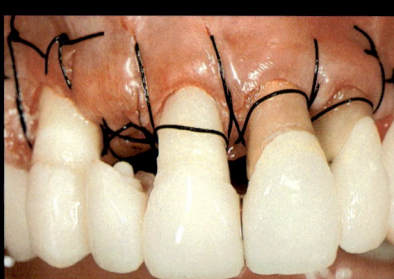

FIG 20 *(a and b)* The patient complains of an esthetic defect, which is especially evident because of the high smile line, caused by the considerable misalignment between the right and the left sides of the rehabilitation at both incisal and cervical levels. The restoration was done some years earlier in another office. *(c)* The view of both arches in an edge-to-edge position reveals a noticeable discrepancy of the occlusal plane as well. *(d)* The radiographic examination highlights the presence of periodontal problems primarily in the anterior sectors on both arches. *(e to i)* After the maxillary rehabilitation has been removed and a first provisional restoration has been positioned, the patient undergoes resective surgery aimed at eliminating the periodontal defects as well as modifying the asymmetry of the gingival levels. (Periodontal surgery by Dr Roberto Pontoriero.) *(j)* The photograph of the smile 10 days after surgery highlights the increase in tooth length (17 to 18 mm) and the formation of wide interproximal spaces. Only after resective surgery in the posterior sectors has been accomplished roughly 10 months after the surgery in the anterior sector will the possibility of shortening the maxillary incisal margins be evaluated from both esthetic and phonetic viewpoints. *(k and l)* The reduction is first previewed with a pencil and then carried out directly in the mouth with the aid of a bur. *(m)* After being shortened by approximately 3 mm and undergoing tissue maturation at the cervical level that has led to their coronal regrowth by another 3 mm or so, the central incisors now measure a little more than 11 mm. *(n)* Alginate impressions are now taken of both arches. *(o)* In the maxillary arch, an impression is taken of the provisional restoration in situ as well as the abutments underneath it to assist the technician in creating the diagnostic wax-up. *(p and q)* In addition to having ideal esthetic characteristics, the provisional restorations derived from the diagnostic wax-up also must ensure optimal occlusal stability. *(r and s)* The comparison between the postoperative photograph of the first maxillary provisional restoration and that of the new provisional restorations in situ shows the excellent integration achieved by the latter from the esthetic-functional and biologic standpoints. *(t to v)* Close-up views of the intrasulcular preparations, the partial insertion of the provisional restoration, and the provisional restoration in situ demonstrate that a good level of tissue maturation has been reached, which is essential before the final stages of the prosthetic rehabilitation are completed.

Fig 3-20j

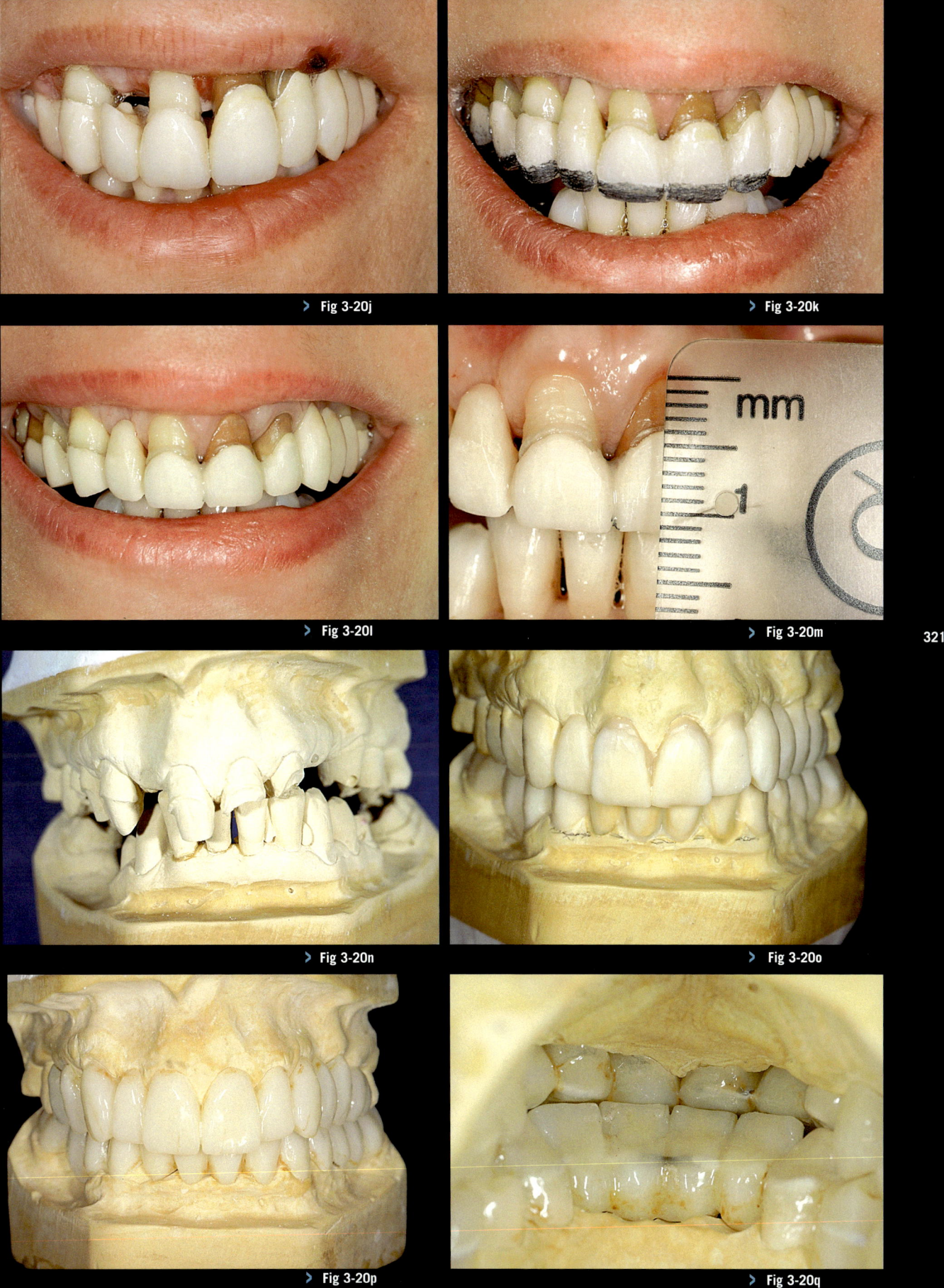

Fig 3-20k

Fig 3-20l

Fig 3-20m

Fig 3-20n

Fig 3-20o

Fig 3-20p

Fig 3-20q

> Fig 3-20r

> Fig 3-20s

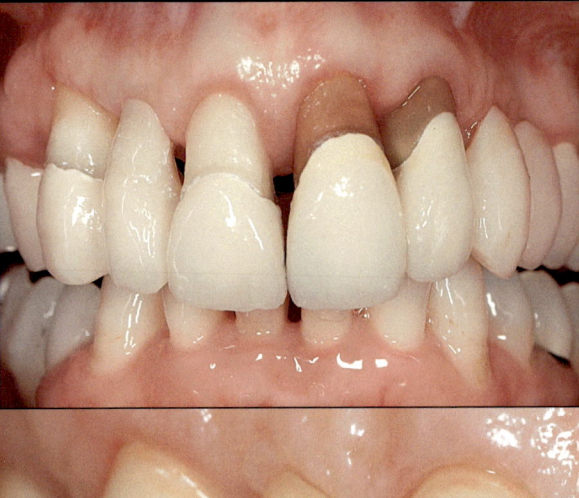

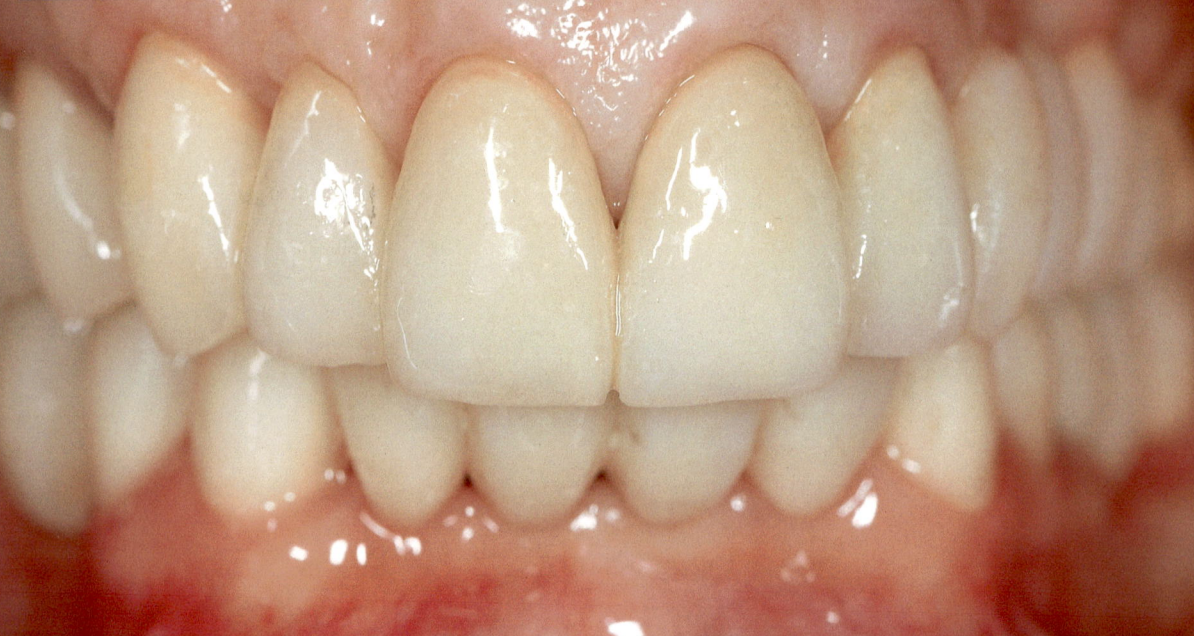

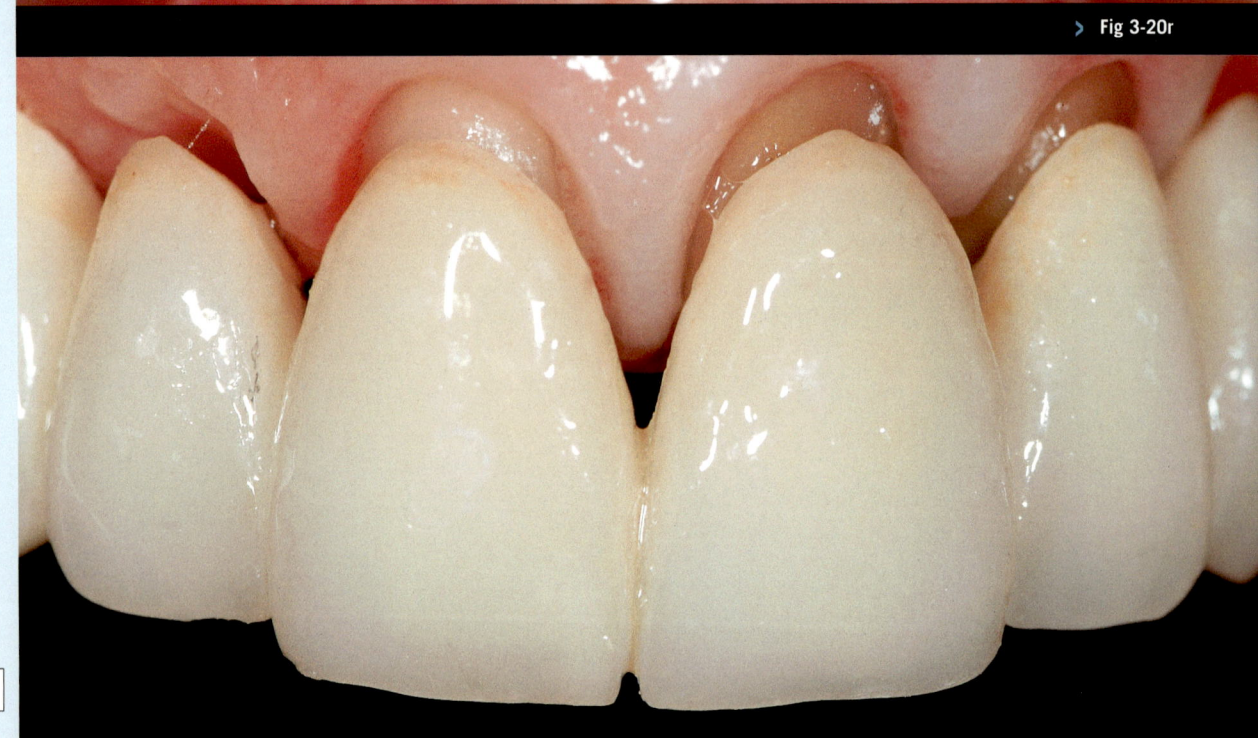

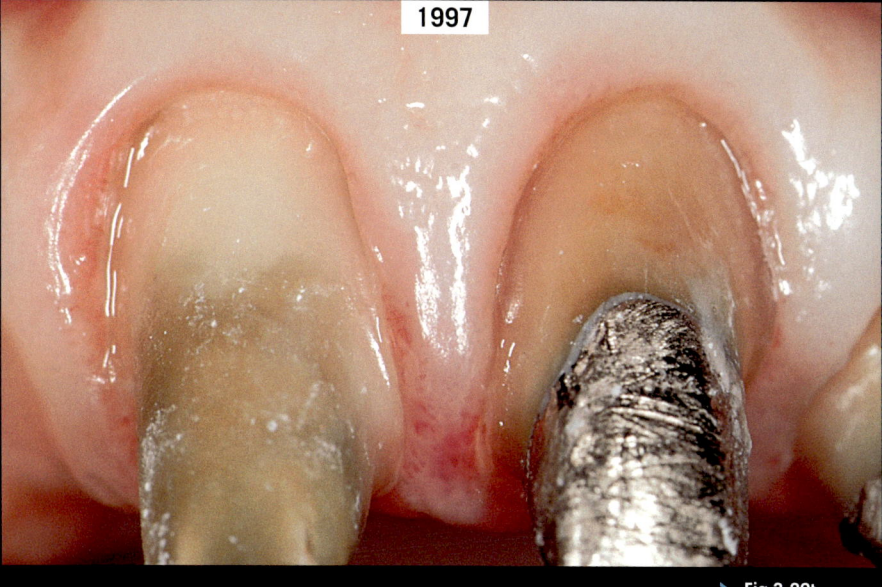

1997

> Fig 3-20t

> Fig 3-20u

> Fig 3-20v

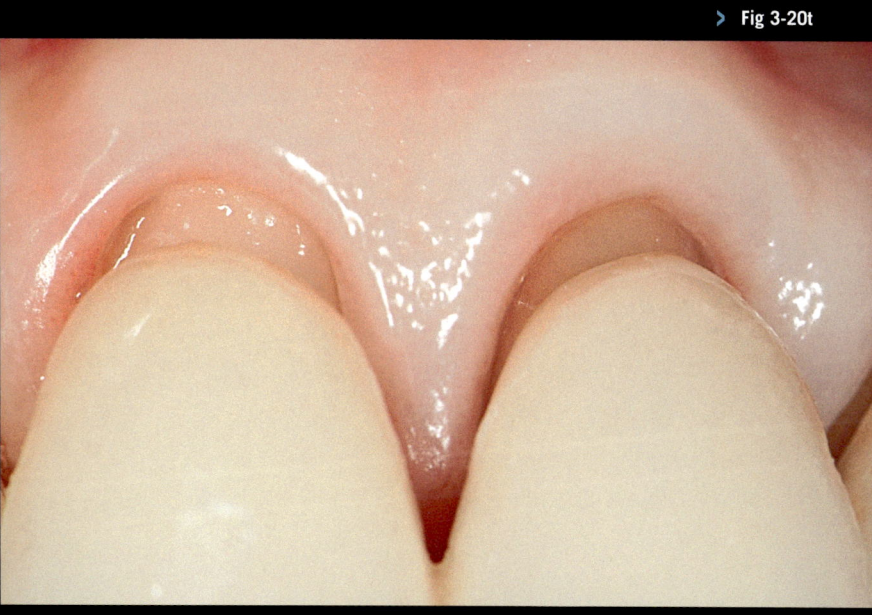

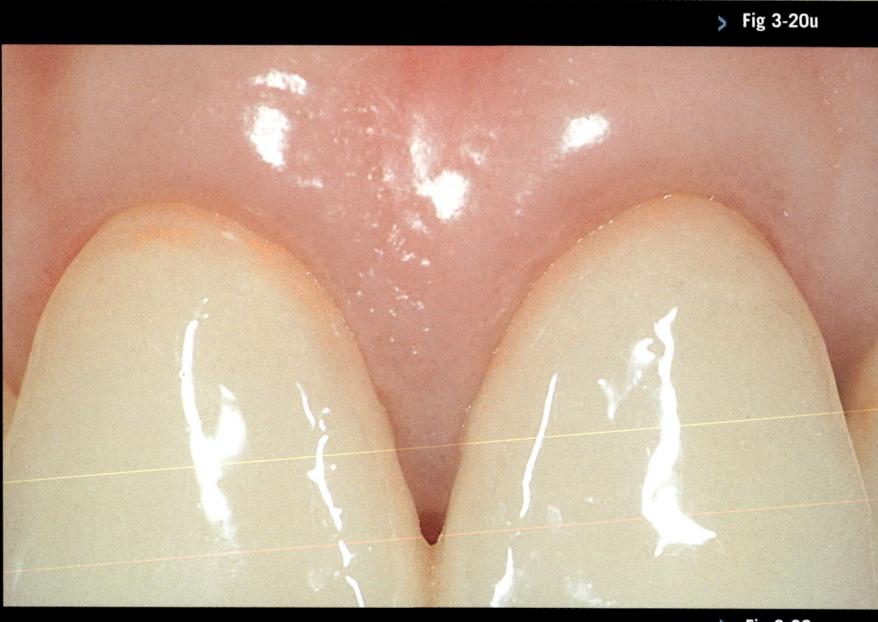

FINAL TOOTH PREPARATION

Tooth preparation is a fundamental and irreversible clinical phase in the prosthetic rehabilitation and therefore requires maximum attention to guarantee retention, resistance, and longevity of the prosthetic restoration.[78-92]

Treating a limited number of teeth allows the clinician to proceed with the preparations, and sometimes the final impressions as well, at the same time as positioning of the provisional restoration. This is possible only if the patient is in a perfect state of gingival health and if the tooth position, tooth length, and/or the restorative contour do not need to be modified.

The need to test the esthetic-functional modifications, their phonetic implications, and/or the tissue response to new restorative contours make it necessary to delay finalizing the definitive work, especially in more extended treatments. In all of these cases, or if other associated surgical therapies are also involved, the clinician very often just completes a preliminary preparation at the time of inserting the provisional restoration (see chapter 2, pages 130–133). This approach tends to reduce the invasiveness of the prosthetic treatment, at least in the initial stages, and allows good structural maintenance of the abutment. It is also particularly useful in periodontal cases where, following resective surgery, a marked apicalization of the gingival levels is often created (Fig 3-20w). The progressively conical shape of the roots, frequently combined with axial modifications found in the root area, could lead to a structural weakening of the abutments at a later phase of tooth preparation.

In the majority of patients, the appointment for the definitive preparations must precede that of the final impressions by at least 3 weeks. This is especially important in cases where the margins of the definitive preparations exhibit intrasulcular positioning. In order to correctly integrate the provisional restoration, the tooth preparations are always performed under the guidance of the acetate or silicone indexes derived from the functional provisional restorations.

Choice of restorative material Final preparation of the abutments must create the spaces necessary to accommodate the chosen definitive material (Figs 3-20x and 3-20y) (see chapter 5, pages 466–479). A transparent matrix or a silicone index derived from the provisional restorations, which have properly functioned for a suitable period of time, gives the clinician the opportunity to optimize the buccal as well as lingual thicknesses.

FIG 20 *(w)* Ten months after periodontal surgery, in addition to restored symmetry of the gingival levels, there is considerable distance between the position of the preparation margins and the current level of the tissues. *(x and y)* The abutments are prepared definitively under the guide of an acetate index derived from the cast of the provisional restorations, which will increase the sulcular depth and the marginal limit.

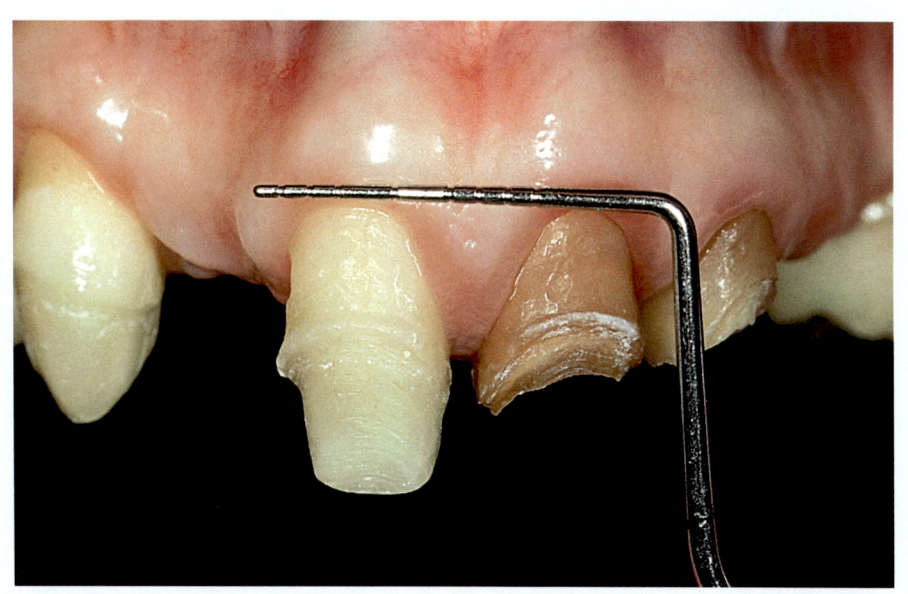

Fig 3-20w

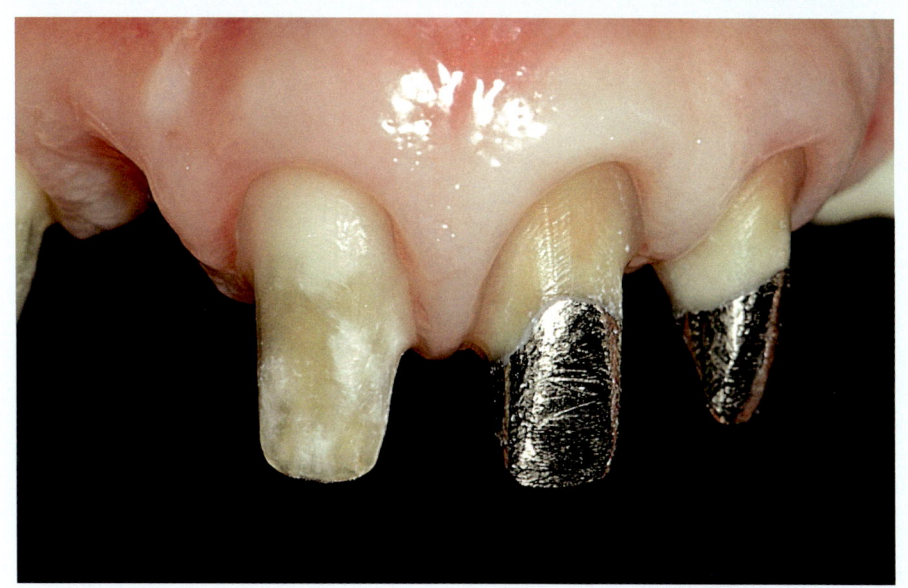

Fig 3-20x

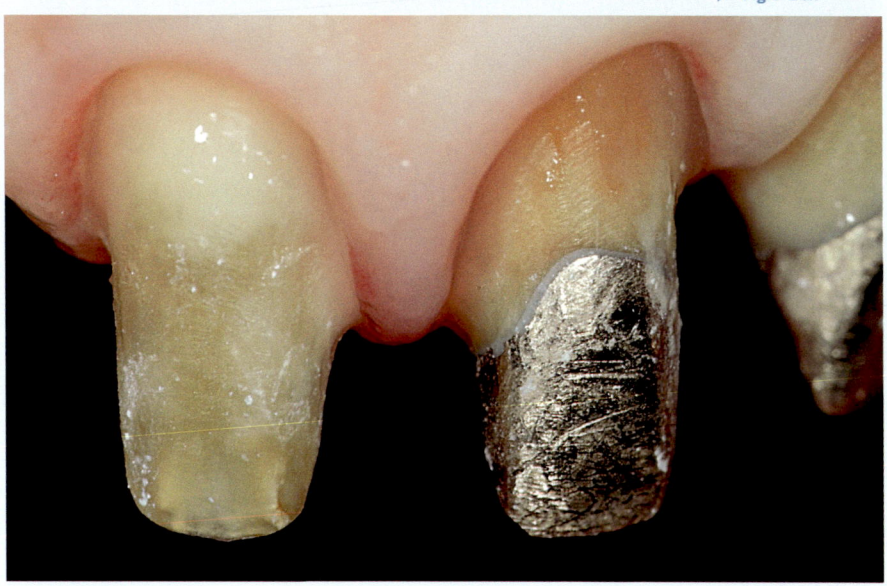

Fig 3-20y

325

TOOTH PREPARATION

PREPARATION THICKNESS

To optimize the esthetics of the definitive restoration, the minimum preparation thickness in the buccal area must be between 1.0 and 1.5 mm depending on the definitive material chosen (Figs 3-20z to 3-20aa).[93–97] To adequately resist the masticatory forces, a minimum lingual thickness of 1.0 mm is necessary in the anterosuperior sector, and an occlusal thickness of approximately 2.0 mm is required in the posterior sectors. Keeping to these values prevents having to prepare the abutments again at the final impressions stage. The spaces created in this way must be found to be exactly the same as the thickness measurements of the functional provisional, relined following the definitive preparations (Fig 3-20bb).

ANTERIOR SECTOR

Buccal area

Reduced incisal thickness If the position of the incisal edge appears to be correct, the buccal thickness is measured at the cervical as well as the incisal level after the provisional restoration is removed from the mouth and before the definitive preparations are carried out. In the absence of sufficient space to contain the final restorative material, the preliminary tooth preparations must be appropriately modified. If the clinician does not notice this lack of space, the technician is left without the necessary thickness for layering the ceramic and will be compelled to buccalize the restoration, hence modifying the incisal profile. This can result in an unpleasant sensation of obstruction for the patient and is detectable during the pronunciation of the F sound from the position of the upper incisal margin, which, going beyond the limit of the vermilion border of the lower lip, causes considerable esthetic-functional discomfort (see volume 1, chapter 4). During the biscuit try-in, in attempting to comply with the patient's requests, the clinician is forced to rectify the excessive buccal convexity at the risk of irreparably compromising the ceramic layering. If, instead, the clinician notices the reduced thickness but deems it unnecessary to deepen the tooth preparation because of the risk of excessively weakening the residual structure, he/she may increase the buccal thickness of the provisional restoration. At this point it is necessary to test the provisional restoration clinically for 3 to 4 weeks before copying it to the definitive, thereby assessing the patient's esthetic and phonetic adaptation to the new situation.

Limited cervical thickness A cervical preparation thickness of less than 1.0 mm is difficult to see by simply looking at the provisional restoration because of the nature of the acrylic resin. If the definitive restoration is made of metal-ceramic, insufficient thickness would inevitably make the restoration appear opaque in this area. If the restorative choice is made to use all-ceramic instead, a limited thickness could in some cases dangerously reduce resistance.

FIG 20 *(z and aa)* With the provisional restoration inserted, it is not easy to evaluate the thicknesses available for the definitive restorations. *(bb)* Once relining is completed, a thickness gauge is used to measure the space available at the buccal/facial level and thereby evaluate its suitability in relation to the restorative material chosen.

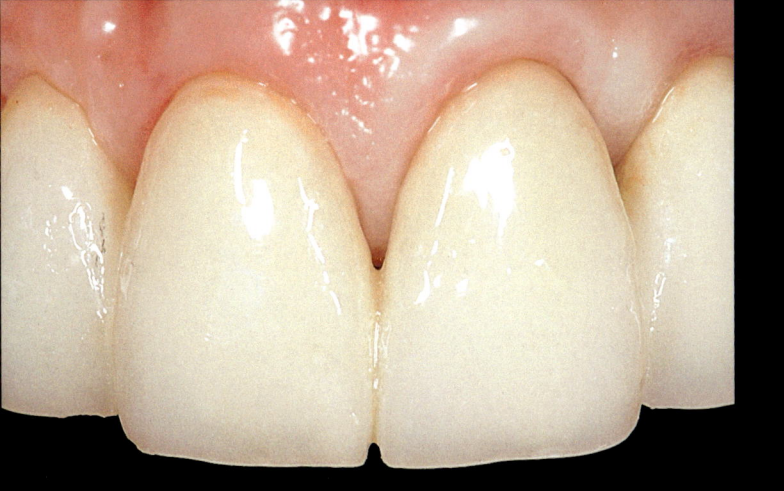

> Fig 3-20z

> Fig 3-20aa

> Fig 3-20bb

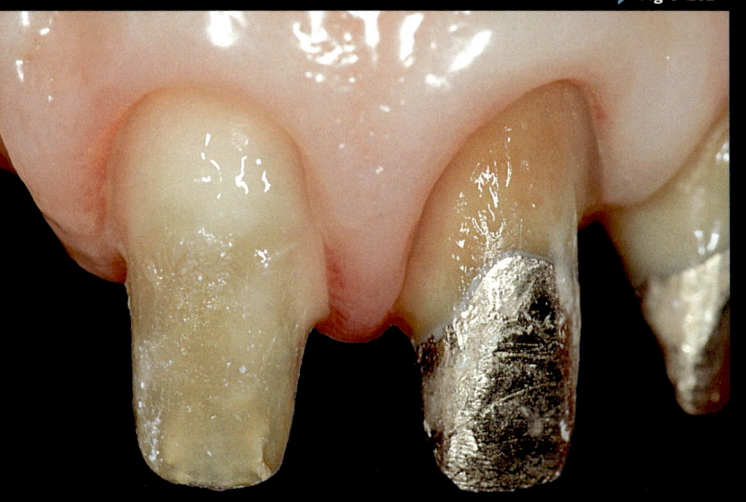

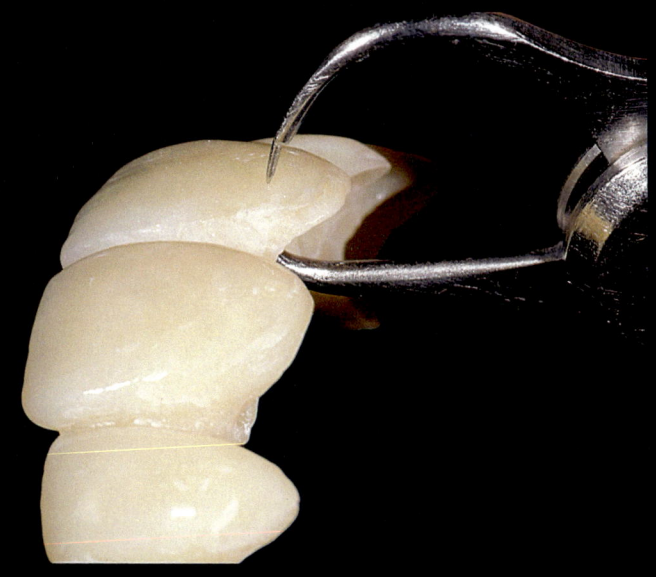

→ Gallery of cases, page 534

ANTEROSUPERIOR SECTOR

Lingual area

Ideally, once the abutment has been prepared, there should be a minimum thickness of 1.0 mm in the maxillary lingual concavity. However, the amount of overjet and overbite often conditions in a determinant manner the achievement of this value. In the anterosuperior sector it is also necessary to evaluate not just the occlusal space in the static phase (MI or CR), but also the space present during the excursive movements, which can change with time. It is not uncommon to find that the lingual concavity, designed to optimize the anterior guidance in the maxillary teeth when the provisional restoration is being positioned, is already inadequate within just a few weeks due to the abrasion of the acrylic resin and/or the supraeruption of the teeth. Only after carefully evaluating the thickness of the provisional restoration in this area (Fig 3-21a) should the clinician then correct the lingual preparation using a football-shaped bur, redefining the space necessary for finalizing the work (Figs 3-21b and 3-21c). In the opposite case, with inadequate thicknesses, since the concavity in the acrylic resin cannot be reproduced with the definitive material, the technician has to thicken the lingual area arbitrarily (Fig 3-21d), therefore completely modifying the disocclusion pattern found in the provisional restoration. This forces the patient to adapt to this new clinical situation with the definitive work, with possible restrictions in the development of function that may cause discomfort, phonetic difficulty, tooth mobility, and joint problems.[98-101] To remedy this inconvenience, often found only after the work has been cemented, the clinician can opt to modify the shape of the lingual concavity of the definitive restorations directly in the mouth. If metal-ceramic has been used, these refinements can easily expose the opaque layer, which is much more abrasive compared with the opposing natural dentition. If, instead, all-ceramic restorations have been used, these modifications could significantly reduce their resistance.

Measuring the thickness of the provisional restoration, which is done after relining it following the definitive tooth preparation, prevents functional problems and structural weakening of the definitive restoration. In addition, this excludes the need to make significant refinements at the appointment for taking the final impressions, 3 to 4 weeks later (Figs 3-21e and 3-21f).

FIG 21 *(a)* The thickness of each of the preliminary preparations is checked before the definitive prosthetic abutment is prepared. *(b)* In the absence of adequate thickness in the lingual area, a football-shaped bur is used to accentuate the curvature of the lingual concavity and thus create a space of at least 1.0 mm for the restoration. *(c and d)* Appropriate preparation of the upper lingual concavity allows an ideal anterior guidance to be developed, which instead proves inadequate if preparation in this area is not completed as illustrated. *(e and f)* The buccolingual thickness of the abutment, on the border between the middle and incisal thirds, must allow a restoration to be created that has a thickness of no more than 3.5 mm in this specific area.

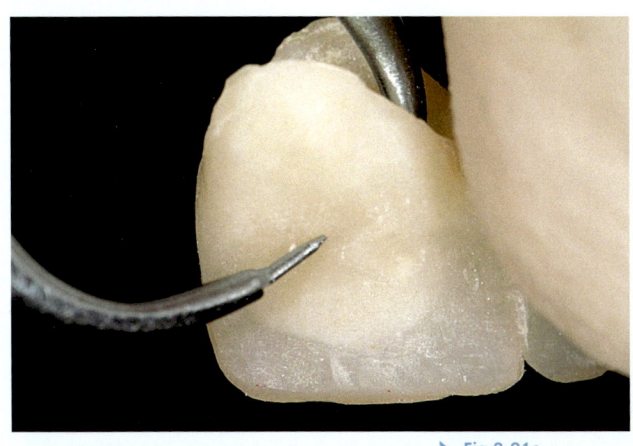

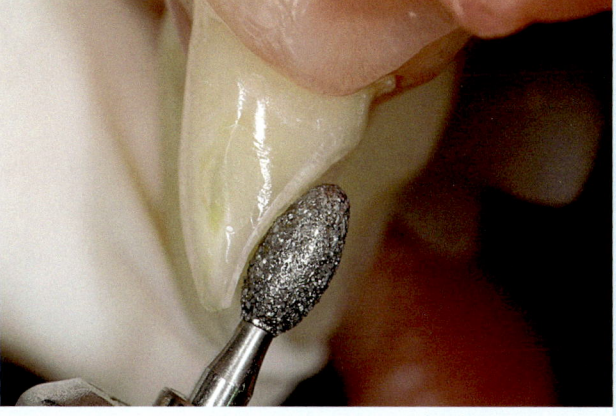

> Fig 3-21a

> Fig 3-21b

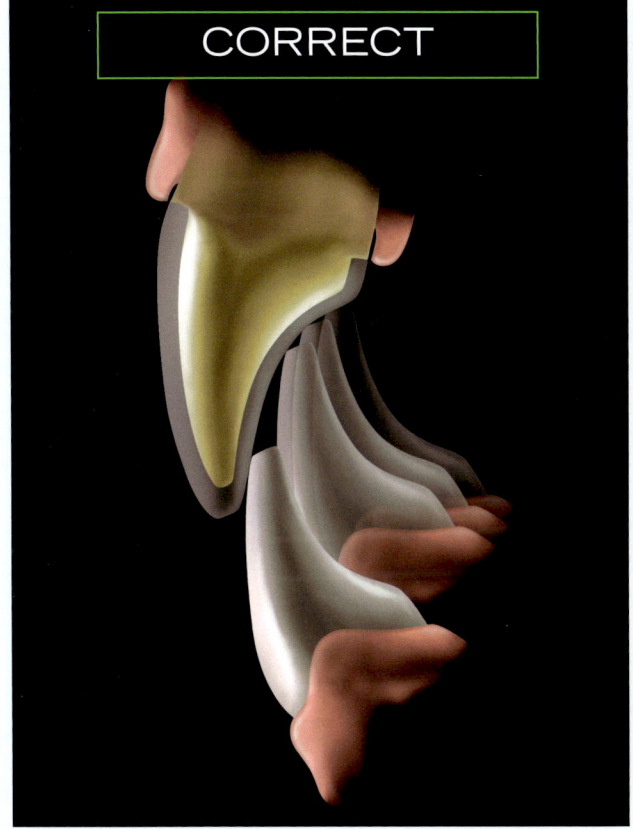

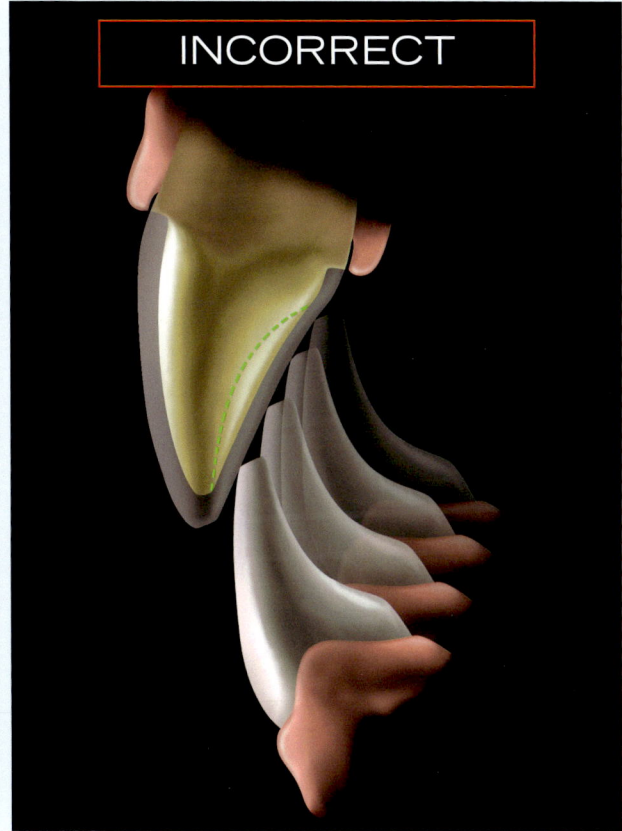

CORRECT

INCORRECT

> Fig 3-21c

> Fig 3-21d

> Fig 3-21e

> Fig 3-21f

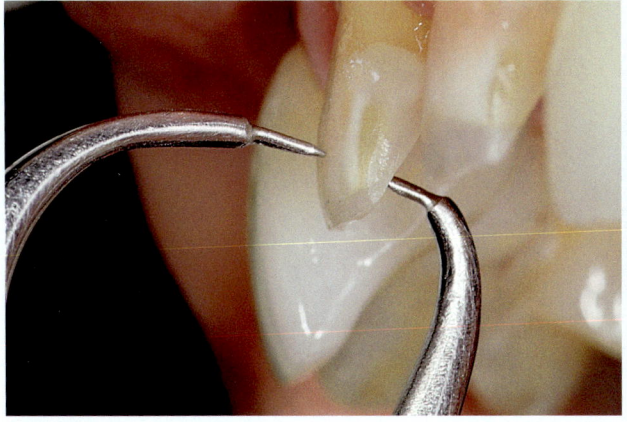

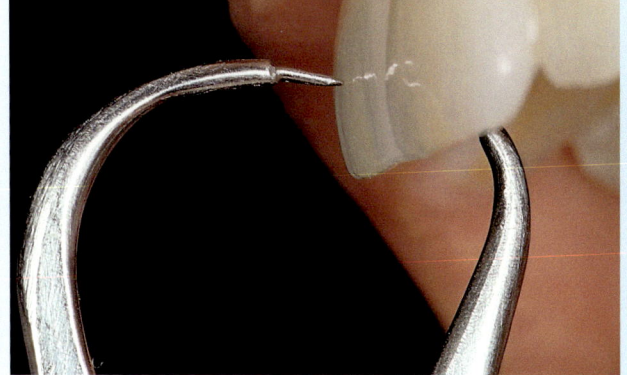

329

TOOTH PREPARATION

MARGINAL CONFIGURATION

The choice of marginal configuration inevitably affects the esthetic result and the degree of resistance of the definitive restoration. It should therefore be selected while considering the restorative goal to be achieved.

The tooth preparations can be described as either *vertical* (knife edge, bevel, slight chamfer) or *horizontal* (deep chamfer, shoulder). The choice of preparation type depends on the restorative objectives and the esthetic needs of the patient.

Vertical preparations These are typically chosen for patients who have no particular esthetic needs (eg, those with a low smile line, posterior restorations, distolingual sites) and especially in cases of complex rehabilitation, where the need to join numerous teeth, particularly if they undergo surgical resection therapy, makes it necessary to seek parallelism and structural preservation of the abutments. The esthetic result is compromised by the limited thickness of the vertical preparations. Despite the wide range of indications for all-ceramics, their use in these cases is not prescribed even today. Instead, the elective material for this type of preparation is metal-ceramic in very reduced thicknesses, which allows adequate marginal closure with a metal collar.

Horizontal preparations These are increasingly used for esthetic reasons in both all-ceramic and metal-ceramic restorations. While the esthetic results are excellent, they require a considerable sacrifice of tooth structure and hence greater risk to the integrity of the pulp.

Differentiated preparation In many cases, to combine esthetic needs and preservation of biologic and structural integrity, a *differentiated* preparation may be chosen. Rather than reducing the circumference of the abutment in a uniform manner, a slightly more aggressive preparation (horizontal) can be carried out in the areas of greatest esthetic value, while more conservative (vertical) preparations that contribute to preservation of the structural integrity of the tooth can be made elsewhere (Fig 3-22).

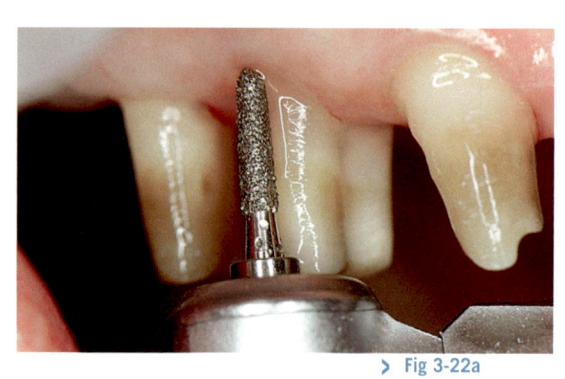

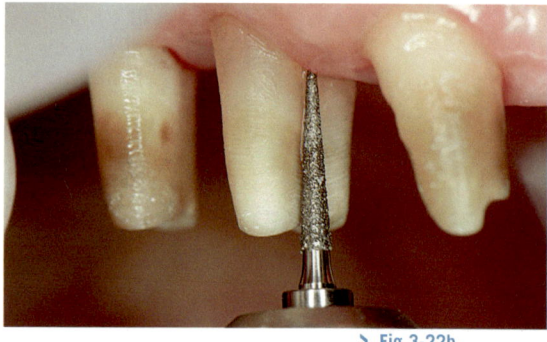

> Fig 3-22a   > Fig 3-22b

FIG 22 It is especially possible in the posterior sectors to vary the ways of reducing the abutment. *(a)* To favor the esthetic appearance, in the most visible areas (buccal) a horizontal type of preparation can be carried out. *(b)* In the interproximal and lingual sites, however, a vertical preparation is useful to preserve the structural integrity of the abutment.

Chapter 3 BIOLOGIC INTEGRATION OF THE PROVISIONAL RESTORATION AND DEFINITIVE PREPARATIONS

TYPE OF MARGIN	ADVANTAGES	DISADVANTAGES
KNIFE EDGE	- Easy execution - Good marginal fit - Preserves tooth structure - Suitable for periodontal cases	- Difficult marginal definition - Unsatisfactory esthetics - Presence of overcontour - Possible raised bite
BEVEL	- Good marginal definition - Preserves tooth structure - Satisfactory esthetics (deep chamfer) - Minimal stress concentration - Easy cement flow	- Difficult execution ("U" shaped margin) - Unsatisfactory esthetics (light chamfer) - Difficult marginal fit (light chamfer)
90-DEGREE SHOULDER	- Excellent marginal definition - Excellent esthetics - Minimal stress concentration (rounded shoulder) - Ideal fitting	- Difficult execution - Not ideal marginal fit - Difficult cement flow
50-DEGREE SHOULDER	- Good marginal definition - Satisfactory esthetics - Satisfactory marginal fit	- Difficult execution - Inner angle not easily identified
BEVEL	- Increased retention and stability - Good marginal fit	- Difficult execution - Unsatisfactory esthetics - Instability during thermal cycle - Possible raised bite

TOOTH PREPARATION

RESPECTING BIOLOGIC INTEGRITY

To guarantee optimal biologic integration of the prosthetic rehabilitation, two fundamental premises during the tooth preparation stages must be observed:

- Maintenance of pulp integrity
- Maintenance of gingival integrity

PARTIAL PREPARATIONS

Veneers and inlays-onlays Over the past 15 to 20 years, in the effort to preserve as much tooth structure as possible, minimally invasive techniques (veneers and inlays) have been developed that reduce the biologic risk associated with tooth preparation phases. In the case of veneers, the reduction, normally confined to the enamel,[102–104] is limited to the buccal-incisal area of the anterior teeth, thus allowing preservation of a considerable amount of tooth structure (Fig 3-23). Besides conserving pulp integrity, the opportunity to design the preparation margin supragingivally in the majority of cases also allows for preservation of the integrity of the gingival tissues. This double advantage can also be seen in partial preparations of the posterior sectors for positioning inlays and onlays.

COMPLETE PREPARATIONS

Coronal restorations If the clinician is instead forced to make a complete coronal restoration, the preparation will involve the entire 360 degrees of tooth circumference. The ever–more pressing esthetic needs of patients today frequently force clinicians to complete horizontal-type preparations not just to optimize the final appearance, but also to design a coronal contour that allows for the removal of plaque.[28,105] All of this requires considerable deepening of the preparation into the dentin, and consequently greater exposure of the dental tubules, which is, obviously, an important risk factor for maintenance of pulp vitality.

The need to conceal the restoration in the cervical third instead threatens the integrity of the gingival margin, especially in metal-ceramic restorations. Deepening the preparation subgingivally can have repercussions on the biologic integration of the restoration with the surrounding tissues. Today, the use of all-ceramic materials for complete coronal restorations in many cases allows the preparation limit to be supragingival, with benefits for the periodontal health.

FIG 23 The patient, who has agenesis of the lateral incisors, consulted with the authors following orthodontic treatment aimed at moving the canines to a lateral position and creating sufficient posterior space to accommodate the placement of implants. *(a)* Closing the interdental spaces requires widening of the central incisors as well as lengthening to achieve optimum dental proportion. From the intraoral examination, however, the possibility emerges of an incisal increment limited to roughly 1.0 to 1.5 mm. *(b and c)* After noting that the cementoenamel junction is located subgingivally, the decision is made to perform a gingivectomy with internal bevel to increase the tooth length at cervical level as well. (Surgery by Dr Stefano Gori.) This is necessary to guarantee congruity in tooth proportions. *(d)* After 8 weeks, the central incisors show an increased length of 1 mm. *(e)* In the photograph of the preparations undertaken for positioning six veneers, the presence of enamel can be seen up to the finish line, which guarantees the restorations ideal adhesion. The impressions for the two crowns on the implants at the first premolars are taken at the same time as the impressions for the veneers. *(f to l)* The view of the definitive restorations (veneers: IPS Empress Esthetic, Ivoclar Vivadent; alumina crowns on abutments in zirconium: Procera, Nobel Biocare) shows good esthetic integration overall and adequate respect for the gingival tissues.

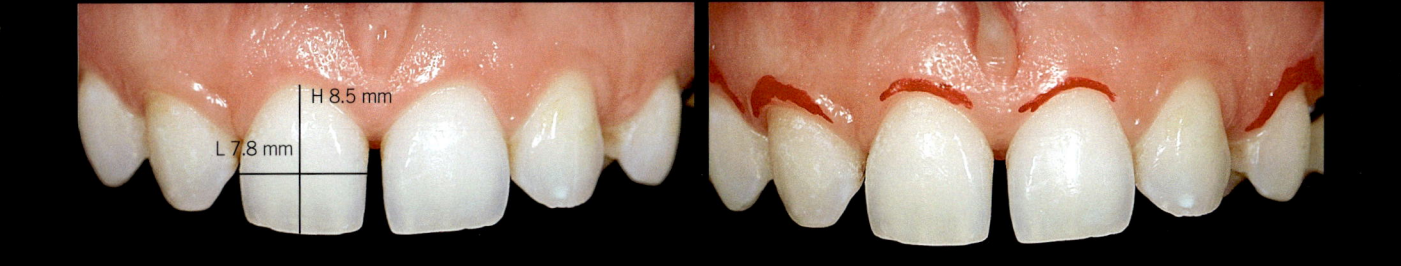

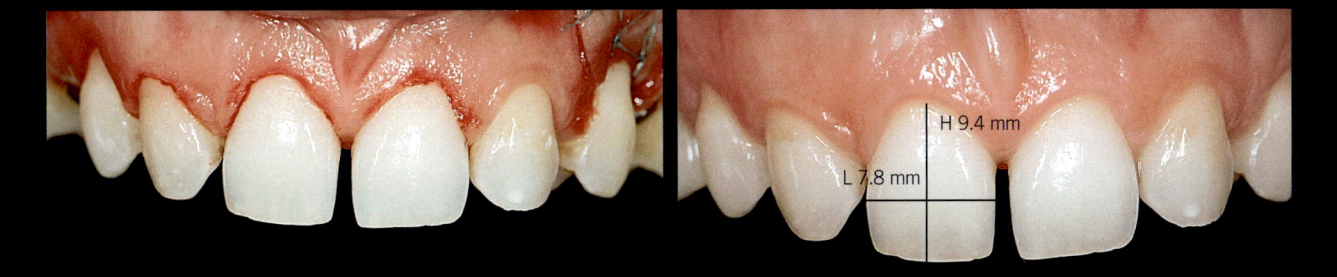

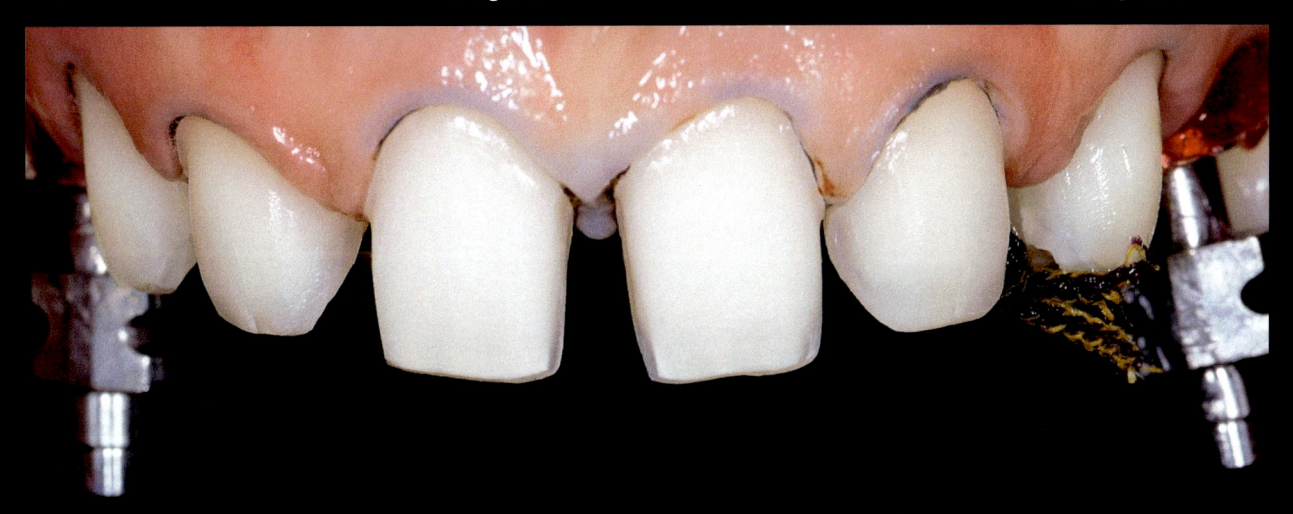

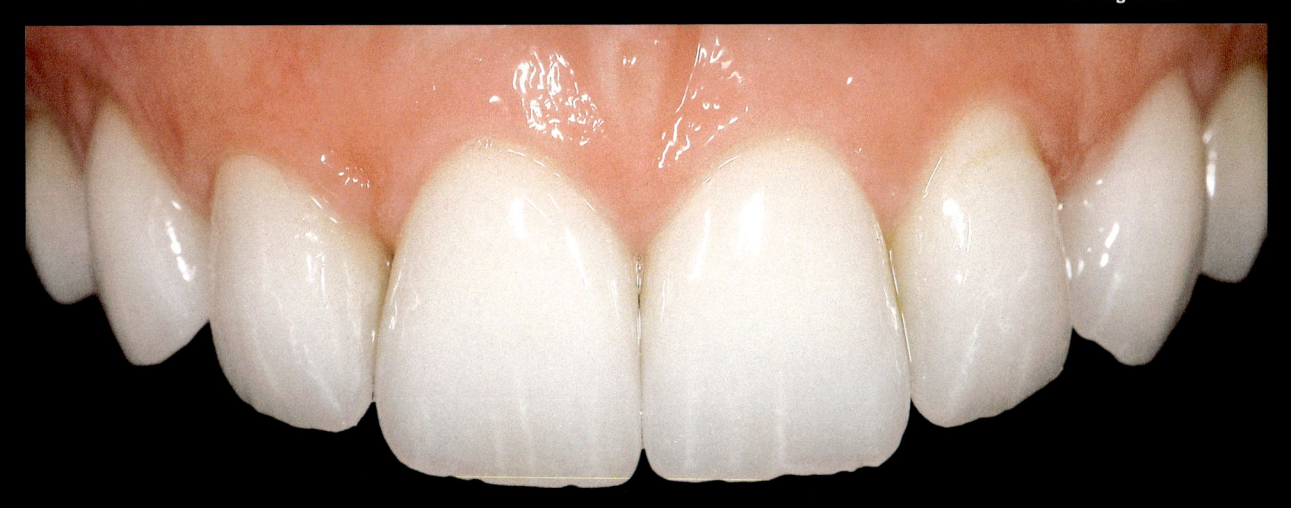

> Fig 3-23a

> Fig 3-23b

> Fig 3-23c

> Fig 3-23d

> Fig 3-23e

> Fig 3-23f

> Fig 3-23g

> Fig 3- 23h

> Fig 3-23i

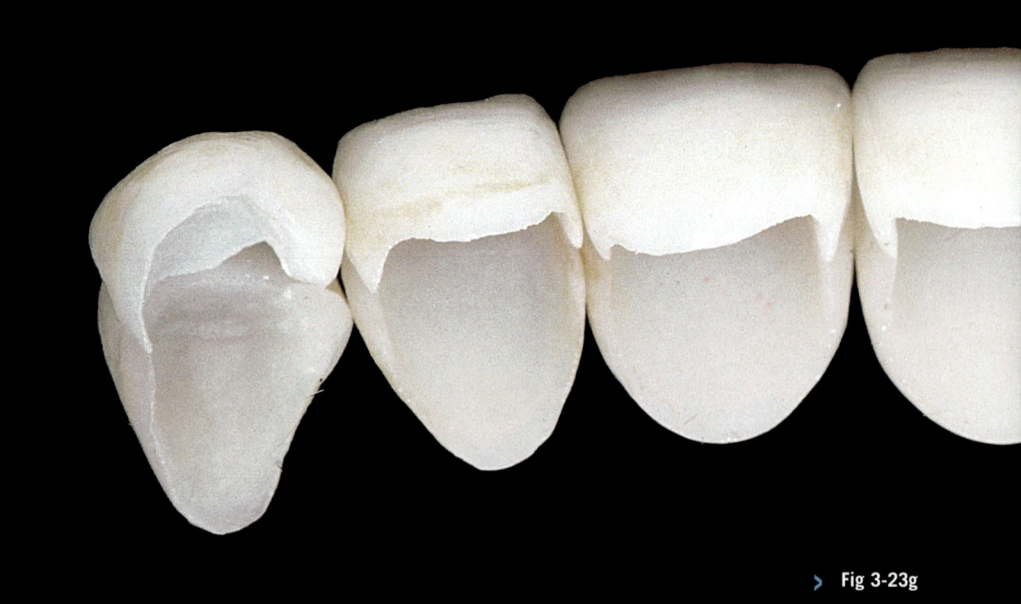

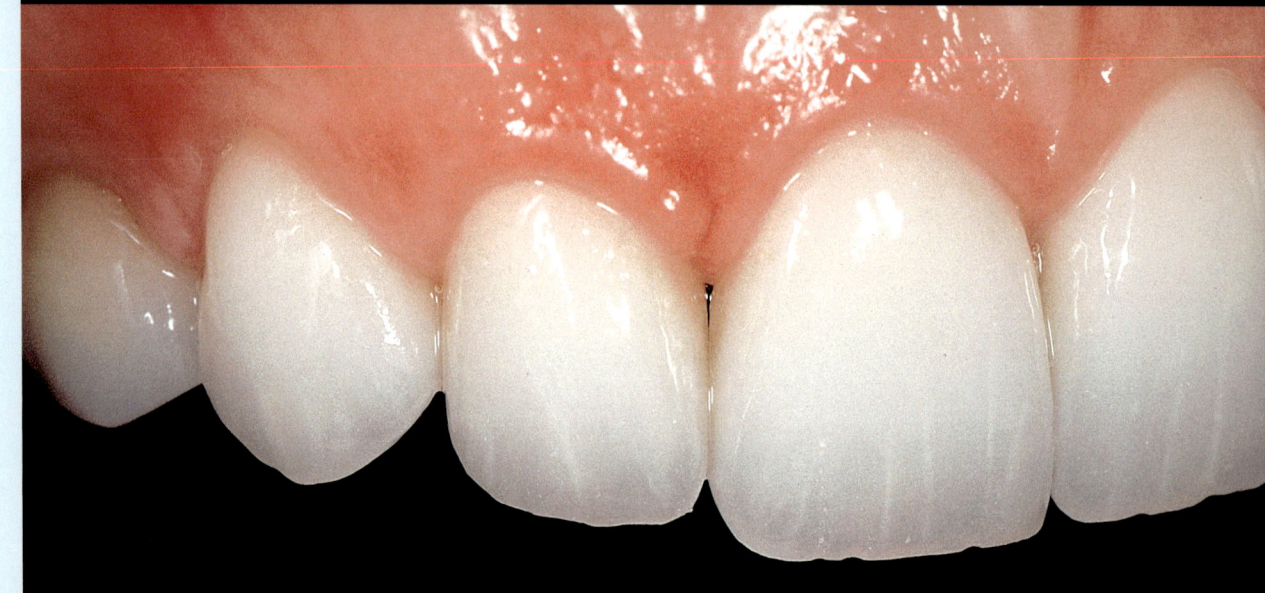

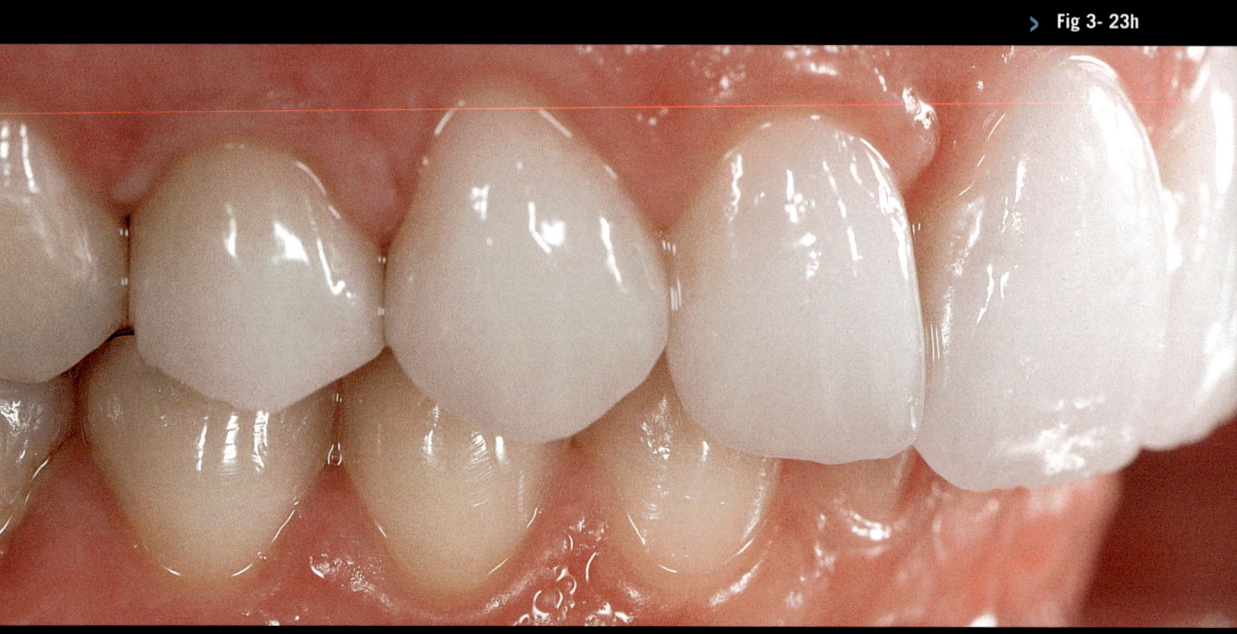

> Fig 3-23j

> Fig 3-23k

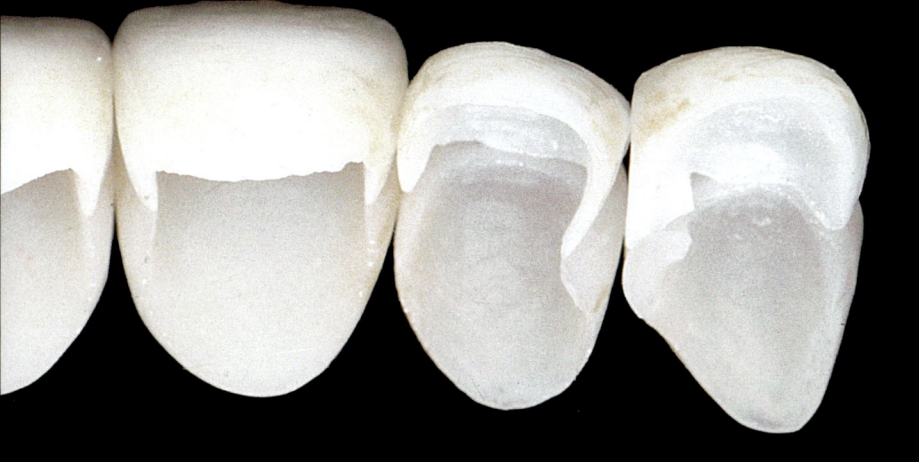

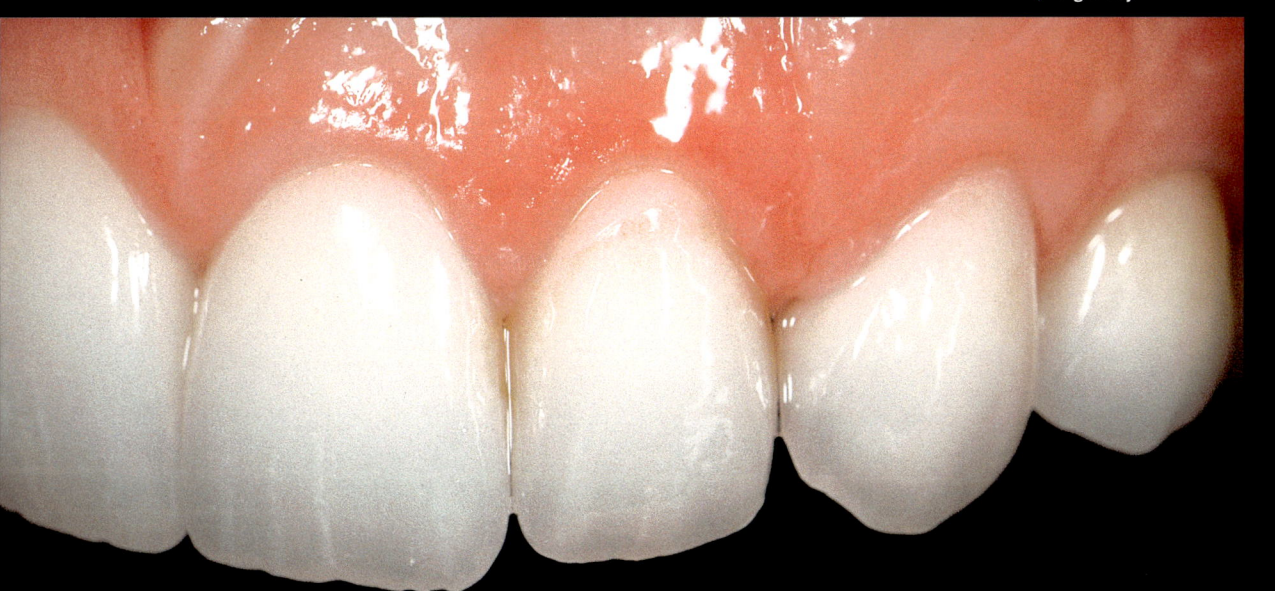

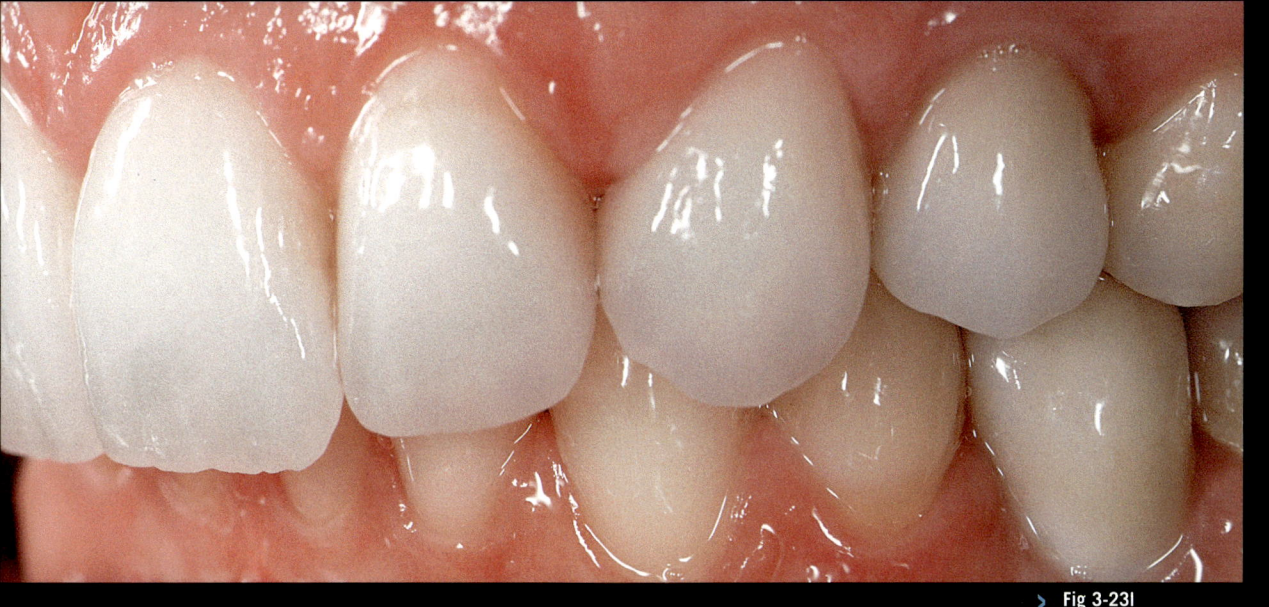

335

> Fig 3-23l

PULP INTEGRITY

Pulp vitality can be compromised by various factors that are directly and indirectly connected to tooth preparation procedures. Among the most frequent culprits are excessive reduction of the abutment with accidental exposure of the pulp, bacterial contamination, chemical agents, and excessive increase in intrapulpal temperature and pressure. The temperature increase to which a vital abutment is exposed during tooth preparation can easily cause pulp damage, stemming from evaporation of the dentinal fluid and variation of the pulp microcirculation. Any temperature increase beyond 41° or 42°C can lead to irreversible damage and even pulp necrosis.[106,107] Following are some useful measures to prevent this occurrence.

Respecting the pulpal anatomy Anatomy and size are aspects of the pulp that vary not only by tooth type but also according to age.[108] In young patients, it is especially advisable not to deepen the preparation by more than 1.0 mm; otherwise, pulp vitality could be compromised because of the reduced thickness of enamel and dentin (Fig 3-24). Consistent incisal/occlusal thickness (2.0 to 2.5 mm) instead allows greater reduction in both anterior and posterior teeth.

In the presence of numerous teeth, it is best to prepare the same sides (eg, the interproximal walls) in sequence on all teeth so as not to concentrate the bur for too long on any one tooth to complete the preparation. This approach makes it easier to reach correct parallelism between the abutments in addition to offsetting the increase in temperature (Fig 3-25).

Irrigating the abutment The atomized jets of air-water spray coming out of the preparation handpiece must be powerful and properly directed onto the tip of the bur (Fig 3-26a). Their job is to limit the rise in temperature and also to prevent the detritus from compacting, which would lead to increased intrapulpal pressure by reducing the cutting efficiency of the fitted tip.[109–113] A further aid can be simultaneous use of the air-water spray by the assistant.

Type of bur If possible, new burs should be used, especially when preparing vital teeth, and they should cut well. The use of diamond burs, which are particularly reliable and efficient at cutting, seems to generate increases in temperature and intrapulpal pressure greater than those produced by the same tools in tungsten carbide.[113] The advantage of the latter type of tool is often cancelled out by its inferior cutting efficiency, however, translating into longer preparation times and greater pressure exerted on the handpiece, with inevitable repercussions to the pulp.

Choosing the handpiece The red-ring handpiece develops a lower temperature increase compared with the turbine, an obvious advantage for pulp integrity.[114] The improved control from the higher torque, combined with greater precision in the finishing stage, makes it the handpiece of choice in fixed prosthodontics (Fig 3-26b).

> Fig 3-24a

> Fig 3-24b

> Fig 3-25a

> Fig 3-25b

> Fig 3-26a

> Fig 3-26b

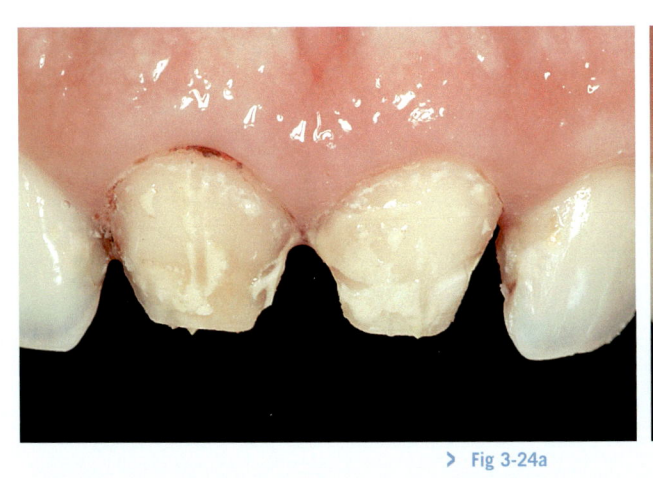

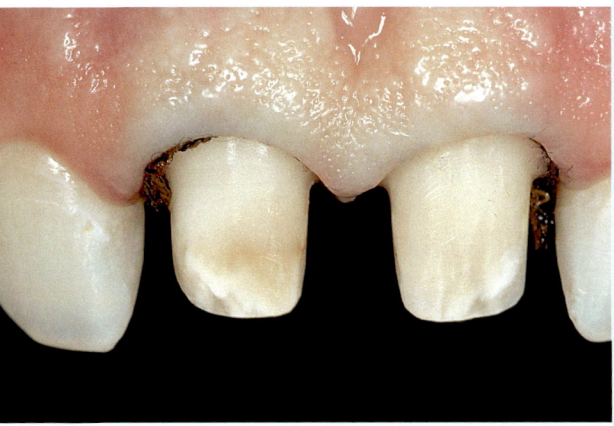

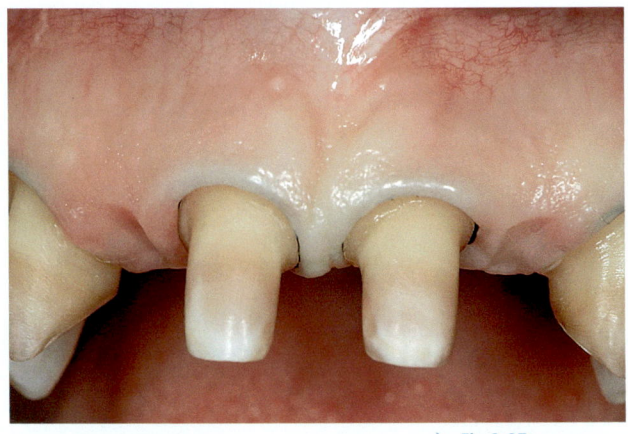

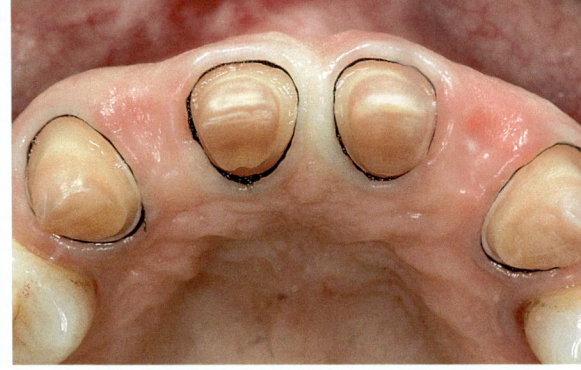

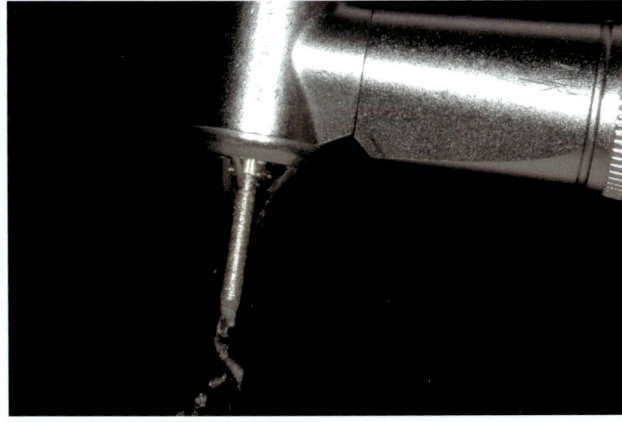

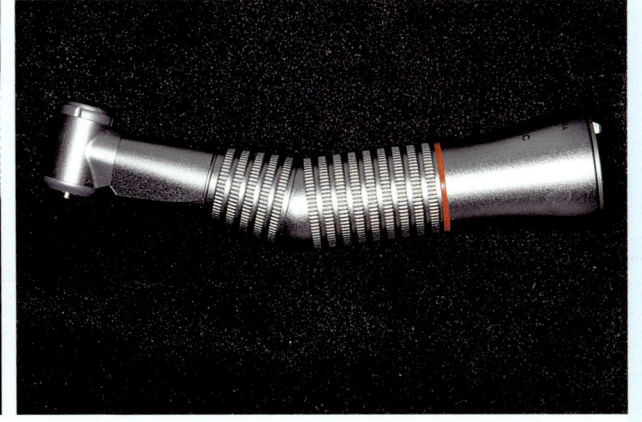

FIG 24 *(a and b)* The insufficient thickness available to accommodate the definitive restorations compels the clinician to modify the abutment preparations of the two central incisors but without causing any biologic compromise of either the pulp or the gingival tissues.

FIG 25 *(a and b)* Interspaced preparation, which counteracts the rise in temperature and thus minimizes the risk of damaging the pulp integrity, is particularly useful for multiple teeth, allowing the parallelism of the abutments to be more easily ascertained.

FIG 26 *(a)* The clinician must check that the handpiece is working properly and above all that the air-water sprays are properly directed onto the end of the bur, to prevent any rise in temperature within the pulp chamber. *(b)* In addition to preventing an excessive increase in temperature, the red-ring contra-angle handpiece is much more efficient and precise than the turbine in the abutment finishing phases.

TOOTH PREPARATION — RESPECTING BIOLOGIC INTEGRITY

GINGIVAL INTEGRITY

The position of the preparation margin in relation to the gingival tissues is a determining factor in maintaining periodontal health. The prosthetic margin can be situated at one of three levels:
- Supragingival
- Gingival crest
- Subgingival

SUPRAGINGIVAL MARGIN

Margins that are positioned supragingivally allow easy inspection of the finishing lines, undoubtedly simplifying all of the operative phases. This type of margin also gives a more favorable biologic response compared with a margin in direct contact with the gingival tissues,[115,116] despite having limitations mainly dealing with esthetics.

Esthetic limitations—Visibility of the prosthetic margin The ever-increasing demands of patients means that visibility of the prosthetic margin can constitute an important esthetic limitation. It should nevertheless be considered that the cervical margin of the restorations is not visible during the patient's normal functions, such as speech and smile (see volume 1, chapter 3).[77,117–125] Furthermore, the use of specific techniques, such as veneers and all-ceramic crowns, today allows the prosthetic margin to be camouflaged effectively even if positioned supragingivally, thanks to the extreme translucency achieved by the most innovative materials. This often makes the margin invisible to the patient's eyes (Fig 3-27).

Esthetic limitations—Presence of large spaces between the anterior teeth Supragingival preparation is not indicated if the patient has large spaces between the anterior teeth that the prosthetic treatment sets out to close. In these cases the clinician must extend the preparation inside the sulcus in order to modify the contour and condition the tissues aimed at resolving the esthetic deficit.

MARGIN AT THE GINGIVAL CREST

Positioning the margin at the gingival crest does not completely eliminate the esthetic limitation because it can still be seen, although not as much as when positioned supragingivally. In addition, it is not an efficient solution for closing large interdental spaces. Positioning the margin at the gingival level is therefore best used in the posterior sectors, where the patient's esthetic demands are not as essential. The skill required in completing all of the prosthetic stages is in this case even more demanding than that required for supragingival positioning. It should be considered that, while no direct periodontal damage is caused because the preparation does not go deep into the sulcus, any imperfect marginal fit and/or overcontours that cause the buildup of plaque can easily lead to gingival inflammation and consequent biologic damage.

FIG 27 *(a)* The young patient has reduced tooth structure caused by chemical erosion from a digestive disorder, which has led to a considerable shortening of the teeth in both arches. *(b and c)* The structural deficit, which is particularly noticeable on the lingual surfaces, means that the teeth involved will need to be covered with crowns.

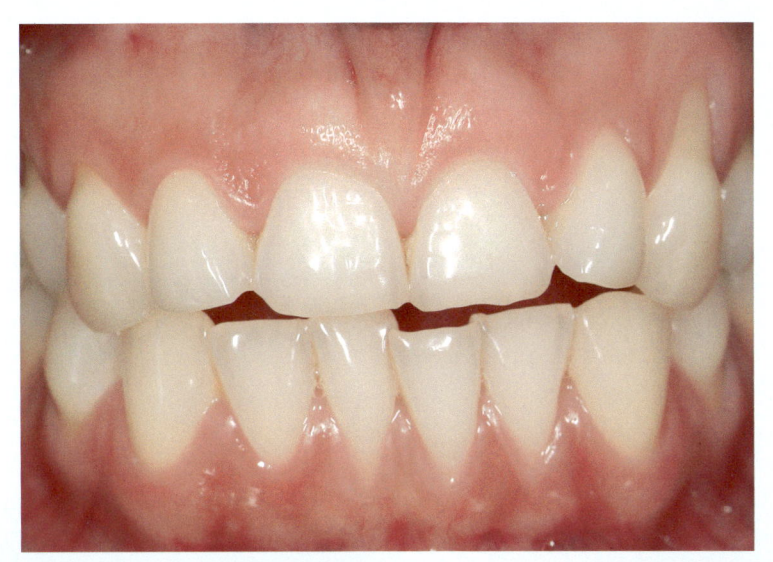

> Fig 3-27a

> Fig 3-27b

> Fig 3-27c

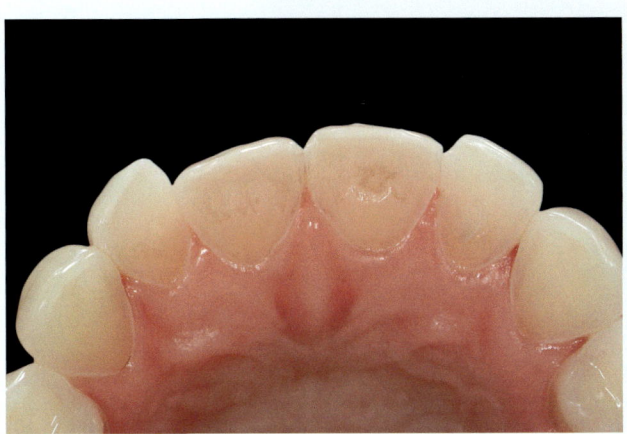

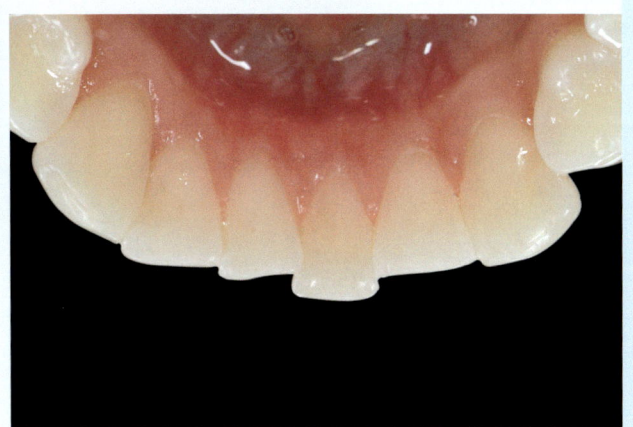

SUPRAGINGIVAL - GINGIVAL MARGIN

INDICATIONS

- Limited esthetic requests
- Cervical margins not visible during speech and smile
- Abutments with sufficient mechanical retention
- Absence of restorations or caries at marginal level
- Use of all-ceramics

ADVANTAGES

- Clinical steps made easier in phases of
  - Tooth preparation
  - Impression taking
  - Relining provisional restorations
  - Checking fit of restoration
- Maintaining periodontal health

DISADVANTAGES

- Visible margin
- Difficult to close interproximal spaces
- Low mechanical retention

> Fig 3-27d

> Fig 3-27e

> Fig 3-27f

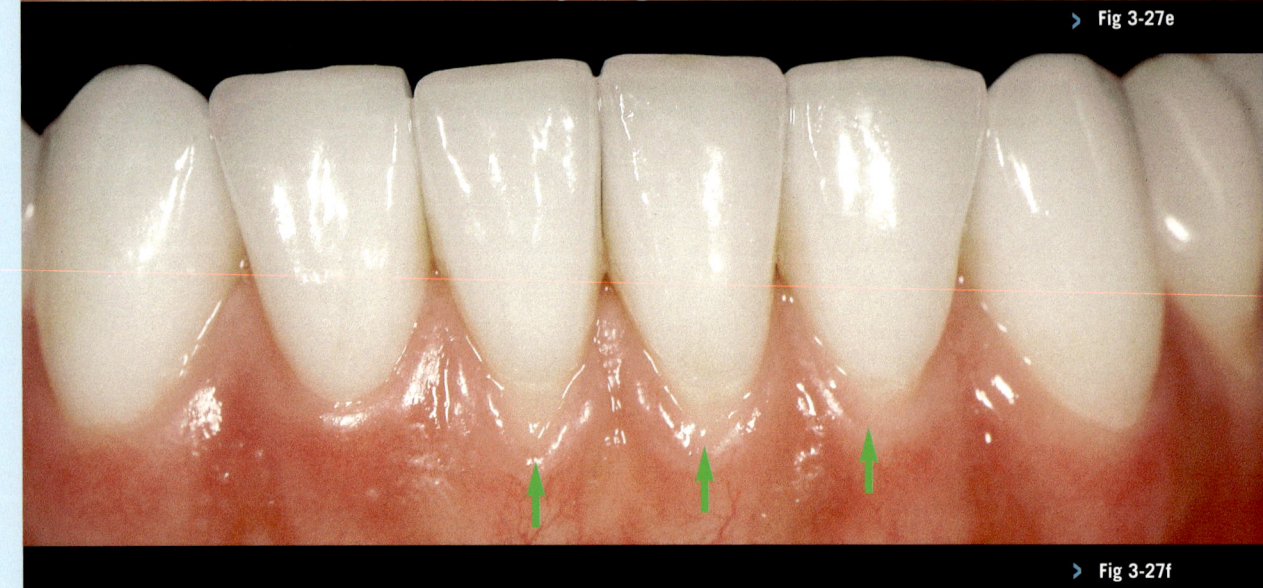

FIG 27 *(d)* The preoperative view of the mandibular teeth highlights the considerable reduction in tooth length. *(e)* The preparations seem particularly conservative, with marginal thicknesses of less than 1 mm. *(f)* In some specific buccal areas, the finish line has been maintained supragingivally *(arrows)* to avoid contact with the extremely thin and delicate soft tissues. Nevertheless, the use of all-ceramics has allowed for definitive restorations that are satisfactorily integrated from the esthetic point of view as well.

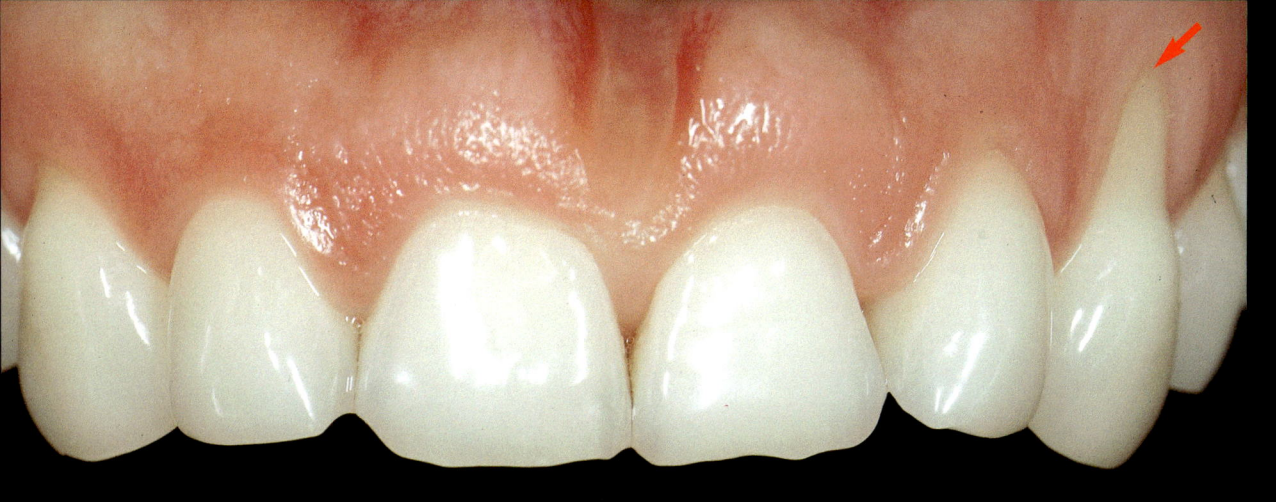

> Fig 3-27g

> Fig 3-27h

> Fig 3-27i

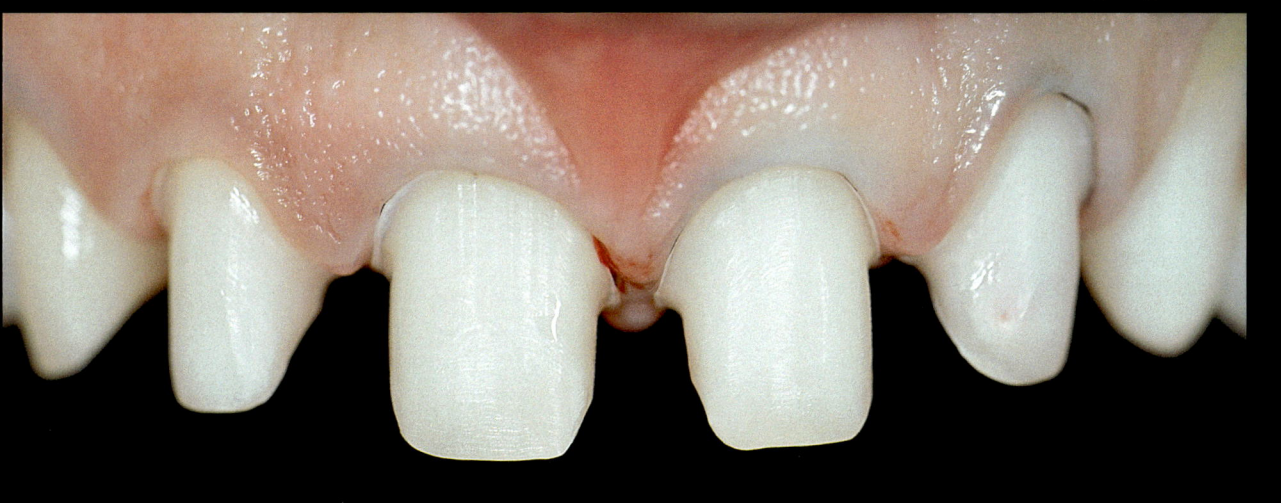

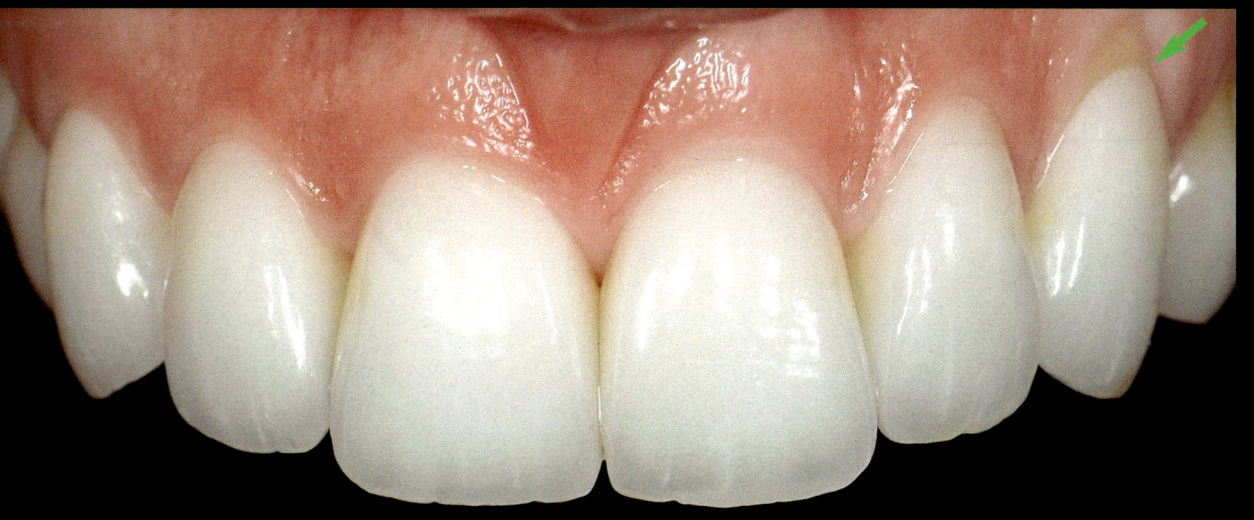

FIG 27 *(g)* In the maxillary arch, in addition to a reduction in the length of the teeth, a substantial gingival recession of the left maxillary canine is also noticeable *(arrow)*. *(h)* Tooth preparations with intrasulcular margins have been completed on all teeth with the exception of the buccal area of the left canine, where the finish line has been purposely maintained in a clearly more supragingival position to prevent any contact with the delicate gingival tissues. *(i)* After cementation, the six anterior restorations show excellent biologic integration and a satisfactory overall esthetic result.

SUBGINGIVAL MARGIN

VIOLATION OF BIOLOGIC INTEGRITY

Today, for esthetic reasons, many clinicians deepen the preparation line into the gingival sulcus to carefully conceal the restoration margin from the eyes of the patient. Although in these cases the esthetic motivation is the justification for the clinical choice made, it has been well-demonstrated that a significant number of individuals do not expose the gingival margins of the anterior teeth even in maximum smile[119–121,125] (see volume 1, chapter 3). Insufficient mechanical retention of the prosthetic abutment, the presence of old restorations, and/or caries lesions that extend beyond the gingival margin often lead the clinician to extend the restoration margin too deep, frequently violating the connective tissue attachment. It is therefore advisable, in these cases, to carry out surgical lengthening of the clinical crown, which ensures sufficient tooth exposure for the prosthetic finalization and thereby avoids excessive deepening of the preparation margin. This is even more appropriate considering the correlation between tissue inflammation and subgingival positioning of the margin, found in many animal as well as human studies.[23,42,61,116,126–138] One of the most common errors is carrying out excessively horizontal tooth preparations in the interproximal areas, which therefore do not follow the natural periodontal architecture that is particularly scalloped in the anterior teeth[4,29] (Fig 3-28) (see volume 1, chapter 6). Valderhaug[139–141] has demonstrated that more than 70% of margins that are subgingival and therefore invisible when the work is delivered are visible after 10 years due to gingival recession. In the presence of an excessively deep preparation margin, irreversible periodontal damage can occur as a result of both violation of the connective tissue attachment and indirect causes such as the following:

- Inadequate marginal closure
- Incorrect coronal contour
- Surface roughness
- Excess cement

These discrepancies and irregularities, which are not easily detected because of concealment by the tissues, encourage the buildup of plaque and therefore an increased pathogenicity that causes inflammation in the subgingival location, damaging the periodontal support. Depending on the thickness of underlying bone and the presence of keratinized gingiva, these restorative defects can lead to different clinical and histologic responses.[28,142] With a thick periodontal biotype, intraosseous pockets can form more easily, accompanied by gingival hyperplasia (Fig 3-29) or slight recession.[8,35] In patients with a thin periodontal biotype, more pronounced gingival recession can instead be observed,[35] which can sometimes limit itself in an apical position.[143]

FIG 28 *(a and b)* One of the most common errors made during abutment preparation is to advance too deep interproximally and not respect the natural dentogingival scalloping.

FIG 29 *(a to d)* Incorrect finish lines or excessive subgingival deepening can easily lead to a pronounced inflammatory reaction.

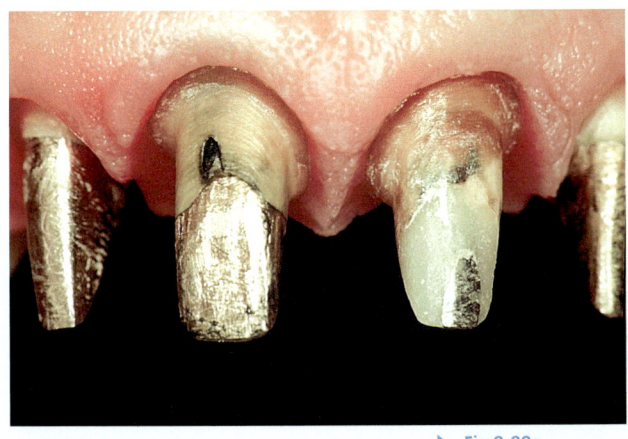

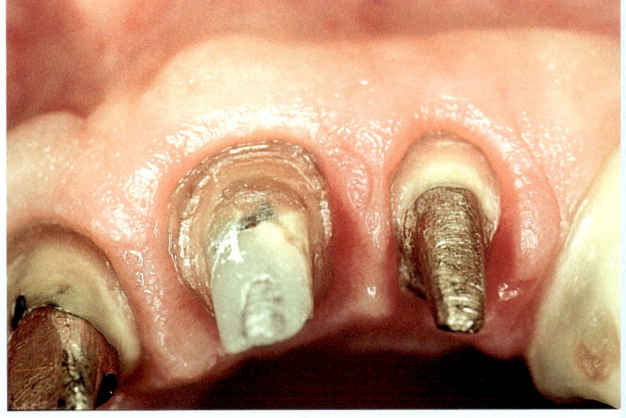

> Fig 3-28a

> Fig 3-28b

> Fig 3-29a

> Fig 3-29b

> Fig 3-29c

> Fig 3-29d

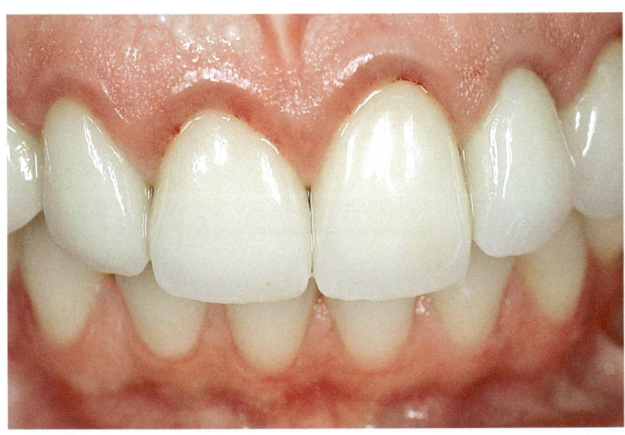

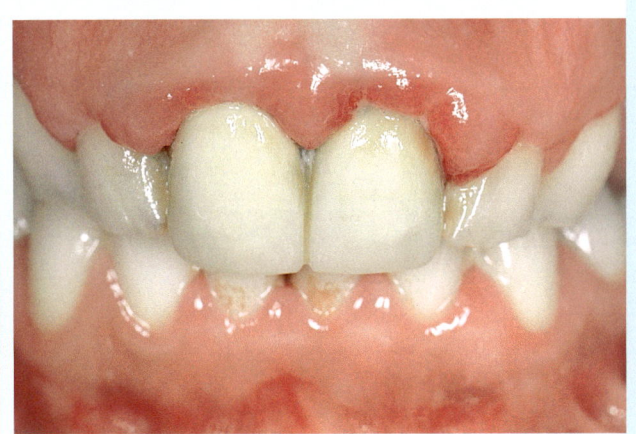

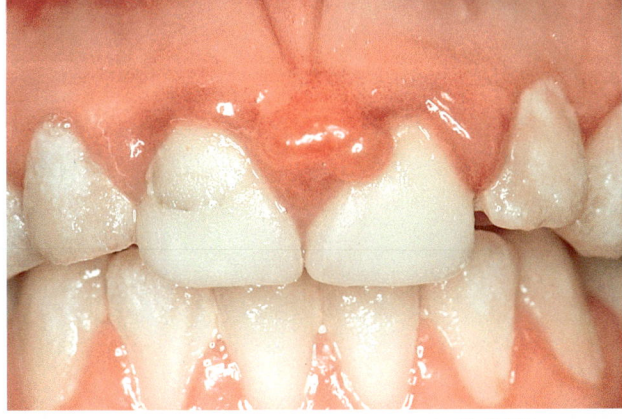

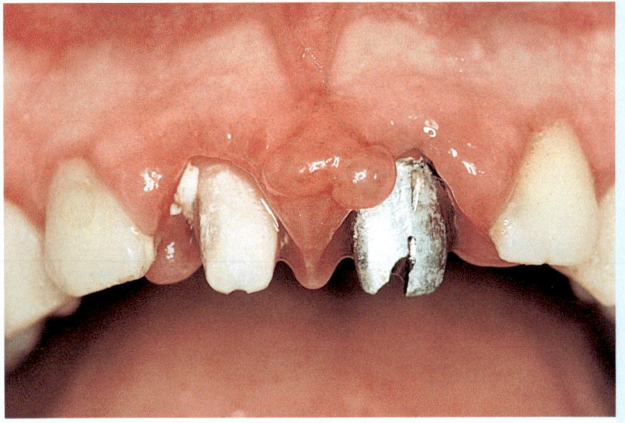

SUBGINGIVAL MARGINS

CONCERNS

- Violation of connective tissue attachment
- Inadequate margins and contours
- Roughness of restorative material to marginal interface
- Presence of excess cement
- Increased pathogenicity of subgingival plaque

SUBGINGIVAL MARGIN

INTRASULCULAR PREPARATION

RESPECT OF BIOLOGIC INTEGRITY

To be able to position the line so it finishes below the gingival margin without causing periodontal damage, the clinician must complete a preparation that, confined within the gingival sulcus, has such an apical extension that it does not damage the epithelial or, more importantly, the connective tissue attachment. The term *intracrevicular* or *intrasulcular margin*[8,62] has been coined to indicate a line that finishes within the gingival sulcus that, while concealing the restoration margin, does not cause any damage to the periodontal structures. During the tooth preparation stages, especially where gingival retraction cords are used, it is not uncommon to find the epithelial attachment inadvertently penetrated. Given the limited number of blood vessels in the epithelial section, this insult to the supporting tissues can usually be reversed[11] as long as the marginal fit of the restorations is appropriate.[127,130,144] Interference with the richly vascularized connective tissue attachment can instead lead to irreversible damage with gingival inflammation, loss of attachment, and the formation of infrabony pockets.[12]

CLINICAL STEPS

The presence of healthy tissue prior to initiation of tooth preparation is essential (see volume 1, chapter 6).[2,8] The procedures described below, which are aimed at achieving a perfectly integrated restoration from an esthetic perspective, must be carried out with total respect for the biologic width, thereby allowing gingival health to be maintained.

MAPPING THE SULCUS

Knowledge of the sulcus depth values makes it possible to establish any intrasulcular extension of the margin needed. The probing depth of each site should be checked (mapping the sulcus) using a periodontal probe, while any bleeding should be noted to exclude current inflammation (Figs 3-30a to 3-30f). A healthy sulcus normally shows a shallow depth (0.5 to 1.0 mm) in the buccal area,[9,10] while greater values are usually found both lingually (1.0 to 2.0 mm) and interproximally (1.0 to 3.0 mm). It is therefore paradoxical that a more shallow probing depth is normally found precisely in the buccal area, where the greatest esthetic demands are recognized, with the consequent difficulty of hiding restorative margins effectively. The increased sulcus depth noticeable in the interproximal areas, however, turns out to be useful in cases where the unesthetic black triangles must be closed.

FIG 30 *(a to f)* Before finalizing the tooth preparation intrasulcularly, a periodontal probe is used to measure the probing depth in order to determine which type and diameter of retraction cord should be used for the specific patient. In addition to verifying the absence of bleeding and hence inflammation, probing at the maxillary central incisor level shows the depth of the sulcus to be approximately 0.5 mm in the buccal areas, deepening by roughly 1.0 mm interproximally. These rather modest values, while assuring the clinician of the patient's periodontal health, should still be taken into consideration to avoid exerting excessive pressure while inserting the cords, in an attempt to fully contain them within the sulcus.

→ ...from page 169

CASE 1

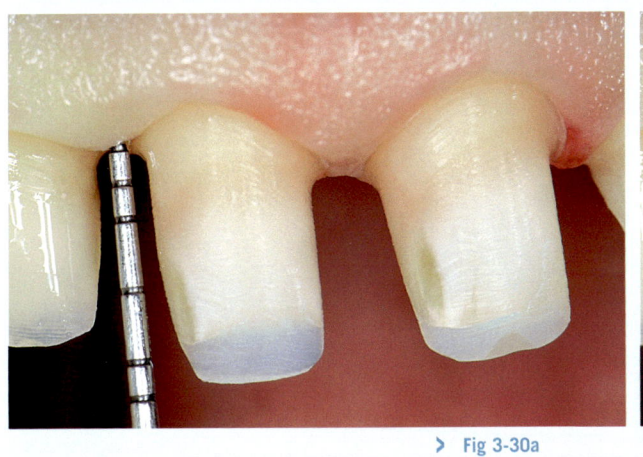

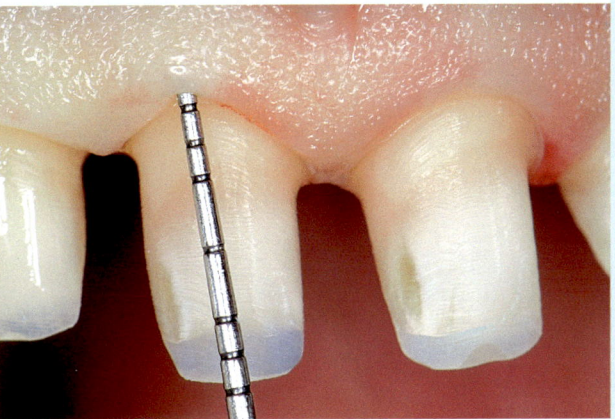

> Fig 3-30a

> Fig 3-30b

> Fig 3-30c

> Fig 3-30d

> Fig 3-30e

> Fig 3-30f

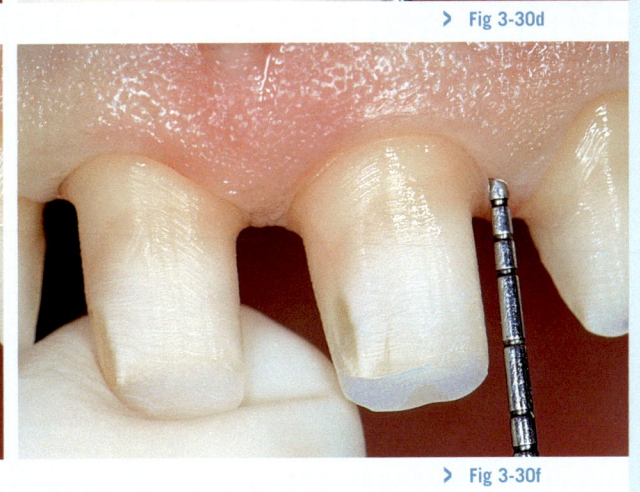

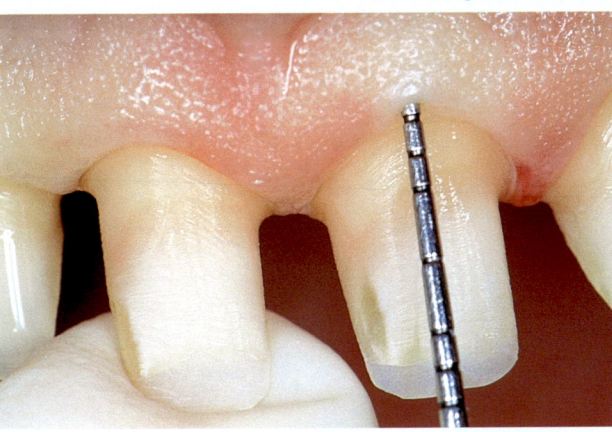

345

INTRASULCULAR PREPARATION

ADVANTAGES

- Esthetic optimization
- Modification of tooth contour and closing interproximal spaces
- Increase in mechanical retention
- Invisible margin

PREPARATION AT THE GINGIVAL LEVEL

Definitive preparation of the prosthetic abutments must be undertaken while scrupulously checking the thicknesses, on the buccal as well as the lingual side, with the aid of a transparent index or silicone matrix (see chapter 2, pages 130–133). The marginal finish line must be positioned at gingival level, almost flush with the sulcular epithelium but without interfering with the tissues underneath (Fig 3-30g).

INSERTING THE CORD

Only after completing the "mapping" is the knitted cord (Ultrapak, Ultradent), of suitable diameter for its size and tonicity, inserted into the sulcus (Fig 3-30h). The healthier the tissues and the more shallow the probing depth, the thinner the cord required. Minimal pressure must be exerted on insertion to avoid injuring the connective tissue attachment.[10,145] Only if the final impression is taken in the same session can the cord be impregnated with chemical agents to encourage the sulcus to expand.[146-151] This expedient is not applied if the purpose of using the retraction cord is strictly to mechanically position the limit of the preparation intracrevicularly, leaving the impression-taking to a later stage. Inserting the cord creates a temporary gingival retraction as well as a slight expansion of the sulcus. The margin in the buccal area should at this point be easily visible because the tissues apicalize by roughly 0.2 to 0.5 mm, directly proportional to the depth of the sulcus and to the diameter of the cord inserted. In the interproximal areas, the greater sulcular depth frequently requires an additional cord to be inserted to achieve greater tissue dislocation in the apical direction, if deepening of the preparation even more is desired to achieve adequate tissue conditioning with the provisional restoration.

PREPARATION AT THE NEW GINGIVAL LEVEL

The margins must, at this point, be prepared again to the new gingival level (Fig 3-30i). This deepening is often limited to the buccal area and, if the restorative contour is to be modified, extended to the interproximal site, often saving the lingual area. During this second marginal preparation, the cord acts as an efficient barrier to protect the base of the sulcus and also to prevent the bur from interfering with the gingival tissues. With a thin periodontal biotype, particular care must be taken to avoid excessive deepening in the buccal areas, which could encourage irreversible recession.

INTRASULCULAR PREPARATION
STEPS

- Prepare at level of gingival crest
- Map the sulcus to select the size and type of cord
- Insert cord appropriate for the depth and tonicity of the sulcus
- Prepare again to the new apicalized gingival level
- Remove the cord and re-margin the provisional restoration

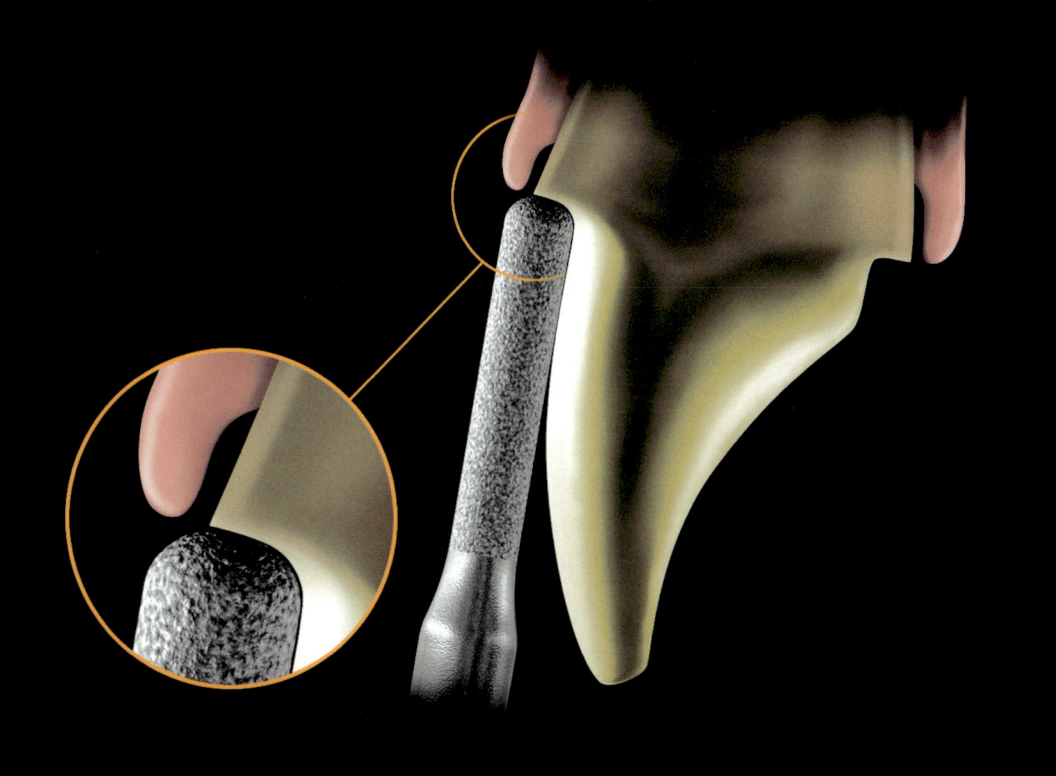

> Fig 3-30g

> Fig 3-30h

> Fig 3-30i

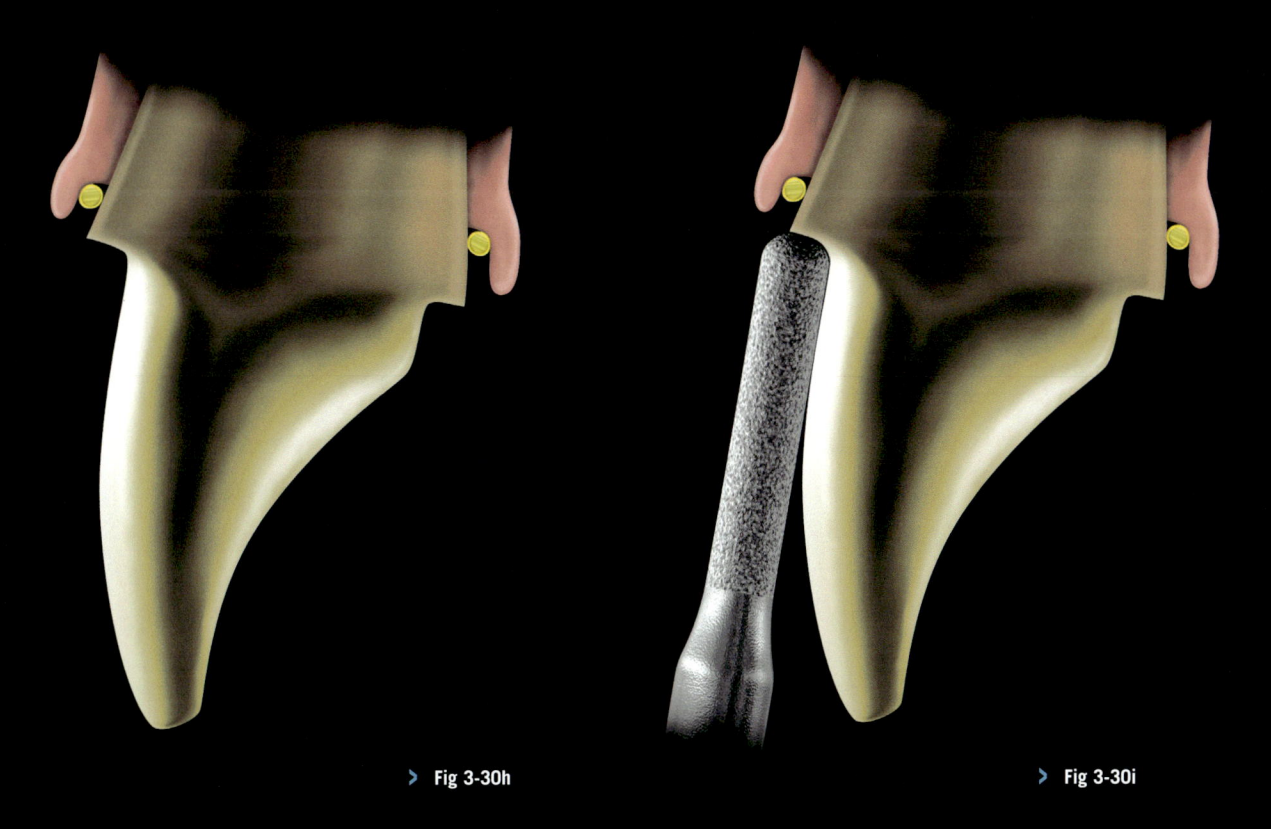

FIG 30 *(g)* The clinician finalizes tooth preparation at the marginal level using a bur of adequate shape and size for the chosen restorative objective, keeping it level with the gingival crest so as not to interfere with the surrounding tissues. *(h)* The cord is then inserted into the sulcus, which causes the gingival levels to shift apically, meaning that the preparation margin will be supragingival. *(i)* The preparation is, at this point, deepened to the new apicalized level of the gingival margin.

In the anterior teeth, the conical shape and the progressive inclination of the roots in the lingual direction frequently cause the buccal margin to shrink following apical deepening of the preparation. This occurrence must be carefully checked and evaluated. The choice to restore the original marginal thickness requires axial adjustment of the preparations, with a further reduction in the diameter of the prosthetic abutment.

FINISHING

The marginal area, at this point, is finished with fine-grained diamond or tungsten carbide burs homologous with those used to reduce the abutment (Figs 3-30j and 3-30k) or using specific rotary or manual instruments that allow cutting to be restricted to the marginal area.

REMOVING THE CORD AND RELINING THE PROVISIONAL RESTORATION

The authors habitually postpone taking the final impressions until a few weeks after the preparations, to check the tissue response to intrasulcular positioning of the prosthetic margins and to exclude inflammatory reactions.[8] Preparation at the new gingival level necessarily involves relining of the provisional restoration, which can be done before or after removing the cords. The cords should not remain in the sulcus for more than 30 minutes, even if they are unmedicated, to avoid tissue damage.[152] Maintaining the cords in situ obviously allows an easier and more precise marginal reading, but this could be impaired by collapse of the tissues when the cords are removed. The number of abutments prepared again using the cords, as well as calculation of the overall time used for deepening the margin and remargining the provisional restoration, indicates to the clinician the most suitable choice between immediate or delayed removal of the cords. Once the cord is removed (Fig 3-30l), the healthy tissue returns to its original level (Fig 3-30m), in a more coronal position than the marginal limit by roughly 0.2 to 0.5 mm in the buccal area, and sometimes by a significantly greater distance at interproximal level, thereby allowing the restorative margin to remain totally invisible (Figs 3-30n to 3-30q).

After relining, the thicknesses of the acrylic prosthesis should be checked with a caliper. Functional parameters such as the occlusal stability and the excursive movements must also be checked again, along with all of the esthetic parameters already optimized when the provisional restoration was inserted. This careful check allows the clinician to avoid substantial refinements before taking the final impressions 3 to 4 weeks later, during the final check on integration of the provisional restoration (see chapter 4, pages 374–381).

FIG 30 *(j to l)* Once deepening is complete and the new prosthetic margin has been defined, the cord is removed. *(m)* In the presence of healthy tissue, the gingival margin will resume its original position, collapsing in a coronal direction beyond the new preparation margin, which will then become intrasulcular and hence invisible. *(n)* After the cord insertion, the gingival levels undergo a slight apicalization. *(o)* The preparations are then deepened to the new gingival level with a finishing bur. *(p)* Once the cord is removed from the sulcus and with the provisional relining complete, it is easy to see the tissues resume a more coronal position in relation to the marginal finishing line. *(q)* From the occlusal view it is easier to see the intrasulcular placement of the preparation margin.

Fig 3-30j

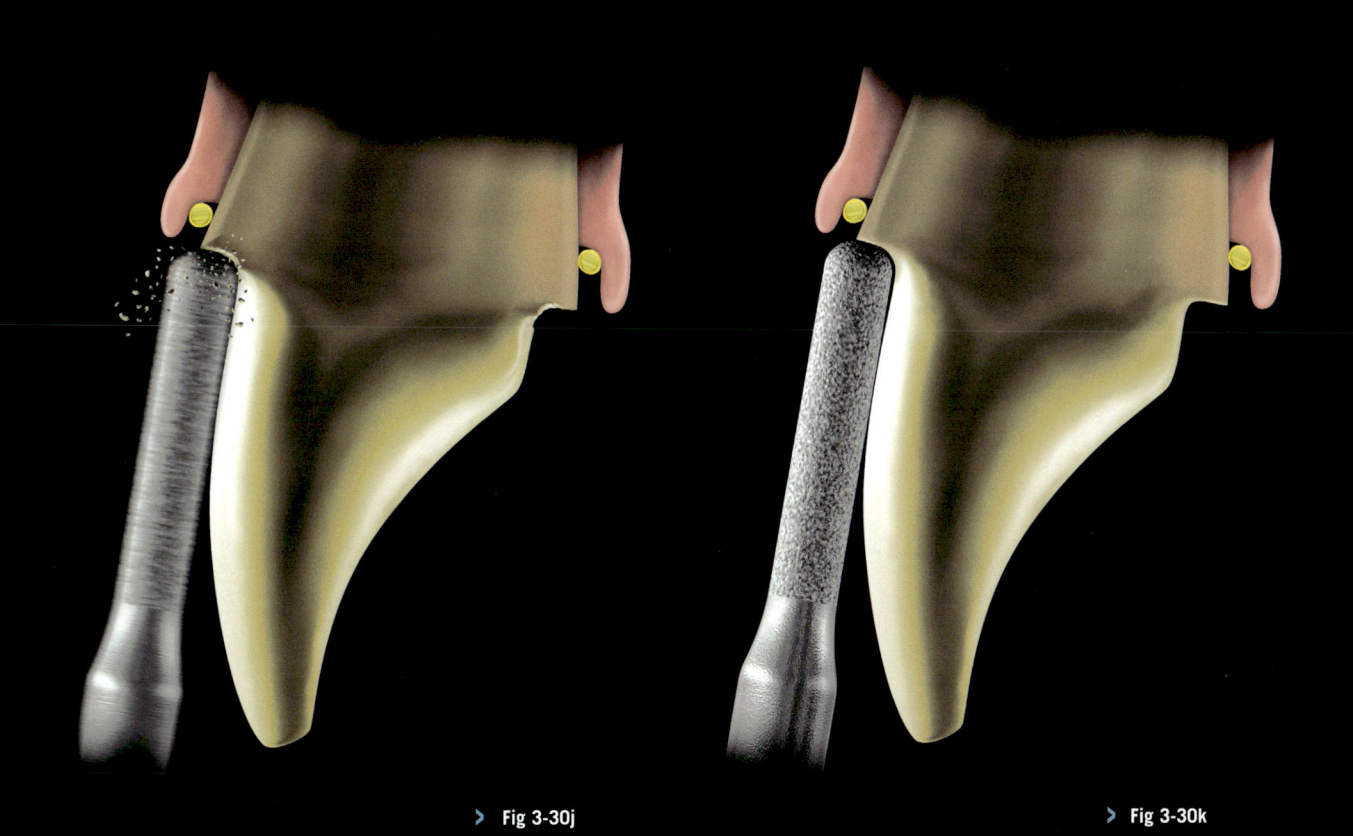

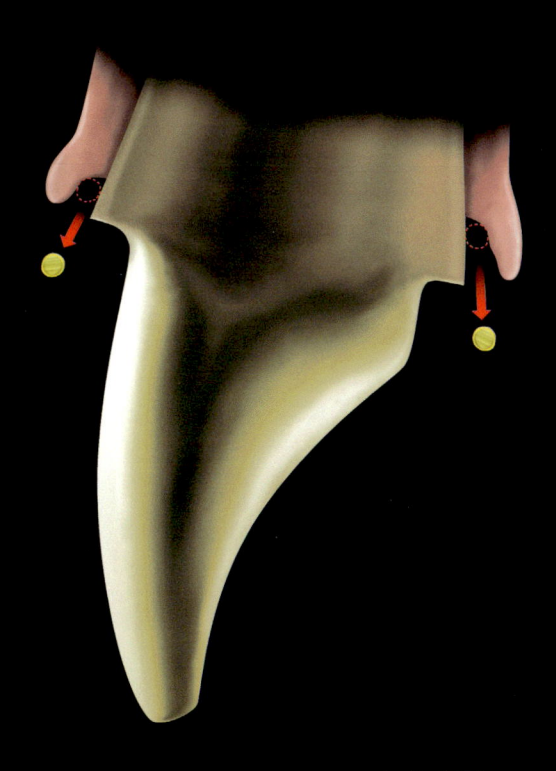

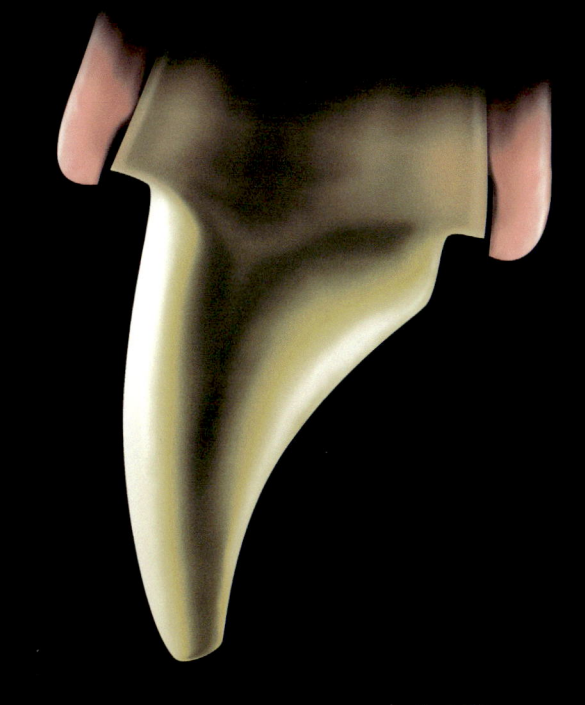

Fig 3-30k

Fig 3-30l

Fig 3-30m

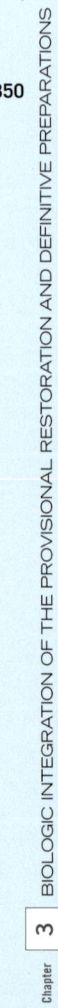

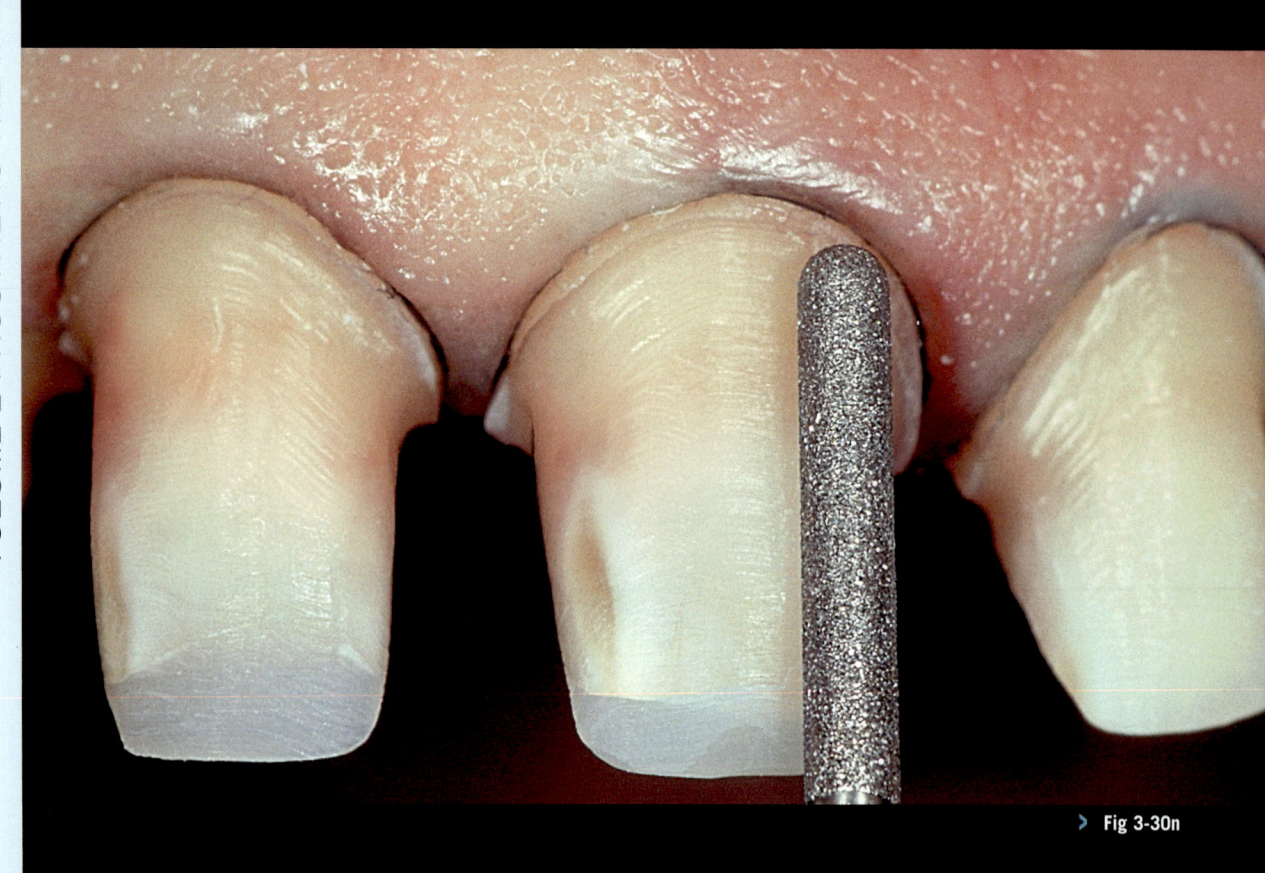

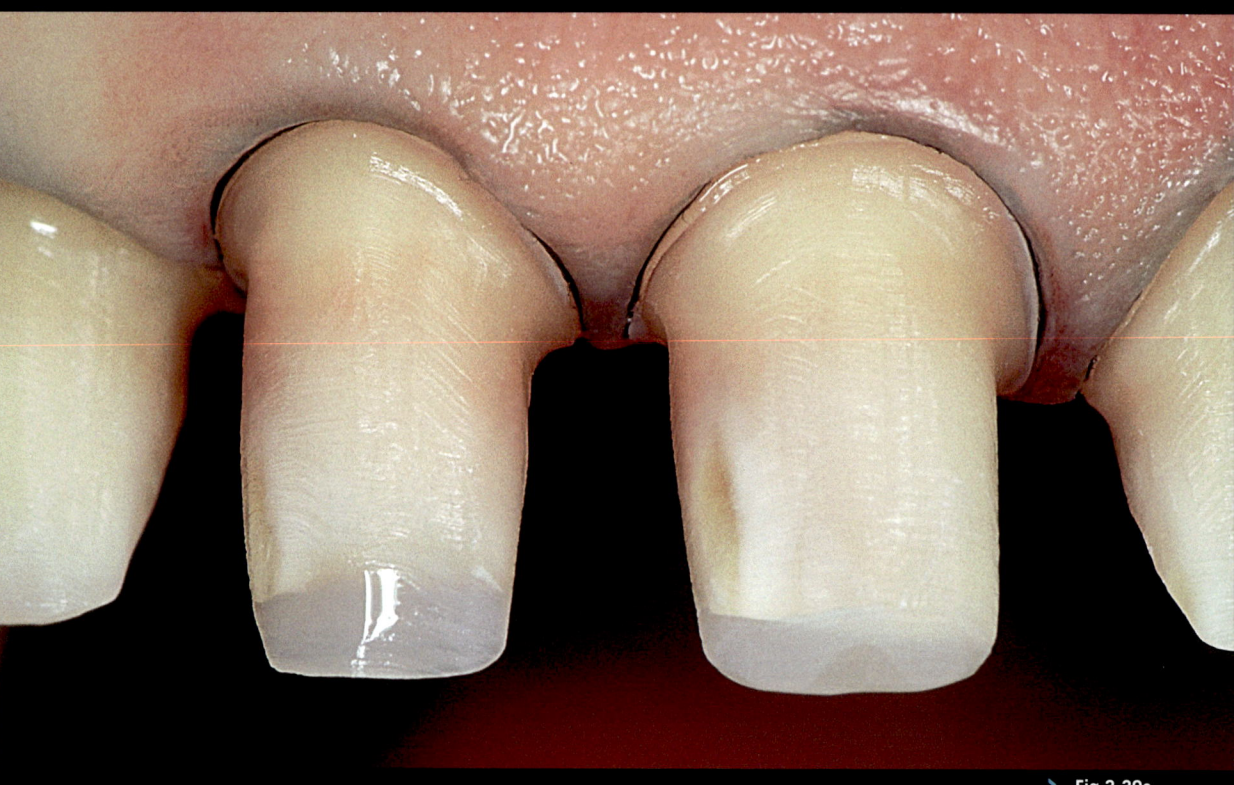

> Fig 3-30n

> Fig 3-30o

> Fig 3-30p

> Fig 3-30q

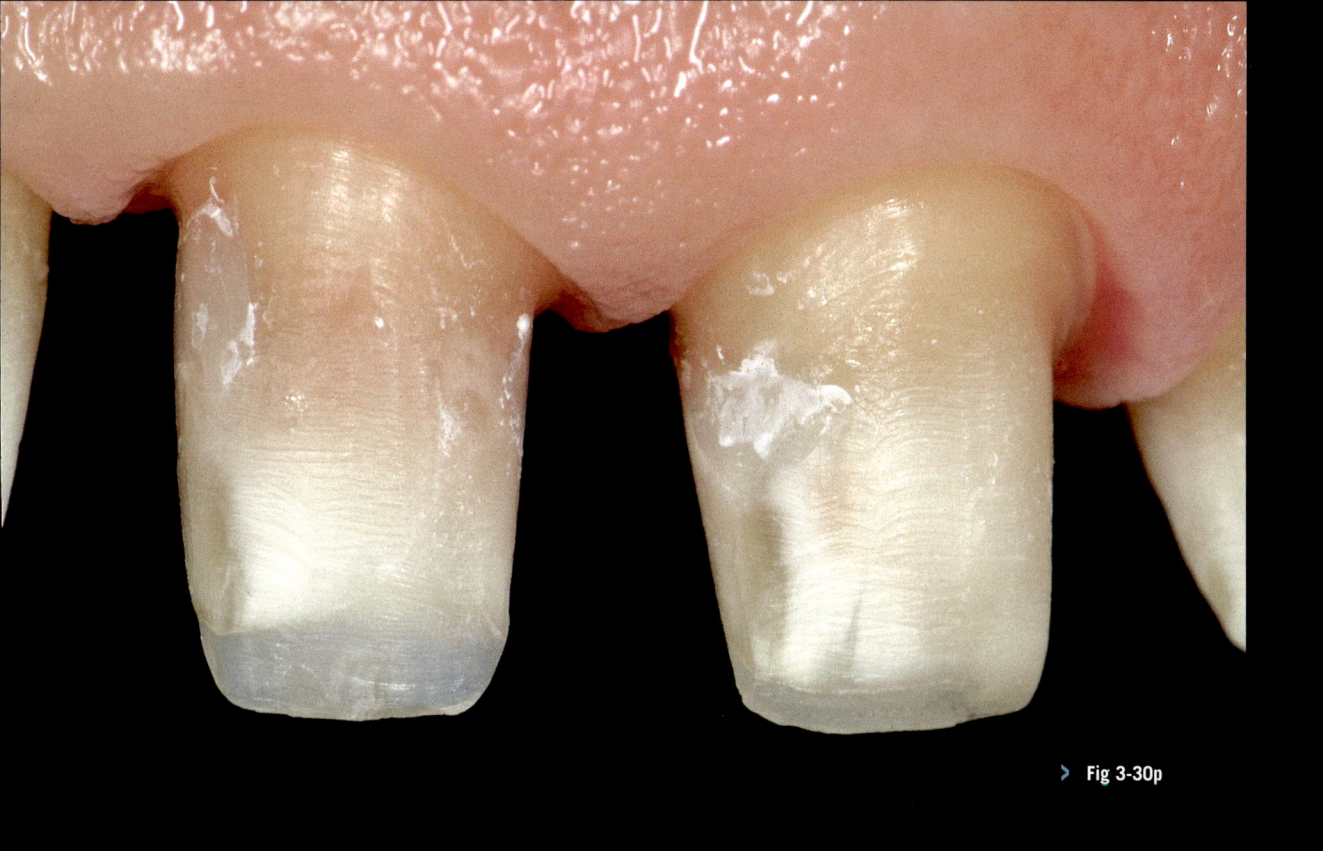

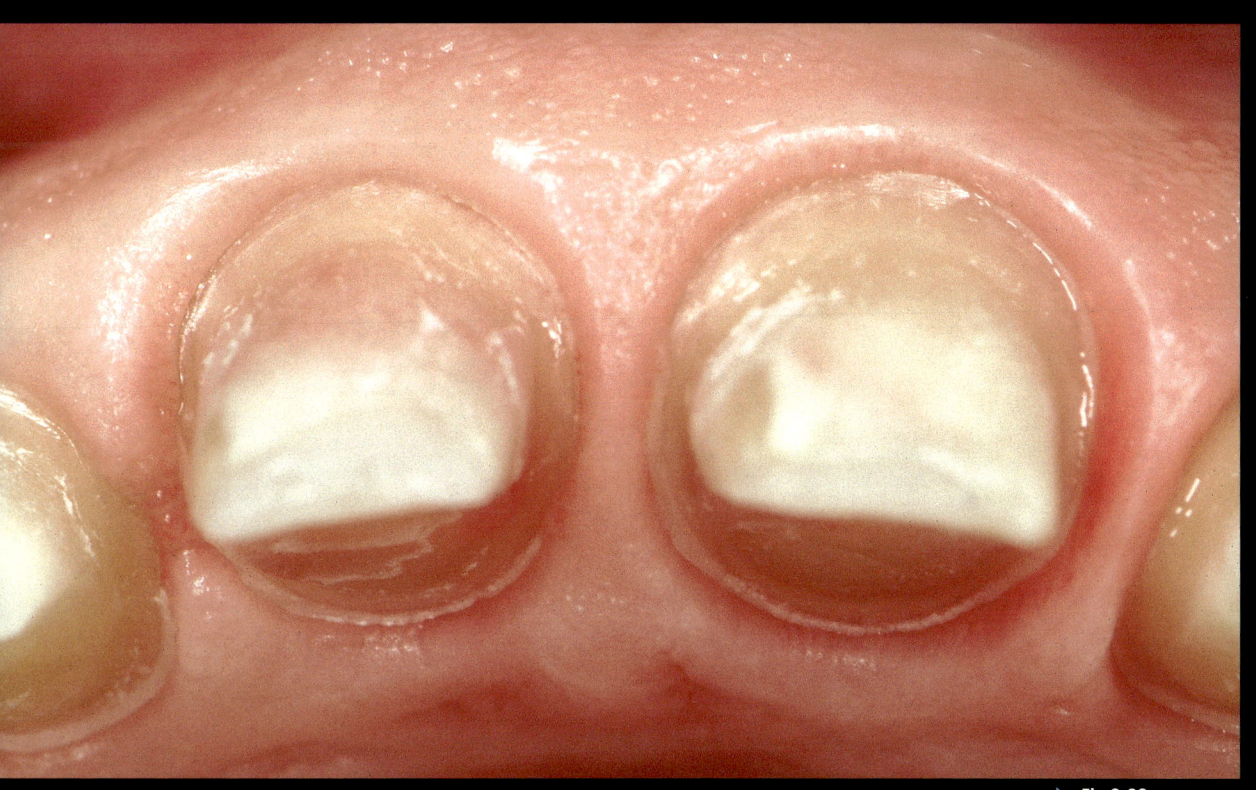

Case 1 → continues on page 377

BIOLOGIC INTEGRATION

IMPLANT-PROSTHETIC THERAPY

PERI-IMPLANT SOFT TISSUES

Maintaining osseointegration and the stability of the marginal alveolar ridge over time assumes that a healthy state of the peri-implant soft tissues has been formed and conserved.[153,154] In addition to playing a primary role in achieving the ideal esthetic outcome, the soft tissues represent a fundamental defensive barrier for preserving the integrity of the bone-implant interface. The peri-implant mucosa serves exactly the same function as that of the supracrestal gingival tissues[155] and, in the same way, it is made up histologically of three different components[156] that collectively occupy a minimum of 3 mm of biologic space coronally to the marginal edge.[157,158] These three histologic entities comprise two structures of an epithelial nature, whose height extension amounts to at least 2 mm, and a connective tissue, whose minimum vertical dimension is about 1 mm.[157] The characteristics of the individual components of what is defined as *peri-implant biologic width* are discussed in more detail below[155] (Figs 3-31 and 3-32).

Sulcular epithelium This component faces the surface of the implant abutment and prosthetic restoration without establishing any type of bond with it.

Junctional epithelium This component is able to establish, through hemidesmosomes, an attachment with surfaces in titanium or in alumina-based sintered ceramic[159] and in zirconium,[160] but not with surfaces in gold alloy or in glass-ceramic.

Supracrestal connective tissue This component is considerably different from the connective tissues of the dentogingival complex since it possesses the following:

- A lower number of fibroblasts (roughly 2% versus about 10%)
- A greater number of collagen fibers (90% versus 65%)
- Collagen fibers that are mainly oriented parallel or circumferential relative to the implant axis. Recently, some authors[161] have also documented the presence of collagen fibrils set out perpendicular to the implant surface and inserted into its micropores. This anchorage, achieved due to the rough surface of titanium oxide (TiUnite, Nobel Biocare), could improve the adhesive capacity of the mucosa.
- Poor vascularization: In particular, the vascular network that originates in the periodontal ligament is missing.[162]

From these histologic observations come important biologic implications that lead toward well-defined clinical behaviors.

FIG 31 A, Sulcular epithelium. B, Junctional epithelium. C, Supracrestal connective tissue. Note the circular collagen fibers in the cross-section.

FIG 32 Clinical photograph of the peri-implant tissues with transmucosal path suitably conditioned by an appropriately designed provisional restoration.

> Fig 3-31

> Fig 3-32

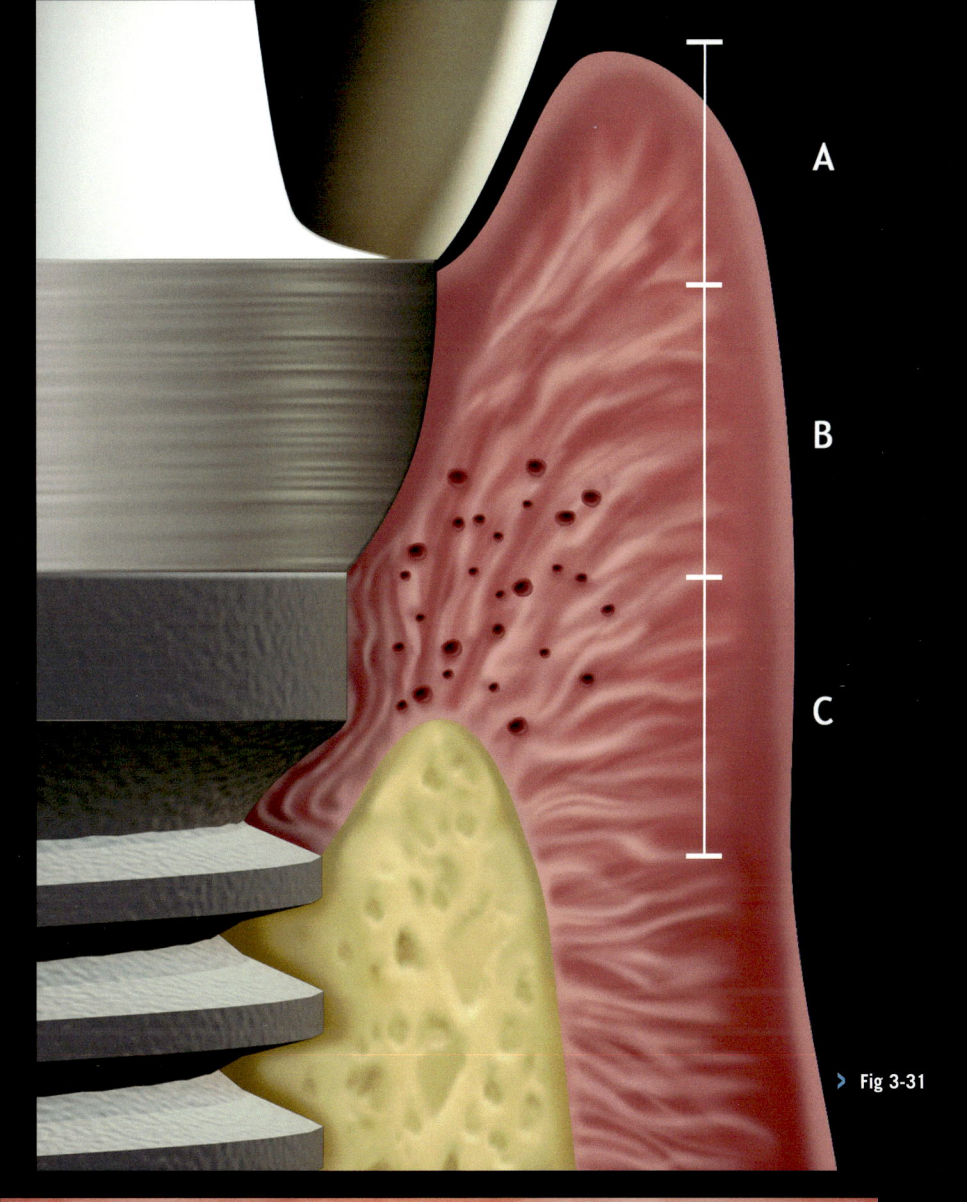

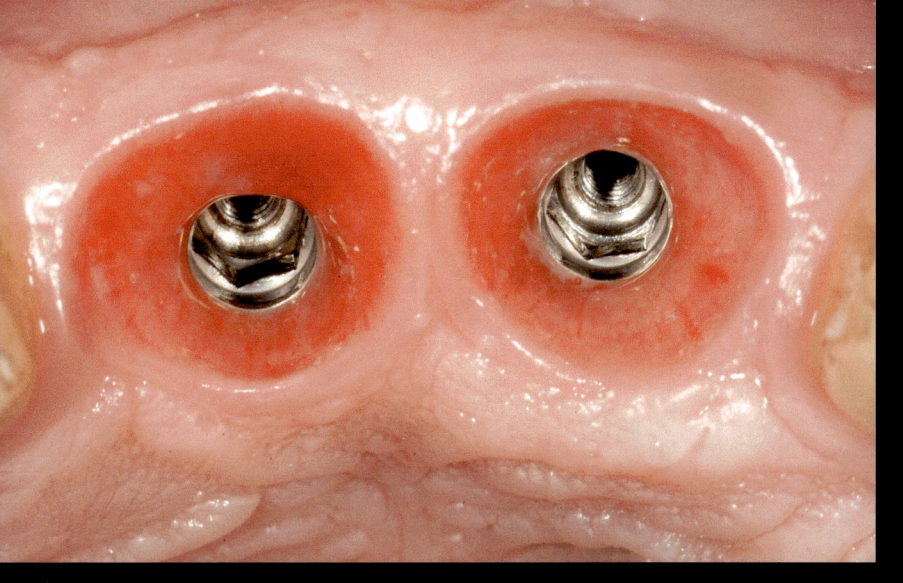

BIOLOGIC IMPLICATIONS

Poor vascularization and reduced cellularity make the peri-implant mucosa less reactive and less efficient regarding damage defense and repair mechanisms.[163] The peri-implant soft tissues respond to the buildup of recently formed plaque in a manner similar to that of the gingival tissues,[164] with the same type of cause-effect relationship and the same microbiologic composition.[165] In the case of persistent buildup of plaque, however, a more apical extension of inflammatory cellular infiltration takes place.[166] According to experimental studies,[167] this inflammatory response is associated with more pronounced tissue destruction, and extends to the bone if the buildup of plaque is associated with a lesion of the peri-implant tissues. With the noxious pathogen removed, the peri-implant tissue does not always manage to encapsulate the inflammatory lesion and render it inactive, in this way demonstrating less capacity for limiting and repairing the damage.[168]

CLINICAL BEHAVIOR

3D management of the implant

Three-dimensional positioning of the implant should involve the retention or regeneration of at least 2.0 mm thickness of the buccal osseous table to prevent possible gingival recession.[169–171] A minimum distance of 3.0 mm between implants[172–174] and a distance of 1.5 mm between tooth and implant also must be maintained[172,173,175,176] (Fig 3-33). Observing these parameters not only prevents interproximal marginal ridge resorption, with consequent papillae recession, but also facilitates interproximal hygiene measures, thereby encouraging appropriate plaque control. For the same reason, it is important during the prosthetic, provisional, or definitive function phase to take maximum care so that the architecture of the soft tissues and the contour of the restorative prostheses permit ideal hygiene maintenance (Figs 3-34a to 3-34d).

FIG 33 Diagram of the minimum natural tooth–implant distance (1.5 mm) and of the minimum distance (3 mm) between implants, which is necessary for maintaining the interproximal osseous peaks.

FIG 34 *(a)* Occlusal view immediately following surgical extraction of the lateral incisor. A postextraction implant is inserted in this site immediately next to the previously positioned implant at the right maxillary central incisor. *(b and c)* The provisional restoration, anchored solely to the central incisor, has a pontic unit on the lateral incisor, which is not in contact with the healing abutment. *(d)* After roughly 6 months, it is apparent that the papilla between the implants has been preserved, promoted by the combination of an adequate distance between the two implants (> 3 mm) and the ideal level of the connective tissue attachment of the lateral incisor present at the time of extraction.

> 1.5 mm   > 3 mm   > 1.5 mm

> Fig 3-33

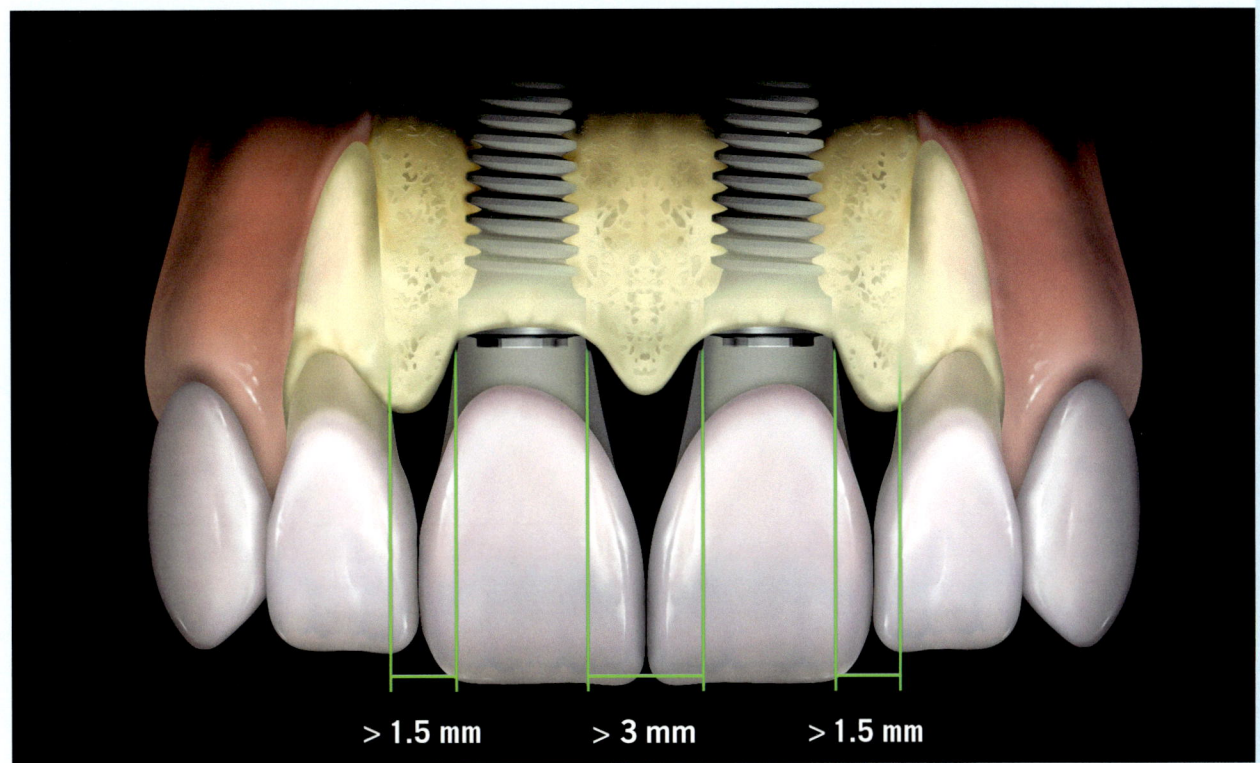

→ ...from page 247

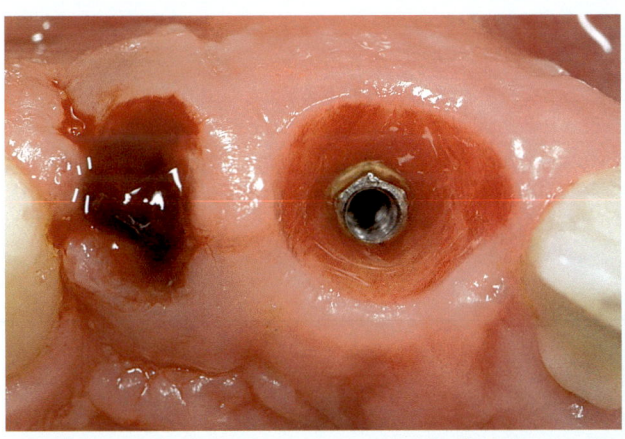

> Fig 3-34a

> Fig 3-34b

> Fig 3-34c

> Fig 3-34d

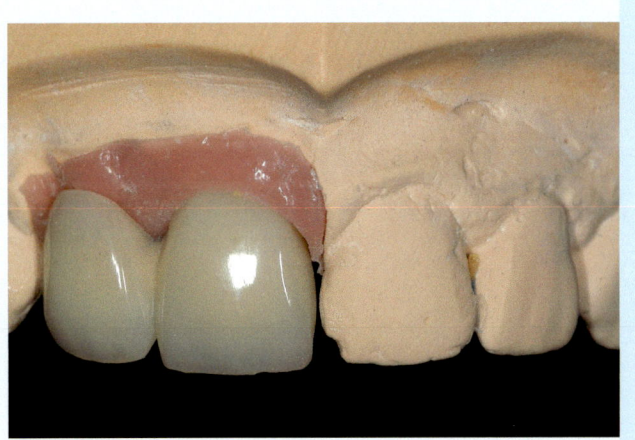

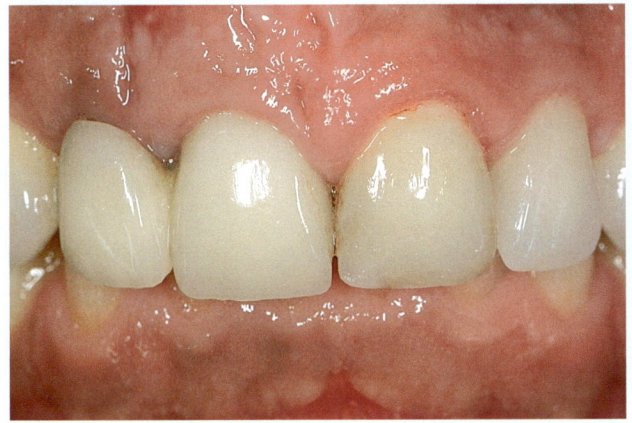

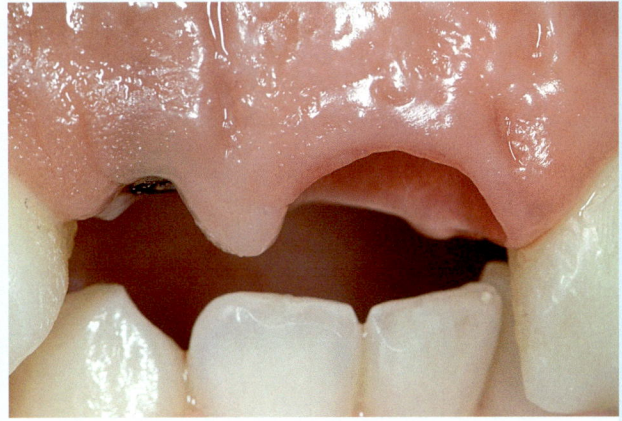

Absence of bleeding during probing This is a clinical factor of essential importance in the periodontal sphere, but it must not be considered excessively reassuring in the case of peri-implant tissues. The presence of fewer blood vessels can be misleading and mask an inflammatory-infective process that has been present for some time clinically undetectable. It has also been demonstrated that the peri-implant mucosa offers less resistance to probe penetration, which can almost reach the level of the marginal crestal bone by moving the junctional epithelium and the connective tissue.[177] As a consequence, probing around the implant is inadvisable.

Therapy for hygiene maintenance of the implant sites Hygiene maintenance of the implant site is equally if not more important than for natural teeth.[165] In patients who are susceptible to periodontal disease, maintenance therapy is fundamental to avoiding the risk of implant failure and/or loss of marginal alveolar support, which these patients can more easily encounter.[178–180]

Screwing in and unscrewing It is advisable to avoid removing the screw-retained healing and/or prosthetic abutments as much as possible so as not to detach the hemidesmosomes of the junctional epithelium from the surface of the abutments themselves. It has been demonstrated[181] that the repetition of these movements causes apical migration of the junctional epithelium and a certain degree of resorption of marginal crestal bone.

Replica of the transmucosal path Once optimal conditioning of the peri-implant soft tissues has been achieved with the provisional restoration, it is possible to make customized prosthetic abutments using a specific technique[182–184] that, by replicating exactly the transmucosal path created with the first provisional restoration, guarantees maintenance of the resulting biologic integration (Figs 3-34e to 3-34l).

FIG 34 *(e to g)* If we wish to replicate the transmucosal path obtained with the provisional restoration, then the latter will have to be joined to an analog from the laboratory and inserted in silicone material until the cervical area is covered. *(h)* After the silicone has completely hardened and the provisional restoration has been unscrewed, an impression coping is screwed into the laboratory analog still immersed in the impression material, around which fluid resin is poured. *(i to k)* When the acrylic resin has polymerized, the impression coping, covered in resin, is unscrewed and positioned in the mouth. A mark previously made on the buccal side allows it to be correctly oriented in the oral cavity. *(l)* The impression to be taken faithfully reproduces the transmucosal path obtained with the provisional restoration.

Fig 3-34e

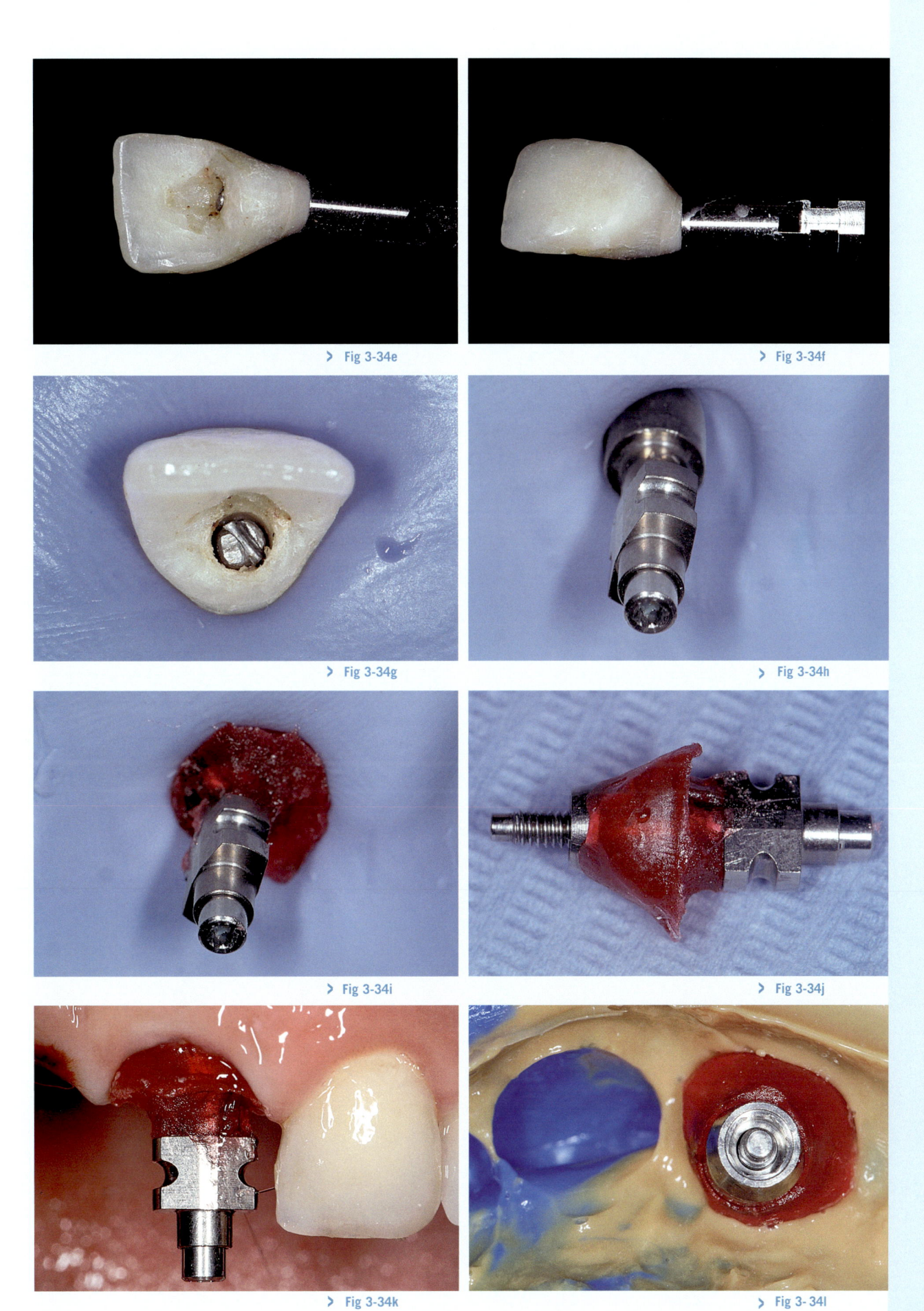

Fig 3-34f

Fig 3-34g

Fig 3-34h

Fig 3-34i

Fig 3-34j

Fig 3-34k

Fig 3-34l

Prosthetic abutment: Choosing the material It is advisable to use biocompatible materials, such as titanium, alumina-based ceramic,[159] or zirconium[160] because of their tissue-integration capacities. The validity of the choice of ceramic abutments, which are determined by esthetic considerations, especially in the anterior sector, also seems to be supported by their trait of adequate resistance[185–188] (Fig 3-34m and 3-34n).

Prosthetic abutment: Choosing the shape Thickening the transmucosal tissue can be attempted by using narrower and more concave abutments to overcome the lack of true anchorage of the connective fiber to the implant abutment surface. This lack of anchorage only weakly seals the soft tissues and therefore imparts a greater chance of tissue recession. Traditional larger abutments with diverging walls can exert excessive compression on the soft tissues, encouraging the appearance of tissue recession. Conversely, the concavity of the transmucosal profile ensures more space for the connective tissue, which is therefore thicker and more stable. This sleeve of tissue gives rise to a kind of connective O-ring that makes the biologic seal of the peri-implant mucosa more efficient, protecting the bone underneath from any marginal resorptions that may inevitably exist in consequent tissue recession.[189] The concave profile also increases the linear distance between the implant platform and the prosthetic margin. The surface available for the supracrestal tissues is thereby increased, in the same way as if the "platform switching" technique is followed.[190] This can allow more superficial implant positioning in relation to the marginal alveolar crest, with consequent reduction of the subsequent bone remodeling.[189] The use of concave abutments does not, however, prevent the peri-implant tissues from being ideally conditioned. Specifically marked countersinking at the more coronal portion of the abutment produces compression on the cervical contour of the transmucosal path that would cause a lengthening of the clinical crown if developed in the buccal area. A similar countersinking in the area between implants should, on the contrary, encourage vertical development of the interproximal papilla (Figs 3-34o to 3-34v and 3-35). This particular design of the abutment nevertheless requires special care to completely remove all of the excess cement.

FIG 34 *(m and n)* Both the definitive abutments in zirconium and the second provisional restorations are made in the laboratory. *(o and p)* The concave design of the abutments at the transmucosal path should guarantee a thickening of the connective tissue section, with consequent improved stability of the gingival tissues. *(q to v)* The intraoral views of the zirconium abutments and the provisional restorations positioned on them demonstrate that good biologic integration has been achieved at this stage, as well as the substantial preservation of the height of the papilla between implants. The patient's original tooth shape (predominantly square) and the periodontal biotype (thick and a bit scalloped) have been distinct advantages for achieving adequate tissue stability. The presence of a thin and scalloped periodontal biotype can more easily lead to tissue instability. In these cases, surgical thickening of the peri-implant tissues by means of a subepithelial connective tissue grafting technique can be indicated.

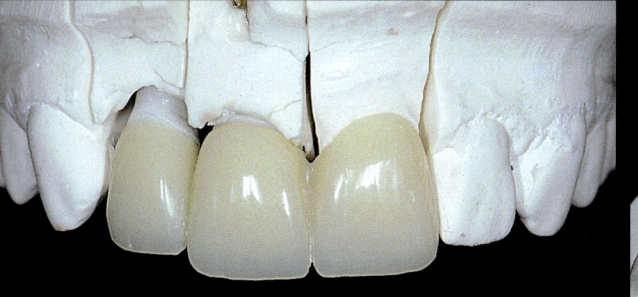

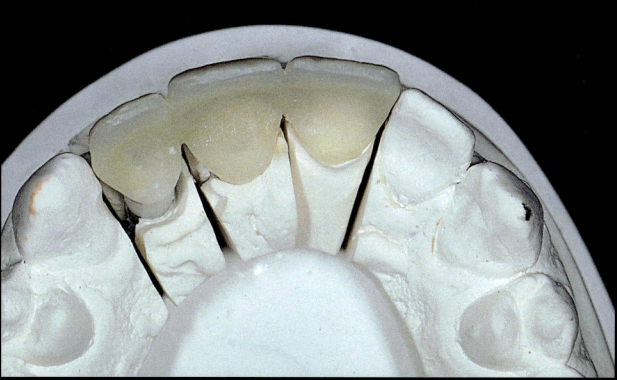

> Fig 3-34m

> Fig 3-34n

> Fig 3-34o

> Fig 3-34p

> Fig 3-34q

> Fig 3-34r

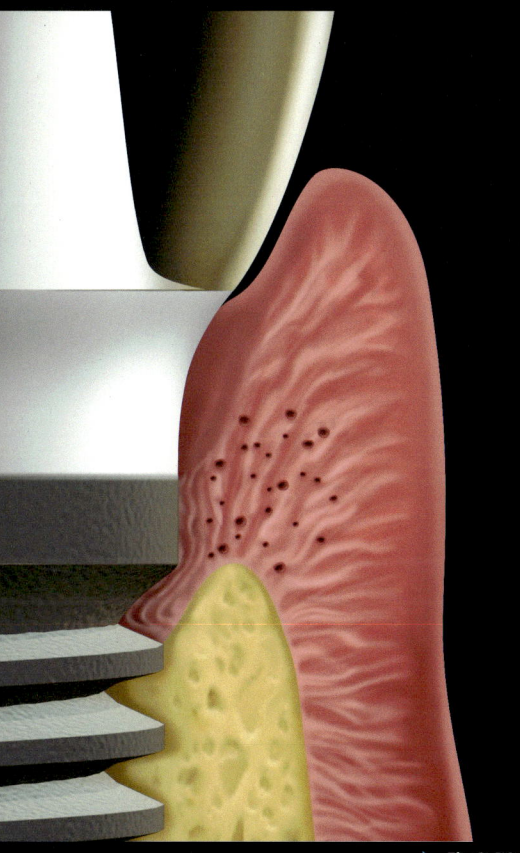

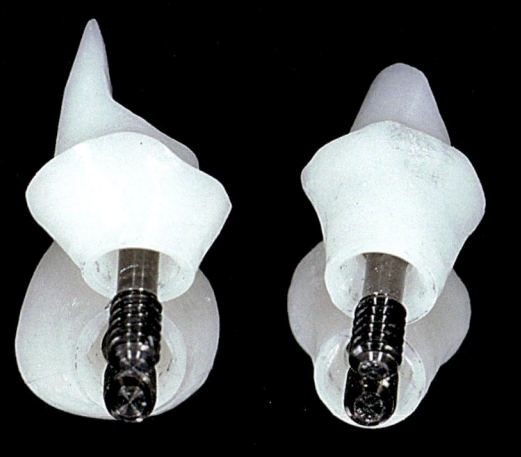

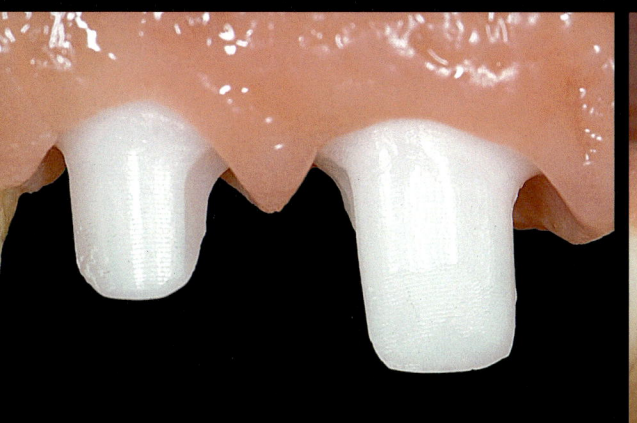

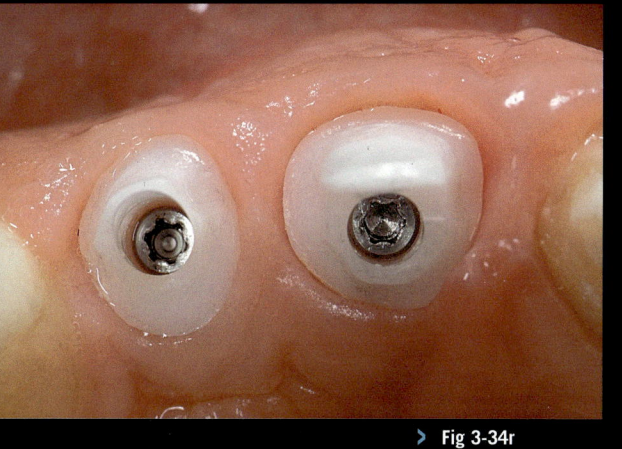

ZIRCONIUM ABUTMENTS

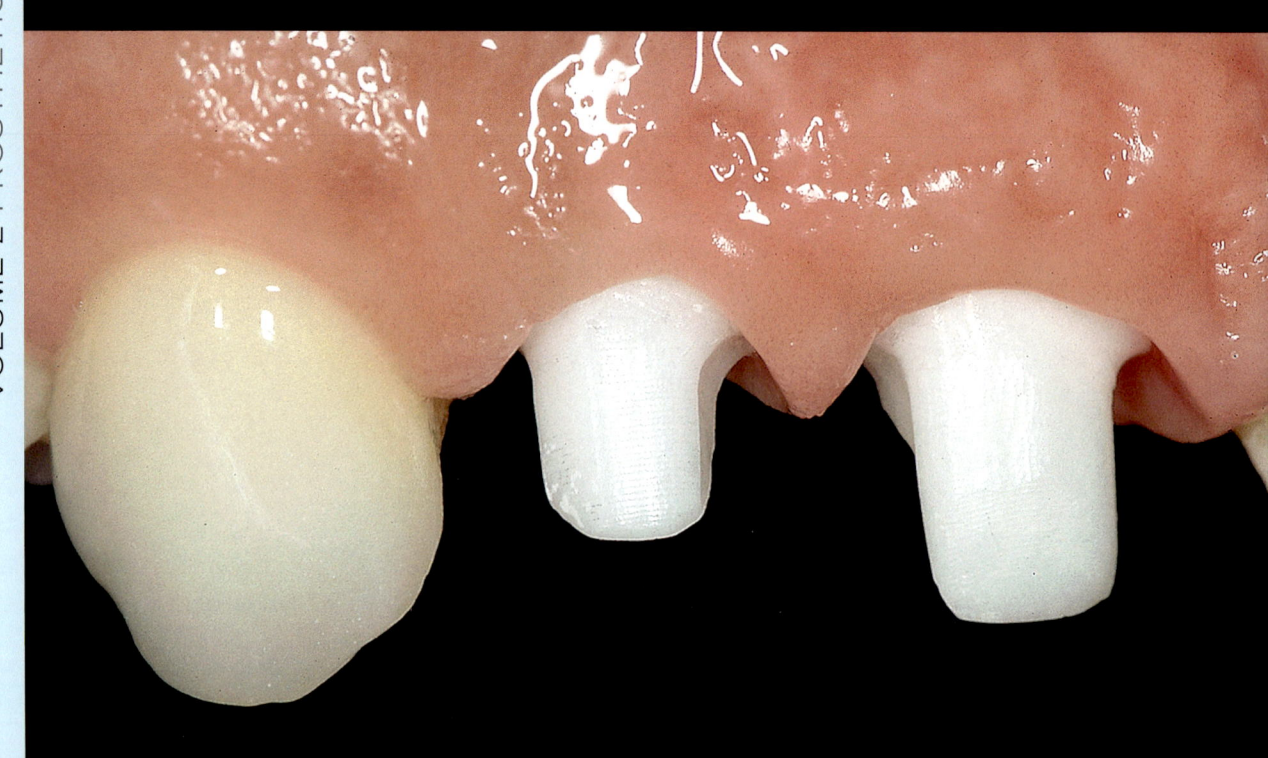

> Fig 3-34s

> Fig 3-34t

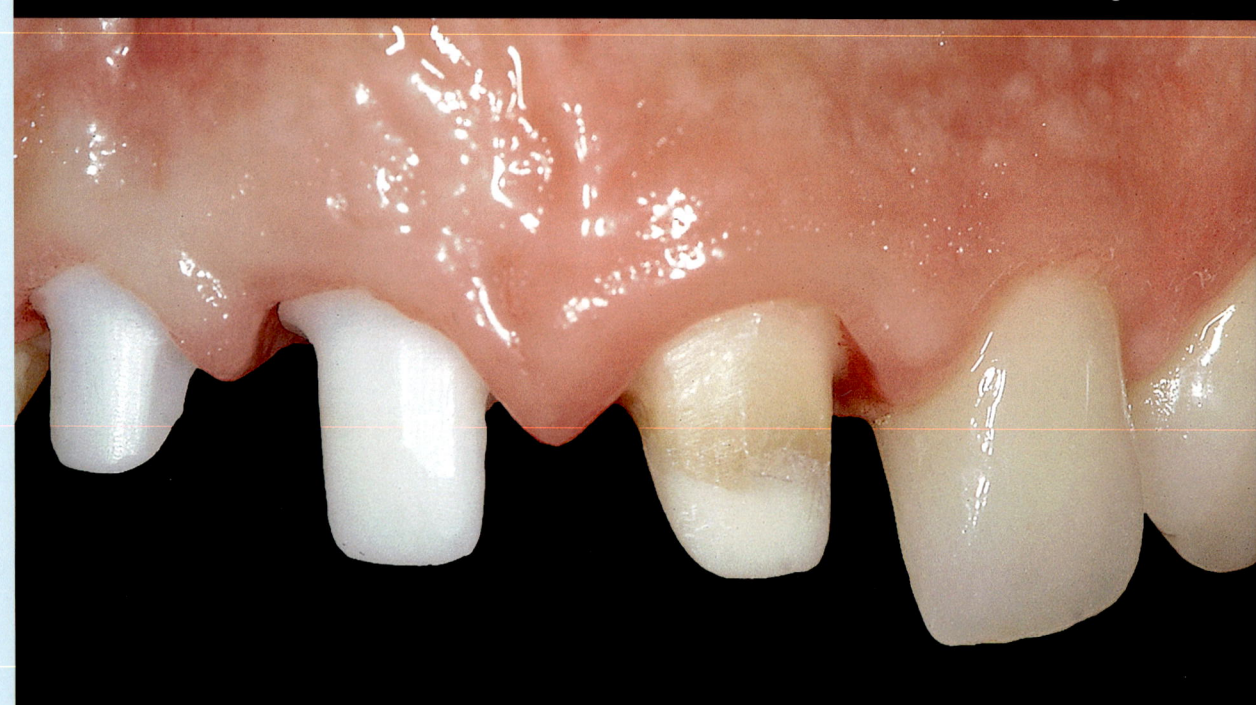

PROVISIONAL RESTORATIONS

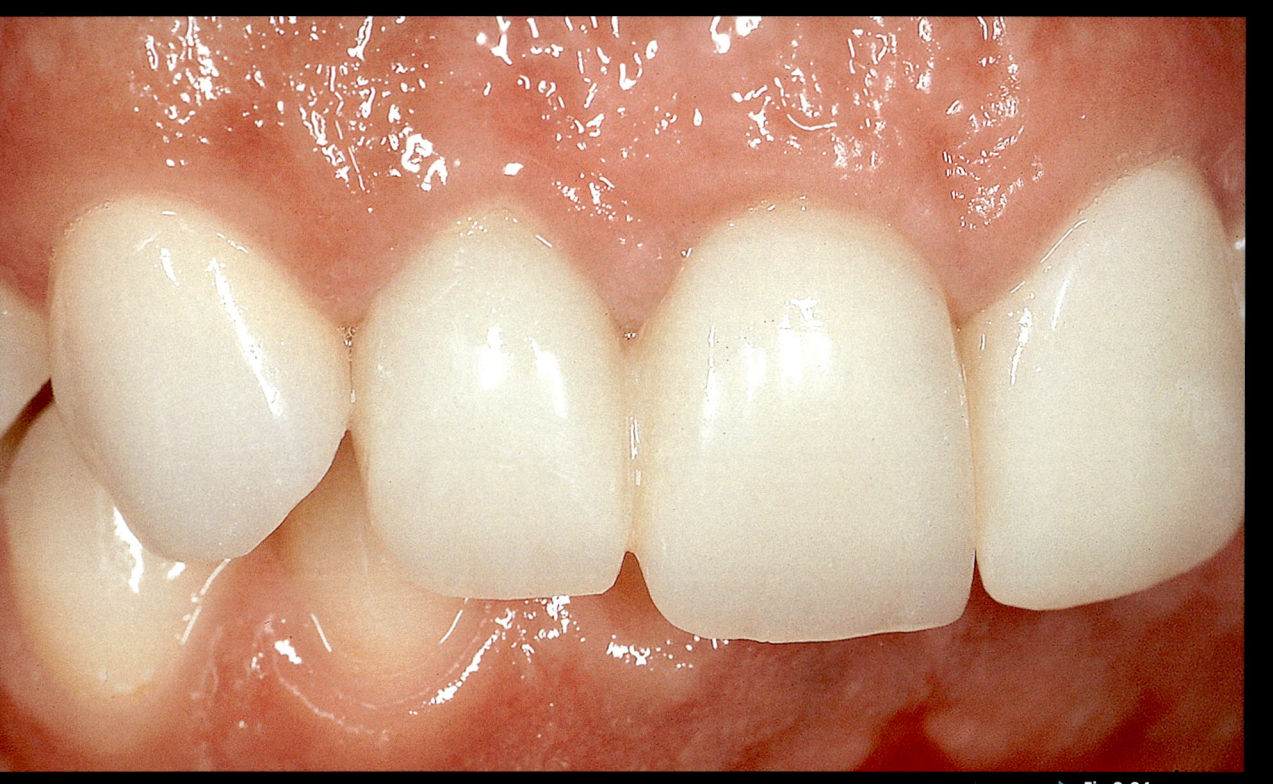

> Fig 3-34u

> Fig 3-34v

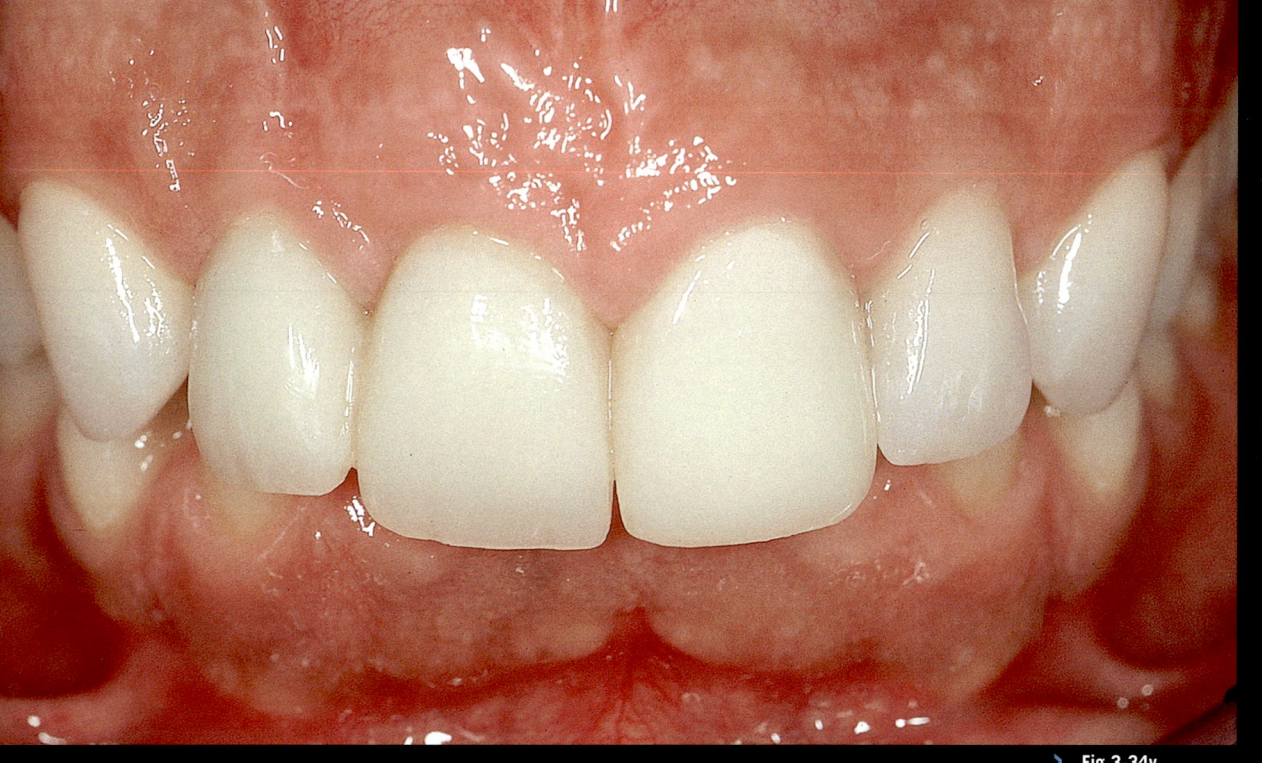

→ Gallery continues on page 586

> Fig 3-35a

> Fig 3-35b

> Fig 3-35c

> Fig 3-35d

> Fig 3-35e

> Fig 3-35f

FIG 35 *(a and b)* The grayish halo found in the cervical area of the left central incisor can be attributed to the presence of the titanium abutment underneath it. *(c and d)* After the wax-up to fabricate the new provisional restorations has been created, the design of the abutment is optimized for the implant on the left central incisor. *(e and f)* The titanium abutment is then taken out of the cast and, after screwing it into another analog, the previously waxed coping is placed on top. The coping has a double margin: the first one closes on the scalloped margin of the implant head, and the second is positioned on the finish line of the crown, which is ideally designed at gingival level. *(g)* The technique requires a double scan procedure (Procera Forte, Nobel Biocare): one scan of the titanium abutment and one of the wax-up of the customized abutment. *(h)* The information obtained by the double scan is transferred electronically to the milling center to make the abutment in zirconium. *(i and j)* An access hole is made for the screw, and then the original titanium abutment and the customized one in zirconium are joined together with a resinous cement. *(k and l)* The comparison between the original titanium abutment and the customized one in titanium-zirconium shows the substantial difference in the respective prosthetic margins. The red arrow shows the finishing line of a crown cemented directly onto the head of the implant (Perfect, Nobel Biocare), which will inevitably cause difficulty in completely removing the excess cement. The green arrow indicates instead the possibility of cementing the crown with the margin at gingival level, which, in this case being roughly 3 mm above the head of the implant, helps enormously in the removal of any residual cement. *(m to p)* The sequence of photographs of the customized zirconium abutment and the adjacent natural abutment, and those with the provisional restorations inserted, highlights the ideal alignment of the gingival margins and the perfect preservation of the interproximal papillae.

Fig 3-35g

Fig 3-35h

Fig 3-35i

Fig 3-35j

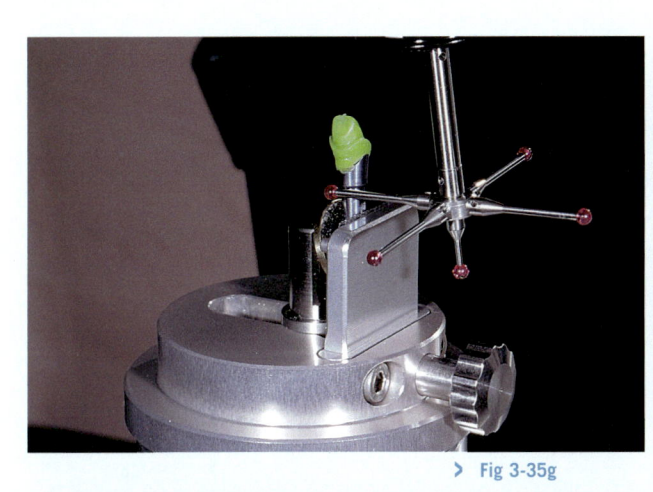

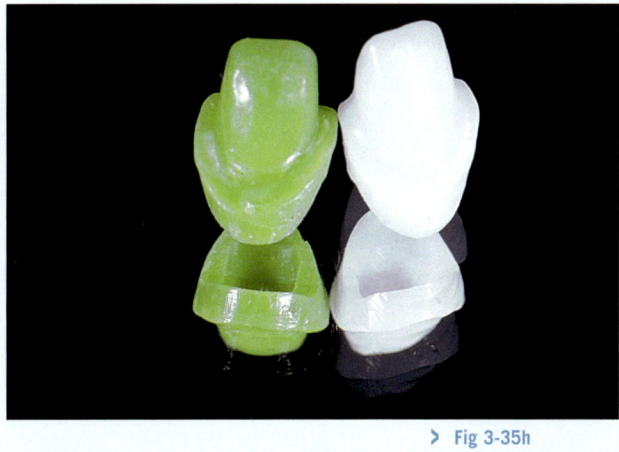

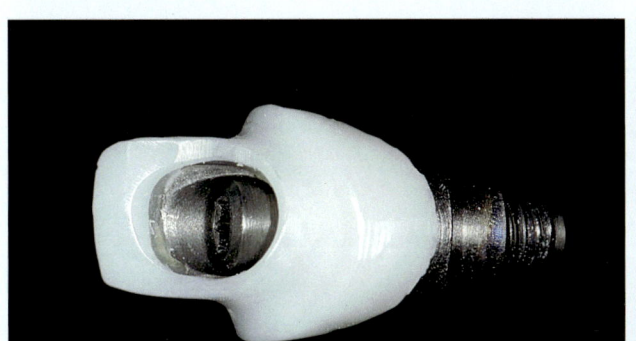

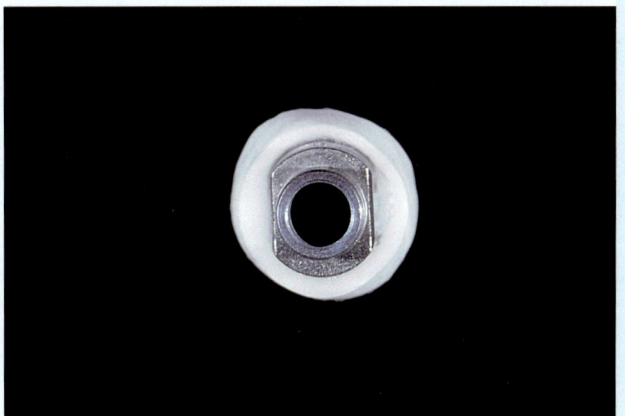

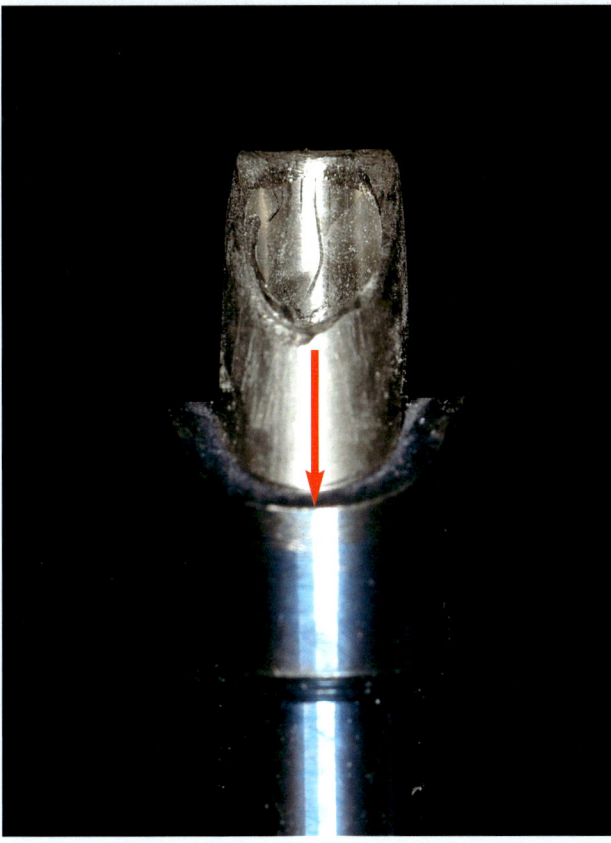

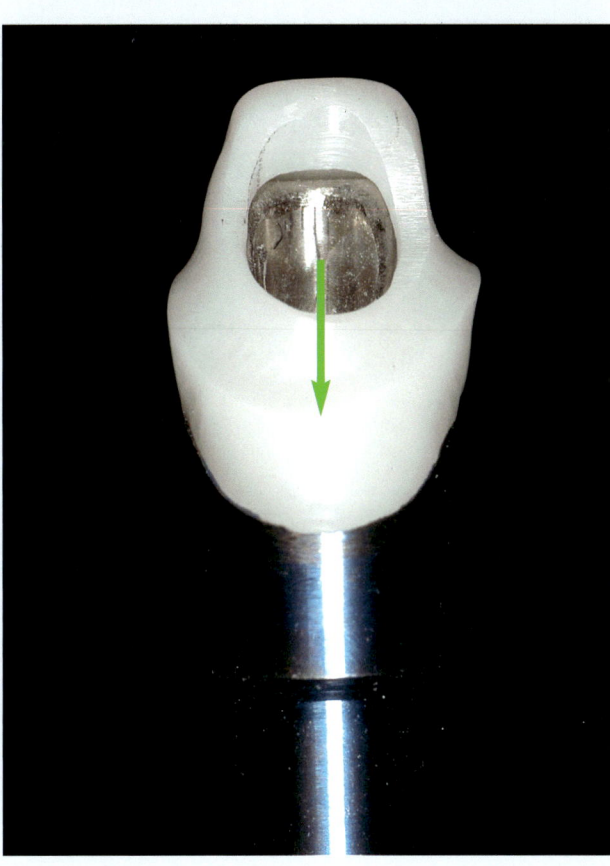

Fig 3-35k

Fig 3-35l

ZIRCONIUM ABUTMENT

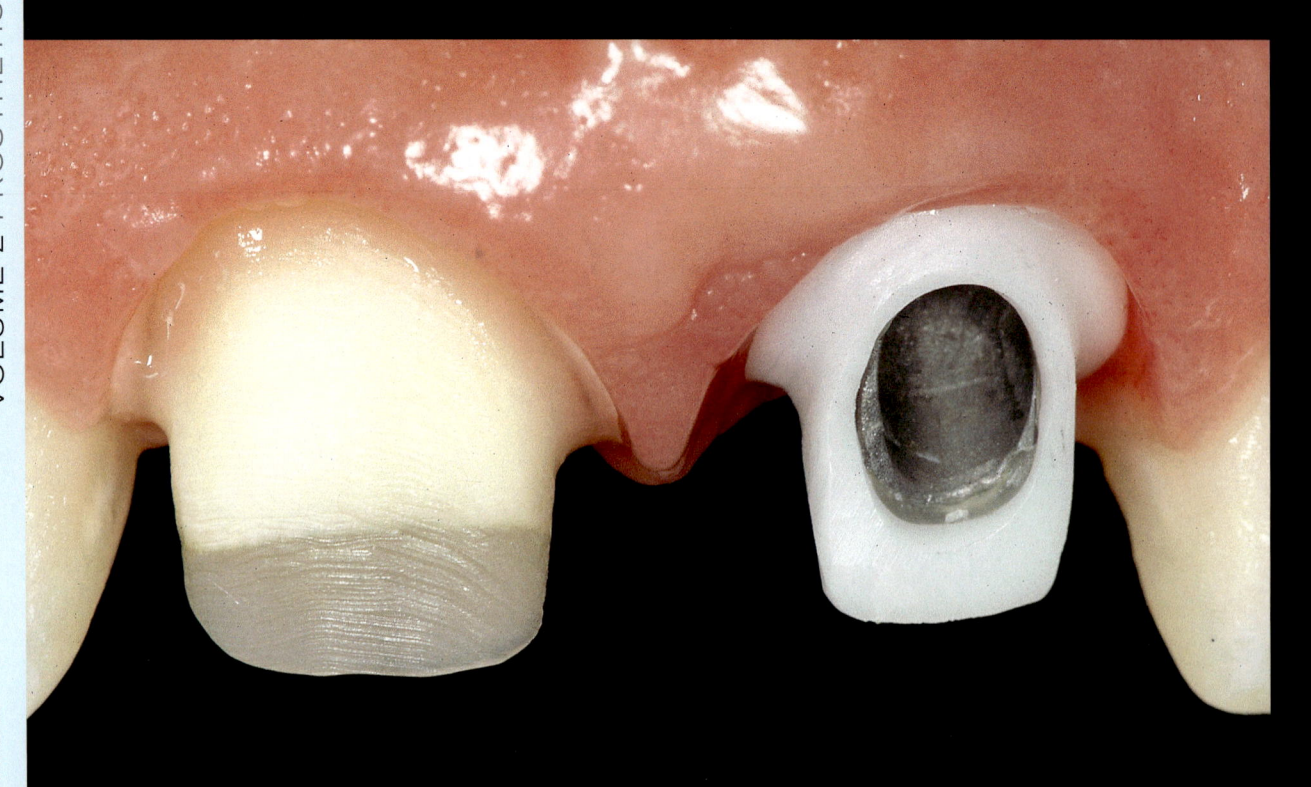

> Fig 3-35m

> Fig 3-35n

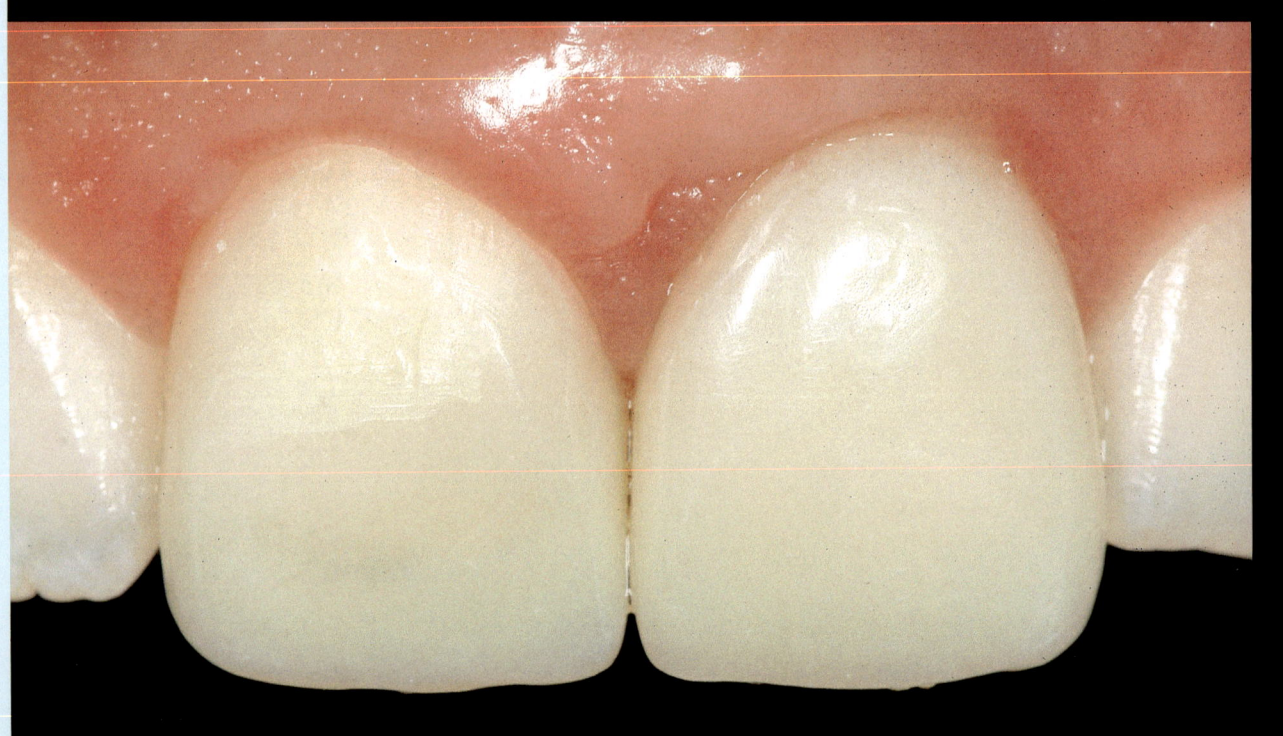

PROVISIONAL RESTORATIONS

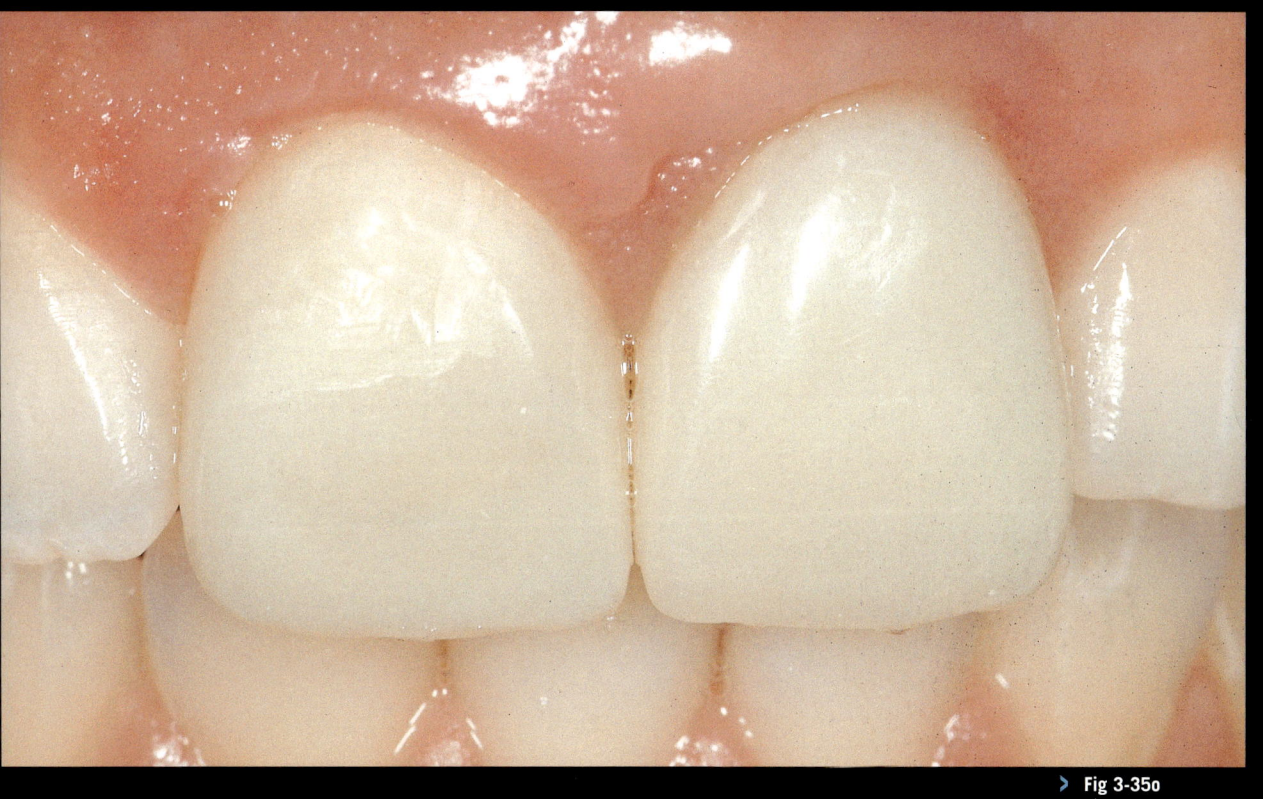

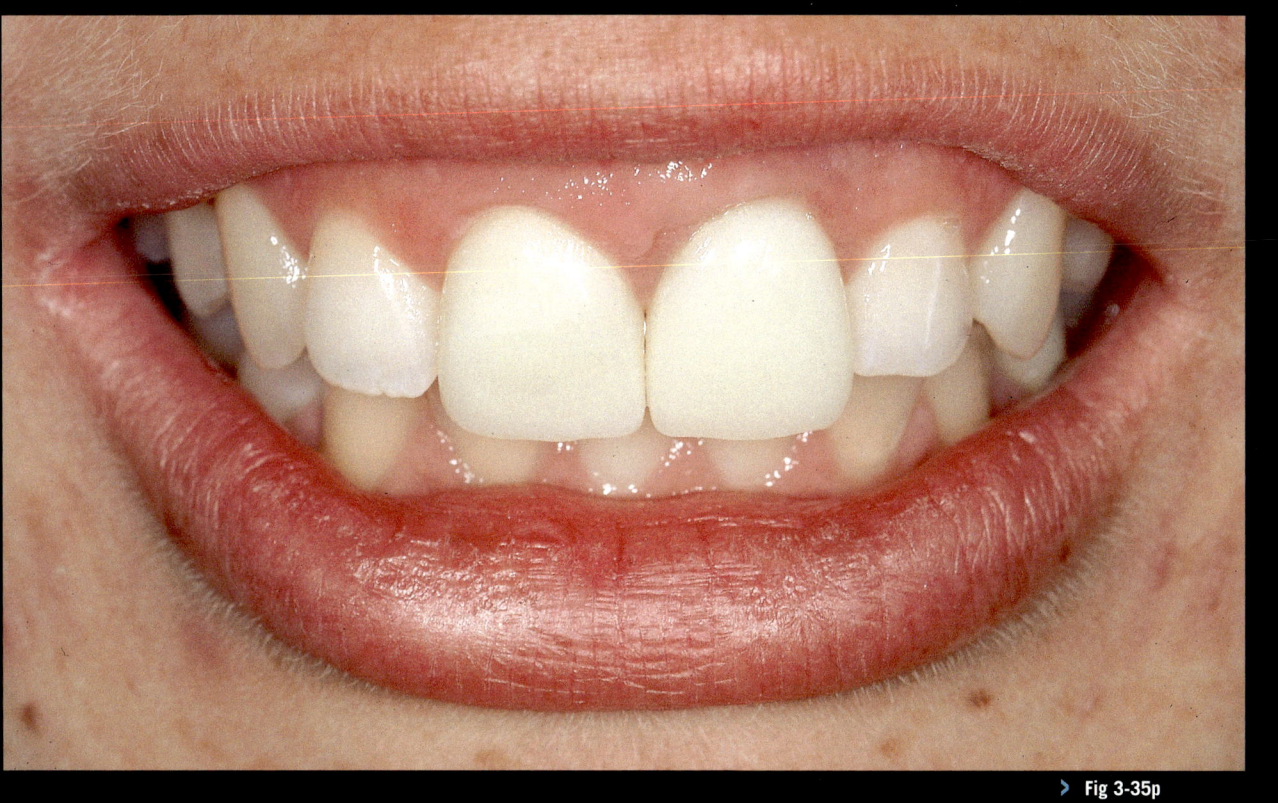

> Fig 3-35o

> Fig 3-35p

→ Gallery continues on page 578

REFERENCES

1. Nemetz H. Tissue management in fixed prosthodontics. J Prosthet Dent 1974;31:628–636.

2. Shavell HM. Mastering the art of tissue management during provisionalization and biologic final impressions. Int J Periodontics Restorative Dent 1988;8:25–43.

3. Maynard JG Jr, Wilson RD. Physiologic dimensions of the periodontium significant to the restorative dentist. J Periodontol 1979;50:170–174.

4. Weisgold AS. Contours of the full crown restorations. Alpha Omegan 1977:70:77–89.

5. Gargiulo AW, Wentz FM, Orban B. Dimension and relations of the dento-gingival junction in humans. J Periodontol 1961;32:261.

6. Ingber JS, Rose LF, Coslet JG. The "biologic width" – a concept in periodontics and restorative dentistry. Alpha Omegan 1977;70:62–65.

7. Vacek JS, Gher ME, Assad DA, Richardson C, Giambarresi LI. The dimensions of the human dentogingival junction. Int J Periodontics Restorative Dent 1994:14:154–165.

8. Wilson RD, Maynard G. Intracrevicular restorative dentistry. Int J Periodontics Restorative Dent 1981;1(4):34–49.

9. Robinson PJ, Vitek RM. The relationship between gingival inflammation and the probe resistance. J Periodontal Res 1975;14:239–243.

10. Dragoo MR, Williams GB. Periodontal tissue reactions to restorative procedures. Int J Periodontics Restorative Dent 1981;1:8–23.

11. Listgarten MA. Normal development, structure, physiology and repair of gingival epithelium. Oral Sci Rev 1972;1:3–67.

12. Parma Benfenati S, et al. The effect of restorative margins on the postsurgical development and nature of the periodontium. Part I: anatomical considerations. J Periodont Rest Dent 1985;6:31–51.

13. Waerhaug J, Zander HA. Reaction of gingival tissues to self-curing acrylic restorations. J Am Dent Assoc 1957;54:760–768.

14. Donaldson D. Gingival recession associated with temporary crowns. J Periodontol 1973;44:691-696.

15. Donaldson D. The etiology of gingival recession associated with temporary crowns. J Periodontol 1974;45:468–71.

16. Garvin PH, Malone WF, Toto PD, Mazur B. Effect of self-curing acrylic resin treatment restorations on the crevicular fluid volume. J Prosthet Dent 1982;47:284-289.

17. Grajower R, Shaharbani S, Kaufman E. Temperature rise in pulp chamber during fabrication of temporary self-curing resin crowns. J Prosthet Dent 1979;41:535–540.

18. Giunta J, Zablotsky N. Allergic stomatitis caused by self-polymerizing resin. Oral Surg Oral Med Oral Pathol 1976;41:631–637.

19. Hochman N, Zalkind M. Hypersensitivity to methyl methacrylate: mode of treatment. J Prosthet Dent 1997;77:93–96.

20. Ramfjord SP, Ash MM. Periodontology and Periodontics. Philadelphia: Saunders, 1979.

21. Wunderlich RC, Caffesse RG. Periodontal aspects of porcelain restorations. Dent Clin North Am 1985;29:693–703.

22. Rodriguez-Ferrer HJ, Strahan JD, Newman HN. Effect on gingival health of removing overhanging margins of interproximal subgingival amalgam restorations. J Clin Periodontol 1980;7:457–462.

23. Waerhaug J. Tissue reactions around artificial crowns. J Periodontol 1953;24:172.

24. Larato DC. Effect of cervical margins on gingiva. J South Calif Dent Assoc 1969;45:19–22.

25. Parkinson CF. Excessive crown contours facilitate endemic plaque niches. J Prosthet Dent 1976;34:424–429.

26. Wagman S. The role of coronal contour in gingival health. J Prosthet Dent 1977;37:280–287.

27. Martignoni M, Schonenberger A. Precision Fixed Prosthodontics: Clinical and Laboratory Aspects. Chicago: Quintessence, 1990.

28. Gracis S, Fradeani M, Celletti R, Bracchetti G. Biological integration of aesthetic restorations: factors influencing appearance and long-term success. Periodontol 2000 2001;27:29–44.

29. Kois JC. The restorative-periodontal interface: biological parameters. Periodontol 2000 1996;11:29–38.

30. Yuodelis RA, Weaver JD, Sapkos S. Facial and lingual contours of artificial complete crown restorations and their effects on the periodontium. J Prosthet Dent 1973;29:61–66.

31. Ehrlich J, Yaffe A, Weisgold AS. Faciolingual width before and after tooth restoration: a comparative study. J Prosthet Dent 1981;46:153–156.

32. Perel ML. Axial crown contours. J Prosthet Dent 1971;25:642–649.

33. Perel ML. Periodontal considerations of crown contours. J Prosthet Dent 1971;26:627–630.

34. Sackett BP, Gildenhuys RR. The effect of axial crown overcontour on adolescents. J Periodontol 1976;47:320–323.

35. Ruben MP, et al. Healing of periodontal surgical wounds. In: Goldman HM, Cohen DW (eds). Periodontal Therapy, ed 6. St Louis: Mosby, 1980:640.

36. Kay HB. Criteria for restorative contours in the altered periodontal environment. Int J Periodontics Restorative Dent 1985;5(3):42–63.

37. Keough BE, Kay HB. Postsurgical prosthetic management. In: Rosenberg MM, Kay HB, Keough BE, Holt RL (eds). Periodontal and Prosthetic Management for Advanced Cases. Chicago: Quintessence, 1998:323–408.

38. Swartz ML, Phillips RW. Comparison of bacterial accumulations on rough and smooth surfaces. J Periodontol 1957;28:304–307.

39. Grasso JE, Nalbandian J, Sanford C, Bailit H. Effect of restoration quality on periodontal health. J Prosthet Dent 1985;53:14–19.

40. Sorensen JA. A rationale for comparison of plaque-retaining properties of crown systems. J Prosthet Dent 1989;62:264–269.

41. Glantz PO. On wettability and adhesiveness: a study of enamel, dentin, some dental restorative materials and dental plaque. Odontol Revy 1969:17 (suppl 20):1–124.

42. Silness J. Periodontal conditions in patients treated with dental bridges. II. The influence of full and partial crowns on plaque accumulation, development of gingivitis and pocket formation. J Periodontal Res 1970;5:219–224.

43. Savitt ED, Malament KA, Socransky SS, Melcer AJ, Backman KJ. Effect on colonization of oral microbiota by a cast glass ceramic restoration. Int J Periodontics Restorative Dent 1987;2:22–35.

44. Adamczyk E, Spiechowics E. Plaque accumulation on crowns made of various materials. Int J Prosthodont 1990;3:285–291.

45. Koidis PT, Schroeder K, Johnston W, Campagni W. Color consistency, plaque accumulation, and external marginal surface characteristics of the collarless metal-ceramic restoration. J Prosthet Dent 1991;65:391–400.

46. Yuodelis RA, Faucher R. Provisional restorations: an integrated approach to periodontics and restorative dentistry. Dent Clin North Am 1980;24:285–303.

47. Trebbi L, Di Febo G, Carnevale G. A technique to obtain a precise functional occlusion using porcelain fused to gold. Int J Periodontics Restorative Dent 1982; 2:44–57.

48. Silness J, Hegdahl T. Area of the exposed zinc phosphate cement surfaces in fixed restorations. Scand J Dent Res 1970;78:163–177.

49. Saltzberg DS, Ceravolo FJ, Holstein F, Groom G, Gottsegen R. Scanning electron microscope study of the junction between restorations and gingival cavosurface margins. J Prosthet Dent 1976;36:517–522.

50. Janenko C, Smales RJ. Anterior crowns and gingival health. Aust Dent J 1979;24:225–230.

51. Waerhaug J. Temporary restorations: advantages and disadvantages. Dent Clin North Am 1980;24:305–316.

52. Trushkowsky RD. Fabrication of a fixed provisional restoration utilizing a light-curing acrylic resin. Quintessence Int 1992;23:415–419.

53. Palomo F, Kopczyk RA. Rationale and methods for crown lengthening. J Am Dent Assoc 1978;96:257–260.

54. Rosenberg ES, Garber DA, Evian CI. Tooth lengthening procedures. Compend Contin Educ Gen Dent 1980; 1:161–172.

55. Wagenberg BD, Eskow RN, Langer B. Exposing adequate tooth structure for restorative dentistry. Int J Periodontics Restorative Dent 1989;9:323–331.

56. Pontoriero R, Carnevale G. Surgical crown lenghtening: a 12-month clinical wound healing study. J Periodontol 2001;72:841–848.

57. Coslet JG, Vanarsdall RL, Weisgold A. Diagnosis and classification of delayed passive eruption of the dentogingival junction in the adult. Alpha Omega 1977;70:24–28.

58. Seibert J, Lindhe J. Esthetics in periodontal therapy. In: Lindhe J, Karring T, Lang NP (eds). Clinical Periodontology and Implant Dentistry, ed 3. Copenhagen: Blackwell Munksgaard, 1997:647–681.

59. Allen EP. Surgical crown lengthening for function and esthetics. Dent Clin North Am 1993;37:163–179.

60. Caudill R, Chiche GJ. Establishing an esthetic gingival appearance. In: Chiche GJ, Pinault A (eds). Esthetics of Anterior Fixed Prosthodontics. Chicago: Quintessence, 1994:177–198.

61. Newcomb GM. The relationship between the location of subgingival crown margins and gingival inflammation. J Periodontol 1974;45:151–154.

62. Nevins M, Skurow HM. The intracrevicular restorative margin, the biologic width, and the maintenance of the gingival margin. Int J Periodontics Restorative Dent 1984;4(3):30–49.

63. Davarpanah M, Jansen CE, Vidjak FM, Etienne D, Kebir M, Martinez H. Restorative and periodontal considerations of short clinical crowns. Periodontics Restorative Dent 1998;18:424–433.

64. Gegauff AG. Effect of crown lengthening and ferrule placement on static load failure of cemented cast post-cores and crowns. J Prosthet Dent 2000;84:169–179.

65. Olsen CT, Ammons WF, van Belle G. A longitudinal study comparing apically repositioned flaps, with and without osseous surgery. Int J Periodontics Restorative Dent 1985;5:10–33.

66. Lindhe J, Socransky SS, Nyman S, Westfelt E. Dimensional alteration of the periodontal tissues following therapy. Int J Periodontics Restorative Dent 1987; 7:9–21.

67. Kaldahl WB, Kalkwarf KL, Patil KD, Dyer JK, Bates RE Jr. Evaluation of four modalities of periodontal therapy. Mean probing depth, probing attachment level and recession changes. J Periodontol 1988;59:783–793.

68. Bragger U, Lauchenauer D, Lang NP. Surgical lengthening of the clinical crown. J Clin Periodontol 1992;19:58–63.

69. Kaldahl WB, Kalkwarf KL, Patil KD, Molvar MP, Dyer JK. Long-term evaluation of periodontal therapy: I. Response to 4 therapeutic modalities. J Periodontol 1996;67:93–102.

70. Smith DH, Ammons WF Jr, van Belle G. A longitudinal study of periodontal status comparing osseous recontouring with flap curettage. I. Results after 6 months. J Periodontol 1980;51:367–375.

71. Tarnow DP, Magner AW, Fletcher P. The effect of the distance from the contact point to the crest of bone on the presence or absence of the interproximal dental papilla. J Periodontol 1992;63:995–996.

72. Wennström J, Heijl L, Lindhe J. Periodontal surgery: access therapy. In: Lindhe J, Karring T, Lang NP (eds.). Clinical Periodontology and Implant Dentistry. Copenhagen: Munksgaard, 1998:508–549.

73. Carnevale G, Pontoriero R, Lindhe J. Treatment of furcation-involved teeth. In: Lindhe J, Karring T, Lang NP (eds). Clinical Periodontology and Implant Dentistry, ed 4. Oxford: Blackwell Munksgaard, 2003:705–730.

74. Goldman HM, Schluger S, Fox L, Cohen DW. Periodontal Therapy, ed 3. St Louis: Mosby, 1964:560.

75. Rosen H, Gitnick PJ. Integrating restorative procedures into the treatment of periodontal disease. J Prosthet Dent 1964;14:343.

76. van der Velden U. Regeneration of the interdental soft tissues following denudation procedures. J Clin Periodontol 1982;9:455–459.

77. Watson JF, Crispin BJ. Margin placement of esthetic veneer crowns. Part III. Attitudes of patients and dentists. J Prosthet Dent 1981;45:499–501.

78. Jorgensen KD. The relationship between retention and convergence angle in cemented veneer crowns. Acta Odontol Scand 1955;13:35–40.

79. Ohm E, Silness J. The convergence angle in teeth prepared for artificial crowns. J Oral Rehabil 1978;5:371–375.

80. Woolsey GD, Matich JA. The effect of axial grooves on the resistance form of cast restorations. J Am Dent Assoc 1978;97:978–980.

81. Dodge WW, Weed RM, Baez RJ, Buchanan RN. The effect of convergence angle on retention and resistance form. Quintessence Int 1985;16:191–194.

82. Maxwell AW, Blank LW, Pelleu GB Jr. Effect of crown preparation height on the retention and resistance of gold castings. Gen Dent 1990;38:200–202.

83. Noonan JE Jr, Goldfogel MH. Convergence of the axial walls of full veneer crown preparations in a dental school environment. J Prosthet Dent 1991;66:706–708.

84. Parker MH, Calverley MJ, Gardner FM, Gunderson RB. New guidelines for preparation taper. J Prosthodont 1993;2:61–66.

85. Wilson AH Jr, Chan DC. The relationship between preparation convergence and retention of extracoronal retainers. J Prosthodont 1994;3:74–78.

86. Annersted AL, Engstrom U, Hansson A, Jansson T, Karlsson S, Liljhagen H, Lindquist E, Rydhammar E, Tyreman-Bandhede M, Svensson P, Wandel U. Axial wall convergence of full veneer crown preparations. Documented for dental students and general practitioners. Acta Odontol Scand 1996;54:109–112.

87. Wiskott HW, Nicholls JI, Belser UC. The relationship between abutment taper and resistance of cemented crowns to dynamic loading. Int J Prosthodont 1996;9:117–139.

88. Shillingburg HT, Hobo S, Whitsett LD, Jacobi R, Brackett SE. Fundamentals of Fixed Prosthodontics, 3rd ed. Chicago: Quintessence, 1997:119–169.

89. Trier AC, Parker MH, Cameron SM, Brousseau JS. Evaluation of resistance form of dislodged crowns and retainers. J Prosthet Dent 1998;80:405–409.

90. Smith CT, Gary JJ, Conkin JE, Franks HL. Effective taper criterion for the full veneer crown preparation in preclinical prosthodontics. J Prosthodont 1999;8:196–200.

91. Goodacre CJ, Campagni WV, Aquilino SA. Tooth preparations for complete crowns: an art form based on scientific principles. J Prosthet Dent 2001;85:363–376.

92. Massironi D, Pascetta R, Romeo G. Estetica e precisione. Procedure cliniche e di laboratorio. Vol I. Milan: Quintessenza Edizioni, 2004:147–179.

93. Jorgenson MW, Goodkind RJ. Spectrophotometric study of five porcelain shades relative to the dimensions of color, porcelain thickness, and repeated firings. J Prosthet Dent 1979;42:96–105.

94. Barghi N, Lorenzana RE. Optimum thickness of opaque and body porcelain. J Prosthet Dent 1982;48:429–431.

95. Seghi RR, Johnston WM, O'Brien WJ. Spectrophotometric analysis of color differences between porcelain systems. J Prosthet Dent 1986;56:35–40.

96. Jacobs SH, Goodacre CJ, Moore BK, Dykema RW. Effect of porcelain thickness and type of metal-ceramic alloy on color. J Prosthet Dent 1987;57:138–145.

97. Terada Y, Maeyama S, Hirayasu R. The influence of different thicknesses of dentin porcelain on the color reflected from thin opaque porcelain fused to metal. Int J Prosthodont 1989;2:352–356.

98. D'Amico A. Functional occlusion of the natural teeth in man. J Prosthet Dent 1961;11:899.

99. Schuyler CH. The function and importance of incisal guidance in oral rehabilitation. J Prosthet Dent 1963;13:1011.

100. Dawson PE. Evaluation, diagnosis and treatment of occlusal problems. St Louis: Mosby, 1974.

101. Farrar WB, McCarthy WL. A Clinical Outline of Temporomandibular Joint Diagnosis and Treatment, ed 7. Normandie Study Group for TMJ Dysfunction. Montgomery: Walker, 1983.

102. Chiche GJ, Pinault A, eds. Esthetics of Anterior Fixed Prosthodontics. Chicago: Quintessence, 1994.

103. Magne P, Belser U. Bonded Porcelain Restorations in the Anterior Dentition. A Biomimetic Approach. Chicago: Quintessence, 2002.

104. Gürel G. The Science and Art of Porcelain Laminate Veneers. Chicago: Quintessence, 2003.

105. Pameijer JHN. Periodontal and Occlusal Factors in Crown and Bridge Procedures. Amsterdam: Dental Center for Postgraduate Courses, 1985.

106. Schubert L. Temperaturmessungen im Zahn während des Schleif-und Bohrvorgangs mittel des Lichtstrichgalvonometers. Zahnarztl Welt 1957;58:768–772.

107. Simon U. Vergleichende Messungen von handelsüblichen Bohrmaschinen und Turbinen. Dtsch Zahnartztl Z 1979;34:768–772.

108. Shillingburg HT Jr, Grace CS. Thickness of enamel and dentin. J South Calif Dent Assoc 1973;41(1):33–36.

109. Zach L, Cohen G. Thermogenesis in operative techniques: comparison of four methods. J Prosthet Dent 1962;12:977–984.

110. Beveridge EE, Brown AC. The measurement of human dental intrapulpal pressure and its response to clinical variables. Oral Surg Oral Med Oral Pathol 1965;19:655–668.

111. Langeland K, Langeland LK. Cutting procedures with minimized trauma. J Am Dent Assoc 1968;76:991–1005.

112 ■ Pashley DH. Smear layer: physiological considerations. Oper Dent Suppl 1984;3:13–29.

113 ■ Christopher DJ, Wilson PR. The effects of tooth preparation on pressure measured in the pulp chamber: a laboratory study. Int J Prosthodont 1999;12:439–443.

114 ■ Lauer HC, Kraft E, Rothlauf W, Zwingers T. Effects of the temperature of cooling water during high-speed and ultrahigh-speed tooth preparation. J Prosthet Dent 1990;63:407–414.

115 ■ Marcum JS. The effect of crown margin depth upon gingival tissue. J Prosthet Dent 1967;17:479–487.

116 ■ Larato DC. The effect of crown margin extension to gingival inflammation. J South Calif Dent Assoc 1969;37:476–478.

117 ■ Aboucaya WA. A classification of smiles. Quintessence Int 1975;10:1–2.

118 ■ Matthews TG. The anatomy of a smile. J Prosthet Dent 1978;39:128–134.

119 ■ Crispin BJ, Watson JF. Margin placement of esthetic veneer crowns. Part I. Anterior tooth visibility. J Prosthet Dent 1981;45:287–292.

120 ■ Crispin BJ, Watson JF. Margin placement of esthetic veneer crowns. Part II. Posterior tooth visibility. J Prosthet Dent 1981;45:389–391.

121 ■ Tjan AH, Miller GD, The JG. Some esthetic factors in a smile. J Prosthet Dent 1984;51:24–28.

122 ■ Peck S, Peck L, Kataja M. The gingival smile line. Angle Orthod 1992;62:91–100.

123 ■ Mackley RJ. An evaluation of smiles before and after orthodontic treatment. Angle Orthod 1993;63:183–189.

124 ■ Morley J, Eubank J. Macroesthetic elements of smile design. J Am Dent Assoc 2001;132:39–45.

125 ■ Owens EG, Goodacre CJ, Loh PL, Hanke G, Okamura M, Jo K, Muñoz CA, Naylor WP. A multicenter interracial study of facial appearance. Part 2: a comparison of intraoral parameters. Int J Prosthodont 2002;15:283–288.

126 ■ Waerhaug J. Histologic considerations which govern where the margins of restorations should be located in relation to the gingiva. Dent Clin North Am 1960;4:161–176.

127 ■ Karlsen K. Gingival reactions to dental restorations. Acta Odontol Scand 1970;28:895–904.

128 ■ Silness J. Periodontal conditions in patients treated with dental bridges. III. The relationship between the location of the crown margin and the periodontal condition. J Periodontal Res 1970;5:255–259.

129 ■ Renggli HH, Regolati B. Gingival inflammation and plaque accumulation by well-adapted supragingival and subgingival proximal restorations. Helv Odontol Acta 1972;16:99–101.

130 ■ Richter WA, Ueno H. Relationship of crown margin placement to gingival inflammation. J Prosthet Dent 1973;30:156–161.

131 ■ Mörmann W, Regolati B, Renggli HH. Gingival reaction to well-fitted subgingival proximal gold inlays. J Clin Periodontol 1974;1:120–125.

132 ■ Waerhaug J. Presence or absence of plaque on subgingival restorations. Scand J Dent Res 1975;83:193–201.

133 ■ Silness J. Fixed prosthodontics and periodontal health. Dent Clin North Am 1980;24:317–329.

134 ■ Ericsson I, Lindhe J. Recession in sites with inadequate width of the keratinized gingiva. An experimental study in the dog. J Clin Periodontol 1984;11:95–103.

135 ■ Parma Benfenati S, Fugazzotto PA, Ferreira PM, Ruben MP, Kramer GM. The effect of restorative margins on the postsurgical development and nature of the periodontium. Part II: anatomical considerations. Int J Periodontics Restorative Dent 1986;6:64–75.

136 ■ Müller HP. The effect of artificial crown margins at the gingival margin on the periodontal conditions in a group of periodontally supervised patients treated with fixed bridges. J Clin Periodontol 1986;13:97–102.

137 ■ Orkin DA, Reddy J, Bradshaw D. The relationship of the position of crown margins to gingival health. J Prosthet Dent 1987;57:421–424.

138 ■ Flores-de-Jacoby L, Zafiropoulos GG, Ciancio S. The effect of crown margin location on plaque and periodontal health. Int J Periodontics Restorative Dent 1989;9:197–205.

139 ■ Valderhaug J, Birkeland JM. Periodontal conditions in patients 5 years following insertion of fixed prostheses. Pocket depth and loss of attachment. J Oral Rehabil 1976;3:237–243.

140 ■ Valderhaug J, Heloe LA. Oral hygiene in a group of supervised patients with fixed prostheses. J Periodontol 1977;48:221–224.

141 ■ Valderhaug J, Birkeland JM. Periodontal conditions and carious lesions following the insertion of fixed prostheses. A 10-year follow-up study. Int Dent J 1981;30:296.

142 ■ De Waal H, Castellucci G. The importance of restorative margin placement to the biologic width and periodontal health. Part I. Int J Periodontics Restorative Dent 1993;13:461–471.

143 ■ Tarnow D, Stahl SS, Magner A, Zamzock J. Human gingival attachment responses to subgingival crown placement. Marginal remodelling. J Clin Periodontol 1986;13:563–569.

144 ■ Lang NP, Kiel RA, Anderhalden K. Clinical and microbiological effects of subgingival restorations with overhanging or clinically perfect margins. J Clin Periodontol 1983;10:563–578.

145 ■ Löe H, Silness J. Tissue reactions to string packs used in fixed restorations. J Prosthet Dent 1963;13:318.

146 ■ Woycheshin FF. An evaluation of the drugs used for gingival retraction. J Prosthet Dent 1964;14:769.

147 ■ Anneroth G, Nordenram A. Reaction of the gingiva to the application of threads in the gingival pocket for taking impressions with elastic material. Odontol Rev 1969;20:301–310.

148 ■ Ramadan FA, Harrison JD. Literature review of the effectiveness of tissue displacement materials. Egypt Dent J 1970;16:271–282.

149 ■ Baharav H, Laufer BZ, Langer Y, Cardash HS. The effect of displacement time on gingival crevice width. Int J Prosthodont 1997;10:248–253.

150. Jokstad A. Clinical trial of gingival retraction cords. J Prosthet Dent 1999;81:258–261.

151. Acka EA, Yildirim E, Dalkiz M, Yavuzyilmaz H, Beydemir B. Effects of different retraction medicaments on gingival tissue. Quintessence Int 2006;37:53–59.

152. Harrison JD. Effect of retraction materials on the gingival sulcus epithelium. J Prosthet Dent 1961;11:514–521.

153. Gould TRL, Brunette DM, Westbury L. The attachment mechanism of epithelial cells to titanium in vitro. J Periodontal Res 1981;16:611–616.

154. Brånemark P-I. Introduction to osseointegration. In: Brånemark P-I, Zarb GA, Albrektsson T (eds). Tissue-Integrated Prostheses: Osseointegration in Clinical Dentistry. Chicago: Quintessence, 1985:11–76.

155. Cochran DL, Hermann JS, Schenk RK, Higginbottom FL, Buser D. Biologic width around titanium implants. A histometric analysis of the implanto-gingival junction around unloaded and loaded nonsubmerged implants in the canine mandible. J Periodontol 1997;68:186–198.

156. Berglundh T, Lindhe J, Ericsson I, Marinello CP, Liljenberg B, Thomsen P. The soft tissue barrier at implants and teeth. Clin Oral Implants Res 1991;2:81–90.

157. Berglundh T, Lindhe J. Dimension of the peri-implant mucosa: biologic width revisited. J Clin Periodontol 1996;23:971-973.

158. American Academy of Periodontology. Dental implants in periodontal therapy. J Periodontol 2000;71:1934–1942.

159. Abrahamsson I, Berglundh T, Glantz PO, Lindhe J. The mucosal attachment at different abutments: an experimental study in dogs. J Clin Periodontol 1998;25:721–727.

160. Degidi M, Artese L, Scarano A, Perrotti V, Gehrke P, Piattelli A. Inflammatory infiltrate, microvessel density, nitric oxide synthase expression, vascular endothelial growth factor expression, and proliferative activity in peri-implant soft tissues around titanium and zirconium oxide healing caps. J Periodontol 2006;77:73–80.

161. Glauser R, Schupbach P, Gottlow J, Hammerle CH. Periimplant soft tissue barrier at experimental one-piece mini-implants with different surface topography in humans: a light-microscopic overview and histometric analysis. Clin Implant Dent Relat Res 2005;7:S44–S51.

162. Berglundh T, Lindhe J, Jonsson K, Ericsson I. The topography of the vascular systems in the periodontal and peri-implant tissues in the dog. J Clin Periodontol 1994;21:189–193.

163. Buser D, Weber HP, Donath K, Fiorellini J, Paquette DW, Williams R. Soft tissue reactions to nonsubmerged unloaded titanium implants in beagle-dogs. J Periodontol 1992;63:226–236.

164. Berglundh T, Lindhe J, Marinello CP, Ericsson I, Liljenberg B. Soft tissue reactions to de novo plaque formation at implants and teeth: an experimental study in the dog. Clin Oral Implants Res 1992;3:1–38.

165. Pontoriero R, Tonelli MP, Carnevale G, Mombelli A, Nyman SR, Lang NP. Experimentally induced peri-implant mucositis. A clinical study in humans. Clin Oral Implants Res 1994;5:254-259.

166. Ericsson I, Berglundh T, Marinello CP, Liljenberg B, Lindhe J. Long-standing plaque and gingivitis at implants and teeth in the dog. Clin Oral Implants Res 1992;3:99–103.

167. Lindhe J, Berglundh T, Ericsson I, Liljenberg B, Marinello CP. Experimental breakdown of peri-implant and periodontal tissues: a study in the beagle-dog. Clin Oral Implants Res 1992;3:9–16.

168. Marinello CP, Berglundh T, Ericsson I, Klinge B, Glantz PO, Lindhe J. Resolution of ligature induced peri-implantitis lesions in the dog. J Clin Periodontol 1995;22:475–480.

169. Adell R, Eriksson B, Lekholm U, Brånemark PI, Jemt T. Long-term follow-up study of osseointegrated implants in the treatment of totally edentulous jaws. Int J Oral Maxillofac Implants 1990;5:347–359.

170. Saadoun AP, LeGall M. Implant positioning for periodontal, functional, and aesthetic results. Pract Periodontics Aesthet Dent 1992;4:43–54.

171. Saadoun AP, Sullivan DY, Krischek M, Le Gall M. Single tooth implant: management for success. Pract Periodontics Aesthet Dent 1994;6:73–80.

172. Salama H, Salama MA, Garber D, Adar P. The interproximal height of bone: a guidepost to predictable aesthetic strategies and soft tissue contours in anterior tooth replacement. Pract Periodontics Aesthet Dent 1998;10:1131–1141.

173. Saadoun AP, LeGall M, Touati B. Selection and ideal tridimensional implant position for soft tissue aesthetics. Pract Periodontics Aesthet Dent 1999;11:1063–1072.

174. Tarnow DP, Cho SC, Wallace SS. The effect of inter-implant distance on the height of inter-implant bone crest. J Periodontol 2000;71:546–549.

175. Paul SJ, Jovanovic SA. Anterior implant-supported reconstructions: a prosthetic challenge. Pract Periodontics Aesthet Dent 1999;11:585–590.

176. Grunder U. Stability of the mucosal topography around single-tooth implants and adjacent teeth: 1-year results. Int J Periodontics Restorative Dent 2000;20:11–17.

177. Ericsson I, Lindhe J. Probing at implants and teeth: an experimental study in the dog. J Clin Periodontol 1993;20:623–627.

178. Hardt CR, Grondahl K, Lekholm U, Wennstrom JL. Outcome of implant therapy in relation to experienced loss of periodontal bone support: a retrospective 5-year study. Clin Oral Implants Res 2002;13:488–494.

179. Wennstrom JL, Ekestubbe A, Grondahl K, Karlsson S, Lindhe J. Oral rehabilitation with implant-supported fixed partial dentures in periodontitis-susceptible subjects. A 5-year prospective study. J Clin Periodontol 2004;31:713–724.

180. Van der Weijden GA, van Bemmel KM, Renvert S. Implant therapy in partially edentulous, periodontally compromised patients: a review. J Clin Periodontol 2005;32:506–511.

181. Abrahamsson I, Berglundh T, Lindhe J. The mucosal barrier following abutment dis/reconnection. An experimental study in dogs. J Clin Periodontol 1997;24:568–572.

182 ■ Hinds KF. Custom impression coping for an exact registration of the healed tissue in the esthetic implant restoration. Int J Periodontics Restorative Dent 1997;17:584–591.

183 ■ Touati B, Guez G, Saadoun A. Aesthetic soft tissue integration and optimized emergence profile: provisionalization and customized impression coping. Pract Periodontics Aesthet Dent 1999;11:305–314.

184 ■ Fradeani M. Esthetic Rehabilitation in Fixed Prosthodontics. Volume 1. Esthetic Analysis: A Systematic Approach to Prosthetic Treatment. Chicago: Quintessence, 2004:304.

185 ■ Yildirim M, Fischer H, Marx R, Edelhoff D. In vivo fracture resistance of implant-supported all-ceramic restorations. J Prosthet Dent 2003;90:325–331.

186 ■ Glauser R, Sailer I, Wohlwend A, Studer S, Schibli M, Schärer P. Experimental zirconia abutments for implant-supported single-tooth restorations in esthetically demanding regions: 4-year results of a prospective clinical study. In J Prosthodont 2004; 17:285–290.

187 ■ Vult von Steyern P. All-ceramic fixed partial dentures. Studies on aluminum oxide- and zirconium dioxide-based ceramic systems. Swed Dent J Suppl 2005:1–69.

188 ■ Att W, Kurun S, Gerds T, Strub JR. Fracture resistance of single-tooth implant-supported all-ceramic restorations: an in vitro study. J Prosthet Dent 2006;95:111–116.

189 ■ Touati B, Rompen E, Van Dooren E. A new concept for optimizing soft tissue integration. Pract Proced Aesthet Dent 2005;17:711-712, 714–715.

190 ■ Lazzara RJ, Porter SS. Platform switching: a new concept in implant dentistry for controlling postrestorative crestal bone levels. Int J Periodontics Restorative Dent 2006;26:9–17.

VOLUME 2 | PROSTHETIC TREATMENT

ESTHETIC REHABILITATION IN FIXED PROSTHODONTICS

FROM THE PROVISIONAL RESTORATION TO THE DEFINITIVE PROSTHESIS: IMPRESSIONS AND DATA TRANSFER

Final verification that the provisional restoration is properly integrated from the esthetic, functional, and biologic viewpoints must be the starting point for transferring all of the data necessary for finalization of the prosthetic rehabilitation. Recording the facebow and occlusal registrations, taking the final impressions, and accurately completing the laboratory checklist allow the technician to replicate in the definitive restoration what has already been successful in the provisional restoration.

OBJECTIVE _ To correctly transfer all of the data needed to replicate the provisional restoration in the definitive rehabilitation.

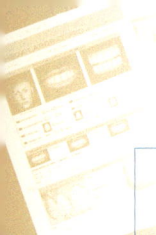

FROM THE PROVISIONAL RESTORATION TO THE DEFINITIVE PROSTHESIS: IMPRESSIONS AND DATA TRANSFER

For too long the provisional restoration has been relegated to a completely secondary role, serving as a temporary placeholder while the technician creates the definitive prosthesis. For this reason, the appearance and functional validity of the provisional restoration have never been a primary objective for many clinicians. Its importance is often undervalued to the extent that, even when it fulfills the patient's expectations, often no systematic approach is employed to transfer its crucial information to the laboratory in an accurate way. This, of course, prevents any faithful reproduction in the definitive work. It is therefore not uncommon to find patients who are dissatisfied with the definitive prosthesis once it is delivered, seeing it as not meeting their expectations because it differs completely from the provisional restorations that they found more pleasing and functional.

INTEGRATED PROVISIONAL RESTORATION

The provisional restoration must take on the role of an instrument used to clinically test the validity of all esthetic-functional modifications prescribed by the clinician in the treatment planning phase and transmitted to the technician to create the diagnostic wax-up. It is essential to fit the provisional restoration in the mouth in the same position in which the technician, after taking it from the diagnostic wax-up, built it on the cast if it is to perform its role as the prototype for the definitive work.[1–7] Depending on the complexity of the case, the provisional restoration must remain in the oral cavity for a sufficient length of time to test the validity of the esthetic-functional modifications and to evaluate the overall biologic integration (Fig 4-1). Only after the provisional restoration has demonstrated in the mouth that it fulfills all of the expectations of the clinician and the patient is it possible to proceed with creating the definitive prosthesis.

OBJECTIVE

It is essential to employ a system that allows all of the characteristics of the functional provisional restoration to be replicated in a simple and effective way. Only in this way can one avoid the risk of errors revealed only in the finished work, which inevitably cause frustration in the clinician and the patient regarding the lack of therapeutic success.

The definitive prosthesis must therefore be a faithful copy of the provisional restoration in order to be equally integrated from the biologic, esthetic, and functional viewpoints, differing only in the restoration material used. It is the clinician's task to adequately transmit all of the information contained in the provisional restoration by means of the laboratory checklist. It is the technician's task to use this information and replicate it faithfully in the definitive work, optimizing, in regard to the spaces developed with the acrylic shell, the anatomy of the individual teeth to give them the required vitality and natural appearance.

CASE 1

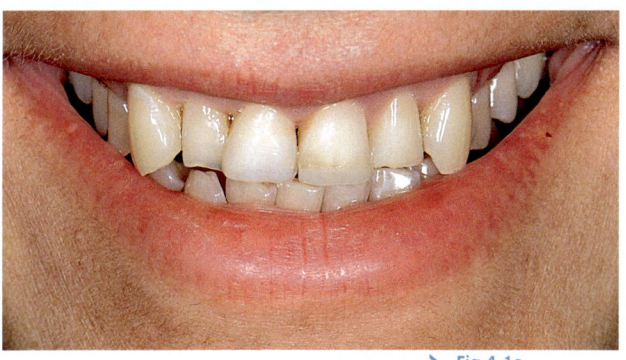

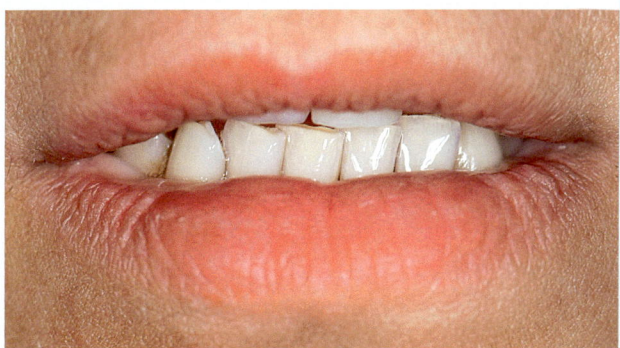

> Fig 4-1a

> Fig 4-1b

> Fig 4-1c

> Fig 4-1d

> Fig 4-1e

> Fig 4-1f

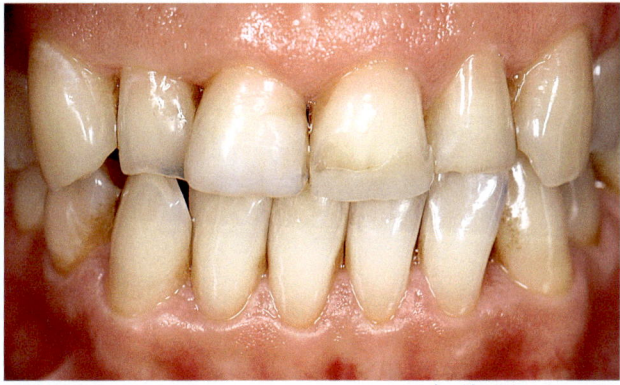

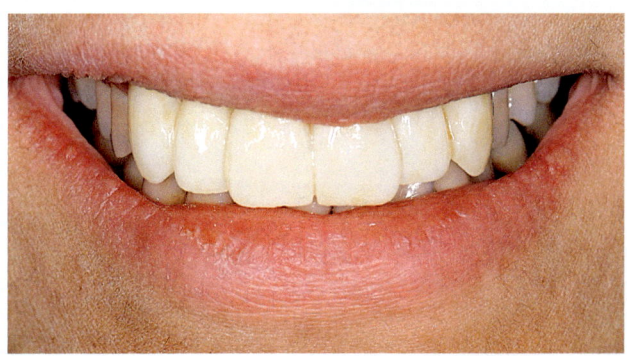

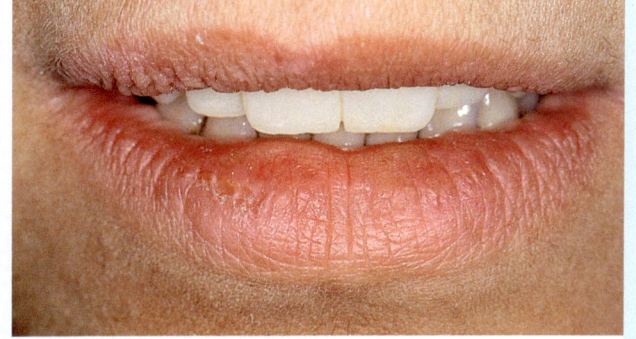

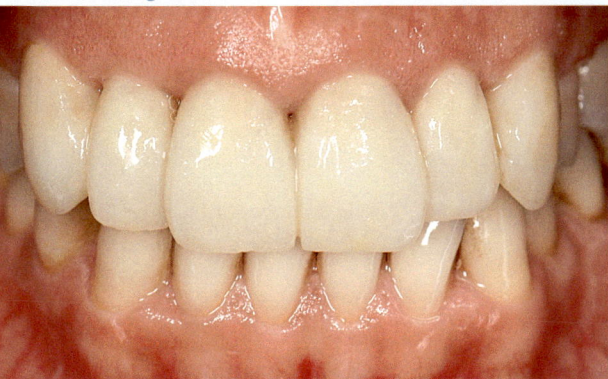

FIG 1 *(a to c)* The preoperative photos show the abraded incisal edges with a marked reduction in the tooth lengths. Note the negative anterior space *(a)*, the lack of visibility of the maxillary teeth *(b)*, and the very limited amount of overbite *(c)*. *(d and e)* The final check of the provisional restorations shows ideal esthetic integration achieved both during smiling and with the lips at rest. *(f)* The increased amount of overbite will encourage good development of the anterior guidance.

PROVISIONAL RESTORATION

■ VERIFYING THE INTEGRATION ■
PROVISIONAL RESTORATION IN SITU

The esthetic, biologic, and functional integration of the provisional restoration is verified once it is positioned in the mouth. If modifications are needed in the future, these can be made during the regular clinical checkups, particularly during the appointment in which the final preparations are made.

The relining carried out after final tooth preparation should not alter the position of the provisional restoration, even if sometimes slight movements occur that do require correction of the occlusal contacts but are so minimal as not to require any further checking.

An appointment is made 3 to 4 weeks after final preparation of the abutments for the specific purpose of carrying out final verification of the overall integration of the provisional restoration. At this time, the provisional restoration is examined again to verify esthetic-functional integration and to assess how the gingival tissues responded to the new crown contours following the intrasulcular deepening carried out earlier (Figs 4-2, 4-3, and 4-4).

If the test shows positive results, the impressions of the functional provisional restorations can be taken in the same session. Together with the final impressions of the abutments and the occlusal registrations, these impressions allow the casts to be cross-mounted in the articulator to proceed with finalizing the restoration.

ESTHETIC PARAMETERS

The parameters that guided the clinician in the initial facial and dentolabial analysis[7,8–19] and were then incorporated by the technician when creating the wax-up and constructing the provisional restoration should now be re-evaluated. These parameters include:

- Tooth exposure at rest
- Incisal edge position
- Smile line
- Smile width
- Labial corridor
- Interincisal line
- Incisal-occlusal plane vs horizontal plane

It is not usually necessary to alter the tooth length or the position of the incisal edge and the inclination of the occlusal plane in this phase. These parameters should have been extensively checked in both the provisional fitting phase and in the subsequent assessments.

FIG 2 3 4 The photographs of three cases show satisfactory overall integration. An ideal state of soft tissue health is essential for taking final impressions that accurately reproduce all of the details of the tooth preparations.

CASE 1

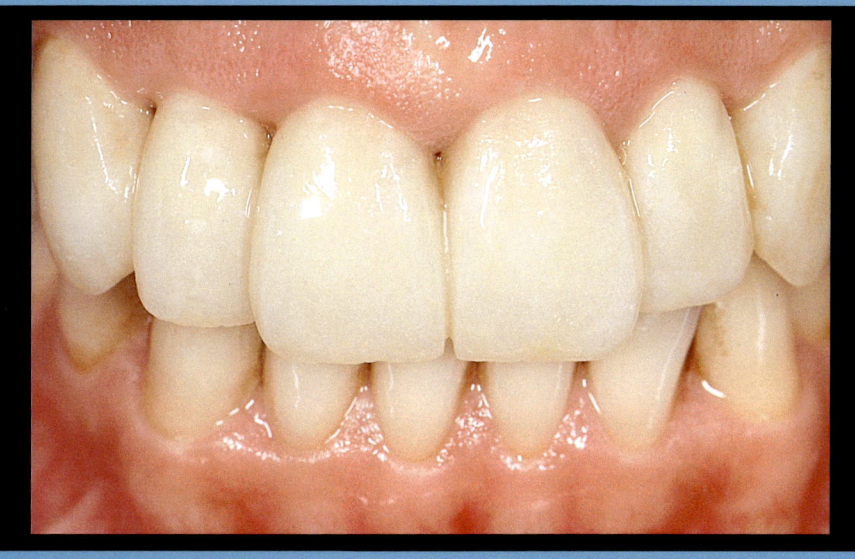

> Fig 4-2

CASE 2

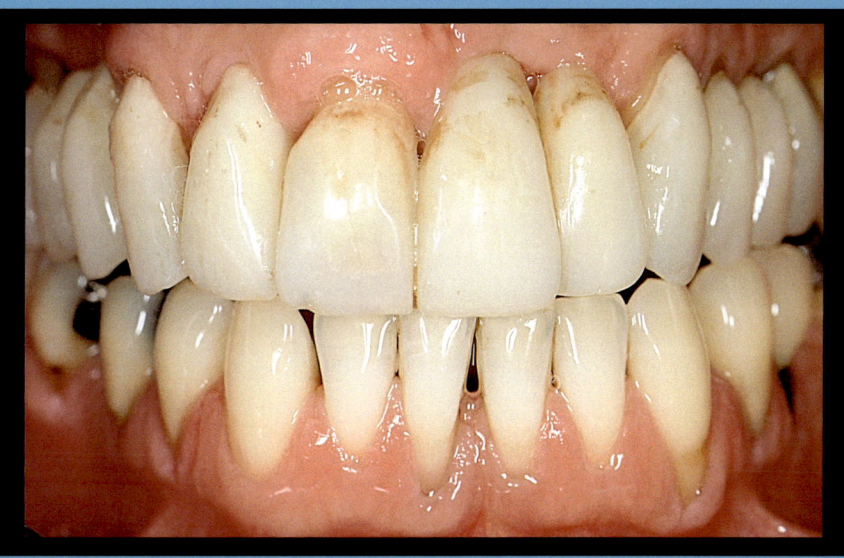

> Fig 4-3

CASE 3

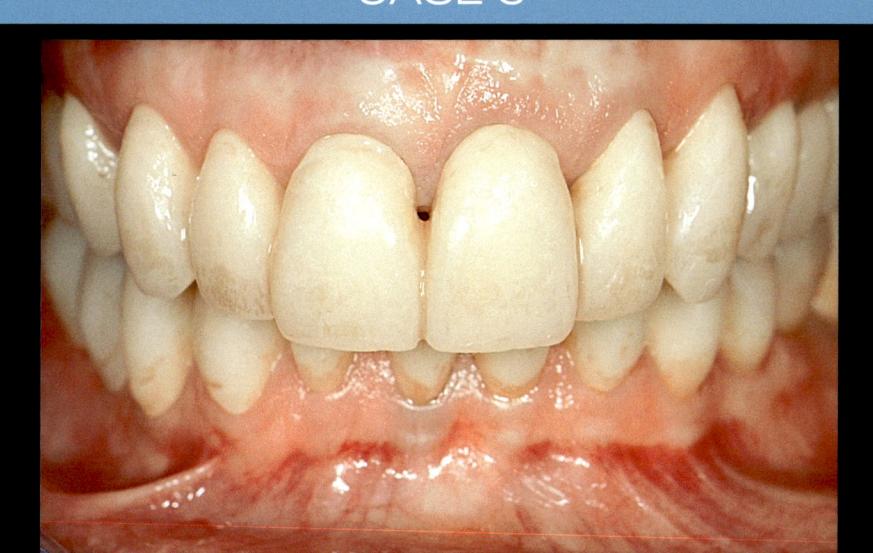

> Fig 4-4

PHONETIC PARAMETERS

Phonetic tests are useful for confirming optimal tooth position and length and for checking the suitability of the VDO in the provisional restoration[1,3,20,21] (see volume 1, chapter 4) (Figs 4-5, 4-6a, and 4-6b).

M sound Having the patient pronounce this sound completely relaxes the lips. Appropriate tooth exposure at rest and the presence of sufficient free space between the arches can thereby be confirmed.[16,22–31]

E sound When the patient pronounces this sound, the tooth length is again evaluated, in the context of the patient's age, by the amount of interlabial space occupied by the maxillary teeth.[32]

F sound The clinician tests the correctness of the incisal profile once again, which, to be adequate, requires that the incisal edge of the maxillary provisional restoration remain inside the vermilion of the bottom lip.[8,33–35]

S sound This sound is used to test the buccolingual position of the anterior teeth[36–38] and to verify the clinical acceptability of the VDO,[36,37,39–42] especially for patients in whom the height between the arches has been significantly varied during positioning of the provisional restoration.[38,43,44]

FUNCTIONAL PARAMETERS

The casts of the provisional restorations are determinants for transmitting the functional information contained in them.[5,45–47]

Overjet-overbite These values must be carefully checked. If they are adequate, anterior guidance will develop correctly.[38,48,49]

Anterior guidance The ease with which the mandible moves during excursive movements (incisal guidance and canine guidance) must be checked[50,51] (Figs 4-6c and 4-6d). Episodes of fractures or decementation of the provisional restoration usually indicate excursive movements that are too steep. The periodic checkups should identify any need for adjustments to be made to the disocclusive path so as to prevent the occurrence of such problems and to avert fractures of the outer ceramic layer in the definitive restoration.[38]

FIG 5 *(a)* The photograph of the smile shows the restored harmony between the incisal outline and the curvature of the lower lip. *(b)* In this phase, the length and position of the incisal edges, which must allow the patient easy excursive movements, are checked again.

FIG 6 *(a and b)* The dentolabial and phonetic analyses show appropriate overall integration. *(c and d)* The lateral excursions on the right and left sides highlight the presence of a canine guidance that, though only slightly inclined, nevertheless allows disocclusion of the posterior sectors in this periodontal patient.

CASE 1

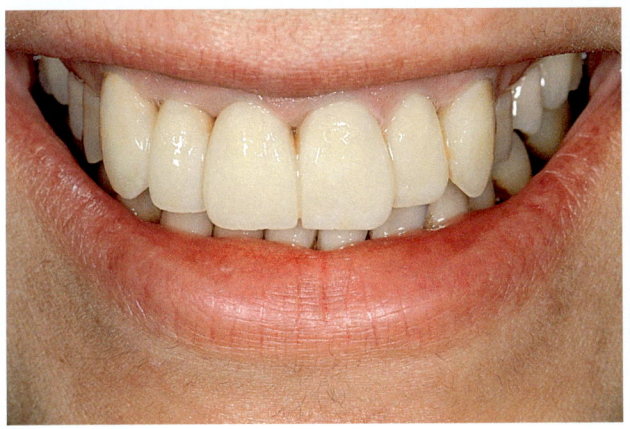

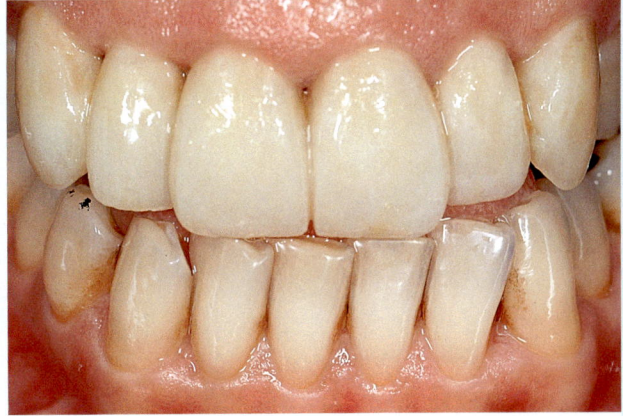

> Fig 4-5a

> Fig 4-5b

CASE 2

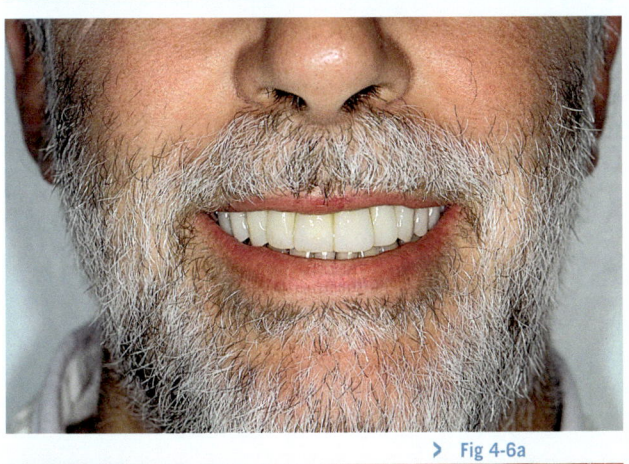

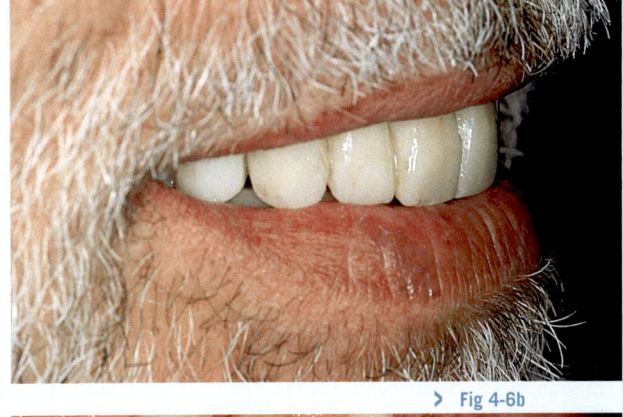

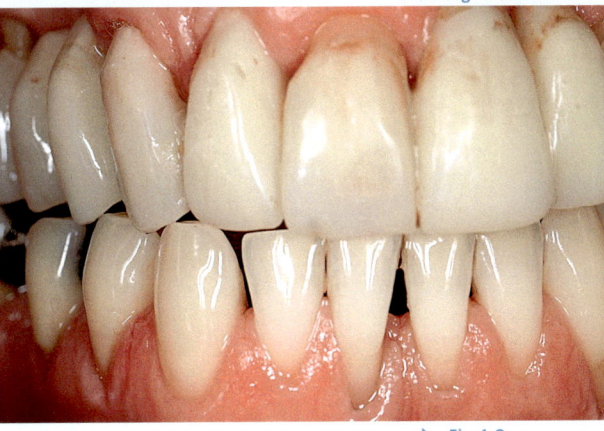

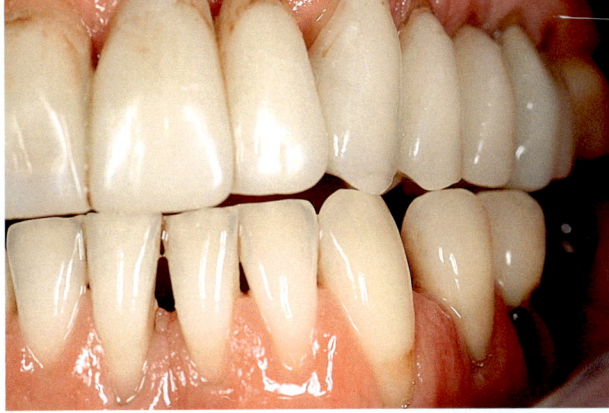

> Fig 4-6a

> Fig 4-6b

> Fig 4-6c

> Fig 4-6d

Vertical dimension of occlusion The value of the VDO during the positioning and relining of the provisional restoration should remain constant throughout the course of treatment. This can be reconfirmed by checking that the value found between two reference points at the dentogingival border (eg, right maxillary canine and right mandibular canine) remains constant over time. In cases where the VDO has been purposely modified by the clinician, the adaptation to this variation should be checked instead. The new clinical situation, which usually requires an adaptation period of roughly 3 to 4 weeks, is then analyzed again to ensure that the patient is in a comfortable position.[38,43,44] If contraction and muscular fatigue are still present, adjustments are made that should then be tested for a few weeks before proceeding with the final phases.

Occlusal stability Whether the case has been finalized in MI or in CR, a check must be made for synchronous and well-distributed punctiform contacts[52–56] (Figs 4-7a and 4-7b). In the anterior sector, light contact between the maxillary and mandibular teeth, in addition to guaranteeing necessary stability, allows any interference in the posterior teeth during excursive movements to be avoided[57] (Figs 4-7c to 4-7f).

Centric relation–centric occlusion The clinician must make sure that the patient, when closing his or her mouth, whether alone or during manipulation, manages to achieve CO with extreme ease.[58–60] The exact definition of this position is crucial in order for the casts of the provisional restorations to be mounted correctly on the articulator and then for carrying out the cross-mounting.

BIOLOGIC PARAMETERS

Biologic integration of the acrylic shell is a determining factor in taking the final impressions correctly. It is therefore essential to ensure that the gingival tissues are adequately supported by the restorative contours and that there are no signs of gingival inflammation.[2,61–63] Confirmation should also be made that the patient is able to correctly clean the areas affected by the prosthetic treatment, especially the interproximal areas.[64–70] For single restorations, the use of dental floss is advised. For the posterior sectors of fixed partial dentures, an interproximal brush is required. For the anterior area, so as not to compromise the height of the papillae, the use of a superfloss is recommended instead. This is much less invasive than the interproximal brush, which can sometimes cause trauma but is still effective.

CASE 3

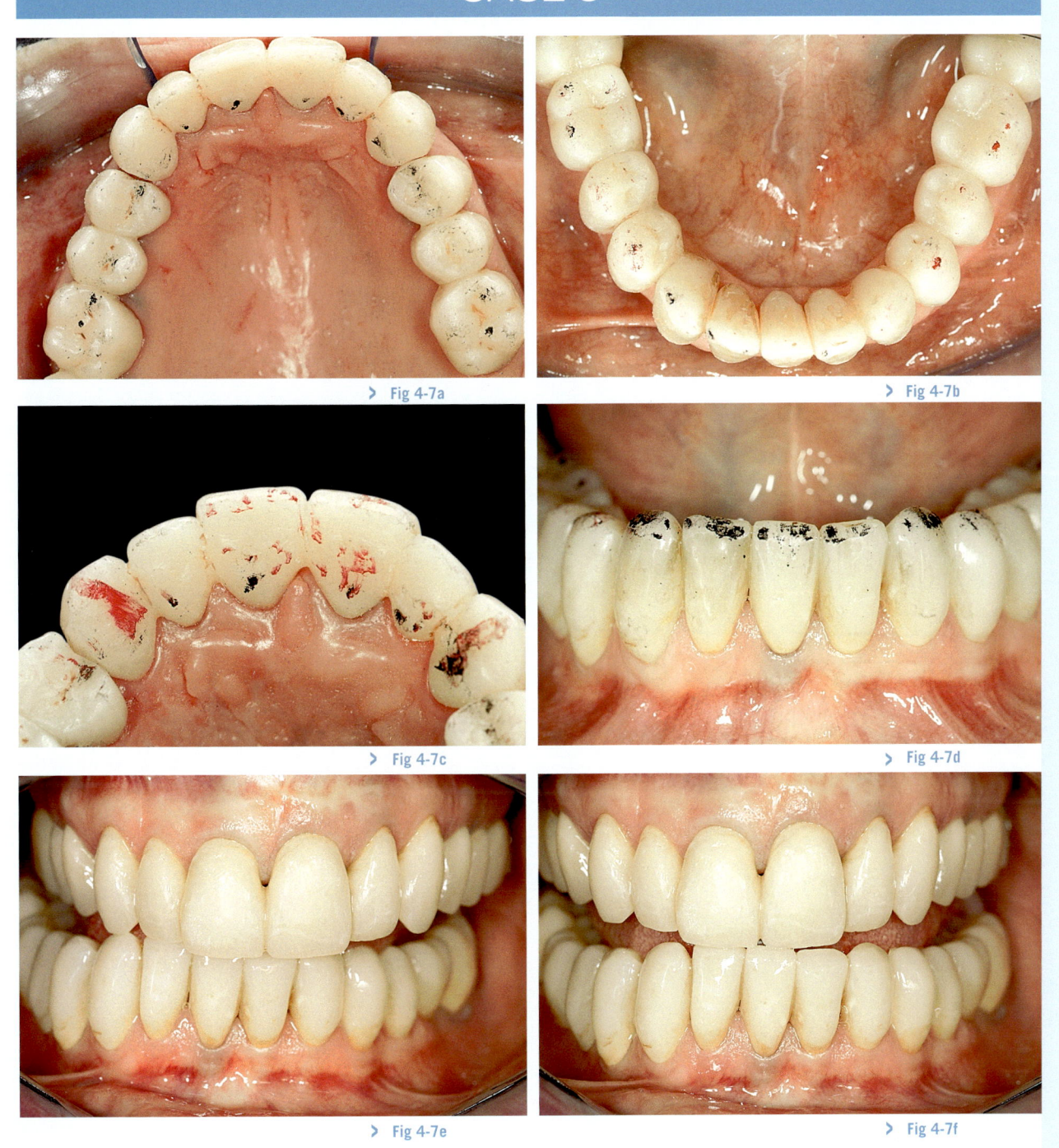

> Fig 4-7a

> Fig 4-7b

> Fig 4-7c

> Fig 4-7d

> Fig 4-7e

> Fig 4-7f

FIG 7 *(a and b)* In the rehabilitation of both arches, punctiform and well-distributed contacts on the cusps can be seen in CR. *(c to f)* The presence of the anterior guidance allows the patient to move the mandible easily without any interference from the posterior teeth.

PROVISIONAL RESTORATION IN SITU

DATA TRANSFER

IMPRESSION OF THE PROVISIONAL RESTORATION AND OF THE OPPOSING ARCH

After carefully verifying the correct integration of the provisional restoration, the clinician, before removing it, must take its impression with that of the opposing arch. In such cases, alginate is normally used. Despite lacking the accuracy typical of elastomers, alginate can nevertheless be considered a reliable material on the condition that it is poured immediately using a vacuum mixer. Unfortunately not all clinicians are properly equipped to pour the impression and develop precise stone casts in their own clinics. In this case it is certainly preferable to use an elastomeric material, which, because of its dimensional stability, allows the clinician to send the impressions to the laboratory without any risk of distortion.

To correctly transfer the information contained in the provisional restoration, the two stone casts must be completely accurate. Any defect or distortion of the impressions, once in the articulator, can alter the occlusal relationship that exists in the mouth, and so prevent replication of the esthetic-functional characteristics of the provisional restoration.

PROTRUSIVE INTEROCCLUSAL RECORD

As already shown (see chapter 1, page 70), protrusive interocclusal record is accomplished by asking the patient to bring the teeth into the edge-to-edge position. In the space that opens between the posterior teeth (Angle Class I and Class II), occlusal registration material must then be inserted until it has hardened or polymerized completely (Fig 4-8). The protrusive interocclusal record carried out in this way allows the technician to determine the condylar inclination in the articulator so that it is not set arbitrarily at 20 degrees[71] (see chapter 1, page 100).

FACEBOW

To mount the maxillary cast on the articulator and orient it correctly, the recording of the facebow plays a decisive role. The use of an arbitrary facebow is reliable in daily clinical use.[76–81] As amply illustrated earlier (see chapter 1, page 80), to reproduce the clinical situation on the articulator, the clinician stands in front of the patient, orienting the arms of the facebow parallel with the horizon[17,72–75] (Fig 4-9). This registration can be recorded identically with either the provisional restorations in situ or by positioning the fork of the facebow on the definitive preparations because, as shown later, the use of a systematic approach allows for interchanging of the casts by means of the occlusal registration wax-ups (cross-mounting).

FIG 8 The patient is asked to open and close the mandible in the edge-to-edge position. The occlusal registration material for recording the patient's protrusive interocclusal record is then inserted between the posterior teeth.

FIG 9 Before the provisional restoration is removed to take the final impressions, the facebow is recorded to correctly orient the maxillary cast on the articulator.

PROTRUSIVE INTEROCCLUSAL RECORD

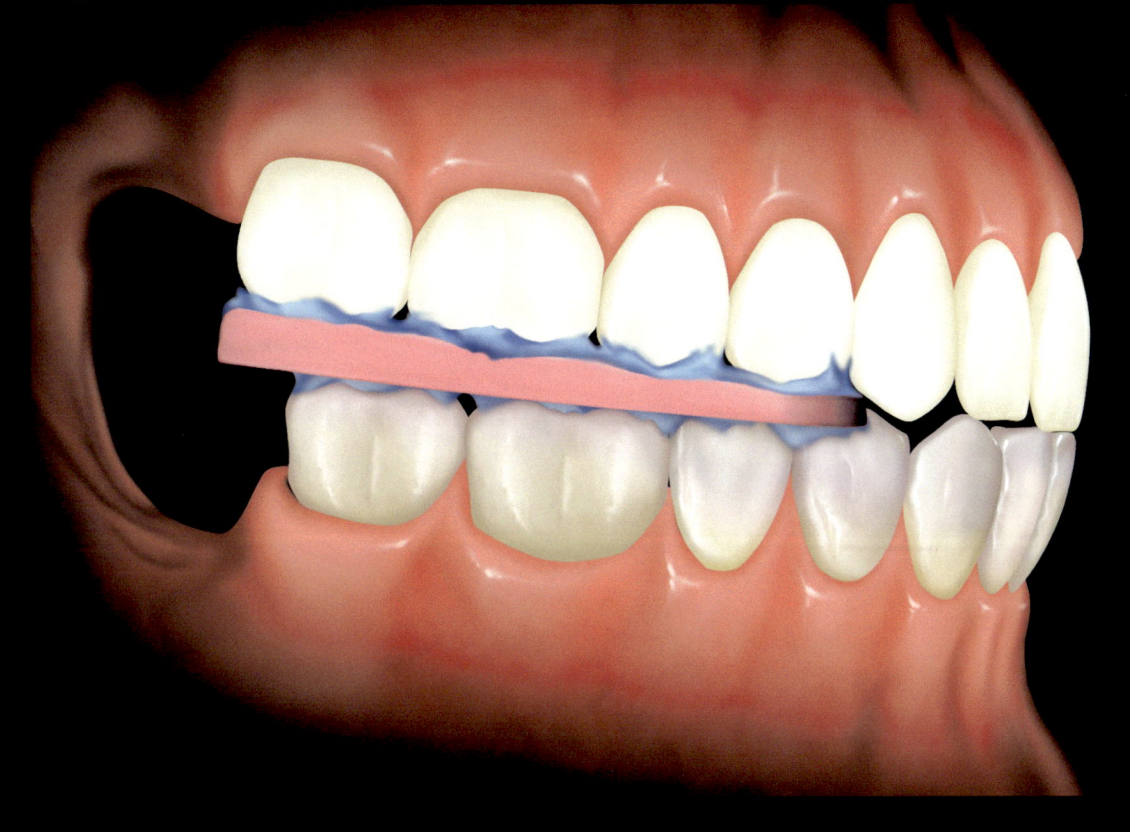

> Fig 4-8

FACEBOW

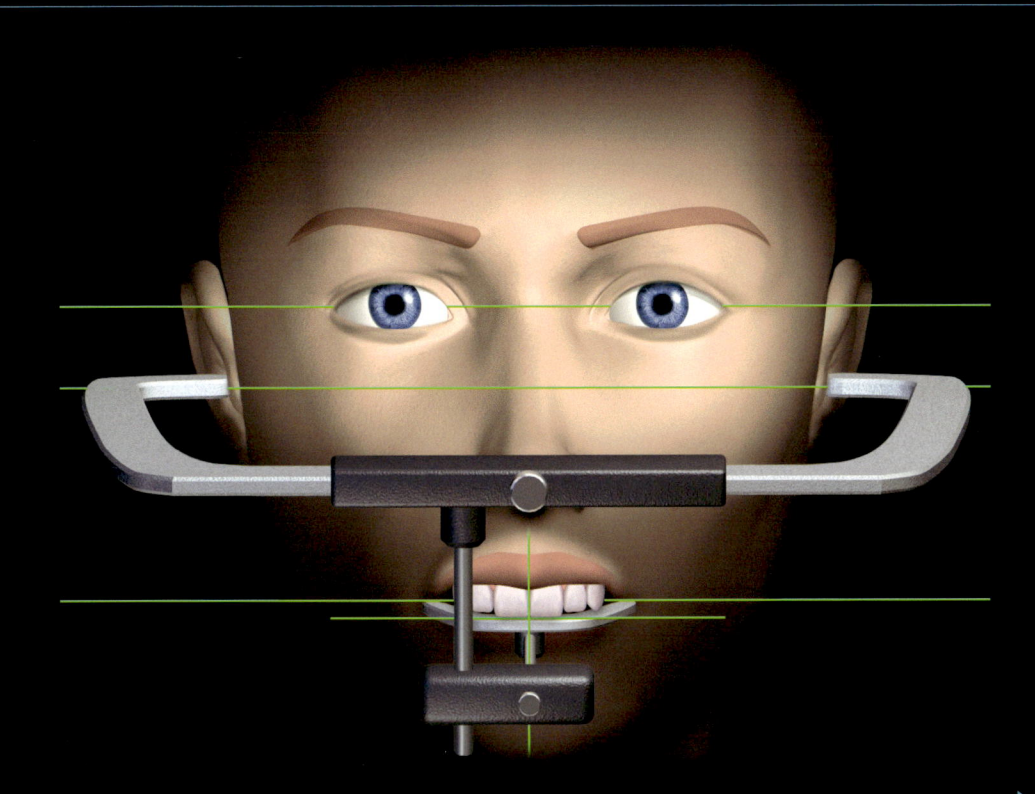

> Fig 4-9

DATA TRANSFER

FINAL IMPRESSIONS

REMOVING THE PROVISIONAL RESTORATION

Once the facebow has been recorded, impressions have been taken of the provisional restorations and of the opposing arch with the provisional restoration in place, and the protrusive interocclusal record has been completed, the provisional restoration is removed for another check of its thicknesses in the various areas.

The position of the prosthetic margins in relation to the gingival levels must also be evaluated, especially in cases where intracrevicular deepening has been carried out during the specific appointment for final preparation of the abutments (see chapter 3, page 324). If the clinician decides to deepen the preparation in a specific site even further, the slight discrepancy that would be created with the provisional margin could be compensated for by simply re-margining the acrylic resin without causing any variation in the position of the provisional restoration.

The accuracy of the marginal fit at the time of relining and the meticulous care taken when the excess cement is removed allow the tissues to maintain an adequate state of gingival health,[64–70] an essential prerequisite for taking the impression. If the state of gingival health is less than adequate, it is necessary to ascertain the cause of the inflammation and to postpone taking the impressions to a later date.

FINAL IMPRESSIONS

The impression represents one of the most important means of communicating with the laboratory, allowing the reproduction of the dentogingival structures involved in the prosthetic rehabilitation to be transmitted in negative. To obtain ideal tissue stability, the impressions are usually taken 3 to 4 weeks after the final preparations have been carried out.[2,82,83] A good "reading" of the impression is essential for fabricating the definitive prosthesis in the laboratory (Figs 4-10 and 4-11). For every abutment, it is necessary to take an impression of a portion of tooth beyond the finish line, which allows the technician to read the finish line perfectly while gaining information on the root anatomy that can prove useful for creating the contour of the restoration.[84] The accuracy of the reproduction depends strongly on the chemical-physical characteristics of the material used[85] as well as the chosen fabrication technique. Especially in cases of extended rehabilitation, it is a good rule to always take two impressions of the same cast in order to be certain that all of the abutment details have been captured (Fig 4-12).

CASE 1

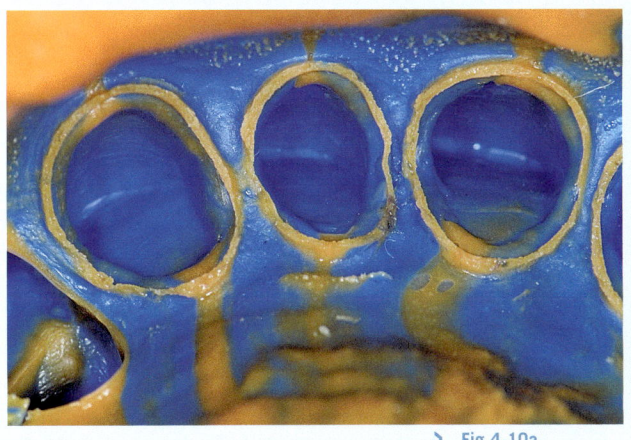

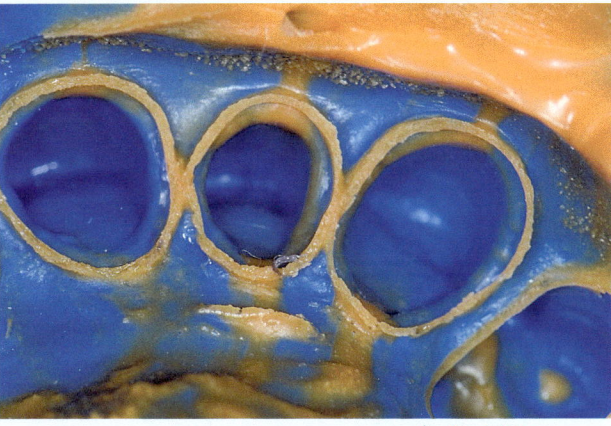

> Fig 4-10a

> Fig 4-10b

CASE 2

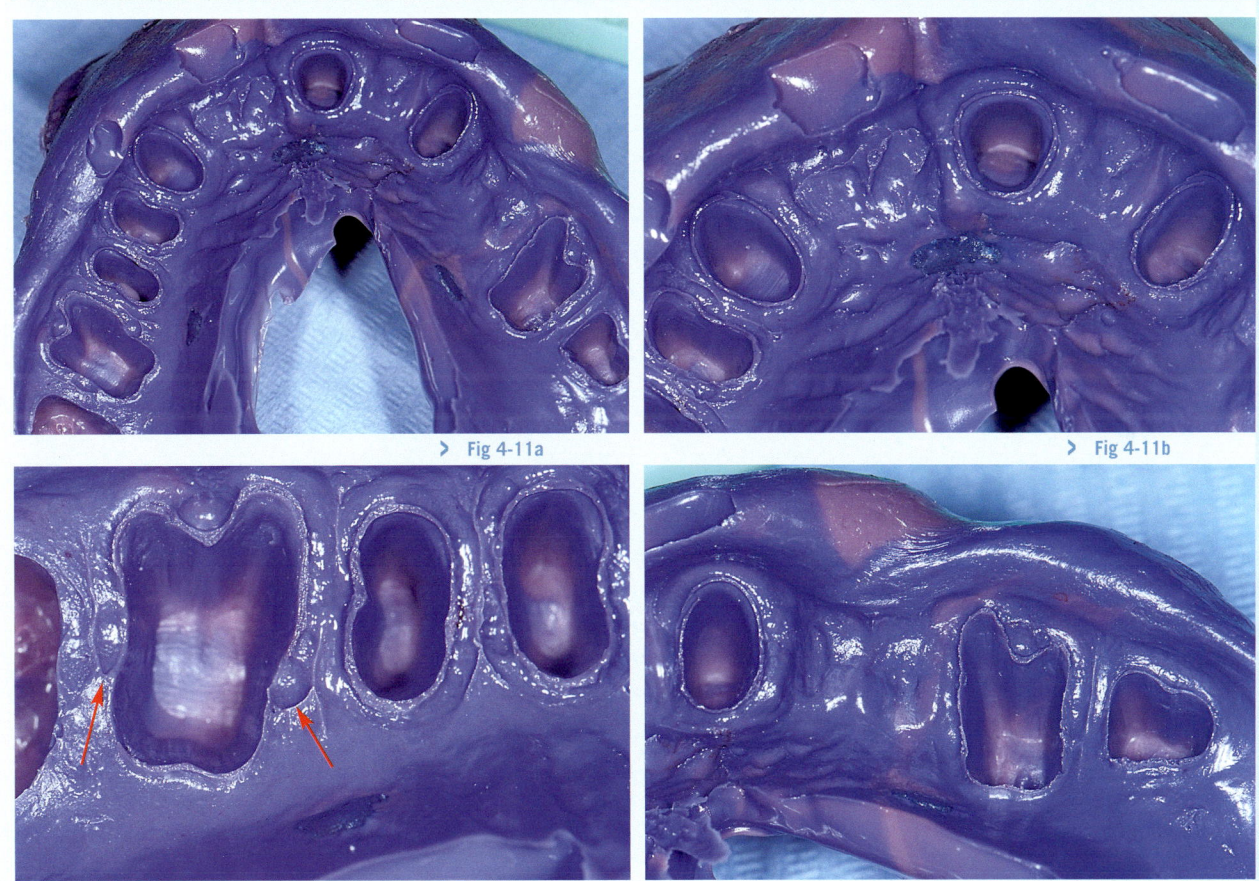

> Fig 4-11a

> Fig 4-11b

> Fig 4-11c

> Fig 4-11d

FIG 10 *(a and b)* The final impression adequately highlights the margins of the six prosthetic abutments.

FIG 11 *(a)* In the rehabilitation of an entire arch, a good reading of the impression of all abutments is essential for correct fabrication of the definitive work. *(b to d)* The close-up photographs display the well-recorded details. Exceptions are the interproximal areas of the right first molar, where two air bubbles *(arrows)* are visible. It should be pointed out, however, that the air bubbles do not compromise the marginal reading because there are knife-edge preparations in these sites, and the defects are localized beneath the gingival margin.

CASE 3

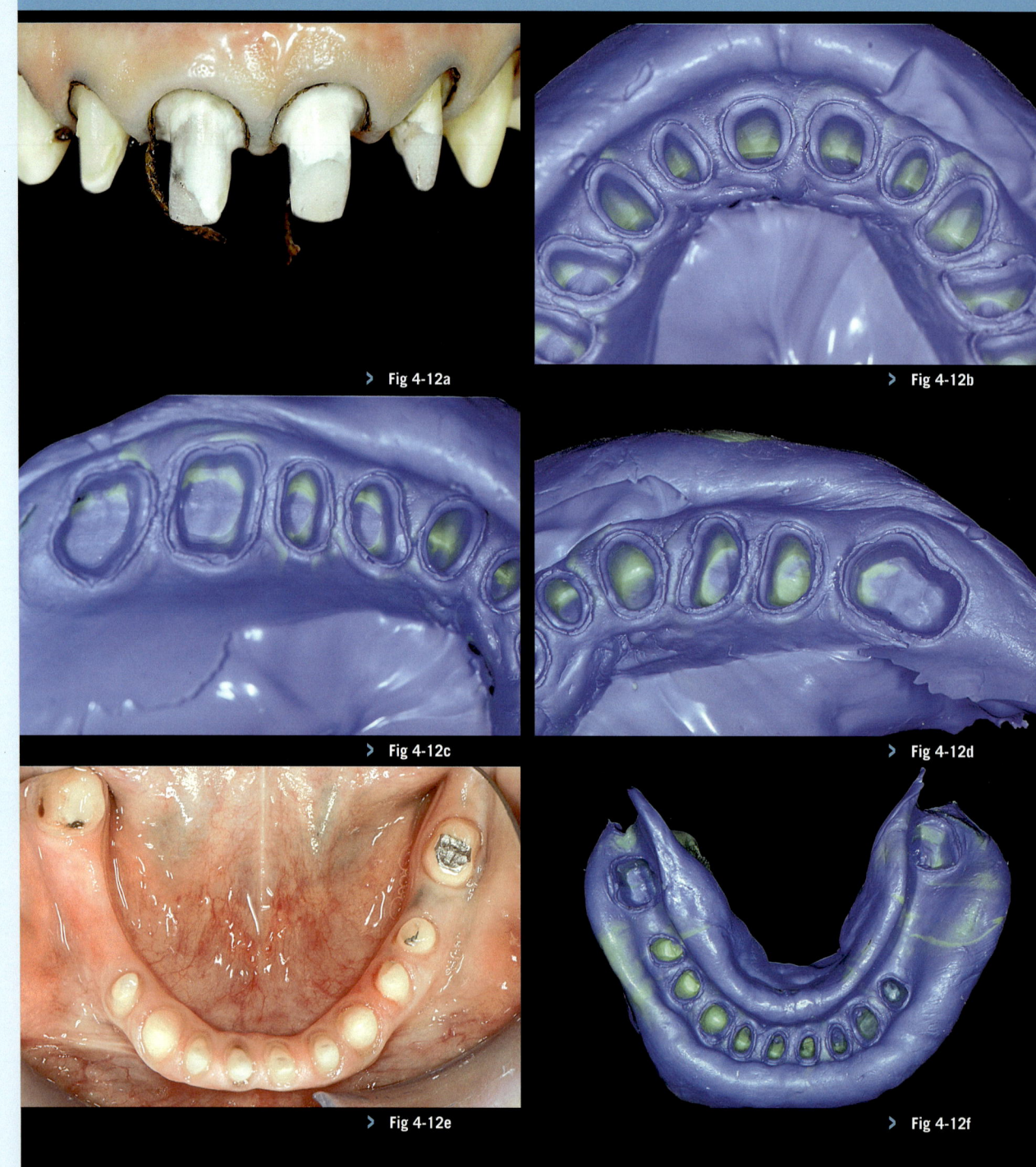

> Fig 4-12a

> Fig 4-12b

> Fig 4-12c

> Fig 4-12d

> Fig 4-12e

> Fig 4-12f

FIG 12 *(a to d)* Insertion of the cord around the abutments allows a particularly detailed impression to be taken in the marginal areas of all the abutments in the maxillary arch. *(e and f)* The cords are then inserted around the prepared teeth of the mandibular arch to obtain a correct impression. *(g to i)* In more complex cases, it is a good rule to take at least two final impressions to ensure that all of the details necessary to guarantee optimum success are captured.

CASE 3

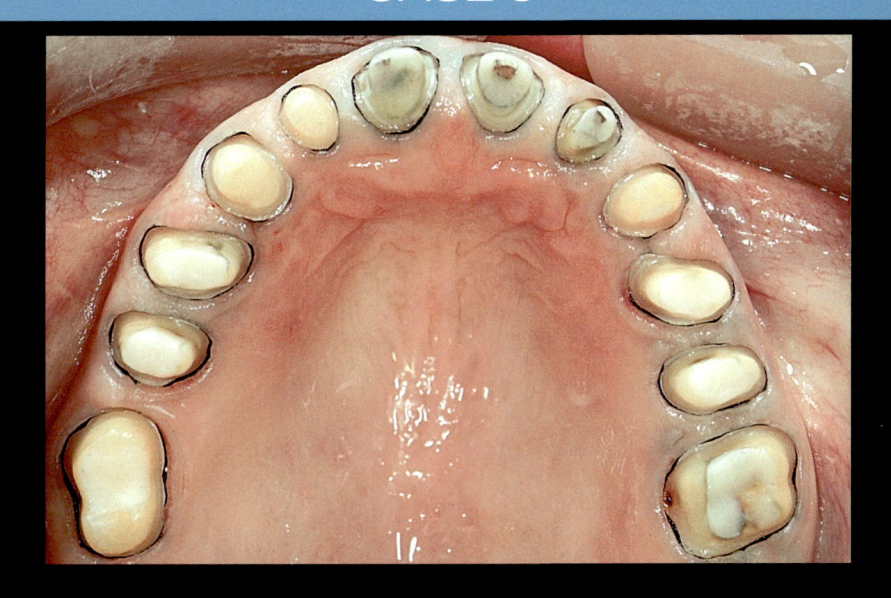

> Fig 4-12g

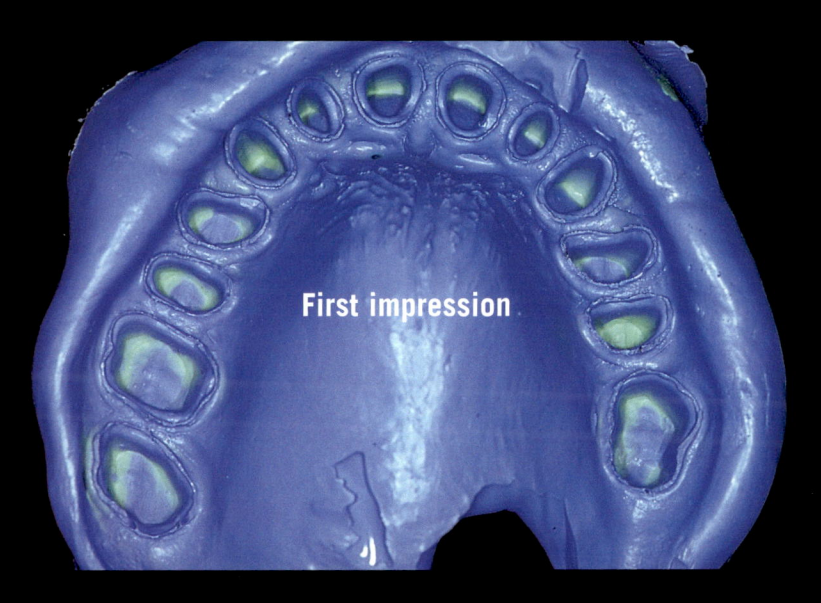

First impression

> Fig 4-12h

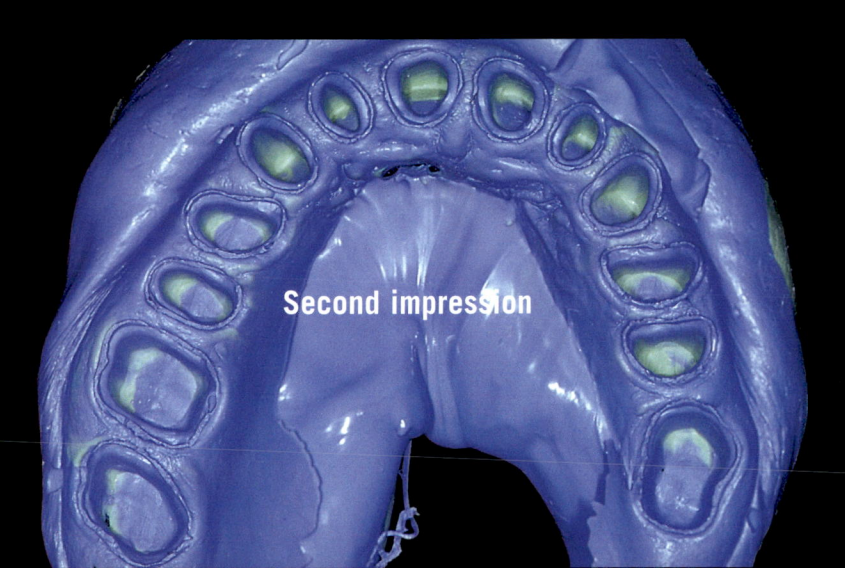

Second impression

> Fig 4-12i

Elastomeric materials are used to take the final impression. Among these, the most commonly used are polyvinyl siloxanes (PVS) and polyethers (PE). Because of their optimal resistance to deformation, excellent accuracy of detail, and good dimensional stability, they can without doubt be considered the materials of choice[86–89] (Figs 4-13a and 4-13b). The dimensional stability, among other factors, allows the pouring of the impression to be delayed by as much as a few days, addressing the needs of many clinicians who send the impressions to an external laboratory.

POLYVINYL SILOXANES and POLYETHERS

Clinic Under dry conditions both materials allow an excellent impression to be taken. However, because they are slightly hydrophilic, the PE materials behave better under moist conditions during the polymerization phases than PVS materials, including the so-called hydrophiles of the latest generation.[90–93] In addition, because of their viscoelastic properties, PE materials seem able to remain in the plastic state for a longer time,[94,95] thereby penetrating deeper into the sulcus and recording the detail more finely. Their extreme rigidity (double that of PVS materials) can create considerable difficulties when the impression is being removed from the mouth, however. The clinician is forced, at times, to use nonaxial disinsertion paths, which can result in permanent deformation of the material.[96] To avoid this serious disadvantage, before taking the impression with a PE material, it is advisable to box all of the dentogingival undercuts with wax. In recent years, to reduce the rigidity of these materials, "soft" PE materials (Impregum Penta DuoSoft, 3M ESPE) have appeared on the market. Possessing greater elasticity, these soft PE materials allow the impression to be extracted from the oral cavity more easily and in an axial manner, thereby reducing the risk of permanently deforming the impression.[97]

The use of PE materials is especially appropriate in cases of complete rehabilitation (Figs 4-13c and 4-13d). The absence of interdental undercuts and the frequent need to join the teeth together require the material to be particularly rigid. It may, however, be preferable to use PVS materials in cases where the work is less extensive and where single teeth are to be restored, especially in the maxillary arch where it is much easier to monitor moisture (Figs 4-13e and 4-13f).

Given the substantial overlap of PE and PVS characteristics, the choice of which elastomer to use relies heavily on the clinician's confidence with each material.

Laboratory The addition of a surfactant in the hydrophilic PVS materials to improve their "wettability" characteristics certainly aids the technician in pouring the stone cast, even if this procedure is still easier with PE materials because of their slight hydrophilia. The rigidity of this material, however, can put at risk the integrity of the plaster abutments taken from the impression, especially in patients with long, thin teeth (eg, mandibular incisors); in these cases the technician is forced to pour the casts with an epoxy or polyurethane resin.

> Fig 4-13a

> Fig 4-13b

> Fig 4-13c

> Fig 4-13d

> Fig 4-13e

> Fig 4-13f

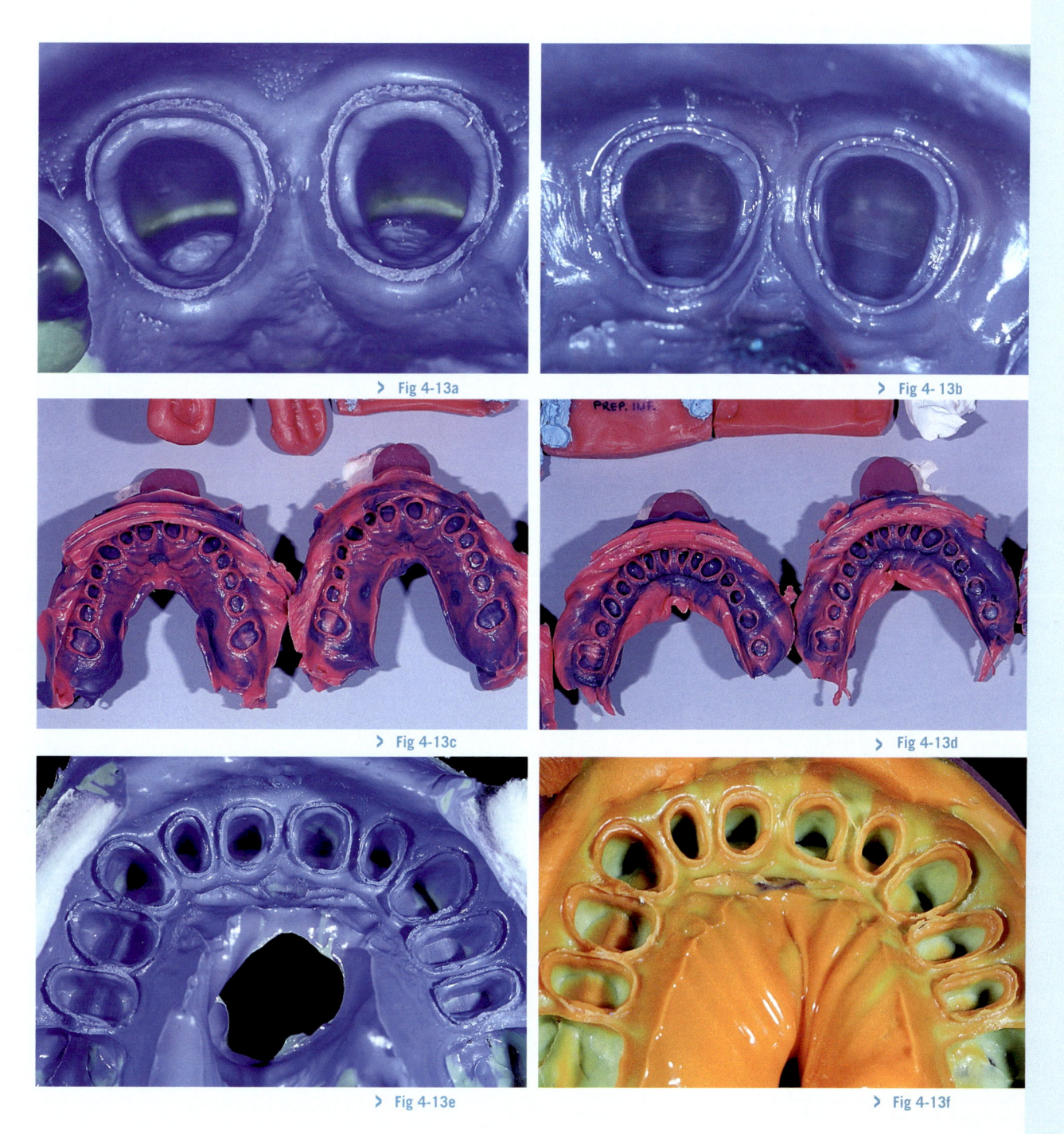

FIG 13 *(a and b)* PVS and PE materials allow excellent details to be obtained. *(c and d)* In cases of complete rehabilitation, the absence of dental undercuts allows even rigid materials such as the PEs to be removed from the mouth. *(e and f)* For single restorations, PVS materials can be used since it is not necessary for the impression material to be extremely rigid. In every patient, it is advisable to take at least two accurate impressions to be sure that all necessary details are captured.

IMPRESSION TECHNIQUE

ONE STEP–DOUBLE MIX

The impression techniques are based on the number of phases and the viscosity of the materials used. Among these, the one that has undoubtedly proved the most reliable over the course of the past 20 years, in the authors' opinion, is the "one step–double mix." This technique consists of the simultaneous polymerization of two pastes of different viscosities. First, a special syringe is used to apply a light body material at the margins of the abutments; to drive it into the sulcus, the syringe is used to gently blow air. After a further layer of light body is applied to the abutments, the individual impression tray is then seated. The material in the impression tray has greater viscosity (heavy body), and its compressive effect helps the light body material penetrate into the sulcus.

RECOMMENDATIONS

The following recommendations are useful for optimizing the recording of the final impression.

Impression tray It is very convenient, especially in complex cases, to use an individual impression tray that, because of the presence of uniform thicknesses, minimizes contraction of the material.[98] An impression tray equipped with side handles aids in its quick removal in the axial direction, thereby preventing permanent deformation of the impression material. The use of a specific tray adhesive for each individual impression material also avoids any possible detachment and/or stretching.[99]

Mixing To minimize the risk of inaccuracies caused by manual mixing, it is advisable to use manual dispensers (Fig 4-14a) or automatic vacuum mixers (Fig 4-14b) that guarantee optimal consistency and union between base paste and catalyzer.[100–103]

Gloves When using PVS materials, vinyl gloves rather than latex should be used during the preparation and impression-taking phases, because of the possible interaction between the latex glove and the added silicone, which might inhibit complete polymerization.[104–108]

Disinfection In recent years the ability of disinfectants to reduce the risk of contamination originating from the impressions has been analyzed.[109–117] Disinfection with appropriate substances (2% glutaraldehyde or 5% hypochlorite for a period of roughly 10 to 15 minutes) does not seem to significantly compromise the physicochemical properties of either PE or PVS materials.[118]

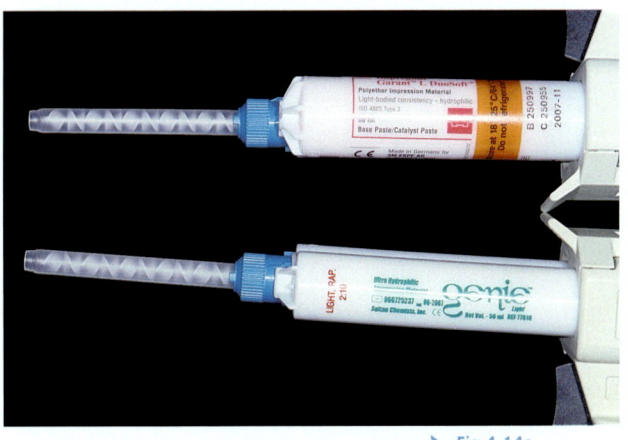

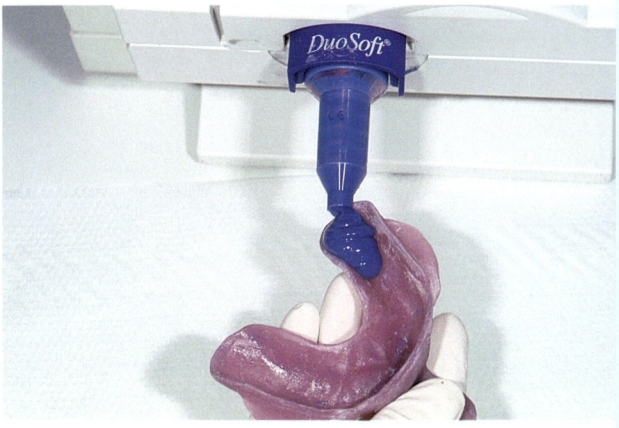

> Fig 4-14a   > Fig 4-14b

POLYETHERS (PE)

ADVANTAGES	DISADVANTAGES
▪ Excellent reproduction of detail ▪ Considerable resistance to deformation ▪ Optimum dimensional stability ▪ Good resistance to tearing ▪ Favorable hydrophilic behavior ▪ Possibility of pouring the impression even after 1 week ▪ Easy development of the stone cast	▪ Excessive rigidity ▪ Impression difficult to remove ▪ Possible fracture of abutments in stone

POLYVINYL SILOXANES (PVS)

ADVANTAGES	DISADVANTAGES
▪ Excellent reproduction of detail ▪ Considerable resistance to deformation ▪ Optimum dimensional stability ▪ Discreet resistance to tearing ▪ Easy removal of the impression from oral cavity ▪ Possibility of pouring the impression even after 1 week ▪ Better wettability characteristics (hydrophilic PVS)	▪ Marginal recording critical in moist area ▪ Interaction with latex gloves ▪ Difficulty in pouring stone cast

FIG 14 *(a and b)* The use of self-mixing dispensers and vacuum mixers guarantees perfect union between the base paste and the catalyzer.

DATA TRANSFER

FINAL IMPRESSIONS

VISUALIZING THE FINISH LINE

Taking the impressions is without a doubt easier when the finish line is supragingival, compared with the specific techniques that need to be used if it is positioned at the gingival crest or intrasulcularly. Especially in the latter case, healthy gingival tissue is essential to obtaining an effective final impression; the gingival condition must be verified 1 or 2 weeks before taking the final impressions in a checkup specifically focused on hygiene.

MAPPING THE SULCUS

When taking the final impressions, it is necessary to carefully map the gingival sulcus to check the condition of the tissues. In addition to verifying the absence of bleeding, mapping also serves to evaluate the tonicity and depth of the sulcus, thus allowing the clinician to select the most suitable cord (Figs 4-15a to 4-15d).

CORDS

Mechanical, mechanical-chemical,[119–132] surgical techniques with rotary tools,[133] or electrosurgery[134] can be used to achieve adequate displacement of the sulcus. To avoid the danger of provoking gingival recession phenomena,[136] the chosen technique must not cause irreversible damage to the supporting structures.[82,120,123,129,135] The method still considered the most practical and effective is to use cords that, when inserted into the sulcus, displace the tissues both horizontally and vertically (Figs 4-15e and 4-15f).[123,127–129,137,138]

The resulting horizontal displacement must make it possible to maintain, until polymerization is complete, a thickness of impression material inside the sulcus that is sufficient to prevent any tearing during removal from the oral cavity.[131] Vertical retraction of the tissues and a clear recording of the abutment also allow a portion of the unprepared tooth to be included in the impression, though more apical compared with the preparation margin.

INSERTION FORCE

The pressure used to insert the cords into the sulcus can be crucial to maintaining periodontal health. The clinician should exert an insertion force delicate enough to avoid any damage to the connective tissue attachment.[139] The presence of bleeding caused by excessive pressure used in inserting the cords, in addition to impairing correct impression taking, does not guarantee maintenance of gingival margin stability, the level of which could prove to be altered at the next appointment.

→ ...from page 281

> Fig 4-15a

> Fig 4-15b

> Fig 4-15c

> Fig 4-15d

> Fig 4-15e

> Fig 4-15f

→ Gallery of cases, page 544

FIG 15 *(a to d)* Use of the periodontal probe should not result in any bloody exudate, which is a clear sign of gingival inflammation. *(e and f)* Mapping the sulcus and measuring the depth of the different sites also gives important indications for an accurate selection of the retraction cord.

MECHANICAL ACTION

The effect of the mechanical action alone, exerted by a nonimpregnated cord inside the gingival sulcus, causes predominantly vertical tissue displacement that can be ideal for intrasulcular deepening during the appointment for final preparations (Figs 4-16a to 4-16c). The mechanical action on its own does not, however, produce adequate displacement of the sulcus, which is necessary to avert the risk of tearing the impression material. A nonimpregnated cord can be inserted into the sulcus for up to a maximum of 30 minutes without causing irreversible damage to the supporting tissues.[119,140]

MECHANICAL-CHEMICAL ACTION

The use of chemical agents to impregnate the gingival retraction cords appears to significantly improve opening of the sulcus, guaranteeing the impression a much higher percentage of success.[121,122] Because of their effectiveness and tolerability,[123] the following substances are most commonly used:

- Aluminum chloride
- Aluminum sulfate
- Potassium sulfate
- Ferric sulfate

These chemical agents, if used correctly, are particularly effective and do not cause any local damage or, more important, systemic damage. The use of 8% racemic epinephrine was very popular in the past, especially for its hemostatic effect, which different studies have shown to be quite effective.[119–121,126] This chemical agent is used less and less, however, because of its potentially dangerous systemic action, which can be recognized by a marked increase in blood pressure and heart rate.[119,121,130,141]

Impregnating cords with buffered aluminum chloride (Hemodent Gingival Retraction Cord, Premier Dental Products) and keeping the cords in the sulcus for a maximum of 15 minutes allows both a good tissue response and prolonged opening of the gingival sulcus, thus guaranteeing a very high percentage of impression success (Figs 4-16d and 4-16e).[119,121,122,124,125,127,142] To try to minimize the potential damage to the periodontal structures, the impregnated cords must only be inserted in the phase that immediately precedes that of final impression-taking (Figs 4-16f to 4-16h).

FIG 16 *(a to c)* Insertion of a nonimpregnated cord causes slight apicalization of the gingival levels. *(d and e)* Soaking the cord in aluminum chloride guarantees the impression a high percentage of success. The impregnated cords must be put in position a few minutes before the final impression is taken. *(f to h)* After the first cord is positioned, the tooth can be prepared again at marginal level before a second cord is inserted. The cords should not be kept in the sulcus for longer than 15 minutes.

NONIMPREGNATED CORD

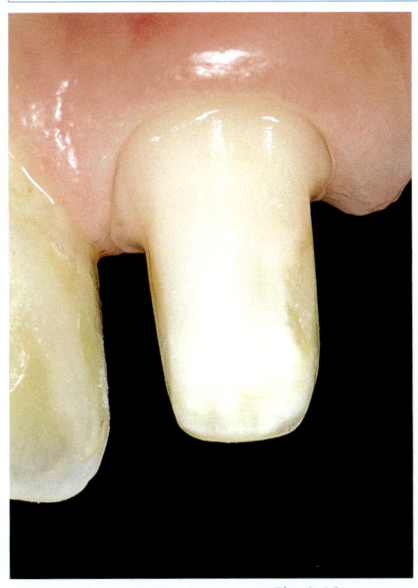

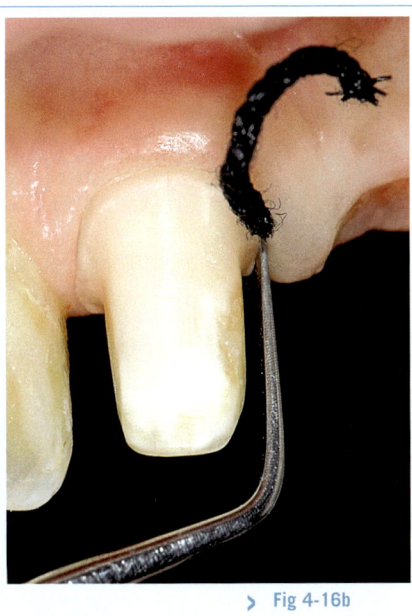

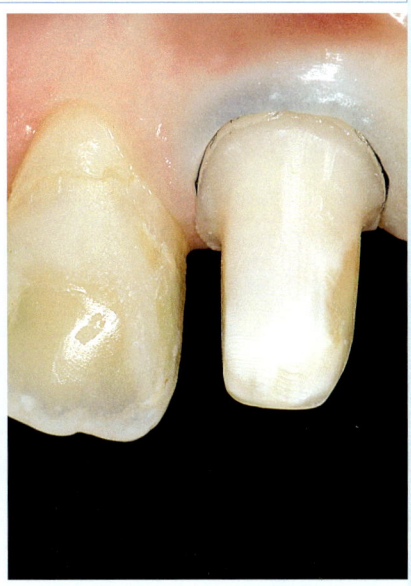

> Fig 4-16a

> Fig 4-16b

> Fig 4-16c

IMPREGNATED CORD

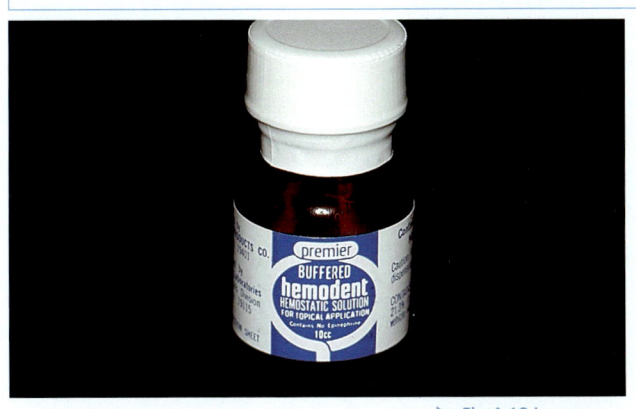

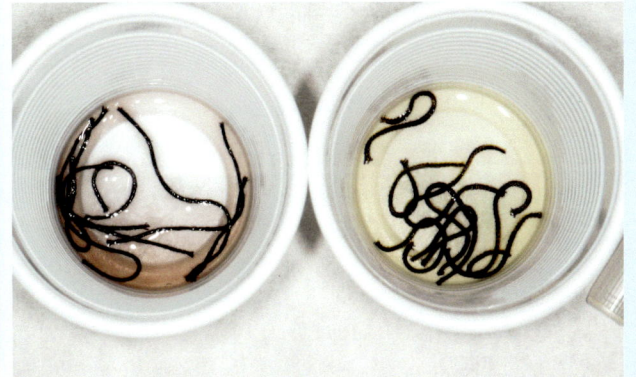

> Fig 4-16d

> Fig 4-16e

> Fig 4-16f

> Fig 4-16g

> Fig 4-16h

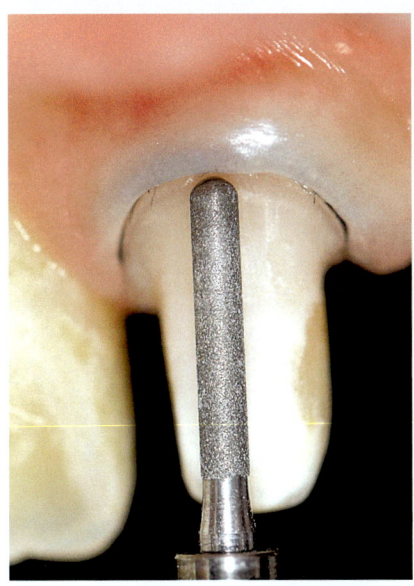

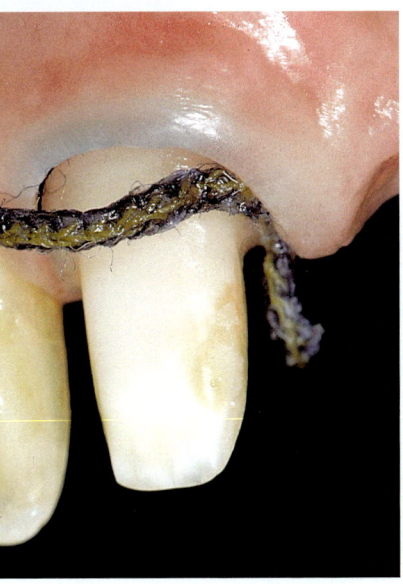

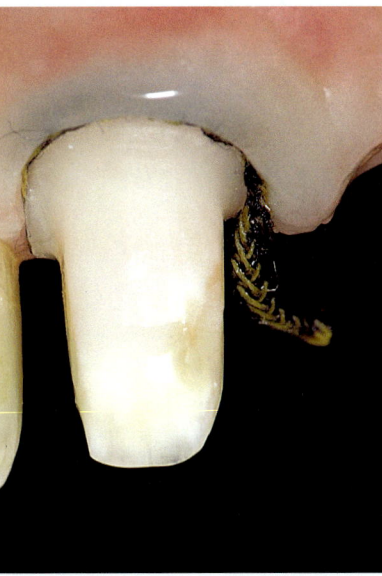

FINAL IMPRESSIONS

■ PREPARATION AT THE GINGIVAL CREST ■
SINGLE-CORD TECHNIQUE

The single-cord technique is traditionally used by many clinicians to minimize trauma to the tissues in the presence of a thin periodontal biotype, and/or when the sulcus is especially shallow. The insertion of a single cord, whether or not it is impregnated with chemical agents, is also quite useful in cases where the final preparations have been completed while maintaining the margins in a position at the dentogingival junction. Inserting one cord, which causes a predominantly vertical tissue displacement, can be very effective in counteracting the presence of crevicular fluid, and, if impregnated, any bloody exudate. The section of the cord is strictly based on the depth and tonicity of the sulcus, as well as the characteristics of the seat in which it will be placed. The cord may be cut to a length longer than the circumference of the abutment and folded back into the interproximal area if a deeper sulcus is present in this zone. The insertion is started at interproximal level because the greater sulcular depth in this area allows the cord to be anchored more easily.[136] The palatal zone is approached and then, only at the end, the delicate buccal area. Special care must be taken not to exert excessive force and, especially if the cord has been impregnated, not to keep it in the sulcus for more than 15 minutes if possible to avoid unpleasant reactions and damage to the periodontal tissues.[124,126,128,143]

IMPRESSION WITH THE CORD INSERTED

In addition to a limited horizontal displacement, the inserted cord also causes a more or less vertical displacement (Figs 4-17a and 4-17b). In cases where it is preferable not to deepen the preparation apically, taking the impression with the cord in situ allows the finish limits to be found easily, since the margin at the gingival crest is temporarily in a supragingival position (Figs 4-17c and 4-17d) and returns to its original position once the cord is removed.

SINGLE-CORD TECHNIQUE
- Carry out mapping to evaluate depth and tonicity of the sulcus.
- Select the appropriate size and type of cord.
- Insert chosen cord into the sulcus.
- Check that a light apicalization of the gingival margins has taken place.
- Take the impression with the cord inserted.

FIG 17 *(a)* After the abutment has been prepared at the level of the gingival crest, a retraction cord suitable for the depth and tonicity of the sulcus is inserted. *(b)* The cord causes an apical displacement of the gingival tissue that temporarily locates the preparation margin supragingivally. *(c and d)* The impression is taken with the cord inserted in the sulcus, making it much easier to highlight the finish line as a result of the coronal displacement.

> Fig 4-17a

> Fig 4-17b

> Fig 4-17c

> Fig 4-17d

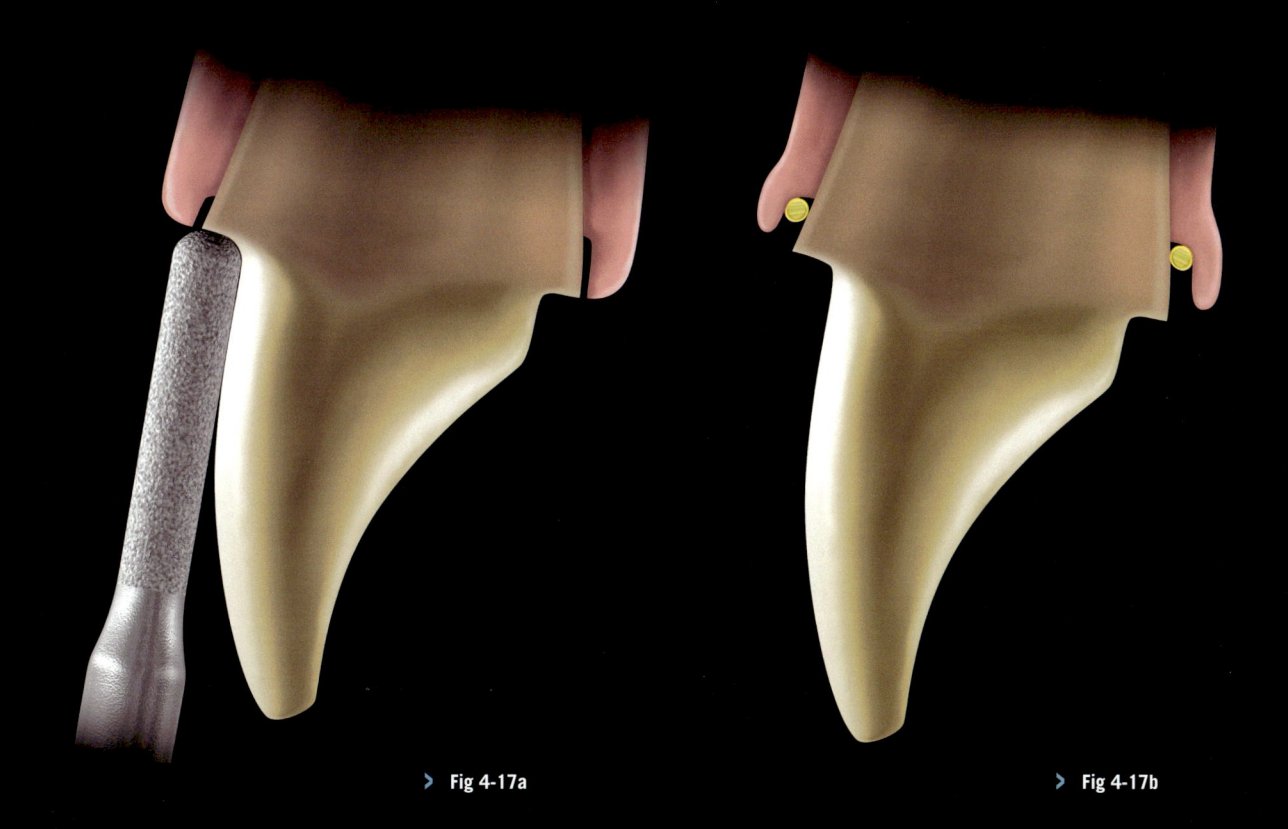

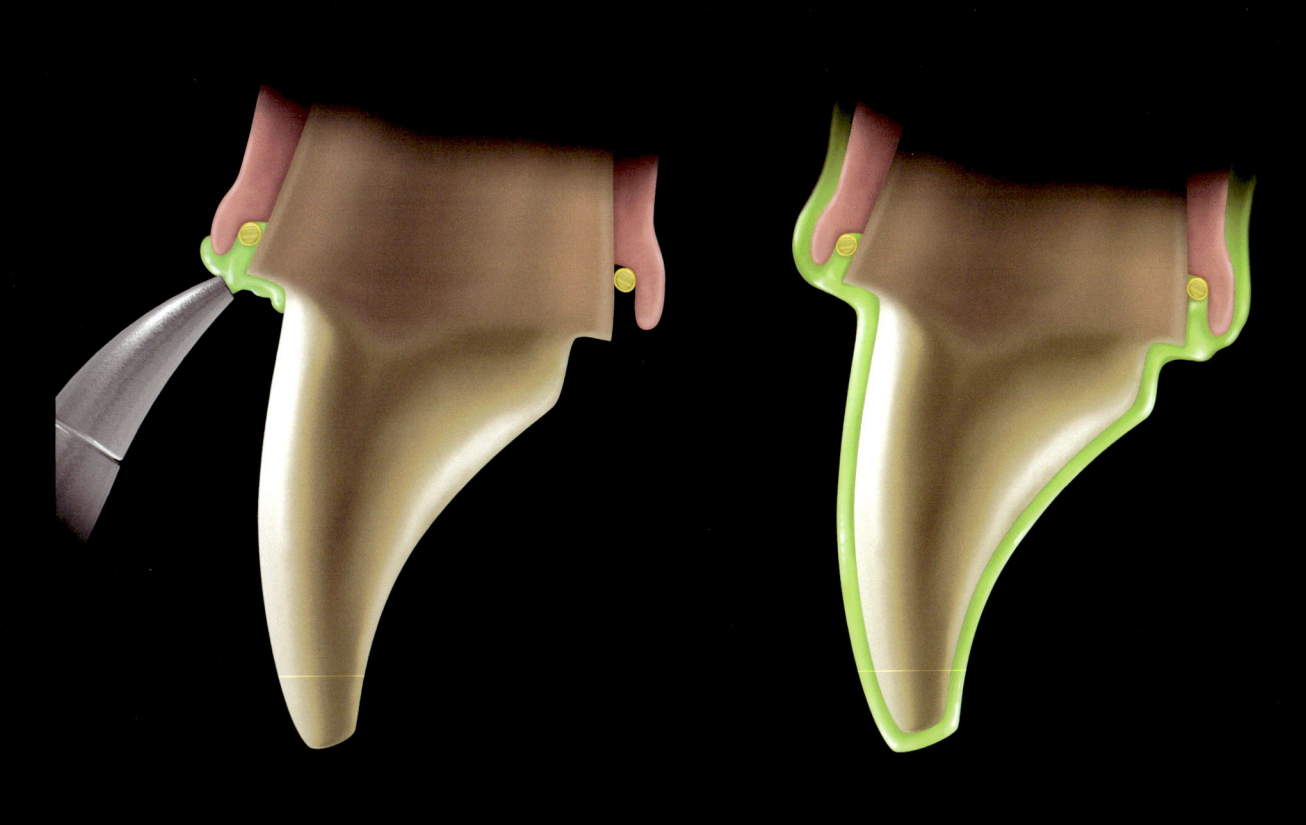

FINAL IMPRESSIONS

■ INTRASULCULAR PREPARATION ■
TWO-CORD TECHNIQUE

In the clinical environment some still question whether one, two, or more cords should be used to take the final impression correctly. As a general rule, the two-cord technique is preferred in the presence of a thick biotype and/or a deeper sulcus or if, to vary the restorative contour, it is decided to apicalize the preparation margin.

The technique in which two cords are inserted is potentially more traumatic than the single-cord technique. However, if all of the passages are completed with necessary care, this method causes no irreparable damage to the soft tissues and allows a wider horizontal displacement of the sulcus.[143] When the impression is taken, the two-cord technique creates an adequate thickness of material (> 2 mm) in the intracrevicular area once polymerization is complete, to prevent tearing when the impression tray is removed.[143]

INSERTING THE FIRST CORD

Before removing the provisional restoration, the clinician must determine whether the intrasulcular deepening carried out a few weeks earlier during the final preparation phases (see chapter 3, page 344) allows the prosthetic margin to be suitably concealed in an intrasulcular position. After the provisional restoration has been removed, further mapping of the sulcus is carried out to select the diameter of the first knitted cord (Ultrapak #000, Ultradent). The diameter of the cord must be appropriate for the dimension and tonicity of the sulcus and usually is not impregnated. If the marginal apicalization caused by inserting the first cord shows the finish line to be in a supragingival position in any specific site, the clinician can deepen the area in question further with a finishing bur to adequately conceal the restorative margin (Figs 4-18a to 4-18d). As it did during the final preparation phases, the cord will act as a barrier to any possible trauma caused by the rotary instrument, thereby preventing interference with the tissue during this extremely delicate phase.

FIG 18 *(a to d)* Once the gingival levels have been temporarily apicalized by positioning of the cord, the preparation margin can be deepened with a fine-grade finishing bur down to the new gingival level.

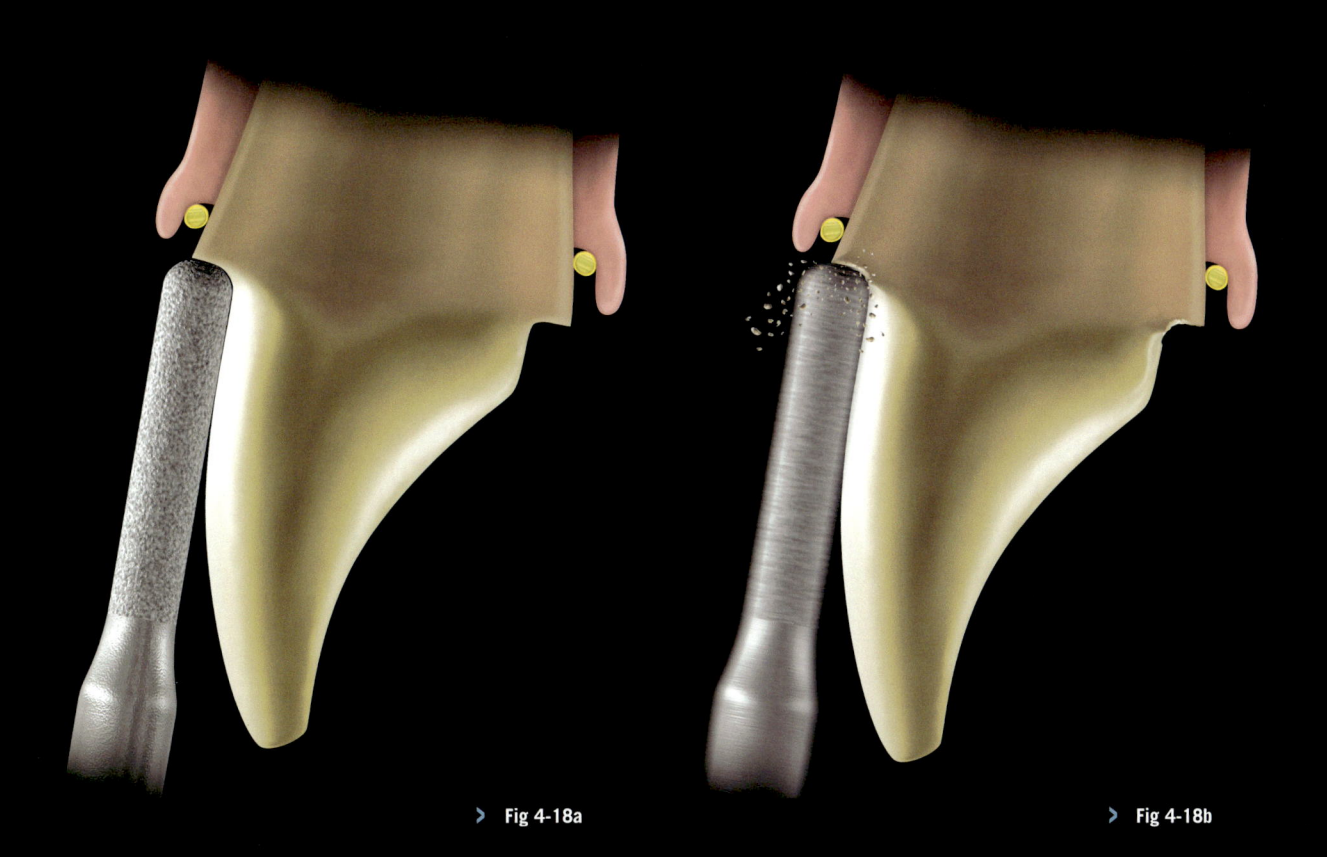

Fig 4-18a

Fig 4-18b

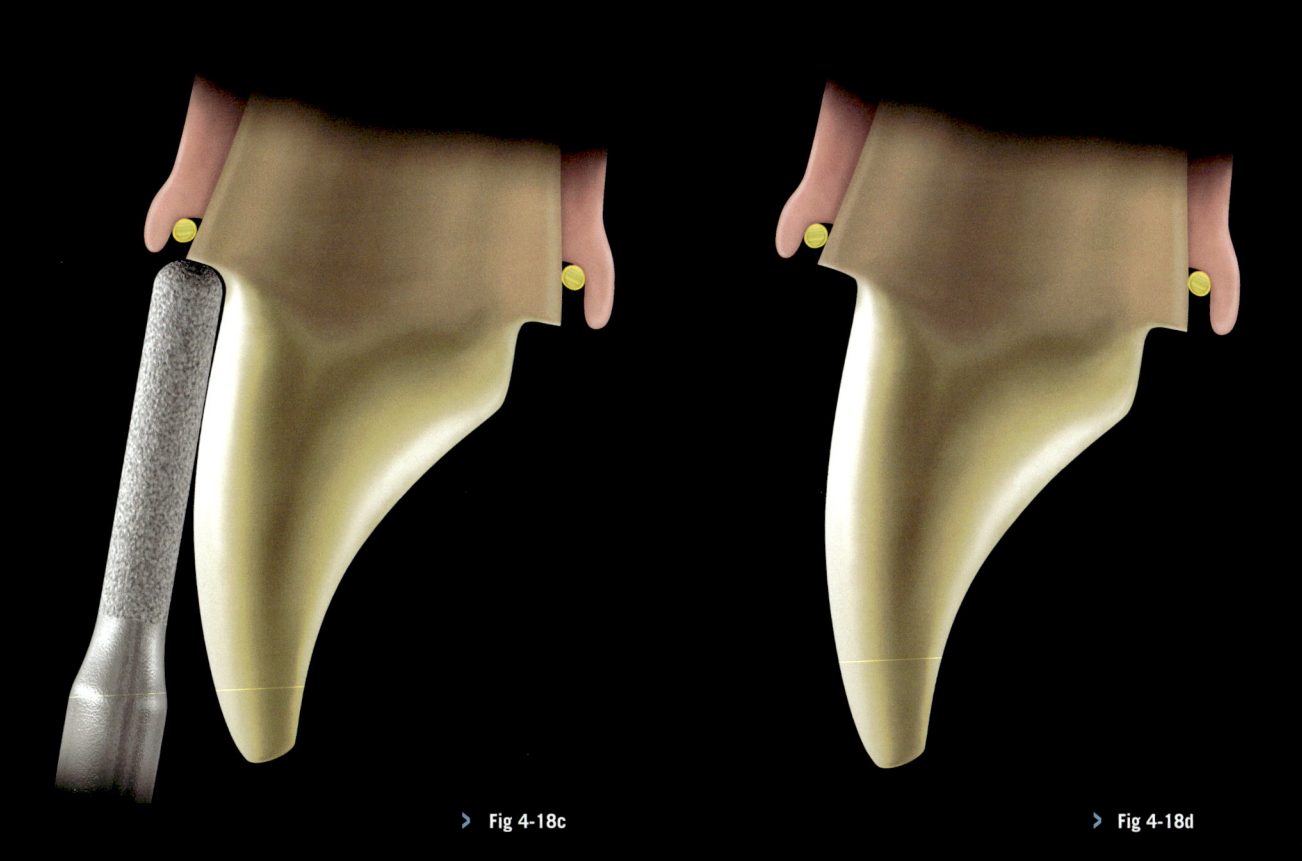

Fig 4-18c

Fig 4-18d

INSERTING THE SECOND IMPREGNATED CORD

After insertion of the first cord, the second, larger one is introduced (Ultrapak #00, Ultradent) after soaking it in a solution of aluminum chloride (Hemodent Gingival Retraction Cord, Premier Dental). In the buccal area of the anterior teeth, however, the depth of a healthy sulcus does not normally exceed 1.0 mm,[135,144] often making it impossible to insert the entire thickness of the second cord (Fig 4-18e).[135,144] To avoid exerting excessive pressure on the second cord, which could result in possible lesions to the connective tissue attachment,[119,120] care must be taken to place the cord delicately without any undue pressure. In the interproximal areas, however, the greater depth of the sulcus in many cases requires a double portion of cord to be inserted and folded back on itself, if adequate displacement is to be achieved. This technique of selective cord insertion therefore often requires the presence of two or more cords in the interproximal areas and just a single cord in the buccal area, upon which the second cord is placed.

Once the second, impregnated cord has been inserted, the clinician must wait a minimum of 4 to 5 minutes for the chemical agent to take effect and for the cord to gradually expand by means of water absorption. Great care should be taken to ensure that the cords are not kept in for an excessive length of time (> 15 minutes), which would have negative consequences on the soft tissues.

REMOVING THE SECOND CORD AND TAKING THE IMPRESSION

After removing the second cord (Fig 4-18f) and cleaning the abutments with an air-water spray to remove any debris left by the impregnated substance,[145] the clinician injects the low-consistency material contained in the syringe into the sulcus and onto the preparations (Figs 4-18g and 4-18h). It is advisable to blow air delicately on the area covered by the fluid material, allowing it to penetrate the intrasulcular areas. The mechanical-type displacing action produced by the second cord is also reinforced by the action of the chemical agent,[127,137,138,146] which is especially obvious when aluminum chloride is used. This means that the fluid material does not need to be injected hurriedly into the sulcus with the syringe at the same time that the cord is removed; the clinician has a few extra seconds to make sure that the margins are visible around the whole circumference of the abutments. A check must also be made for any partial disconnection of the first cord that overlaps the prosthetic margins. Last, to minimize the risk of air bubble formation, before the impression tray is inserted into the oral cavity, the heavier material placed on the impression tray must be covered with a layer of light body material where the prosthetic abutments are located.

Once the impression has been taken, the first cord is removed (Fig 4-18i). Where healthy tissue is present, the gingival margin, which initially had contracted due to the cord's action, returns to its original more coronal position so that the finish line is concealed inside the sulcus (Figs 4-18j, 4-18k, 4-19, and 4-20).

> Fig 4-18e

> Fig 4-18f

> Fig 4-18g

> Fig 4-18h

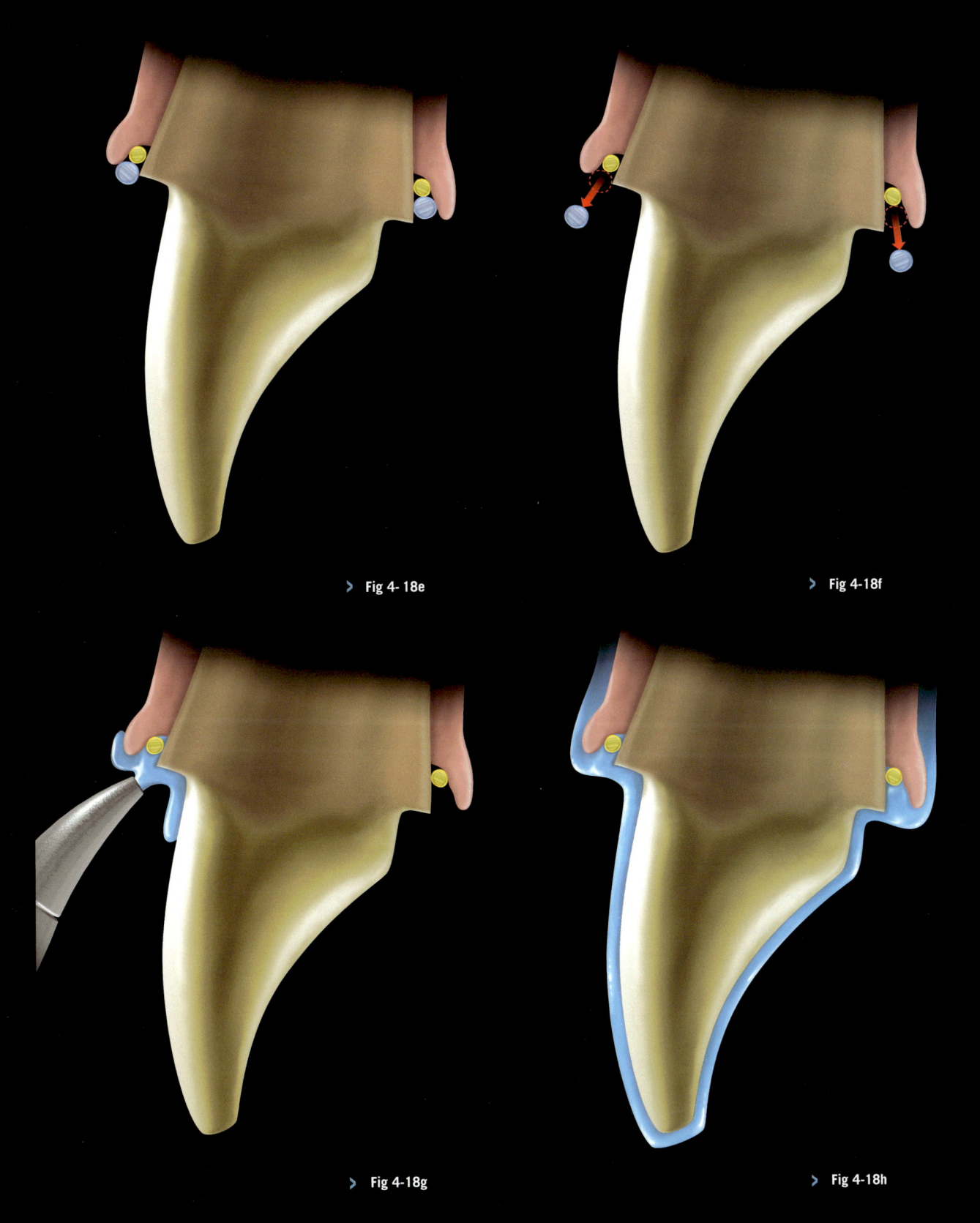

FIG 18 *(e)* Complete insertion of the second impregnated cord can often be hindered in the buccal area by the shallow sulcular depth. *(f to h)* When the final impression is taken, the second cord is removed just before insertion of the low-viscosity impression material around the abutments, which allows the preparation margins to be recorded properly.

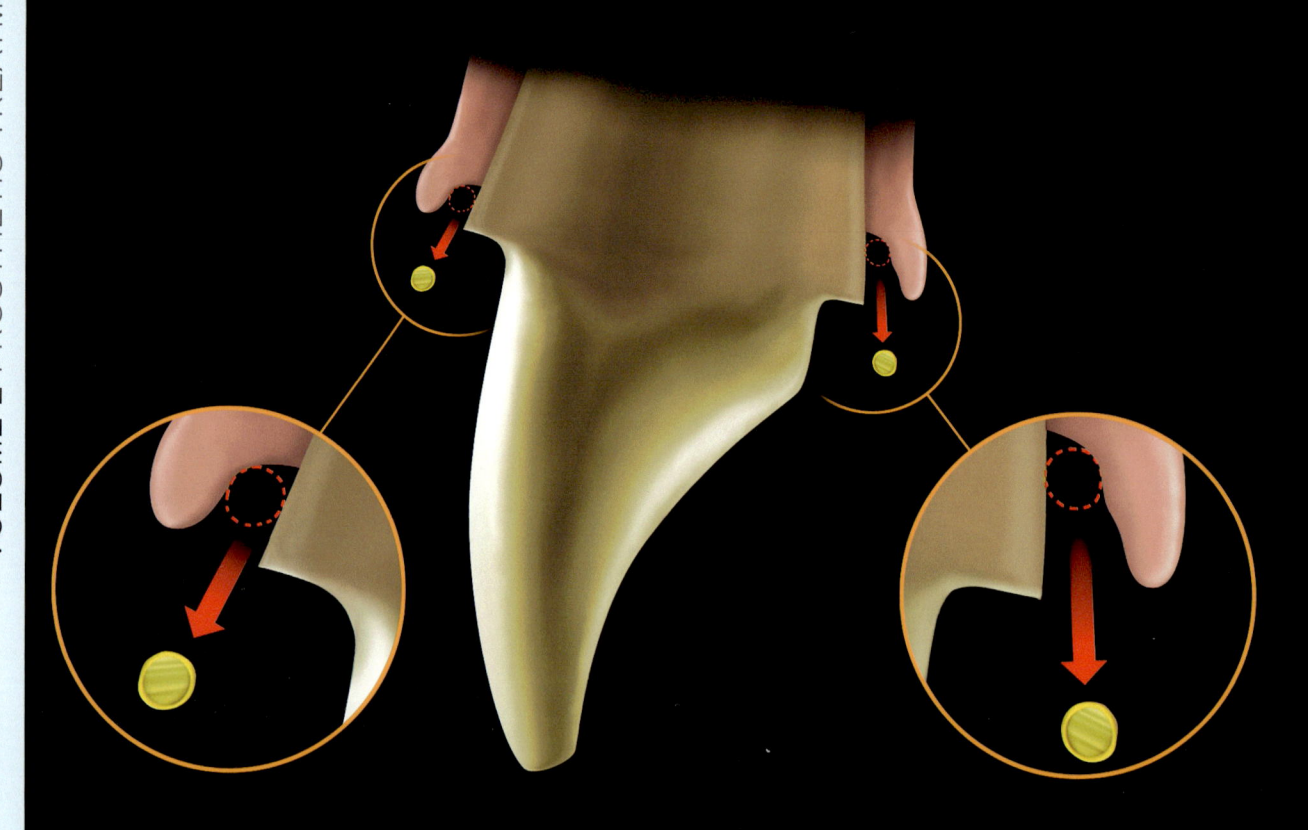

> Fig 4-18i

> Fig 4-18j

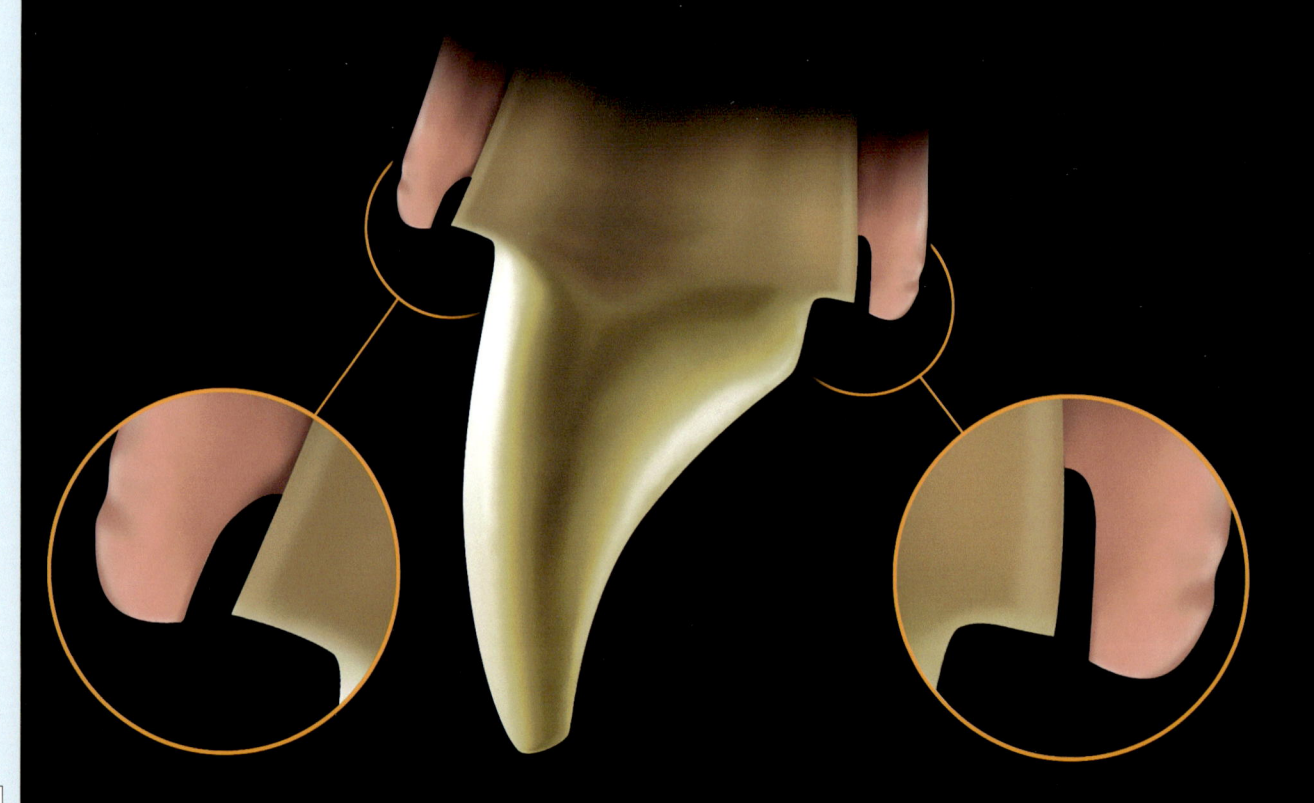

› Fig 4-18k

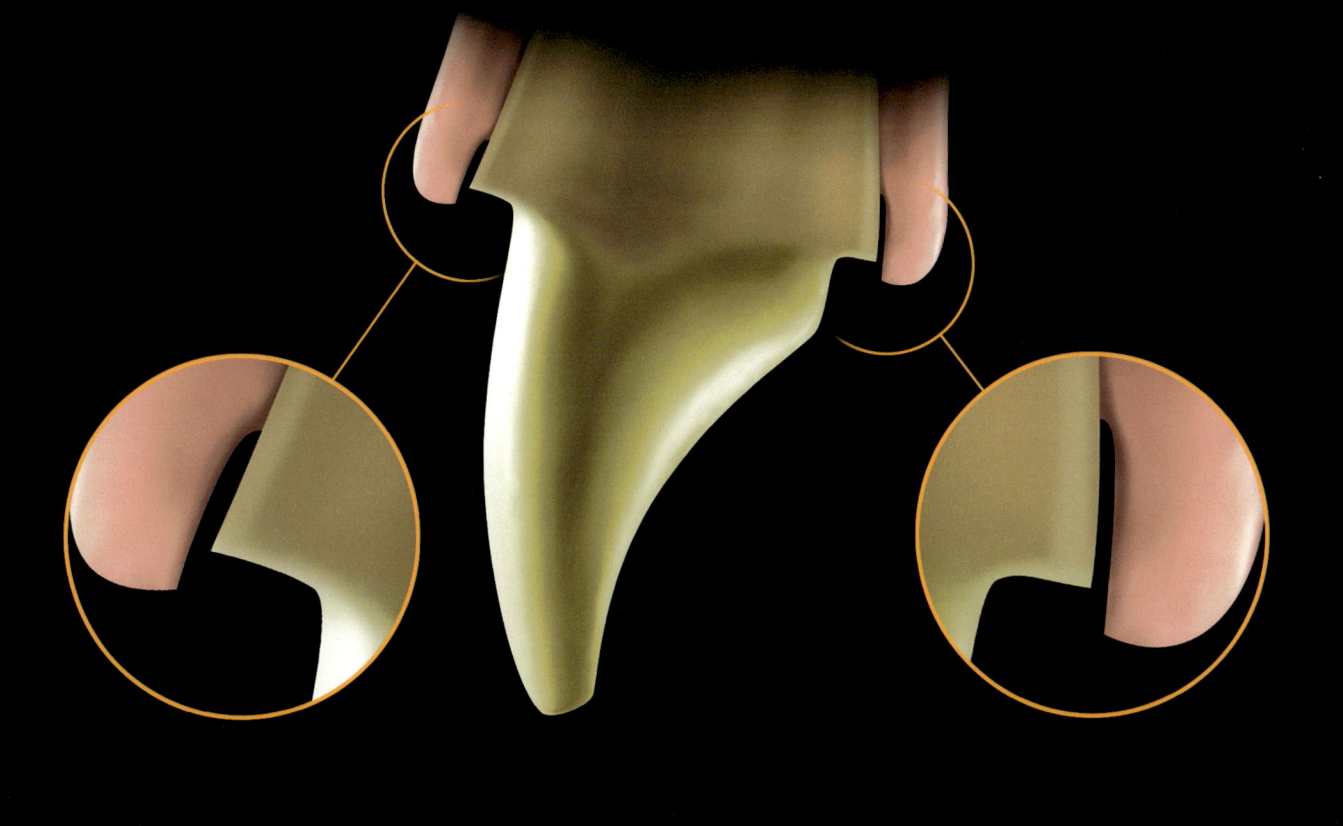

TWO-CORD TECHNIQUE

- Carry out mapping to evaluate depth and tonicity of the sulcus.
- Select cords with appropriate diameters.
- Insert the first nonimpregnated cord into the sulcus.
- Deepen the preparation margin in specific sites if necessary.
- Position the second cord impregnated with buffered aluminum chloride.
- For more than one abutment, first insert the impregnated cords into the distal areas, squeezing them tighter.
- Wait at least 4–5 minutes after positioning the last cord before taking the impression.
- Do not keep the impregnated cords in place for more than 10–15 minutes. Remove the second impregnated cord when the impression is taken.
- Inject the light body impression material into the marginal areas with a syringe.
- Blow air with the syringe and then apply a new layer of light body material.
- Superimpose the light body material over the heavy body material on the impression tray to make the fluid material flow more easily.
- Take the impression.

FIG 18 *(i and j)* After the first cord has also been removed, the gingival tissue, contracted by the mechanical action of the cord and by the chemical action of the impregnating agent, gradually regains its original, more coronal position if it is healthy. *(k)* The preparation margin, as a result, automatically takes up an intrasulcular position.

CASE 1

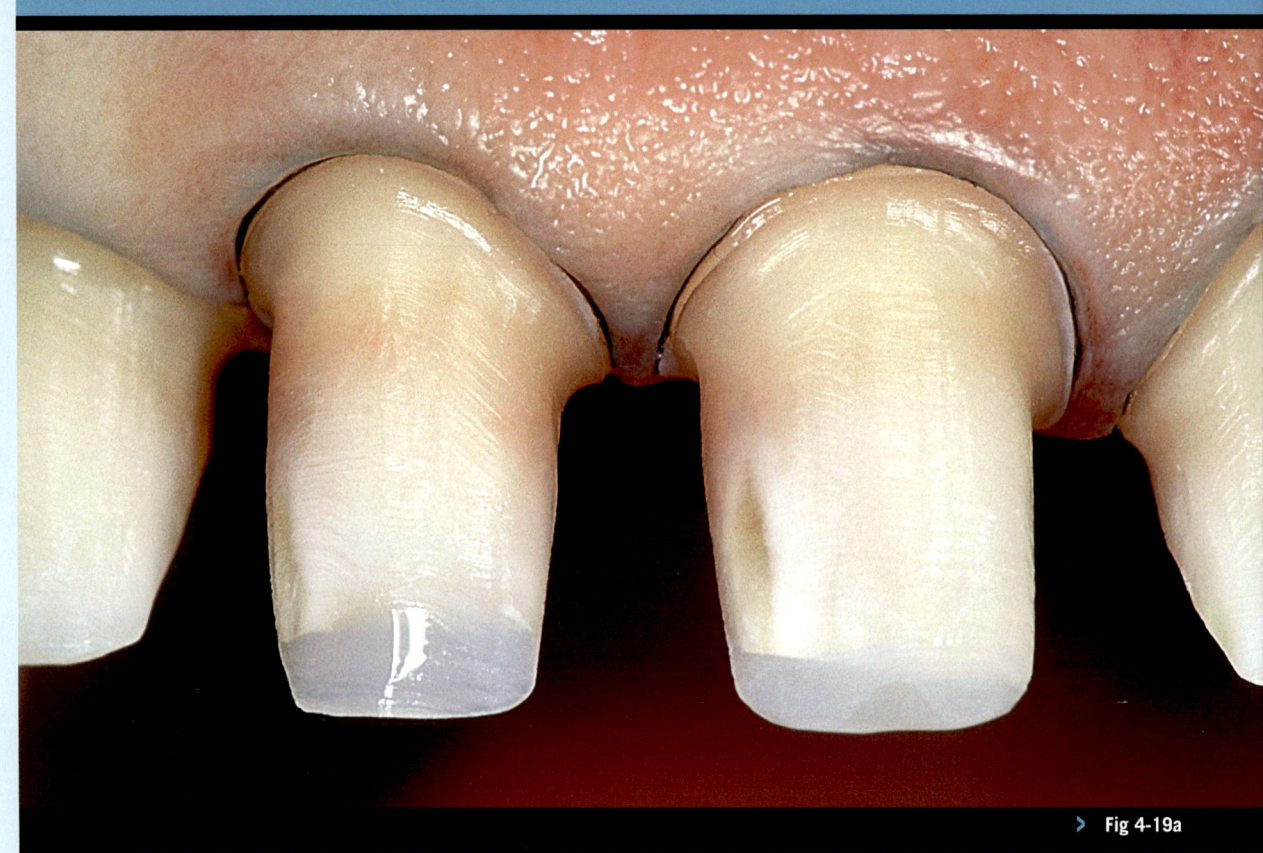

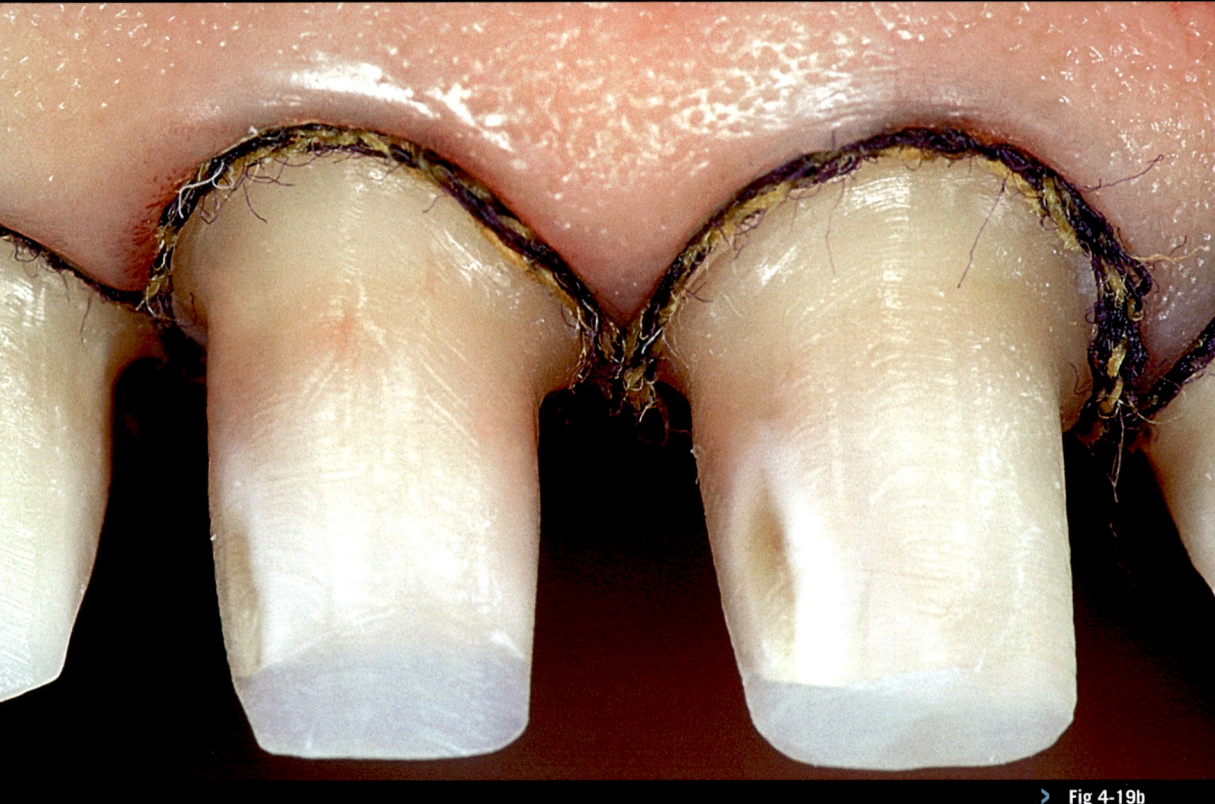

> Fig 4-19a

> Fig 4-19b

FIG 19 *(a and b)* After the first cord is inserted, the marginal area is prepared again before positioning of the second cord, which may not be completely inserted on the buccal side due to the shallow depth of the sulcus.

CASE 1

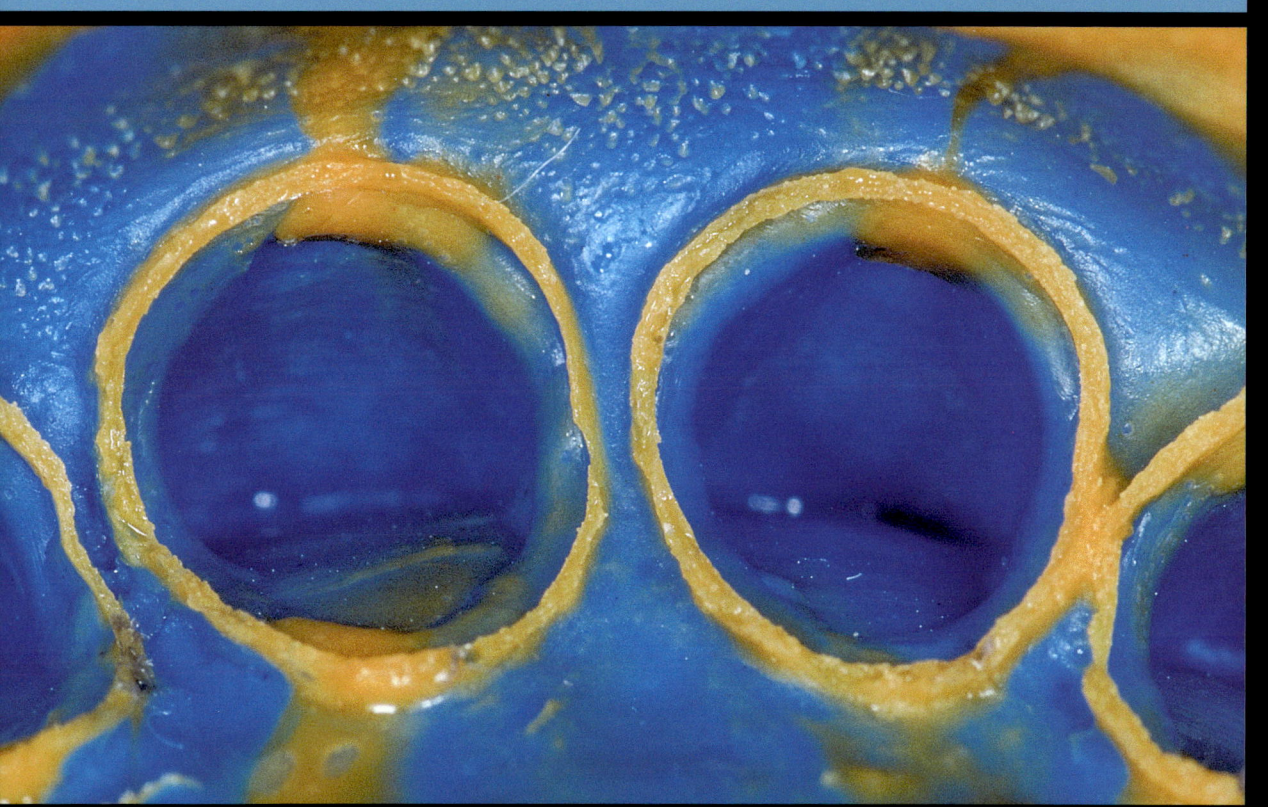

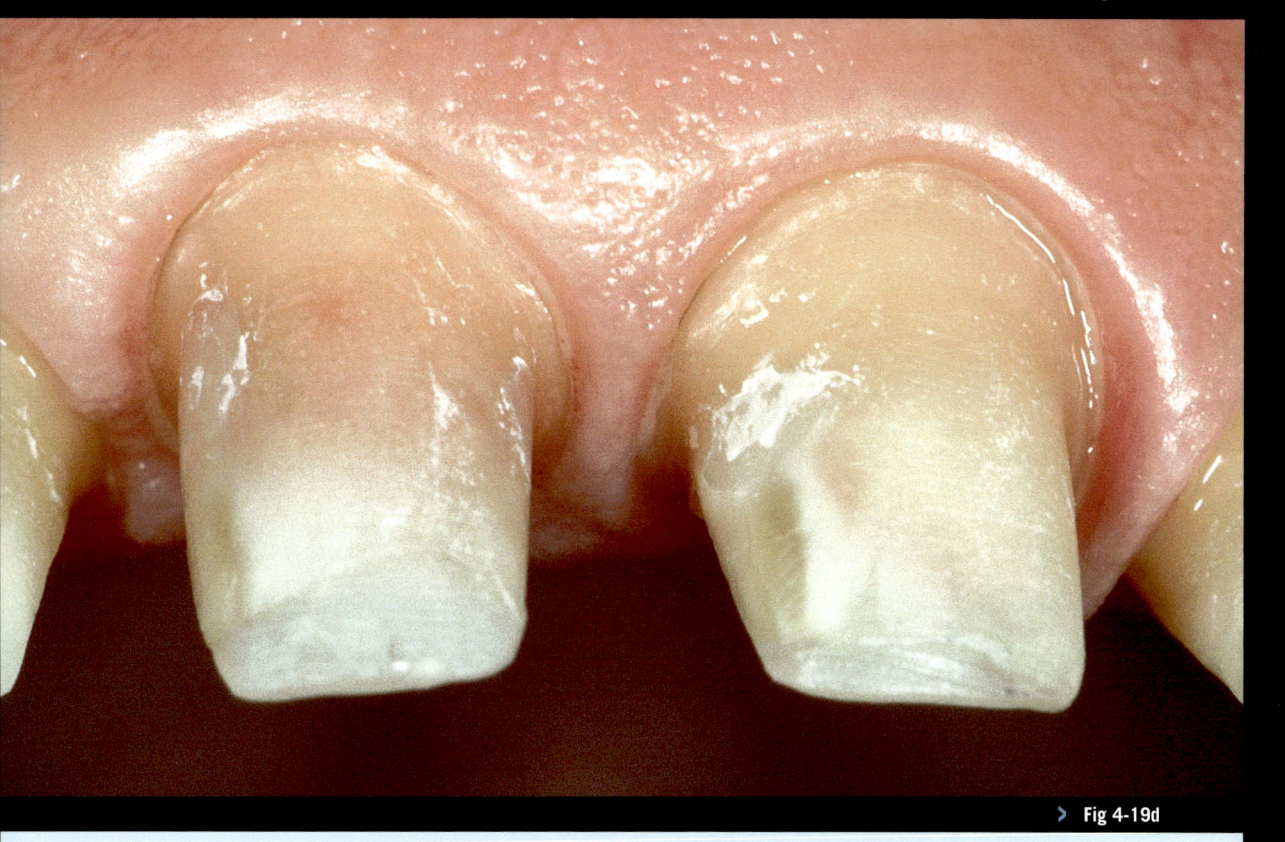

> Fig 4-19c

> Fig 4-19d

FIG 19 *(c)* After the second cord is removed, the impression is taken, which appears to be well defined. *(d)* Upon removal of the provisional restoration 2 months later, the preparation margins appear to be positioned intrasulcularly with healthy tissues.

> Fig 4-20a

> Fig 4-20b

> Fig 4-20c

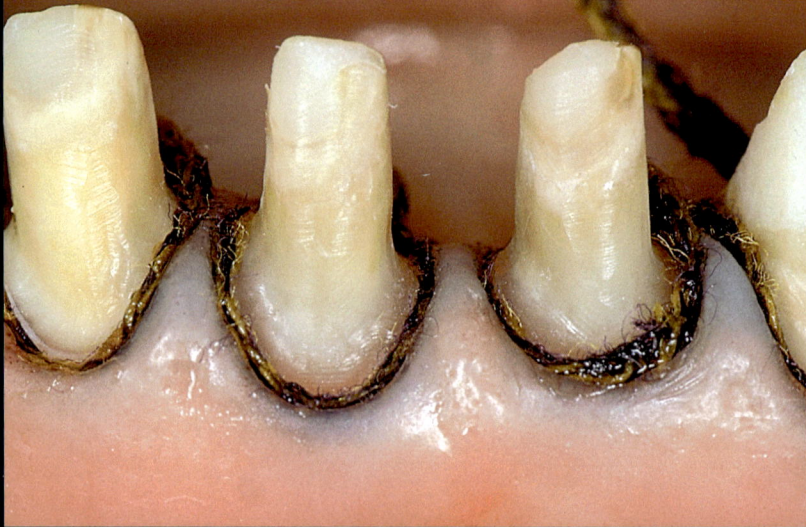

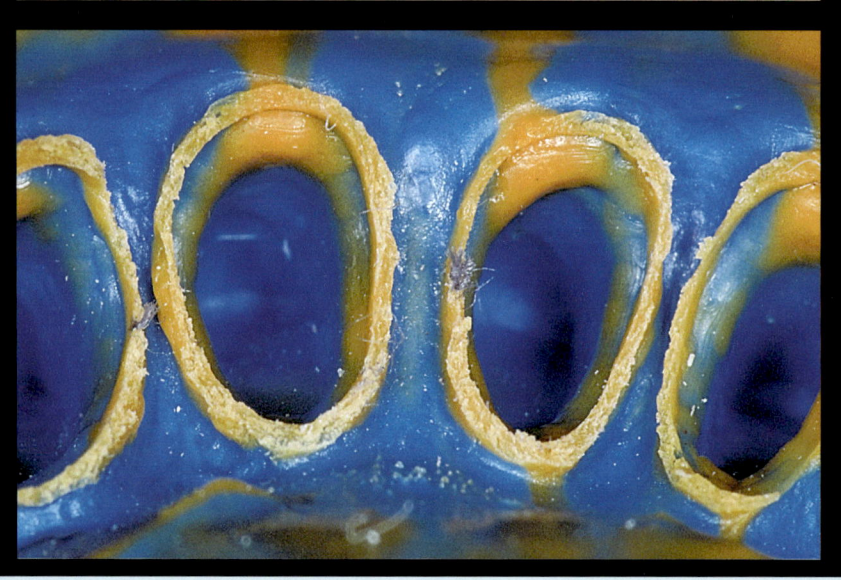

FIG 20 *(a)* After the first cord is positioned, the preparation margins clearly appear to be supragingival. *(b)* Once the abutments have been prepared down to the new gingival level, the second cord is inserted. *(c)* Once the cords are removed, the impression is taken; the margins appear to be adequately readable.

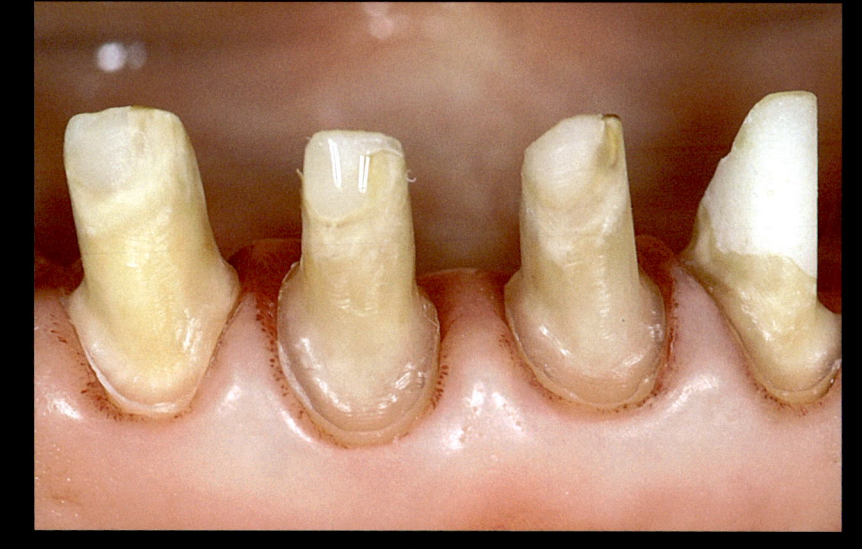

> Fig 4-20d

> Fig 4-20e

> Fig 4-20f

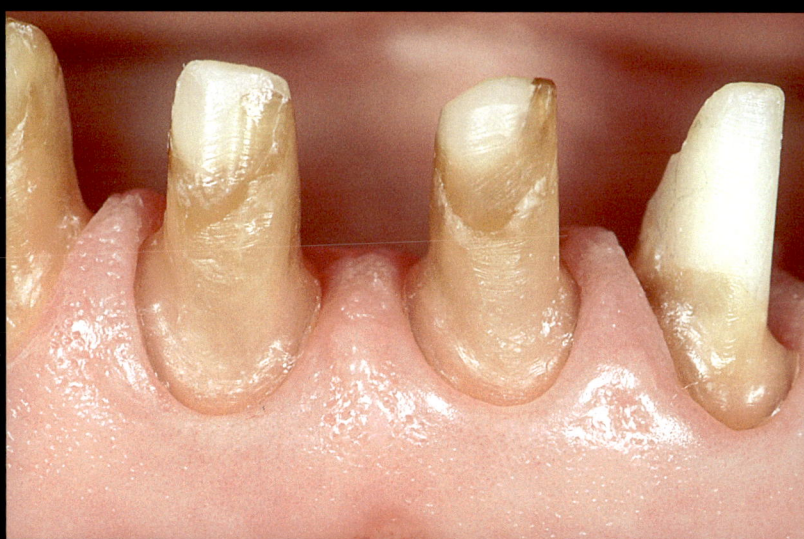

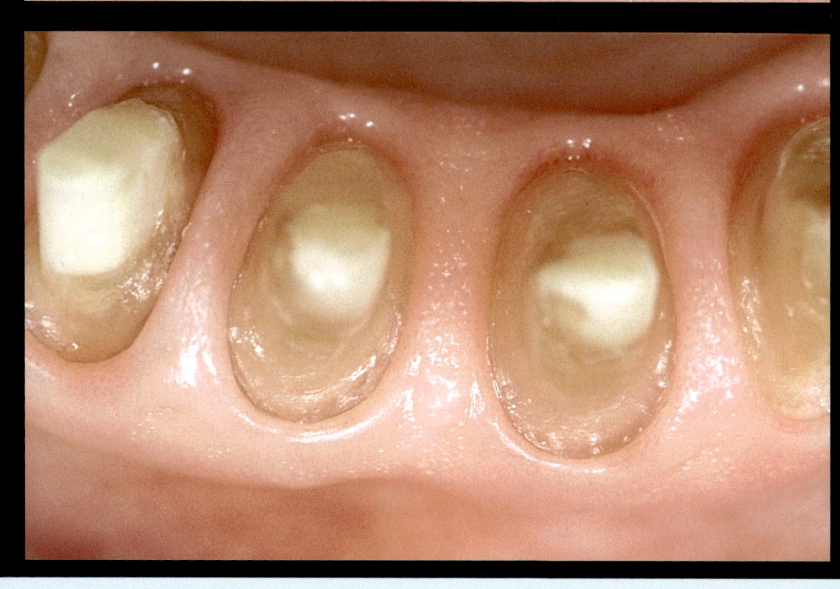

FIG 20 *(d)* As soon as the first cord is removed, it is apparent that the prosthetic margins appear in a slightly supragingival position. *(e)* The tissue was slightly reddened from the prosthetic maneuvers carried out while the impression was taken; this redness has completely disappeared at a checkup 1 month later. *(f)* The preparation margins are now positioned intrasulcularly. It is clear that, in the presence of a healthy sulcus, the operating methods described above allow esthetic needs to be combined with respect for all of the biologic parameters.

IMPRESSION TECHNIQUES AND MATERIALS

VENEERS AND INLAYS-ONLAYS

Taking the final impression is easier for partial restorations than for complete crowns; in the latter, the extent of the tooth preparation is reduced and the location of the finish margin is predominantly supragingival. However, to modify the emergence profile of the restorations in the anterior sector (in the case of veneers) or to capture a particularly deep margin in the posterior sectors (in the case of inlays or onlays), it can sometimes be necessary to extend the margin intrasulcularly using the two-cord technique. For partial restorations, an addition silicone from the PVS family is normally used, which can be easily removed from the oral cavity because of its increased flexibility. This addition silicone prevents the numerous undercuts often found between the natural teeth in these cases, which force the clinician to remove the impression with an oblique disinsertion axis, thereby causing distortion.

PROBLEMS

VENEERS

Interproximal undercuts One specific problem encountered when taking the impression for veneers is the presence of undercuts in interproximal areas, which occur if the interdental contacts are kept intact during preparation (Figs 4-21 and 4-22). It is advisable in these cases to cover the undercut areas with soft wax that has a high resistance to tearing, positioning it from the palatal side.[147] Once the stone cast is poured, a thin disk is used to cut it, starting in the palatal area, to create the removable dies. In this way, the technician can detach the teeth in the plaster without the resulting fracture affecting the tooth preparation area.

INLAYS-ONLAYS

Polymerization inhibition As normally prepared, the tooth surfaces expose a considerable quantity of dentin that needs to be adequately treated before the final impressions are taken and the case is subsequently finalized. To prevent the collagen fibers from collapsing, which significantly reduces the power of the adhesive,[148–150] some authors propose applying the tooth adhesive before taking the final impressions.[150–153] The presence of the adhesive could, however, inhibit polymerization of the impression material, with inevitable repercussions to the final adaptation of the restoration. To prevent this problem, it is advisable to polymerize the layer of adhesive for a longer period by coating it with glycerine gel.[154]

FIG 21 *(a and b)* Preparations for veneers require the interproximal contact areas to be maintained as much as possible.

FIG 22 *(a to d)* The significant undercuts highlighted by the arrows can cause lacerations of the impression material; these undercuts, however, seem to be outside the areas affected by tooth preparation. *(e and f)* Positioning of the definitive restorations demonstrates satisfactory overall integration.

> Fig 4-21a

> Fig 4-21b

> Fig 4-22a

> Fig 4-22b

> Fig 4-22c

> Fig 4-22d

> Fig 4-22e

> Fig 4-22f

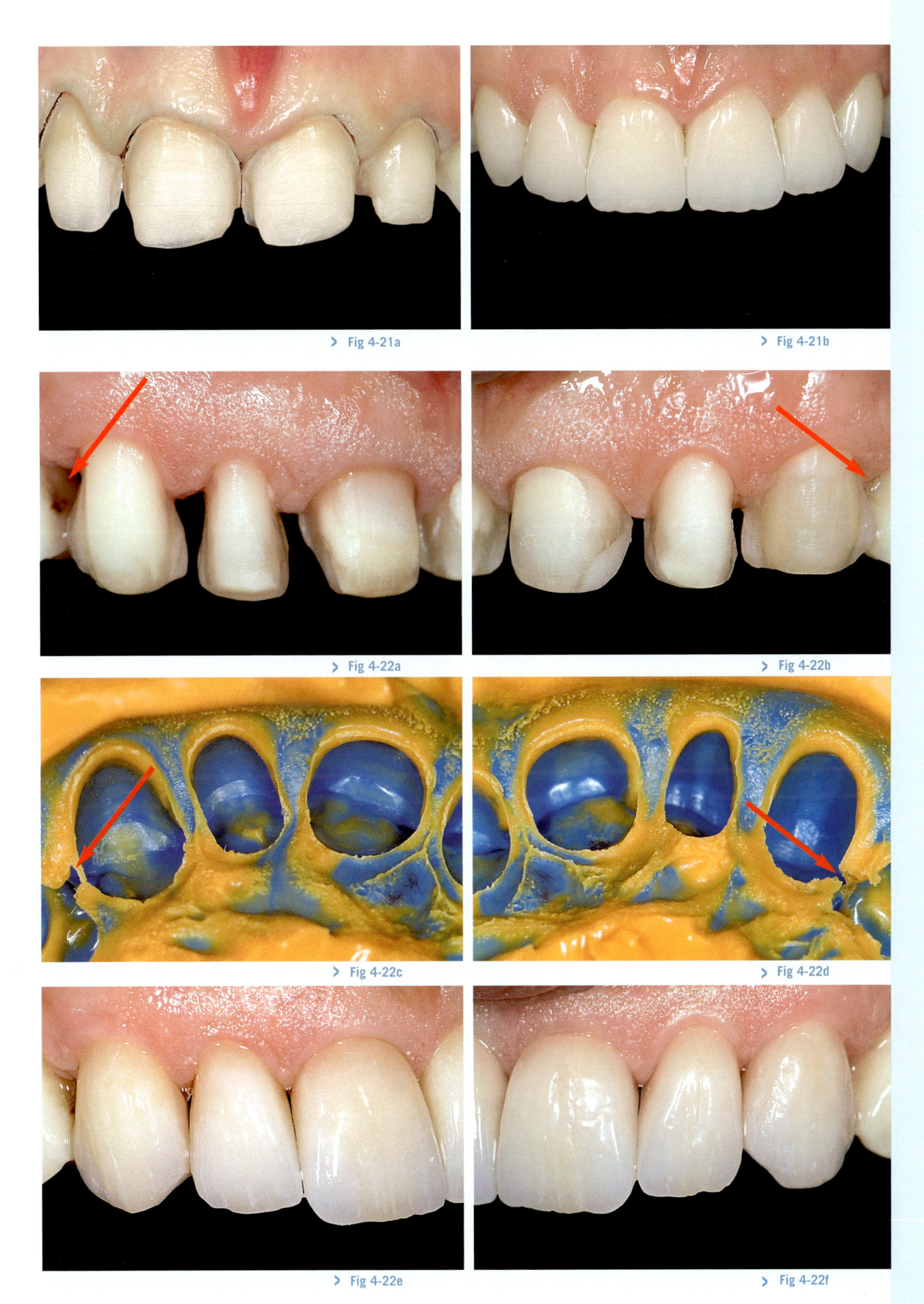

409

IMPRESSION MATERIALS AND TECHNIQUES

IMPLANTS

The objective of taking the impression in implant cases is to record the three-dimensional spatial position of the implants. The impression can be recorded both on the head of the implant, transferring its replica to the master cast,[155] and on the abutment fabricated on the implant head. This approach is always necessary unless prefabricated abutments, replicated on the master cast, are used.[156]

TAKING THE IMPRESSION ON THE HEAD OF THE IMPLANTS

Repositioning technique Once the impression is taken, the copings are removed from the oral cavity and connected to the laboratory analogs. Then, using a design that makes repositioning easier, they are reinserted in the impression before it is poured.

Pick-up technique This technique involves removing the impression with the copings still captured inside it. To apply this technique, a customized impression tray must be used, with suitable windows cut out where the copings are so they can be unscrewed before the impression is removed (Figs 4-23a and 4-23b).[157,158]

Splinted pick-up technique Compared with the pick-up technique, this technique ensures greater positioning accuracy by requiring the copings to be joined together with the acrylic resin or solidified with the individual impression tray.

None of the three techniques described here, however, can be said to be completely error-proof in the transfer process.[159-171]

TAKING THE IMPRESSION ON THE ABUTMENTS

Once the impression has been taken on the head of the implants, customized abutments can be fabricated in the laboratory; these abutments can be treated in the same way as natural teeth once they are positioned in the mouth (Figs 4-24a to 4-24c). If, for example, their margins are supragingival and this constitutes an esthetic problem for the patient, the finish line can be deepened with a bur on the stone cast as well as directly in the oral cavity before the impression is taken. If, on the other hand, the margins are subgingival, retraction cords can be gently inserted into the sulcus, taking the utmost care not to push them excessively and cause damage to the delicate peri-implant structure[172-175] (see chapter 3, page 352).

> Fig 4-23a

> Fig 4-23b

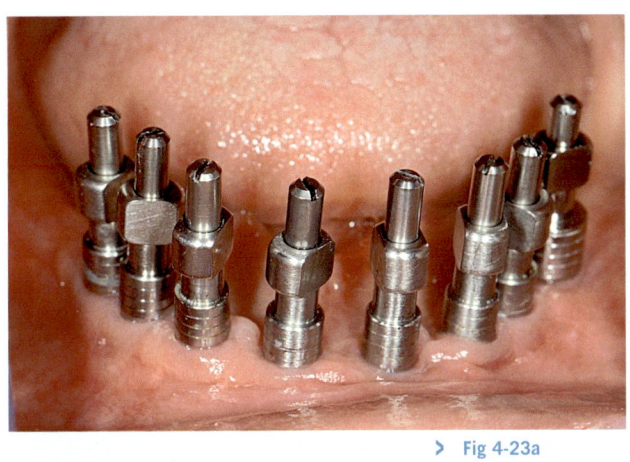

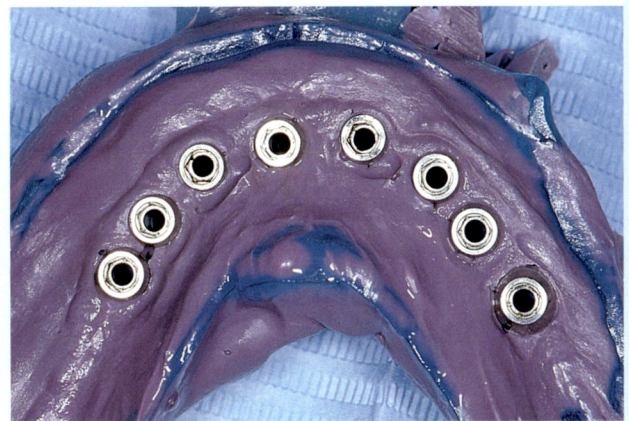

→ ...from page 239

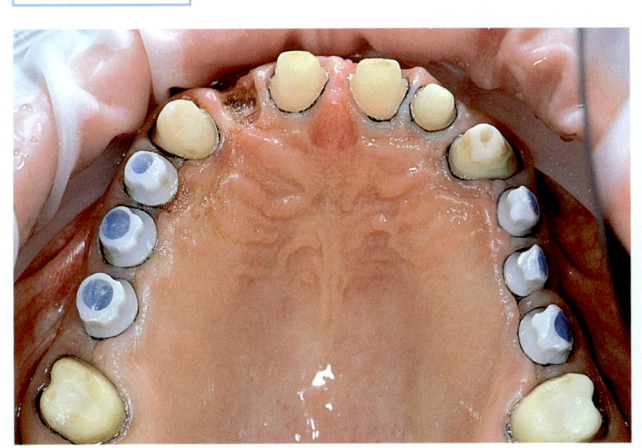

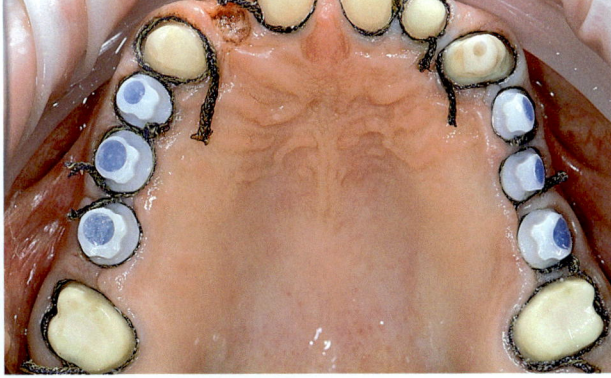

> Fig 4-24a

> Fig 4-24b

> Fig 4-24c

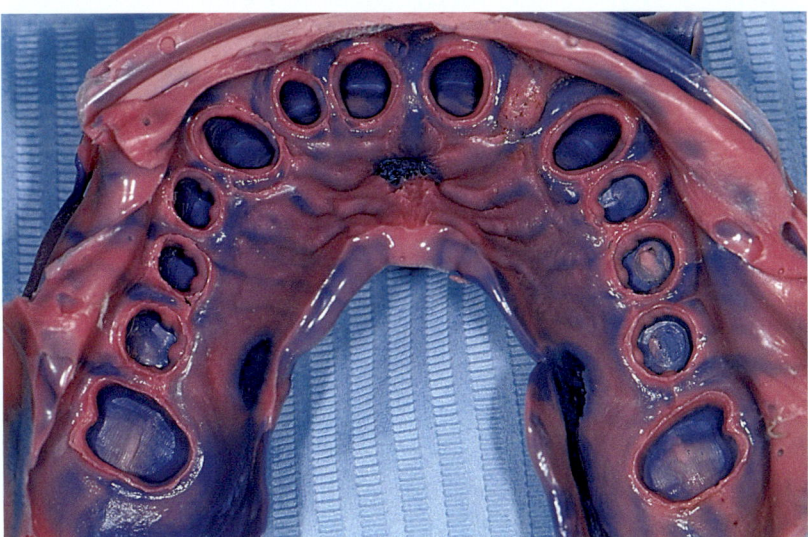

→ Gallery of cases, page 562

FIG 23 *(a)* The pick-up technique involves capturing the copings inside the impression the moment it is removed from the mouth. *(b)* After the fixing screws are removed, the copings are stable as captured in the polymerized material. Because of their particular design, which requires the presence of specific undercuts, the copings allow accurate positioning.

FIG 24 The zirconium abutments, screwed onto the implant heads, are treated as natural abutments. *(a and b)* After the first cord is inserted, a second one is put in place for a few minutes. *(c)* Once the second cord is removed, the final impression is taken, and it shows a good recording of the prosthetic margins on the natural teeth as well as on the implant abutments.

DATA TRANSFER

■ OCCLUSAL REGISTRATION ■
ANTERIOR REHABILITATION

OCCLUSAL REGISTRATION IN PARTIAL CASES

The occlusal registration is done to ensure that, when mounted on the articulator, the plaster casts are in the same position as the arches in the oral cavity. The registration does not need to be recorded in cases where the extent of the prosthetic work is particularly limited (eg, a single crown) or in relatively simple cases if the occlusal contacts in the untreated teeth guarantee the casts a stable position.

ANTERIOR REHABILITATION

When treating the entire anterior sector (ie, from canine to canine), where there is adequate intercuspation (in MI or in CR–CO), it may not be necessary to take an occlusal registration. If, to obtain a precise position of the stone casts, the clinician still prefers to take an interocclusal record, the registration material must under no circumstances be extended to the unprepared posterior teeth to avoid the risk of any imprecision during positioning.

REGISTRATION BETWEEN ABUTMENTS AND OPPOSING ARCH

To allow the technician to mount the casts correctly on the articulator, it is preferable to record an occlusal registration that is positioned exactly between the prepared abutments and the corresponding area in the opposing arch (Fig 4-25a). The registration is carried out by positioning adequately warmed wax between the abutments and the opposing arch, and asking the patient to close the mouth until the two arches are completely closed, reaching their normal occlusion.

For its extreme practicality, a rigid wax (Beauty Pink X-Hard, Miltex) is preferred. The wax is kept in the mouth until it has completely hardened. To make the record more accurate, the wax must be relined with a zinc oxide–eugenol paste (Superbite Paste, Harry J. Bosworth) as soon as it is removed from the oral cavity (Fig 4-25b). So as not to interfere with the existing occlusion, maximum care must be taken to prevent the registration from extending to areas with unprepared teeth. Any material placed between the occlusal surfaces of the unprepared teeth can very easily cause an alteration to the existing occlusal relationship (MI).

FIG 25 *(a)* When the rehabilitation involves only the anterior sector, the occlusal registration is taken between the prepared teeth and the opposing arch. The rigid wax, suitably heated in a thermostatic tank (54°C), is inserted into the mouth and cooled before being removed. *(b)* It is then relined using a zinc oxide–eugenol paste that guarantees the registration greater accuracy.

CASE 1

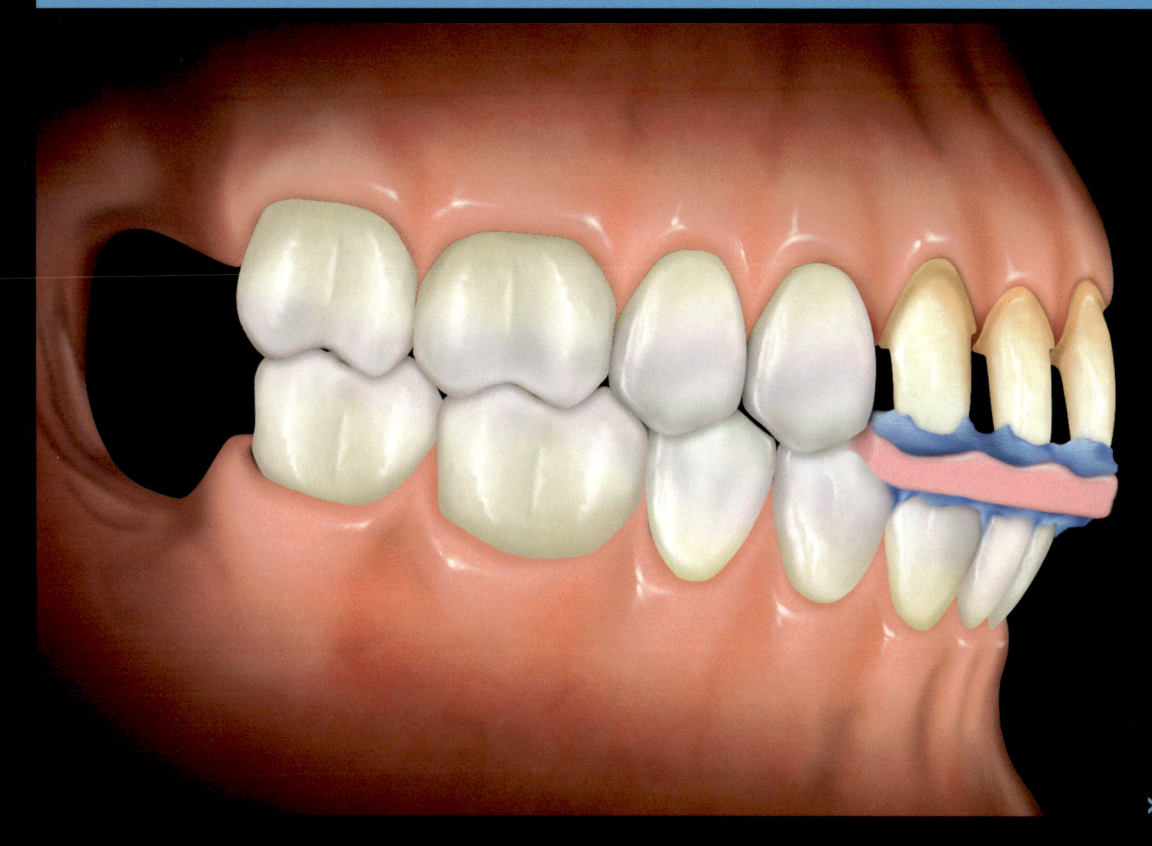

> Fig 4-25a

> Fig 4-25b

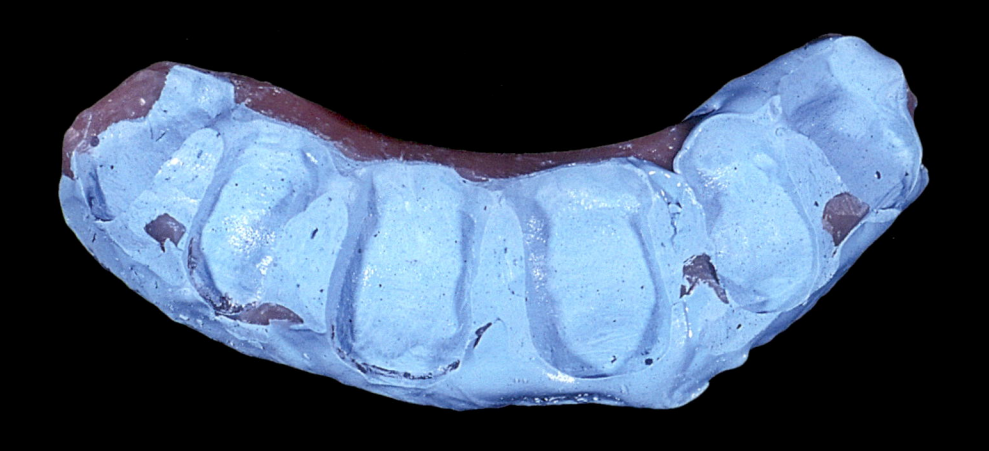

DATA TRANSFER

■ OCCLUSAL REGISTRATION ■
REHABILITATION OF ONE ARCH

When rehabilitating an entire arch, the clinician can no longer rely on the occlusal key provided by the natural unprepared teeth. Therefore, a registration must be taken between the abutments of the arch to be treated and the natural teeth of the opposing arch in CR. To replicate in the definitive work all of the esthetic-functional characteristics contained in the provisional restoration, which also is positioned in CR, the registration must be completed at the same VDO as the provisional restoration.

For this purpose, two reference points are established at the dentogingival limit (ie, cervical margin of the maxillary and mandibular canines) (Fig 4-26a); these points are used to verify that the height between the arches is the same for the provisional restoration and opposing arch as it is for the prepared teeth and the opposing arch.

REGISTRATION BETWEEN PREPARED TEETH AND OPPOSING ARCH

While the position of the provisional restoration is guaranteed in the articulator by the synchronized, punctiform, and adequately distributed contacts with the cast of the opposing arch, the relationship between these and the abutments must be ensured by means of a single occlusal registration, recorded in CR and at the correct VDO.

This procedure is done by guiding the patient into CR (see chapter 1, pages 66 through 69),[176–179] and placing an extra-hard wax (Beauty Pink X-Hard) heated to 54°C, between the prepared abutments and the opposing arch. The wax should be extended over the entire arch with the exception of the anterior teeth to avoid stimulating an instinctive protrusive movement. With the wax applied, the clinician must verify that the VDO is the same as the height previously recorded between the arches with the provisional restoration in position. To guarantee the registration greater accuracy and reliability, the wax is relined with zinc oxide–eugenol (Superbite Paste) (Fig 4-26b) after it is hardened and removed from the mouth.

When rehabilitating one arch where a significant number of abutments allow separate provisional restorations, the clinician may be tempted to keep just one of the provisional restorations (eg, right and left sides alternately) in place, positioning the wax each time only on the remaining prepared abutments. However, recording several registrations obtained by this method is not recommended. The occlusal stabilization of just one side can cause a condylar distraction with significant occlusal inaccuracies.

FIG 26 *(a) Two reference points are set, one between the provisional restoration positioned in the maxillary arch (maxillary right canine) and one on the natural teeth in the opposite arch (mandibular right canine). When the provisional restoration is removed from the maxillary arch, measurement of the distance between the reference points allows a single occlusal registration to be taken in CR and at the same VDO as the acrylic resin shell. After being properly heated to reach a malleable state and to allow the operator sufficient working time in the patient's mouth, the wax must demonstrate adequate rigidity and stability once cooled. (b) To guarantee optimal accuracy, it is then relined with zinc oxide–eugenol paste.*

CASE 2

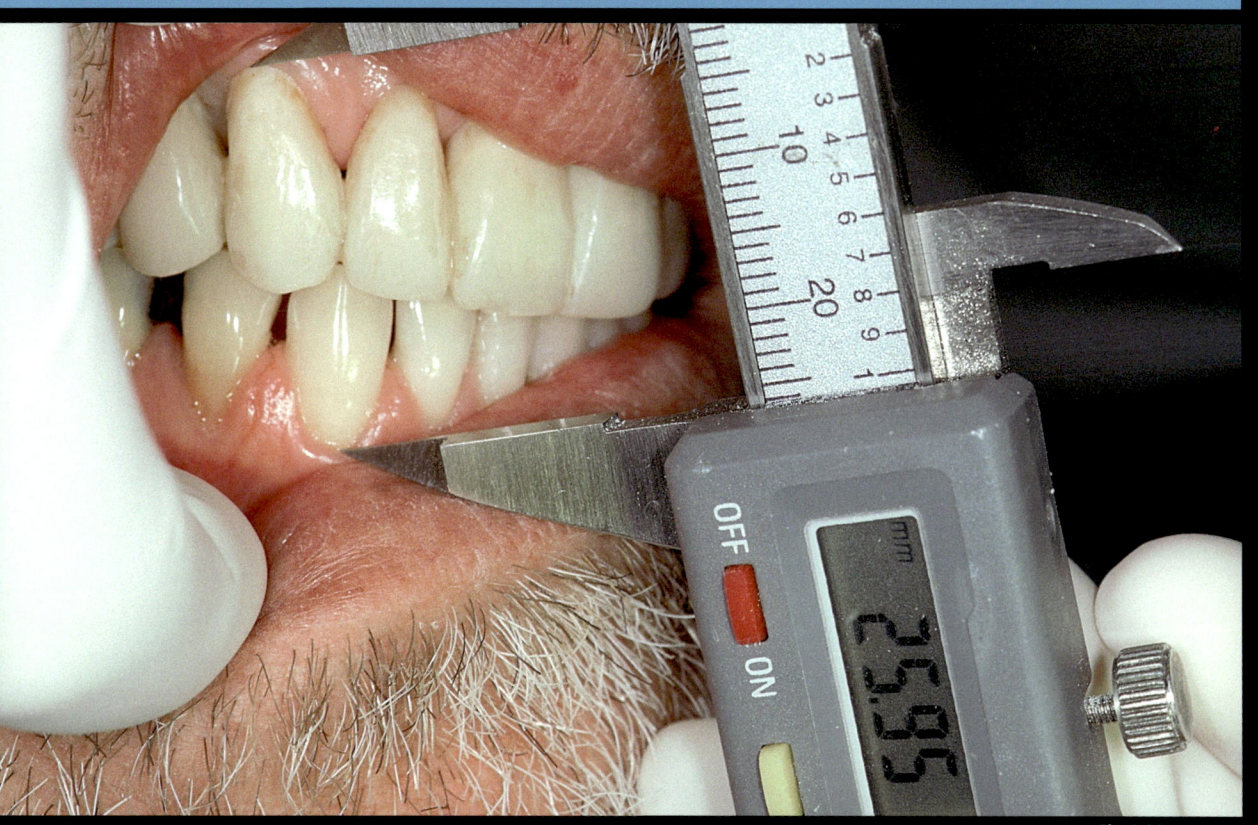

> **Fig 4-26a**

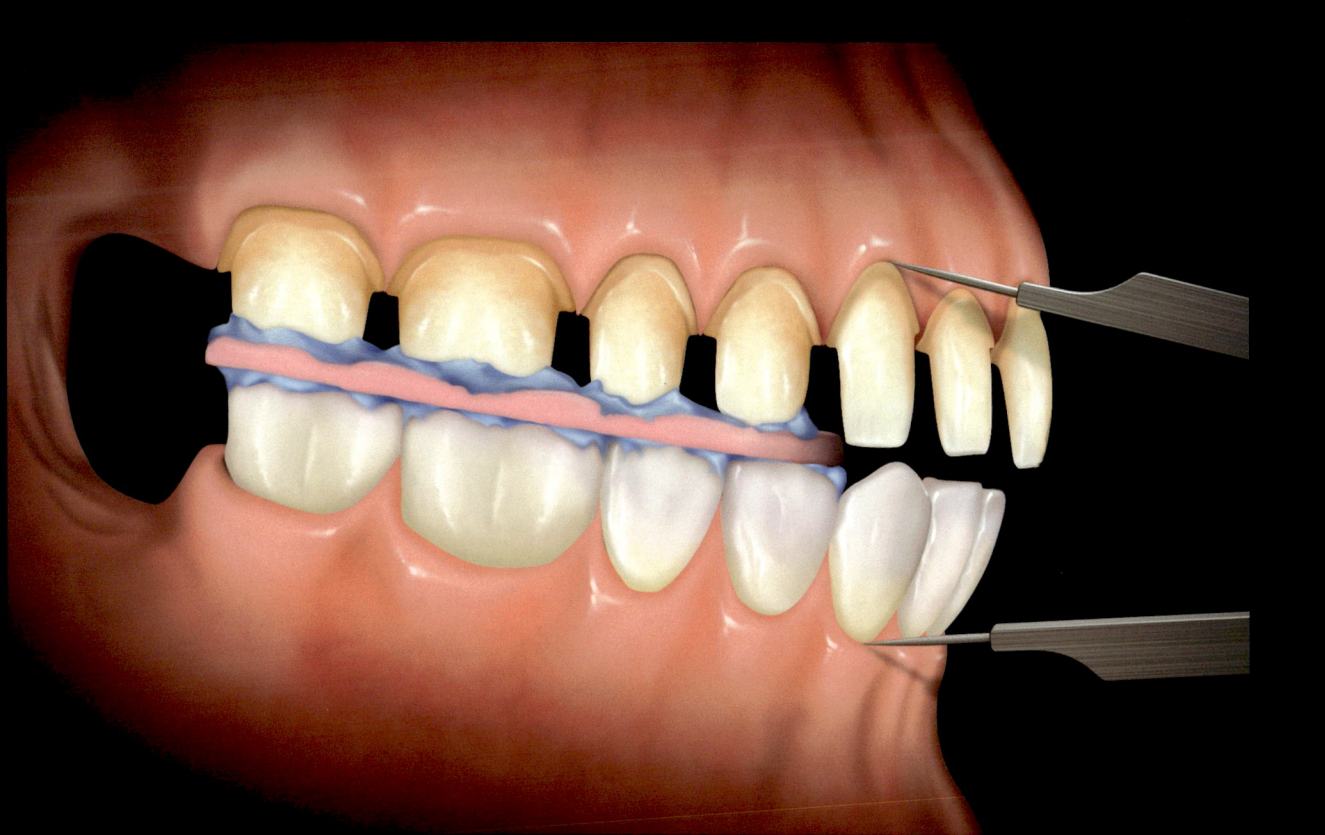

DATA TRANSFER

■ OCCLUSAL REGISTRATION ■
REHABILITATION OF TWO ARCHES

In cases where both arches are rehabilitated, the stability between the two provisional restorations should be checked again in CO before proceeding with the occlusal registrations. Even if satisfactory occlusal stability is found in the oral cavity, the clinician must ensure that the existing occlusal contacts guarantee a key to secure placement, especially in extended cases, before sending the casts of the provisional restorations to the laboratory with the rest of the documentation.

CROSS-MOUNTING OF THE MAXILLARY AND MANDIBULAR CASTS

To ensure that the casts are correctly mounted on the articulator and to be able to interchange them, two registrations must be recorded: one between the final maxillary preparations and the mandibular provisional restorations, and one between the final mandibular preparations and the maxillary provisional restorations. Both of these occlusal registrations, carried out with an extra-hard wax (Beauty Pink X-Hard), must be recorded in CR and at the same VDO.

Before the wax is relined with zinc oxide–eugenol (Superbite Paste), the height between the arches must be carefully checked using the dentogingival reference points (Fig 4-27), as described in the procedures for rehabilitation of a single arch.

REGISTRATION BETWEEN MAXILLARY AND MANDIBULAR ABUTMENTS

For further verification of the position of the casts, a recording also is made of the registration between the maxillary and mandibular abutments using the procedures described previously.

To use the cross-mounting system, it is essential that all of the registrations are recorded in the same spatial position (CR) and at the same height (VDO). Otherwise, it is impossible to replicate the esthetic and functional aspects of the rehabilitation that were created and tested with the provisional restoration, and hence the systematic approach followed to this point would be rendered useless.

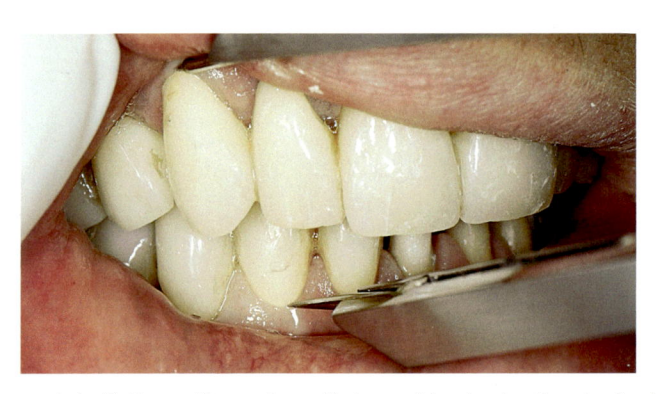

> Fig 4-27a

FIG 27 (a) After the VDO has been recorded with the maxillary and mandibular provisional restorations in situ, three occlusal registrations must be taken: (b) the first between the mandibular provisional restoration and the maxillary abutments; (c) the second between the maxillary provisional restoration and the mandibular abutments; (d) the third between the maxillary and mandibular abutments. For correct cross-mounting of the casts, the three registrations must be recorded in the same articular position (CR) and at the same VDO.

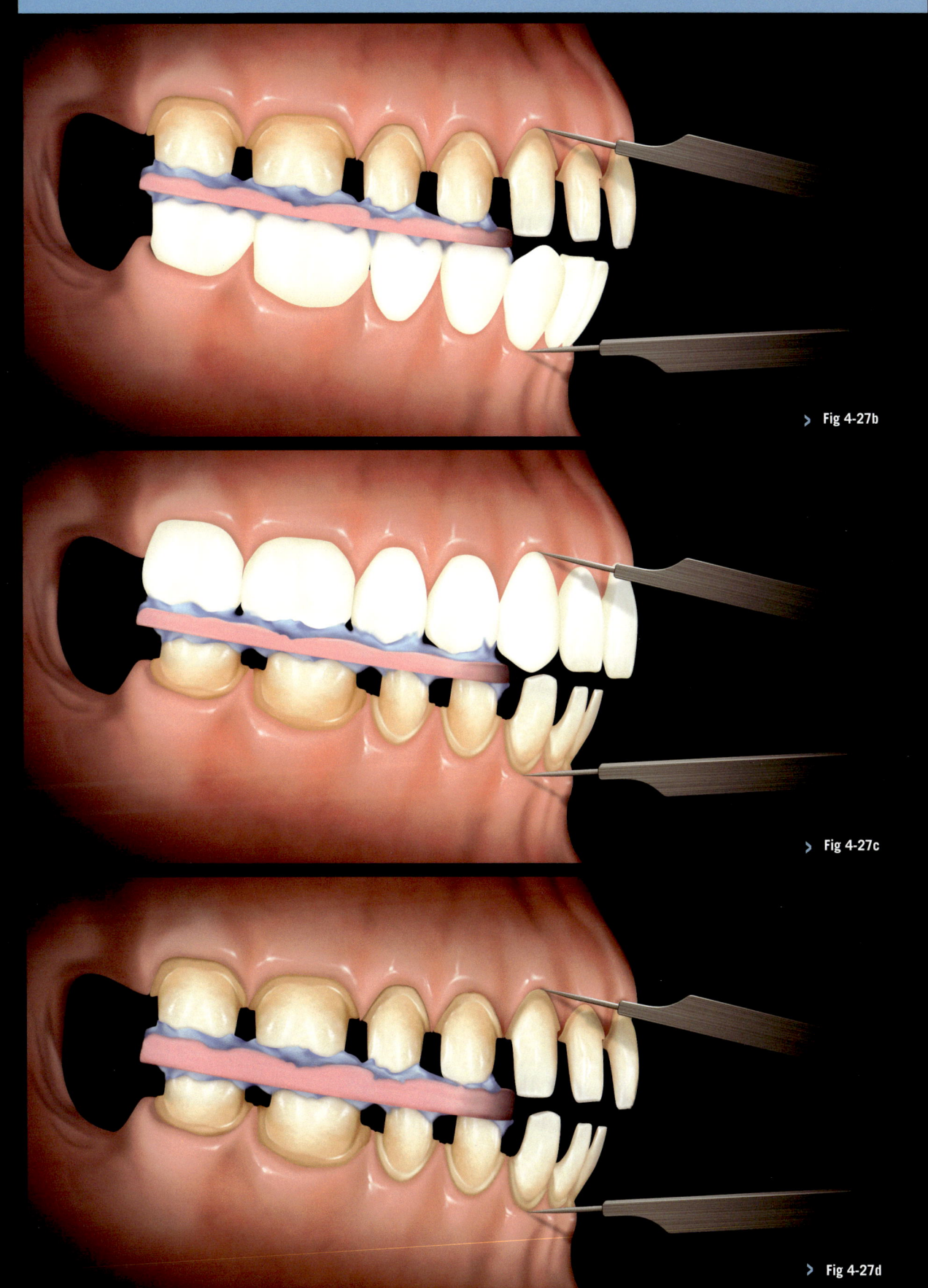

CASE 3

> **Fig 4-27b**

> **Fig 4-27c**

> **Fig 4-27d**

DATA TRANSFER

RECORDING AND TRANSMITTING THE COLOR

The scope of this text is limited to providing the clinical indications for recording and transferring the color to the laboratory, leaving the reader to investigate further aspects of color through other texts.[180–191]

RECORDING THE COLOR

The color can be perceived, recorded, and transmitted differently from one person to another according to the knowledge, experience, and sensitivity of the individual.[192–194] It is important to identify the light sources with which the patient comes into contact most frequently, even if the color is to be recorded under different lighting conditions. The patient should always be examined in daylight (Fig 4-28a) as well as under artificial light. For this purpose, it is essential for the clinician and technician to work under the same light source (5,500° K), using specific lights (Fig 4-28b).

In recording the color, the choice of shade guide plays an important role. A considerable number of these are commercially available (Figs 4-28c and 4-28d), but the authors' preference, after more than 25 years of communication between clinician and technician, is the traditional VITA Lumin Vacuum shade guide (Vita Zahnfabrik). It can be very useful, however, to create a customized scale with the ceramics used every day in the laboratory (Figs 4-28e and 4-28f). In recent years, electronic instruments have been developed (spectrophotometers and colorimeters) for dental use that are of undeniable assistance to the clinician in recording the color correctly.[191,195–202]

RECORDING THE COLOR

- Clean the teeth to be compared with pumice paste.
- Wet with water both the teeth and the sample chosen.
- Examine the patient under different light sources (natural and artificial).
- Highlight the differences in hue, chroma, value, translucency, and opacity.
- Choose the sample with the hue closest to the one required.
- If in doubt, select the hue with the highest value.
- Position the sample next to the natural tooth, first in the same arrangement, then in the opposite one.
- If possible, use a customized shade guide.
- Use the unit lamp and the photographic flash, tilting them to 45 degrees in relation to the tooth.
- Do not record the color in strongly chromatic settings.
- Half close your eyes to differentiate the value better.
- Observe the overall effect both with the lips relaxed and during smile.
- Do not look at the teeth to be compared for more than 8 seconds.
- To prevent visual habituation, turn your gaze to a light blue card every 5–10 seconds.
- If necessary, use a gingival shade guide.
- Where possible, record the color using electronic instruments, too.

> Fig 4-28a

> Fig 4-28b

> Fig 4-28c

> Fig 4-28d

> Fig 4-28e

> Fig 4-28f

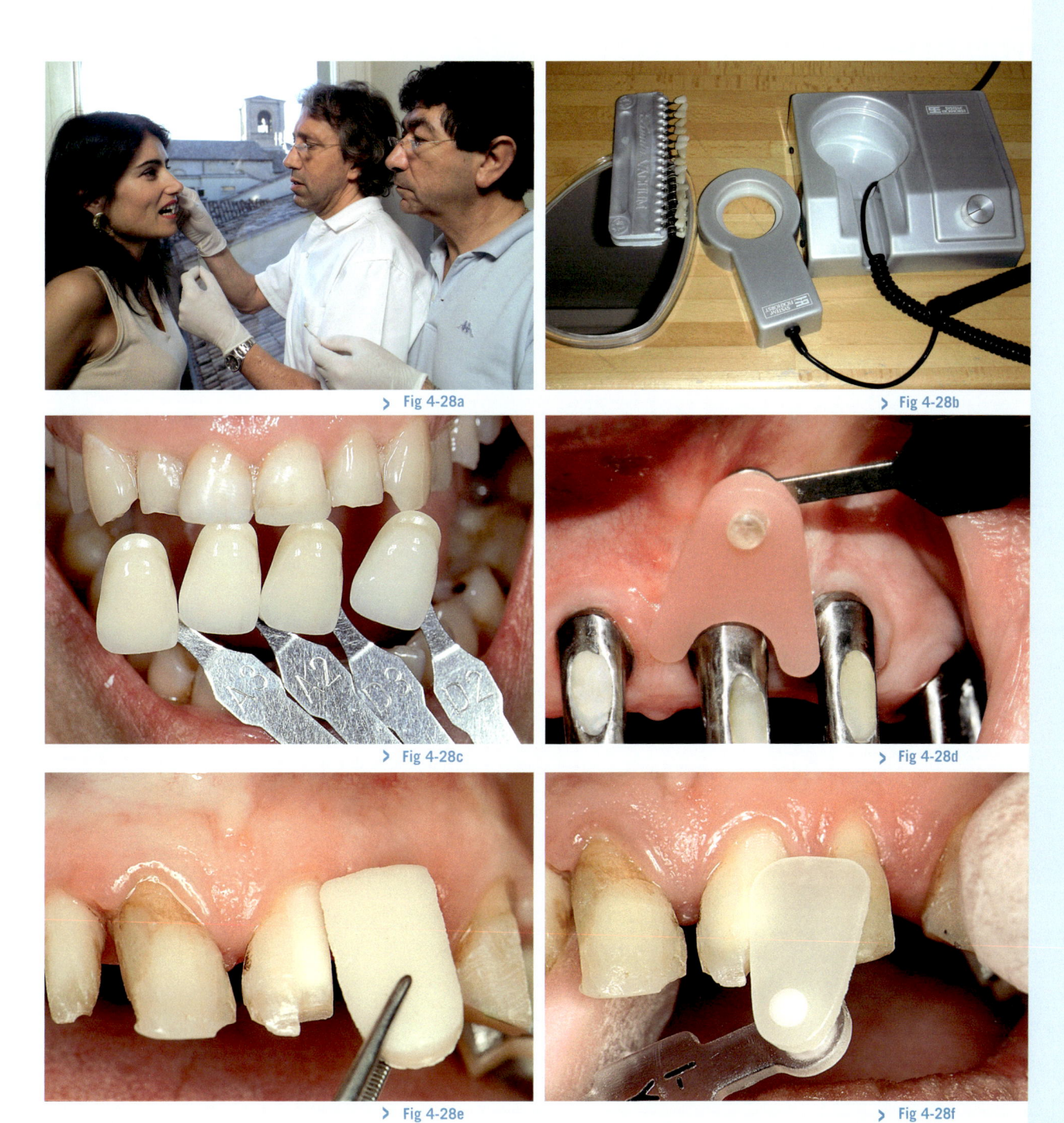

FIG 28 The color is normally recorded by the clinician and transmitted to the laboratory on a designated section of the checklist. Only in a few special cases will the technician's presence be required in the clinic to achieve optimal results. *(a and b)* Color recording must be carried out in daylight as well as under artificial lighting systems that must be identical for both the clinician and the technician. *(c and d)* Commercially available shade guides are routinely used, including those for reproducing the gingival tissue. This is necessary when significant apicocoronal losses of the alveolar ridge force the technician, especially in implant cases, to design specific flanges that reproduce gingival appearance. *(e and f)* In addition to the above, it can be very convenient to use customized shade guides to select the color of the dentin and the enamel.

TRANSMITTING THE COLOR

After accurately recording the color, the clinician can transmit it to the laboratory in various ways.[187,188,191,196,197] Digital cameras make it simple and quick to e-mail the images. For a comprehensive evaluation, it is preferable to compare the chromatic intensity of samples that have a similar disposition to those in the mouth in order to assess the chromatic intensity of the cervical areas (Figs 4-28g and 4-28h), as well as inverting them to compare their translucency with the incisal part of the natural tooth (Fig 4-28i). The photographs must be taken in different positions, with the sample teeth from the shade guide set next to the natural ones chosen as a reference (Figs 4-28i and 4-28j). If the clinician is using all-ceramics, manufacturers also offer ceramic ingot shade guides (Ivoclar Vivadent, Schaan, Liechtenstein) that can be specifically selected for each case (Fig 4-28k). A shade guide is also very useful for the abutments (Ivoclar Vivadent), which are reproduced in the laboratory with light-curing resin of the same shade (Fig 4-28l). The clinician must create a chromatic map containing information on the hue, chroma, and value and showing any characterizations that are present and where they are located (Figs 4-29 to 4-31). In this way, areas that are particularly translucent will be highlighted, especially in the incisal and interproximal areas.

As mentioned earlier, when recording the color, electronic instruments that are able to process the hue, chroma, and value with extreme accuracy can be used to transmit the information to the laboratory. The spectrophotometer used by the authors (SpectroShade, MHT Optic Research) processes the reading by means of special software and provides a chromatic map of the various tooth areas based on the shade guide used (Fig 4-32). The file sent to the laboratory provides the technician with precise data to recreate the correct color in the restoration. After the first ceramic firing, an intermediate color trial can be carried out by means of a simulator that reproduces the conditions of the oral cavity.

These instruments, though they are an indisputable aid to both clinician and technician, especially when the laboratory is not near to the dental clinic, and are reliable for faithfully recording and conveying the three dimensions of color, cannot in the authors' opinion be a substitute for the human eye. They should therefore be considered a valid auxiliary to more traditional methods of recording the color.

FIG 28 *(g and h)* To accurately evaluate the hue and the chroma of the cervical areas and the tooth body, it is preferable to orient the color samples in the same position as the natural tooth. *(i and j)* It is equally important to arrange them edge to edge to check the translucency of the incisal third. In this way, the laboratory will receive photographs that reproduce teeth and samples from different angles. *(k)* When all-ceramics are used, it is possible in some cases to choose the color of the ceramic ingots for constructing the copings (substructure). *(l)* Similarly, use of a suitable shade guide allows custom resin abutments that reproduce the same hue of the natural abutments to be fabricated in the laboratory.

> Fig 4-28g

> Fig 4-28h

> Fig 4-28i

> Fig 4-28j

> Fig 4-28k

> Fig 4-28l

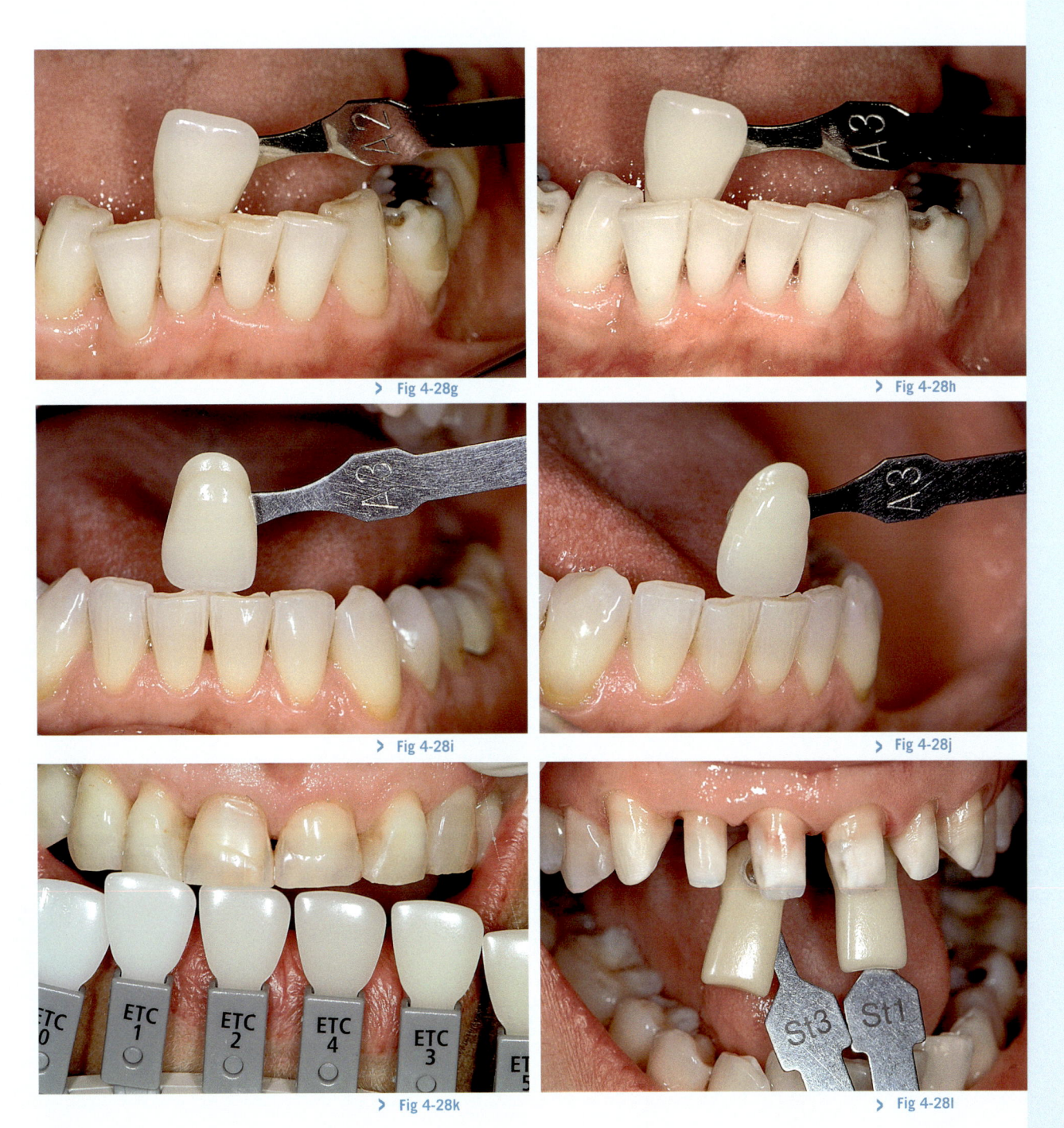

TRANSMITTING THE COLOR

- Send the laboratory photos of the chosen samples with different arrangements and from different angles.
- Set out the photos to compare them at a distance.
- If using all-ceramics, send photos of the abutments with the relative shade guide.
- Create and send a chromatic map with hue, chroma, value, and characterizations.
- If possible, also send photos taken with electronic instruments.

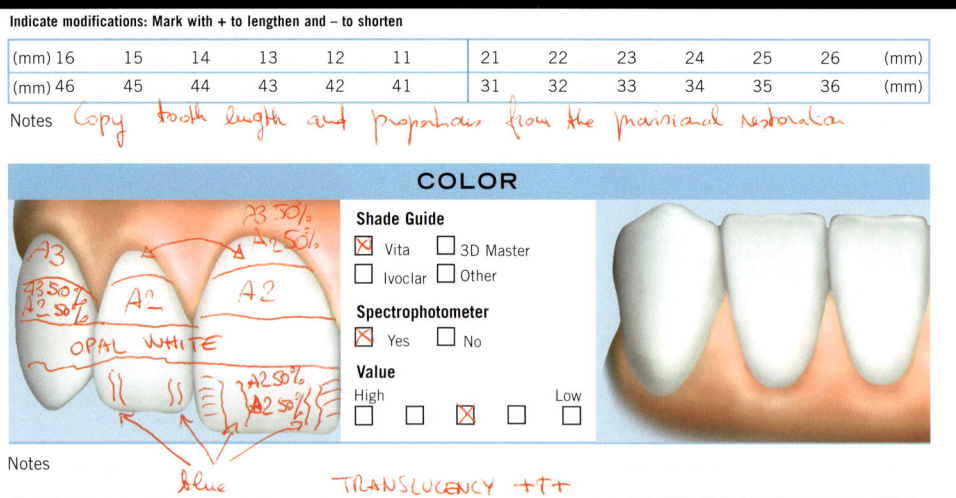

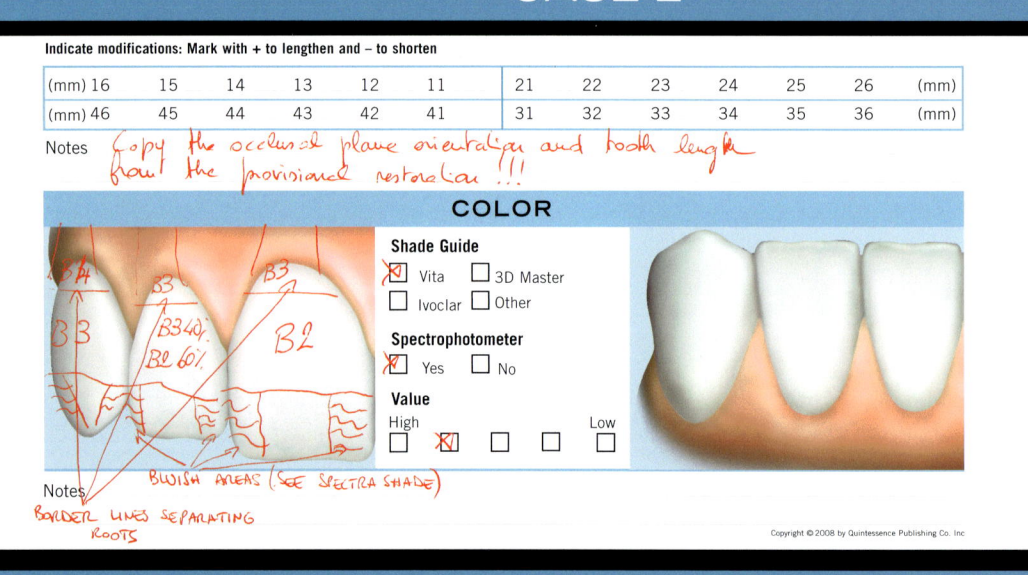

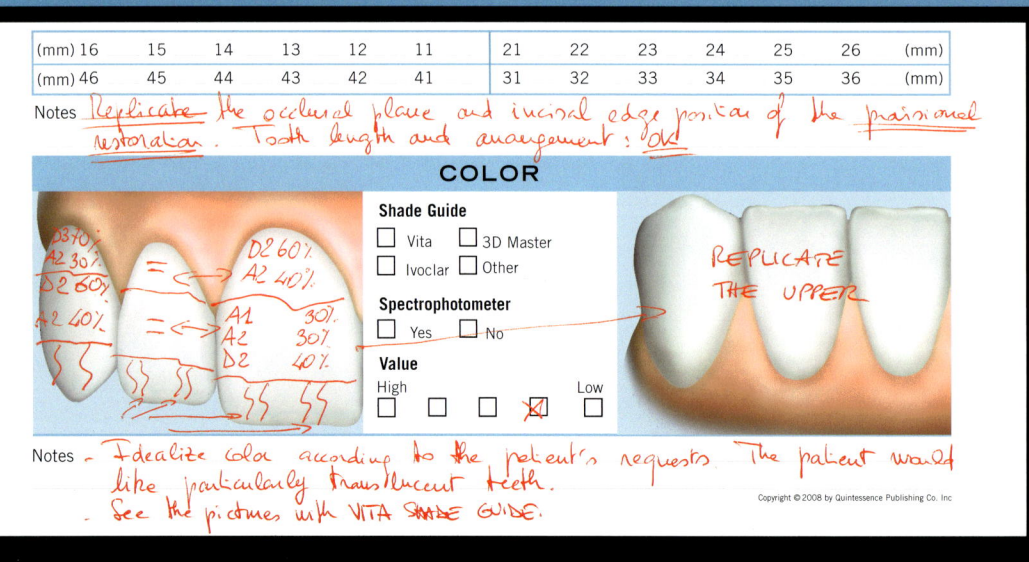

> Fig 4-29

> Fig 4-30

> Fig 4-31

> Fig 4-32a

> Fig 4-32b

> Fig 4-32c

> Fig 4-32d

> Fig 4-32e

> Fig 4-32f

> Fig 4-32g

> Fig 4-32h

FIG 29 30 31 Compiling the color chart.

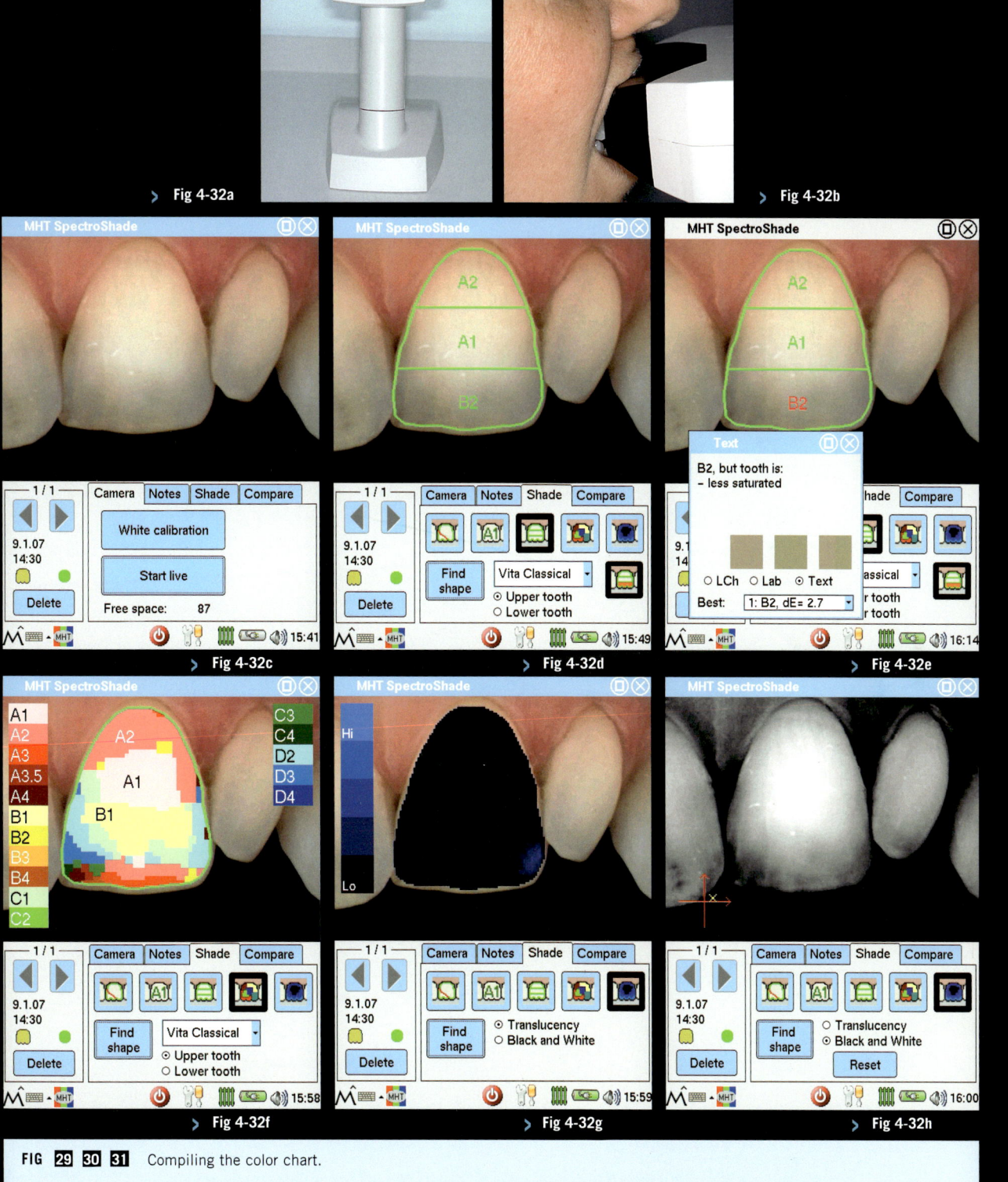

FIG 32 *(a and b)* Using a spectrophotometer to record the color. *(c)* Polarized light image. *(d)* Recording the color of the buccal surface, with the areas divided into: cervical, middle, and incisal. *(e)* Checking the corrections to be made in the incisal area. *(f)* Detail of the color distribution. *(g)* Checking the translucency. *(h)* Distribution of the value with a view of the tooth in black and white.

DATA TRANSFER

■ DEFINITIVE RESTORATION ■
LABORATORY CHECKLIST

As discussed earlier in the section on fabricating the wax-up (see chapter 1, page 58), when transmitting the information for the definitive prosthesis, the technician is provided with a new laboratory checklist containing the photos of the patient's face, smile, and teeth with the provisional restorations in situ. Sometimes there may be a difference in the smile line, with greater tooth and gingival exposure compared with when the esthetic checklist was first compiled. This can be a result of the increased confidence acquired by the patient after positioning of the provisional restoration, especially when, in the presence of serious esthetic deficits, significant modifications to appearance have been made.

Effectively fine-tuning and testing all of the modifications to the provisional restoration over time ensures, from the esthetic, biologic, and functional viewpoints, that the definitive prosthesis is a faithful reproduction of what has already been tried and deemed successful. No further modifications other than minor ones mainly to do with variations in shape should be necessary, and these revisions should be restricted to the spaces tested with the provisional restoration. As a result, compiling the laboratory checklist for constructing the definitive work is less laborious than the one provided for creating the diagnostic wax-up. The checklist should be concentrated on the section regarding the registrations and work directions, with specifications for the techniques and materials to be used. Along with the impressions, the facebow, and the occlusal keys, the color chosen for the definitive restorations is also transmitted, with greater attention to detail than that given to construction of the provisional restoration.

FROM THE PROVISIONAL TO THE DEFINITIVE RESTORATION

DATA TRANSFER Chapter 4	FINALIZATION Chapter 5
CLINIC	LABORATORY
■ Impression of the provisional restoration ■ Impression of the antagonist ■ Protrusive interocclusal record ■ Facebow ■ Final impression ■ Occlusal registrations ■ Color transmission ■ Laboratory checklist	■ Mounting on the articulator with a facebow ■ Setting the articulator ■ Customized anterior guidance ■ Silicone indexes ■ Constructing the substructure ■ Preventive simulation ■ Finalization

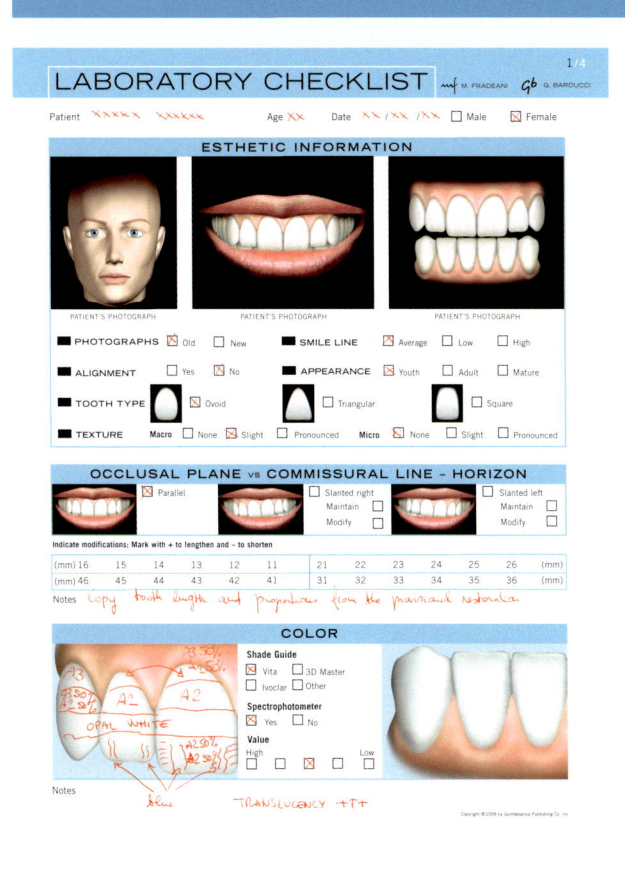

CASE 1

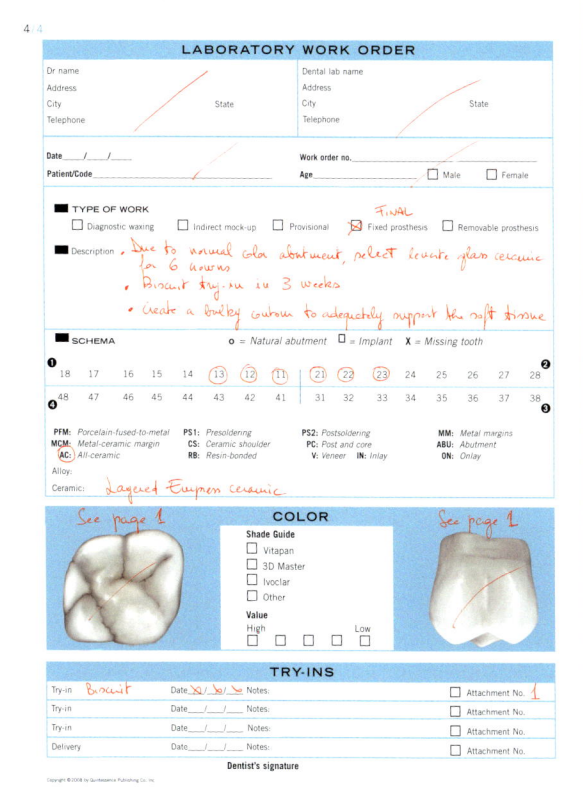

> Fig 4-33

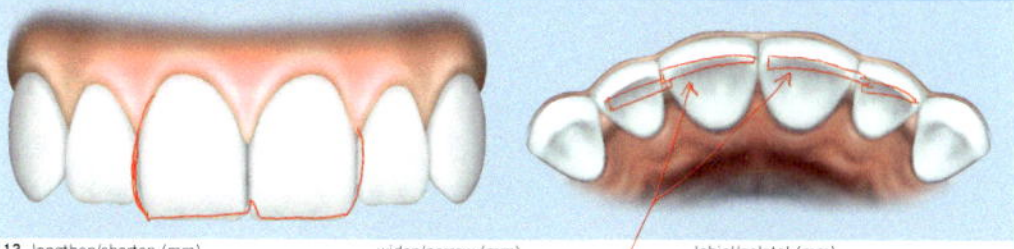

Case 1 → continues on page 437

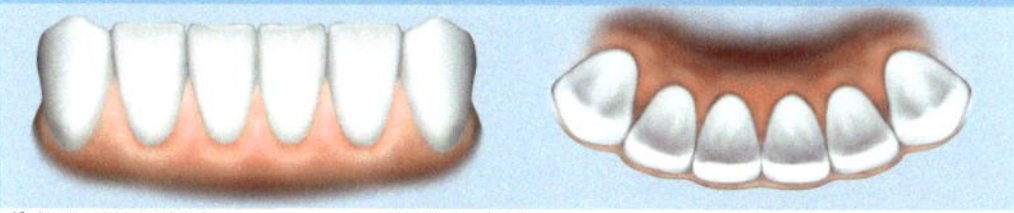

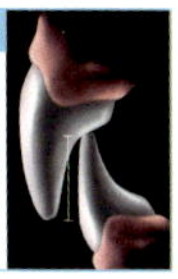

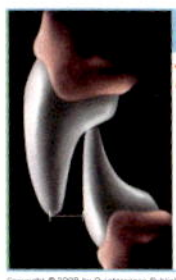

CASE 2

Fig 4-34

Case 2 → continues on page 437

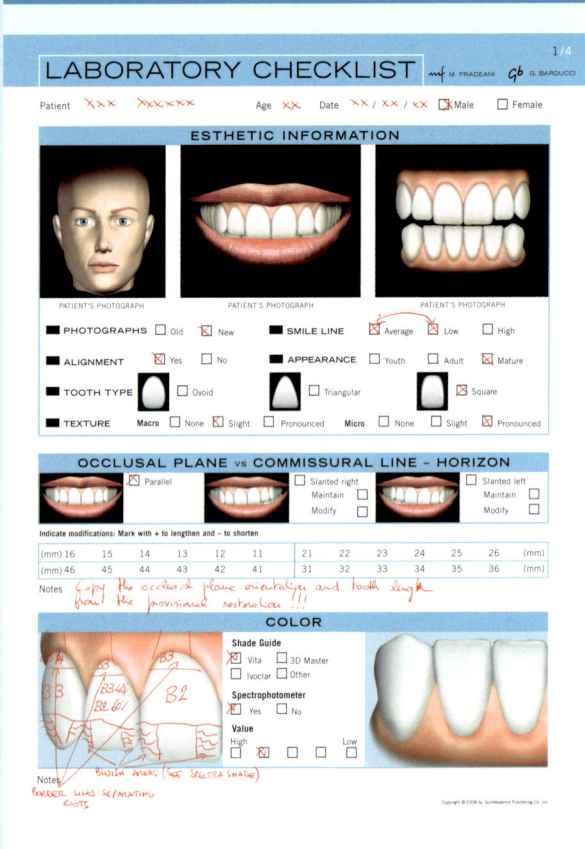

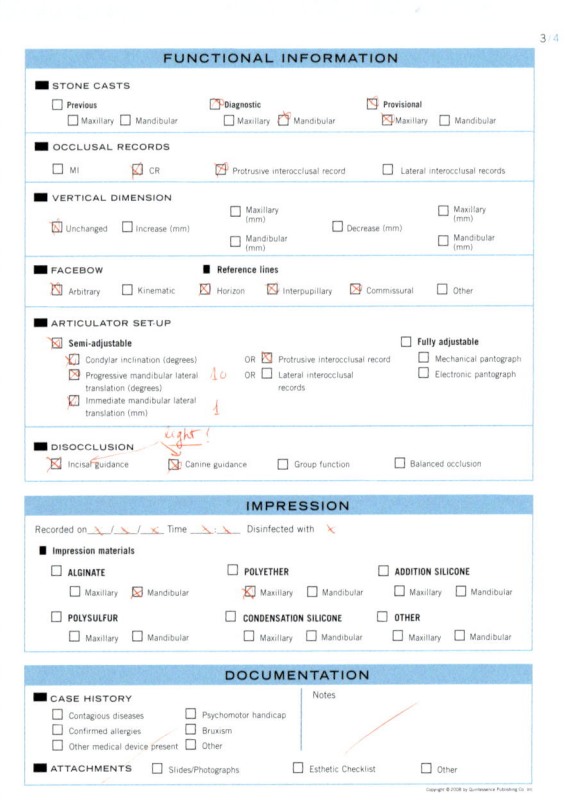

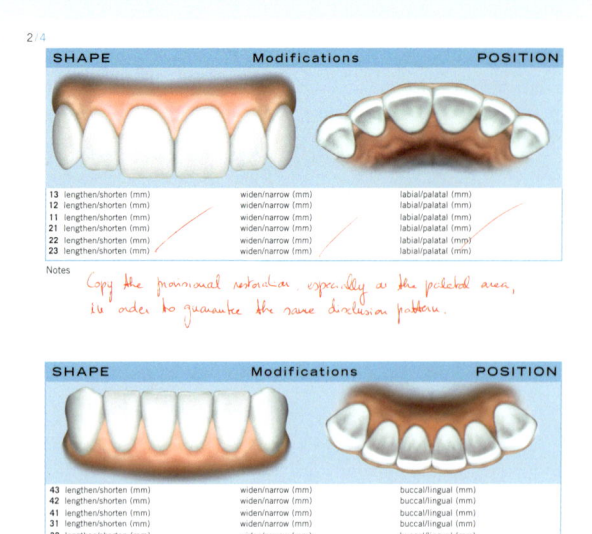

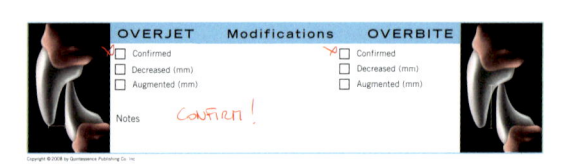

CASE 3

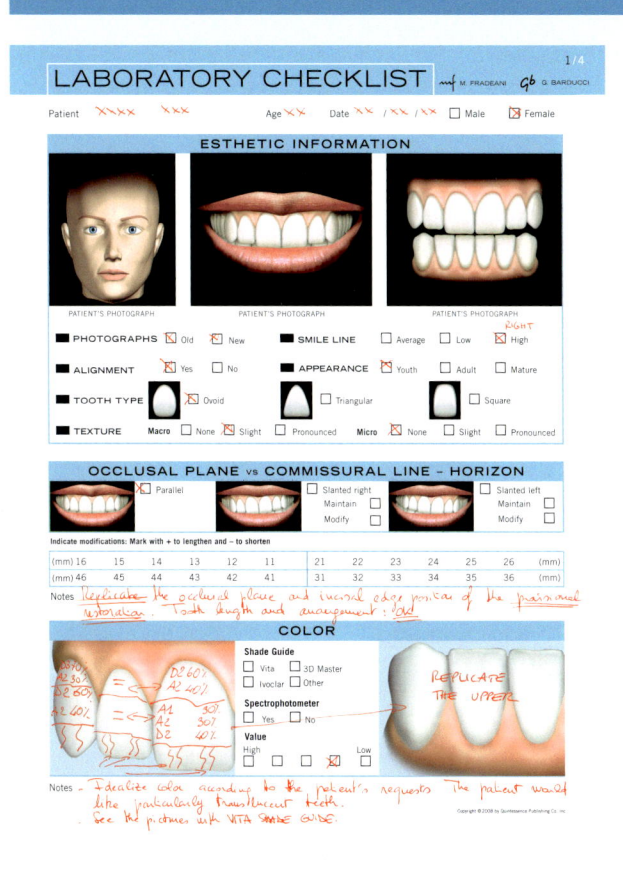

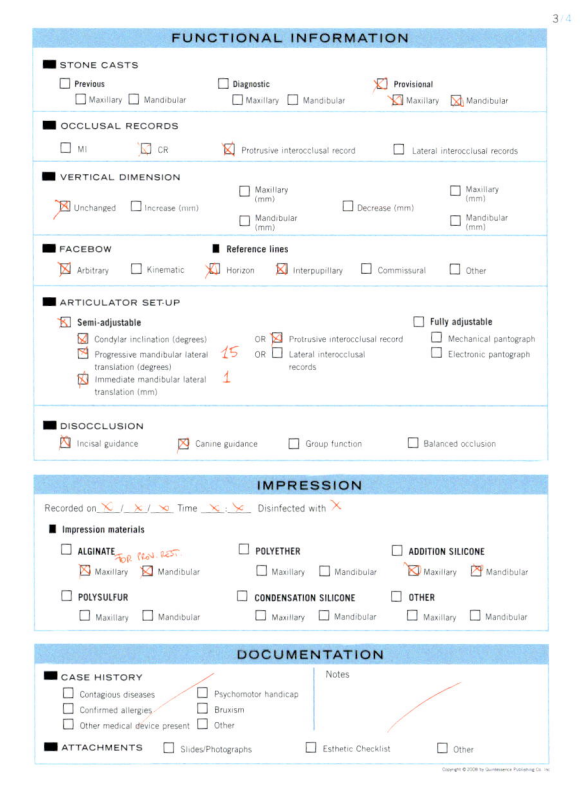

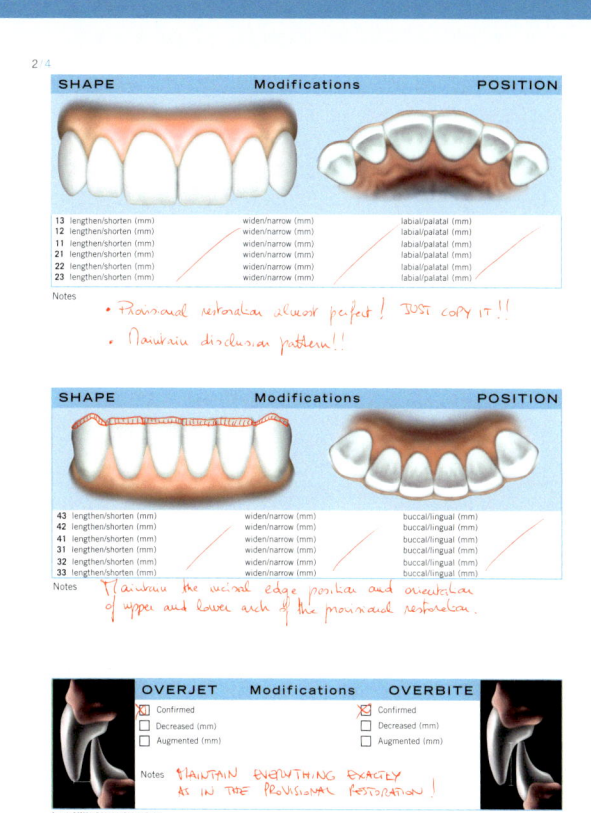

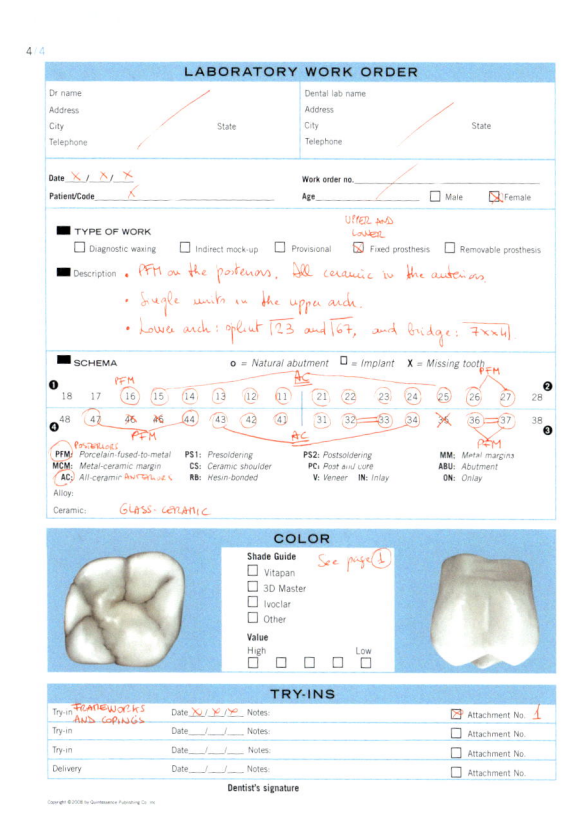

> Fig 4-35

Case 3 → continues on page 437

REFERENCES

1. Capp NJ. The diagnostic use of provisional restorations. Restorative Dent 1985;1:92–94.

2. Shavell HM. Mastering the art of tissue management during provisionalization and biologic final impressions. Int J Periodontics Restorative Dent 1988;8:24–43.

3. Zinner ID, Trachtenberg DI, Miller RD. Provisional restorations in fixed partial prosthodontics. Dent Clin North Am 1989;33:355–377.

4. Bral M. Periodontal considerations for privisional restorations. Dent Clin North Am 1989;33:457–477.

5. Higginbottom FL. Quality provisional restorations: a must for successful restorative dentistry. Compend Contin Educ Dent 1995;16:442–444.

6. Nemcovsky CE. Transferring the occlusal and esthetic anatomy of the provisional to the final restoration in full-arch oral rehabilitations. Compend Contin Educ Dent 1996;17:72-74 76, 78.

7. Donovan TE, Cho GC. Diagnostic provisional restorations in restorative dentistry: the blueprint for success. J Can Dent Assoc 1999;65:272–275.

8. Pound E. Personalized Denture Procedures. Dentist's Manual. Anaheim: Denar, 1973.

9. Preston JD. A systematic approach to the control of esthetic form. J Prosthet Dent 1976;35:393–402.

10. Vig RG, Brundo GC. The kinetics of anterior tooth display. J Prosthet Dent 1978;39:502–504.

11. Clements WG. Predictable anterior determinants. J Prosthet Dent 1983;49:40–45.

12. Goldstein RE. Change Your Smile. Chicago: Quintessence, 1984.

13. Tjan AH, Miller GD, The JG. Some esthetic factors in a smile. J Prosthet Dent 1984;51:24–28.

14. Rufenacht CR. Fundamentals of Esthetics. Chicago: Quintessence, 1990:67–134.

15. Arnett GW, Bergman RT. Facial keys to orthodontic diagnosis and treatment planning. Part I. Am J Orthod Dentofacial Orthop 1993;103:299–312.

16. Chiche JG, Pinault A. Esthetics of Anterior Fixed Prosthodontics. Chicago: Quintessence, 1994:13–32.

17. Roach RR, Muia PJ. Communication between dentist and technician: an esthetic checklist. In: Preston JD (ed). Perspectives in Dental Ceramics: Proceedings of the Fourth International Symposium on Ceramics. Chicago: Quintessence, 1998:445–455.

18. Fradeani M. Esthetic Rehabilitation in Fixed Prosthodontics. Volume 1. Esthetic Analysis: A Systematic Approach to Prosthetic Treatment. Chicago: Quintessence, 2004:35–61.

19. Fradeani M. Esthetic Rehabilitation in Fixed Prosthodontics. Volume 1. Esthetic Analysis: A Systematic Approach to Prosthetic Treatment. Chicago: Quintessence, 2004:63–114.

20. Pound E. Esthetic dentures and their phonetic values. J Prosthet Dent 1951;1:98–112.

21. Fradeani M. Esthetic Rehabilitation in Fixed Prosthodontics. Volume 1. Esthetic Analysis: A Systematic Approach to Prosthetic Treatment. Chicago: Quintessence, 2004:117–134.

22. Boos RH. Intermaxillary relation established by biting power. J Am Dent Assoc 1940;27:1192–1199.

23. Pleasure MA. Correct vertical dimension and freeway space. J Am Dent Assoc 1951;43:160–163.

24. Landa JS. The free-way space and its significance in the rehabilitation of the masticatory apparatus. J Prosthet Dent 1952;2:756–779.

25. Garnick JJ, Ramfjord SP. Rest position. An electromyographic and clinical investigation. J Prosthet Dent 1962;12:895–911.

26. Mehringer EJ. The use of speech patterns as an aid in prosthodontic reconstruction. J Prosthet Dent 1963;13:825–836.

27. Gibbs CH, Messerman T, Reswick JB, Derda HJ. Functional movements of the mandible. J Prosthet Dent 1971;26:604–620.

28. Mansour RM, Reynik RJ. In vivo occlusal forces and moments: 1. Forces measured in terminal hinge position and associated moments. J Dent Res 1975;54:114–120.

29. Pound E. Applying the vertical dimension of speech to restorative procedures. In: Lefkovitz W (ed). Proceedings of the Second International Prosthodontic Congress. St Louis: Mosby, 1979.

30. Rugh JD, Drago CJ, Barghi N. Comparison of electromyographic and phonetic measurements of vertical rest position [abstract]. J Dent Res 1979;58(special issue):316.

31. MacGregor AR. Fenn, Liddelow and Gimson's Clinical Dental Prosthetics. London: Wright, 1989:89.

32. Spear FM. Achieving the harmony between esthetics and function. Presented at the XIV Italian Academy of Prosthetic Dentistry International Congress, Bologna, Italy, November 9th, 1995.

33. Robinson SC. Physiological placement of artificial anterior teeth. J Can Dent Assoc 1969;35:260–266.

34. Dawson PE. Determining the determinants of occlusion. Int J Periodontics Restorative Dent 1983;3:8–21.

35. Dawson PE. Evaluation, Diagnosis, and Treatment of Occlusal Problems, ed 2. St Louis: Mosby, 1989:321–352.

36. Pound E. The mandibular movements of speech and their seven related values. J Prosthet Dent 1966;16:835–843.

37. Rivera-Morales WC, Mohl ND. Variability of closest speaking space compared with interocclusal distance in dentulous subjects. J Prosthet Dent 1991;65:228–232.

38. Spear FM. Fundamental occlusal therapy considerations. In: McNeill C (ed). Science and Practice of Occlusion. Chicago: Quintessence, 1997:421–434.

39. Pound E. Let /S/ be your guide. J Prosthet Dent 1977;38:482–489.

40. Manns A, Miralles R, Palazzi C. EMG, bite force, and elongation of the masseter muscle under isometric voluntary contractions and variations of vertical dimension. J Prosthet Dent 1979;42:674–682.

41. Dawson PE. Evaluation, Diagnosis, and Treatment of Occlusal Problems, ed 2. St Louis: Mosby, 1989: 298–319.

42. Silverman SI. Biology of esthetics. In: Goldstein RE (ed). Esthetics in Dentistry. 2nd ed, Vol 1. Principles, Communications, Treatment Methods. Hamilton, London: BC Decker, 1998:101–121.

43. Silverman ET. Speech rehabilitation: habits and myofunctional therapy. In: Seide L (ed). Restorative Procedures in Dynamic Approach to Restorative Dentistry. Philadelphia: Saunders, 1980.

44. Strub JR. Gingival and dental esthetics. Mimiching mother nature. Presented at the Study Club ACE 2001, Pesaro, Italy, November 10th, 2001.

45. Federick DR. The provisional fixed partial denture. J Prosthet Dent 1975;34:520–526.

46. Vahidi F. The provisional restoration. Dent Clin North Am 1987;31:363–381.

47. Alpert RL. A method to record optimum anterior guidance for restorative dental treatment. J Prosthet Dent 1996;76:546–549.

48. Katona TR. The effect of cusp and jaw morphology on the forces on teeth and the temporomandibular joint. J Oral Rehabil 1989;16:211–219.

49. Weinberg LA, Kruger B. A comparison of implant/prosthesis loading with four clinical variables. Int J Prosthodont 1995;8:421–433.

50. D'Amico A. Functional occlusion of the natural teeth of man. J Prosthet Dent 1961;11:899–915.

51. Thornton LJ. Anterior guidance: group function/canine guidance. A literature review. J Prosthet Dent 1990; 64:479–482.

52. Krough-Poulson WG, Olsson A. Management of the occlusion of the teeth: background, definitions, rationale. In: Schwartz L, Chayes C (eds). Facial Pain and Mandibular Dysfunction. Philadelphia: WB Saunders, 1968.

53. Dawson PE, Arcan M. Attaining harmonic occlusion through visualized strain analysis. J Prosthet Dent 1981;46:615–622.

54. Ramfjord S, Ash MM. Occlusion, ed 3. Philadelphia: WB Saunders, 1983.

55. Dawson PE. Evaluation, Diagnosis, and Treatment of Occlusal Problems, ed 2. St Louis: Mosby, 1989:14–17.

56. Castellani D. Elements of Occlusion. Bologna, Italy: Edizioni Martina, 2000:37–54.

57. MacDonald JW, Hannam AG. Relationship between occlusal contacts and jaw-closing muscle activity during tooth clenching. Part. 1. J Prosthet Dent 1984;52:718–728.

58. Dawson PE. Optimum TMJ condyle position in clinical practice. Int J Periodontics Restorative Dent 1985; 5:10–31.

59. Dawson PE. Evaluation, Diagnosis, and Treatment of Occlusal Problems, ed 2. St Louis: Mosby, 1989: 28–55.

60. McKee JR. Comparing condylar position repeatability for standardized versus nonstandardized methods of achieving centric relation. J Prosthet Dent 1997; 77:280–284.

61. Nemetz H. Tissue management in fixed prosthodontics. J Prosthet Dent 1974;31:628–636.

62. Weisgold AS. Contours of the full crown restorations. Alpha Omegan 1977:70:77–89.

63. Maynard JG Jr, Wilson RD. Physiologic dimensions of the periodontium significant to the restorative dentist. J Periodontol 1979;50:170–174.

64. Waerhaug J, Zander HA. Reaction of gingival tissues to self-curing acrylic restorations. J Am Dent Assoc 1957;54:760–768.

65. Donaldson D. Gingival recession associated with temporary crowns. J Periodontol 1973;44:691–696.

66. Donaldson D. The etiology of gingival recession associated with temporary crowns. J Periodontol 1974; 45:468–471.

67. Giunta J, Zablotsky N. Allergic stomatitis caused by self-polymerizing resin. Oral Surg Oral Med Oral Pathol 1976;41:631–637.

68. Grajower R, Shaharbani S, Kaufman E. Temperature rise in pulp chamber during fabrication of temporary self-curing resin crowns. J Prosthet Dent 1979;41: 535–540.

69. Garvin PH, Malone WF, Toto PD, Mazur B. Effect of self-curing acrylic resin treatment restorations on the crevicular fluid volume. J Prosthet Dent 1982;47: 284–289.

70. Hochman N, Zalkind M. Hypersensitivity to methyl methacrylate: mode of treatment. J Prosthet Dent 1997;77:93–96.

71. Dawson PE. Evaluation, Diagnosis, and Treatment of Occlusal Problems, ed 2. St Louis: Mosby, 1989: 206–237.

72. Preston JD. A reassessment of the mandibular transverse horizontal axis theory. J Prosthet Dent 1979; 41:605–613.

73. Dawson PE. Evaluation, Diagnosis, and Treatment of Occlusal Problems, ed 2. St Louis: Mosby, 1989: 238–260.

74. Chiche GJ, Kokich VG, Caudill R. Diagnosis and treatment planning of esthetic problems. In: Chiche GJ, Pinault A (eds). Esthetics of Anterior Fixed Prosthodontics. Chicago: Quintessence, 1994:33–52.

75. Chiche GJ, Aoshima H. Functional versus aesthetic articulation of maxillary anterior restorations. Pract Periodontics Aesthet Dent 1997;9:335–342.

76. Schallhorn RG. A study of the arbitrary center and the kinematic center of rotation for face-bow mountings. J Prosthet Dent 1957;7:162–169.

77. Lauritzen AG, Bodner GH. Variations in location of arbitrary and true hinge axis points. J Prosthet Dent 1961;11:224–229.

78. Teteruck WR, Lundeen HC. The accuracy of an ear face-bow. J Prosthet Dent 1966;16:1039–1046.

79. Walker PM. Discrepancies between arbitrary and true hinge axes. J Prosthet Dent 1980;43:279–285.

80. Simpson JW, Hesby RA, Pfeifer DL, Pelleu GB Jr. Arbitrary mandibular hinge axis locations. J Prosthet Dent 1984;51:819–822.

81. Palik JF, Nelson DR, White JT. Accuracy of an earpiece face-bow. J Prosthet Dent 1985;53:800–804.

82. Wilson RD, Maynard G. Intracrevicular restorative dentistry. Int J Periodontics Restorative Dent 1981;1:34–49.

83. Harrison JD, Chiche GJ, Pinault A. Tissue management for the maxillary anterior region. In: Chiche GJ, Pinault A (eds). Esthetics of Anterior Fixed Prosthodontics. Chicago: Quintessence, 1994:143–159.

84. Martignoni M, Schonenberger A. Precision Fixed Prosthodontics: Clinical and Laboratory Aspects. Chicago: Quintessence, 1990:49–66.

85. Sydiskis RJ, Gerhardt DE. Cytotoxicity of impression materials. J Prosthet Dent 1993;69:431–435.

86. Clancy JM, Scandrett FR, Ettinger RL. Long-term dimensional stability of three current elastomers. J Oral Rehabil 1983;10:325–333.

87. Craig RG. Review of dental impression materials. Adv Dent Res 1988;2:51–64.

88. Chai J, Takahashi Y, Lautenschlager EP. Clinically relevant mechanical properties of elastomeric impression materials. Int J Prosthodont 1998;11:219–223.

89. Piwowarczyk A, Ottl P, Buchler A, Lauer HC, Hoffmann A. In vitro study on the dimensional accuracy of selected materials for monophase elastic impression making. Int J Prosthodont 2002;15:168–174.

90. Petrie CS, Walker MP, O'mahony AM, Spencer P. Dimensional accuracy and surface detail reproduction of two hydrophilic vinyl polysiloxane impression materials tested under dry, moist, and wet conditions. J Prosthet Dent 2003;90:365–372.

91. Mondon M, Ziegler C. Changes in water contact angles during the first phase of setting of dental impression materials. Int J Prosthodont 2003;16:49–53.

92. Blatz MB, Sadan A, Burgess JO, Mercante D, Hoist S. Selected characteristics of a new polyvinyl siloxane impression material—A randomized clinical trial. Quintessence Int 2005;36:97–104.

93. Walker MP, Petrie CS, Haj-Ali R, Spencer P, Dumas C, Williams K. Moisture effect on polyether and polyvinylsiloxane dimensional accuracy and detail reproduction. J Prosthodont 2005;14:158–163.

94. McCabe JF, Arikawa H. Rheological properties of elastomeric impression materials before and during setting. J Dent Res 1998;77:1874–1880.

95. McCabe JF, Carrick TE. Rheological properties of elastomers during setting. J Dent Res 1989;68:1218–1222.

96. Shulz HH, Schwickerath H. Die Abformung In Der Zahnheilkunde. Köln: Deutscher Ärzte-Verlag, 1989.

97. Hondrum SO. Tear and energy properties of three impression materials. Int J Prosthodont 1994;7:517–521.

98. Phillips RW. Science of Dental Materials, ed 9. Philadelphia: Saunders, 1991.

99. Bindra B, Heath JR. Adhesion of elastomeric impression materials to tray. J Oral Rehabil 1997;24:63–69.

100. Keck SC. Automixing: a new concept in elastomeric impression material delivery systems. J Prosthet Dent 1985;54:479–483.

101. Chong YH, Soh G, Wickens JL. The effect of mixing method on void formation in elastomeric impression materials. Int J Prosthodont 1989;2:323–326.

102. Lee EA. Predictable elastomeric impressions in advanced fixed prosthodontics: a comprehensive review. Pract Periodontics Aesthet Dent 1999;11:497–504.

103. Di Felice R, Scotti R, Belser UC. The influence of the mixing technique on the content of voids in two polyether impression materials. Schweiz Monatsschr Zahnmed 2002;112:12–16.

104. Cook WD, Thomasz F. Rubber gloves and addition silicone materials. Current note No. 64. Aust Dent J 1986;31:140–145.

105. Kahn RL, Donovan TE. A pilot study of polymerization inhibition of poly(vinyl siloxane) materials by latex gloves. Int J Prosthodont 1989;2:128–130.

106. Kahn RL, Donovan TE, Chee WW. Interaction of gloves and rubber dam with poly(vinyl siloxane) impression material: a screening test. Int J Prosthodont 1989;2:342–346.

107. Baumann MA. The influence of dental gloves on the setting of impression materials. Br Dent J 1995;179:130–135.

108. Matis BA, Valadez D, Valadez E. The effect of the use of dental gloves on mixing vinyl polysiloxane putties. J Prosthodont 1997;6:189–192.

109. Matyas J, Dao N, Caputo AA, Lucatorto FM. Effects of disinfectants on dimensional accuracy of impression materials. J Prosthet Dent 1990;64:25–31.

110. Kern M, Rathmer RM, Strub JR. Three-dimensional investigation of the accuracy of impression materials after disinfection. J Prosthet Dent 1993;70:449–456.

111. Davis BA, Powers JM. Effect of immersion disinfection on properties of impression materials. J Prosthodont 1994;3:31–34.

112. Lepe X, Johnson GH, Berg JC. Surface characteristics of a polyether and addition silicone impression materials after long-term disinfection. J Prosthet Dent 1995;74:181–186.

113. Rios M, Morgano SM, Stein RS, Rose L. Effects of chemical disinfectant solutions on the stability and accuracy of the dental impression complex. J Prosthet Dent 1996;76:356–362.

114. Thouati A, Deveaux E, Iost A, Behin P. Dimensional stability of seven elastomeric impression materials immersed in disinfectants. J Prosthet Dent 1996;76:8–14.

115. Lepe X, Johnson GH. Accuracy of polyether and addition silicone after long-term immersion disinfection. J Prosthet Dent 1997;78:245–249.

116. Johnson GH, Chellis KD, Gordon GE, Lepe X. Dimensional stability and detail reproduction of irreversible hydrocolloid and elastomeric impressions disinfected by immersion. J Prosthet Dent 1998;79:446–453.

117. Abado GL, Zanarotti E, Fonseca RG, Cruz CA. Effect of disinfectant agents on dimensional stability of elastomeric impression materials. J Prosthet Dent 1999;81:621–624.

118. Adabo GL, Zanarotti E, Fonseca RG, Cruz CA. Effect of disinfectant agents on dimensional stability of elastomeric impression materials. J Prosthet Dent 1999;81:621–624.

119. Harrison JD. Effect of retraction materials on the gingival sulcus epithelium. J Prosthet Dent 1961;11:514–521.

120. Löe H, Silness J. Tissue reactions to string packs used in fixed restorations. J Prosthet Dent 1963;13:318.

121. Woycheshin FF. An evaluation of the drugs used for gingival retraction. J Prosthet Dent 1964;14:769.

122. Anneroth G, Nordenram A. Reaction of the gingiva to the application of threads in the gingival pocket for taking impressions with elastic material. An experimental histological study. Odontol Revy 1969;20:301–310.

123. Ramadan FA, Harrison JD. Literature review of the effectiveness of tissue displacement materials. Egypt Dent J 1970;16:271–282.

124. Ramadan FA, el-Sadeek M, Hassanein el-S. Histopathologic response of gingival tissues to hemodent and aluminum chloride solutions as tissue displacement materials. Egypt Dent J 1972;18:337–352.

125. Mokbel AM, Mohamed YR. Local effect of applying aluminum chloride on the dento-gingival unit as a tissue displacement material. Part I. Egypt Dent J 1973;19:35–48.

126. de Gennaro GG, Landesman HM, Calhoun JE, Martinoff JT. A comparison of gingival inflammation related to retraction cords. J Prosthet Dent 1982;47:384–386.

127. Weir DJ, Williams BH. Clinical effectiveness of mechanical-chemical tissue displacement methods. J Prosthet Dent 1984;51:326–329.

128. Donovan TE, Gandara BK, Nemetz H. Review and survey of medicaments used with gingival retraction cords. J Prosthet Dent 1985;53:525–531.

129. Nemetz EH, Seibly W. The use of chemical agents in gingival retraction. Gen Dent 1990Mar-Apr;38:104–108.

130. Jokstad A. Clinical trial of gingival retraction cords. J Prosthet Dent 1999;81:258–261.

131. Kopac I, Cvetko E, Marion L. Gingival inflammatory response induced by chemical retraction agents in beagle dogs. Int J Prosthodont 2002;15:14–19.

132. Csempesz F, Vág J, Fazekas Á. In vitro kinetic study of absorbency of retraction cords. J Prosthet Dent 2003;89:45–49.

133. Azzi R, Tsao TF, Carranza FA Jr, Kennedy EB. Comparative study of gingival retraction methods. J Prosthet Dent 1983;50:561–565.

134. Ruel J, Schuessler PJ, Malament K, Mori D. Effects of retraction procedures on the periodontium in humans. J Prosthet Dent 1980;44:508–515.

135. Dragoo MR, Williams GB. Periodontal tissue reactions to restorative procedures. Int J Periodontics Restorative Dent 1981;1(1):8–23.

136. Chiche GJ, Pinault A. Impressions for the anterior dentition. In: Chiche GJ, Pinault A (eds). Esthetics of Anterior Fixed Prosthodontics. Chicago: Quintessence, 1994:161–175.

137. Baharav H, Laufer BZ, Langer Y, Cardash HS. The effect of displacement time on gingival crevice width. Int J Prosthodont 1997;10:248–258.

138. Adams HF. Managing gingival tissues during definitive restorative treatment. Quintessence Int 1981;12:141–149.

139. Parma Benfenati S, et al. The effect of restorative margins on the postsurgical development and nature of the periodontium. Part I: anatomical considerations. Int J Periodontics Restorative Dent 1985;6:31–51.

140. Feng J, Aboyoussef H, Weiner S, Singh S, Jandinski J. The effect of gingival retraction procedures on periodontal indices and crevicular fluid cytokine levels: a pilot study. J Prosthodont 2006;15:108–112.

141. Malamed SF. Handbook of Local Anesthesia, ed 3. St Louis: Mosby Year Book, 1990.

142. Albers HF. Impressions. A Text for Selection of Materials and Techniques. Santa Rosa, CA: Alto, 1990:21.

143. Nemetz H, Donovan T, Landesman H. Exposing the gingival margin: a systematic approach for the control of hemorrhage. J Prosthet Dent 1984;51:647–651.

144. Robinson PJ, Vitek RM. The relationship between gingival inflammation and resistance to probe penetration. J Periodontal Res 1979;14:239–243.

145. O'Mahony A, Spencer P, Williams K, Corcoran J. Effect of 3 medicaments on the dimensional accuracy and surface detail reproduction of polyvinyl siloxane impressions. Quintessence Int 2000;31:201–206.

146. Bowles WH, Tardy SJ, Vahadi A. Evaluation of new gingival retraction agents. J Dent Res 1991;70:1447–1449.

147. Garber DA, Goldstein RE, Feinman RA. Porcelain Laminate Veneers. Chicago: Quintessence, 1988.

148. Dietschi D, Magne P, Holz J. Bonded to tooth ceramic restorations: in vitro evaluation of the efficiency and failure mode of two modern adhesives. Rev Mens Suisse Odontostomatol 1995;105:299–305.

149. Dietschi D, Herzfeld D. In vitro evaluation of marginal and internal adaptation of class II resin composite restorations after thermal and occlusal stressing. Eur J Oral Sci 1998;106:1033–1042.

150. Magne P, Douglas WH. Porcelain veneers: dentin bonding optimization and biomimetic recovery of the crown. Int J Prosthodont 1999;12:111–121.

151. Bertschinger C, Paul SJ, Luthy H, Schärer P. Dual application of dentin bonding agents: effect on bond strength. Am J Dent 1996;9:115–119.

152. Paul SJ, Schärer P. The dual bonding technique: a modified method to improve adhesive luting procedures. Int J Periodontics Restorative Dent 1997;17:536–545.

153. Paul SJ. Adhesive Luting Procedures. Berlin: Quintessence, 1997:89–98.

154. Magne P, Belser U. Bonded Porcelain Restorations in the Anterior Dentition. A Biomimetic Approach. Chicago: Quintessence, 2002:272–290.

155. Parel SM, Sullivan DY. Esthetics and Osseointegration. Osseointegration Seminars, 1989.

156. Wee AG. Comparison of impression materials for direct multi-implant impressions. J Prosthet Dent 2000; 83:323–331.

157. Briley TF. Master cast implant impression: using the open-tray technique. Dent Implantol Update 2002 Oct;13:73–80.

158. Calderini A, Redemagni M, Garlini G, Maschera E, D'Amato S. Le impronte in implanto-protesi. Il Dentista Moderno, Maggio 2004 (aggiornamento monografico): 25–51.

159. Brånemark P-I, Zarb GA, Albrektsson T. Tissue-integrated Prostheses: Osseointegration in Clinical Dentistry. Chicago: Quintessence, 1985.

160. Craig RG. Restorative Dental Materials, ed. 7. St Louis, Mosby, 1985:469.

161. Humphries RM, Yaman P, Bloem TJ. The accuracy of implant master casts constructed from transfer impressions. Int J Oral Maxillofac Implants 1990;5:331–336.

162. Mojon P, Oberholzer JP, Meyer JM, Belser UC. Polimerization shrinkage of index and pattern acrylic resins. J Prosthet Dent 1990;64:684–688.

163. Spector MR, Donovan TE, Nicholls JI. An evaluation of impression techniques for osseointegrated implants. J Prosthet Dent 1990;63:444–447.

164. Assif D, Fenton A, Zarb G, Schmitt A. Comparative accuracy of implant impression procedures. Int J Periodontics Restorative Dent 1992;12:112–121.

165. Ness EM, Nicholls JI, Rubenstein JE, Smith DE. Accuracy of the acrylic resin pattern for the implant retained prosthesis. Int J Prosthodont 1992;5:542–549.

166. Hsu CC, Millstein PL, Stein RS. A comparative analysis of the accuracy of implant transfer techniques. J Prosthet Dent 1993;69:588–593.

167. Inturregui JA, Aquilino SA, Ryther JS, Lund PS. Evaluation of three impression techniques for osseointegrated oral implants. J Prosthet Dent 1993;69:503–509.

168. Liou AD, Nicholls JI, Yuodelis RA, Brudvik JS. Accuracy of replacing three tapered transfer impression copings in two elastomeric impression materials. Int J Prosthodont 1993;6:377–383.

169. Assif D, Nissan J, Varsano I, Singer A. Accuracy of implant impression splinted techniques: effect of splinting material. Int J Oral Maxillofac Implants 1999;14:885–888.

170. Gregory-Head B, LaBarre E. Two-step pick-up impression procedure for implant-retained overdentures. J Prosthet Dent 1999;82:615–616.

171. Burns J, Palmer R, Howe L, Wilson R. Accuracy of open tray implant impressions: an in vitro comparison of stock versus custom trays. J Prosthet Dent 2003;89:250–255.

172. American Academy of Periodontology. Dental implants in periodontal therapy. J Periodontol 2000;71:1934–1942.

173. Berglundh T, Lindhe J, Ericsson I, Marinello CP, Liljenberg B, Thomsen P. The soft tissue barrier at implants and teeth. Clin Oral Implants Res 1991;2:81–90.

174. Berglundh T, Lindhe J. Dimension of the peri-implant mucosa: biological width revisited. J Clin Periodontol 1996;23:971–973.

175. Cochran DL, Hermann JS, Schenk RK, Higginbottom FL, Buser D. Biologic width around titanium implants. A histometric analysis of the implanto-gingival junction around unloaded and loaded nonsubmerged implants in the canine mandible. J Periodontol 1997;68:186–198.

176. Dawson PE. Temporomandibular joint pain-dysfunction problems can be solved. J Prosthet Dent 1973;29:100–112.

177. Weinberg LA. The role of muscle deconditioning for occlusal corrective procedures. J Prosthet Dent 1991;66:250–255.

178. Tripodakis AP, Smulow JB, Mehta NR, Clark RE. Clinical study of location and reproducibility of three mandibular positions in relation to body posture and muscle function. J Prosthet Dent 1995;73:190–198.

179. Academy of Prosthodontics. The Glossary of Prosthodontic Terms, ed 7. St Louis, Mosby, 1999.

180. Munsell AH. A Grammar of Color. New York: Van Nostrand Dreinhold, 1969.

181. Sproull RC. Color matching in dentistry. Part I. The three-dimensional nature of color. J Prosthet Dent 1973;29:416–424.

182. Yamamoto M. Metal-Ceramics. Tokyo: Quintessence, 1982.

183. Preston JD. Currrent status of shade selection and color matching. Quintessence Int 1985;16:47–58.

184. Miller L. Organizing color in dentistry. J Am Dent Assoc 1987;Spec No:26E–40E.

185. Miller LL. A scientific approach to shade matching. In: Preston JD (ed). Perspectives in Dental Ceramics: Proceedings of the Fourth International Symposium on Ceramics. Chicago: Quintessence, 1988:193:208.

186. Miller MD, Zaucha R. Color and tones. In: The Color Mac: Design Production Techniques. Carmel, IN: Hayden, 1992:23–39.

187. Miller LL. Shade matching. J Esthet Dent 1993;5:143–153.

188. Miller LL. Shade selection. J Esthet Dent 1994;6:47–60.

189 ■ Chu SJ. Precision shade technology: contemporary strategies in shade selection. Pract Proced Aesthet Dent 2002;14:79–83.

190 ■ Chu SJ. The science of color and shade selection in aesthetic dentistry. Dent Today 2002;21:86–89.

191 ■ Chu SJ, Devigus A, Mieleszko A. Fundamentals of Color: Shade Matching and Communication in Esthetic Dentistry. Chicago: Quintessence, 2004.

192 ■ Ecker GA, Moser JB. Visual and instrumental discrimination steps between two adjacent porcelain shades. J Prosthet Dent 1987;58:286–291.

193 ■ Lichter JA, Solomowitz BH, Sher M. Shade selection. Communicating with the laboratory technician. NY State Dent J 2000;66:42–46.

194 ■ Sim CP, Yap AU, Teo J. Color perception among different dental personnel. Oper Dent 2001;26:435–439.

195 ■ Ishikawa-Nagai S, Sato R, Furukawa K, Ishibashi K. Using a computer color-matching system in color reproduction of porcelain restorations. Part 1: application of CCM to the opaque layer. Int J Prosthodont 1992;5:495–502.

196 ■ Ishikawa-Nagai S, Sawafuji F, Tsuchitoi H, Sato RR, Ishibashi K. Using a computer color-matching system in color reproduction of porcelain restorations. Part 2: color reproduction of stratiform-layered porcelain samples. Int J Prosthodont 1993;6:522-527.

197 ■ Ishikawa-Nagai S, Sato RR, Shiraishi A, Ishibashi K. Using a computer color-matching system in color reproduction of porcelain restorations. Part 3: a newly developed spectrophotometer designed for clinical application. Int J Prosthodont 1994;7:50–55.

198 ■ Okubo SR, Kanawati A, Richards MW, Childress S. Evaluation of visual and instrument shade matching. J Prosthet Dent 1998;80:642–648.

199 ■ Chu SJ, Tarnow DP. Digital shade analysis and verification: a case report and discussion. Pract Proced Aesthet Dent 2001;13:129–136.

200 ■ Paul S, Peter A, Pietrobon N, Hammerle CH. Visual and spectrophotometric shade analysis of human teeth. J Dent Res 2002;81:578–582.

201 ■ Tung FF, Goldstein GR, Jang S, Hittelman E. The repeatability of an intraoral dental colorimeter. J Prosthet Dent 2002;88:585–590.

202 ■ Dancy WK, Yaman P, Dennison JB, O'Brien WJ, Razzoog ME. Color measurements as quality criteria for clinical shade matching of porcelain crowns. J Esthet Restorative Dent 2003;15:114–121.

VOLUME 2 | PROSTHETIC TREATMENT

ESTHETIC REHABILITATION IN FIXED PROSTHODONTICS

Chapter 5

PRODUCING AND FINALIZING THE PROSTHETIC REHABILITATION

Cross-mounting of the casts on the articulator is a fundamental step for replicating in the definitive restoration all of the esthetic and functional characteristics tested in the provisional restoration. Silicone indices allow for construction of a suitable substructure for obtaining uniform thickness of ceramic, which will give the prosthetic rehabilitation not only adequate resistance but an excellent esthetic appearance as well.

OBJECTIVE _ Adopt a systematic approach for ideal integration of the prosthetic rehabilitation.

Chapter 5
PRODUCING AND FINALIZING THE PROSTHETIC REHABILITATION

PRODUCING THE DEFINITIVE RESTORATION

CLINIC

Primary objectives must be to scrupulously take all of the necessary registrations and faithfully replicate the esthetic-functional characteristics present in the provisional restoration. It is equally important to observe the meticulously achieved biologic integration and maintain it in all of the therapeutic phases.[1–14] The gingival tissues should be in perfect health in order to cement the definitive restorations under ideal conditions. In light of this, the removal of excess cement represents a delicate clinical step, and it often takes place at the end of a particularly demanding session. One option is to reinsert the provisional restoration on the abutments at the end of the final impression-taking session without proceeding with further cementation. This is an option only if, when the provisional restoration is removed, the cement inside is intact and shows no color change, and if no new tooth preparation was necessary before the final impressions were taken. The integrity of the cement demonstrates adequate retention and resistance of the restoration to masticatory forces, as well as the absence of any marginal leakage, thereby preventing both pulpal damage and gingival inflammation. In these cases the appointment for the try-in of the definitive substructure must be scheduled to take place within 2 to 3 weeks.

LABORATORY

In addition to the laboratory checklist, which transfers all of the information necessary for finalizing the prosthetic rehabilitation, the technician will also receive the impressions of the provisional restoration, the impressions of the prepared abutments, and the cast of the opposing arch. Included with these are the facebow and all of the occlusal registrations essential for correct cross-mounting of the casts on the articulator (Figs 5-1 to 5-3). Using special silicone indices taken from the provisional restoration, it is possible to replicate all of the characteristics of the provisional restoration in the definitive restoration.[15] The only difference between the acrylic index and the definitive restoration is the type of material used, and this is selected at the time of final tooth preparations (see chapter 3, page 324). The final preparations were carried out according to the volume of the provisional restoration and taking into account the thickness of the definitive restorations. It is the technician's task to improve the anatomy, shape, and proportion of the individual teeth while maintaining the position, tooth arrangement, and inclination of the occlusal plane. The registrations allow the laboratory to reproduce all of the functional characteristics of the provisional restoration, thus ensuring occlusal stability and an ideal disocclusive path, the latter of which is due to the use of a customized anterior guidance.

FIG 1 2 3 To proceed with finalizing the restoration, impressions, registrations, and the laboratory checklist are all sent to the technician.

CASE 1

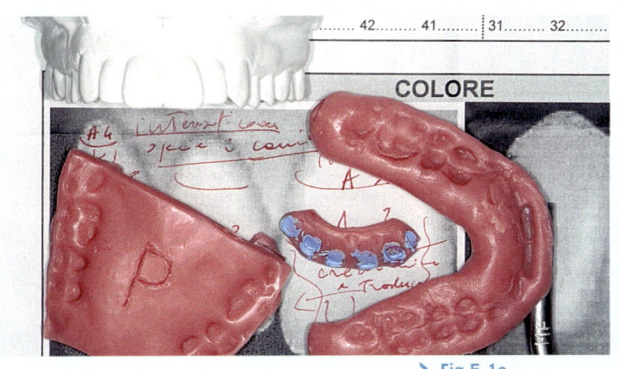

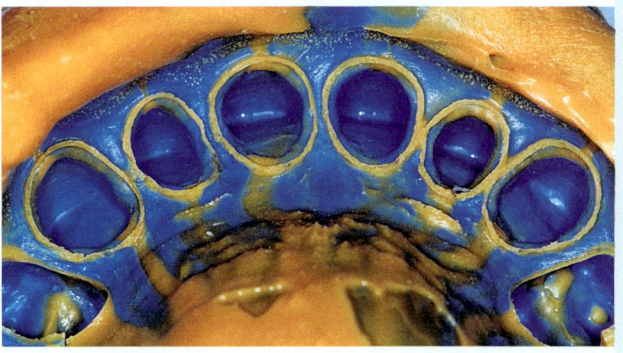

> Fig 5-1a

> Fig 5-1b

CASE 2

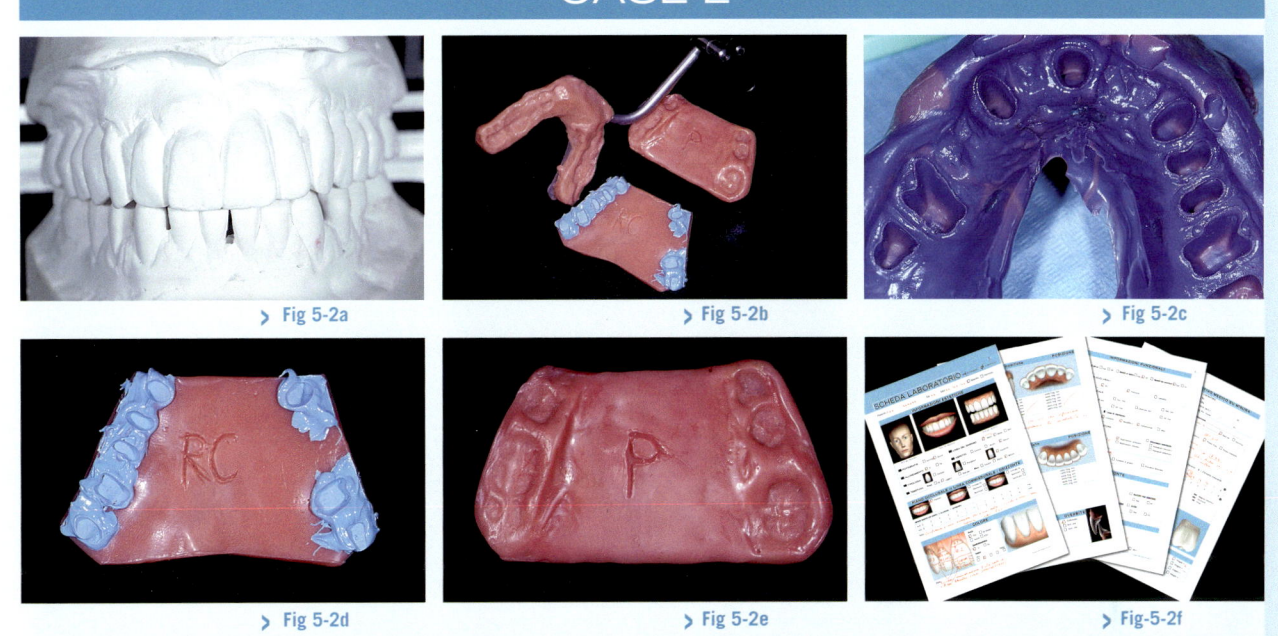

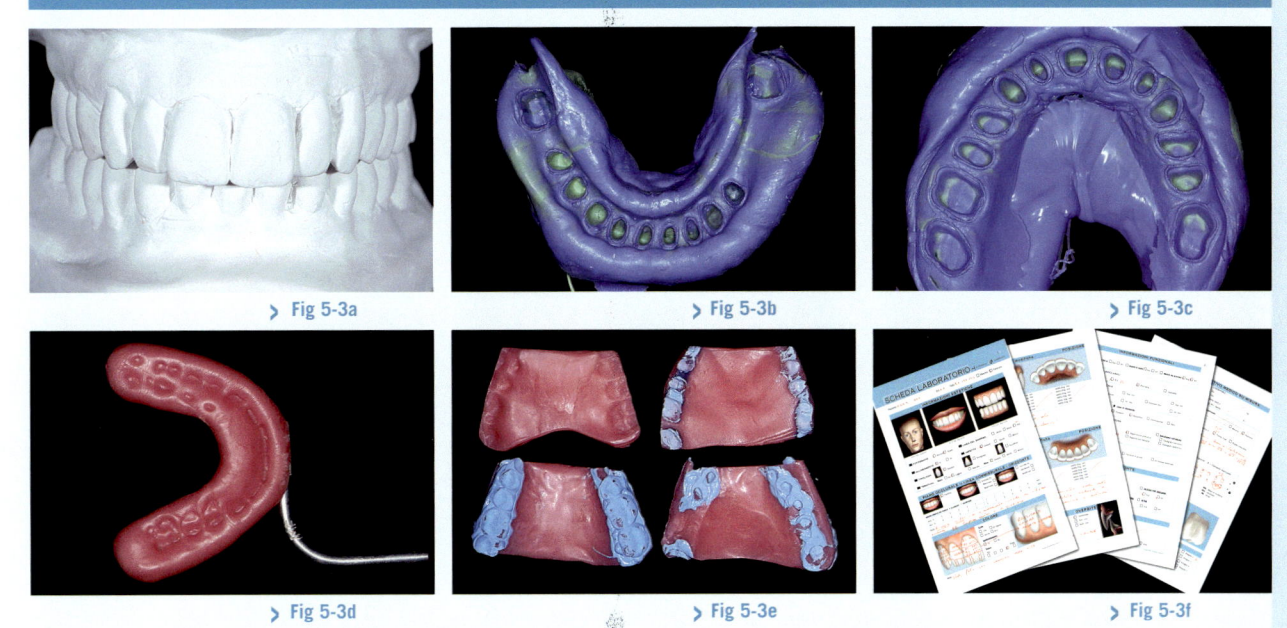

> Fig 5-2a

> Fig 5-2b

> Fig 5-2c

> Fig 5-2d

> Fig 5-2e

> Fig-5-2f

CASE 3

> Fig 5-3a

> Fig 5-3b

> Fig 5-3c

> Fig 5-3d

> Fig 5-3e

> Fig 5-3f

437

PRODUCING THE DEFINITIVE RESTORATION   LABORATORY

MASTER CAST (MC)

REMOVABLE ABUTMENTS

It is essential to take more than one final impression to give the technician the opportunity to choose, with the help of a stereomicroscope, the one most suitable for creating the master cast (MC) to be used for constructing the removable abutments with double precision pins. Extra-hard stone (type IV)[16] is normally used to pour this final cast even if, when faced with very thin abutments (mandibular incisors or hemisections), the use of epoxy or polyurethane resins can be advised. It is important that there are no striations and/or irregularities on the surfaces of the abutments and that all of the preparation margins are clearly visible. Once the cast has been poured (Fig 5-4a), it is necessary to discard the plaster, removing the portion that represents the gingival tissues (Figs 5-4b to 5-4e), taking care not to touch the preparation limits. To achieve ideal design of the emergence profile, it is important to highlight a portion of integral tooth beyond the finish margin.[17]

DIE SPACER

To visualize the finish line, the technician uses a pencil to mark the preparation limit (Figs 5-4f and 5-4g). The markings are fixed by spreading a layer of cyanoacrylate over the abutment, limited only to the marginal area. In addition to giving the plaster greater resistance, this expedient protects this very delicate area, in every phase of the work, from the abrasion that could take place while the definitive restorations are being constructed (Figs 5-4h to 5-4m).[18] To compensate for any inaccuracies in the marginal fit of the definitive restorations, attributable to the use of the various materials (impression, plasters or resins, waxes, investment, alloy),[19-26] the abutments are coated with a die spacer (Fig 5-4n).[27] Its application must be approximately 20 to 25 µm thick to create a space in the definitive restoration useful for accommodating the luting cement, thus allowing the restoration a better fit and a more accurate marginal closure. The die spacer must only be applied once the casts have been mounted on the articulator, so as not to interfere with the correct positioning of the registration waxes. An initial layer will cover only the occlusal surfaces of the posterior teeth and the incisal and cingulum surfaces of the anterior teeth (Figs 5-4o to 5-4q). To reach the final thickness required, one or two additional layers will be applied in succession, which should also cover the axial walls but exclude the marginal area by 1.0 or 1.5 mm (Figs 5-4r and 5-4s). This variation in the thickness allows the clinician to make only minimal touchups to the substructure, especially in the border areas between the axial and the occlusal/incisal walls.

FIG 4 *(a)* The MC made from the final impression, is used to construct removable dies. *(b and c)* Each die is examined with the aid of a magnification system. *(d)* With a crosscut bur, used because it prevents chipping the stone, the gingival portion is then removed, taking care not to damage the preparation limit. *(e)* The unprepared part of the tooth, which is highlighted by this process, allows for an ideal marginal reading and can be useful for constructing a correct emergence profile. *(f and g)* The preparation limit is then defined with a blue pencil while the unprepared portion of the tooth is located with a red line.

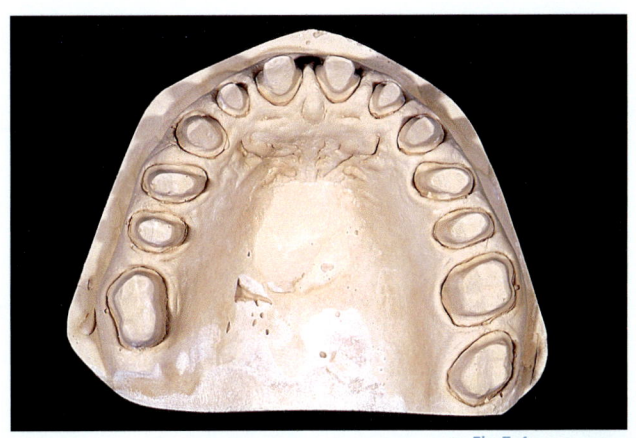

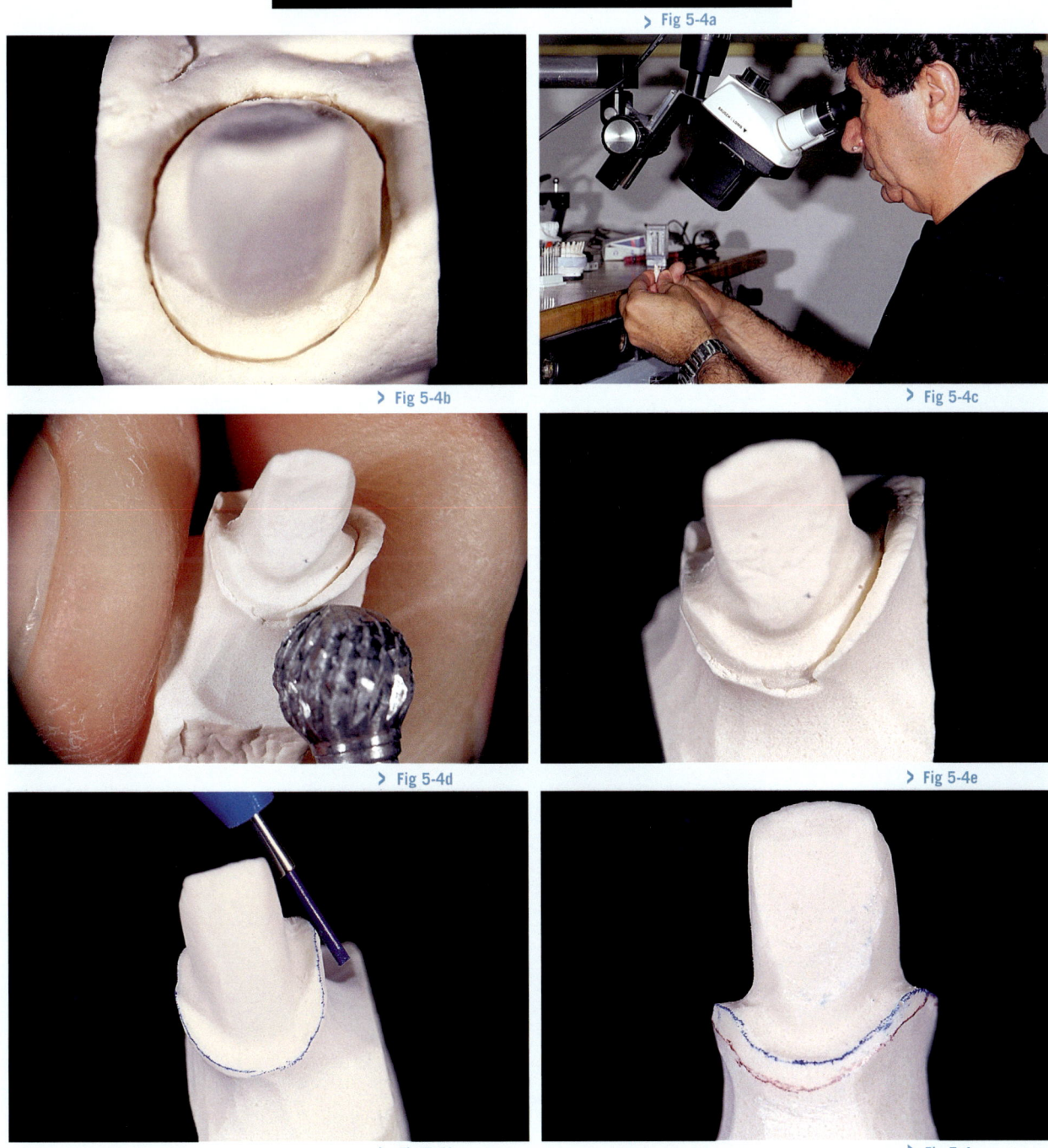

> Fig 5-4a

> Fig 5-4b

> Fig 5-4c

> Fig 5-4d

> Fig 5-4e

> Fig 5-4f

> Fig 5-4g

> Fig 5-4h

> Fig 5-4i

> Fig 5-4j

> Fig 5-4k

> Fig 5-4l

> Fig 5-4m

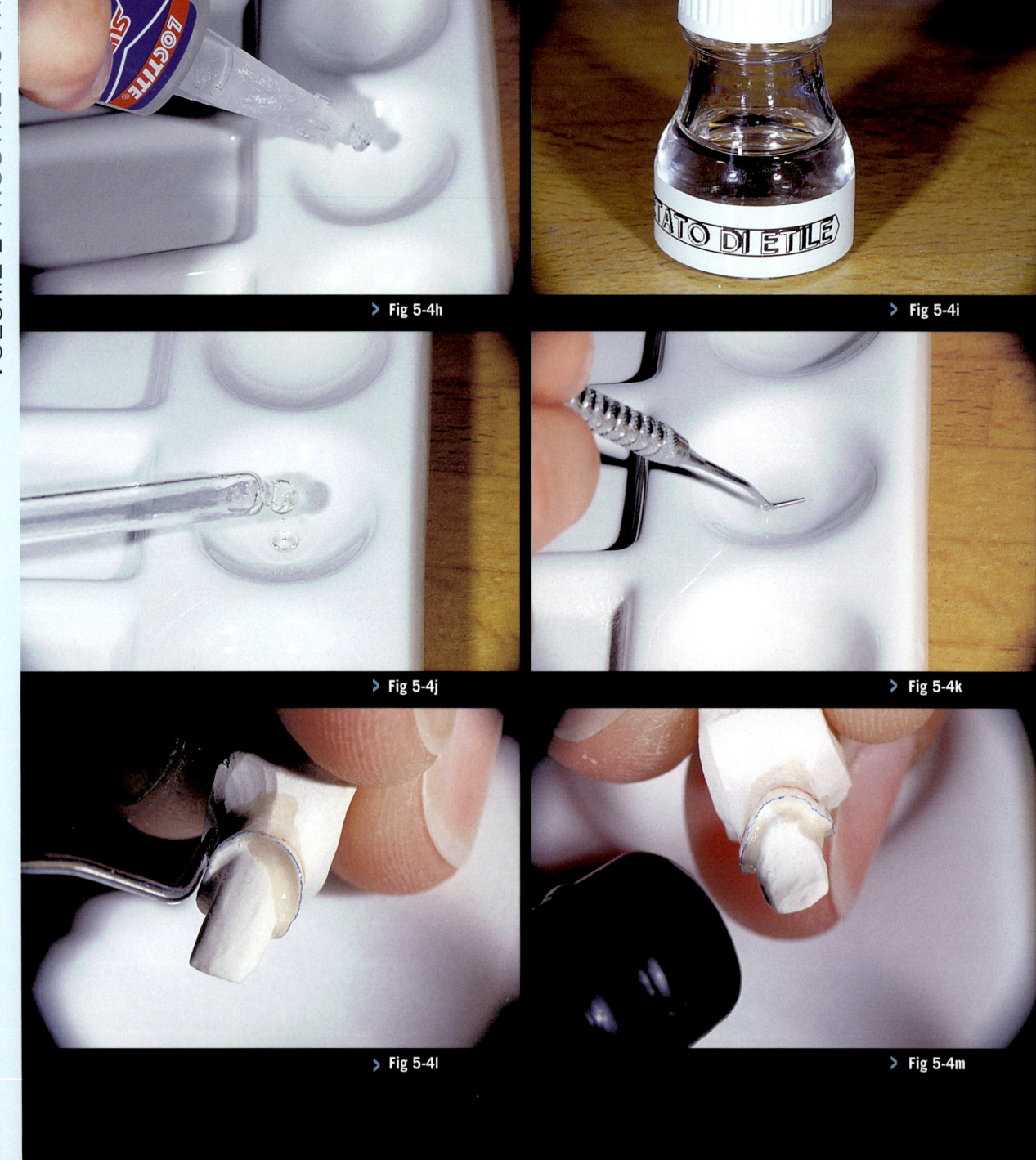

FIG 4 *(h to j)* In a ceramic dish, cyanoacrylate is diluted with ethyl acetate (3:1 ratio) to make it more fluid, thereby preventing it from becoming undesirably thick during application. *(k to m)* The composite thus obtained is applied to the margin with the tip of a metal instrument, and compressed air is used immediately to remove the excess. In addition to preserving the marginal area from deterioration, this procedure also allows the pencil marks to be retained on the plaster until the work is finished.

> Fig 5-4n

> Fig 5-4o

> Fig 5-4p

> Fig 5-4q

> Fig 5-4r

> Fig 5-4s

FIG 4 *(n to q)* An initial layer of die spacer is applied with a brush, limiting it to the incisal angles and to the cingulum area. The application is then repeated, extending the varnish over the entire surface of the abutment, until a thickness of 20 to 25 μm is reached. *(r and s)* So as not to interfere with the marginal closure, the varnish must avoid the cervical area by roughly 1.5 mm.

PRODUCING THE DEFINITIVE RESTORATION

SECONDARY CAST (SC)

REPLICATING GINGIVAL TISSUES

From the impression already used for constructing the MC the secondary cast (SC) is created with a second pouring, which maintains all of the details of the gingival contours that make it possible to optimize the cervical areas of the definitive prosthesis. When the MC is created, portions of impression material often remain trapped in the sulcus area of the plaster, making the reproduction of certain details in that area impossible. However, the tissue morphology in the SC can be reproduced and transferred to the MC by means of a silicone impression into which elastomeric material is injected[28] (Figs 5-5 to 5-7). This will allow for creation of a cast that combines both the preparation margins and the anatomy of the soft tissues.

OPTIMIZING THE RESTORATIVE CONTOUR

Overcontour Because the final impressions were taken with the aid of retraction cords, the restorative contours obtained do not represent the true clinical situation of the tissues fitted with the provisional restorations. Restorations created from this impression would be overcontoured because of the compression exerted by the cords on the gingival tissues.

Undercontour Conversely, if the final impressions of the soft tissue morphology are taken when the substructure is tried in (once the provisional restorations have been removed), it would show collapsed tissues, because they would no longer be supported by the contours of the provisional or the acrylic restorations. The definitive restorations would therefore be undercontoured.

Since an accurate impression of the tissue morphology cannot be obtained by either means, experience urges us to prefer the first option. Adjusting the restorative contours by subtraction, as previously demonstrated with the MIT for fabricating the provisional restorations (see chapter 2, page 154), is easier and more reliable than adjusting by addition.

DESIGN OF THE CONNECTING AREAS

When fixed partial dentures are being constructed, information about the tissue morphology on the SC and on the MC modified in this way is essential for correct design of the connecting areas. The height of these areas is a determining factor in achieving a good level of resistance in the prosthesis.[29-33] If the connection extends too apically, however, the interproximal space is substantially reduced, preventing adequate cleaning in these very delicate areas.

CASE 1

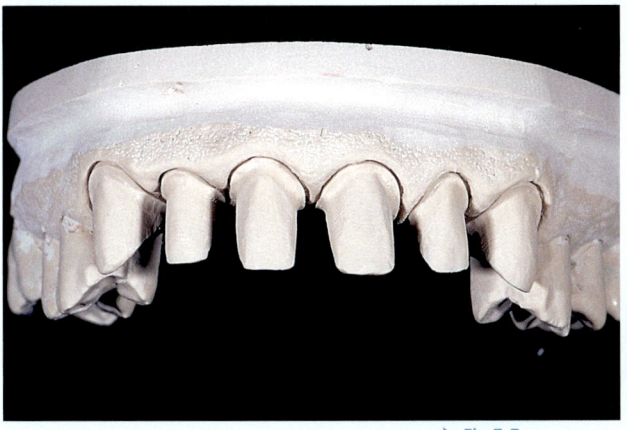

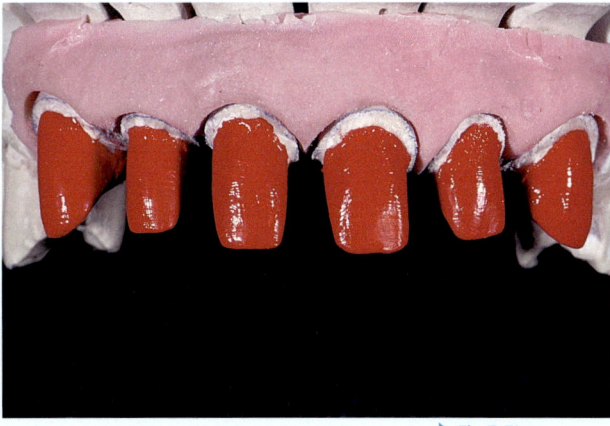

> Fig 5-5a

> Fig 5-5b

CASE 2

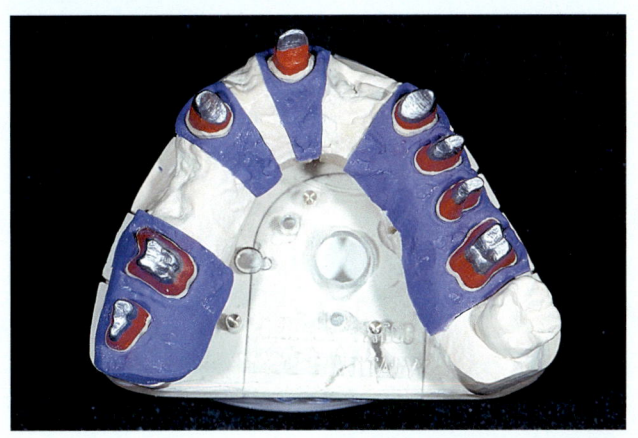

> Fig 5-6a

> Fig 5-6b

> Fig 5-6c

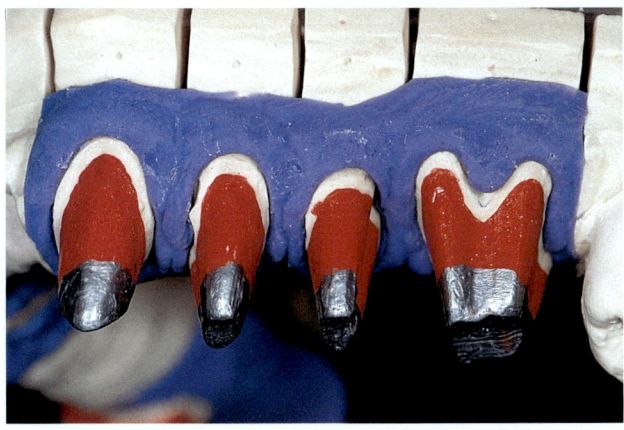

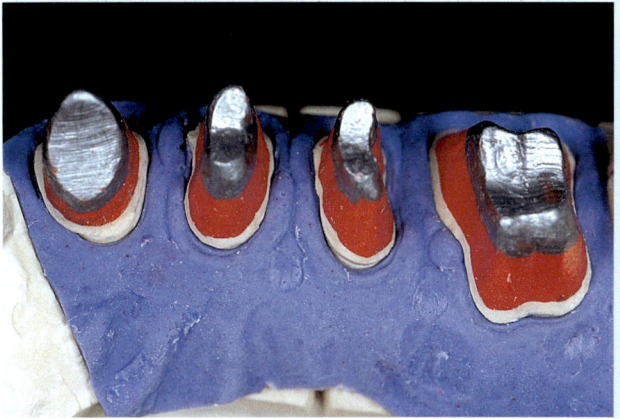

FIG 5 *(a and b)* On the SC kept intact, the morphology of the gingival tissues can be seen and can also be reproduced on the MC using an elastomeric material.

FIG 6 *(a to c)* The reproduction of the tissue morphology on the MC with an elastomeric material allows the design of the connective areas to be correctly defined and, therefore, an ideal closure of the interproximal spaces in the cervical areas to be obtained.

CASE 3

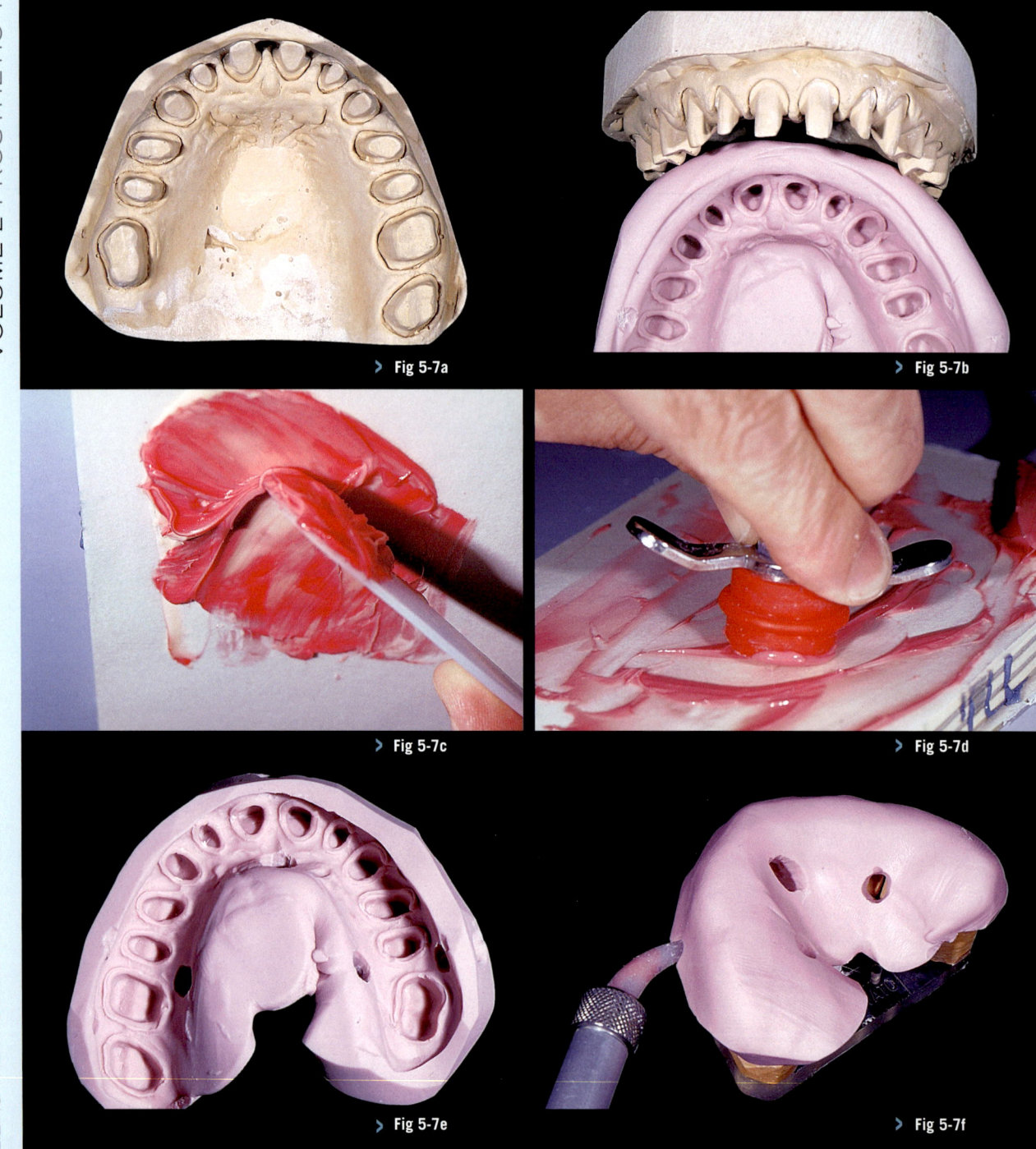

> Fig 5-7a

> Fig 5-7b

> Fig 5-7c

> Fig 5-7d

> Fig 5-7e

> Fig 5-7f

FIG 7 *(a and b)* On the SC, a silicone impression is taken that faithfully reproduces the tissue morphology. *(c to e)* While the PE material is being mixed (Permadyne Garant, 3M ESPE), the silicone index is positioned on the MC. *(f)* Elastomeric material is injected with a syringe through the holes made in the index for that purpose, until the spaces between the MC and the silicone index are filled and the gingival appearance is thus reproduced.

CASE 3

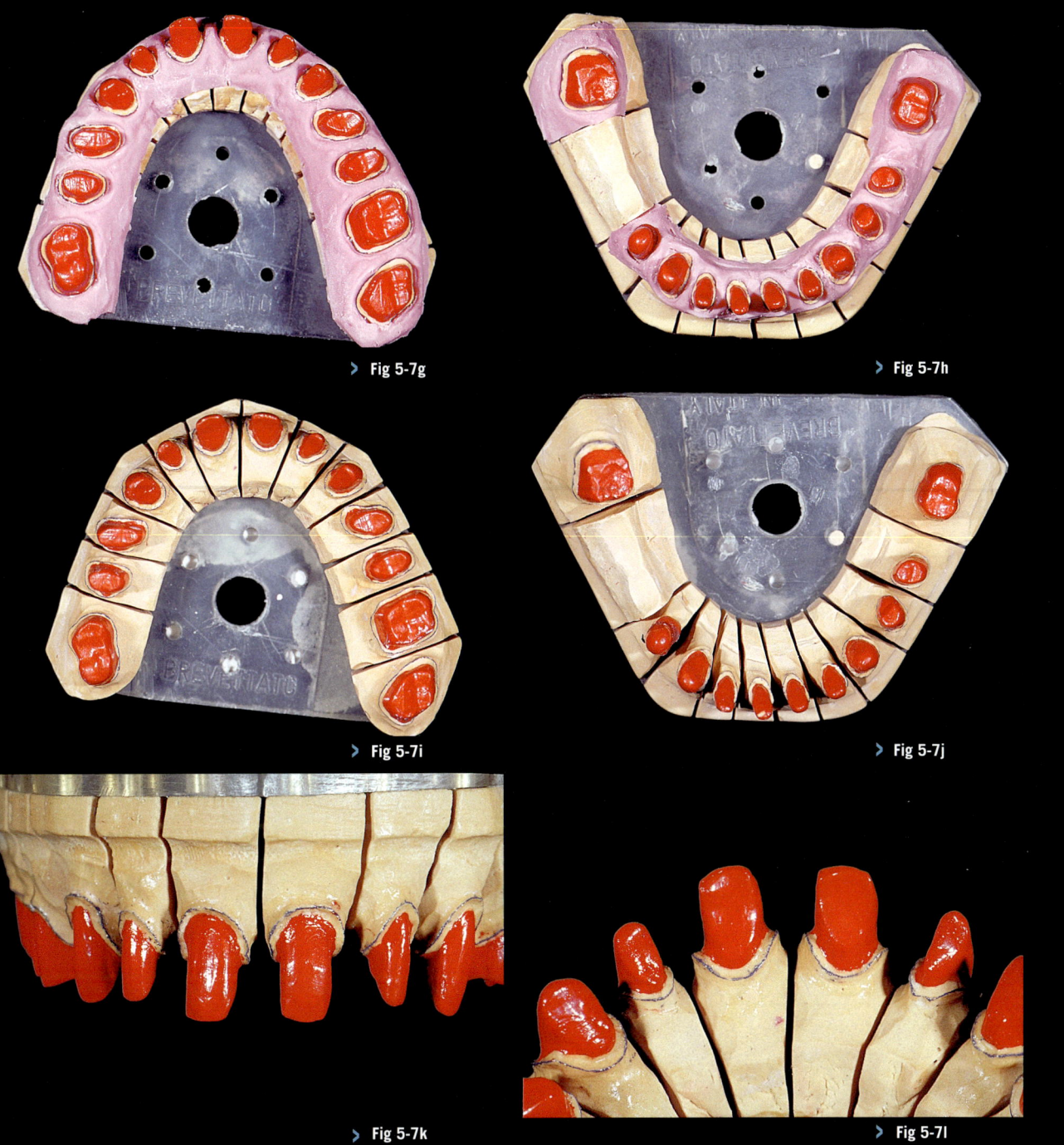

> Fig 5-7g

> Fig 5-7h

> Fig 5-7i

> Fig 5-7j

> Fig 5-7k

> Fig 5-7l

FIG 7 *(g and h)* View of the gingival indices, as taken from the SC, positioned on the MCs of the maxillary and mandibular arches. *(i to l)* So that the technician can suitably highlight the marginal limit of each prosthetic abutment, the previously made gingival indices should be removed.

LABORATORY

■ CROSS-MOUNTING TECHNIQUE ■
ANTERIOR REHABILITATION

The semi-adjustable articulator, which was used (see chapter 1, page 98) for adjusting the condylar eminence, the immediate mandibular lateral translation value, and the progressive lateral translation value, is a reliable instrument for treating both simple and complex cases.[34–37]

In the method illustrated below, faithful replication of the esthetic-functional characteristics of the integrated provisional restoration requires interchanging of the various casts on the articulator (provisional restorations, MCs, and cast of the opposing arch), known as cross-mounting. To correctly record the occlusal registrations, the casts must be positioned alternately in the same articular position (CR) and at the same VDO.

ANTERIOR REHABILITATION

MOUNTING THE CAST OF THE PROVISIONAL RESTORATION WITH THE CAST OF THE OPPOSING ARCH

The facebow can be recorded on tooth preparations as well as on the occlusal surfaces of the provisional restoration. The second option guarantees greater stability (Fig 5-8a) of the cast on the bite fork, allowing it to be adequately mounted on the articulator. The mandibular cast is mounted following the patient's occlusal key (Fig 5-8b). The technician must verify in advance that good stability exists between the two stone casts, which should be free of air bubbles, sufficiently extended, and have good detail definition.

MOUNTING THE MASTER CAST WITH THE CAST OF THE OPPOSING ARCH

Once the cast of the maxillary provisional restoration has been removed using the specific registration taken exclusively between the prepared teeth and the mandibular arch, the cast with the tooth preparations (MC) is mounted on the opposing cast (cross-mounting) (Fig 5-8c).

In partial rehabilitation cases as well, where in theory no occlusal refinements should be necessary on the definitive restorations, there can sometimes be slight discrepancies between the casts mounted on the articulator and the patient's clinical situation. These variations, which can be caused by minimal inaccuracies associated with the impression material, the occlusal registration, or the plaster used to construct the casts, compel the clinician to intervene on the occlusal table.[38–40]

FIG 8 (a) The technician uses the facebow to mount the stone cast of the maxillary arch on the articulator. (b) The adequate intercuspation between the stone casts makes it possible to mount the opposing cast. (c) Because of the registration taken between the abutments and the opposing arch, the MC can then be mounted.

CASE 1

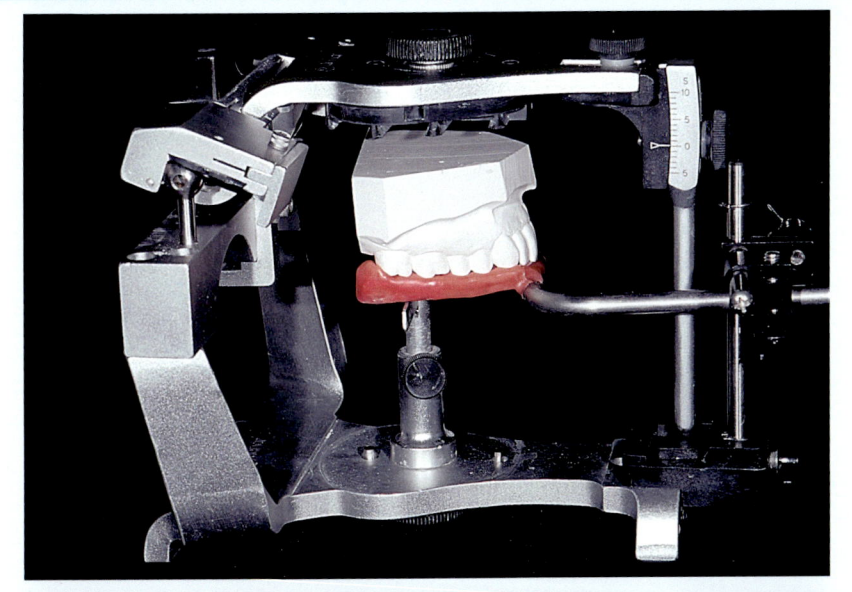

> Fig 5-8a

> Fig 5-8b

> Fig 5-8c

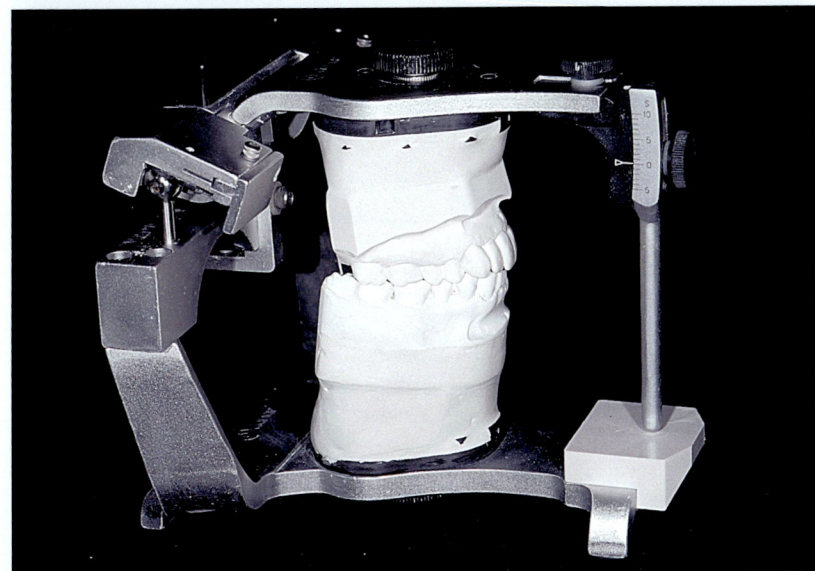

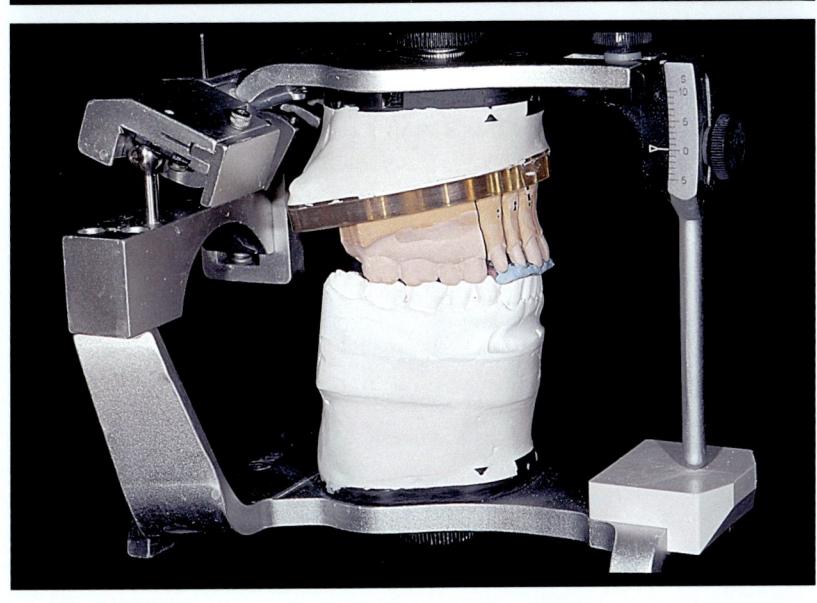

LABORATORY

CROSS-MOUNTING TECHNIQUE
SINGLE-ARCH REHABILITATION

MOUNTING THE CAST OF THE PROVISIONAL RESTORATION WITH THE CAST OF THE OPPOSING ARCH

The two casts must be precise and detailed in both the occlusal and the buccal areas, especially at the dentogingival level, which represents a crucial point of reference for checking the VDO. As noted earlier for the anterior rehabilitation, it is essential that the clinician has verified the occlusal stability between the two stone casts.

With rehabilitation of a complete arch, it is even more important that the provisional restorations possess appropriate development of the anatomy of the posterior sectors to avoid the possibility of finding more than one occlusal position. If there are any uncertainties regarding the correct positioning of the casts, the clinician must provide the technician with a registration taken between the provisional restoration and the opposing cast in CR, which must not be perforated to prevent any possible tooth contact.

Placing wax between the two casts unavoidably increases the VDO in the articulator and must be compensated for, in the casting phase, by raising the incisal pin by an amount equal to the thickness of the registration. This modification can create a difference between the arc of closure of the articulator and the patient's true one, which would necessitate an occlusal refinement, however minimal, in the definitive restoration. To minimize this imprecision, the thickness of the registration must be as low as possible, even though it must not be perforated.

MOUNTING THE MASTER CAST WITH THE CAST OF THE OPPOSING ARCH

The cast with the tooth preparations (MC) is then mounted in CR and at the same VDO, using a single registration extended over the entire arch and taken between prepared teeth and the opposing arch.

Centric relation The mandibular position in CR must coincide exactly between the provisional restoration and the opposing arch, as well as between the tooth preparations (MC) and the opposing arch. This is the only way to realistically interchange the casts while maintaining the same articular position, allowing the technician to copy the functional provisional restoration.

Vertical dimension The technician can verify the correspondence of the VDO between the two maxillary casts (MC and the provisional restoration cast) (Fig 5-9), alternately mounted with the opposing cast because of the coincident measurement between the selected dentogingival reference points.

CASE 2

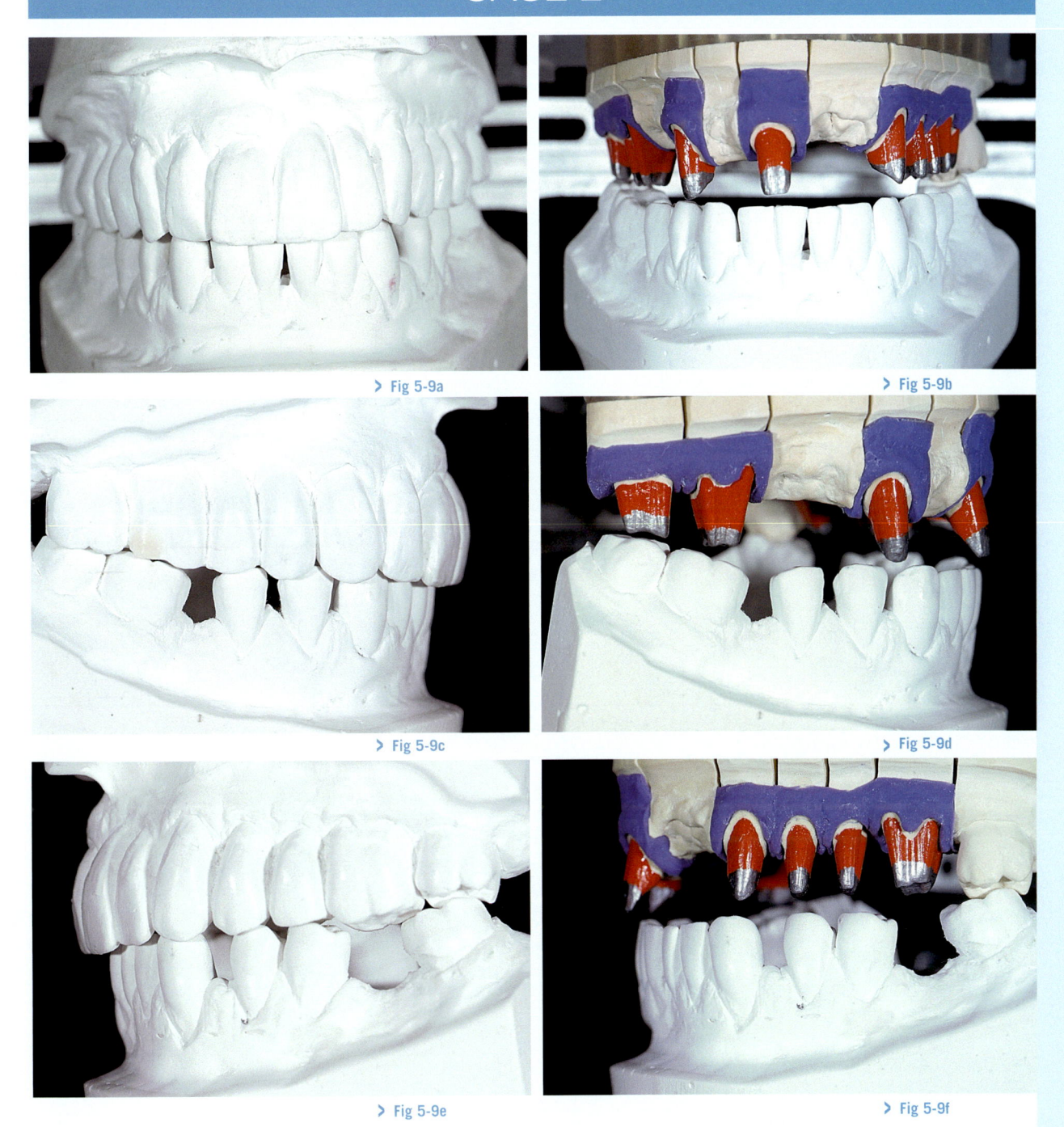

> Fig 5-9a

> Fig 5-9b

> Fig 5-9c

> Fig 5-9d

> Fig 5-9e

> Fig 5-9f

FIG 9 *(a to f)* In order to carry out cross-mounting, the maxillary cast with the provisional restorations must be in the same mandibular position (CR) and at the same VDO as the MC.

LABORATORY

CROSS-MOUNTING TECHNIQUE FOR TWO-ARCH REHABILITATIONS

MOUNTING THE CASTS OF THE MAXILLARY AND MANDIBULAR PROVISIONAL RESTORATIONS

After mounting the cast of the maxillary provisional restoration using the facebow (Fig 5-10a), the technician has all of the registrations necessary for cross-mounting (Fig 5-10b). In the first phase, the cast of the maxillary provisional restoration is counter-positioned with that of the mandibular provisional restoration, making sure they are stable in the CO position (Figs 5-10c to 5-10e).

CROSS-MOUNTING OF THE MAXILLARY AND MANDIBULAR CASTS

The two registrations, taken between the maxillary prepared teeth and the mandibular provisional restoration, and between the mandibular prepared teeth and the maxillary provisional restoration, respectively, were taken in CR and at the same VDO, as described earlier, to correctly interchange the working casts. It is the clinician's responsibility to scrupulously check, on the patient, the coincidence of the height between the reference points recorded with the provisional restorations (Fig 5-10f) and those taken alternately between abutment and provisional restorations (Figs 5-10g and 5-10h). The repeatability of the Dawson maneuver[41–43] is fundamental for obtaining correct registrations and completing precise and reliable cross-mounting.

CHECKING CROSS-MOUNTING WITH MAXILLARY MC AND MANDIBULAR MC

Taking an occlusal registration between prepared maxillary and mandibular teeth allows the technician to confirm that the mountings carried out previously with the two registrations between the MC and the provisional restorations (Figs 5-10i to 5-10k) were done correctly.

If, when carrying out cross-mounting, the technician finds a discrepancy in the VDO in one of the registrations, this inaccuracy must be corrected by adjusting the pin before mounting. If the VDO registration is higher than the one found between the two provisional restorations, the pin must be raised by the same amount before the MC is fabricated. If it is lower, the adjustment must be made in the opposite direction. In both cases, the pin must be taken back to zero once the casts have been fabricated. Without this adjustment, the teeth, especially in the anterior areas, would be shorter in the first instance and longer in the second. These arbitrary variations, carried out in the laboratory on the incisal pin, can cause occlusal inaccuracies that are slight and hence easily corrected during the try-ins in the oral cavity, but only if the height adjustment stays within the range of 1 to 2 mm. To avoid problems of this sort, it is important to take all of the occlusal registrations at the correct VDO.

CASE 3

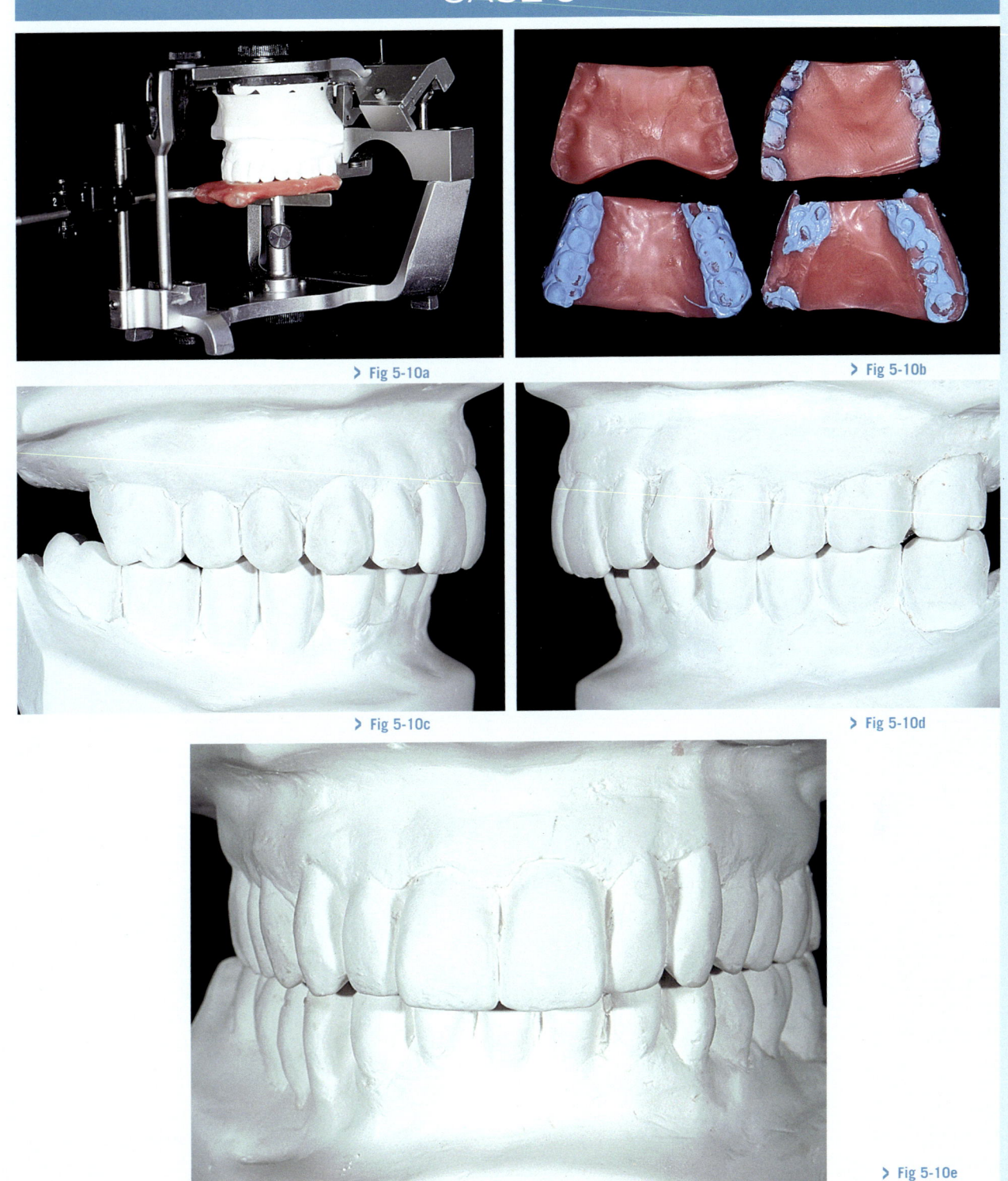

> Fig 5-10a

> Fig 5-10b

> Fig 5-10c

> Fig 5-10d

> Fig 5-10e

FIG 10 *(a and b)* After mounting the maxillary cast of the provisional restoration using the facebow, the technician has all of the necessary registrations available to complete cross-mounting between the various casts. *(c to i)* After ascertaining the effective stability of the casts of the provisional restorations and recording the VDO, the technician checks that there is agreement between this measurement and those taken in all of the possible mounting combinations for the various casts of both arches (casts of the provisional restoration and MC). The VDO must be checked before the mounting on the articulator. *(j and k)* Only at this point is it possible to remove the maxillomandibular relationship records and to apply the die spacer, to ensure that the thickness of the varnish does not interfere with the insertion of the waxes.

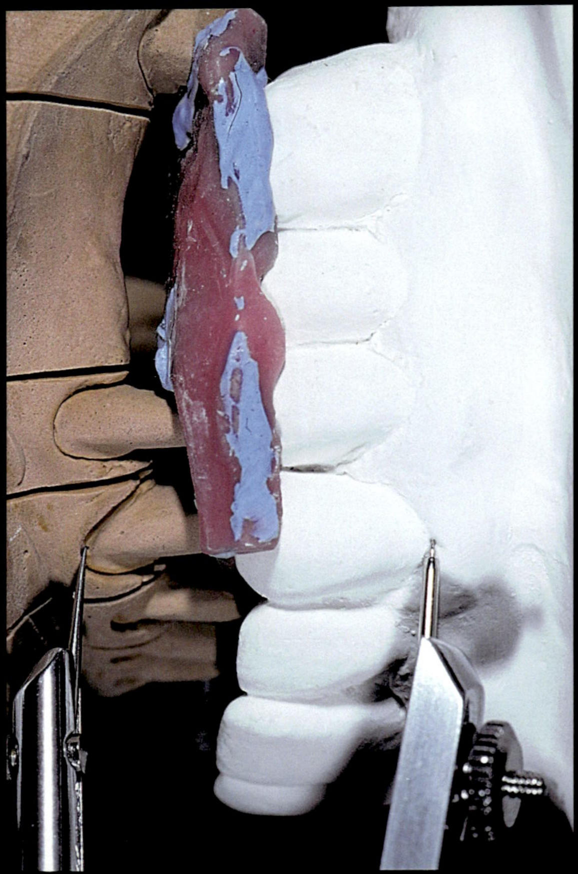

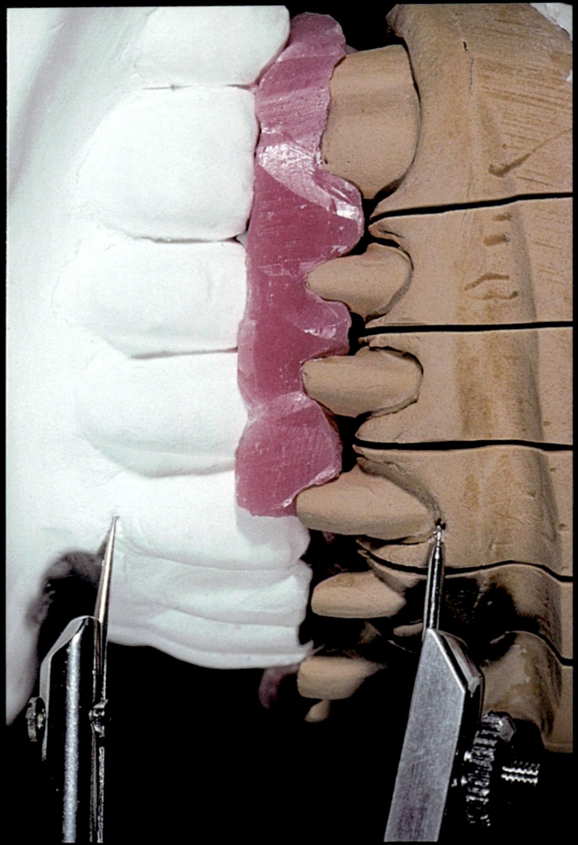

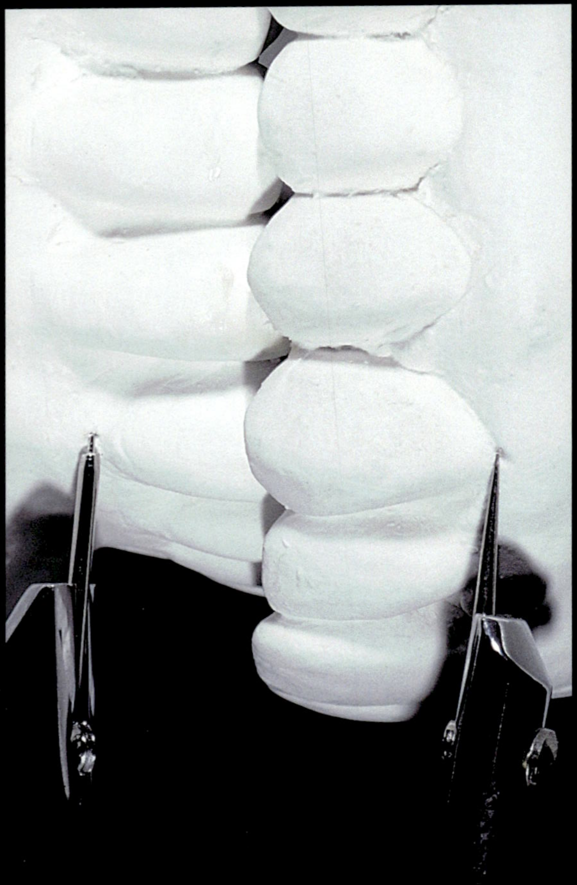

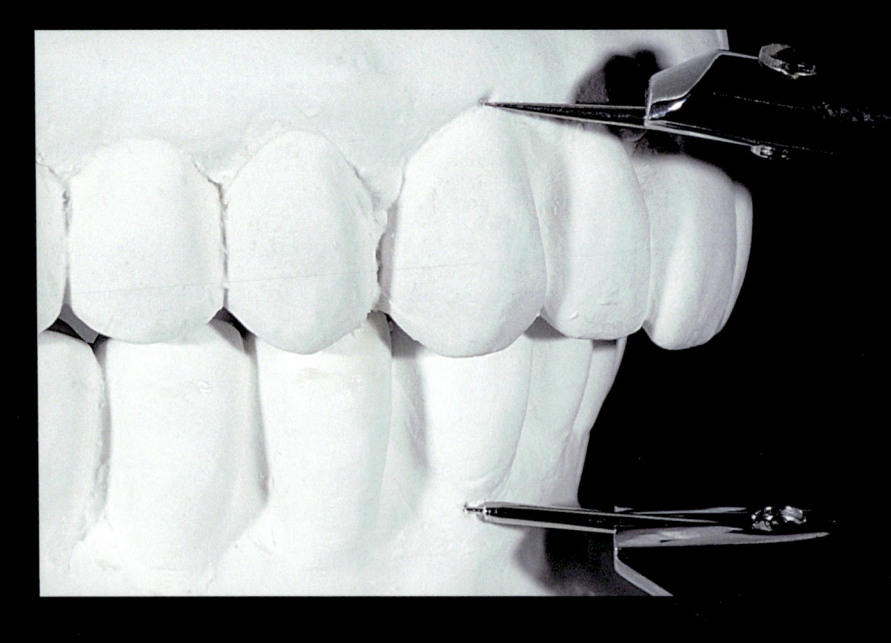

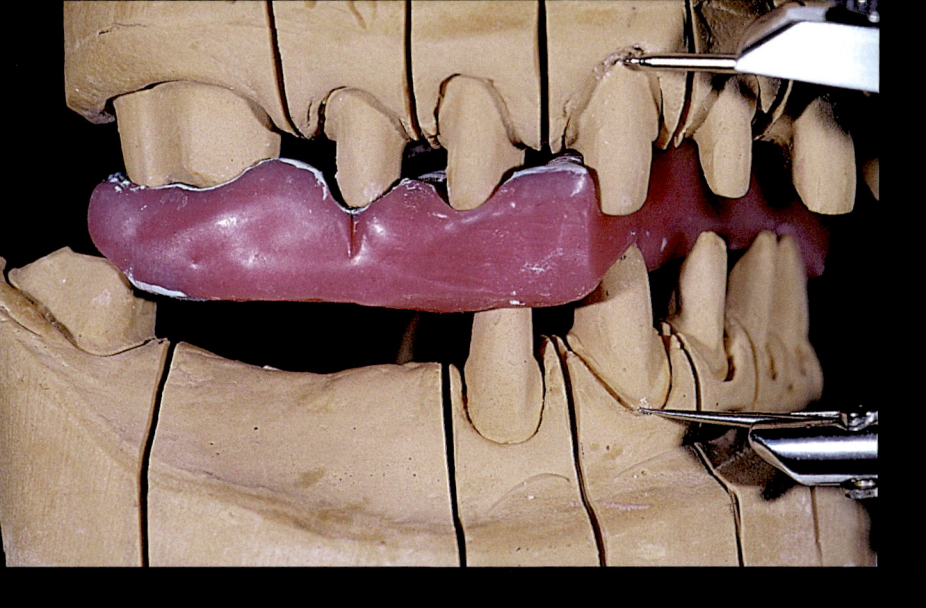

> Fig 5-10i

> Fig 5-10j

> Fig 5-10k

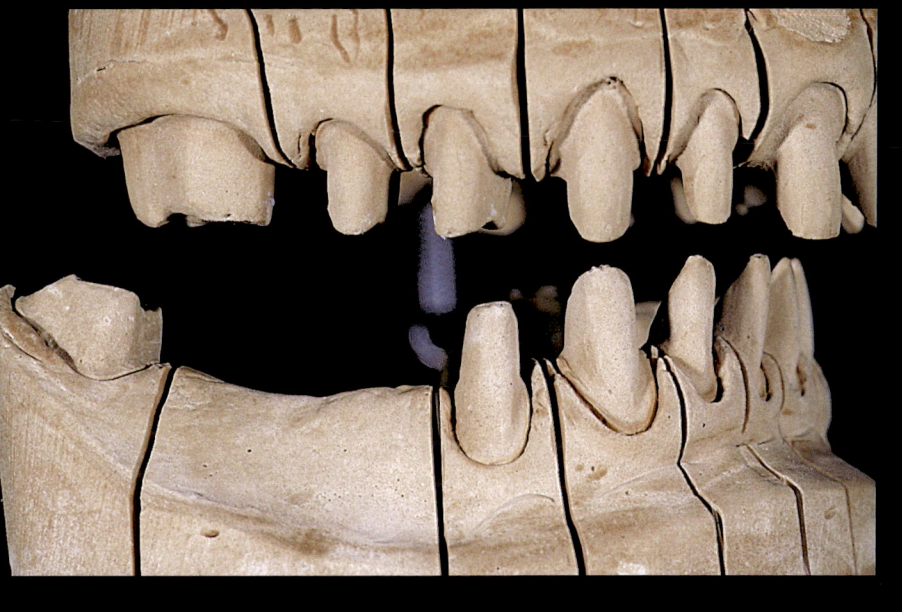

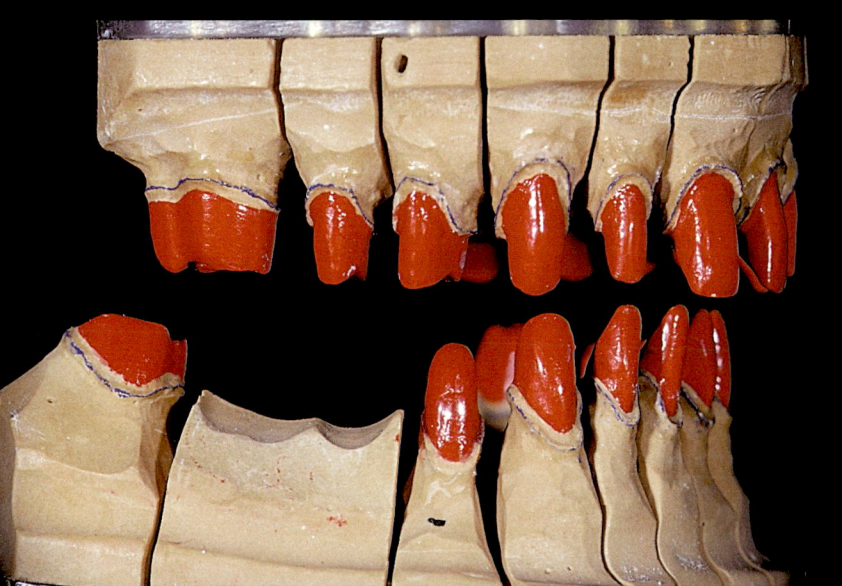

ADJUSTING THE ARTICULATOR — LABORATORY

CUSTOMIZED ANTERIOR GUIDANCE

Protrusive occlusal registration In partial as well as in complete rehabilitations, the protrusive occlusal registration must be taken between the provisional restoration and the opposing arch, whether it is natural teeth (eg, in the case of anterior teeth and rehabilitation of one arch), or a functionalized provisional occlusal restoration (eg, in the case of rehabilitation of two arches). After mounting the cast of the provisional restoration with the cast of the opposing arch, the technician inserts the protrusive occlusal registration, which makes the casts take an edge-to-edge occlusal position and causes the arches to separate in the posterior sectors (Figs 5-11a and 5-11b). This separation also occurs between the condyles and the condylar fossae. After undoing the locking screws on the articulator, the technician angles the fossae until contact is made with the condyles (Figs 5-11c and 5-11d). In this way the articulator is programmed with a condylar inclination that copies that of the patient. If the protrusive occlusal registration is not taken, the technician must program the condylar fossae with an arbitrary setting. In these cases an angle between 20 and 25 degrees is selected,[35,36,44,45] which, considering the normally higher values found in nature, should be sufficient to ensure disocclusion of the posterior teeth in all patients. This adjustment, however, will lead the technician to construct an occlusal table with only a slightly accentuated anatomy, with probable repercussions on the masticatory efficiency.[46]

Constructing the customized anterior guidance After adjusting the condylar inclination (posterior determinant) according to the protrusive occlusal registration, the technician will place light-curing resin, still in the plastic state, on the incisal plate (Fig 5-11e). Starting the casts from the edge-to-edge position (Figs 5-11f and 5-11g), the mandibular cast is slid along the lingual concavity of the maxillary incisors until it reaches the centric position (Fig 5-11h), taking care to maintain the condyles in intimate contact with the relative condylar fossae.[47] This movement, first carried out in the protrusive position, is then repeated in the same way for the path of the lateral excursions (Figs 5-11i and 5-11j). The resin, cast from the incisal pin (Figs 5-11k to 5-11q), is light-cured, then removed from the incisal plate (Fig 5-11r) and placed in a specific furnace to complete its light-curing process.

This procedure makes it possible, by creating a customized anterior guidance, to replicate the lingual concavity of the maxillary anterior teeth of the provisional restoration, thereby reproducing the same disocclusion in the posterior sectors tested in the patient's mouth for a suitable period of time.

CASE 3

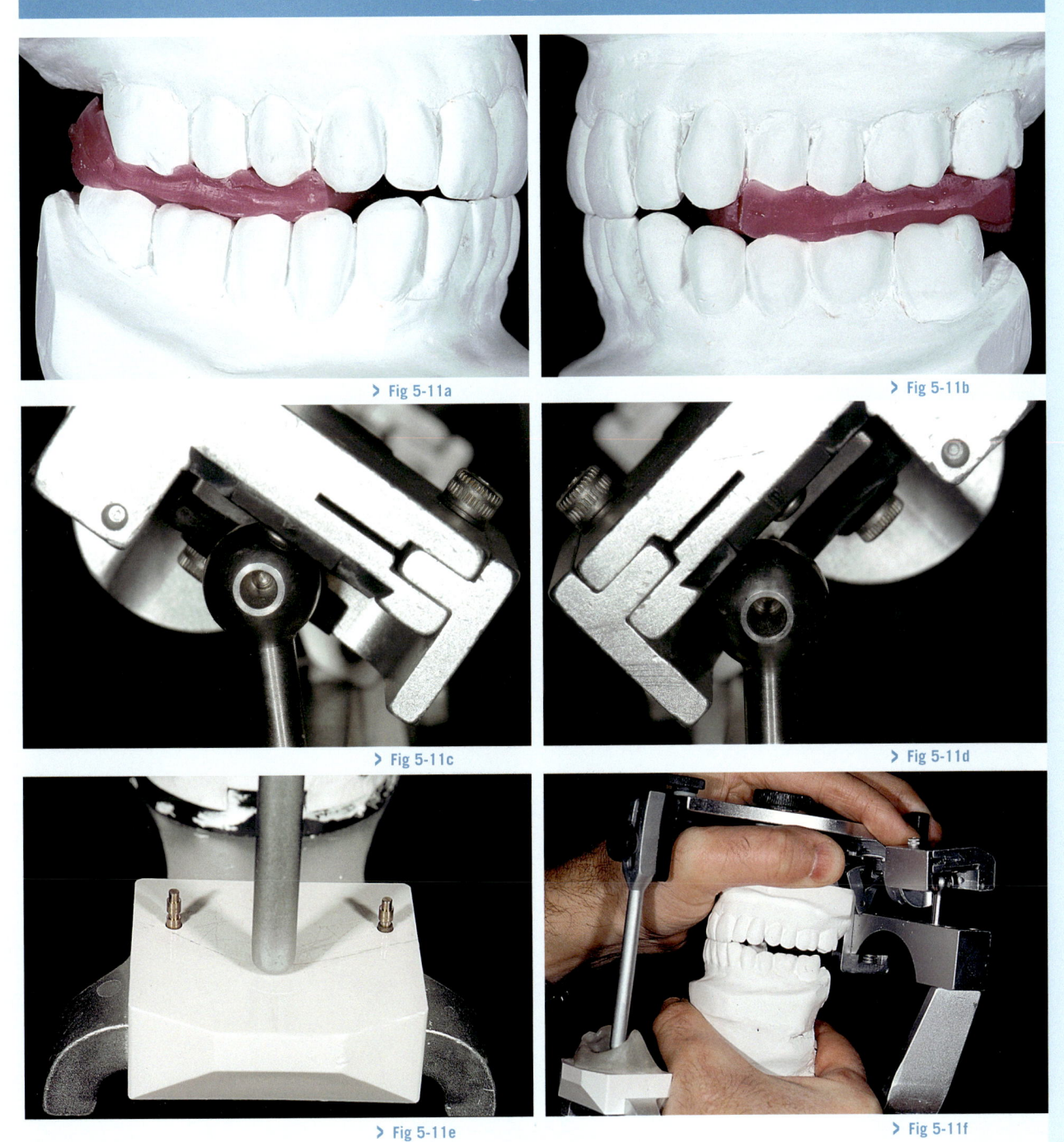

> Fig 5-11a

> Fig 5-11b

> Fig 5-11c

> Fig 5-11d

> Fig 5-11e

> Fig 5-11f

FIG 11 *(a and b)* Lateral view of the casts of the provisional restorations mounted under the guidance of the protrusive occlusal registration. *(c and d)* With the anterior teeth in the edge-to-edge occlusal position, the condyles move down and forward; at this point, the condylar fossae rest on the end of the condyles, making it possible to adjust the inclination of the condylar path. *(e and f)* The pins fitted into the incisal plate allow anchoring of the light-curing resin, which is sculpted as the casts of the provisional restorations are made to perform all of the functional movements. *(g and h)* The incisal pin must be duly insulated to make sure that the resin does not attach to it. Starting from an edge-to-edge position, the casts are made to slip into CO. Particular care must be taken to keep the articulator well anchored so that the condyles always remain in contact with the condylar fossae. *(i and j)* Because of the guidance provided by the anatomy of the anterior teeth (anterior determinant) and adjustment of the condylar slants (posterior determinant), it is possible to sculpt a customized anterior guidance into the acrylic resin by moving the casts in all directions. *(k to p)* The anterior guidance is then refined, to faithfully replicate in the definitive restorations the disocclusive path present in the provisional restorations. *(q)* In all of the phases described, the incisal pin, perforating the acrylic resin, must be in direct contact with the incisal plate. *(r)* The two pins initially inserted into the incisal plate to anchor the resin allow the customized guidance to be removed and refitted whenever necessary.

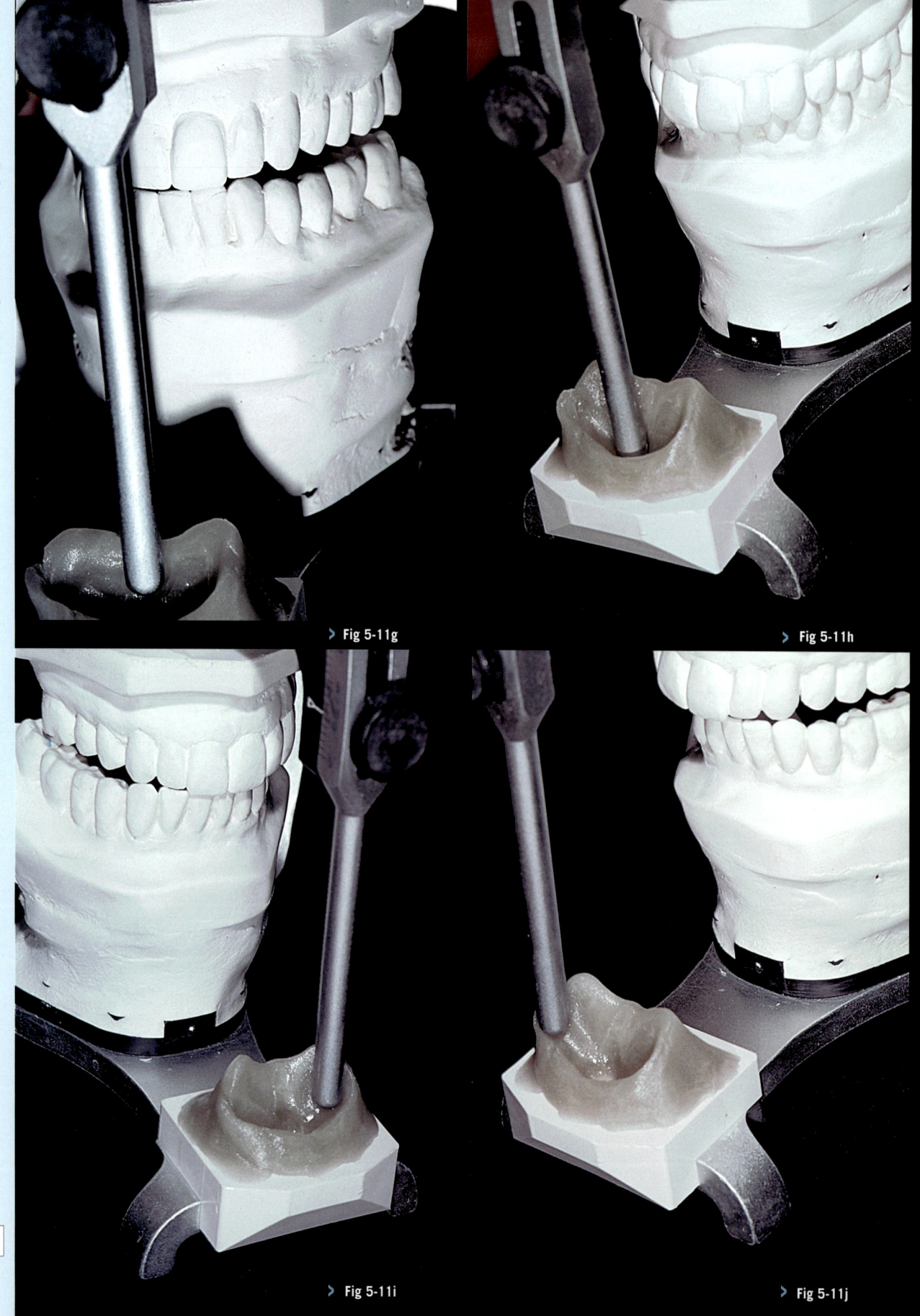

> Fig 5-11g

> Fig 5-11h

> Fig 5-11i

> Fig 5-11j

> Fig 5-11k

> Fig 5-11l

> Fig 5-11m

> Fig 5-11n

> Fig 5-11o

> Fig 5-11p

> Fig 5-11q

> Fig 5-11r

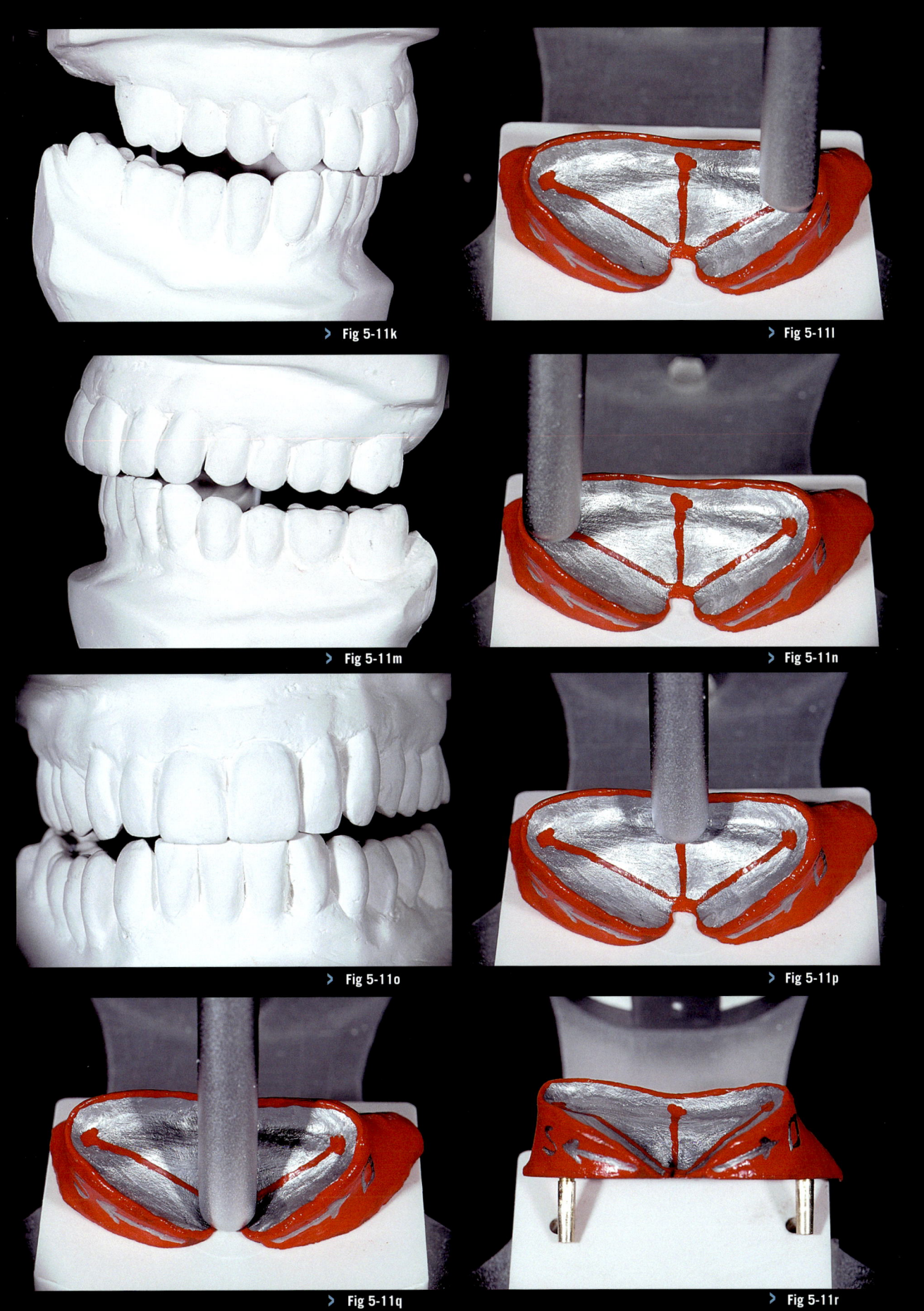

457

CONSTRUCTING THE DEFINITIVE RESTORATION — LABORATORY

SILICONE INDEX

The indices, or silicone matrices, are taken from the casts of the provisional restorations, copying their shape and, more importantly, the tooth arrangement. The technician uses these as a guide to create the definitive prosthesis, reproducing the esthetic and functional characteristics tested in the provisional restoration.[47]

OCCLUSOPALATAL INDEX

The occlusopalatal index is mainly used to copy the position of the incisal margins, the volumes, and the tooth lengths tested in the provisional restoration (Fig 5-12a).

Partial rehabilitations In partial rehabilitation cases, the integral teeth alongside the tooth preparations allow the clinician to use the unprepared pontic elements as an anchor for an occlusal index that, once it is built on the cast of the provisional restorations, is then transferred to the MC (Fig 5-12b).

Complete rehabilitations In complete rehabilitation cases, where it is not possible to find reference points for repositioning, the indices must be constructed by raising the pin of the articulator by two notches. This rise must obviously be maintained when the cast of the provisional restoration is replaced with that of the preparations (MC). In all of the working phases, the silicone index must be anchored to the cast of the opposing arch (Fig 5-13). This procedure is essential for creating an adequate thickness of silicone material that would otherwise puncture because of the intercuspation. The silicone is placed between the arches in its plastic phase. The articulator is then closed until the incisal pin makes contact with the anterior plate, and is kept in position until polymerization is complete. The negative image of the occlusal table is thus captured in the posterior sectors, and negative images of the incisal edge and the lingual concavity are captured in the anterior sectors (Fig 5-14). All excess silicone must be removed so that the peripheral reference margins, which are essential for constructing the definitive restorations, can be seen. It is helpful to mark the tooth limits with a pencil to make their identification easier.

OCCLUSOPALATAL INDEX (ONE OR TWO ARCHES)

STEPS

- Mount the casts of the provisional restorations on the articulator.
- Raise the articulator pin by two notches.
- Place the silicone between the two arches while still soft.
- Close the articulator until the pin stops on the incisal plate.
- Remove all excesses and mark the tooth limits with a pencil.

CASE 1

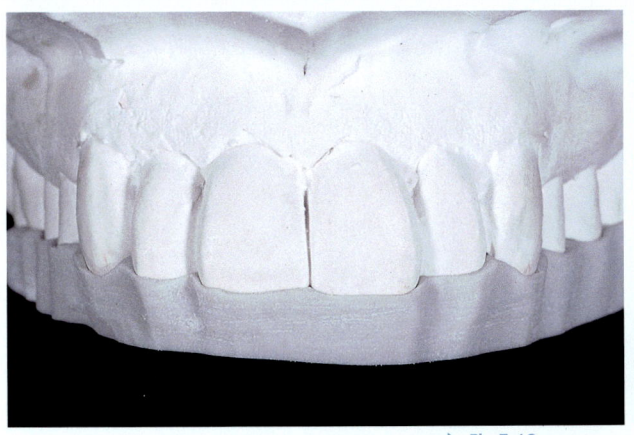

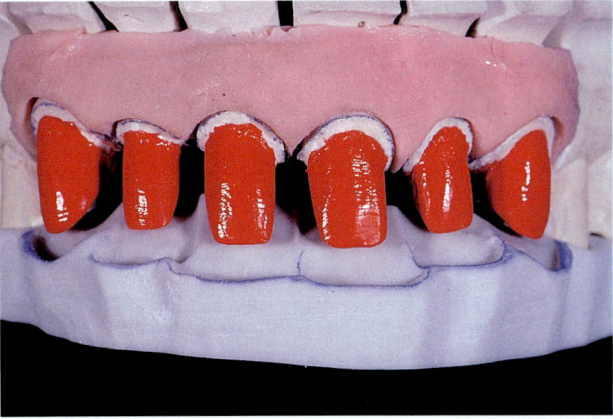

> Fig 5-12a

> Fig 5-12b

CASE 2

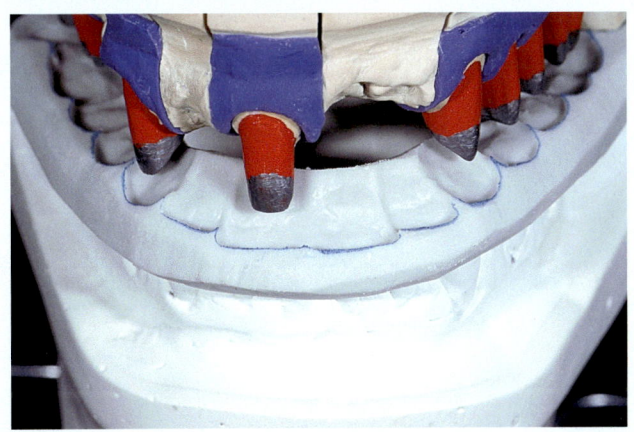

> Fig 5-13a

> Fig 5-13b

> Fig 5-13c

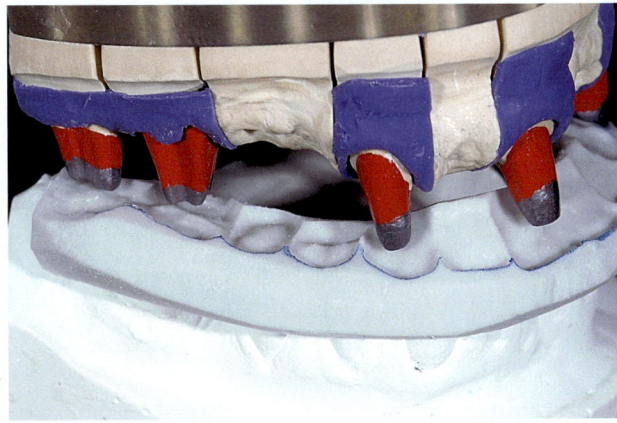

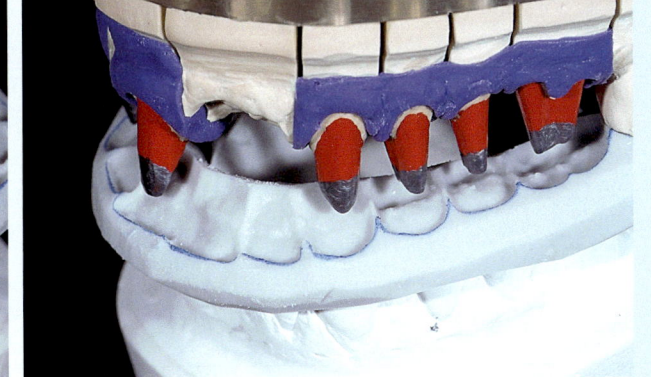

FIG 12 *(a and b)* The occlusopalatal silicone index is recorded on the cast of the provisional restoration. In partial rehabilitation cases, the posterior teeth that are not involved in the treatment are used as reference points to reproduce this identical position of the index on the cast of the final preparations as well.

FIG 13 *(a to c)* In the rehabilitation of an entire maxillary arch, the occlusopalatal silicone index, which reproduces the cast of the provisional restoration, must be anchored to the opposing arch. To prevent the silicone from being perforated by intercuspation, it is necessary to raise the articulator incisal pin by two notches. To properly construct the definitive restoration, the same increase must be maintained when the MC is mounted.

CASE 3

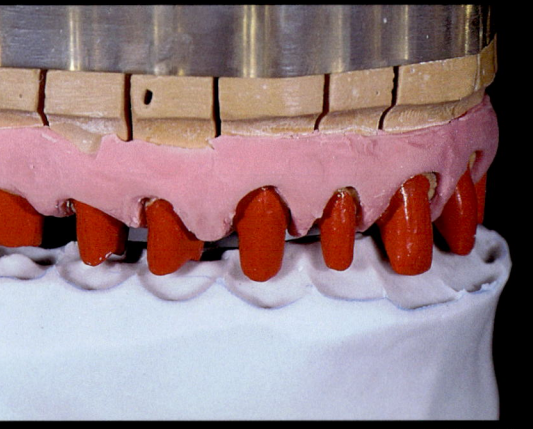

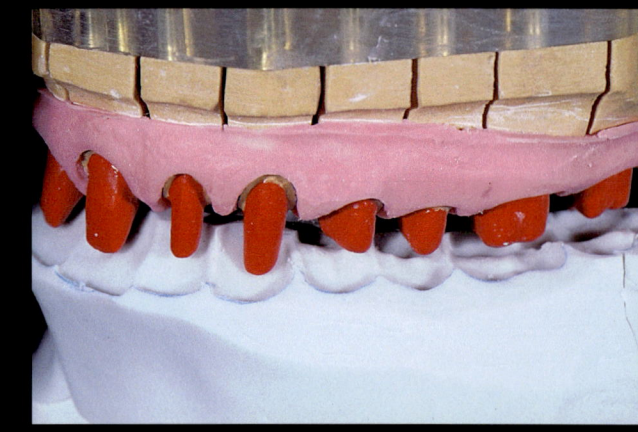

> Fig 5-14a

> Fig 5-14b

> Fig 5-14c

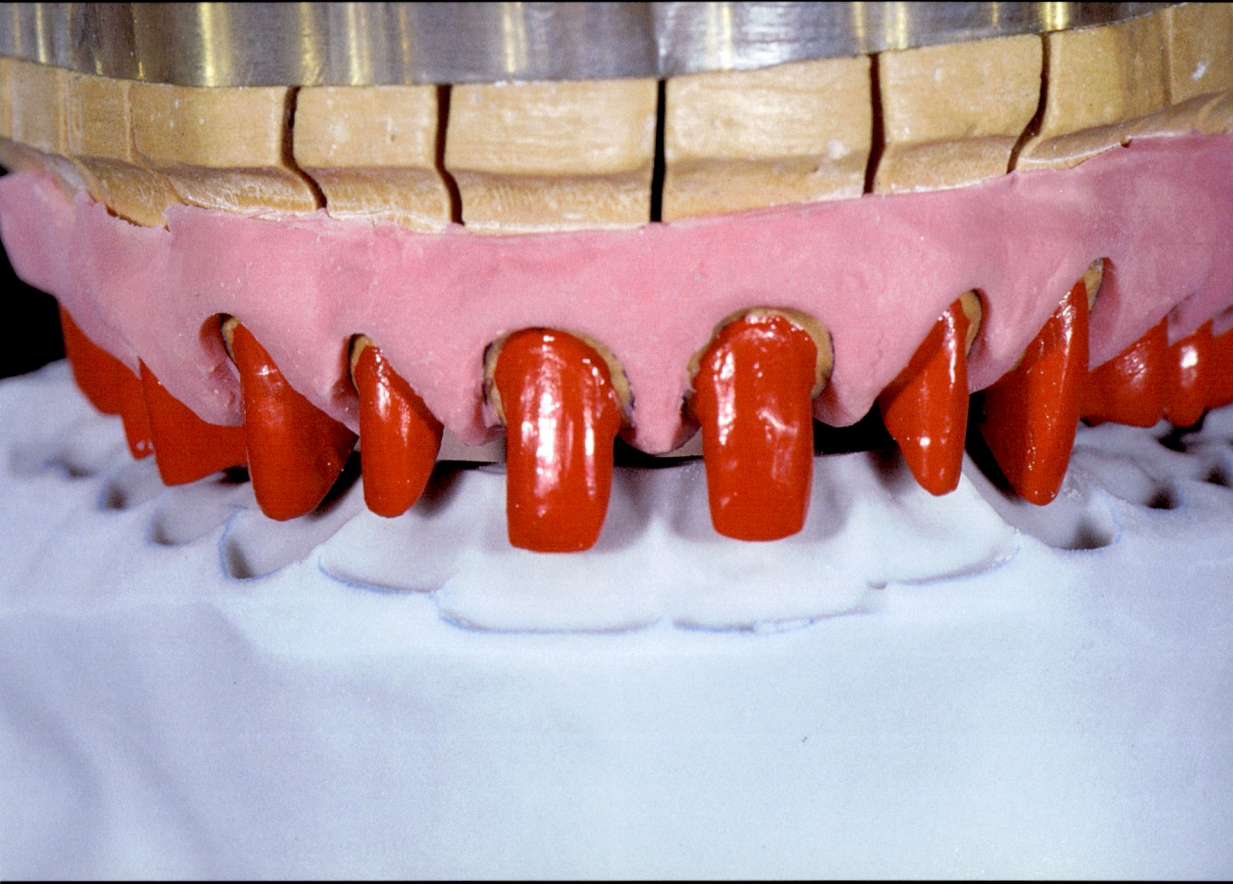

FIG 14 In the case of a complete rehabilitation, the occlusopalatal indices are made in silicone on both arches using the same method illustrated for the treatment of just one arch. *(a to c)* Once anchored to the cast of the mandibular provisional restoration, the maxillary occlusopalatal index shows the congruity of the spaces available to the technician for constructing the definitive prosthesis.

CASE 3

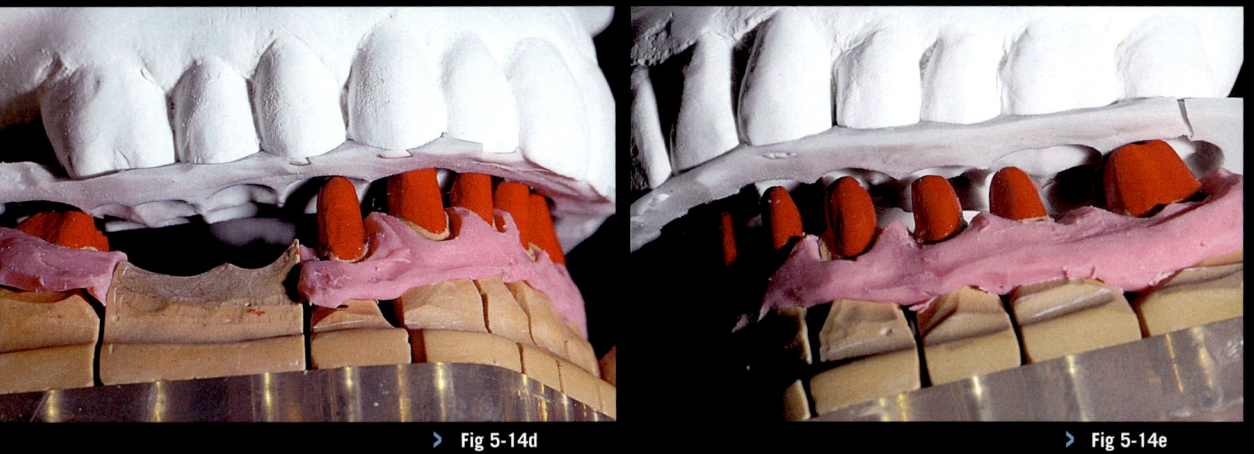

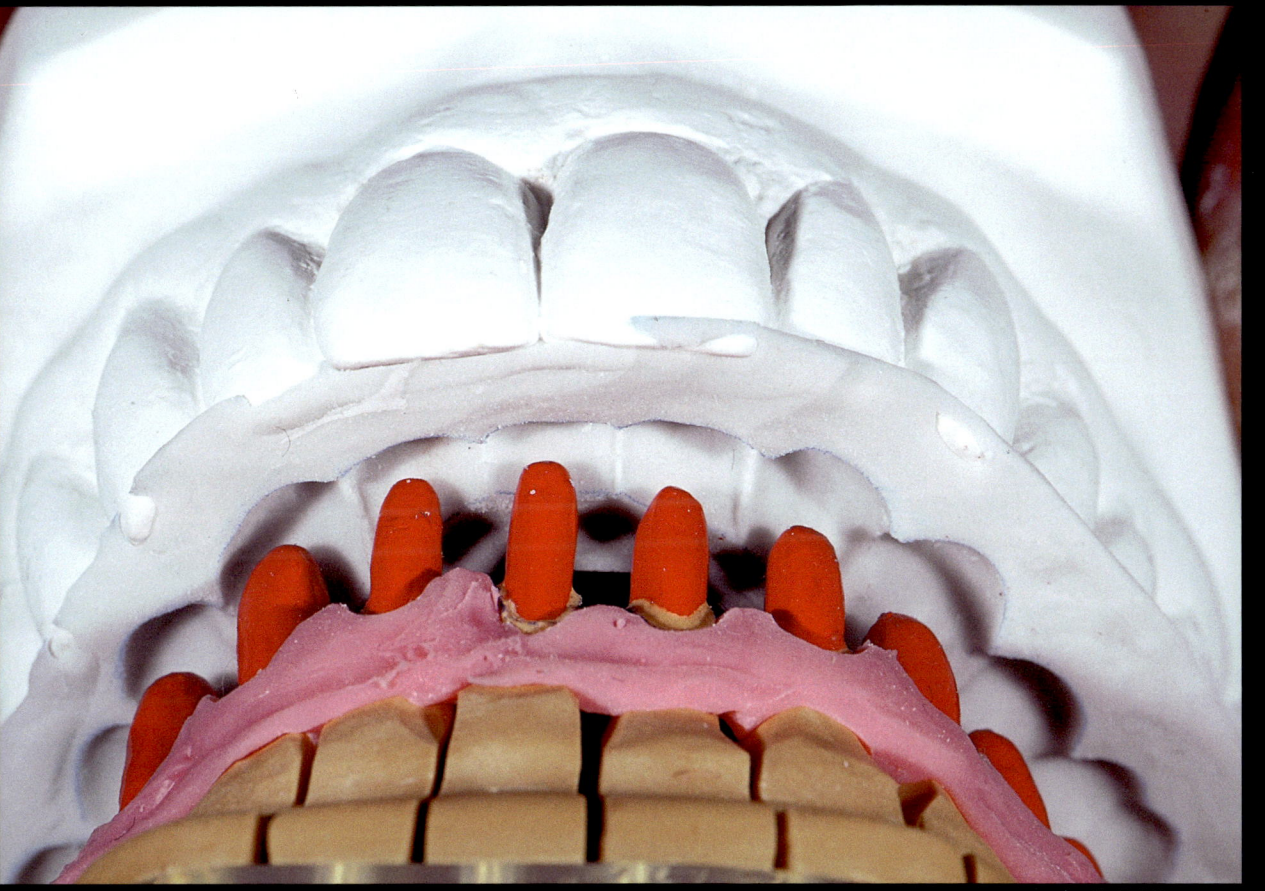

> Fig 5-14d

> Fig 5-14e

> Fig 5-14f

FIG 14 *(d to f)* After the occlusolingual index of the mandibular arch is anchored on the cast of the maxillary provisional restoration, it is possible to make a similar assessment for the mandibular arch, analyzing the final volumes of the rehabilitation as dictated by the index in relation to the final preparations of the MC.

BUCCAL INDEX

The buccal index is used to check the buccal thicknesses while constructing the substructure. To create the buccal index, the occlusopalatal index must be constructed, with the silicone spread up to the fornix of the opposing arch (Fig 5-14g). This extension is necessary to make vertical grooves and recesses in the thickness of the silicone using a football-shaped bur (Fig 5-14h). The matrix must be insulated with liquid petroleum jelly or other lubricating substance before the impression is taken in silicone to construct the buccal index (Fig 5-14i). Once polymerization is complete, the two indices are separated. With the cast of the provisional restoration removed, their stability is checked by repositioning them on the reference points made previously (Figs 5-14j and 5-14k). Through the vertical incisions, the buccal index is then separated into different segments (Figs 5-14l and 5-14m). When these are positioned alternately on the MC, the technician can use the lateral view to check that there is enough space to construct the substructure and layer the ceramic (Figs 5-14n and 5-14o). If the clinician requests an accurate reproduction of the provisional restoration, the buccal matrices can be used to copy the same anatomy of the acrylic resin index during the layering phases. Regarding the spaces identified by the buccal index: Without varying the position of the incisal edge and the tooth lengths adequately tested with the provisional restoration, it is sometimes possible to give the technician the freedom to optimize tooth shapes and proportions, thereby making small esthetic improvements in the definitive prosthesis.

BUCCAL INDEX (ONE OR TWO ARCHES)

STEPS

- Raise the articulator pin by two notches.
- Place the silicone between the two arches while still soft to create the occlusopalatal index up to the buccal fornix of the opposing arch.
- Sculpt the reference points for repositioning the buccal index.
- With the cast of the provisional restoration in situ, take the silicone impression of the provisional restoration and the reference points.
- Detach the buccal index after polymerization.
- Remove the cast from the provisional restoration and check the stability between the two matrices.
- Dissect the matrices to check the buccal thicknesses.

FIG 14 Constructing the buccal index involves extending the occlusopalatal index to the fornix of the opposing arch. *(g to i)* This makes it possible to sculpt reference keys (vertical grooves and circular holes) in the external portion of the index. These reference keys are indispensable for checking the stability of the buccal index. The impression of the buccal index is taken in silicone only after the surfaces of the occlusopalatal index have been appropriately insulated with petroleum jelly. *(j to o)* The silicone index can then be separated into distinct portions to check that the spaces between the preparations and the buccal profile of the provisional restorations are adequate for creating an accurate substructure and for layering the ceramic coating material.

CASE 3

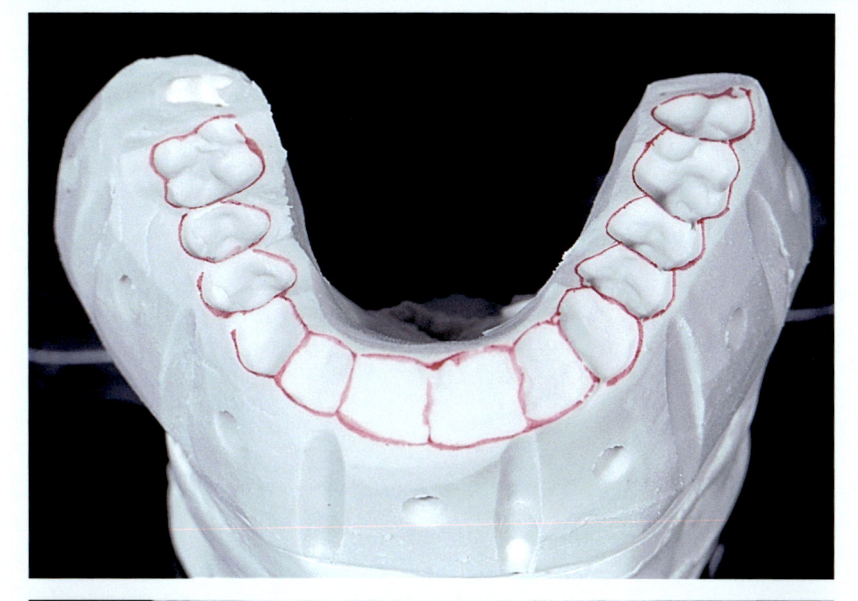

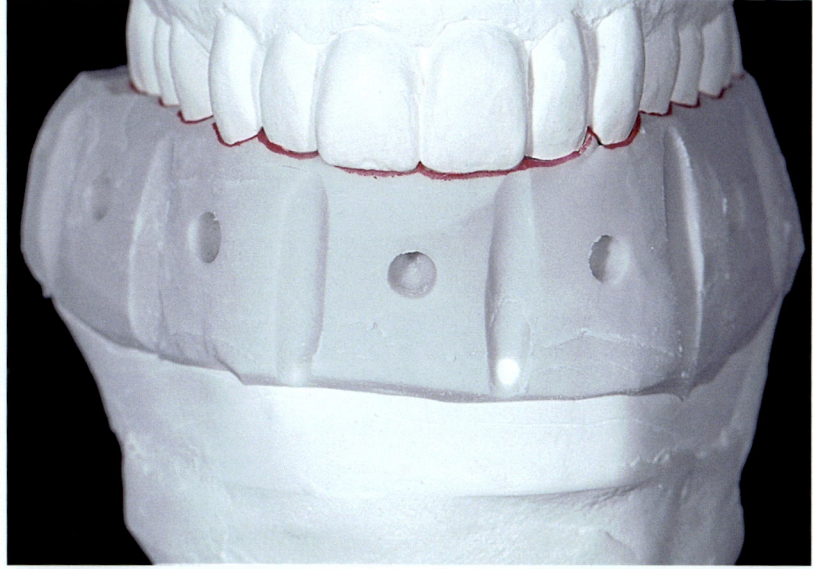

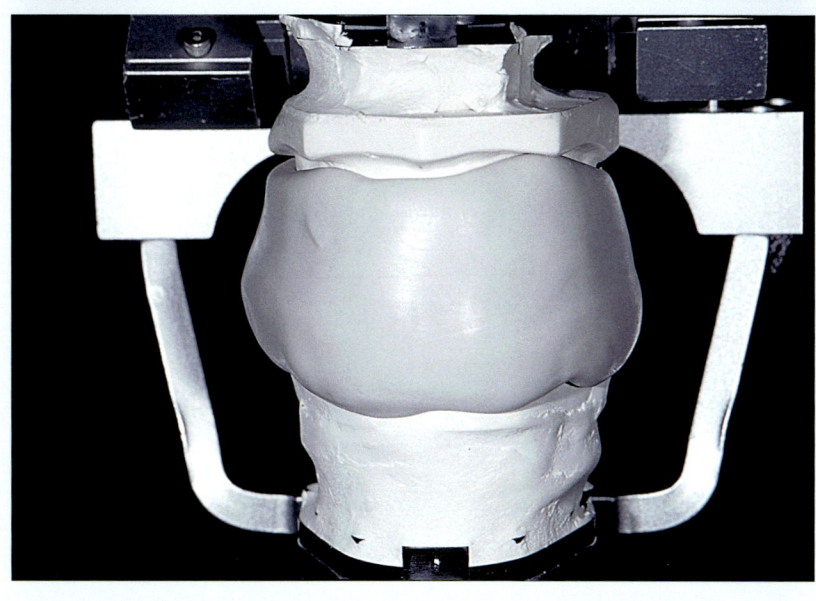

> Fig 5-14g

> Fig 5-14h

> Fig 5-14i

> Fig 5-14j

> Fig 5-14k

> Fig 5-14l

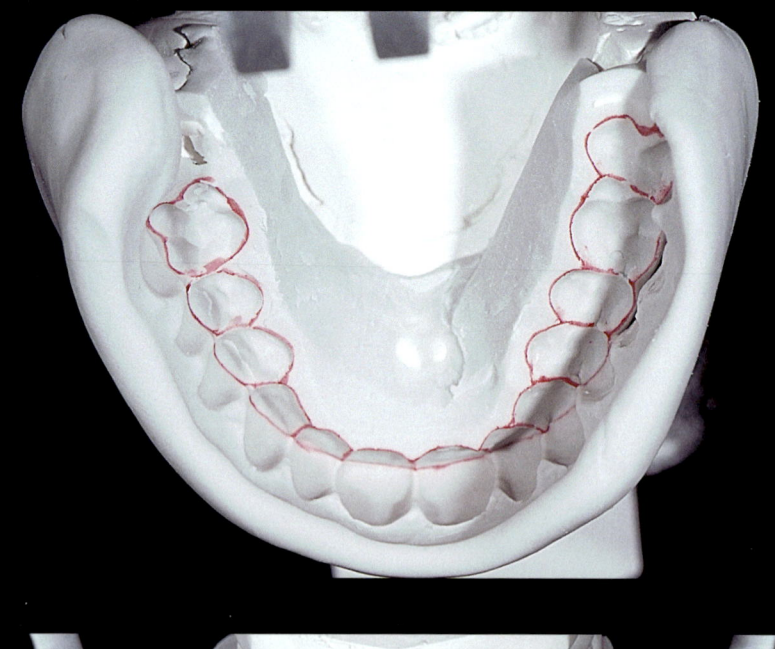

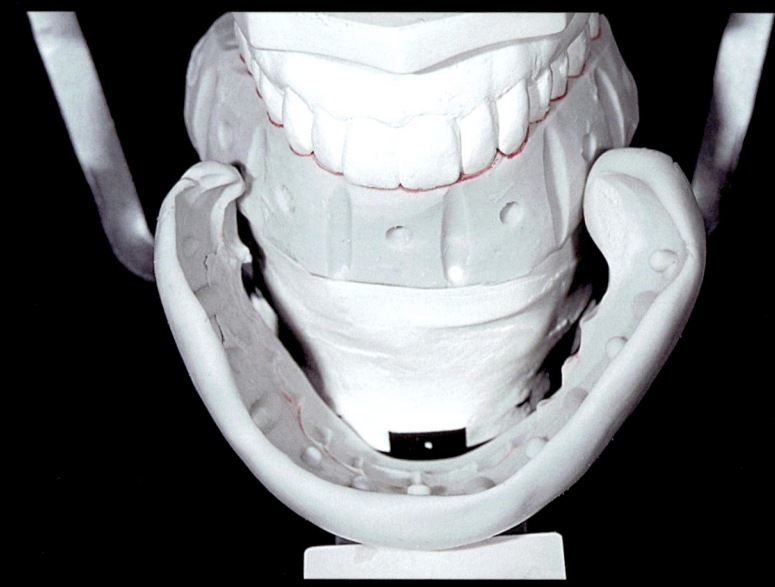

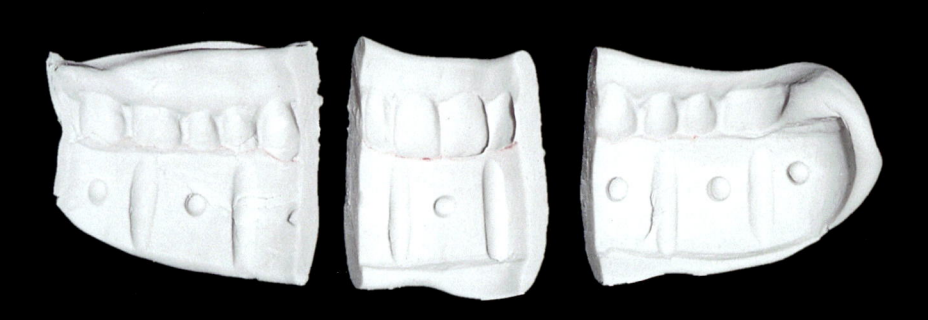

> Fig 5-

> Fig 5-

> Fig 5-

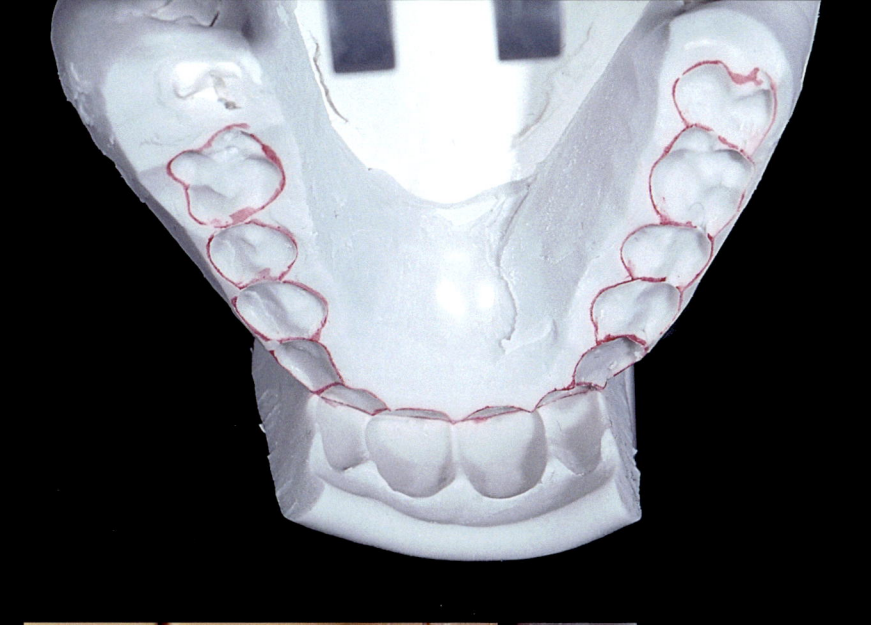

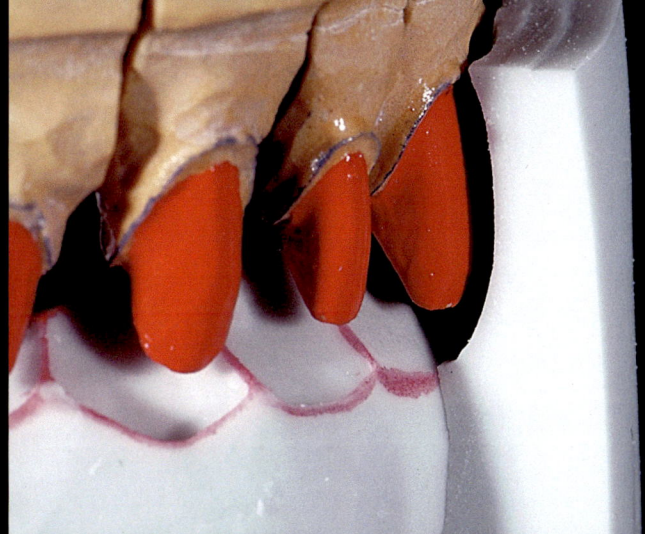

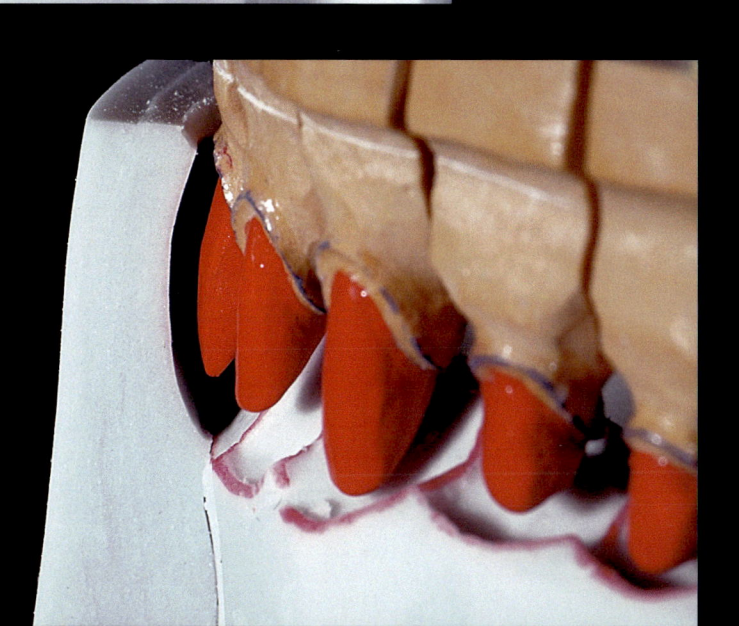

SUBSTRUCTURE

DESIGN

Wax-up guided by the silicone index

The basic role of the substructure is to adequately support the ceramic material that covers it so the prosthesis can resist the masticatory forces and, through layering with an appropriate ceramic thickness, satisfy patients' esthetic needs. This is only possible if the technician can make use of a uniform space of at least 1 mm between the outer limit of the silicone matrix and the substructure (Figs 5-15a and 5-15b).

Keeping the incisal pin in the same position in which the occlusolingual index was constructed (two notches higher), the technician is able to replace the cast of the provisional restorations with that of the preparations (MC), because of the interchangeability of the casts. The support structure is then waxed under the guidance of the occlusopalatal and buccal indices, varying, where necessary, the thickness of the wax to obtain a uniform residual space for layering the ceramic. A definitive prosthesis can then be created, which will allow the technician to express some creativity in optimizing the shapes and chromatic effects while faithfully observing the final volumes of the provisional restoration.

CHOOSING THE RESTORATIVE MATERIAL

The substructure can be fabricated using different methods and different restorative materials.

METAL-CERAMIC

Metal-ceramic is still the most commonly used restorative system. While the presence of the metallic substructure guarantees substantiated resistance for the prosthesis, hence ensuring unquestionable longevity,[48-51] it can also interfere in light transmission, which can cause greater difficulty in reaching an optimal esthetic result.[52]

Lost-wax casting technique The substructure of a metal-ceramic restoration is usually made using a lost-wax casting technique. First, the coping is made by immersion of the abutment in hot wax and ensuring that it reaches the required thickness (Figs 5-15c to 5-15e). After the shape of the coping is perfected, the marginal fit is completed under the stereomicroscope (Figs 5-15f to 5-15h) and the alloy is cast. Despite being covered with ceramic up to the margin,[53,54] the presence of metal can cause a notable opacity and give the surrounding tissues a grayish color due to the shade that the metallic substructure, impenetrable by the light, produces in the cervical area (Fig 5-16a). When single crowns or small fixed partial dentures are created, given adequate preparation (chamfer or shoulder), a ceramic shoulder can be made after the metal margin has been shortened (Fig 5-16b), thus allowing an ideal passage of light.

> Fig 5-15a

> Fig 5-15b

> Fig 5-15c

> Fig 5-15d

> Fig 5-15e

> Fig 5-15f

> Fig 5-15g

> Fig 5-15h

> Fig 5-16a

> Fig 5-16b

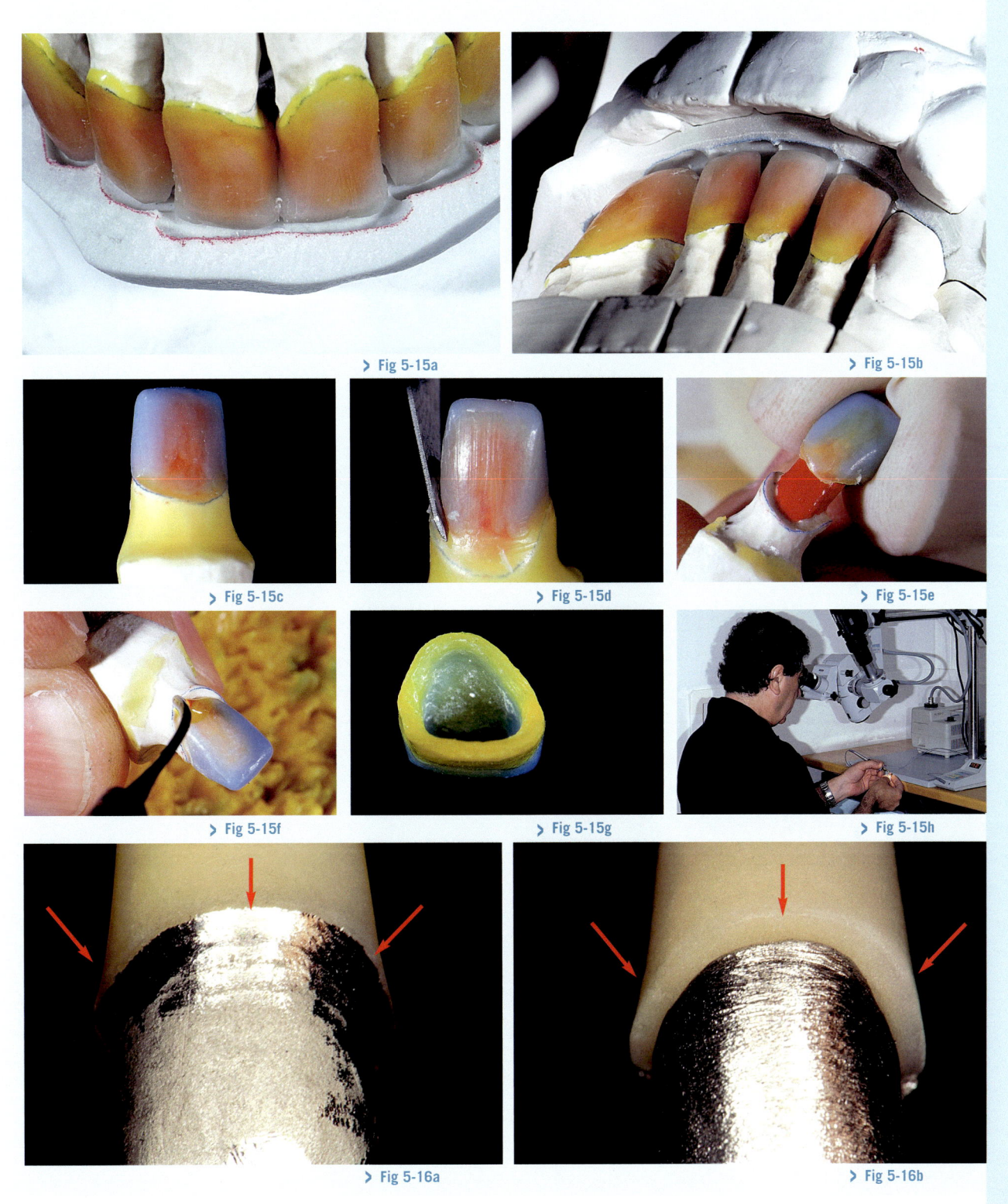

FIG 15 *(a and b)* The substructure is fabricated using the silicone index guide derived from the functionalized provisional restoration. Insulation for wax is applied to each abutment in plaster and, only after it is dry, the abutment is dipped in melted wax and covered beyond the finish margin of the preparation to prevent unwanted shrinkage. *(c and d)* Once the molding is complete, the wax coping can be cut approximately 1 mm inside the margin, inclining the blade of the scalpel toward the abutment. *(e)* The coping is slipped off and the excess wax removed from the abutment beyond the margin. *(f)* When the coping has been repositioned on the abutment, wax is added to the margin again using an electric spatula. *(g)* Once the wax is hardened, an appropriate instrument is used to remove the excess until the blue pencil mark defining the preparation limit is reached. *(h)* In these phases the use of a stereomicroscope is necessary.

FIG 16 *(a)* Extending the metal up to the finish margin creates a shadowed area in the submarginal area, giving a grayish appearance. *(b)* Reducing the metal margin by approximately 1 mm allows ideal passage of light in this area, which now appears much brighter and free of any areas in shadow.

SUBSTRUCTURE

ALL-CERAMICS

Without the metal coping, the restoration allows excellent passage of light and hence has a more natural appearance. Each type of all-ceramic substructure, however, has different optical and mechanical properties. In metal-ceramics as well as all-ceramics, a coping is needed to support uniform layering of the ceramic material and to guarantee that the definitive prosthesis has maximum resistance.

SILICATE-BASED CERAMICS

The most valuable feature of silicate-based ceramics is an extremely natural appearance owing to the translucency of the material.[55,56] The advantages of this feature are unfortunately offset by rather low resistance values.[57–59]

FELDSPATHIC CERAMICS

Traditionally used as a layering material in metal-ceramics, feldspathic ceramics are also excellent for fabricating veneers using the platinum foil or the refractory technique. The system does not involve the use of a substructure; instead, because it adheres perfectly to enamel, the etched abutment tooth serves as a natural substructure. Therefore, although feldspathic ceramics have low flexural resistance in vitro (approximately 100 MPa), they offer a high level of clinical reliability.[60–64]

GLASS-CERAMICS

Because they are reinforced with specific crystals put into the glass matrix, such as leucite (IPS Empress, Ivoclar Vivadent) or lithium disilicate (IPS Empress 2 and E-Max, Ivoclar Vivadent), glass-ceramic materials can be used both to create full-thickness restorations and to fabricate copings covered with layering ceramic or created by pressure. The good resistance values of copings fabricated with these materials (120 MPa for Empress,[57–59] 350 to 400 MPa for Empress 2 and E-Max)[65] guarantees excellent reliability when used for single-tooth restorations, especially in the anterior sector.[66–71]

Heat pressing The lost-wax casting technique is typically used to construct the substructure (Figs 5-17a to 5-17d). The ceramic ingot is then pressed under vacuum (Figs 5-17e and 5-17f) at a specific temperature to ensure adequate marginal adaptation. The wax-up can be developed by designing the restoration in its final shape and contour (Figs 5-17g and 5-17h) as well as creating a coping that acts as a substructure for a specific layering ceramic. Today these restorations can be fabricated using a computer-aided design/computer-assisted manufacture (CAD/CAM) technique. The information is transferred to a milling machine that uses a specific ceramic ingot to form a substructure over which the ceramic is then layered to achieve the definitive restoration (E-Max CAD, Ivoclar Vivadent).

> Fig 5-17a

> Fig 5-17b

> Fig 5-17c

> Fig 5-17d

> Fig 5-17e

> Fig 5-17f

> Fig 5-17g

> Fig 5-17h

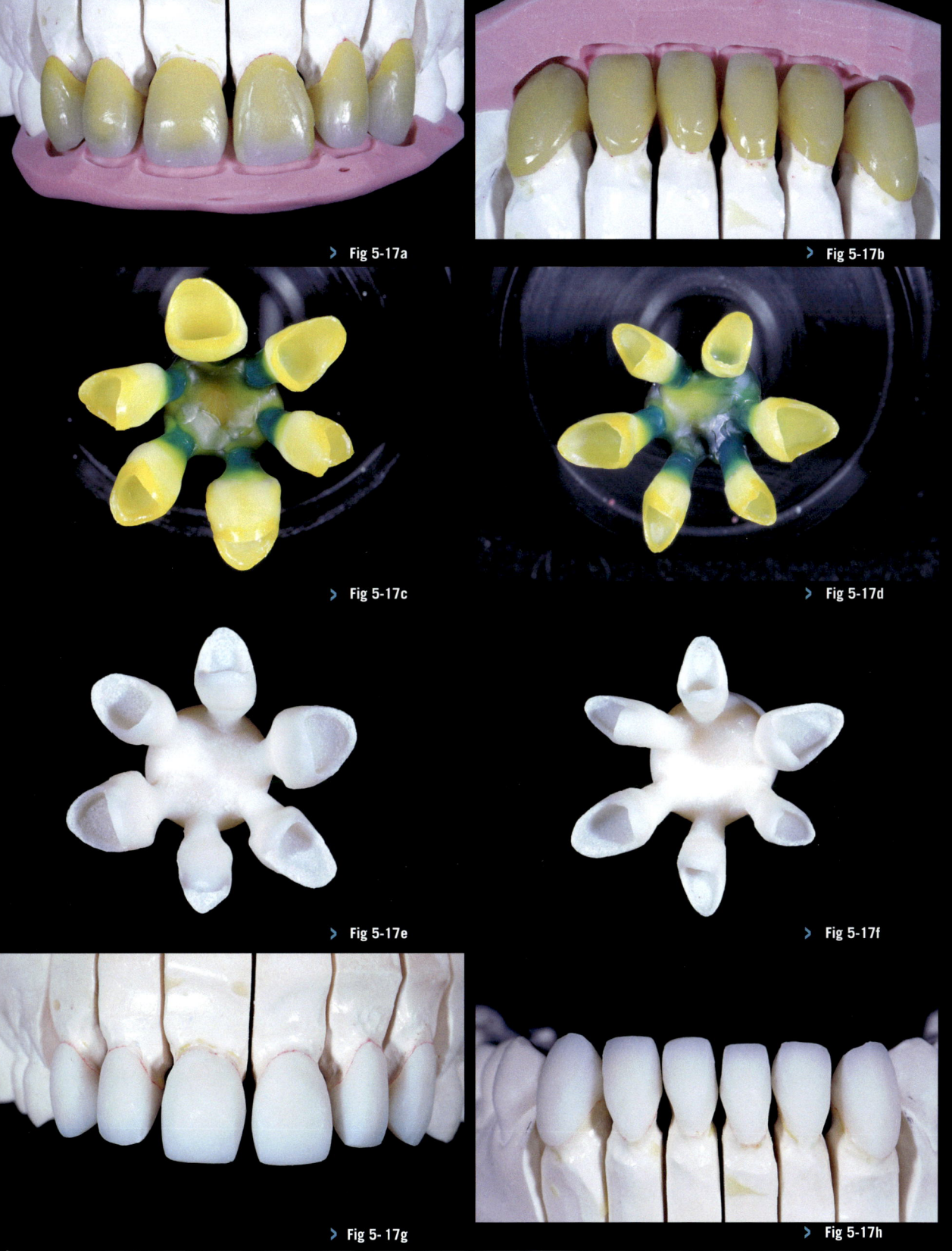

FIG 17 *(a and b)* The wax substructure is constructed with the aid of the silicone index guide taken from the functionalized provisional restorations. *(c to f)* On completion of the lost-wax casting technique, the substructure of the units in the selected ceramic material is obtained. *(g and h)* Once separated from the pressing sprues, the substructures are checked on the MC before moving on to layering.

SUBSTRUCTURE

HIGH-STRENGTH CERAMICS

The high-strength ceramics group comprises systems based on aluminum oxide (Al_2O_3) and zirconium oxide (ZrO_2). These are widely used in the construction of substructures that, though more opaque, are sufficiently tough to withstand substantial occlusal forces such as those developed in the posterior sectors.

ALUMINA

Because of the considerable flexural strength in vitro of its substructure in vitro[72,73] (500 to 650 MPa), pure densely sintered alumina (Procera, Nobel Biocare) can be used for fabricating posterior as well as anterior restorations.[74-76] An inherent balance between opacity and translucency has improved the esthetic results that can be obtained with other alumina systems (VITA In-Ceram Alumina, VITA Zahnfabrik). It can also be recommended for use in cases of discolored teeth, since in many situations it conceals the discoloration without appearing opaque.

CAD/CAM The use of CAD/CAM to create a substructure is rising. The procedure starts with a computerized scan of the stone abutment developed in the laboratory, which is then digitally reprocessed to create a three-dimensional model.[77,78] In the planning phase, the technician uses a digital wax-up technique to define the finish line on the monitor (Fig 5-18a) and then creates a virtual coping (Fig 5-18b). Based on the volume of the silicone index, the coping is designed with a shape that evenly supports the layering ceramic, especially in the incisal and occlusal areas. If the decision is made to create a ceramic shoulder, the finish line must be designed in a position 1 to 2 mm more internal than the preparation margin (Figs 5-18c and 5-18d). The file containing all of the data for the coping is then sent electronically to an external production center, where widened abutments are created to compensate for the shrinkage that takes place during the final sintering. The alumina is pressed onto the coping at a temperature similar to that used before sintering ("green stage"). After it is pressed, the external surface of the alumina is milled to obtain a substructure of the required thickness (0.2 mm, 0.4 mm, 0.6 mm) according to the type and location of the restoration. The coping is removed from the widened abutment and then placed in the sintering furnace to reach its final dimension (Fig 5-19).

FIG 18 *(a)* The preparation margin is identified on the screen image of the computerized scan of the abutment. *(b)* The substructure to be applied must be designed in such a way as to allow uniform ceramic layering. *(c)* In cases where, for esthetic reasons, a ceramic shoulder is required at cervical level, it is necessary to design the finish margin of the coping on the border between the axial and marginal walls, in a more internal position than the preparation limit (dotted line). *(d)* The substructure, expressly shortened, would therefore be able to accommodate the ceramic shoulder.

> Fig 5-18a

> Fig 5-18b

> Fig 5-18c

> Fig 5-18d

> Fig 5-19a

> Fig 5-19b

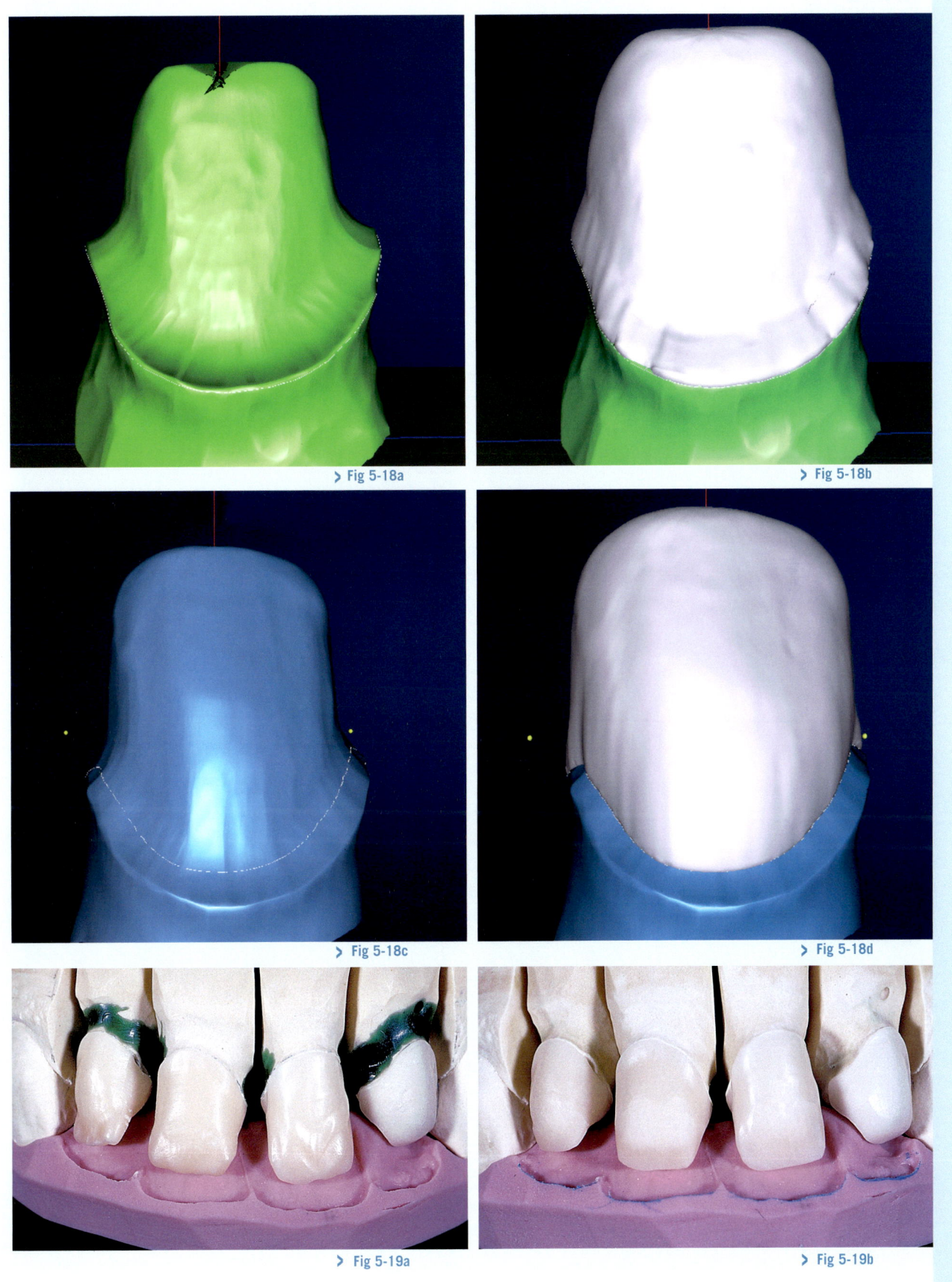

FIG 19 The copings positioned on the MC have been created by means of a double scanning process; the objective is to record both the marginal fit and the final volume of the substructure suggested by the silicone index. *(a)* Green wax is placed beyond the preparation margins with the purpose of removing the undercuts and making it easier for the scanner sensor to read. *(b)* Before layering, the copings are refined.

SUBSTRUCTURE

ZIRCONIUM

Zirconium oxide–based systems, because of their remarkable toughness and high flexural strength in vitro (1,100 MPa), prove suitable for fabricating single crowns to posterior fixed partial dentures[79] and even for bridges extending over an entire arch.

CAD/CAM As already described for alumina, the software for working with zirconium involves reading the prosthetic abutment and computerized design of the substructure (Fig 5-20). Once they are made, the copings (Fig 5-21) are given to the ceramist, who begins the layering procedure.

The substructure can be made using two different methods: The first involves milling a block of densely sintered material (DCS Precident, DC Zirkon, Dentsply Austenal; Smartfit 3D, Kotem Technologies). While this material will not undergo shrinkage, it does have other disadvantages, such as a particularly long milling time, and possible formation of microfractures in the substructure.[79] The second method uses blocks of zirconium oxide that are partially sintered ("green stage"). The structure must be milled with a programmed level of widening (> 25% to 30%, depending on the system), which calculates the amount that the zirconium will shrink during sintering, to obtain an ideal adaptation on the working cast. The following systems are used for this technique: Procera (Nobel Biocare), Lava (3M ESPE), Everest (KaVo Dental), Cercon (Dentsply Ceramco), and Cerec InLab (Sirona). Compared with the first method, this technique involves a much shorter milling time.[80]

Pressing onto the substructure The technique of pressing silicate-based ceramics onto substructures made of alumina and zirconium, as is now commonly done, allows one to finalize the work by pressing the complete volume of the restoration, which is then covered with a surface-coloring technique, or by pressing the dentin (to which the enamel will be applied), allowing the restoration to receive the necessary characterizations and translucency (layering technique) (Fig 5-22). To optimize the esthetic result, the cervical margin of the substructure can be shortened in the anterior sector to allow room for the pressed material. When the silicate-based ceramic, pressed over the coping, is etched, an adhesive cementation technique can be used. Because of the translucency of the material, this technique creates ideal esthetics on the cervical third of the restoration.

FIG 20 *(a to f)* After the margins have been read, the coping is then optimized with the use of a digital spatula that allows the necessary modifications to be made to support the uniform layering of the ceramic.

FIG 21 *(a and b)* Creating substructures in zirconium.

FIG 22 *(a and b)* Both the ceramic layering and the surface coloring material, first waxed and then pressed, can be laid over the substructure in zirconium or in alumina.

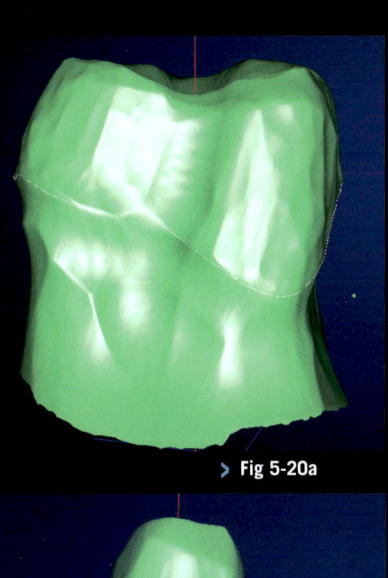

> Fig 5-20a 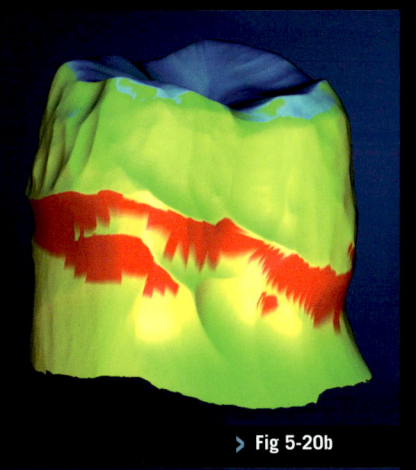 > Fig 5-20b 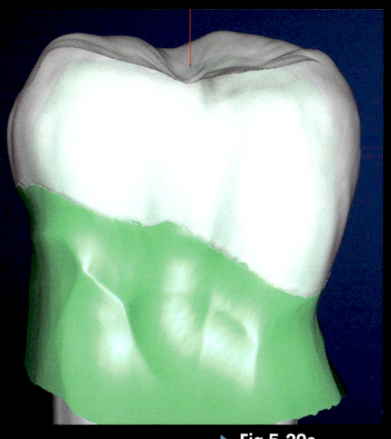 > Fig 5-20c

> Fig 5-20d 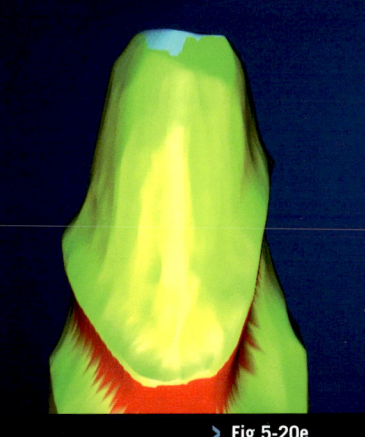 > Fig 5-20e 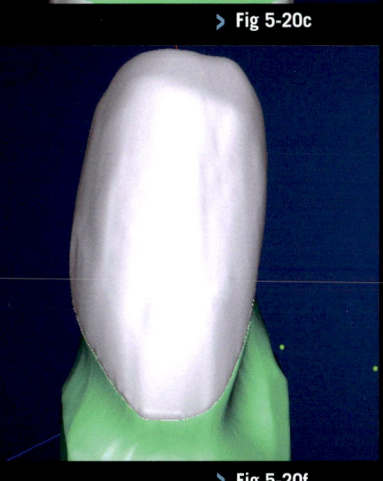 > Fig 5-20f

> Fig 5-21a 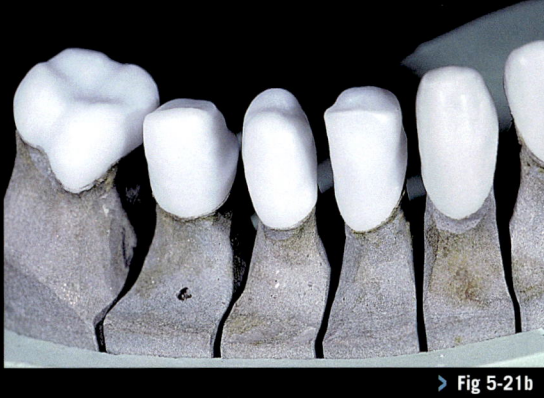 > Fig 5-21b

> Fig 5-22a > Fig 5-22b

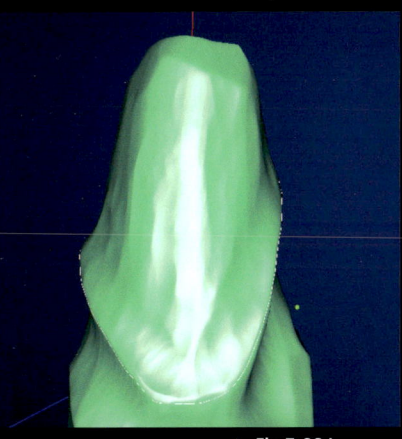

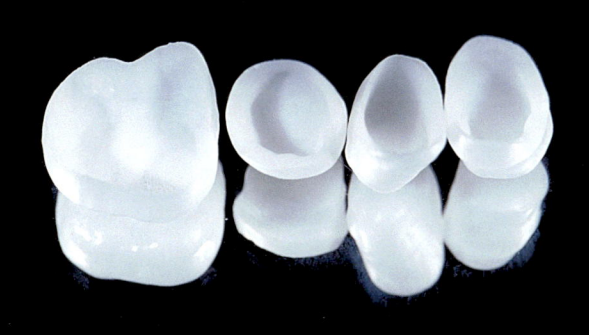

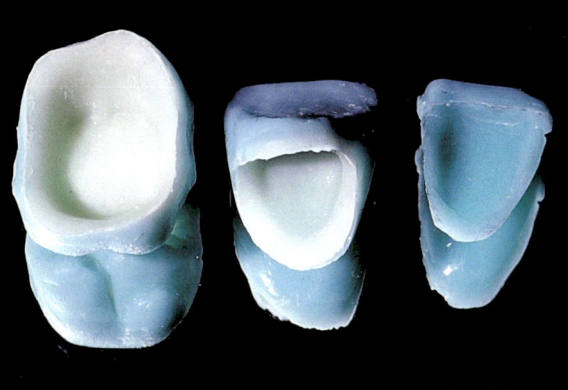

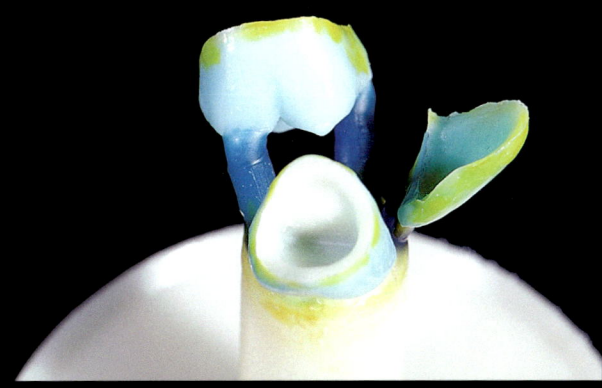

SUBSTRUCTURE FIXED PARTIAL DENTURES

Planning the connecting areas is one of the most delicate phases in the construction of the substructure. These areas must be of a sufficient size to resist fracturing of the framework but must be designed in such a way as to maintain, at the cervical level, interdental spaces that allow appropriate hygiene.

METAL-CERAMIC

Metal-ceramic is undoubtedly the most thoroughly tested system for constructing fixed partial dentures, making the procedure extremely reliable and free of surprises.[31,81,82] To guarantee resistance of the metal pontic elements, a connector that is 6- to 9-mm^2 thick between the elements is considered sufficient (Fig 5-23). It should be remembered that if the interproximal space is insufficient to allow effective cleaning, the connection area can be designed in a more coronal direction because of the ductility of the alloy used, with the consequent exposure of a metallic area in occlusion. It is also important to point out that in the event of rocking, the metal pontic element can be cut and soldered without the need to take new final impressions and construct a new substructure, unlike all-ceramic materials.

ALL-CERAMICS

The increased toughness of all-ceramic materials means they can now be used in the fabrication of substructures for fixed partial dentures, depending to some extent on the type of system chosen. Regardless of the material used, certain common rules must be observed:

- The substructure must be cooled with adequate water irrigation during the finishing phase
- Sharp corners and undercuts must be avoided

Glass-ceramics The glass-ceramics with a lithium disilicate base (e.max, Ivoclar Vivadent) can be used to construct three-element anterior fixed partial dentures that do not extend beyond the first premolar (Fig 5-24). Though these materials guarantee an extremely natural appearance, patients should be carefully selected so as to avoid the risk of fractures caused by excessive masticatory forces.[71] Also, the size of the connection area needed to ensure sufficient resistance (12 to 16 mm^2) may be excessively large, preventing ideal separation between the elements and hence restricting proper hygienic maintenance of the interproximal areas as well as the esthetics of the restorations.

FIG 23 *(a to d)* After ensuring, in the wax-up of the substructure, an adequate height for the connecting areas and an even thickness for the covering ceramic, the technician then proceeds with casting the pontic elements both on natural teeth and on implants in the chosen metal alloy.

FIG 24 *(a to d)* Once the wax-up has been made under the guidance of the silicone index, the next step is sprueing the elements of the fixed partial denture to construct the substructure in glass-ceramic, maintaining adequate space for layering the enamel.

> Fig 5-23a

> Fig 5-23b

> Fig 5-23c

> Fig 5-23d

> Fig 5-24a

> Fig 5-24b

> Fig 5-24c

> Fig 5-24d

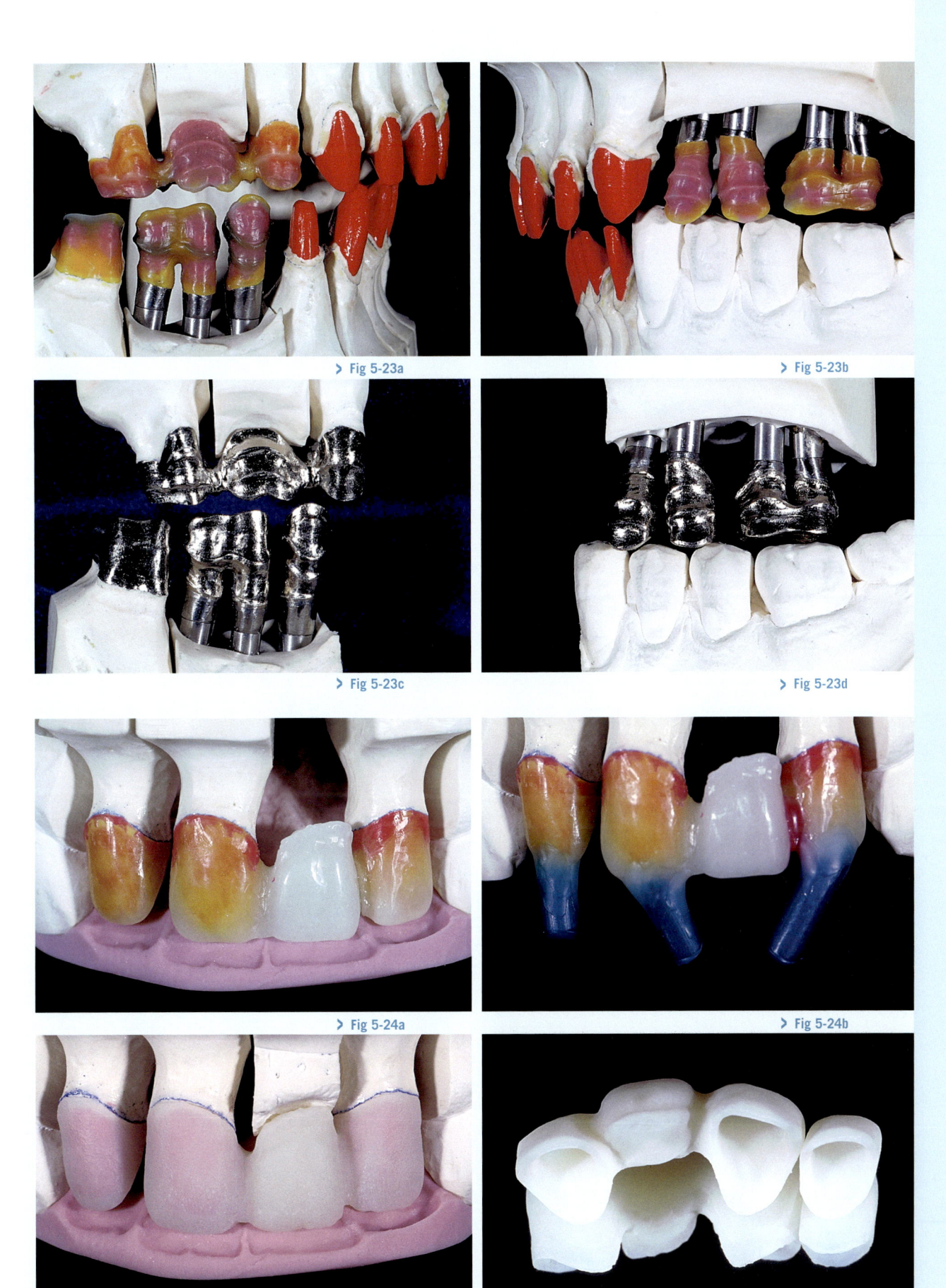

475

SUBSTRUCTURE FIXED PARTIAL DENTURES

Alumina ceramics Densely sintered alumina ceramic (Procera AllCeram, Nobel Biocare) is only applicable in the anterior area for constructing three- or four-unit fixed partial dentures with a single pontic element. Its high resistance values permit a limited extension of the interdental connection (6 to 9 mm^2) that, being particularly confined, allows excellent hygienic maintenance and ideal separation between the elements (Fig 5-25). Optimum esthetic results plus high resistance mean that this ceramic system can be considered ideal for treating the anterior sectors. The data on survival of alumina restorations in the mouth, already very encouraging for glass-infiltrated alumina[83] (VITA In-Ceram Alumina, VITA Zahnfabrik), would indicate that excellent results can also be achieved with the Procera for fixed partial dentures, even if its recent appearance on the market has not allowed for adequate clinical follow-up.

Zirconium-based ceramics These systems have gained enormous popularity in the past few years because of their reputation for high resistance and hence suitability for all areas of the oral cavity, even in the construction of fixed partial dentures extended to an entire arch. They are thus a valid alternative to metal-ceramics in anterior and posterior sectors alike (Fig 5-26). They boast particularly limited connectors (6 to 9 mm^2) that allow good separation between the pontic elements and therefore promote a natural appearance for the restorations. Especially in anterior sectors, however, a certain opacity of the substructure can affect the final esthetic result, reducing the naturalness of these restorations compared with alumina ceramics and glass-ceramics. In fact, the light transmission properties of zirconium-based substructures are significantly less than those of alumina,[77,84] limiting their use in the anterior sectors for discolored teeth or abutments with extended metal restorations (posts or amalgams).

FIG 25 *(a to e)* After the two abutments are scanned, the three pontic elements are designed and then joined with connectors that, because of their limited extension made possible by the use of alumina (9 mm^2), allow for an optimal esthetic result in the anterior sectors.

FIG 26 *(a to c)* To construct fixed partial dentures in zirconium for the posterior sectors, the procedure involves scanning the abutments, designing the connecting areas, and fabricating a substructure ready for application of ceramic layering.

> Fig 5-25a

> Fig 5-25b

> Fig 5-25c

> Fig 5-25d

> Fig 5-25e

> Fig 5-26a

> Fig 5-26b

> Fig 5-26c

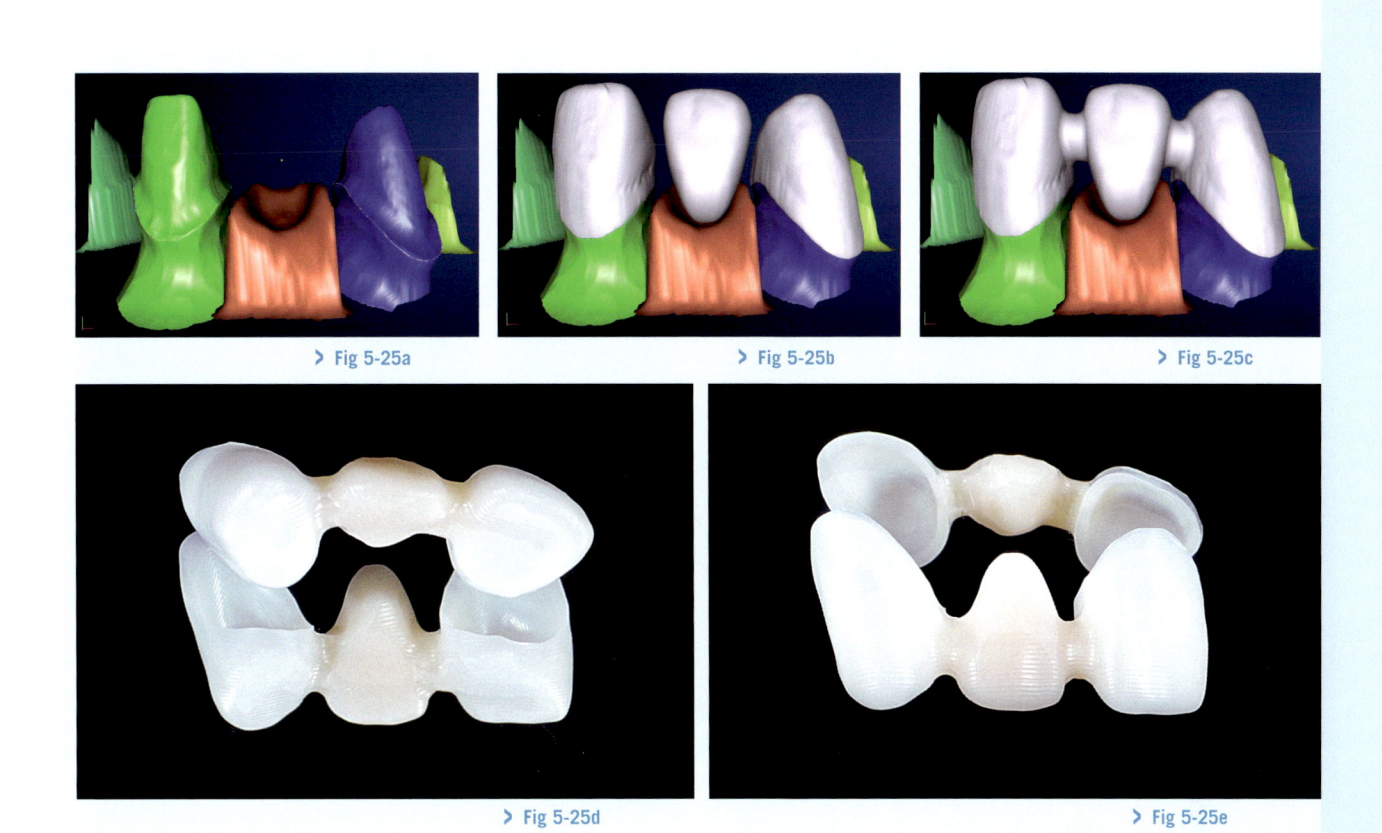

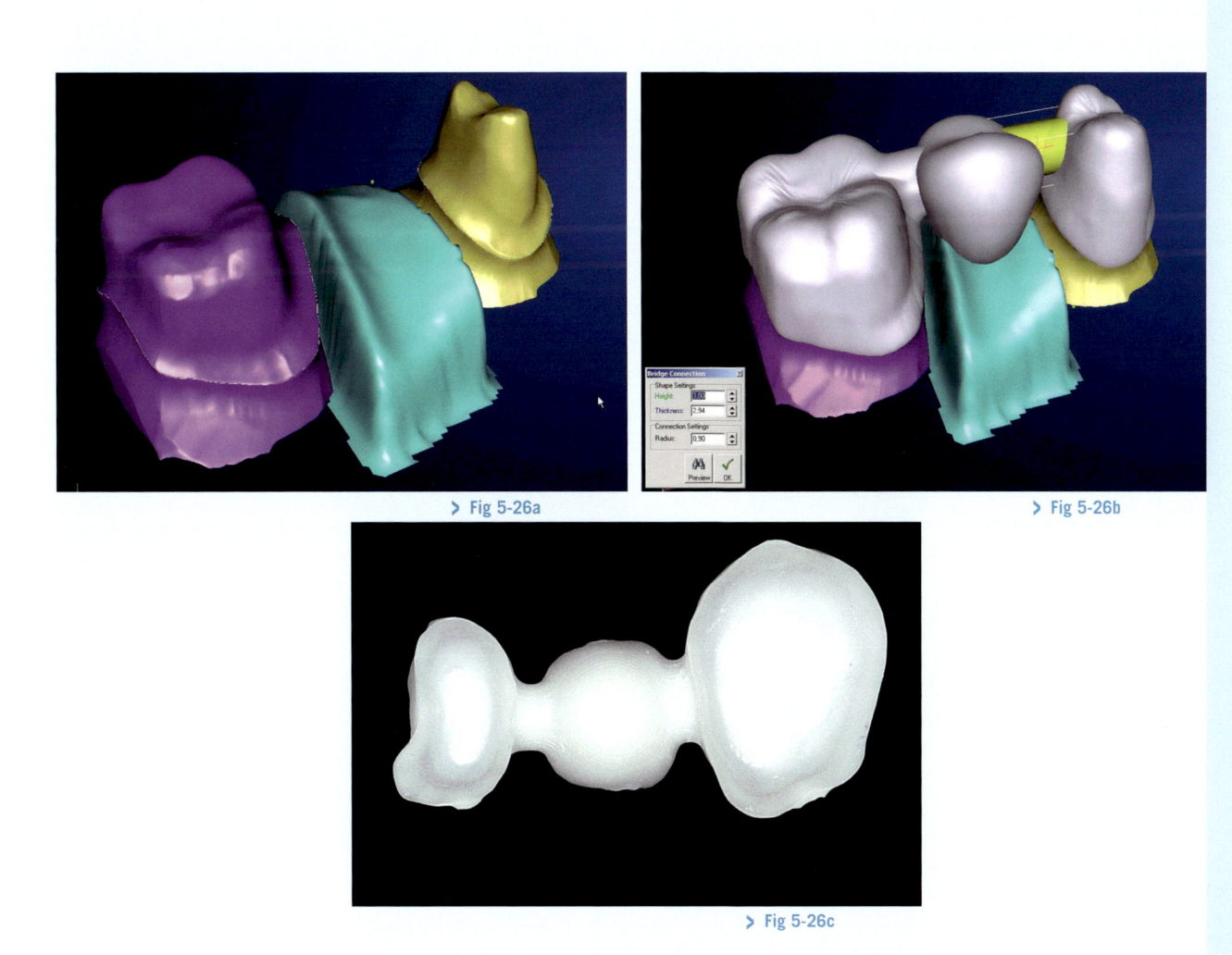

477

■ SUBSTRUCTURE ■
METAL-CERAMIC, ALL-CERAMICS

CLINICAL CONSIDERATIONS

Tooth preparation The versatility and reliability of metal-ceramics allow the preparation methods to be varied, alternating between metal margins on vertical tooth preparations and margins covered with ceramic material on horizontal preparations (shoulder, chamfer), even within the same tooth. This differentiated reduction of the abutment allows greater preservation of the tooth structure compared with all-ceramics, which normally require a circumferential shoulder or chamfer preparation and are therefore less conservative. Although there are not yet enough data to support it, one exception may be the zirconium substructure that could also be configured with visible white collars instead of being covered with layering ceramic, because of its high resistance (Fig 5-27).

Rocking motion One factor to be considered in assessing the inherent advantages and disadvantages of each system when rocking motion is present in a fixed partial denture is the possibility of separating it with a disk and then soldering it again. This solution is offered exclusively by metal-ceramics; the same is not possible with all-ceramics. Any rocking motion in the substructure in all-ceramic materials requires a new impression to be taken, followed by the work being completed again.

Fracture modality Unlike metal-ceramics, in which a cohesive or adhesive fracture is limited to the thickness of the ceramic, thereby safeguarding the metal substructure, the fractures in all-ceramics often occur through the whole thickness, requiring construction of a new restoration (Figs 5-28a and 5-28b).

It should be noted, however, that in the case of alumina and even more so for zirconium, the fracturing trends are similar to those of the metal-ceramics: They do not usually affect the substructure, but are almost always confined to the covering material[85] (Figs 5-28c and 5-28d).

FIG 27 *(a)* In the marginal area, it is sometimes preferable to create the preparations with limited thicknesses (slight chamfer, knife edge), so that the tooth structure can be preserved as much as possible. *(b to d)* In these cases it can be useful to design the substructure with a zirconium collar extended to the point where the thickness of the tooth preparation is sufficient to contain both the coping and the layering material, without an overcontour being created.

FIG 28 *(a and b)* Silicate-based ceramics fracture in ways that usually affect the coping as well as the covering material. *(c and d)* Where a more resistant substructure (alumina and zirconium) is present, the fracture is normally limited to the layering material instead.

> Fig 5-27a

> Fig 5-27b

> Fig 5-27c

> Fig 5-27d

> Fig 5-28a

> Fig 5-28b

> Fig 5-28c

> Fig 5-28d

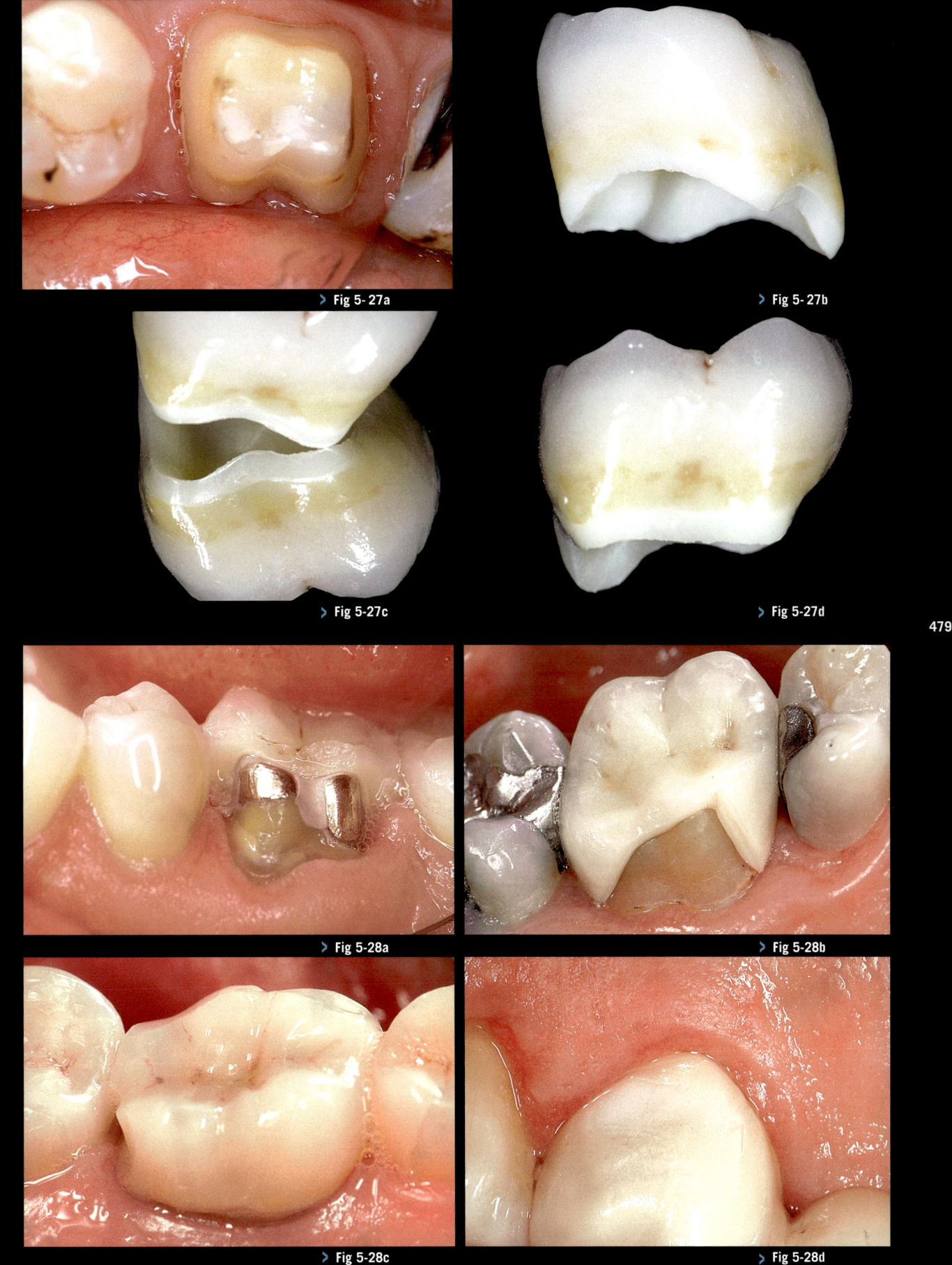

CONSTRUCTING THE SUBSTRUCTURE

CASE 1, CASE 2, CASE 3

Three clinical cases are illustrated step by step to demonstrate the diagnostic evaluations that led to the choice of restorative materials and, hence, the appropriate substructures. In the appropriate section of the laboratory checklist, the clinician must clearly communicate the chosen materials and systems to the technician. In these cases, as indeed in all similar treatments carried out by the authors, the substructures are designed using the silicone index, which accurately reproduces the volumes of the provisional restoration tested on the patient over a sufficient period.

CASE 1

In this rehabilitation of the maxillary anterior sextant, the decision was made to position six all-ceramic crowns (Fig 5-29). The normal chromatic appearance of the abutments directed the authors' choice toward the use of glass-ceramics (Empress, Ivoclar Vivadent). Although glass-ceramics do not possess particularly high resistance values in vitro, they allow excellent esthetics and a natural appearance. Before the prosthetic treatment was initiated, the patient attended a few preliminary occlusal adjustment sessions to ensure adequate occlusal stability in CR and minimize the risk of occlusal overload in the anterior area.

CASE 2

Rehabilitation of the entire maxillary arch in this periodontal case required splinting of the residual teeth with an extended fixed partial denture in metal-ceramics (Fig 5-30). Using this system makes it possible to vary the tooth preparation procedure according to the esthetic needs of specific sites with horizontal-type preparations, or according to the need to preserve the tooth structure with vertical preparations. Another advantage of this system is the option to solder in the event of the substructure rocking, something that can sometimes occur as a result of the possible residual mobility of the abutments, especially in periodontal cases.

CASE 3

For construction of single restorations in the anterior sectors, all-ceramics are recommended to optimize the esthetic appearance (Fig 5-31). Considering the need to create not only crowns but also fixed partial dentures in the maxillary arch, the choice was made to use metal-ceramics in the posterior sectors of the mandibular arch. When this treatment commenced, high-resistance all-ceramics, which would now be a valid alternative, were not yet available.

CASE 1

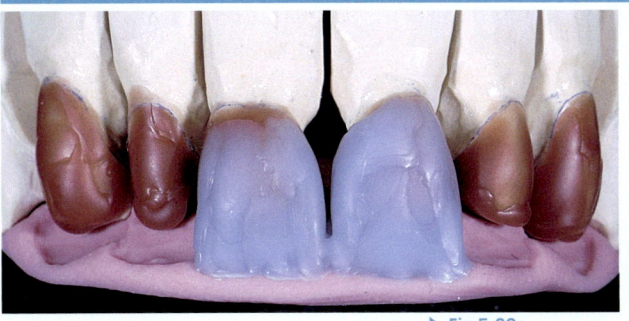

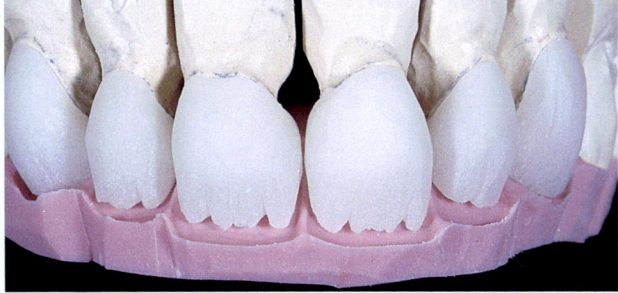

> Fig 5-29a

> Fig 5-29b

CASE 2

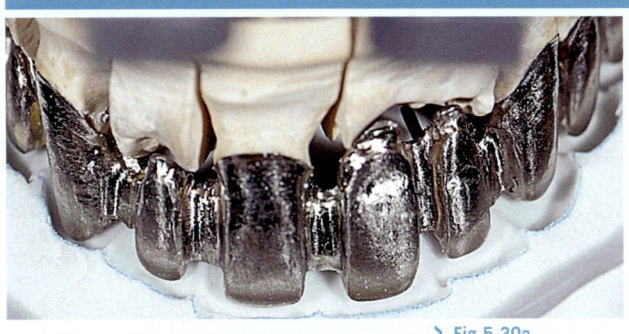

> Fig 5-30a

> Fig 5-30b

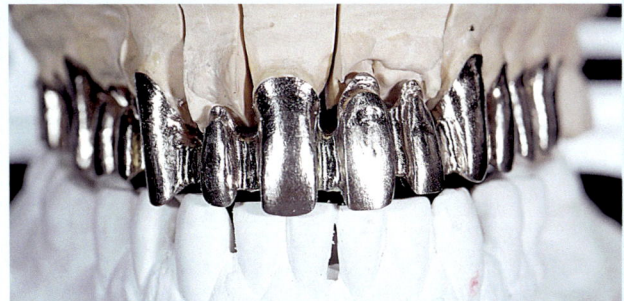

CASE 3

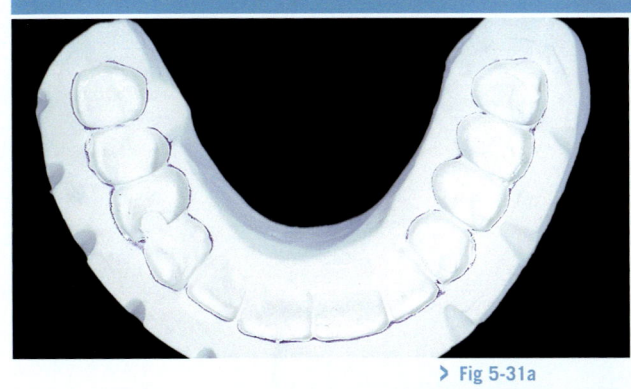

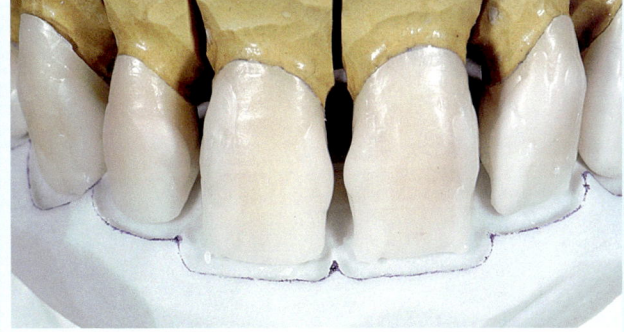

> Fig 5-31a

> Fig 5-31b

> Fig 5-31c

> Fig 5-31d

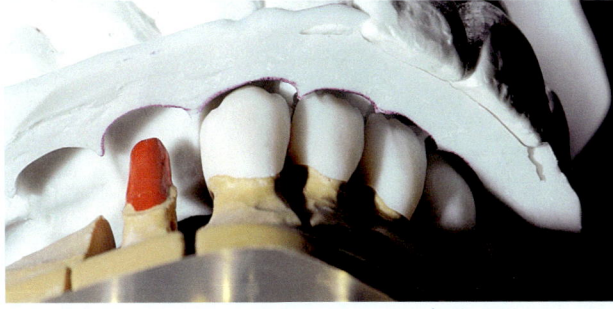

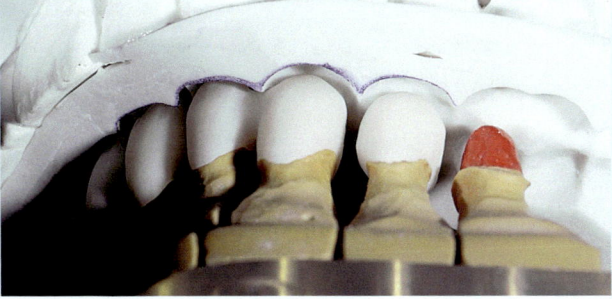

FIG 29 *(a and b)* Substructure made initially in wax, then converted to glass-ceramic under the guidance of the silicone index taken from the functionalized provisional restoration.

FIG 30 *(a and b)* The metal substructure is constructed, leaving an even space for the ceramic layering.

FIG 31 *(a and b)* The occlusopalatal index of the maxillary arch must guide the technician in completing the wax-up of the copings. *(c and d)* After the silicone index is anchored to the opposing arch, the substructures of the mandibular arch are constructed.

CLINIC

SUBSTRUCTURE TRY-IN

MARGINAL ADAPTATION: FIXED PARTIAL DENTURES

After confirming the absence of any rocking motion and an adequate marginal closure on the working cast, the clinician must also check the same parameters in the oral cavity.

Metal-ceramics If, with the aid of a magnification system, a slight rocking of the metal substructure is noted, attempts must be made using a silicone paste to localize the friction areas that are preventing a perfect fit (Figs 5-32a and 5-32b). These areas are normally identified especially at the border between the axial and occlusal walls. In these cases, to prevent excessive thinning or even perforation of the metal structure, the adjustments are mainly carried out on the prosthetic abutment using a fine-grade football-shaped bur and are confined to the friction areas highlighted on the metal. If the rocking motion cannot be eliminated, the fixed partial denture must be separated with a thin diamond disk. Once all of the elements of the substructure have been correctly inserted, verification must be made on the internal as well as the marginal adaptation, using silicone paste for each abutment (Figs 5-32c and 5-32d). This is not always easy to accomplish clinically, especially in the interproximal area.[86] The use of the Fit Checker (GC Dental) can make it possible, after any touch-ups, to achieve a significant improvement in the fit.[87–89] When the elements have been rejoined with a minimal amount of acrylic resin, a registration key for the presoldering must be made and sent to the technician. The soldered structure is then returned to the clinician for another try-in before proceeding with the ceramic layering steps.

All-ceramics To prevent propagation of a fracture, the restorations in all-ceramics, unlike those in metal-ceramic, must not show any friction on the prosthetic abutment (Fig 5-33), either on the cast or in the mouth. To better identify any areas of intimate contact, it is advisable to use a dark-colored silicone paste. If any rocking motion is present, it is not possible to cut the fixed partial denture and solder it back together again, as is the case with a metal substructure.

MARGINAL ADAPTATION: SINGLE RESTORATION

Taking an accurate impression in most cases allows the technician to fabricate a sufficiently accurate substructure that, for single restorations, will usually prevent the need to test its adaptation in the mouth. The reliability achieved by the materials and techniques now makes it possible to prevent possible discrepancies discovered between the working cast and the clinical situation that would compromise the definitive adaptation of a single restoration, which is therefore usually checked directly at the biscuit try-in.

CASE 2

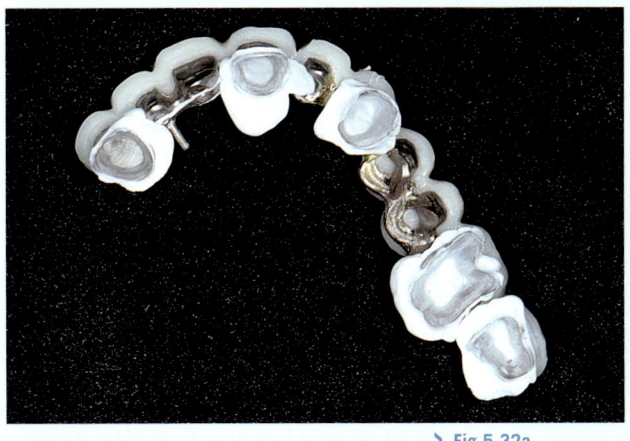

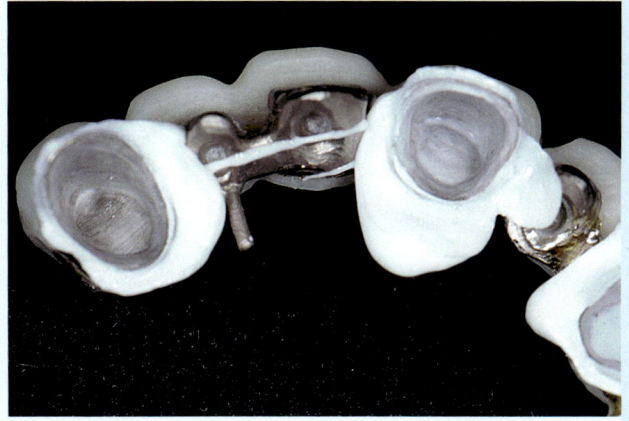

> Fig 5-32a

> Fig 5-32b

> Fig 5-32c

> Fig 5-32d

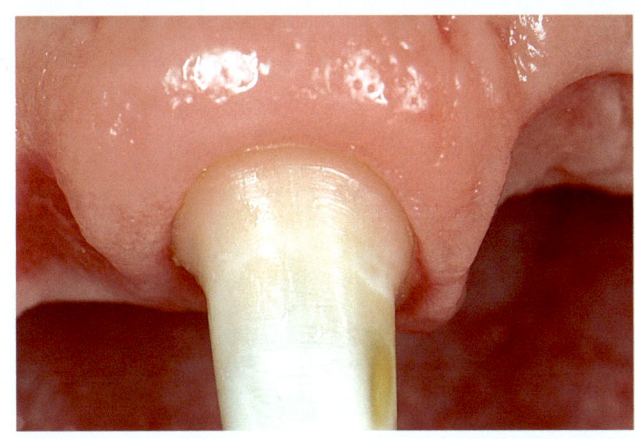

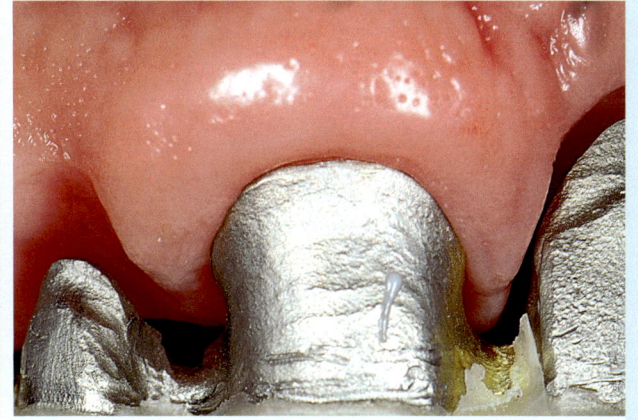

CASE 3

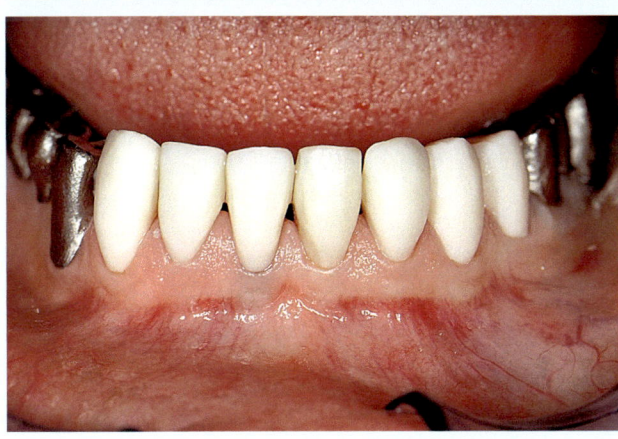

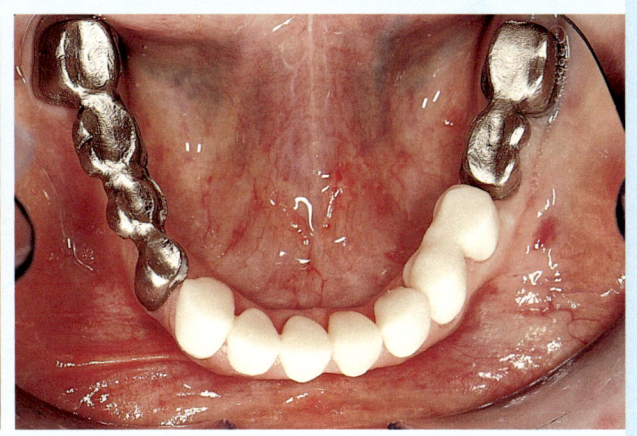

> Fig 5-33a

> Fig 5-33b

FIG 32 *(a and b)* The use of a silicone paste helps reveal any areas of resistance that may obstruct complete insertion of the substructure. *(c and d)* The clinical intraoral photographs demonstrate the good marginal adaptation achieved.

FIG 33 *(a and b)* Testing of the substructures of the mandibular arch reveals the choice of restorative material made for the anterior sector, treated with all-ceramics, versus the posterior sectors, where metal-ceramic was used instead.

CLINICAL CHECK OF THE MOUNTING

■ SUBSTRUCTURE ■
PREVENTIVE SIMULATION (PS)

After fabricating the substructure using the silicone indices but before commencing the ceramic layering procedures, the technician can provide the clinician with a preventive simulation (PS) of the definitive restoration for checking the accuracy of the cast mounting. To make the simulation, self-polymerizing resin is poured into a new silicone matrix (Fig 5-34a) and then applied up to the incisal/occlusal third of the substructure, taking care not to reach the cervical area (Fig 5-34b). This cut-back of the cervical area allows the clinician to properly check the marginal closures, especially in the interproximal areas.

The PS can be used in both metal-ceramics and all-ceramics. Its primary function is to provide the clinician and technician with confirmation of the accurate mounting of the casts with each other (cross-mounting). It also allows them to check the adequacy of the occlusal relationship between the arches, the position of the incisal edge, and the length of the anterior teeth. Preventive simulation reveals any discrepancies in the provisional restoration that would indicate inaccuracies in the positioning of the casts. The ability to identify errors in the cross-mounting at this phase will prevent the team from proceeding until the biscuit try-in stage before they realize the problem and then have to make substantial refinements to the already layered ceramic framework. It therefore seems evident that PS of the substructure is of inestimable value in terms of time as well as quality of the work.

The discovery of only slight occlusal discrepancies on the patient, which are attributable to shrinkage of the resin used for the PS and the variables inevitably connected with the prosthetic steps, acts as clinical confirmation that the substructure has been constructed in the same position as the provisional restoration (Figs 5-34c to 5-34j). At this point the substructure must be sent back to the laboratory, where, once the acrylic resin has been removed, the technician can start the ceramic layering process with the certainty that, at the biscuit try-in, the clinician has only to make a few refinements until the definitive restoration is perfectly integrated from both esthetic and functional viewpoints.

In the event that, due to incorrect mounting of the casts, substantial discrepancies should inauspiciously be found in the occlusal contacts, it is the clinician's task to take new occlusal registrations in CR and then proceed with remounting of the casts on the articulator. In these cases the PS will obviously have to be repeated before work on the definitive restoration can proceed.

CASE 2

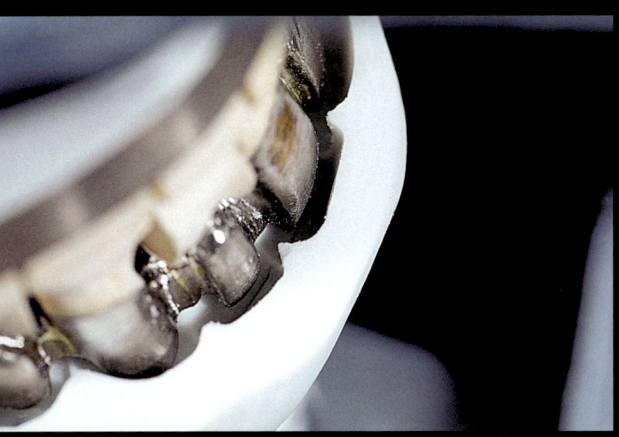

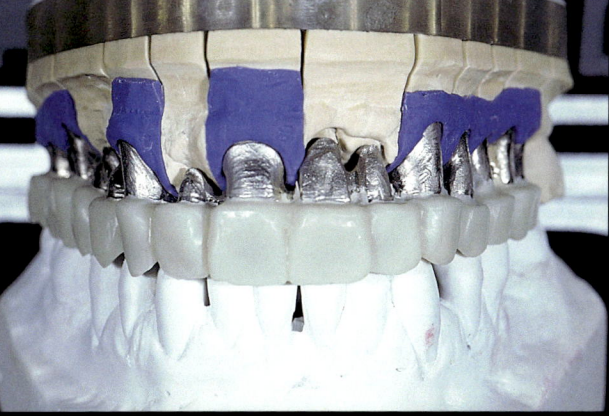

> Fig 5-34a

> Fig 5-34b

> Fig 5-34c

> Fig 5-34d

> Fig 5-34e

> Fig 5-34f

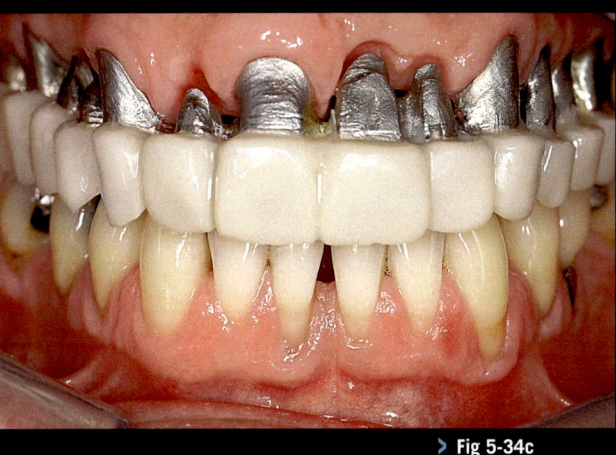

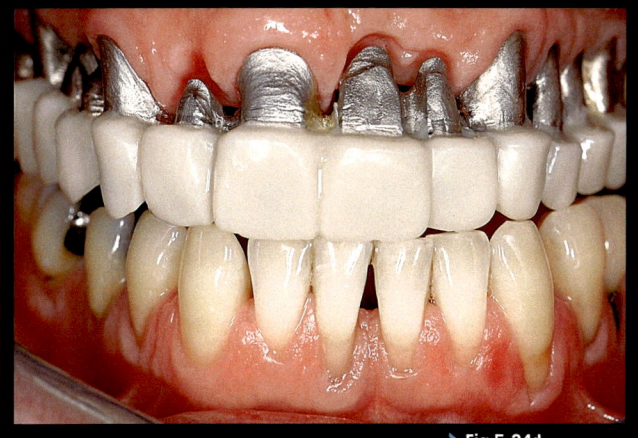

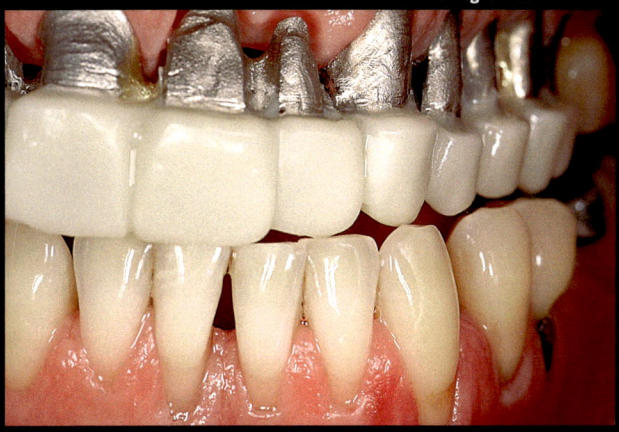

FIG 34 *(a and b)* To check that the casts are correctly mounted on the articulator, the technician, using a new silicone matrix, pours self-polymerizing resin into the space between the index and the substructure. *(c to f)* In this way, the clinician can verify that the occlusal relationships, in both the static (CR) and dynamic (excursive movements) phases, substantially overlap those in the provisional restorations, demonstrating that the casts are positioned correctly. *(g to j)* This can be further confirmed by the correspondence of the values of the VDO and the tooth length, recorded on the provisional restorations and on the PS.

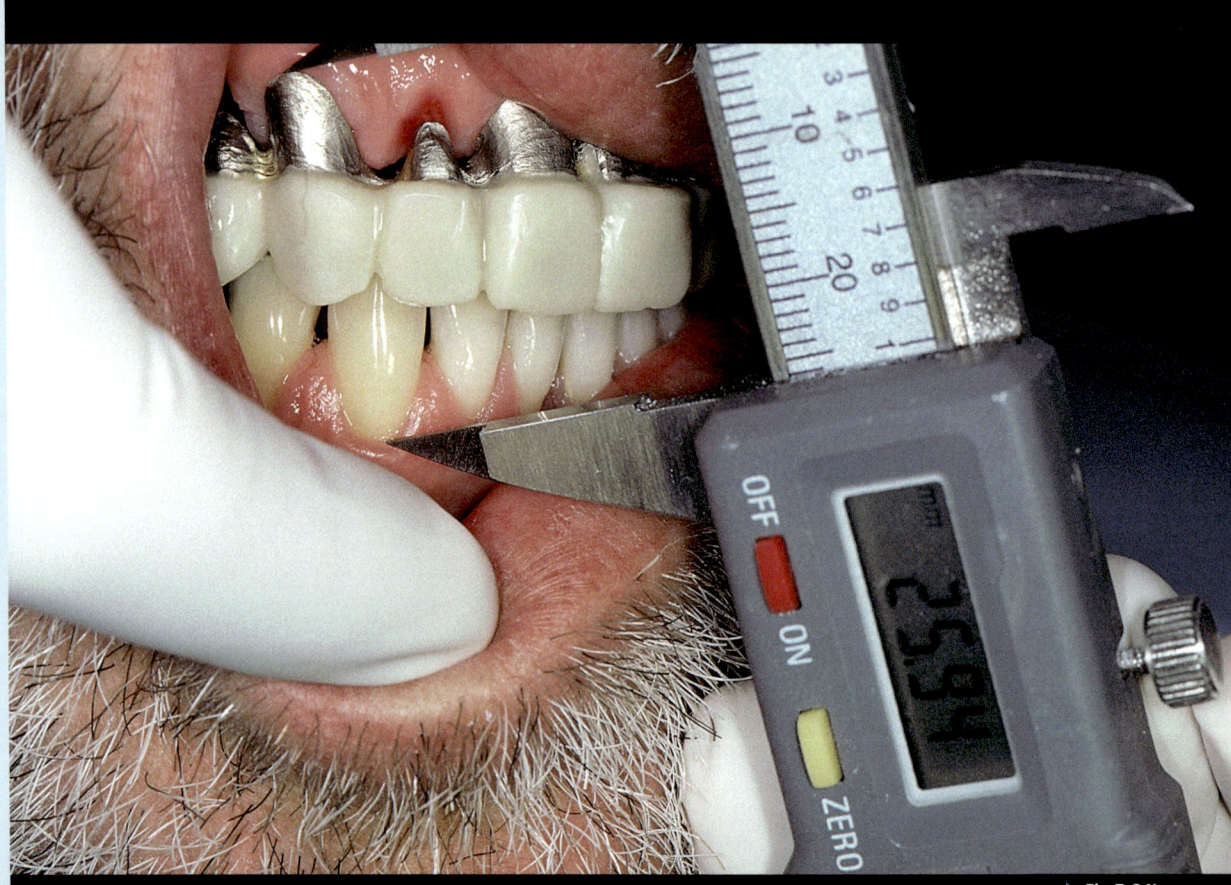

> Fig 5-34g

> Fig 5-34h

> Fig 5-34i

> Fig 5-34j

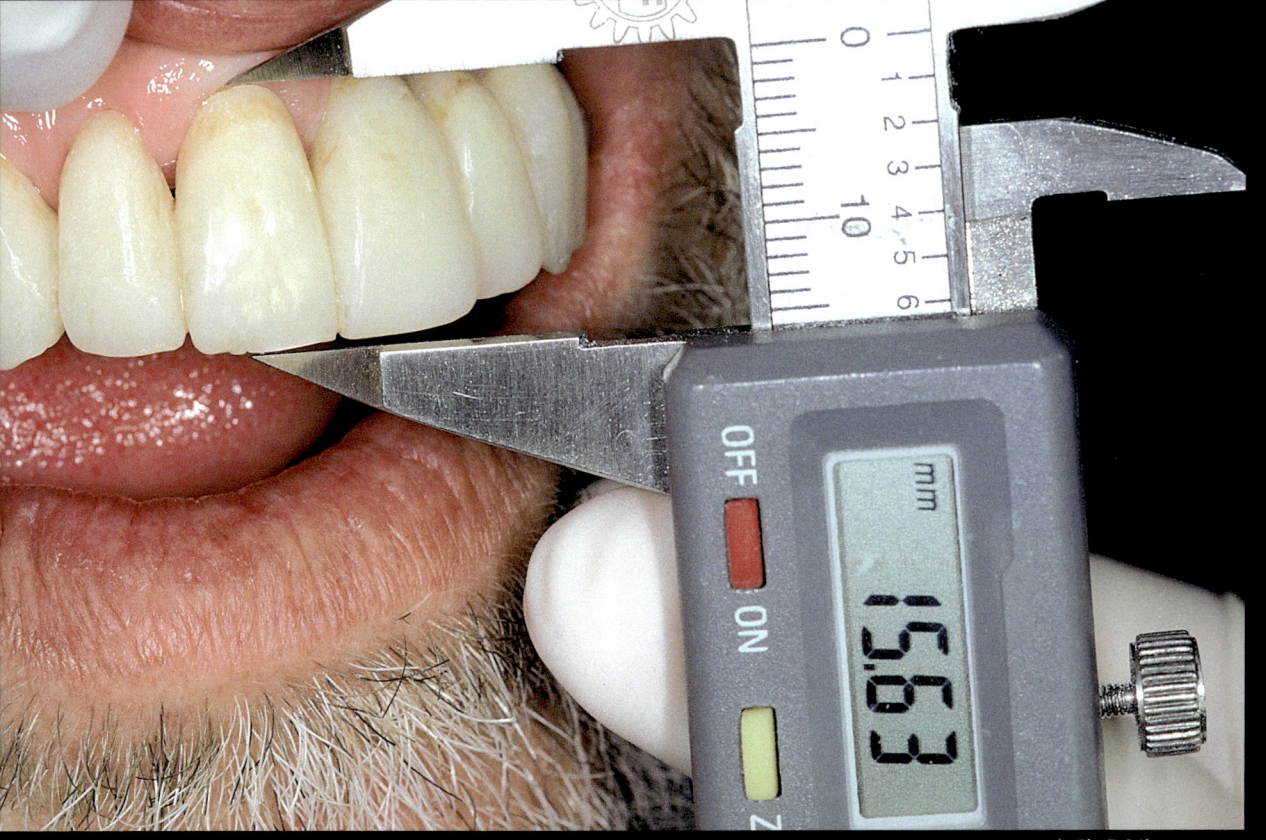

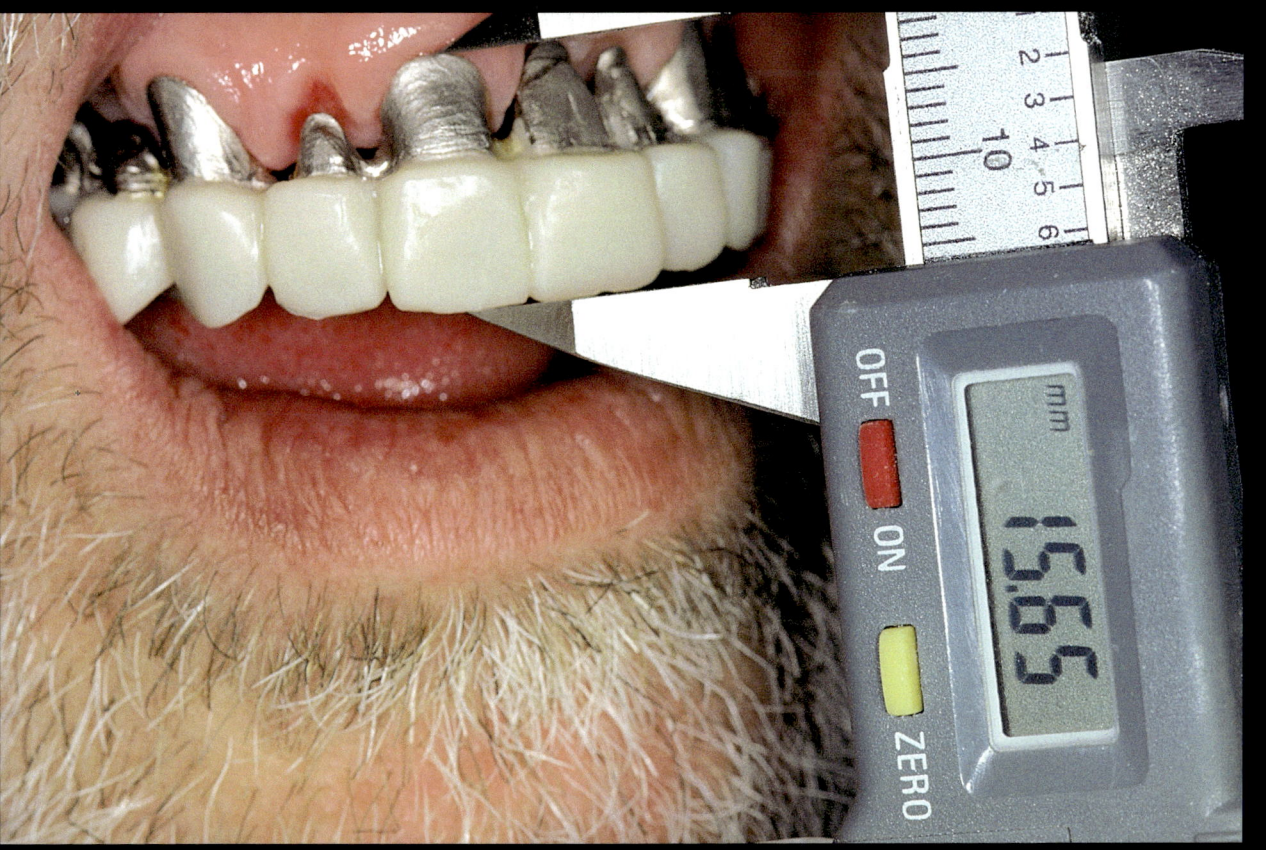

TREATING THE SUBSTRUCTURE

METAL-CERAMIC

The metal surface must be treated to ensure perfect bonding with the ceramic. This is only possible by elimination of all of the impurities caused by the lost-wax casting method: small residues of investment, porosity, irregularly distributed oxides, and other imperfections. In consideration of this requirement, the choice of rotary instruments for grinding the metal surface is of fundamental importance. The use of abrasive burs with bonding agents (eg, cement and Bakelite) or the creation of grooves and excessive roughness while processing the alloy can entrap impurities. By releasing gas during the subsequent ceramic firing, these impurities lead to the appearance of bubbles in the interface, ultimately weakening the bonding between the alloy and ceramic.[90] For this reason it is preferable to use tungsten carbide burs, which can create highly smooth surfaces that are normally free of contamination (Figs 5-35a to 5-35c). When this type of instrument is used, it is unnecessary to sand-blast the metal framework, as is essential when burs with a bonding agent (eg, carborundum, corundum, ceramic burs) have been used. To remove any impurities and grease residue accumulated during the grinding, it is always advisable to clean the metal structure with a solvent or to treat it with saturated steam generated from a specific piece of equipment (Fig 5-35d) before proceeding with the heat treatment (oxidation).

Oxidation of the metal framework

The heat treatment consists of warming the metal substructure in the ceramic furnace, gradually increasing the temperature until it reaches that of opaque firing, and then maintaining that temperature for roughly 10 minutes.[91] Depending on the type of alloy used, the temperatures and the times necessary for optimal oxidation must be checked beforehand, following the manufacturer's instructions. The purpose of this procedure is to create a uniform layer of oxide on the metal surface of a specific thickness and color that will ensure a strong chemical bond with the ceramic. To obtain a qualitatively and quantitatively adequate oxidation, it is sometimes necessary to repeat the heat treatment before proceeding with the application of the first layer of opaque.

ALL-CERAMICS

To minimize the risk of creating microfractures, any touch-ups on the substructure must be carried out by irrigating the area abundantly with water (Fig 5-36). Whether or not the copings are ground, they must be cleaned with saturated steam to eliminate the residue remaining on the surface. The practice of sand-blasting the substructure with 50 μm aluminum oxide before layering the ceramic, though recommended by some authors and manufacturers, today remains controversial.[78,92–94]

> Fig 5-35a

> Fig 5-35b

> Fig 5-35c

> Fig 5- 35d

> Fig 5-36a

> Fig 5-36b

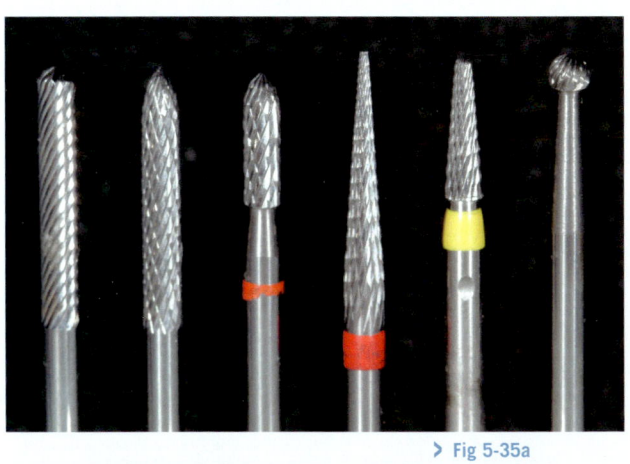

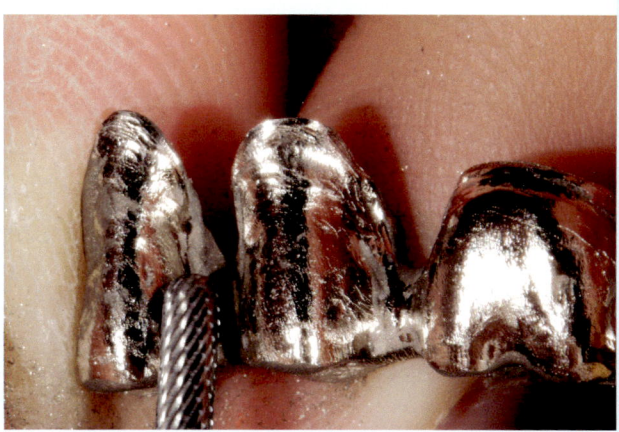

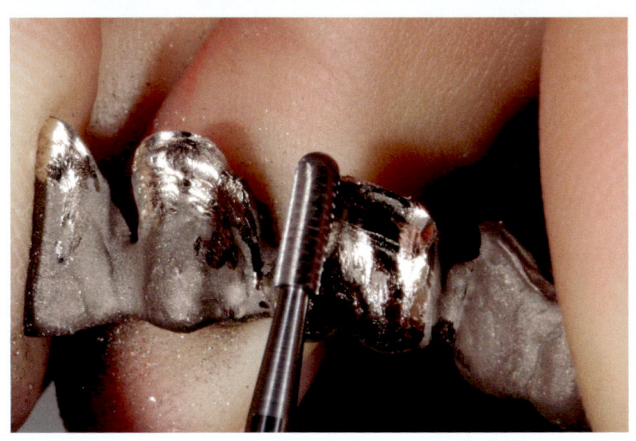

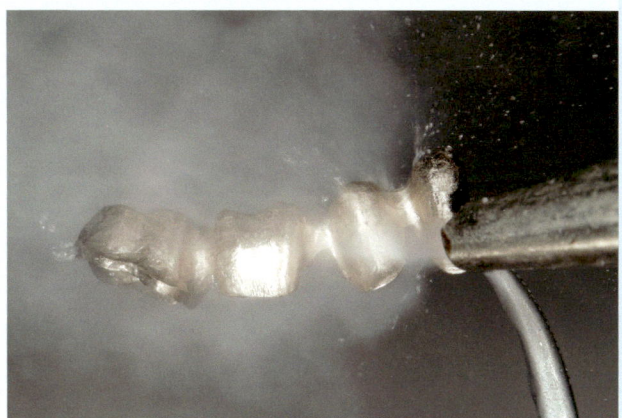

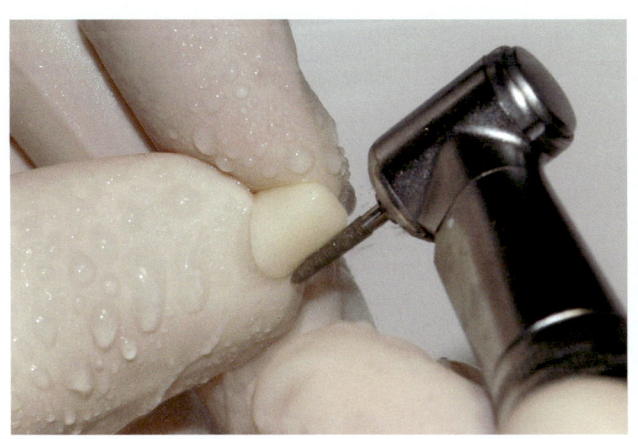

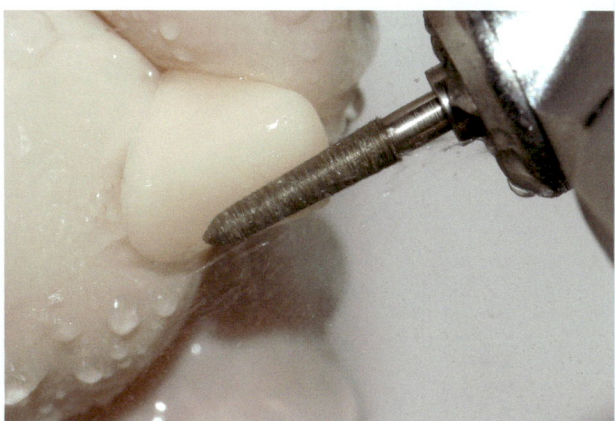

FIG 35 *(a and b)* Tungsten carbide burs of various shapes and sizes are especially useful for refining the metal substructure. *(c and d)* The use of saturated steam is effective in eradicating any impurities in the substructure.

FIG 36 *(a and b)* If the ceramic coping needs modification, rotary instruments must be used with abundant water irrigation to minimize the risk of microfractures in the material.

CONSTRUCTING THE DEFINITIVE RESTORATION   LABORATORY

LAYERING THE CERAMIC

Occlusal index The silicone index derived from the cast of the provisional restoration allows the technician, while layering the ceramic, to transfer all of the functional and esthetic parameters present in the acrylic matrix to the definitive restoration (Fig 5-37a). Using as much skill and creativity as required, the ceramist can now concentrate on the layering process (Fig 5-37b)[31,81,82,95] under the guidance of the occlusal matrix. In addition to confidently reproducing incisal margins and the tooth axes in the same arrangement found in the provisional restoration, the ceramist can also identify the correct location of the mamelons, the translucencies, the colored enamels, and the transparents (Figs 5-37c and 5-39h). Once the matrix has been removed, the tooth morphology and contours can be optimized through slight refinements. The silicone index is extremely useful, from a functional viewpoint, for providing important indications on the occlusal table and, more important, for reproducing the lingual concavity of the maxillary anterior teeth. In the latter case, since the area is not esthetically relevant, it is possible to use a single layer of body porcelain in the first ceramic firing that, with the help of the matrix guide, can reproduce the anterior guidance clinically tested in the provisional restoration. The inevitable shrinkage from ceramic sintering resulting from the first firing is easily compensated for by the subsequent application of enamels until an accurate reproduction of the disocclusive path is achieved. The last of the layering phases is completed without the help of the matrix, and with the articulator incisal pin placed on zero. At this point the lingual concavity is checked and optimized, reproducing in the articulator the excursive movements on the base of the path traced by the previously constructed customized anterior guidance.

Buccal index The buccal index can be used in the initial phases of layering the dentin. It is not recommended while layering the internal effects (enamels and mamelons), because the contact with the silicone index could cause a shift, with the consequent remixing of the body, enamel, and translucent porcelains, which would lead to less-than-ideal esthetic results. Final application of the enamels, for defining the contour and the tooth shape, is therefore done by the technician. The index is used merely as a final check of the tooth position.

FIG 37 *(a)* Positioned on the MC, the occlusopalatal index acts as a guide for the layering. *(b)* The powders retain an appropriate level of humidity by means of a special plate that contains a water circuit. *(c and d)* After the base dentin has been layered, the various effects are applied. *(e)* The enamels and opalescents are then added. The matrix support also aids in stabilization of the materials once they have been positioned in their ideal location.

CASE 1

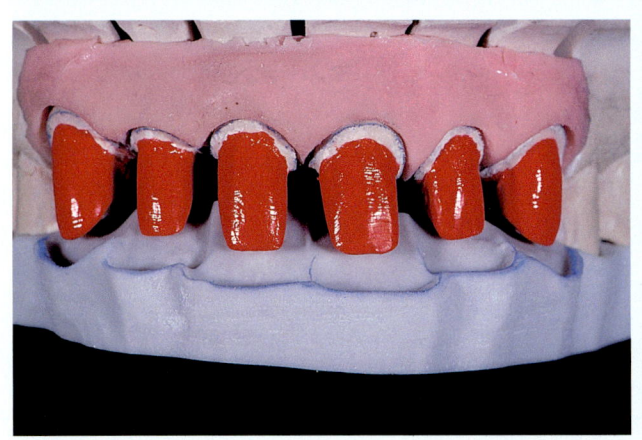

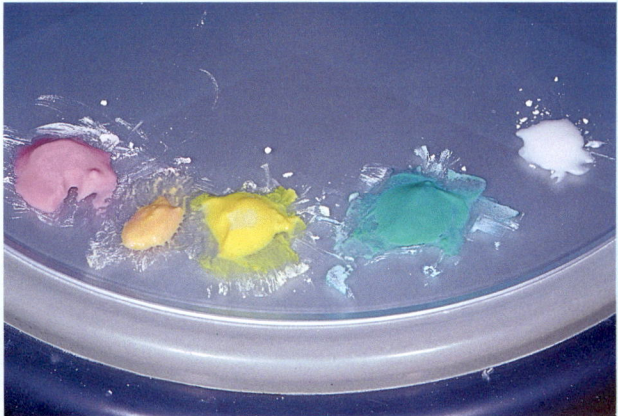

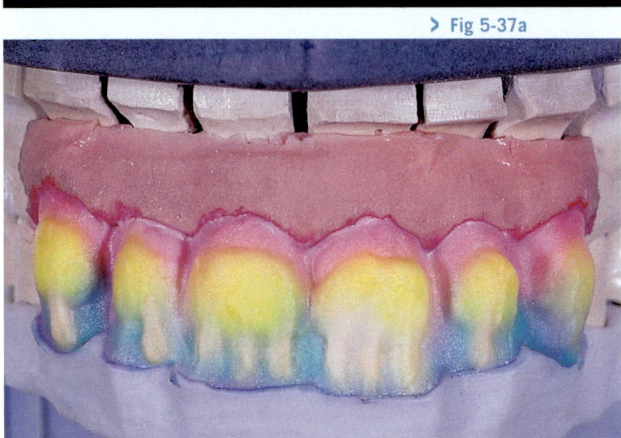

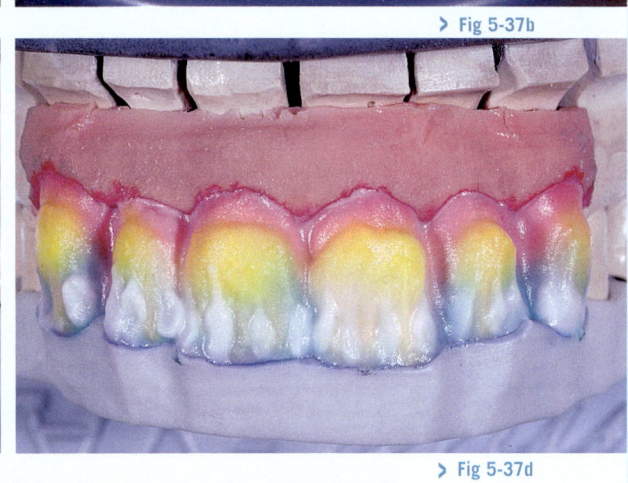

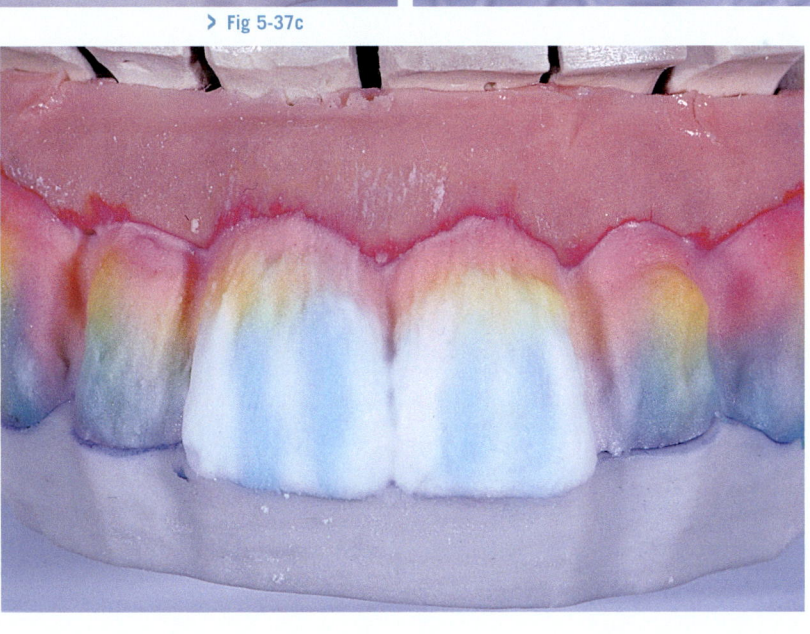

> Fig 5-37a

> Fig 5-37b

> Fig 5-37c

> Fig 5-37d

> Fig 5-37e

CASE 2

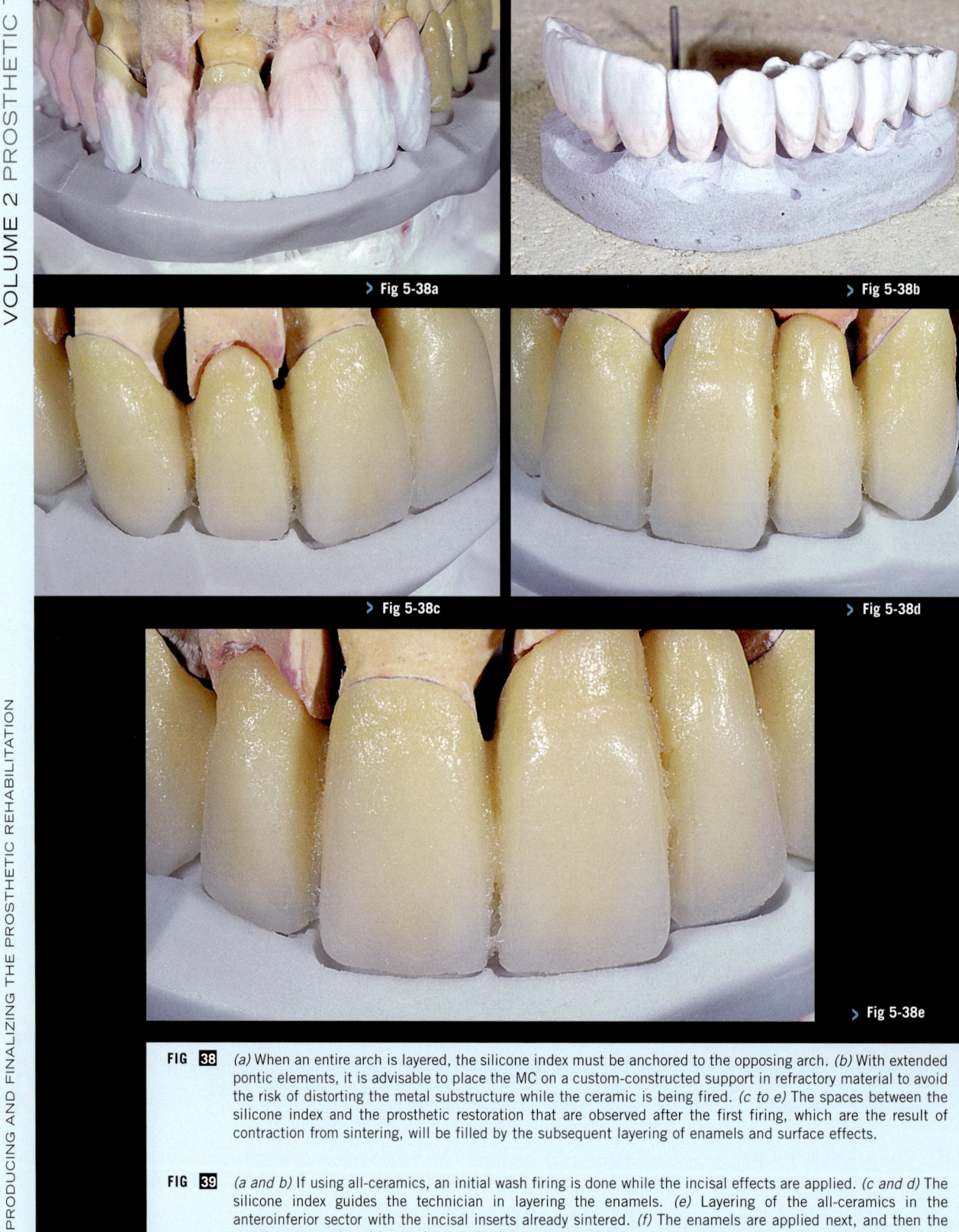

> Fig 5-38a

> Fig 5-38b

> Fig 5-38c

> Fig 5-38d

> Fig 5-38e

FIG 38 *(a)* When an entire arch is layered, the silicone index must be anchored to the opposing arch. *(b)* With extended pontic elements, it is advisable to place the MC on a custom-constructed support in refractory material to avoid the risk of distorting the metal substructure while the ceramic is being fired. *(c to e)* The spaces between the silicone index and the prosthetic restoration that are observed after the first firing, which are the result of contraction from sintering, will be filled by the subsequent layering of enamels and surface effects.

FIG 39 *(a and b)* If using all-ceramics, an initial wash firing is done while the incisal effects are applied. *(c and d)* The silicone index guides the technician in layering the enamels. *(e)* Layering of the all-ceramics in the anteroinferior sector with the incisal inserts already sintered. *(f)* The enamels are applied next, and then the prostheses are placed in the furnace for firing. *(g and h)* Because the tooth position is now defined, the final firings can be accomplished without the aid of the matrices, making use of the occlusal key dictated by the articulator and using the index solely as a check before sintering.

CASE 3

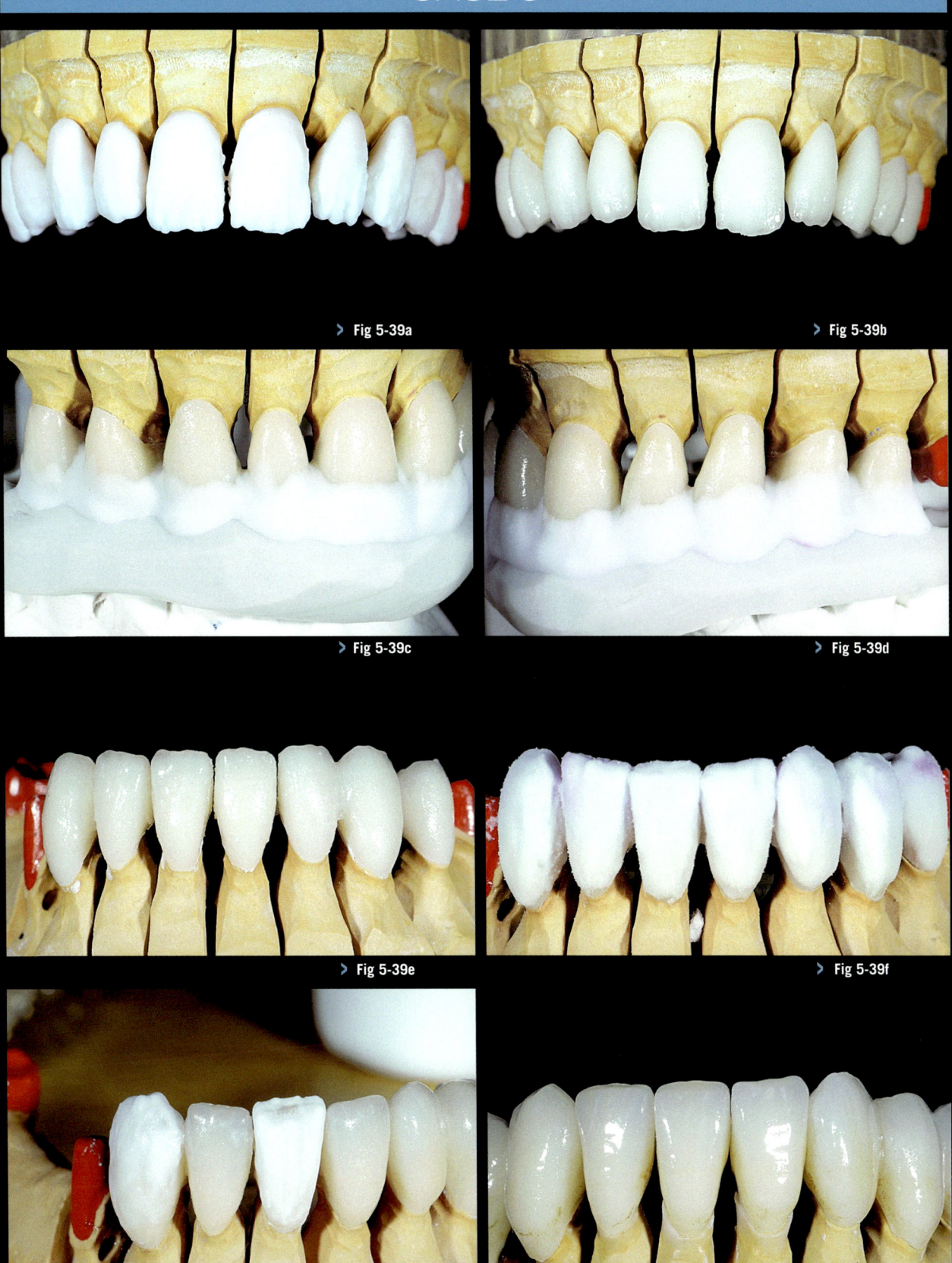

> Fig 5-39a

> Fig 5-39b

> Fig 5-39c

> Fig 5-39d

> Fig 5-39e

> Fig 5-39f

> Fig 5-39g

> Fig 5-39h

CONSTRUCTING THE DEFINITIVE RESTORATION — CLINIC

BISCUIT TRY-IN

ESTHETIC PARAMETERS

This chapter has previously described the ways in which, under the guidance of the silicone indices, the technician constructs the substructure that is subsequently layered by ceramic material.

The result of the biscuit try-in on the patient should correspond, in volume and tooth position, with the situation achieved with the provisional restoration in function, which must therefore represent the prototype of the definitive prosthesis in all aspects.

It is the clinician's task to carefully check the position of the incisal edge and the tooth length with the lips at rest, during speech, and smiling (see volume 1, chapter 3), assessing whether a simple correction in the chair is sufficient for remedying any slight discrepancies that are found. In the oral cavity as in the laboratory, the tooth shape and proportion of each element are evaluated, separating the buccal surfaces through the use of the transition line angle (see volume 1, chapter 5) (Figs 5-40a to 5-40d). After checking the adequacy of the interproximal contact, the restorations are temporarily fixed with silicone paste, to allow the clinician to check the facial and dentolabial esthetic parameters (Fig 5-40e). The lack of surface gloss in the biscuit try-in phase can be compensated for by the simple apposition of glazing liquid (Fig 5-40f) or even more simply by water (Fig 5-40g), to better evaluate the shade of the restoration and its translucency, and to be able to identify any modifications for the laboratory so that they can be made before the final firing.

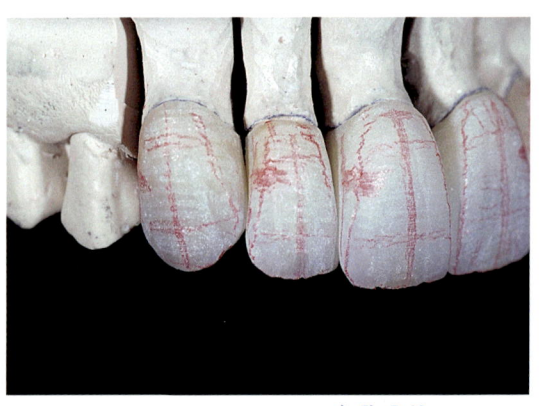

> Fig 5-40a

> Fig 5-40b

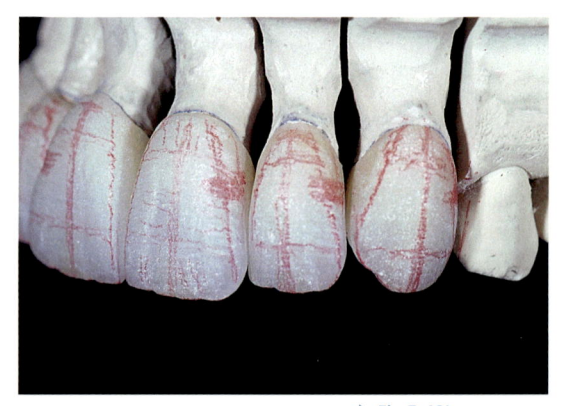

FIG 40 *(a to d)* During the ceramic refining phases, the tooth surface is divided at the transition line angles to optimize the esthetic appearance of the restorations. *(e to g)* The restorations are then checked in the mouth with a silicone paste to verify their marginal fit as well as the esthetic, occlusal, and chromatic aspects (with and without the glaze applied).

CASE 1

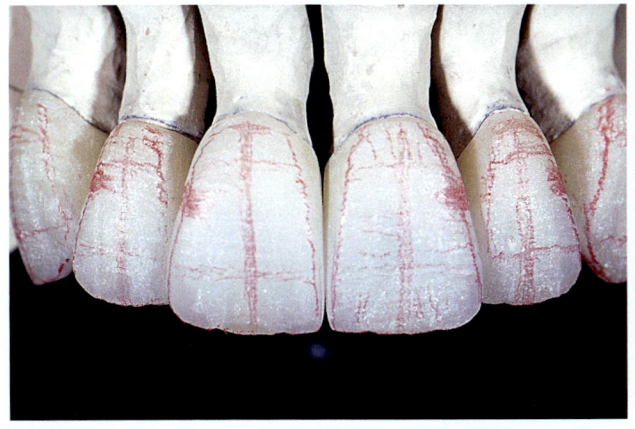

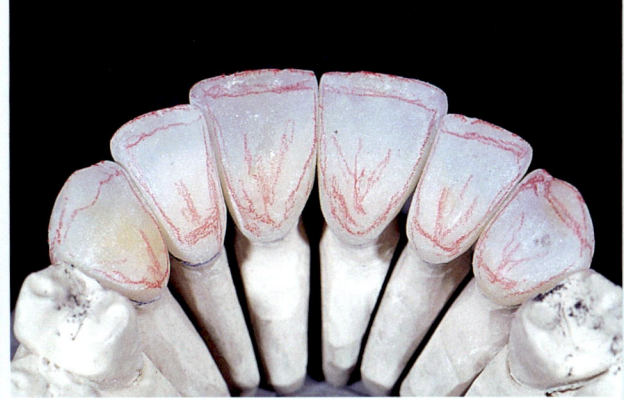

> Fig 5-40c

> Fig 5-40d

> Fig 5-40e

> Fig 5-40f

> Fig 5-40g

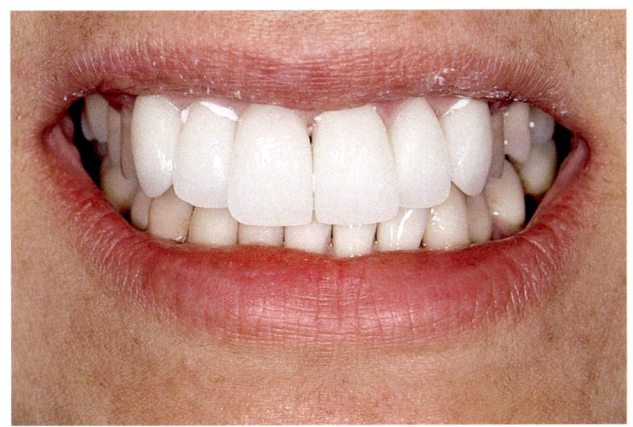

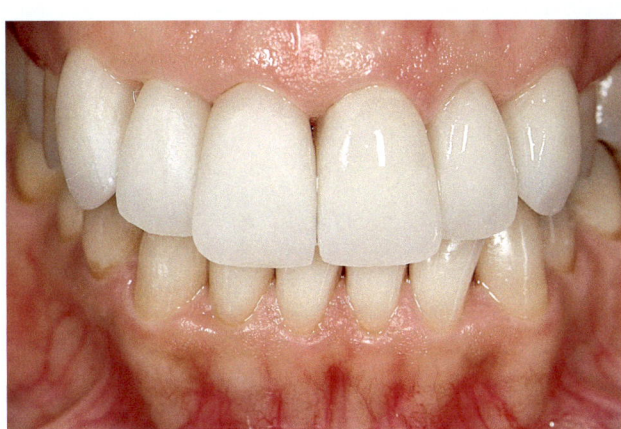

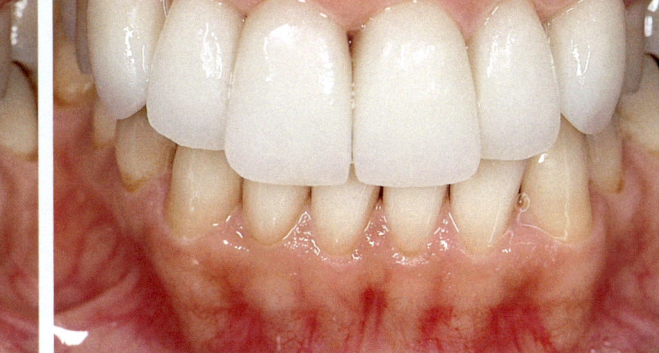

BISCUIT TRY-IN

FUNCTIONAL PARAMETERS

The need to modify the occlusal table at the biscuit try-in phase can be considered normal, but only if the adjustments necessary to achieve satisfactory occlusal stability are slight (Fig 5-41a). The contacts on the tips of the cusps and in the corresponding fossae or marginal ridges, in both MI and CR, must be well distributed, punctiform, synchronized,[96–99] and achieved at the same VDO found in the provisional restorations. To check the adequacy of the contacts, appropriate articulating paper (AccuFilm II, Parkell) as well as metal strips a few microns in thickness (Hanel Shimstock Foil, Coltène/Whaledent) can be used. To prevent the formation of microfractures in the ceramic, extreme care must be taken in the oral cavity using an air-water spray handpiece.

Maximal intercuspation If the definitive restorations have been made in MI, the clinician should check the occlusal contacts by asking the patient to close the mouth in the habitual position. Once the occlusion has been adjusted, it is necessary to check for any interference in the restorations when the patient is guided into CR. During function the patient may move the mandible into CR, thereby interfering with the restorations just checked in MI. Unlike the proprioceptors of contiguous elements, which immediately inform the central nervous system of the presence of any interference, the proprioceptors of the abutments just restored cannot immediately process this information and are therefore initially unable to prevent troublesome premature contacts during function, which are immediately felt by the patient.

Centric relation In cases where the patient has instead been rehabilitated in CR, the clinician must check the occlusal stability achieved by the restorations in centric occlusion (CO–CR). The contacts that are present when the patient is guided by the operator with the bimanual Dawson maneuver must coincide with those that occur when the patient closes the mouth spontaneously[100] (Fig 5-41b). In every case involving treatment of the posterior sectors, it is very important that the clinician ascertain the presence of stable and well-defined contacts in the molar region, to alleviate the load on the temporomandibular joint articulation, especially in patients who complain or have complained of dysfunction.[101]

Anterior guidance In patients who have been restored in MI and CR alike, the eccentric movements must also be checked to ensure the presence of anterior guidance, the consequential disocclusion of the posterior sectors,[102–106] and an excursion similar to the one recorded with the provisional restorations, all of which must be easy and free of any impediments.

CASE 2

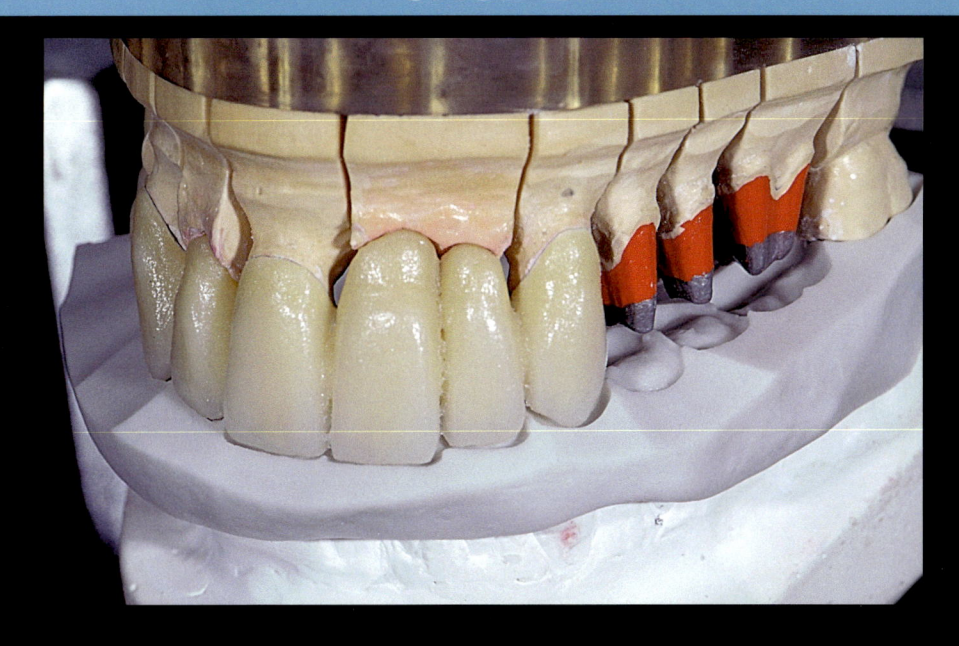

> Fig 5-41a

> Fig 5-41b

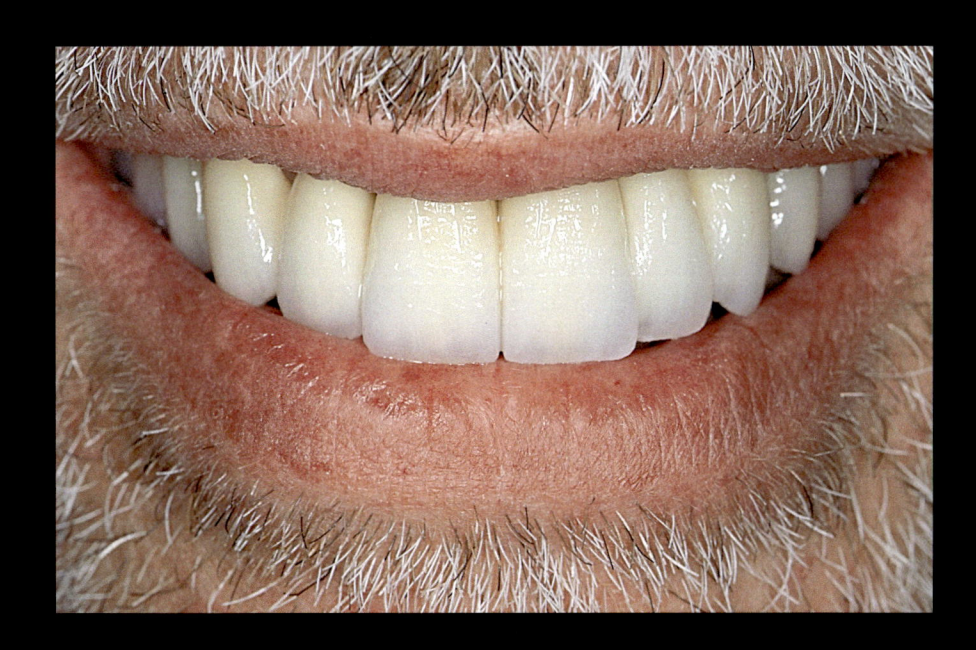

FIG 41 The photograph of the rehabilitation after the first firing of the ceramic shows the need to fire it again to fill the space that still exists and to achieve the volumes defined by the silicone index. *(a)* Note how the index shows the ideal design of the occlusal morphology of the provisional restorations in the left posterior area, without the fixed partial denture. *(b)* In patients rehabilitated in CR, there must be correspondence between the occlusal relationships achieved by guiding the patient with the Dawson maneuver, and those obtained when the patient spontaneously closes the mouth.

BISCUIT TRY-IN

BIOLOGIC PARAMETERS

Contour One of the primary objectives is to maintain the biologic integrity achieved with the provisional restoration in the definitive restoration. To this end, it is necessary to scrupulously replicate the coronal contour in the cervical area of the acrylic index, even if, as already seen (see page 442), its exact transfer to the definitive restorations proves extremely difficult. Once the provisional restorations have been removed, the gingival tissues collapse, which is recorded in the position impression taken in the substructure trial session. This inevitably leads the technician to create subcontoured restorations. The information inferred from the final impression, however, does not permit a faithful reproduction of the design of the cervical third of the provisional restoration, since the use of retraction cords for reading the intrasulcular margins causes the tissues to compress and induces the technician to fabricate overcontoured restorations (Figs 5-42a to 5-42c). This second option is preferable because, during the biscuit try-in, the clinician can make the necessary adjustments by subtraction directly on the patient. Close application of the same principles that guided the operator's hand to achieve ideal biologic integration of the acrylic index now allows the same results to be achieved at the biscuit try-in (Figs 5-42d to 5-42f). If these are judged excessive, the contour is reduced with a bur directly in the mouth, altering the emergence profile in each site and thus promoting biologic integration and an optimal esthetic result, especially in the interproximal areas.

Marginal closure Before the accuracy of the marginal closure can be verified, it must be ensured that the restorations are correctly positioned and that there is no excessive resistance in the areas in contact with contiguous elements that could prevent them from fitting perfectly. The validity of the marginal fit is checked once again in the biscuit try-in using silicone pastes (FitChecker) that allow both the internal and the marginal adaptations to be properly assessed. This fit, compared with the substructure test, may undergo modifications after the layering phases, especially when metal-ceramic is used.[107-111] Richter and Ueno[112] have demonstrated that a good marginal closure is more important in maintaining periodontal health than the position of the margin (supragingival, at the gingival crest, or subgingival), even if the level of marginal opening that can be considered acceptable from the clinical point of view still needs to be established.[13,14] It should nevertheless be pointed out that marginal discrepancies, even those of 200 to 300 µm, are not always directly correlated with recurrent caries lesions and/or the progression of periodontal disease,[113,114] since microbial virulence and individual resistance to infection often play a more important role than the intrinsic value of the marginal closure.[13]

CASE 3

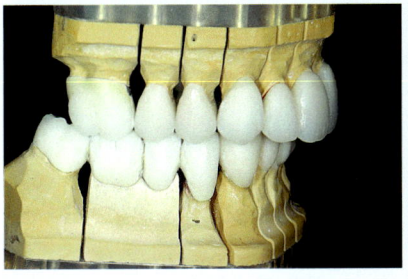

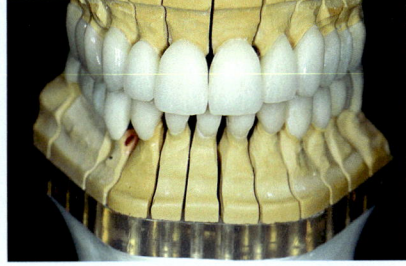

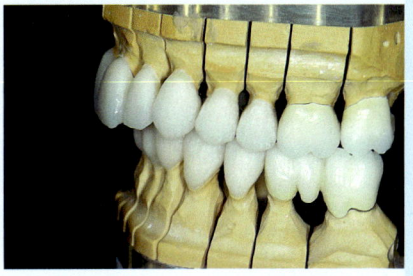

> Fig 5-42a

> Fig 5-42b

> Fig 5-42c

> Fig 5-42d

> Fig 5-42e

> Fig 5-42f

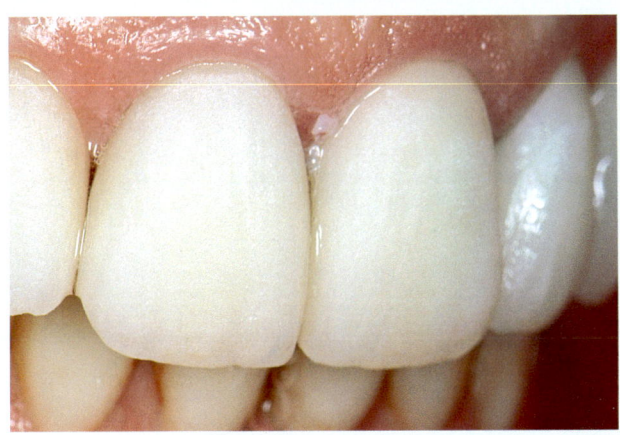

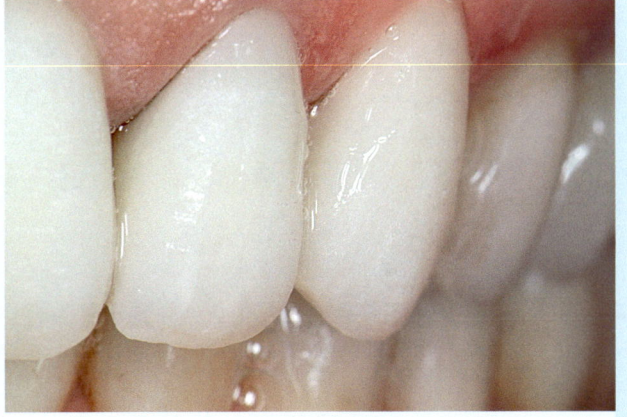

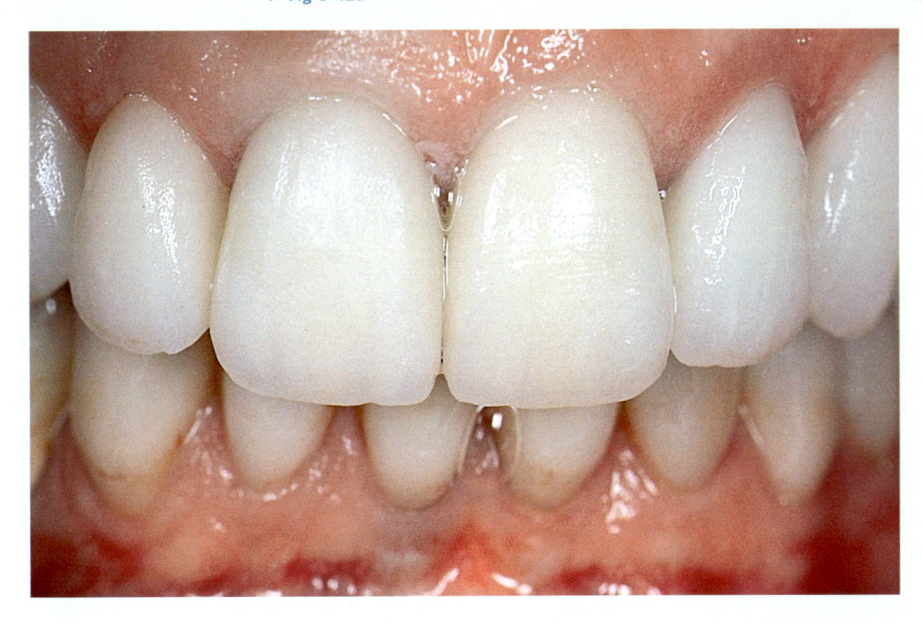

FIG 42 *(a to c)* Following ceramization, the restoration is sent to the clinician still in the biscuit phase. *(d to f)* In addition to evaluating the esthetic-functional appearance of the maxillary and mandibular rehabilitation, the dentist clinically checks both the marginal fit and the validity of the restorative contours, especially in the interproximal areas.

Edentulous ridges The slight collapse in the tissues around the edentulous areas that occurs once the provisional restoration has been removed can initially prevent the definitive prosthesis from fitting perfectly (Figs 5-43a and 5-43b). This difficulty can be accentuated if the technician, to form the ideal tooth shape and contour, creates a slight overextension at the cervical level. Before any fine adjustments are carried out, or assuming that the fixed partial denture is rocking, it is a good idea to position the prosthetic restoration on the abutments and have the patient gently tighten the bite with cotton rolls in place. After a few minutes, if the compression is light, the fixed partial denture will seem to fit perfectly. If the compression is excessive and the clinician therefore needs to make fine adjustments, these must be carried out by merely shortening the root extensions slightly, avoiding at all costs any change to the emergence that was optimized by the technician and leaving the tissues to adapt to the new morphology of the restorations. Last, it is necessary to verify that superfloss will move freely around the pontic elements, to ensure that the patient can maintain adequate hygiene in these areas, too.

GLAZING

Upon receiving the prosthesis after the biscuit try-in, the technician cleans it scrupulously using steam at high pressure and then immersing it in distilled water in an ultrasonic tank. With the aid of the images of the biscuit try-in done in the clinic, the technician makes any remaining corrections regarding morphology and color as requested by the clinician, adding ceramic material to specific sites if requested. Before being glazed in the furnace, the appropriate burs and silicone rubber cups will be used to give the surfaces of the ceramic elements the necessary macro- and microtextures. After glazing, any areas of exposed metal are polished, and the ceramic restorations are treated manually in the buccal aspects with brushes and diamond pastes to make their appearance as natural as possible (Figs 5-43c and 5-43d).

POSTSOLDERING

With metal-ceramics, especially on complex rehabilitations, the definitive restoration is often broken down into different fixed partial dentures of reduced size and then joined back together with *postsoldering* (Figs 5-43e and 5-43f). In addition to minimizing the risk of deforming the metal substructure when the ceramic is sintered, this expedient also makes the technician's work easier; fewer elements at a time can be layered without running the risk of the ceramic material drying out progressively, which could happen if the fixed partial denture were maintained in one piece. After it is glazed, the prosthesis must be returned to the clinician to take a key for positioning in the mouth. The technician requires an accurate recording of this position to complete the postsoldering.

CASE 2

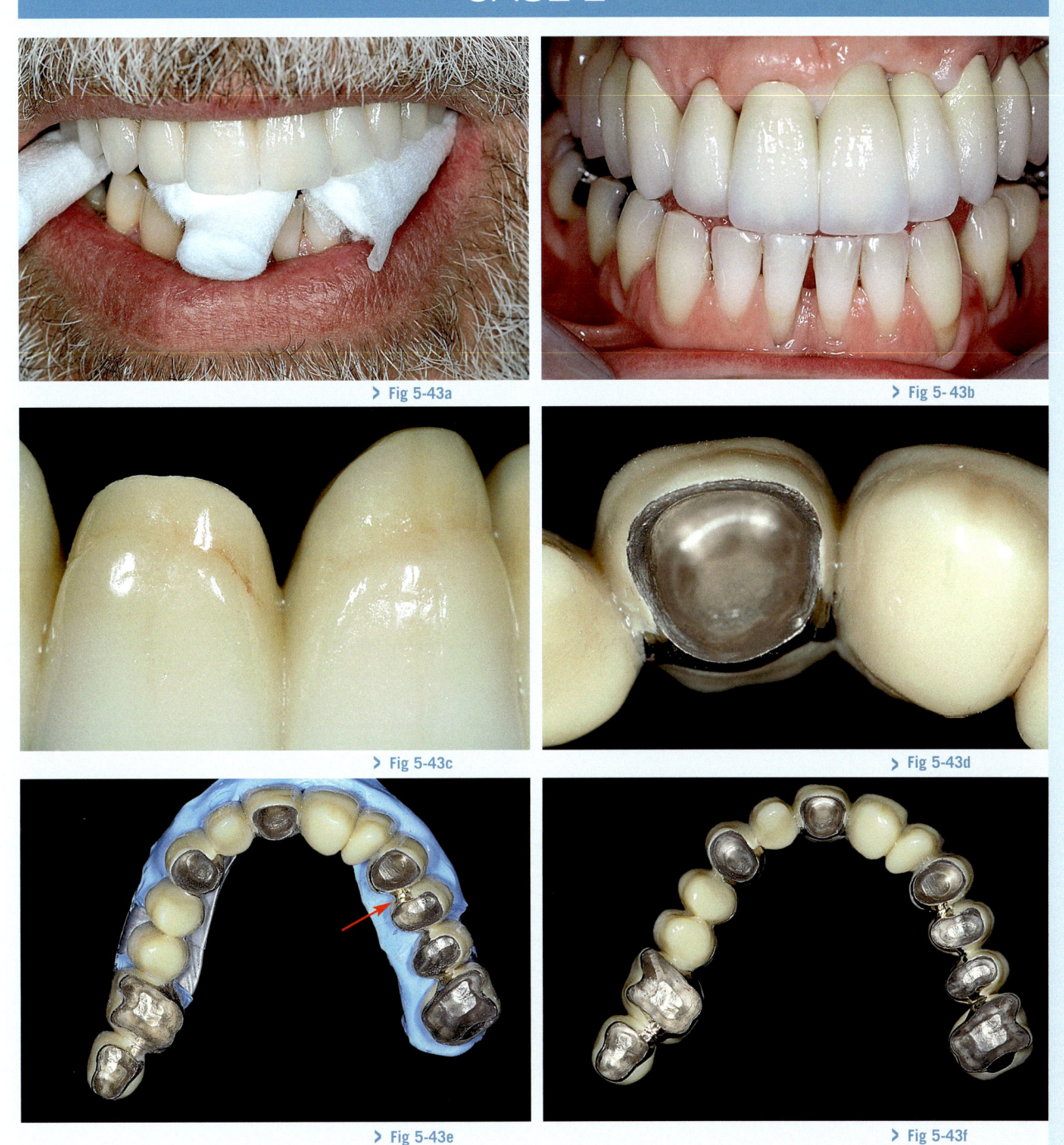

> Fig 5-43a

> Fig 5-43b

> Fig 5-43c

> Fig 5-43d

> Fig 5-43e

> Fig 5-43f

FIG 43 The clinician must ensure that the rehabilitation fits into the mouth perfectly; initially it may seem obstructed by its excessive compression on the tissues, especially where there are edentulous ridges. *(a)* If this happens, the patient must be asked to close the mouth with rolls of cotton placed between the arches, and to hold this position for a few minutes. *(b)* The intraoral view shows the areas of ischemia due to excessive compression of the gingival tissues. *(c and d)* After the biscuit try-in, the rehabilitation is glazed. Despite the limited buccal thickness of the tooth preparation, an effective coating of the metal was obtained in the marginal area of the right central incisor by the application of opaque, dentin, and enamel in succession, while avoiding any overcontour. *(e and f)* Only after glazing is complete, an occlusal key is taken in zinc oxide–eugenol, then used by the technician to join the two parts of the maxillary rehabilitation by means of postsoldering *(arrow)*.

DELIVERING THE DEFINITIVE RESTORATION

With the ability to reproduce in the definitive prosthesis all of the characteristics present in the functional provisional restoration, the clinician can often cement the prosthetic rehabilitation without running the risk of having to make modifications once it has been placed. Any discrepancies between the definitive prosthesis and the provisional restoration should have been addressed already and, if necessary, remedied at the biscuit try-in stage. Only if postsoldering has been done will the clinician need to check that no rocking motion is present and that the marginal closures are accurate.

Even if the restorations simply need glazing after the biscuit try-in, before positioning them in the oral cavity it is still a good rule to recheck the adequacy of the definitive restoration on the master cast (Figs 5-44 to 5-46).

Before selecting the cement that will be used to fix the prosthesis in place, the clinician must ensure, especially in the presence of single elements, that the interdental contact areas on the MC and in the mouth are similar. Sometimes the interproximal areas are too tight on the patient, hence representing a potential obstacle to a perfect fit of the restorations in the cementation phase.

In addition, it is essential to re-evaluate whether or not the spaces are sufficient to allow proper cleaning of the interproximal areas, especially in cases where fixed partial dentures have been constructed. The patient's ability to use the instruments recommended by the clinician for hygiene at home should then be tested. Last, it is necessary to make sure that the ceramic surfaces, and especially the metal surfaces if present, are perfectly polished to avoid the buildup of plaque, which is a possible cause of gingival inflammation.

It is a good rule, particularly in more complex cases, to ask the technician to provide a nighttime occlusal appliance for the patient. The appliance must be used on a routine basis to control neuromuscular activity and to prevent the onset of any fractures that may occur more easily during the night.

FIG 44 *(a and b)* The gingival matrix enabled the technician to optimize the restorative contours of the six anterior crowns.

FIG 45 *(a and b)* Removing the gingival matrix from the MC allows the clinician to properly check the suitability of the marginal fit on the working cast.

FIG 46 *(a and b)* Before they are carefully checked in the oral cavity, the occlusal relationships are verified on the MCs.

CASE 1

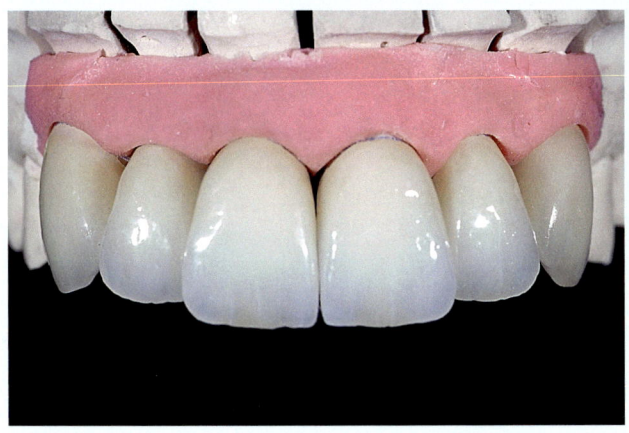

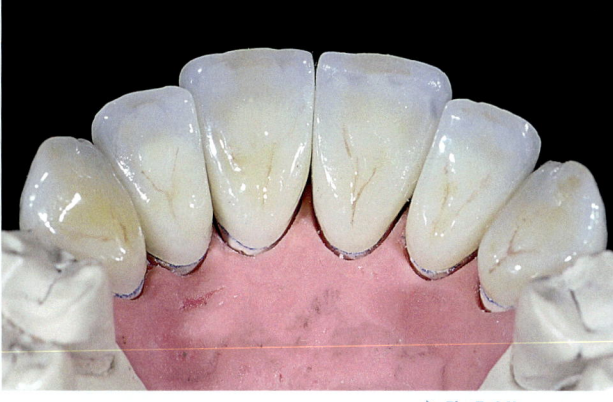

> Fig 5-44a

> Fig 5-44b

CASE 2

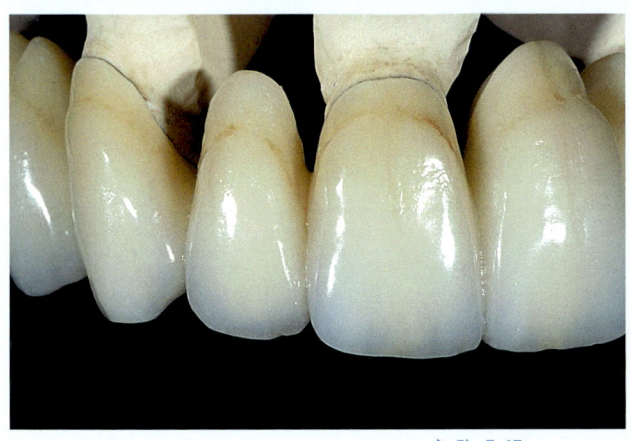

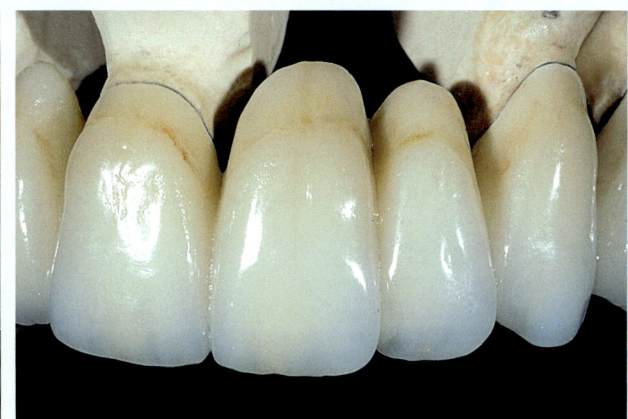

> Fig 5-45a

> Fig 5-45b

CASE 3

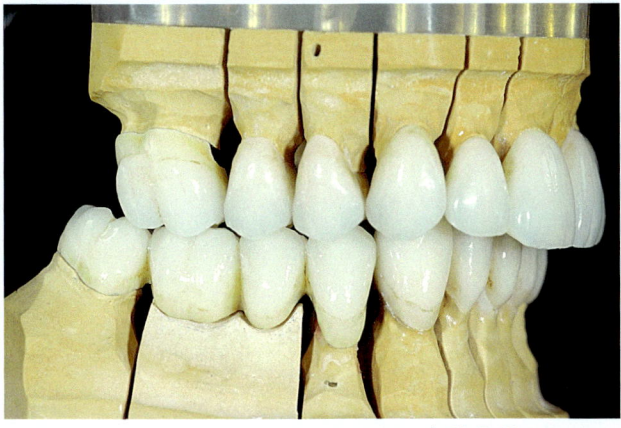

> Fig 5-46a

> Fig 5-46b

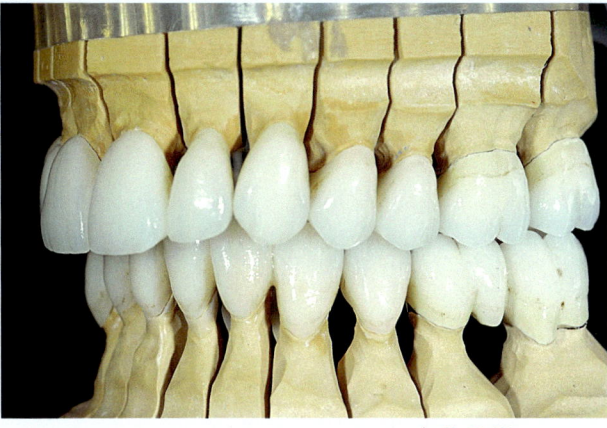

LUTING

TEMPORARY LUTING

Single restorations The temporary luting of single restorations is strongly discouraged, whether metal-ceramics or all-ceramics are used. In the presence of a satisfactory marginal adaptation, removal of the prosthesis would not only be extremely difficult, but could easily damage the restoration's structural integrity.

Fixed partial dentures If the decision is made to lute a fixed partial denture temporarily, certain problems can occur when it is removed (a necessary action for proceeding with the definitive luting). The presence of the materials used for reconstructing the abutments and/or endodontic posts, just as in cases of reduced periodontal support, require extreme care to be taken during the operation to prevent possible structural damage. While the clinician must act with extreme delicacy in the situations described above, removal of a fixed partial denture with structurally integral and particularly retentive abutments can prove extremely difficult, if not impossible.

DEFINITIVE LUTING

Faithful reproduction in the definitive restoration of all of the characteristics in the functionalized provisional restoration more often than not makes it possible to proceed directly to definitive luting. In these cases the luting agent is selected with consideration of the type of materials used for reconstructing the abutments and the nature of the restorative material used. With metal-ceramics, traditional techniques and cements (oxyphosphate, glass ionomer, hybrids) can be used (Figs 5-47a to 5-47d), whereas all-ceramics usually require adhesive techniques. The use of resinous cement is obligatory for the silicate-based ceramics (feldspathic and glass-ceramic) because they can be etched, but this is only one option for alumina- and zirconium-based ceramics (Fig 5-47e). These also can be luted with traditional cements with the exception of oxyphosphates, whose opacity would counteract the esthetic advantage of choosing a ceramic without any metal.[76,78,92] After cementation, all excess must be removed with great care and precision. Even the slightest cement residue in the sulcus can lead to gingival inflammation,[115] although this may also be caused by other factors such as the unevenness of the surfaces of the prosthesis or the presence of roughness in the tooth-restoration interface.[116,117]

After radiographs have been taken of the areas involved in the treatment, an appointment is made for an initial checkup shortly after delivery. In addition to revealing any excess cement residue, the session offers a chance to check the patient's ability to maintain an adequate level of oral hygiene (Figs 5-48 to 5-50).

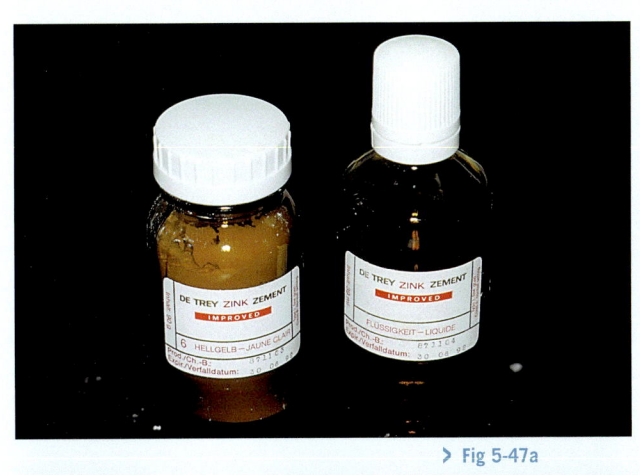

> Fig 5-47a

> Fig 5-47b

> Fig 5-47c

> Fig 5-47d

> Fig 5-47e

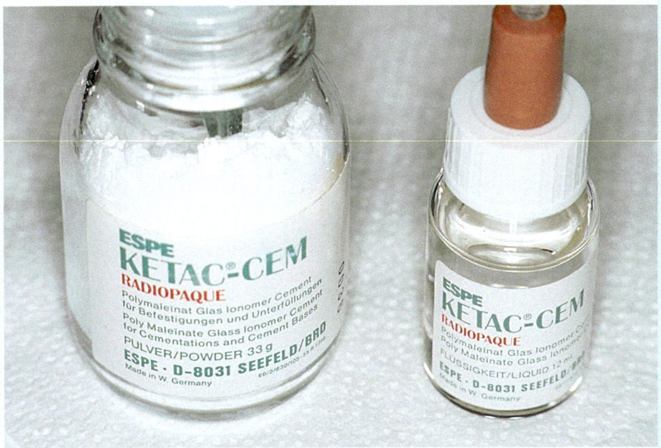

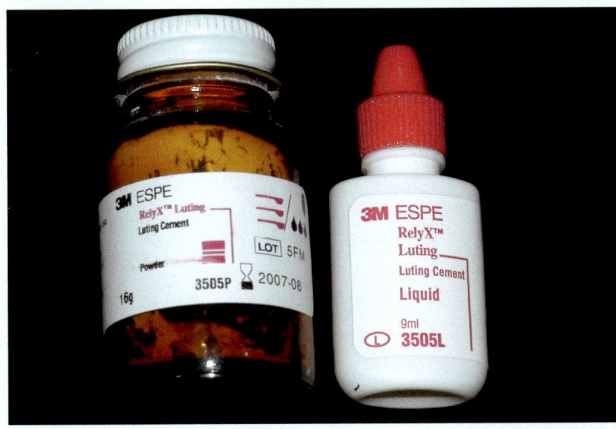

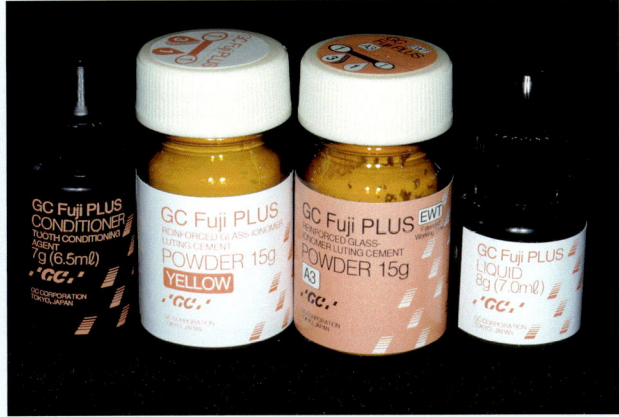

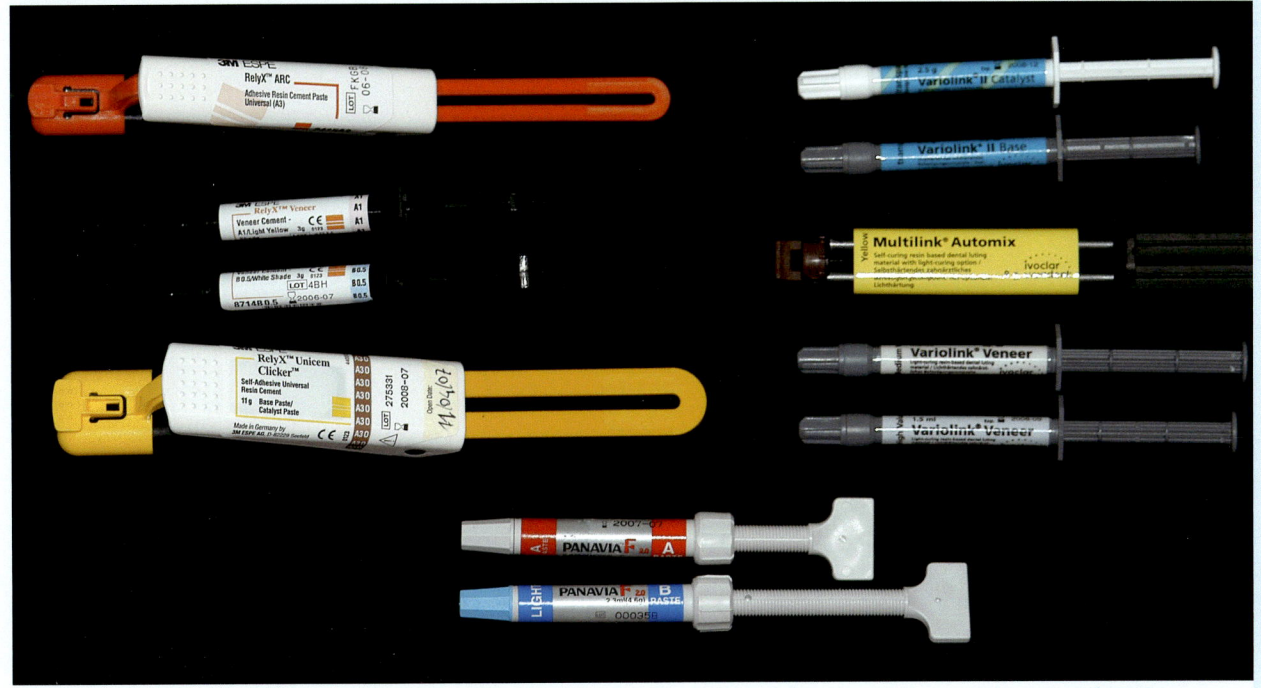

FIG 47 *(a)* Oxyphosphate cement is still used widely in the cementation of gold or metal-ceramic restorations. *(b)* Glass ionomers gained considerable popularity during the 1980s. *(c and d)* Recently their use has been reduced because of the arrival of hybrid materials (resin ionomers), which are used in the cementation of both metal-ceramic and all-ceramic restorations, especially those that are alumina- and zirconium-based. *(e)* Today it is possible to choose from a wide range of resin cements: light-, self-, or dual-curing.

CASE 1

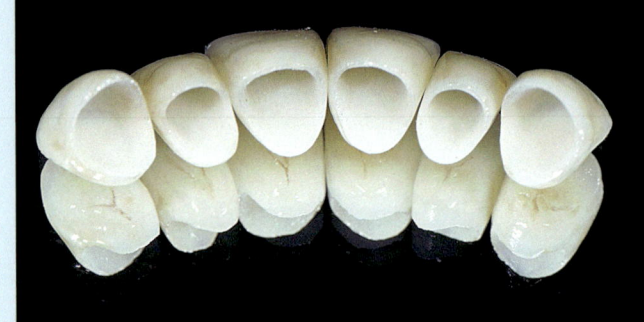

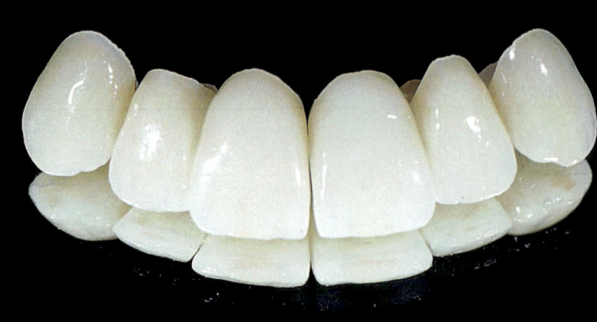

> Fig 5-48a

2003

> Fig 5-48b

> Fig 5-48c

> Fig 5-48d

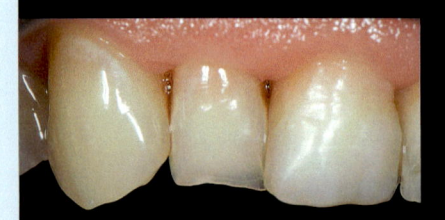

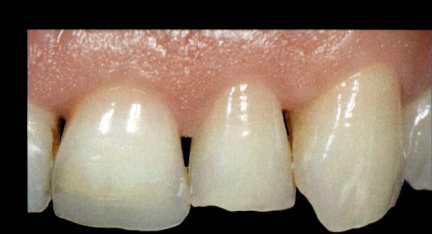

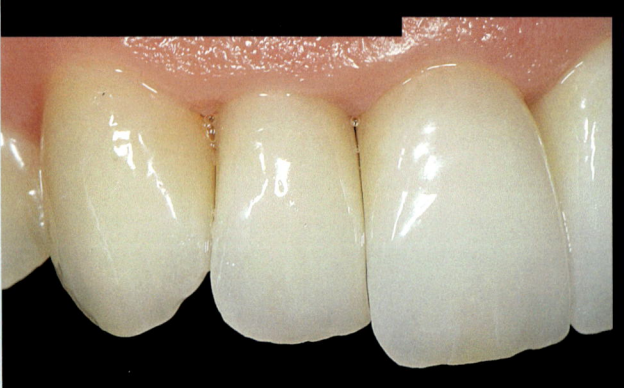

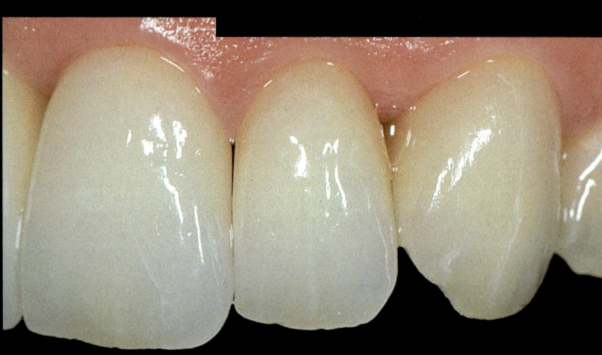

FIG 48 *(a and b)* In the photographs of the restorations placed on a mirror it can be seen how the ceramic is particularly thin at the marginal level, attesting to the conservative tooth preparations. *(c to g)* The pretreatment and posttreatment views demonstrate a significant improvement in the patient's esthetic appearance. *(h to k)* Ideal esthetic and biologic integration of the six anterior restorations can also be seen in the lateral views, both intraoral and during smiling.

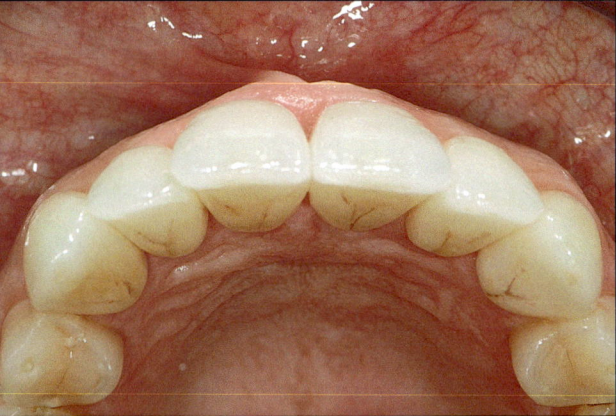

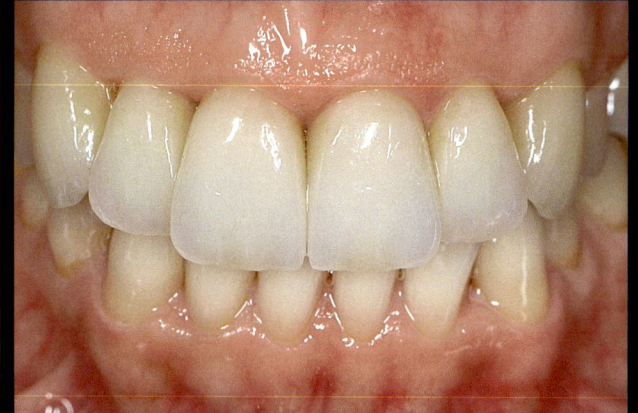

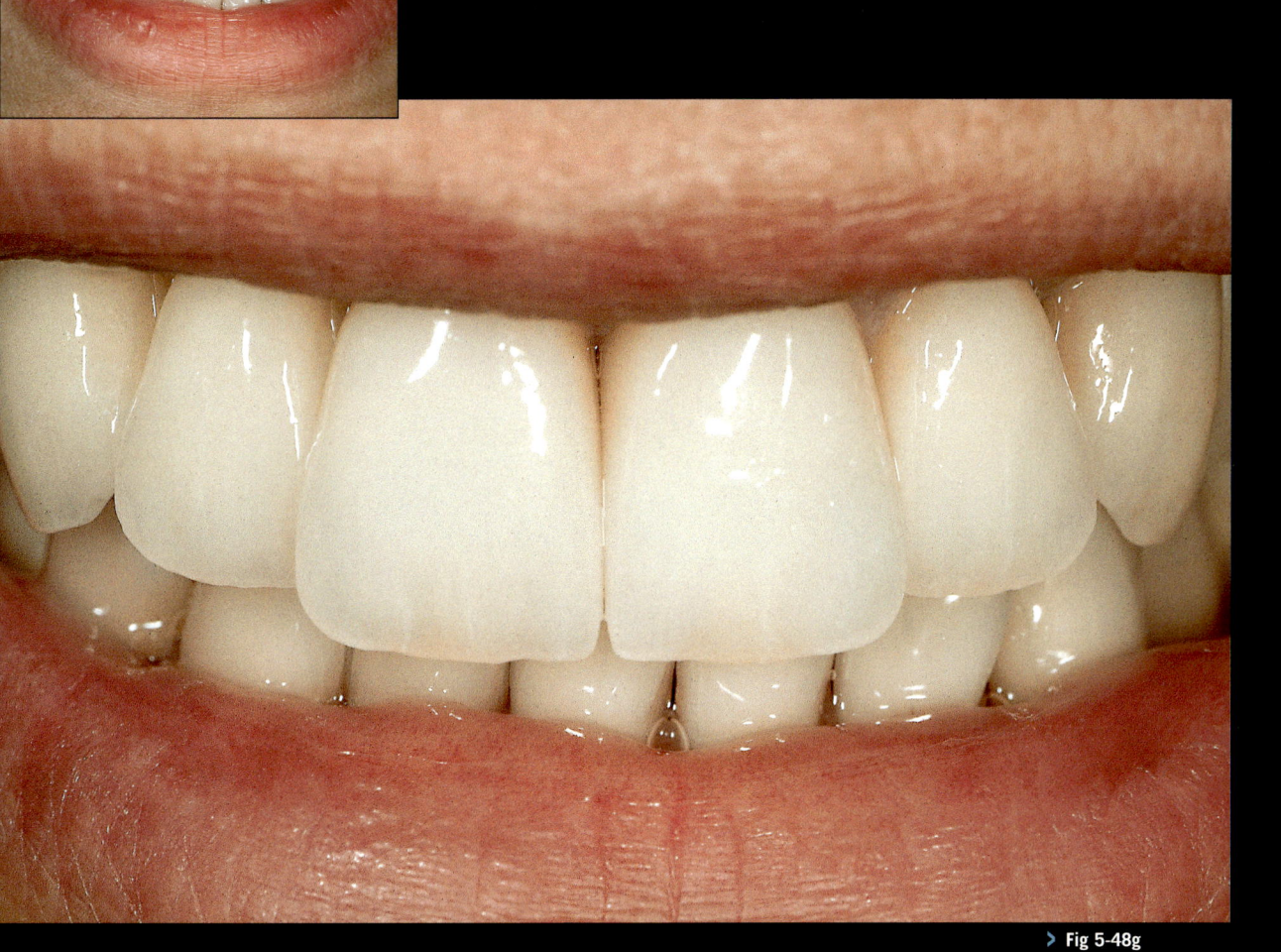

> Fig 5-48e

> Fig 5-48f

> Fig 5-48g

> Fig 5-48h

> Fig 5-48i

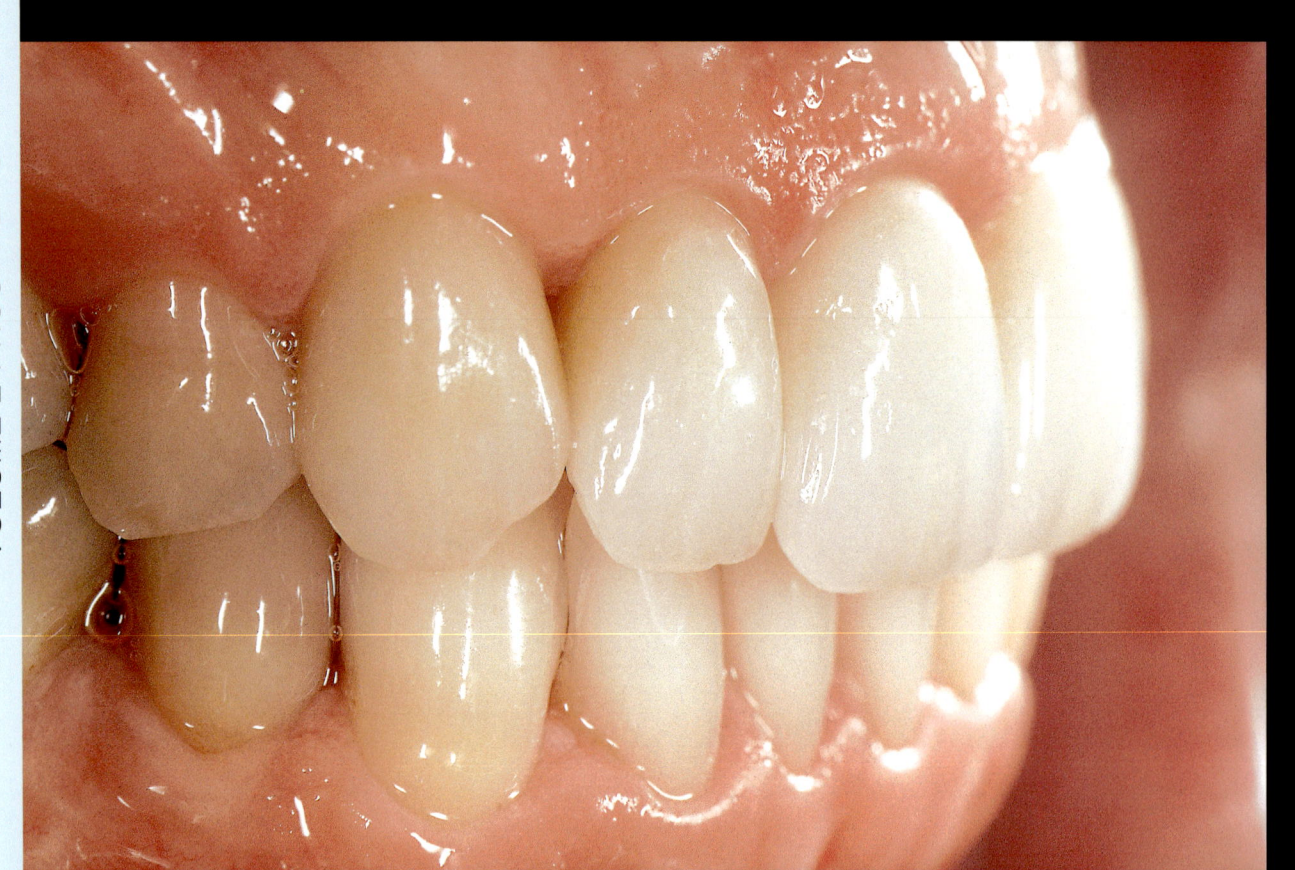

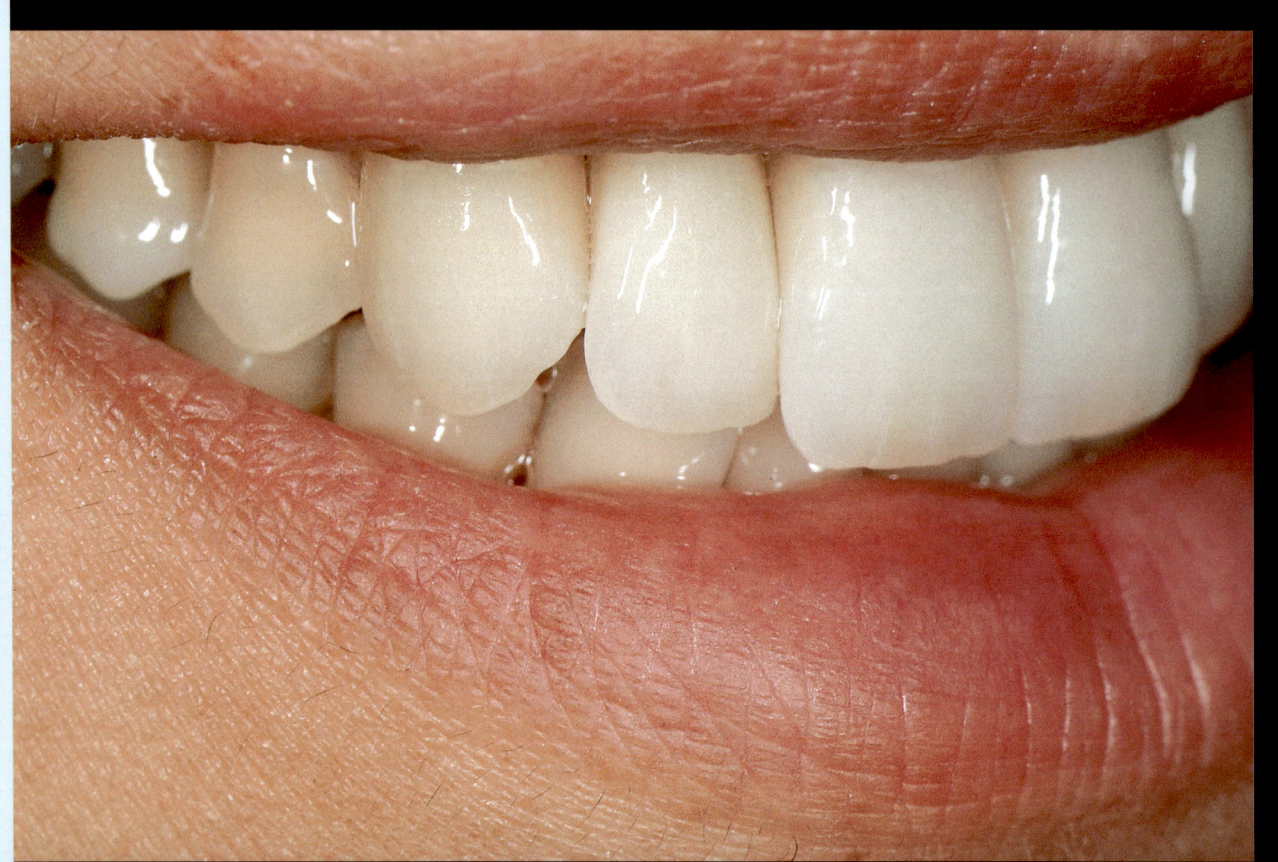

> Fig 5-48j

> Fig 5-48k

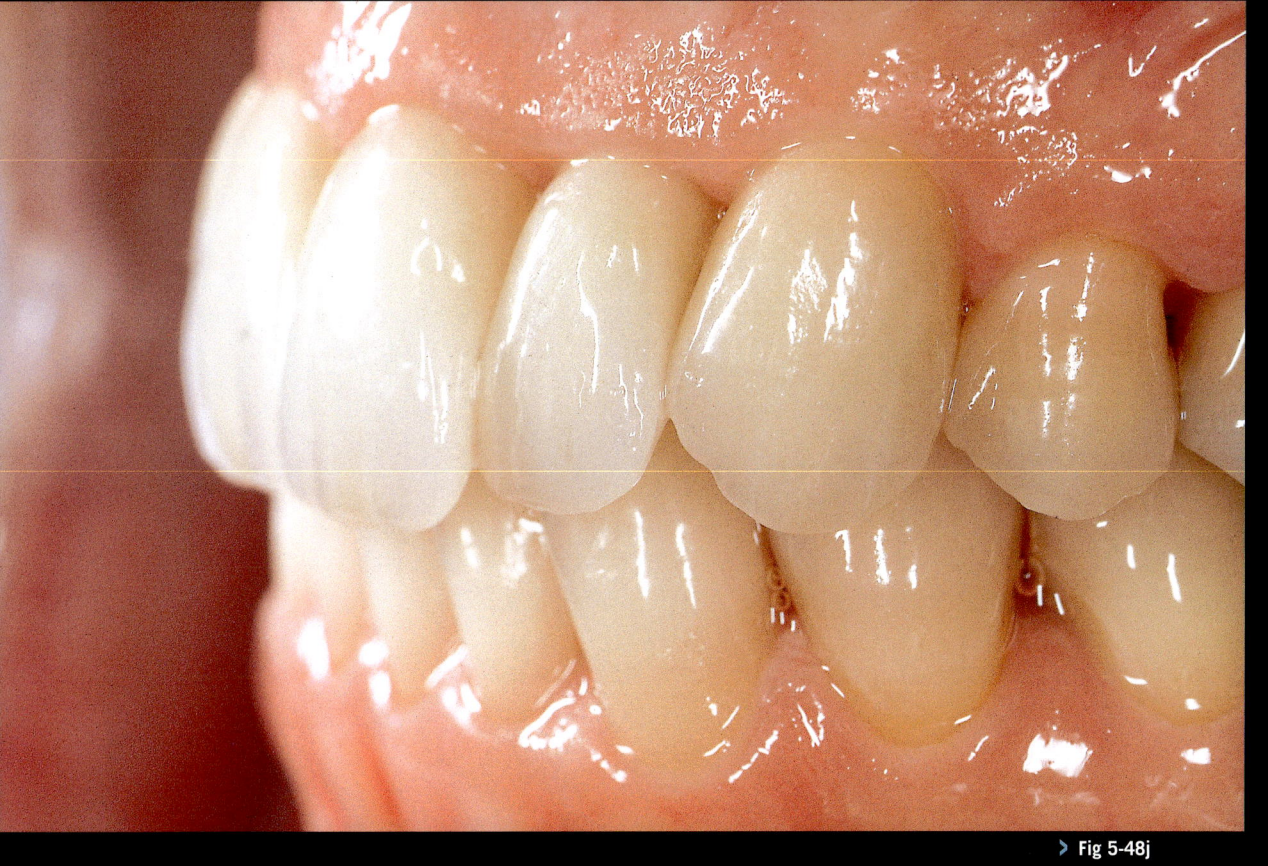

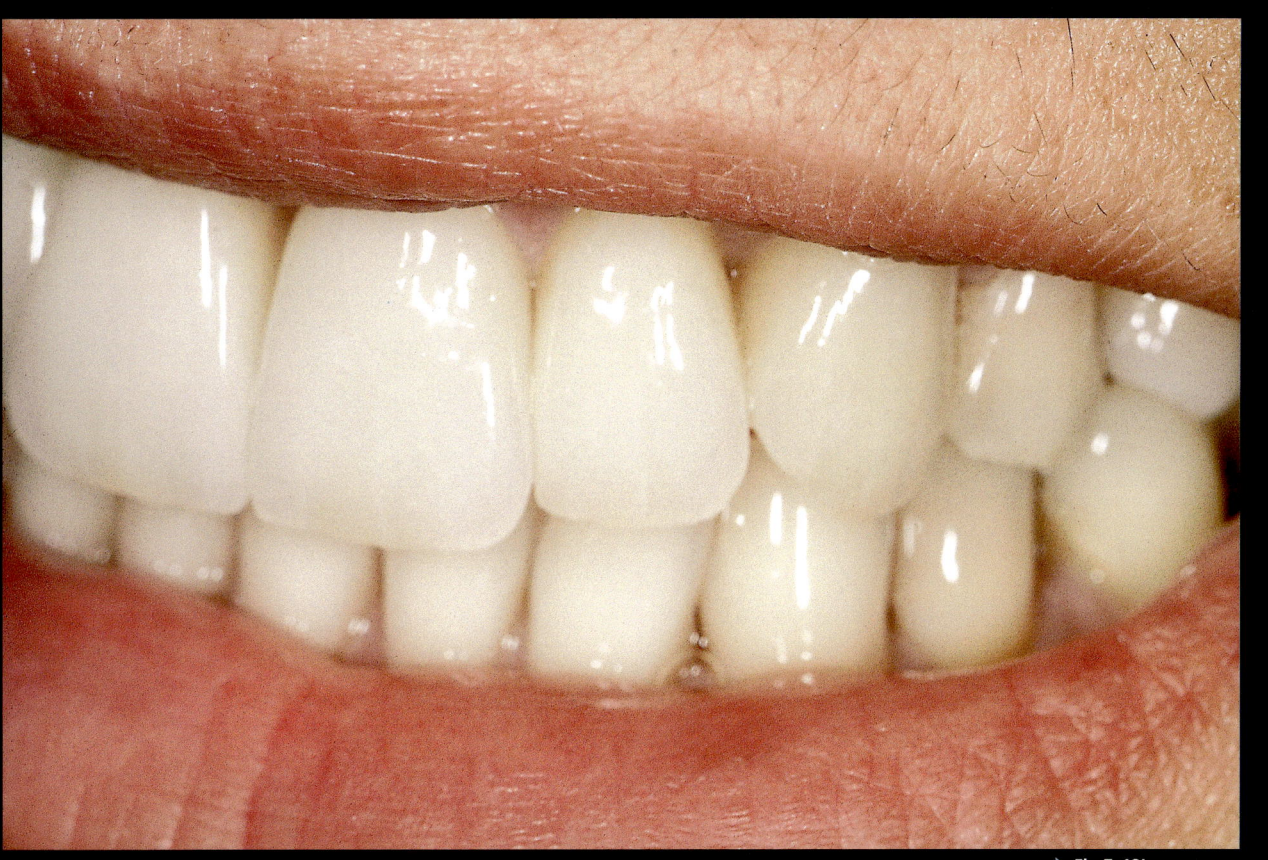

CASE 2

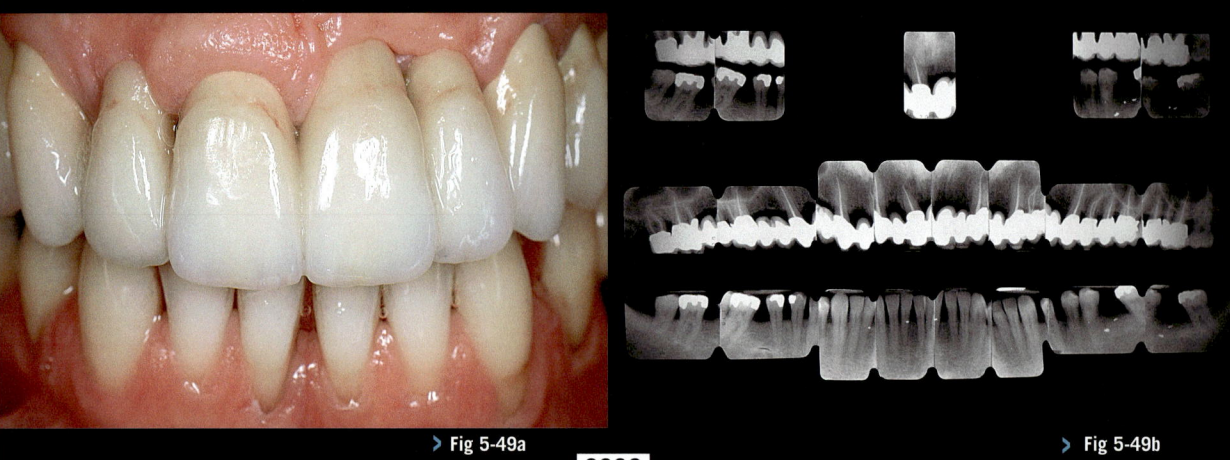

> Fig 5-49a

> Fig 5-49b

2000

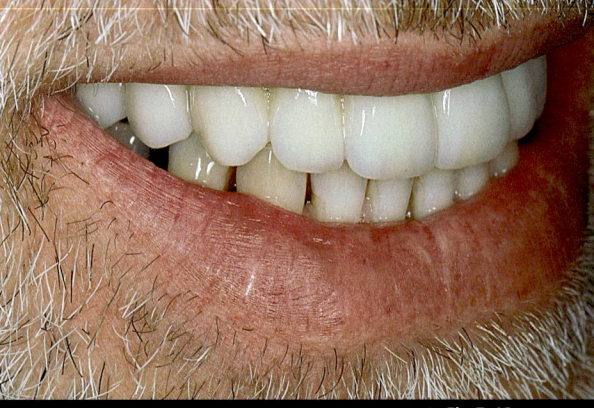

> Fig 5-49c

> Fig 5-49d

> Fig 5-49e

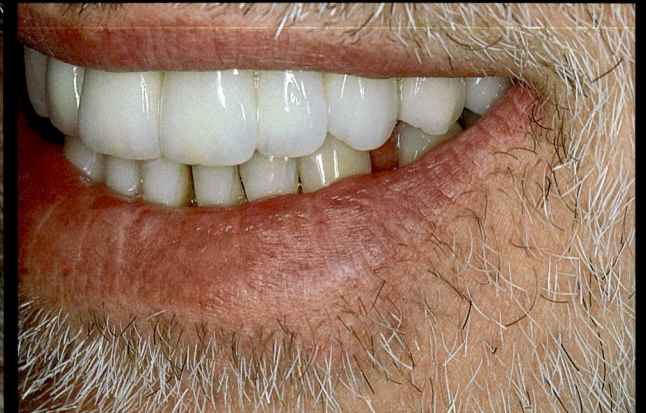

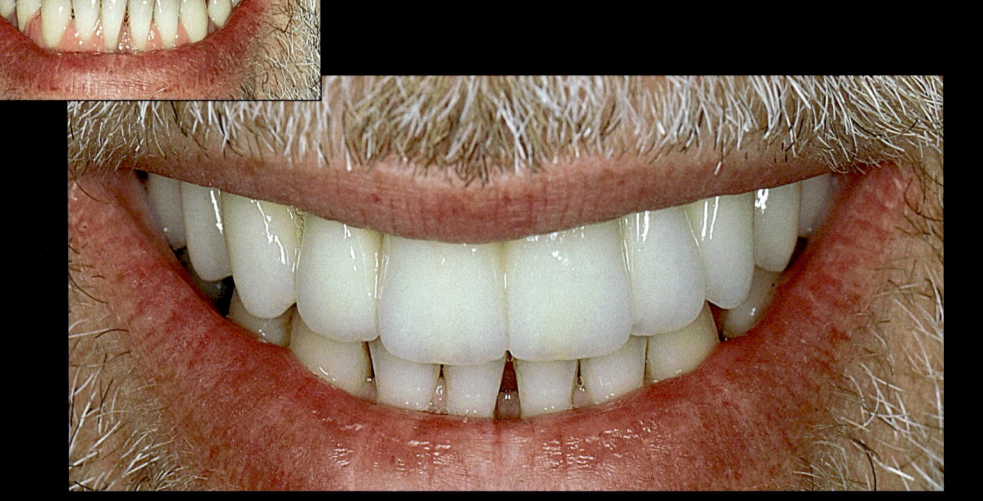

FIG 49 *(a to d)* On completion of the prosthetic-periodontal treatment of the maxillary arch, satisfactory integration has been achieved from the biologic and esthetic viewpoints. *(e)* This is especially evident in the comparison of the preoperative and postoperative photos. *(f to h)* From the functional point of view, the perfect coincidence of the VDO values can be seen between the provisional restorations, the PS, and the definitive restoration, achieved by following the systematic approach described in the text.

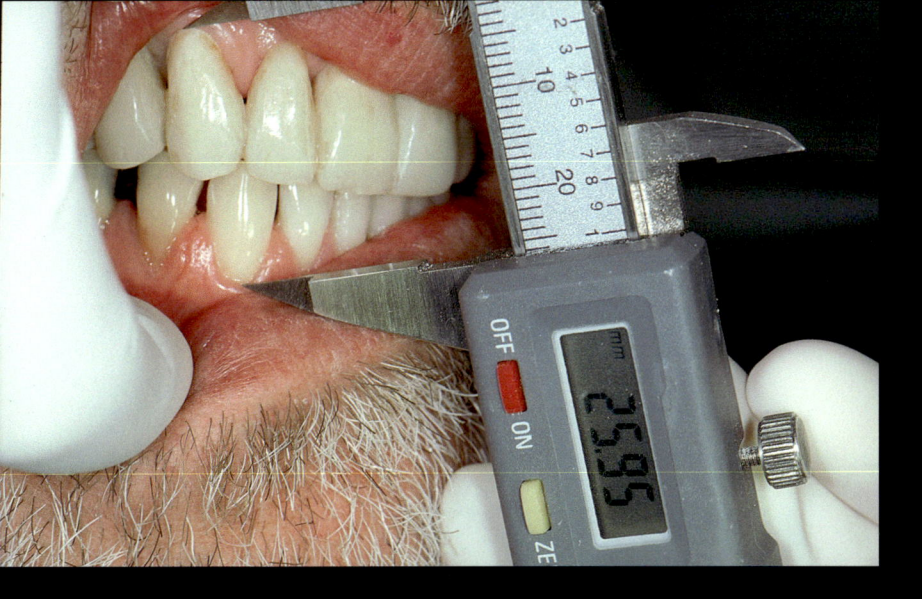

> Fig 5-49f

> Fig 5-49g

> Fig 5-49h

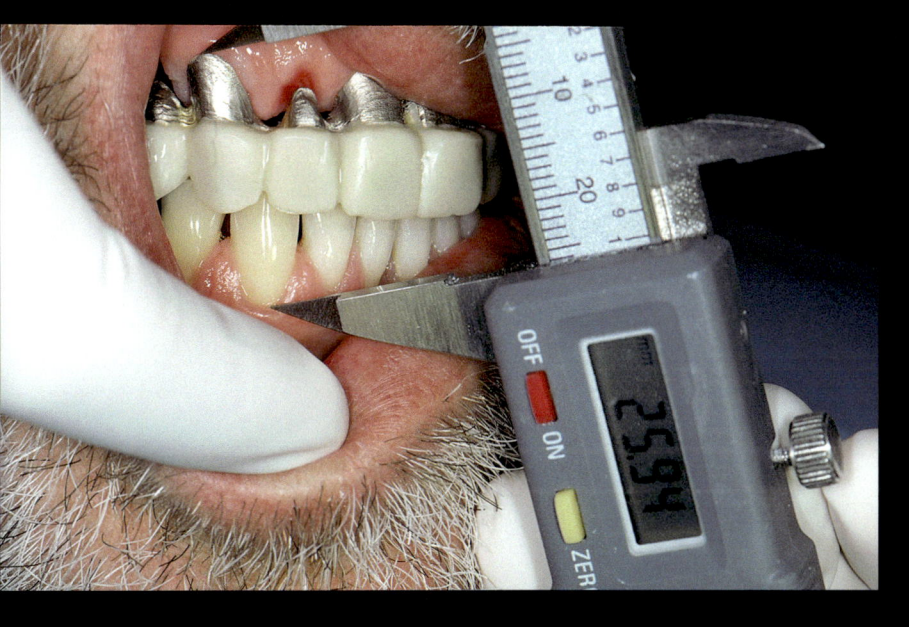

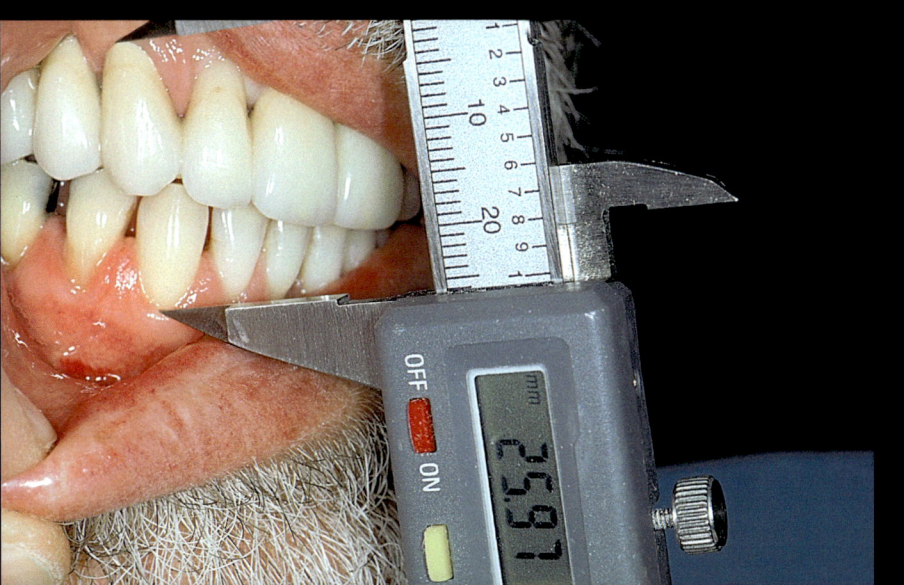

CASE 3

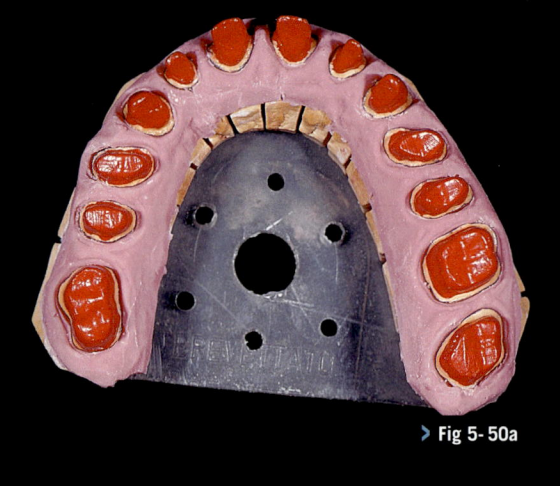

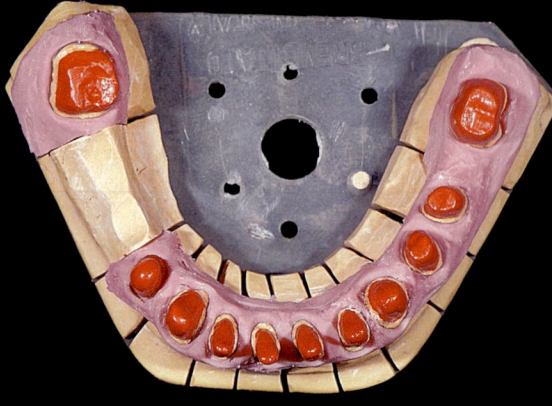

> Fig 5-50a

> Fig 5-50b

1999

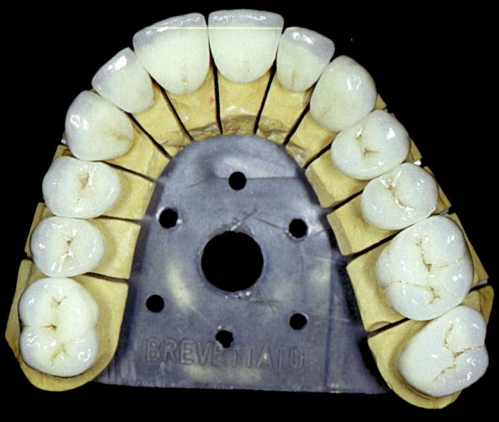

> Fig 5-50c

> Fig 5-50d

> Fig 5-50e

> Fig 5-50f

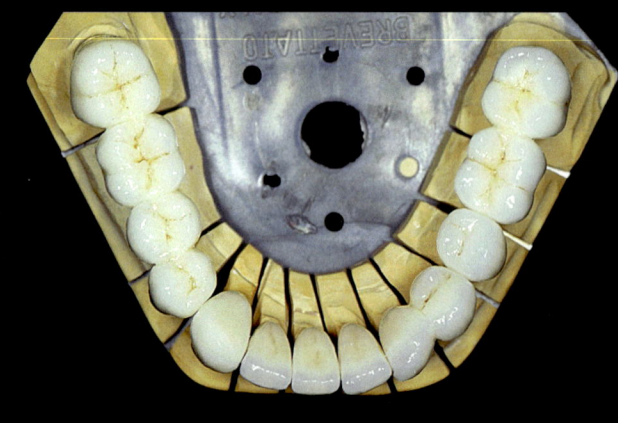

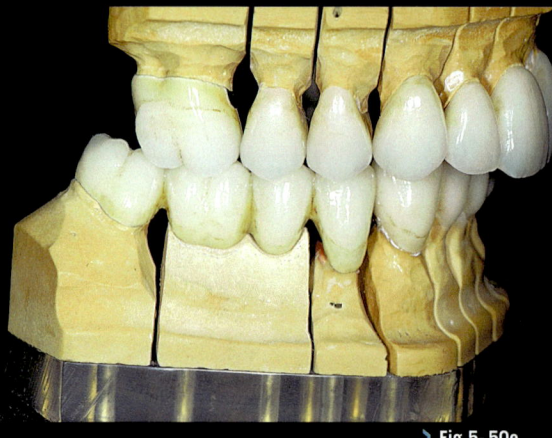

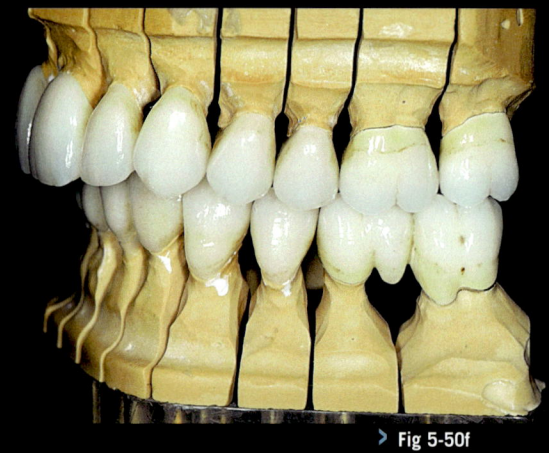

FIG 50 *(a and b)* The gingival matrices positioned on the MCs helped the technician design the restorative contours correctly. *(c to f)* After removing the gingival matrices, the clinician can carefully check for adequate marginal fits and ideal occlusal relationships. The occlusal registrations, recorded alternately between the abutments of one arch and the provisional restorations of the opposing arch, allow correct cross-mounting to be carried out. *(g to i)* It is therefore possible to invariably correlate the casts of the provisional restorations as well as the definitive restorations positioned on the MCs.

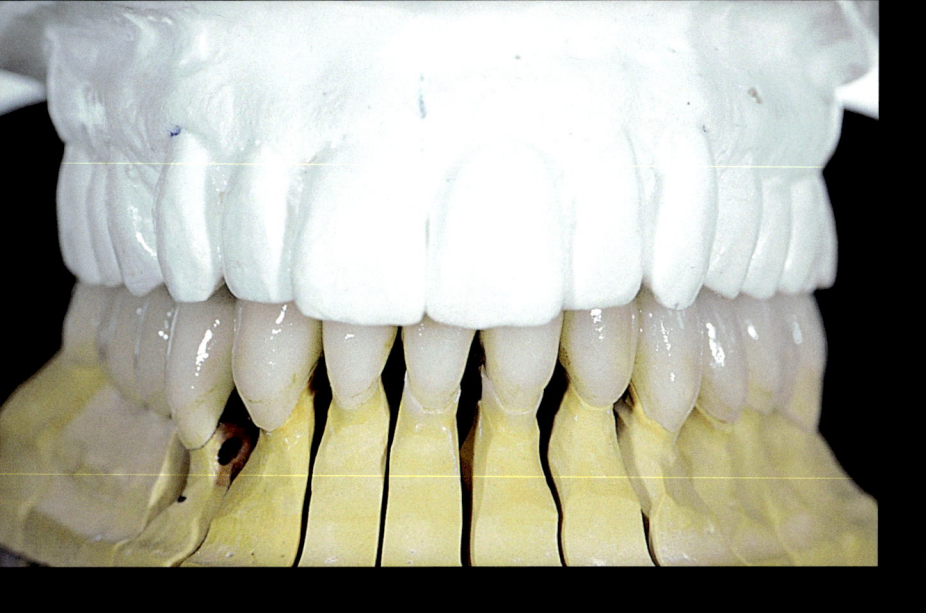

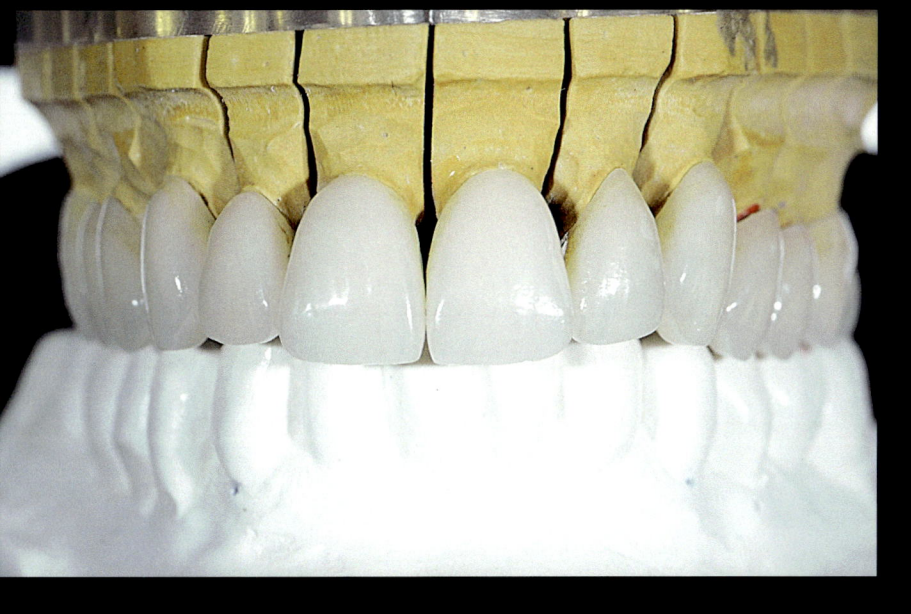

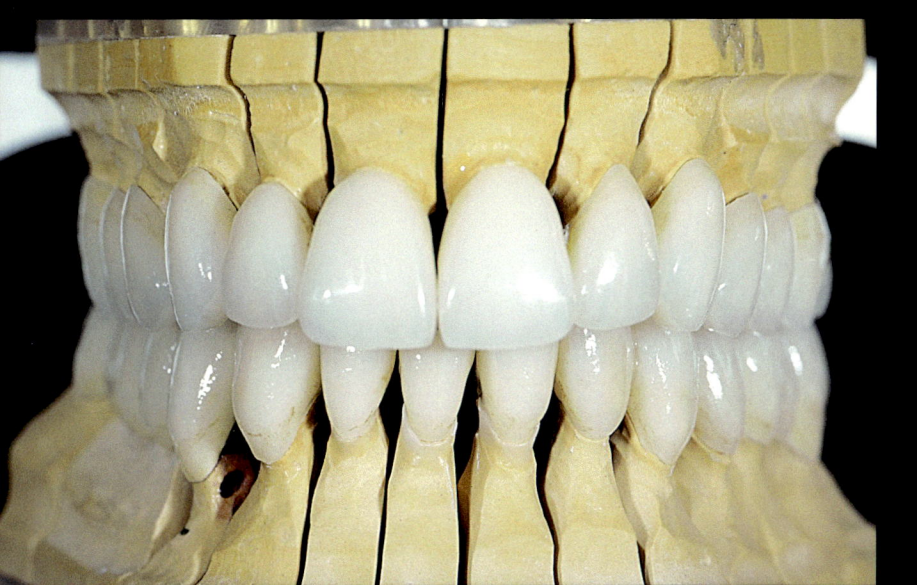

> Fig 5-50g

> Fig 5-50h

> Fig 5-50i

> Fig 5-50j

> Fig 5-50k

> Fig 5-50l

> Fig 5-50m

> Fig 5-50n

> Fig 5-50o

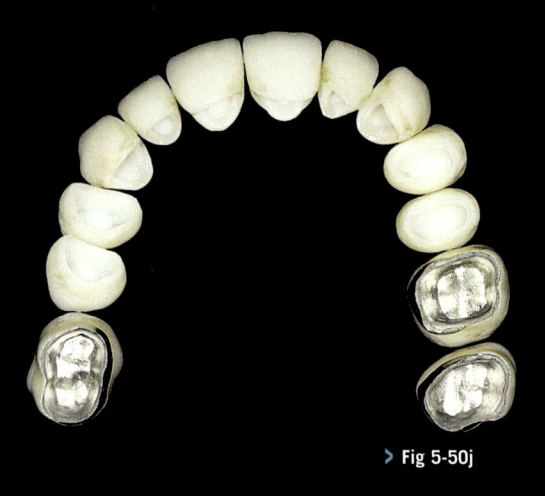

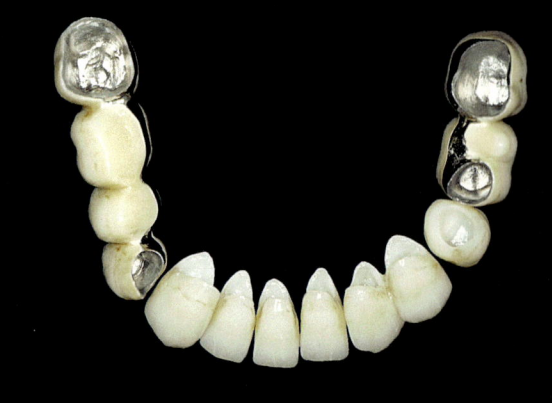

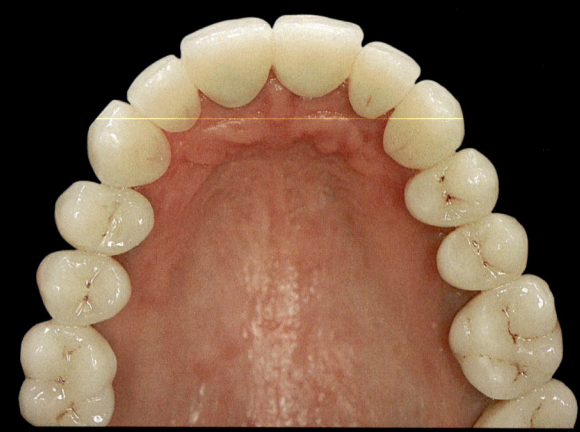

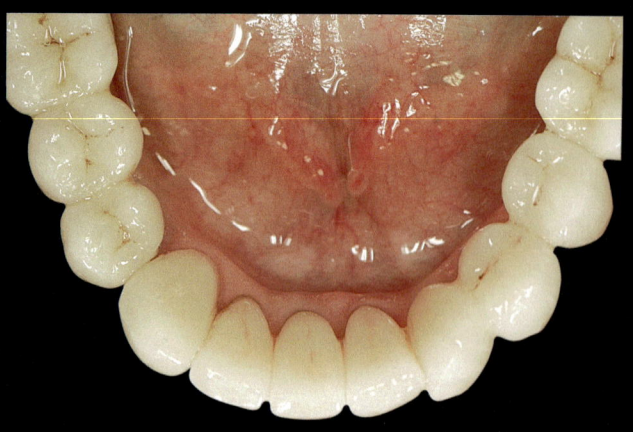

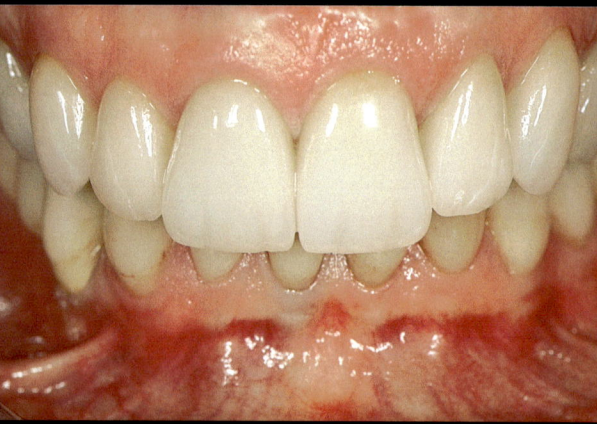

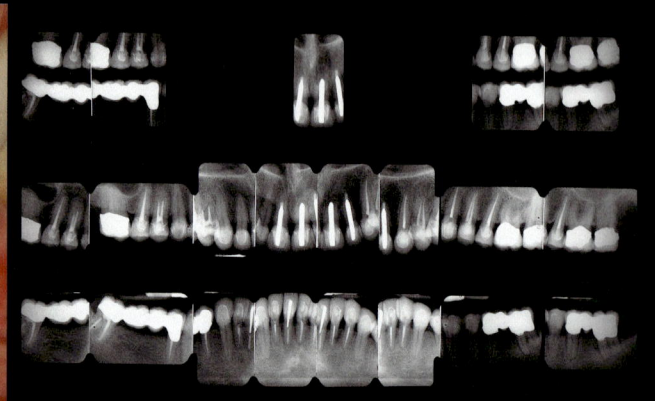

FIG 50 *(j to t)* The view of the two rehabilitations highlights the different materials chosen (all-ceramics in the anterior sector, metal-ceramics in the posterior sectors) and the satisfactory integration achieved, from the biologic, esthetic, and functional viewpoints.

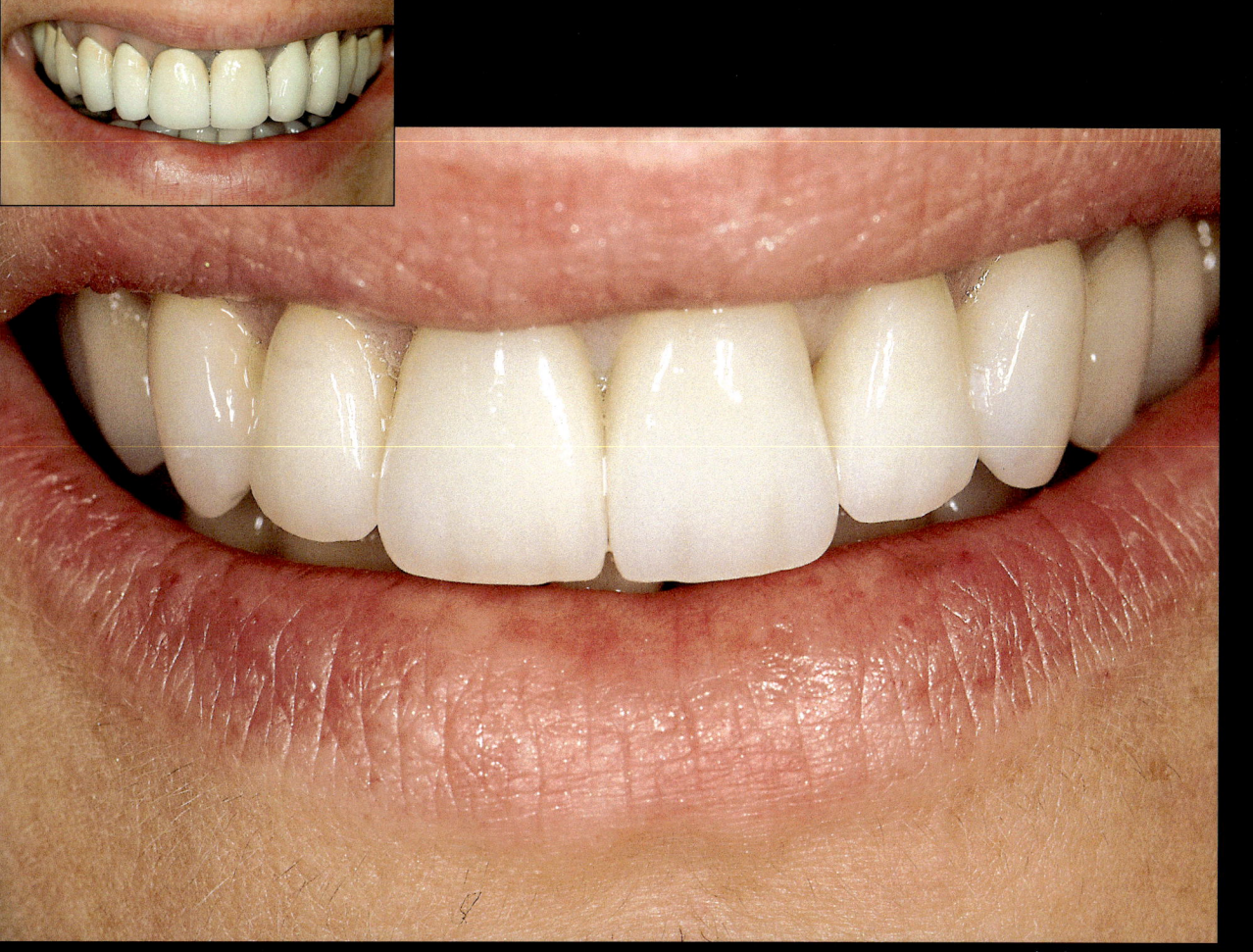

> Fig 5-50p

FROM THE PROVISIONAL TO THE DEFINITIVE RESTORATION

DATA TRANSFER Chapter 4	FINALIZATION Chapter 5
CLINIC	**LABORATORY**
▪ Impression of the provisional restoration	▪ Mounting the articulator with a facebow
▪ Impression of the antagonist	▪ Setting the articulator
▪ Protrusive occlusal registration	▪ Customized anterior guidance
▪ Facebow	▪ Silicone indices
▪ Final impression	▪ Constructing the substructure
▪ Occlusal registrations	▪ Preventive simulation
▪ Color transmission	▪ Finalization
▪ Laboratory checklist	

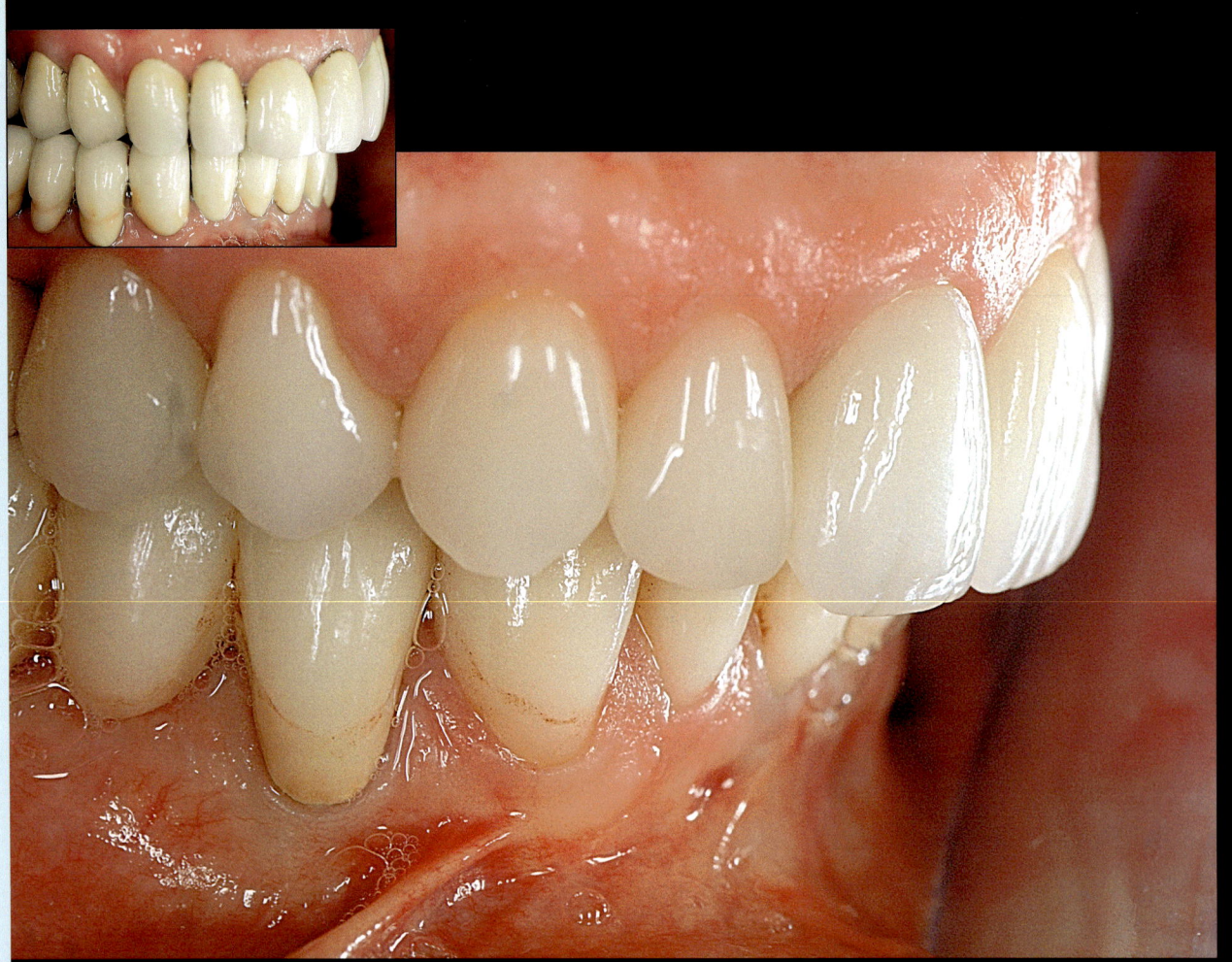

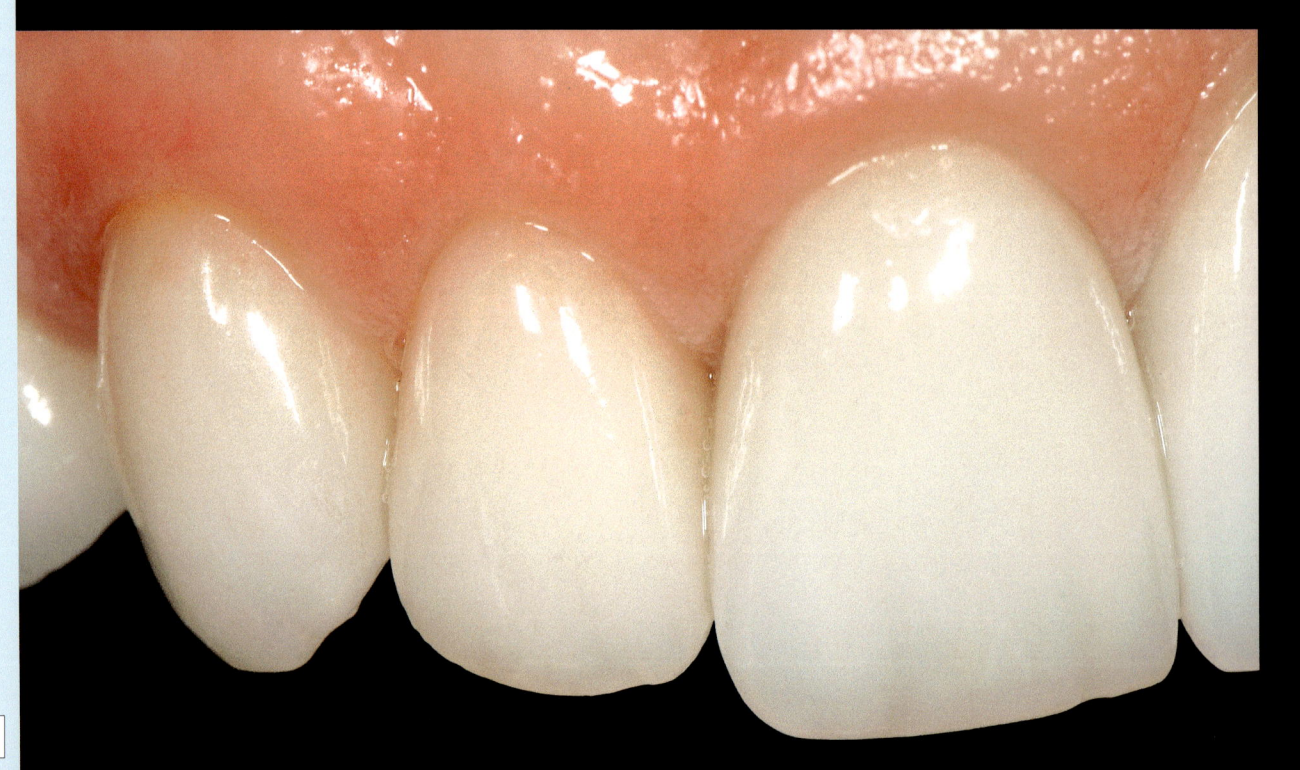

> Fig 5-50q

> Fig 5-50r

> Fig 5-50s

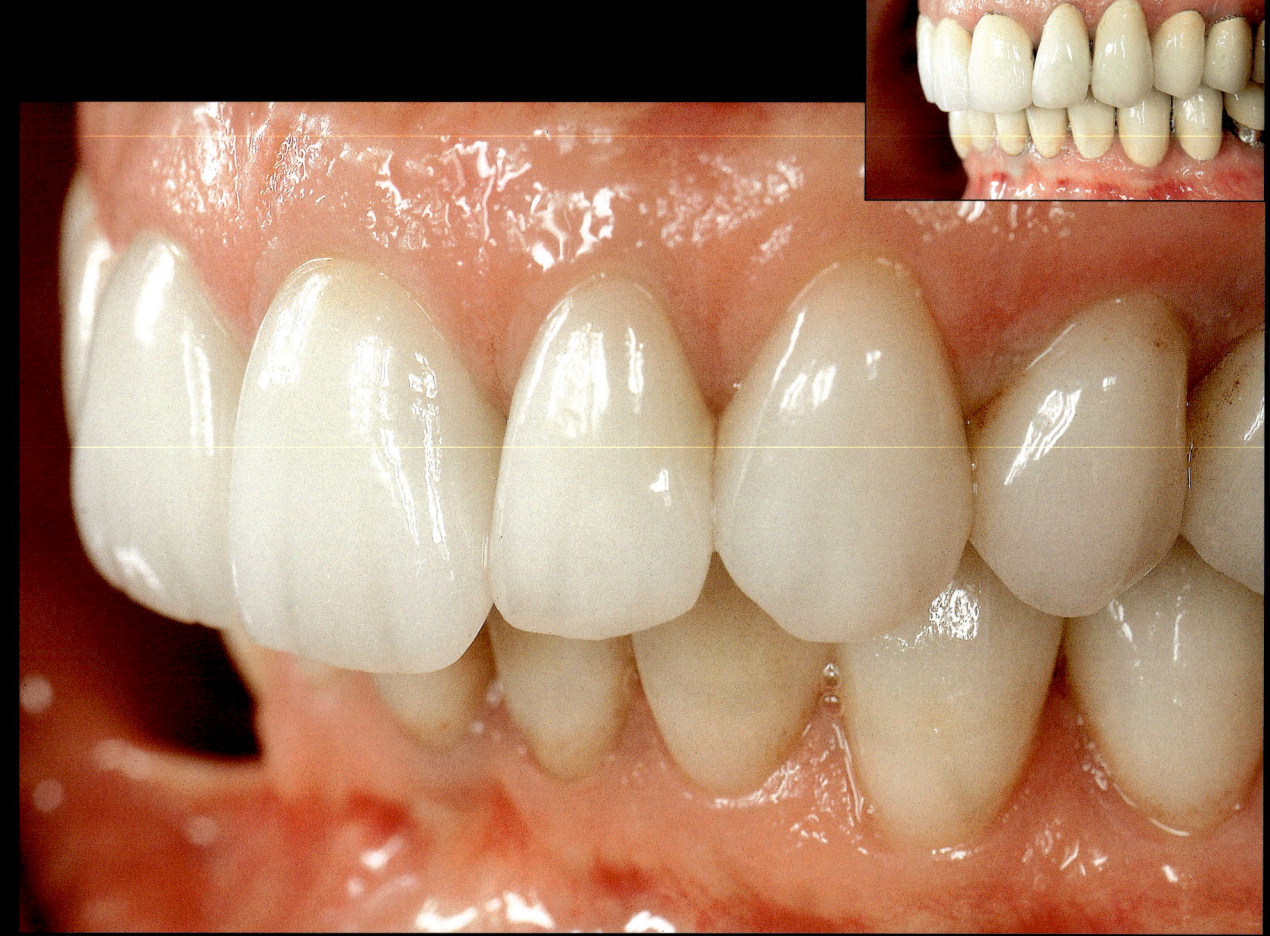

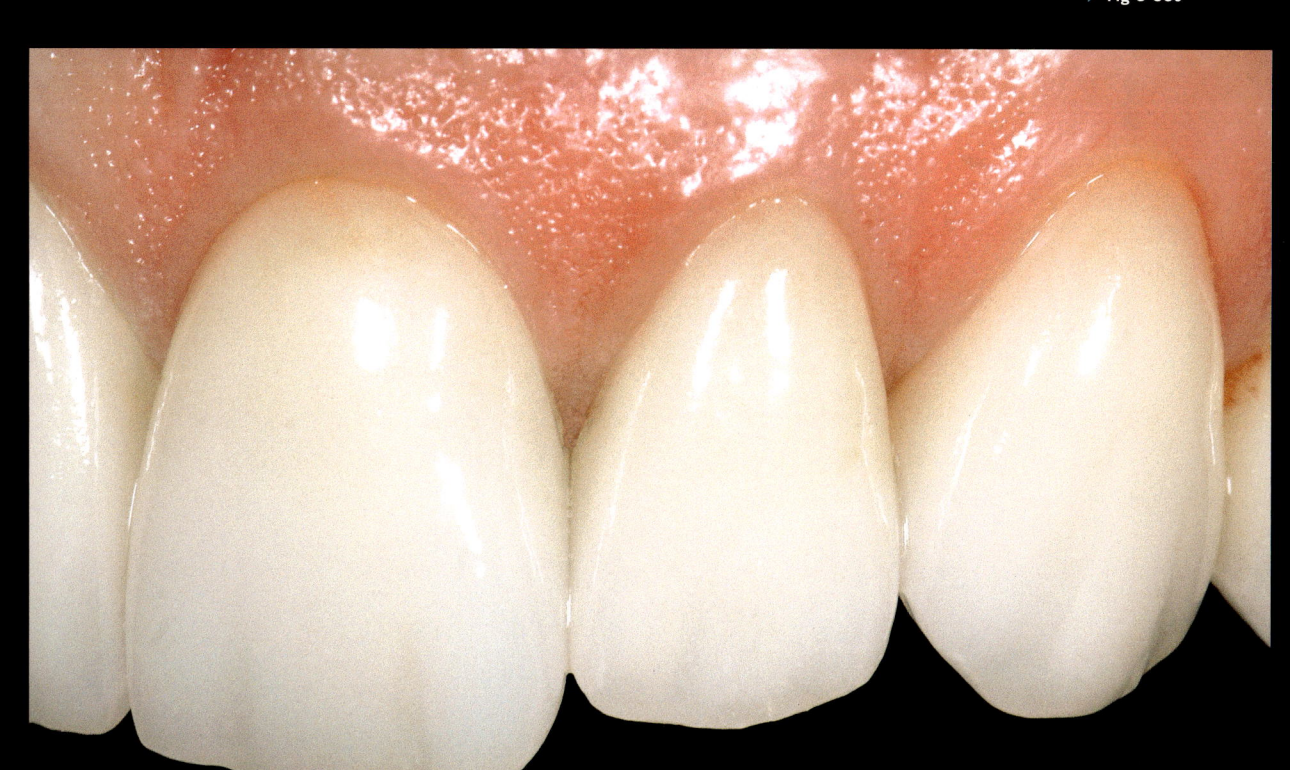

MAINTENANCE

Periodic checkups following delivery of the definitive restoration allow the clinician to monitor the patient's occlusal, neuromuscular, and articular status. If, in these checkups, slight fine adjustments on the occlusal table are considered, care must be taken to refine and polish the altered ceramic surfaces.

The clinician must also check for appropriate health of the gingival tissues. In the majority of cases, a good marginal adaptation and a correct coronal contour of the definitive restorations allow for an effective plaque-control regimen, thereby providing long-term prevention, either mostly[111,118,119] or completely,[120,121] of gingival inflammation. While with single restorations the use of a simple dental floss ensures good hygienic maintenance in all sectors of the oral cavity, posterior fixed partial dentures require the routine use of an interproximal brush that makes it possible to detect adequate integration of the restorations from a biologic viewpoint, even after the passage of time. In anterior fixed partial dentures, the use of superfloss is recommended; the interproximal brush could traumatize the papillae in these cases, flattening them and thus encouraging the onset of unattractive black triangles that are especially evident in the anterior sector. Once the restoration has been delivered, the patient must embark upon a series of professional hygiene recalls performed through periodic office appointments, especially in periodontally involved cases.[122–131] In these sessions it is advisable to avoid the use of ultrasonic instruments and cleaning systems that use an abrasive air jet. Even manual instruments (scalers and scrapers) must be handled with extreme care to prevent any roughening of the metal surface, if exposed, or microfracturing of the ceramic margins.[132,133]

A full-mouth radiographic series should be carried out periodically (every 2 years) to evaluate the periodontal and endodontic situation and to check for the presence of occlusal trauma[114] (Figs 5-51 to 5-53).

Only by completing regular checkups in the office is it possible to formulate an early diagnosis for intercepting any problems that may arise, thereby avoiding any possible failure of the prosthetic rehabilitation.

FIG 51 52 53 Even a few years after delivery, the restorations continue to demonstrate good biologic and esthetic-functional integration.

CASE 1

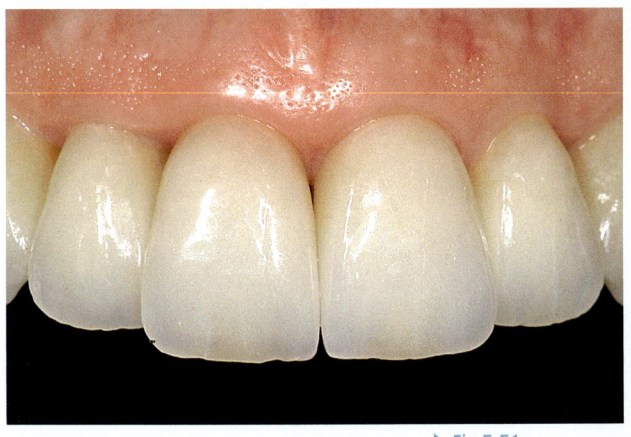

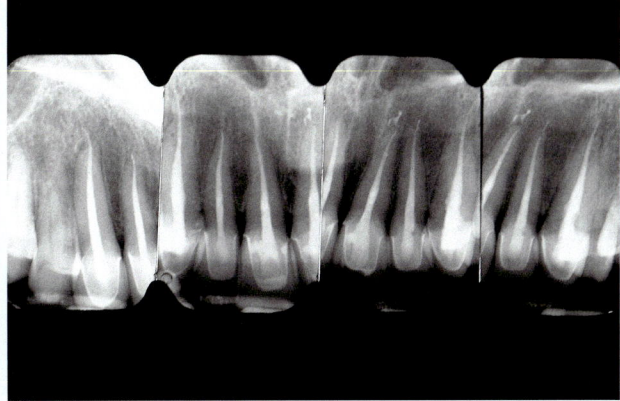

> Fig 5-51a 2007

> Fig 5-51b

CASE 2

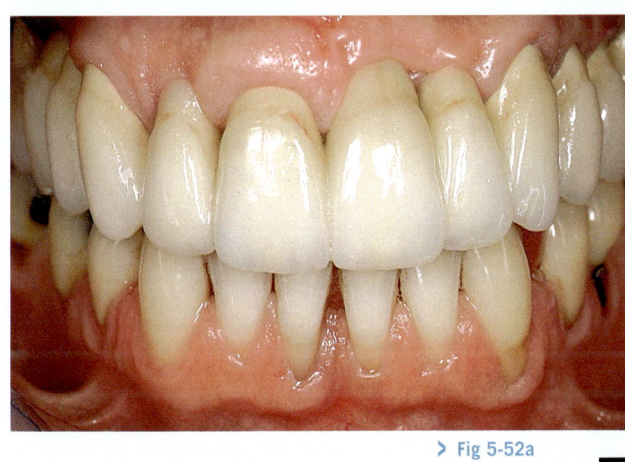

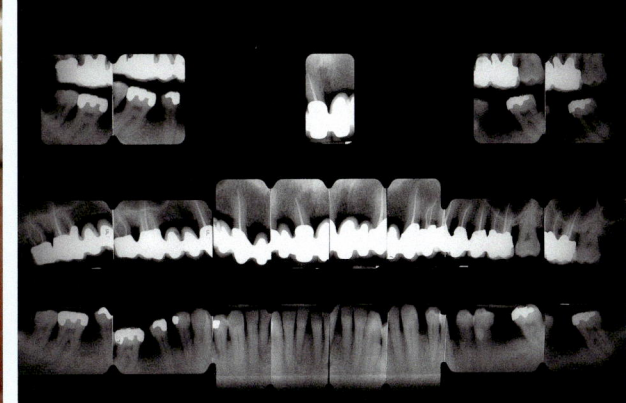

> Fig 5-52a 2007

> Fig 5-52b

CASE 3

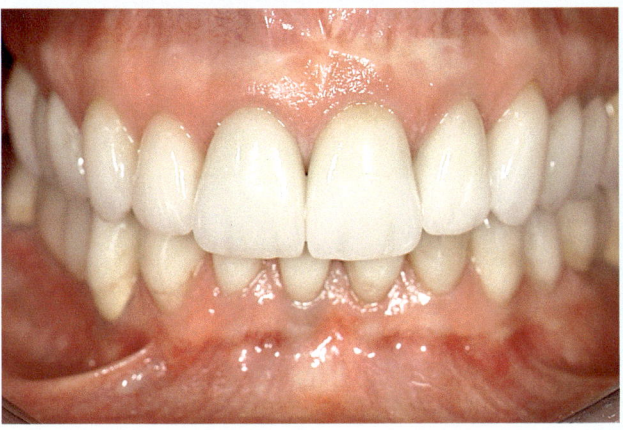

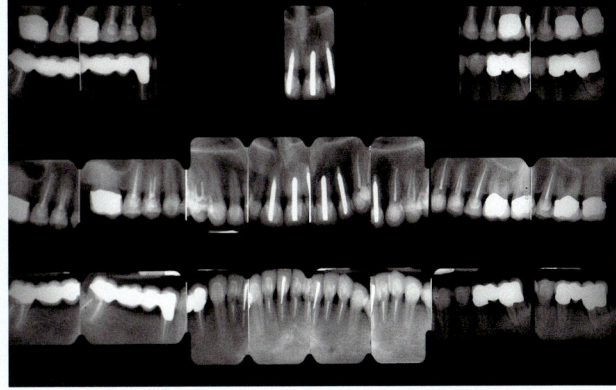

> Fig 5-53a 2007

> Fig 5-53b

519

REFERENCES

1. Waerhaug J, Zander HA. Reaction of gingival tissues to self-curing acrylic restorations. J Am Dent Assoc 1957; 54:760–768.

2. Perel ML. Axial crown contours. J Prosthet Dent 1971; 25:642–649.

3. Perel ML. Periodontal considerations of crown contours. J Prosthet Dent 1971;26:627–630.

4. Donaldson D. Gingival recession associated with temporary crowns. J Periodontol 1973;44:691–696.

5. Yuodelis RA, Weaver JD, Sapkos S. Facial and lingual contours of artificial complete crown restorations and their effects on the periodontium. J Prosthet Dent 1973;29:61–66.

6. Donaldson D. The etiology of gingival recession associated with temporary crowns. J Periodontol 1974; 45:468–471.

7. Weisgold AS. Contours of the full crown restorations. Alpha Omegan 1977:70:77–89.

8. Maynard JG Jr, Wilson RD. Physiologic dimensions of the periodontium significant to the restorative dentist. J Periodontol 1979;50:170–174.

9. Dragoo MR, Williams GB. Periodontal tissue reactions to restorative procedures. Int J Periodontics Restorative Dent 1981;1:8–23.

10. Ehrlich J, Yaffe A, Weisgold AS. Faciolingual width before and after tooth restoration: a comparative study. J Prosthet Dent 1981;46:153–156.

11. Garvin PH, Malone WF, Toto PD, Mazur B. Effect of self-curing acrylic resin treatment restorations on the crevicular fluid volume. J Prosthet Dent 1982;47: 284–289.

12. Parma Benfenati S, et al. The effect of restorative margins on the postsurgical development and nature of the periodontium. Part I: anatomical considerations. Int J Periodontics Restorative Dent 1985;6:31–51.

13. Kois JC. The restorative-periodontal interface: biological parameters. Periodontol 2000 1996;11: 29–38.

14. Gracis S, Fradeani M, Celletti R, Bracchetti G. Biological integration of aesthetic restorations: factors influencing appearance and long-term success. Periodontol 2000 2001;27:29–44.

15. Chiche GJ, Pinault A. Communication with the dental laboratory: try-in procedures and shade selection. In: Chiche GJ, Pinault A (eds). Esthetics of Anterior Fixed Prosthodontics. Chicago: Quintessence, 1994: 115–142.

16. O'Brien WJ. Dental Materials and Their Selection, 2nd ed. Chicago: Quintessence, 1997:51–77.

17. Martignoni M, Schonenberger A. Precision Fixed Prosthodontics: Clinical and Laboratory Aspects. Chicago: Quintessence, 1990.

18. Ghahremannezhad HH, Mohamed SE, Stewart GP, Weinberg R. Effects of cyanoacrylates on die stone. J Prosthet Dent 1983;49:639–646.

19. Eames WB, Wallace SW, Suway NB, Rogers LB. Accuracy and dimensional stability of elastomeric impression materials. J Prosthet Dent 1979;42:159–162.

20. Marcinak CF, Draughn A. Linear dimensional changes in addition curing silicone impression materials. J Prosthet Dent 1982;47:411–413.

21. Williams PT, Jackson G, Bergman W. An evaluation of time-depedent dimensional stability of eleven elastomeric impression materials. J Prosthet Dent 1984;52:120–125.

22. Gordon GE, Johnson GH, Drennon DG. The effect of tray selection on the accuracy of elastomeric impression materials. J Prosthet Dent 1990;63:12–15.

23. Wassel RW, Ibbetson RJ. The accuracy of polyvinyl siloxane impressions made with standard and reinforced stock trays. J Prosthet Dent 1991;65: 748–757.

24. Price RB, Gerrow JD, Sutow EJ, MacSween R. The dimensional accuracy of 12 impression material and die stone combinations. Int J Prosthodont 1991;4:169–174.

25. Panichuttra R, Jones RM, Goodacre C, Munoz CA, Moore BK. Hydrophilic Poly(vinyl siloxane) impression materials: dimensional accuracy, wettability, and effect on gypsum hardness. Int J Prosthodont 1991;4: 240–248.

26. Hung SH, Purk JH, Tira DE, Eick JD. Accuracy of one-step versus two-step putty wash addition silicone impression technique. J Prosthet Dent 1992;67: 583–589.

27. Campbell SD. Comparison of conventional paint-on die spacers and those used with the all-ceramic restorations. J Prosthet Dent 1990;63:151–155.

28. Kuwata M. Color Atlas of Ceramo-Metal Technology. St Louis: Ishiyaku EuroAmerica. 1986.

29. Miller LL. Framework design in ceramo-metal restorations. Dent Clin North Am 1977;21:699–716.

30. Stein RS, Kuwata M. A dentist and a dental technologist analyze current ceramo-metal procedures. Dent Clin North Am 1977;21:729–749.

31. McLean JW. The Science and Art of Dental Ceramics. Vol II: Bridge Design and Laboratory Procedures in Dental Ceramics. Chicago: Quintessence, 1980.

32. Miller L. A clinician's interpretation of tooth preparation and the design of metal substructures for metal-ceramic restorations. In: McLean JW (ed). Dental Ceramics: Proceedings of the First International Symposium on Ceramics. Chicago: Quintessence, 1983:153–206.

33. Berger RP. Esthetic considerations in framework design. In: Preston JD (ed). Perspectives in Dental Ceramics: Proceedings of the Fourth International Symposium on Ceramics. Chicago: Quintessence, 1998:237–249.

34. Pameijer JHN. Periodontal and Occlusal Factors in Crown and Bridge Procedures. Amsterdam: Dental Center for Postgraduate Courses, 1985:331–345.

35. Dawson PE. Evaluation, Diagnosis, and Treatment of Occlusal Problems, ed 2. St Louis: Mosby, 1989: 206–237.

36. Weiner S. Biomechanics of occlusion and the articulator. Dent Clin North Am 1995;39:257–284.

37. Gracis S. Clinical considerations and rationale for the use of simplified instrumentation in occlusal rehabilitation. Part 1: mounting of the models on the articulator. Int J Periodontics Restorative Dent 2003;23:57–67.

38. Linke B, Nicholls JI, Faucher R. Distortion analysis of stone casts made from impression materials. J Prosthet Dent 1985;54:794–802.

39. Boyarsky HP, Loos LG, Leknius C. Occlusal refinement of mounted casts before crown fabrication to decrease clinical time required to adjust occlusion. J Prosthet Dent 1999;82:591–594.

40. Gracis S. Clinical considerations and rationale for the use of simplified instrumentation in occlusal rehabilitation. Part 2: setting of the articulator and occlusal optimization. Int J Periodontics Restorative Dent 2003;23:139–145.

41. Dawson PE. Temporomandibular joint pain-dysfunction problems can be solved. J Prosthet Dent 1973;29:100–112.

42. McKee JR. Comparing condylar position repeatability for standardized versus nonstandardized methods of achieving centric relation. J Prosthet Dent 1997;77:280–284.

43. Tarantola GJ, Becker IM, Gremillion H. The reproducibility of centric relation: a clinical approach. J Am Dent Assoc 1997;128:1245–1251.

44. Lundeen HC, Wirth CG. Condylar movement patterns engraved in plastic blocks. J Prosthet Dent 1973;30:866–875.

45. Lundeen HC, Shryock EF, Gibbs CH. An evaluation of mandibular border movements: their character and significance. J Prosthet Dent 1978;40:442–452.

46. Molina M. Concetti Fondamentali di Gnatologia Moderna. Milan, Italy: Riccardo Ilic Editrice, 1988:199–241.

47. Dawson PE. Evaluation, Diagnosis, and Treatment of Occlusal Problems, ed 2. St Louis: Mosby, 1989:321–352.

48. Leempoel PJ, Eschen S, De Haan AF, Van't Hof MA. An evaluation of crowns and bridges in a general dental practice. J Oral Rehabil 1985;12:515–528.

49. Kerschbaum T, Paszyna C, Klapp S, Meyer G. Failure time and risk analysis of fixed partial dentures. Dtsch Zahnarztl Z 1991;46:20–24.

50. Walton TR. A 10-year longitudinal study of fixed prosthodontics: clinical characteristics and outcome of single-unit metal-ceramic crowns. Int J Prosthodont, 1999;12:519–526.

51. Walton TR. An up to 15-year longitudinal study of 515 metal-ceramic FPDs: Part 1. Outcome. Int J Prosthodont 2002;15:439–445.

52. Yamamoto M. Metal-Ceramics. Chicago: Quintessence, 1985:219–291.

53. Kuwata M. Gingival margin design of abutments for ceramo-metal restorations. Quintessence Dent Tech 1979;10:27.

54. Kuwata M. Dental metal-ceramics and their clinical application. Metal-ceramic binding sites. Quintessenz Zahntech 1984;10:1005–1015.

55. Heffernan MJ, Aquilino SA, Diaz-Arnold AM, Haselton DR, Stanford CM, Vargas MA. Relative traslucency of six all-ceramic systems. Part II: core materials. J Prosthet Dent 2002;88:4–9.

56. Heffernan MJ, Aquilino SA, Diaz-Arnold AM, Haselton DR, Stanford CM, Vargas MA. Relative translucency of six all-ceramic systems. Part II: core and veneer materials. J Prosthet Dent 2002;88:10–5.

57. Campbell SD. A comparative strength study of metal ceramic and all-ceramic esthetic materials: modulus of rupture. J Prosthet Dent 1989;62:476–479.

58. Seghi RR, Sorensen JA, Engelman MJ, et al. Flexural strength of new ceramic materials. J Dent Res 1990;69:299 (Abstract No. 1348).

59. Seghi RR, Sorensen JA. Relative flexural strength of six new ceramic materials. Int J Prosthodont 1995;8:239–246.

60. Friedman MJ. A 15-year review of porcelain veneer failure: a clinician's observations. Compend Contin Educ Dent 1998;19:625–632.

61. Peumans M, Van Meerbeek B, Lambrechts P, Vuylsteke-Wauters M, Vanherle G. Five-year clinical performance of porcelain veneers. Quintessence Int 1998;29:211–221.

62. Magne P, Perroud R, Hodges JS, Belser U. Clinical performance of novel-desing porcelain veneers for the recovery of coronal volume and length. Int J Periodontics Restorative Dent 2000;20:440–457.

63. Dumfahrt H, Schaffer H. Porcelain laminate veneers. A retrospective evaluation after 1 to 10 years of service: Part II – Clinical results. Int J Prosthodont 2000;13:9–18.

64. Fradeani M, Redemagni M, Corrado M. Porcelain laminate veneers: 6-to 12-year clinical evaluation—a retrospective study. Int J Periodontics Restorative Dent 2005;25:9–17.

65. Schweiger M, Höland W, Frank M, et al. IPS Empress 2: a new pressable high-strength glass-ceramic restoration. Quintessence Dent Technol 1999;22:143–151.

66. Fradeani M, Aquilano A. Clinical experience with Empress crowns. Int J Prosthodont 1997;10:241–247.

67. Sorensen JA, Choi C, Fanuscu MI, Mito WT. IPS Empress crown system: three-year clinical trial results. J Calif Dent Assoc 1998;26:130–136.

68. Sjogren G, Lantto R, Granberg A, Sundstrom BO, Tillberg A. Clinical examination of leucite-reinforced glass-ceramic crowns (Empress) in general practice: a retrospective study. Int J Prosthodont 1999;12:122–128.

69. Fradeani M, Redemagni M. An 11-year clinical evaluation of leucite-reinforced glass-ceramic crowns: a retrospective study. Quintessence Int 2002;33:503–510.

70. El-Mowafy O, Brochu JF. Longevity and clinical performance of IPS-Empress ceramic restorations – a literature review. J Can Dent Assoc 2002;68:233–237.

71. Marquardt P, Strub JR. Survival rates of IPS Empress 2 all-ceramic crowns and fixed partial dentures: Results of a 5-year prospective clinical study. Quintessence Int 2006;37:253–259.

72. White SN, Caputo AA, Li ZC, Zhao XY. Modulus of rupture of the Procera All-Ceramic System. J Esthet Dent 1996;8:120–126.

73. Zeng K, Oden A, Rowcliffe D. Flexure tests on dental ceramics. Int J Prosthodont 1996;9:434–439.

74. Oden A, Andersson M, Krystek-Ondracek I, Magnusson D. Five-year clinical evaluation of Procera AllCeram crowns. J Prosthet Dent 1998;80:450–456.

75. Odman P, Andersson B. Procera AllCeram crowns followed for 5 to 10.5 years: a prospective clinical study. Int J Prosthodont 2001;14:504–509.

76. Fradeani M, D'Amelio M, Redemagni M, Corrado M. Five-year follow-up with Procera all-ceramic crowns. Quintessence Int 2005;36:105–113.

77. Sadan A, Blatz MB, Lang B. Clinical considerations for densely sintered alumina and zirconia restorations: part 1. Int J Periodontics Restorative Dent 2005;25:213–219.

78. Sadan A, Blatz MB, Lang B. Clinical considerations for densely sintered alumina and zirconia restorations: part 2. Int J Periodontics Restorative Dent 2005;25:343–349.

79. Luthardt RG, Holzhuter MS, Rudolph H, Herold V, Walter MH. CAD/CAM-machining effects on Y-TZP zirconia. Dent Mater 2004;20:655–662.

80. Raigrodski AJ. Contemporary materials and technologies for all-ceramic fixed partial dentures: a review of the literature. J Prosthet Dent 2004;92:557–562.

81. McLean JW. The Science and Art of Dental Ceramics. Vol I. Chicago: Quintessence, 1979.

82. Yamamoto M. Metal-ceramics. Tokyo: Quintessence, 1982.

83. Segal BS. Retrospective assessment of 546 all-ceramic anterior and posterior crowns in a general practice. J Prosthet Dent 2001;85:544–550.

84. Costello RV, Thompson J, Sadan A, Burgess JO, Blatz MB. Light transmission of high-strength ceramics with four curing lights [Abstract 1813]. J Dent Res 2004;83(Spec Issue A).

85. Sailer I, Feher A, Filser F, Luthy H, Gauckler LJ, Scharer P, Franz Hammerle CH. Prospective clinical study of zirconia posterior fixed partial dentures: 3-year follow-up. Quintessence Int 2006;37:685–693.

86. Christensen GJ. Marginal fit of gold inlay castings. J Prosthet Dent 1966;16:297–305.

87. Davis SH, Kelly JR, Campbell SD. Use of an elastomeric material to improve the occlusal seat and marginal seal of cast restorations. J Prosthet Dent 1989;62:288–291.

88. Sorensen JA. Improved seating of ceramic inlays with a silicone fit-checking medium. J Prosthet Dent 1991;65:646–649.

89. White SN, Sorensen JA, Kang SK. Improved marginal seating of cast restorations using a silicone disclosing medium. Int J Prosthodont 1991;4:323–326.

90. Yamamoto M. Metal-ceramics. Chicago: Quintessence, 1985:15–202.

91. McLean JW. The Science and Art of Dental Ceramics. Vol II: Bridge Design and Laboratory Procedures in Dental Ceramics. Chicago: Quintessence, 1980:242.

92. Blatz MB, Sadan A, Kern M. Resin-ceramic bonding: a review of the literature. J Prosthet Dent 2003;89:268–274.

93. Zhang Y, Lawn BR, Rekow ED, Van Thompson P. Effect of sandblasting on the long-term performance of dental ceramics. J Biomed Mater Res 2004;15:71B:381–386.

94. Zhang Y, Lawn BR, Malament KA, Thompson VP, Rekow ED. Damage accumulation and fatigue life of particle-abraded ceramics. Int J Prosthodont 2006;19:442–448.

95. Muya PJ. The Four-Dimensional Tooth Color System. Chicago: Quintessence, 1982.

96. Krough-Poulsen WG, Olsson A. Management of the occlusion of the teeth: background, definitions, rationale. In: Schwartz L, Chayes C (eds). Facial Pain and Mandibular Dysfunction. Philadelphia: WB Saunders, 1968.

97. Dawson PE, Arcan M. Attaining harmonic occlusion through visualized strain analysis. J Prosthet Dent 1981;46:615–622.

98. Ramfjord S, Ash MM. Occlusion, ed 3. Philadelphia: WB Saunders, 1983.

99. Dawson PE. Evaluation, Diagnosis, and Treatment of Occlusal Problems, ed 2. St Louis: Mosby, 1989:14–17.

100. Weinberg LA. The role of muscle deconditioning for occlusal corrective procedures. J Prosthet Dent 1991;66:250–255.

101. Spear FM. Occlusal considerations for complex restorative therapy. In: McNeill C (ed). Science and Practice of Occlusion. Chicago: Quintessence, 1997:437–456.

102. D'Amico A. The canine teeth-normal functional relation of the natural teeth of man. J South Calif Dent Assoc 1958;26:6–23,49–60,127–142,175–182,194–208,239–241.

103. D'Amico A. Functional occlusion of the natural teeth of man. J Prosthet Dent 1961;11:899–915.

104. MacDonald JW, Hannam AG. Relationship between occlusal contacts and jaw-closing muscle activity during tooth clenching. Part. 1. J Prosthet Dent 1984;52:718–728.

105. Thornton LJ. Anterior guidance: group function/canine guidance. A literature review. J Prosthet Dent 1990;64:479–482.

106. Spear FM. Creating and communicating the ideal gingival profile around teeth, pontics, and implants. Presented at the 20th Anniversary International Symposium on Ceramics, San Diego, California, June 21st, 2002.

107. Shillingburg HT Jr, Hobo S, Fisher DW. Preparation design and margin distortion in porcelain-fused-to-metal restorations. J Prosthet Dent 1973;29:276–284.

108. Faucher RR, Nicholls JI. Distortion related to margin design in porcelain-fused-to-metal restorations. J Prosthet Dent 1980;43:149–155.

109. Hamaguchi H, Cacciatore A, Tueller VM. Marginal distortion of the porcelain-bonded-to-metal complete crown: an SEM study. J Prosthet Dent 1982;47:146–153.

110. Belser UC, MacEntee MI, Richter WA. Fit of three porcelain-fused-to-metal marginal designs in vivo: a scanning electron microscope study. J Prosthet Dent 1985;53:24–29.

111. Richter-Snapp K, Aquilino SA, Svare CW, Turner KA. Change in marginal fit as related to margin design, alloy type, and porcelain proximity in porcelain-fused-to-metal restorations. J Prosthet Dent 1988;60:435–439.

112. Richter WA, Ueno H. Relationship of crown margin placement to gingival inflammation. J Prosthet Dent 1973;30:156–161.

113. Bjorn AL, Bjorn H, Grkovic B. Marginal fit of restorations and its relation to periodontal bone level. I. Metal fillings. Odontol Revy 1969;20:311–321.

114. White SN, Ingles S, Kipnis U. Influence of marginal opening on microleakage of cemented artificial crowns. J Prosthet Dent 1994;71:257–264.

115. Di Febo G. La protesi nella malattia parodontale. In: Calandriello M, Carnevale G, Ricci G (eds). Parodontologia. Torino, Italy: Editrice Cides Odonto Edizioni Internazionali, 1986:589–661.

116. Waerhaug J. Histologic considerations which govern where the margins of restorations should be located in relation to the gingiva. Dent Clin North Am 1960;4:161–176.

117. Renggli HH, Regolati B. Gingival inflammation and plaque accumulation by well-adapted supragingival and subgingival proximal restorations. Helv Odontol Acta 1972;16:99–101.

118. Koth DL. Full crown restorations and gingival inflammation in a controlled population. J Prosthet Dent 1982;48:681–685.

119. Lang NP, Kiel RA, Anderhalden K. Clinical and microbiological effects of subgingival restorations with overhanging or clinically perfect margins. J Clin Periodontol 1983;10:563–578.

120. Waerhaug J. Tissue reactions around artificial crowns. J Periodontol 1953;24:172.

121. Karlsen K. Gingival reactions to dental restorations. Acta Odontol Scand 1970;28:895–904.

122. Rosling B, Nyman S, Lindhe J, Jernt B. The healing potential of the periodontal tissues following different techniques of periodontal surgery in plaque-free dentitions. A 2-year clinical study. J Clin Periodontol 1976;3:233–250.

123. Nyman S, Lindhe J, Rosling B. Periodontal surgery in plaque-infected dentitions. J Clin Periodontol 1977;4:240–249.

124. Axelsson P, Lindhe J. Effect of controlled oral hygiene procedures on caries and periodontal disease in adults. Results after 6 years. J Clin Periodontol 1981;8:239–248.

125. Lindhe J, Nyman S. Long-term maintenance of patients treated for advanced periodontal disease. J Clin Periodontol 1984;11:504–514.

126. Westfelt E, Bragd L, Socransky SS, Haffajee AD, Nyman S, Lindhe J. Improved periodontal conditions following therapy. J Clin Periodontol 1985;12:283–293.

127. Lang NP, Tonetti MS. Periodontal diagnosis in treated periodontitis. Why, when and how to use clinical parameters. J Clin Periodontol 1996;23:240–250.

128. Tonetti MS, Steffen P, Muller-Campanile V, Suvan J, Lang NP. Initial extractions and tooth loss during supportive care in a periodontal population seeking comprehensive care. J Clin Periodontol 2000;27:824–831.

129. Axelsson P, Nystrom B, Lindhe J. The long-term effect of a plaque control program on tooth mortality, caries and periodontal disease in adults. Results after 30 years of maintenance. J Clin Periodontol 2004;31:749–757.

130. Carnevale G, Cairo F, Tonetti MS. Long-term effects of supportive therapy in periodontal patients treated with fibre retention osseous resective surgery. I: recurrence of pockets, bleeding on probing and tooth loss. J Clin Periodontol 2007;34:334–341.

131. Carnevale G, Cairo F, Tonetti MS. Long-term effects of supportive therapy in periodontal patients treated with fibre retention osseous resective surgery. II: tooth extractions during active and supportive therapy. J Clin Periodontol 2007;34:342–348.

132. Miller LM. Porcelain veneer protection plan: maintenance procedures for all porcelain restorations. J Esthet Dent 1990;2:63–66.

133. Magne P, Belser U. Bonded Porcelain Restorations in the Anterior Dentition. A Biomimetic Approach. Chicago: Quintessence, 2002:374.

We thought it useful to present a step-by-step summary of the most significant clinical cases featured in the chapters of this volume; they are organized according to the year they were treated, starting with the complete rehabilitations and finishing with the single restorations on natural teeth and implants in the anterior sector. The sequence of introductory illustrations on the first two pages with a light blue background, in which the photographs already published can be identified by the original numbering of the chapter they belong to, provides a summary of the initial treatment phases. The photos that follow illustrate finalization of the prosthetic rehabilitation; the purpose of these is to show how the systematic approach can be reproduced in both the simplest of cases as well as in more complex treatments.

CLINICAL CASE GALLERY

PROSTHETIC TREATMENT

VOLUME 2

ESTHETIC REHABILITATION IN FIXED PROSTHODONTICS

Patient: D.O.   Gender: F   Age: 59 years

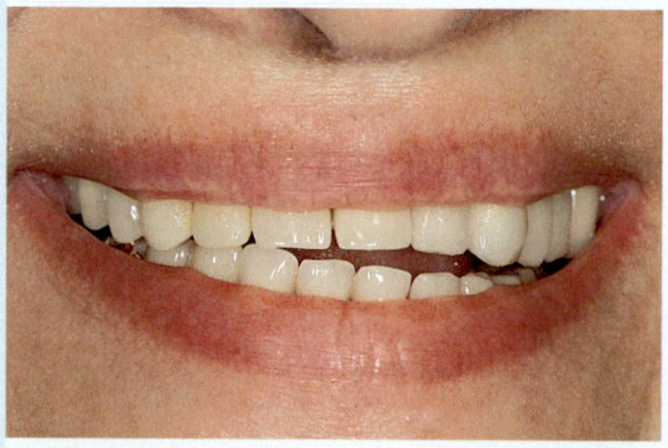

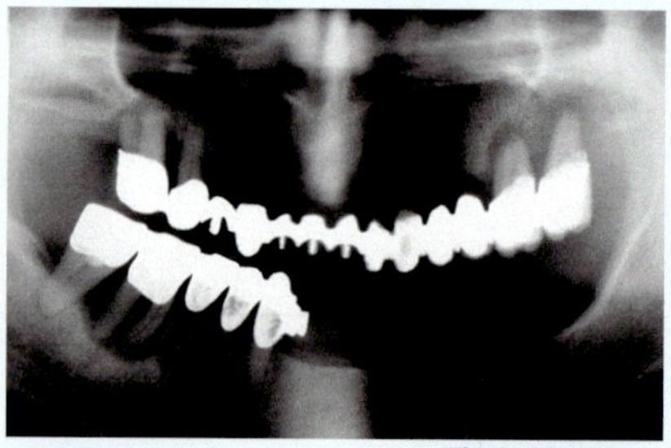

> Fig 2-40b

> Fig 2-40a

> Fig 2-40c

> Fig 2-40f

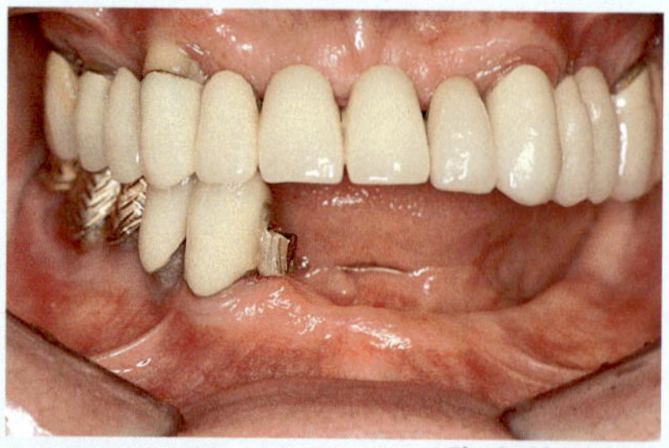

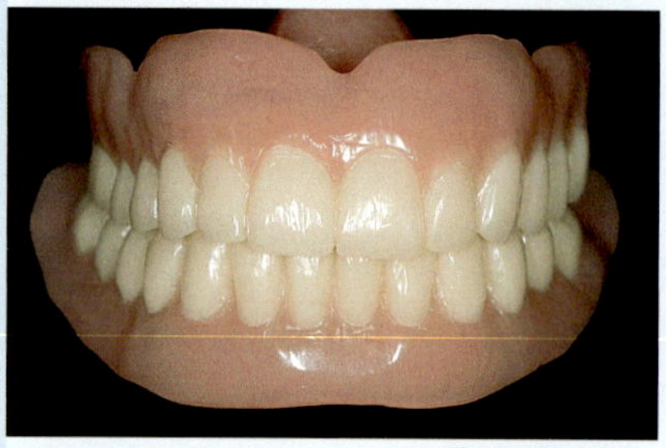

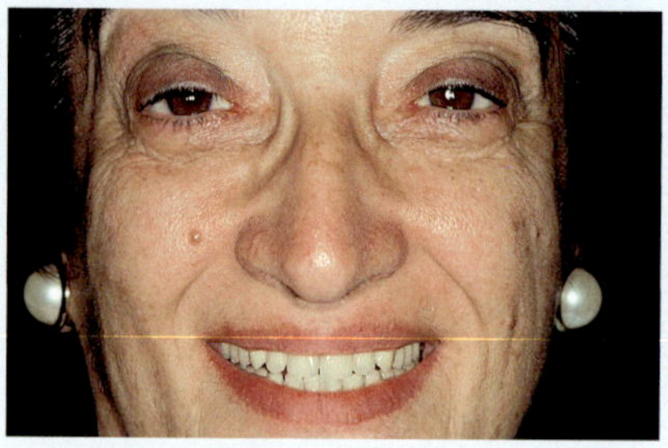

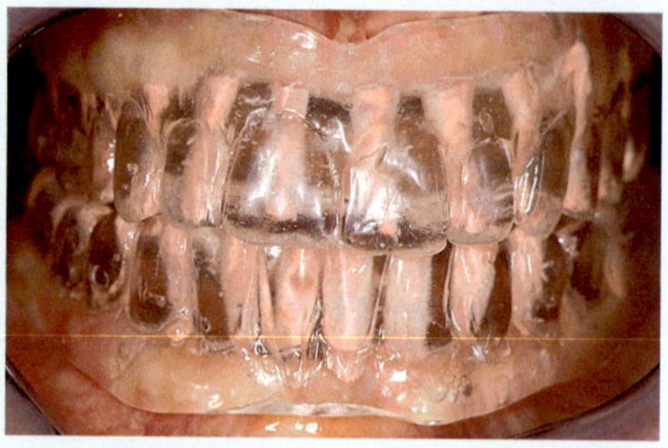

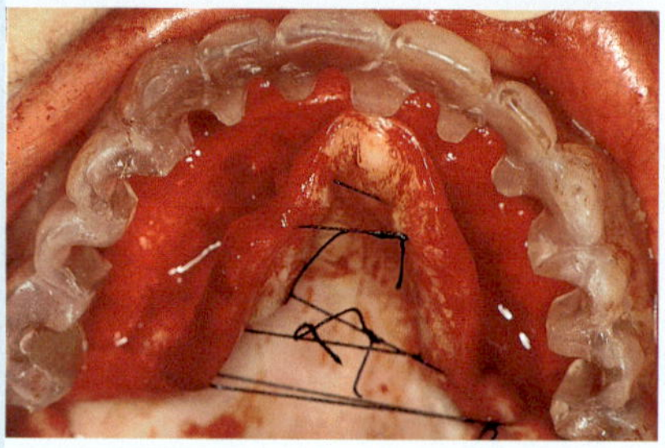

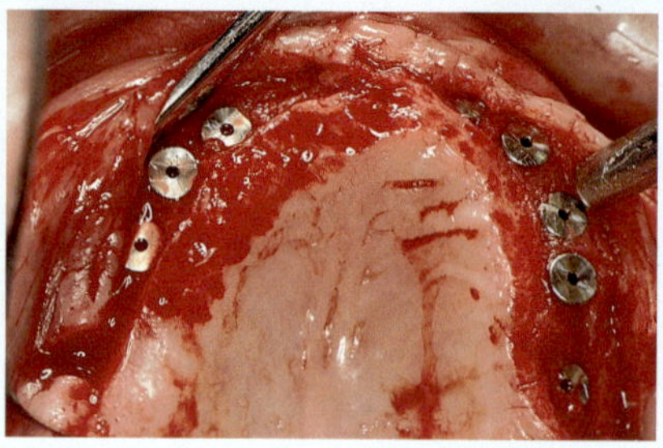

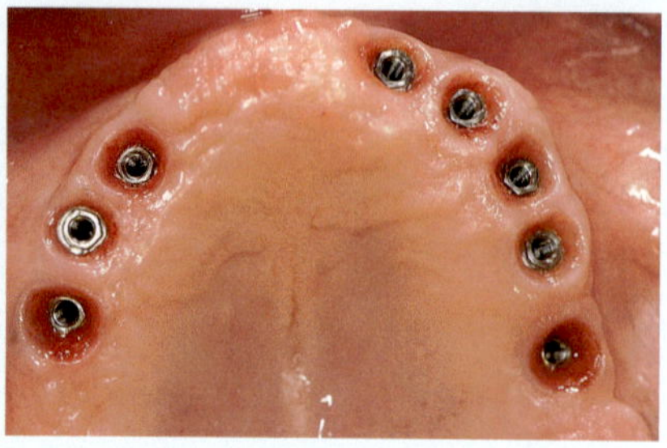

PAGES 526–527   After the extraction of all dentition, initially two complete dentures were created, followed by osseointegrated implants positioned in both arches. After inserting an initial screw-retained provisional restoration, a second was created and then cemented onto customized abutments.

PAGES 528–529   Under the guidance of the silicone indices derived from the provisional restoration, the metal substructures were made. Preventive simulation (PS) makes it possible to obtain a preview of the final esthetic appearance and to check that the casts are correctly fitted before proceeding with ceramic layering.

PAGES 530–531   The cast cross-mounting technique makes it possible to achieve an ideal functional aspect in the definitive work, also demonstrated by the presence of punctiform, synchronized, and well-distributed contacts on the centric canines.

PAGES 532–533   A comparison of the initial and final appearance, 12 years after delivery of the definitive work, demonstrates the esthetic-functional integration successfully achieved by the implant-supported prosthetic rehabilitation.

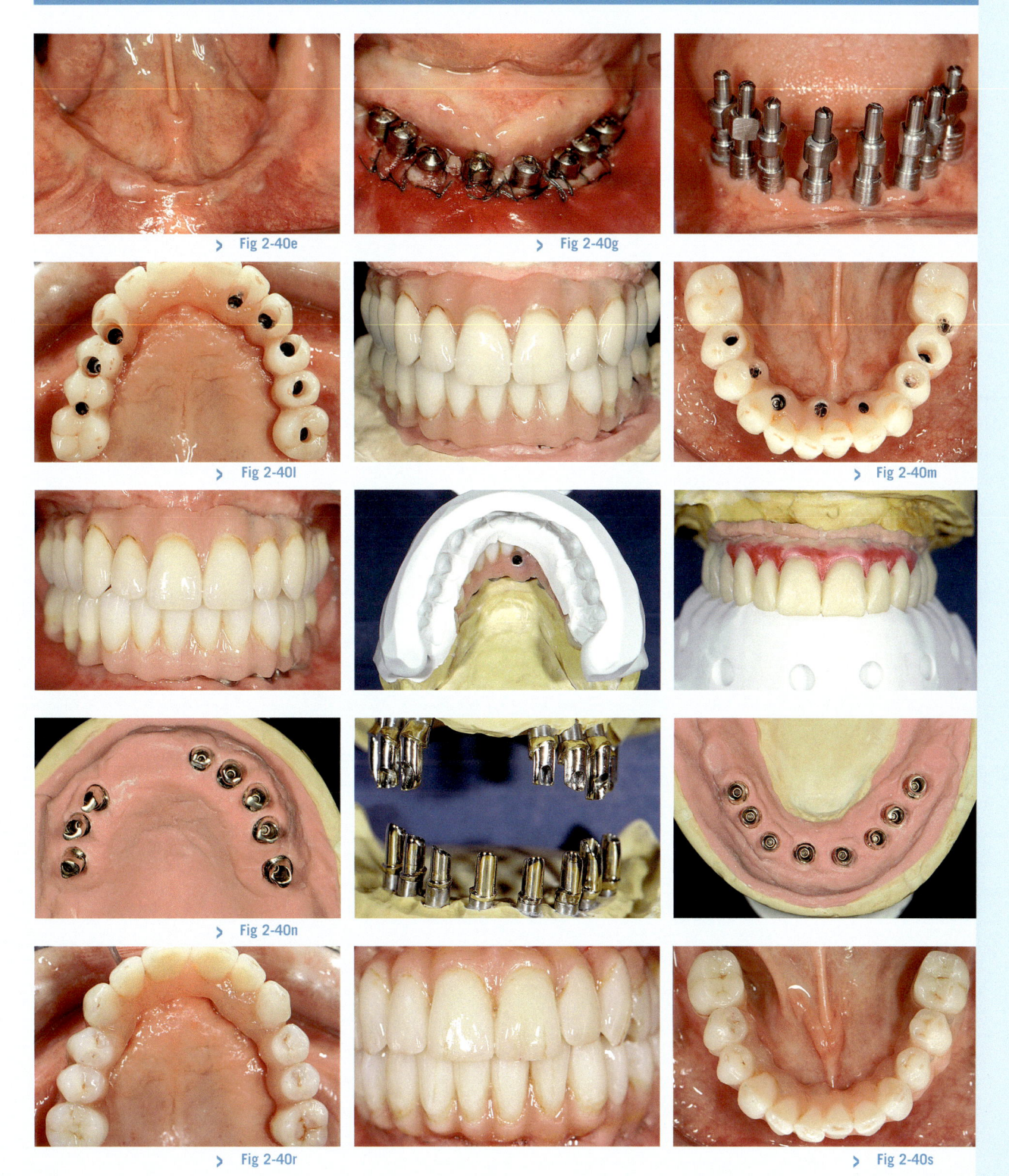

Rehabilitation on implants — Treatment: 1994–1995

> Fig 2-40e

> Fig 2-40g

> Fig 2-40l

> Fig 2-40m

> Fig 2-40n

> Fig 2-40r

> Fig 2-40s

527

528

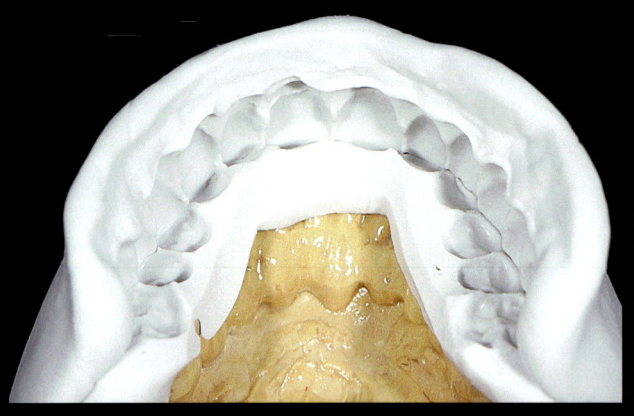

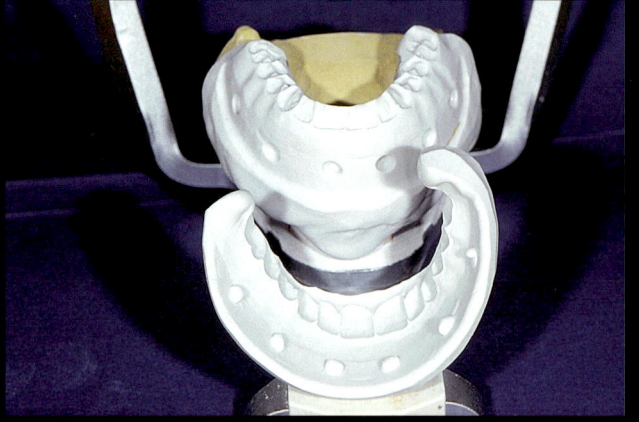

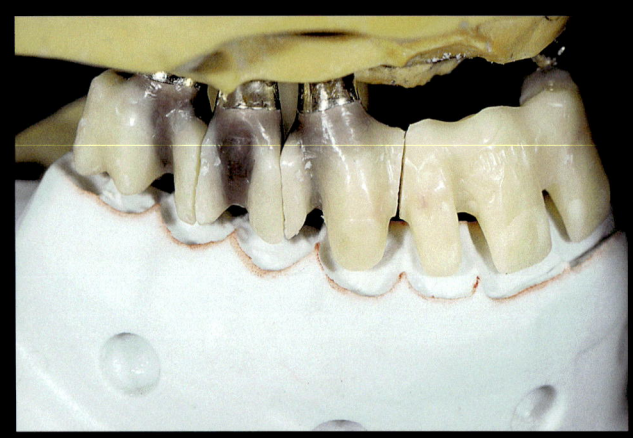

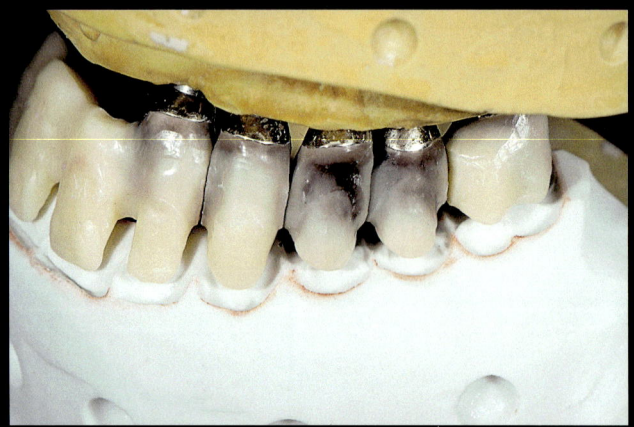

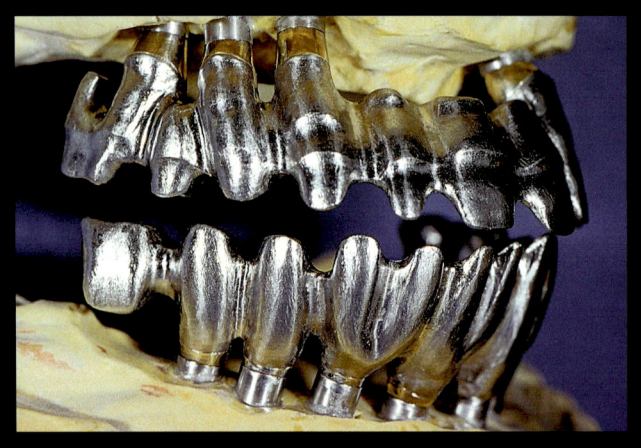

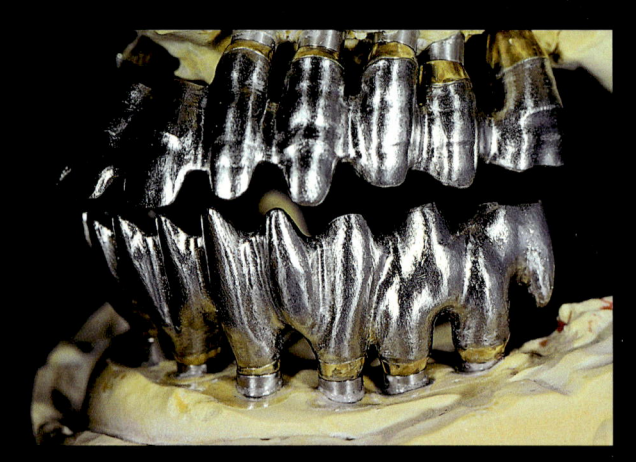

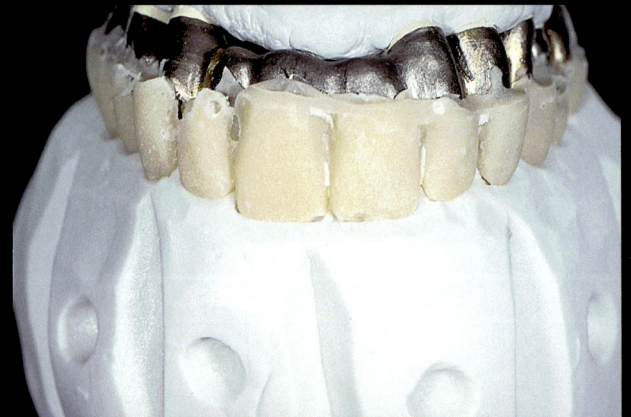

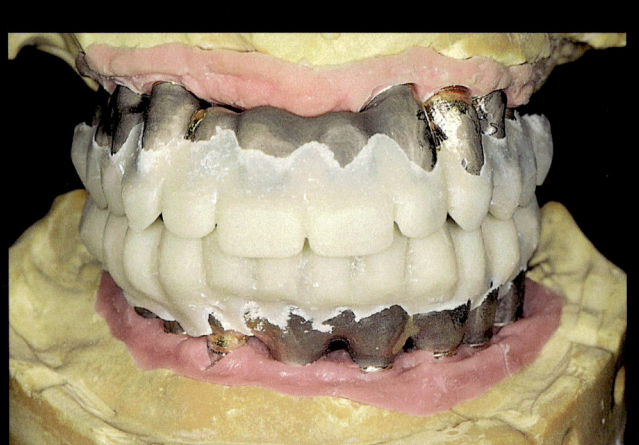

529

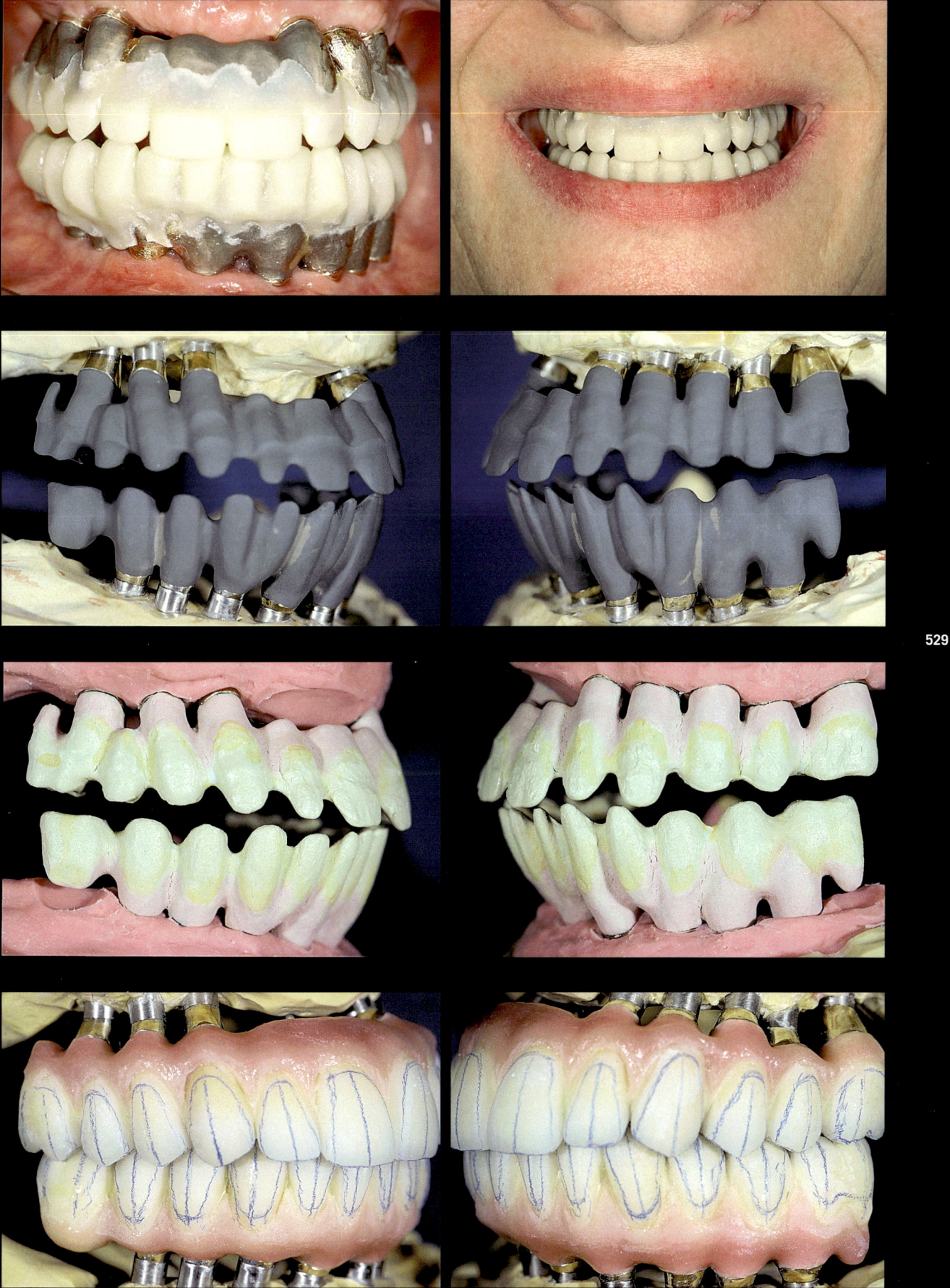

1995

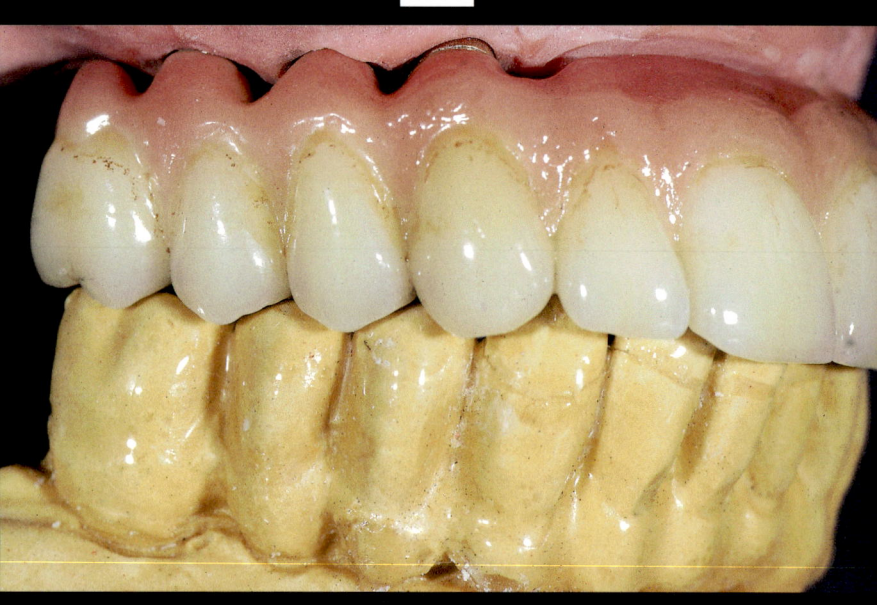

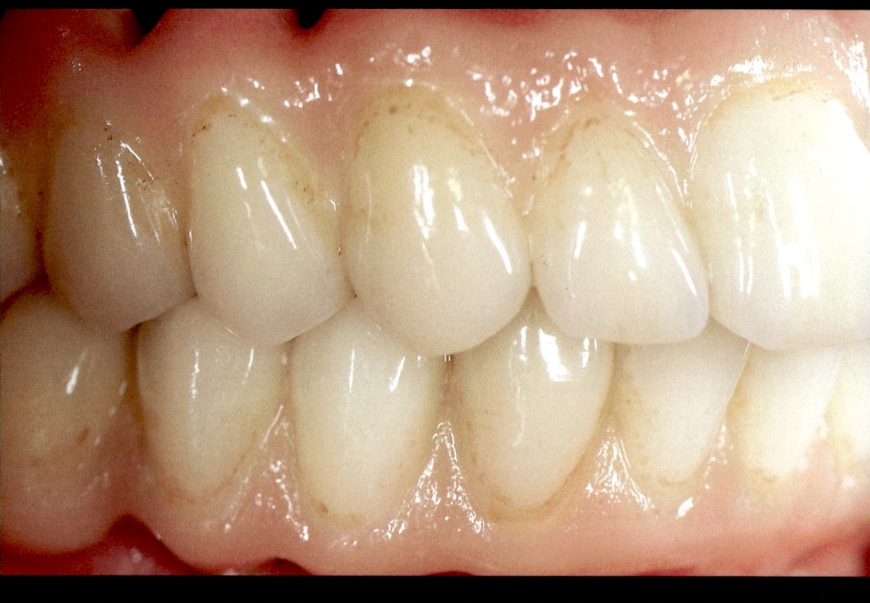

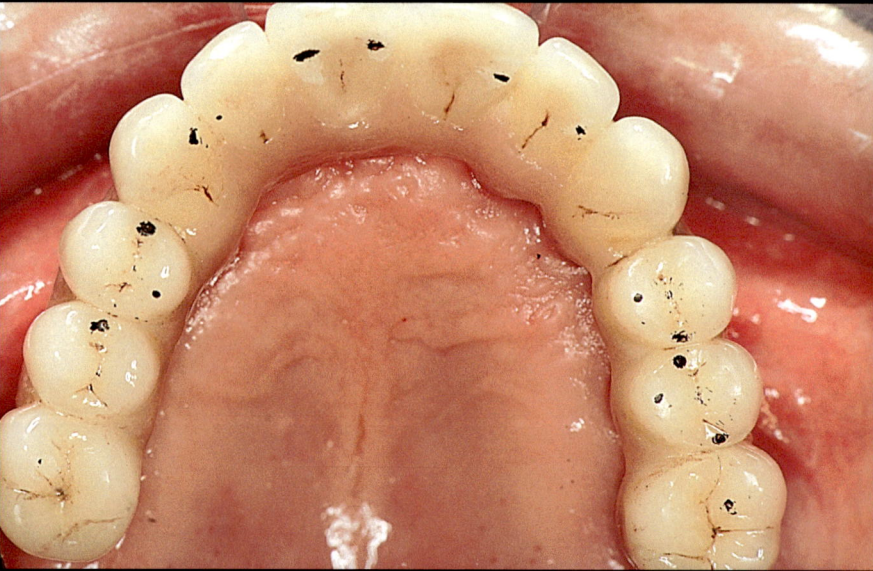

1995

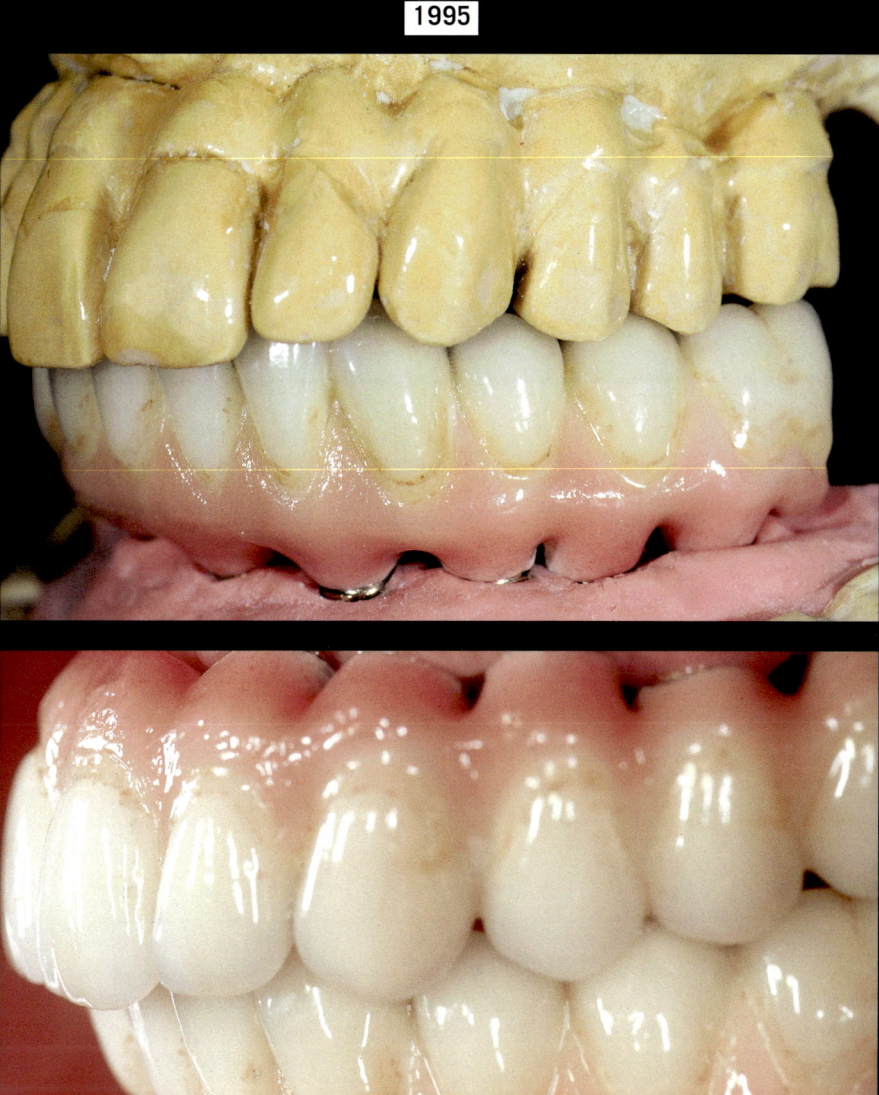

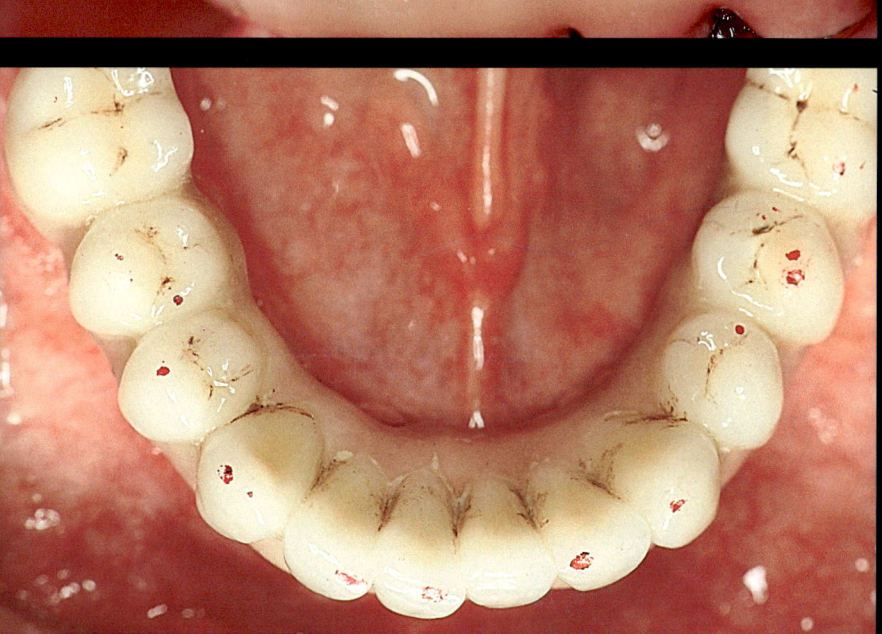

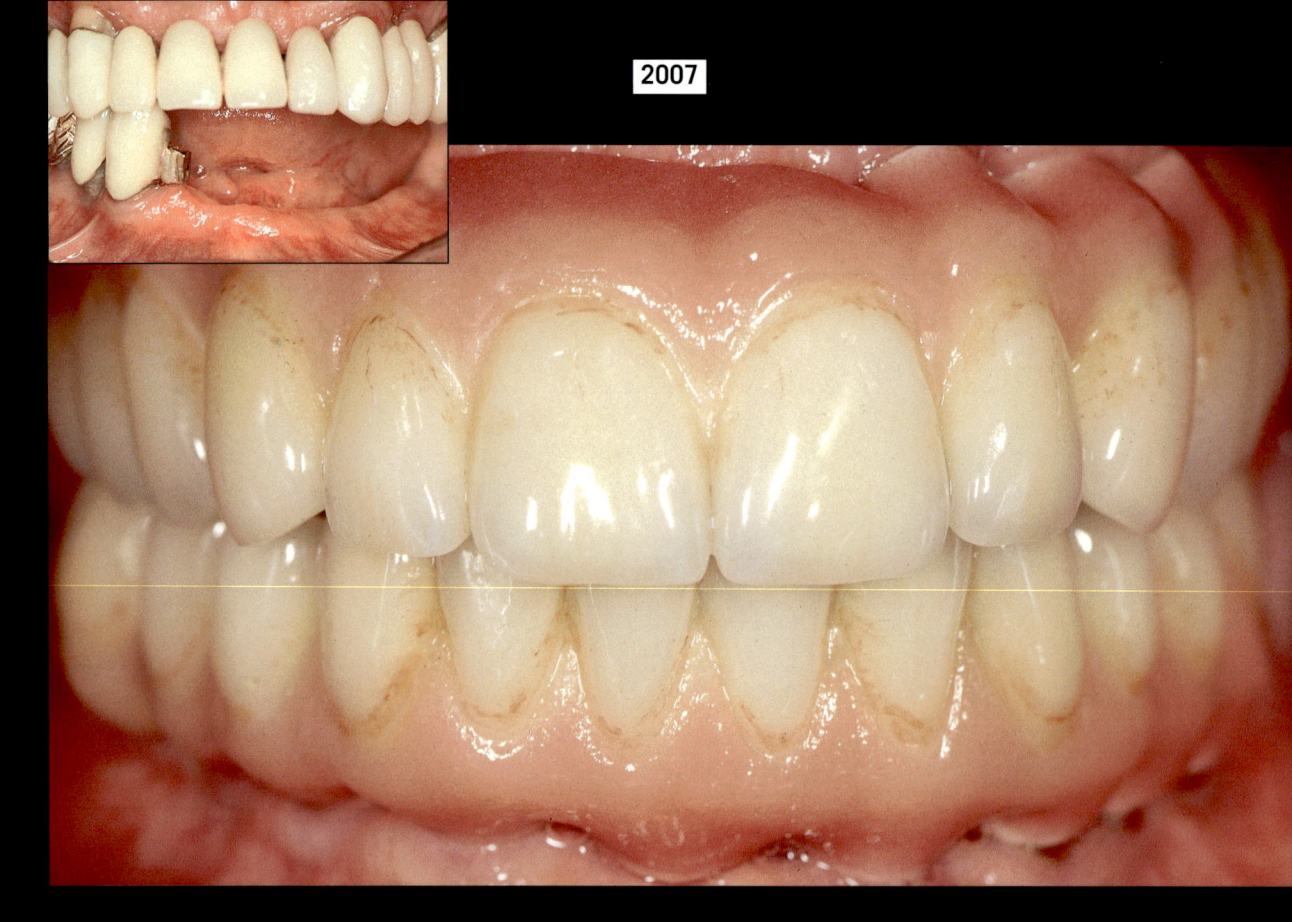

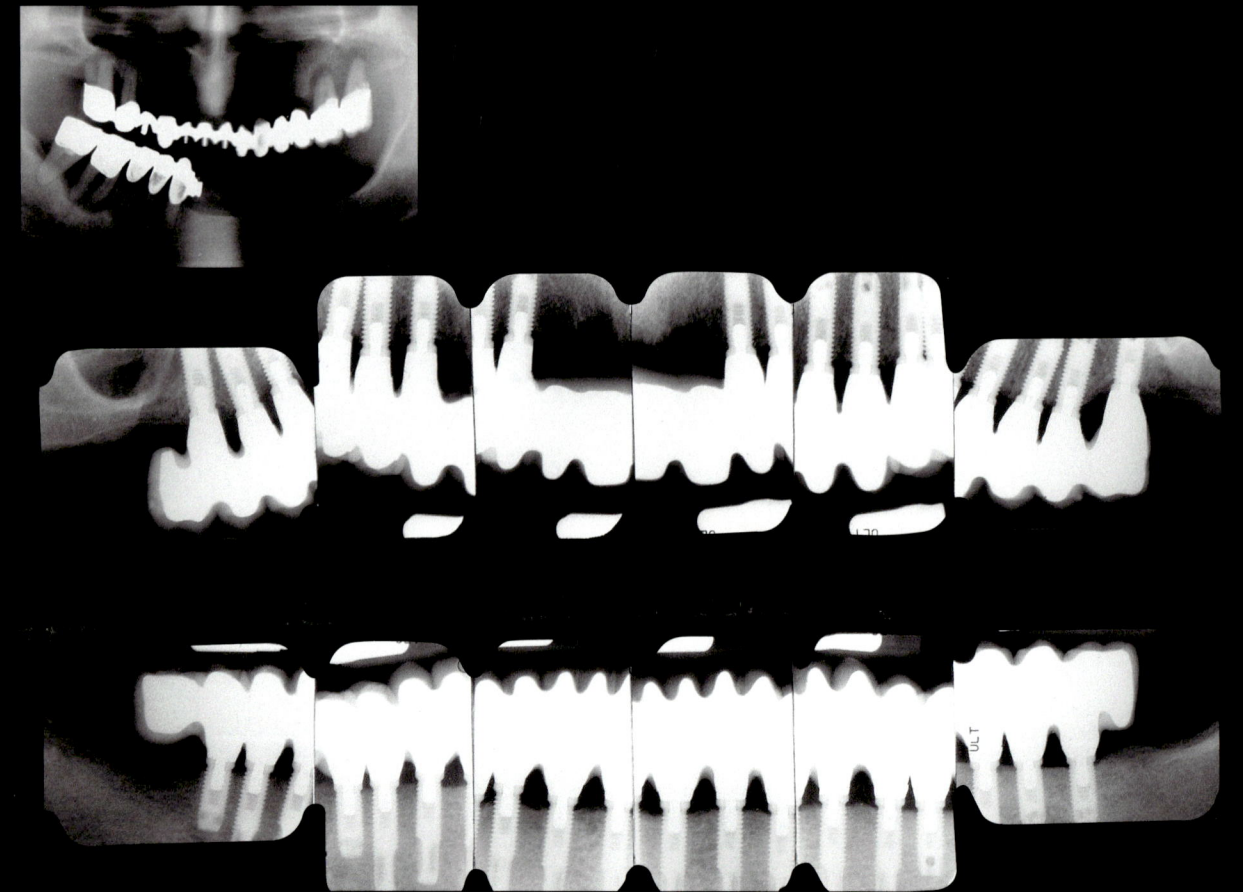

2007

532

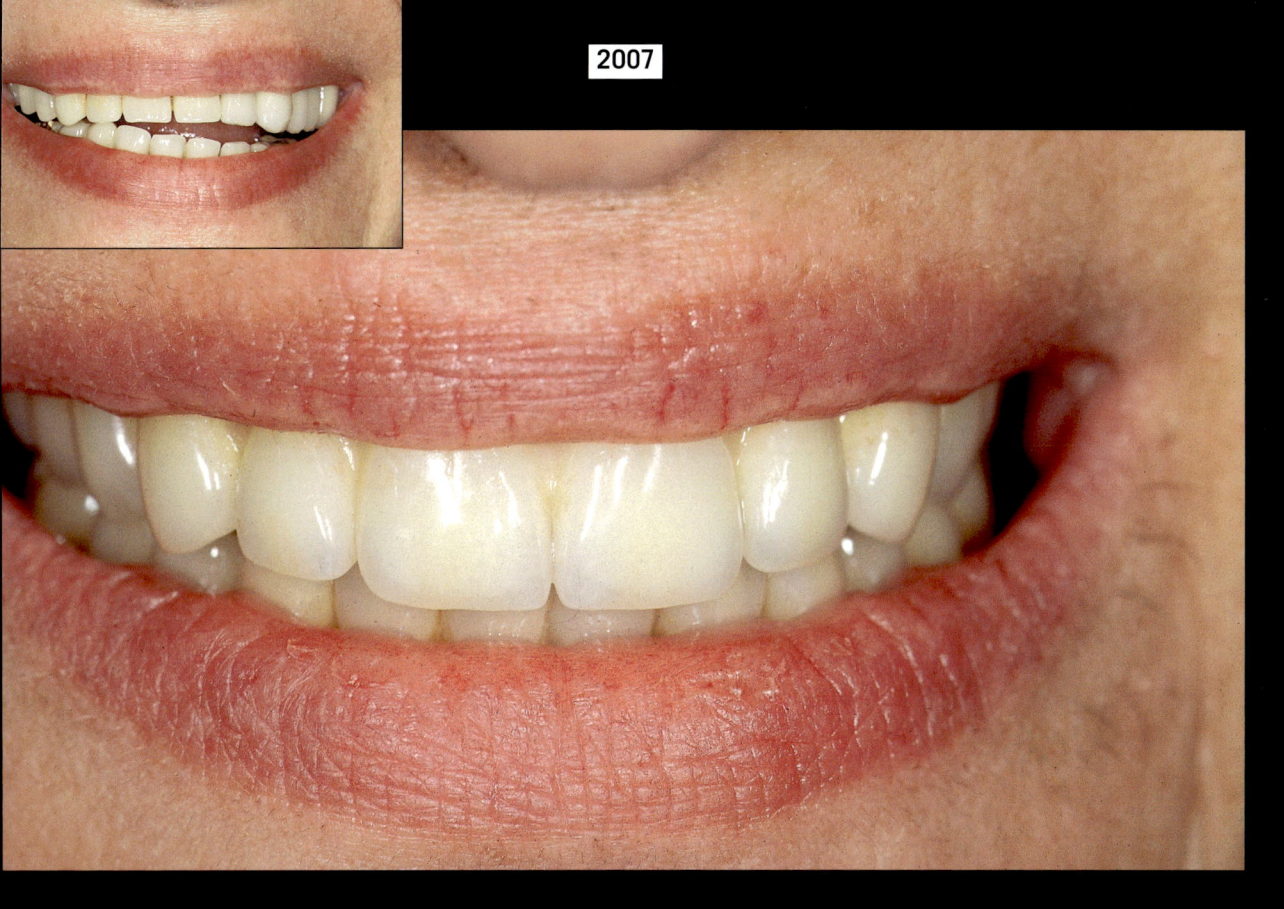

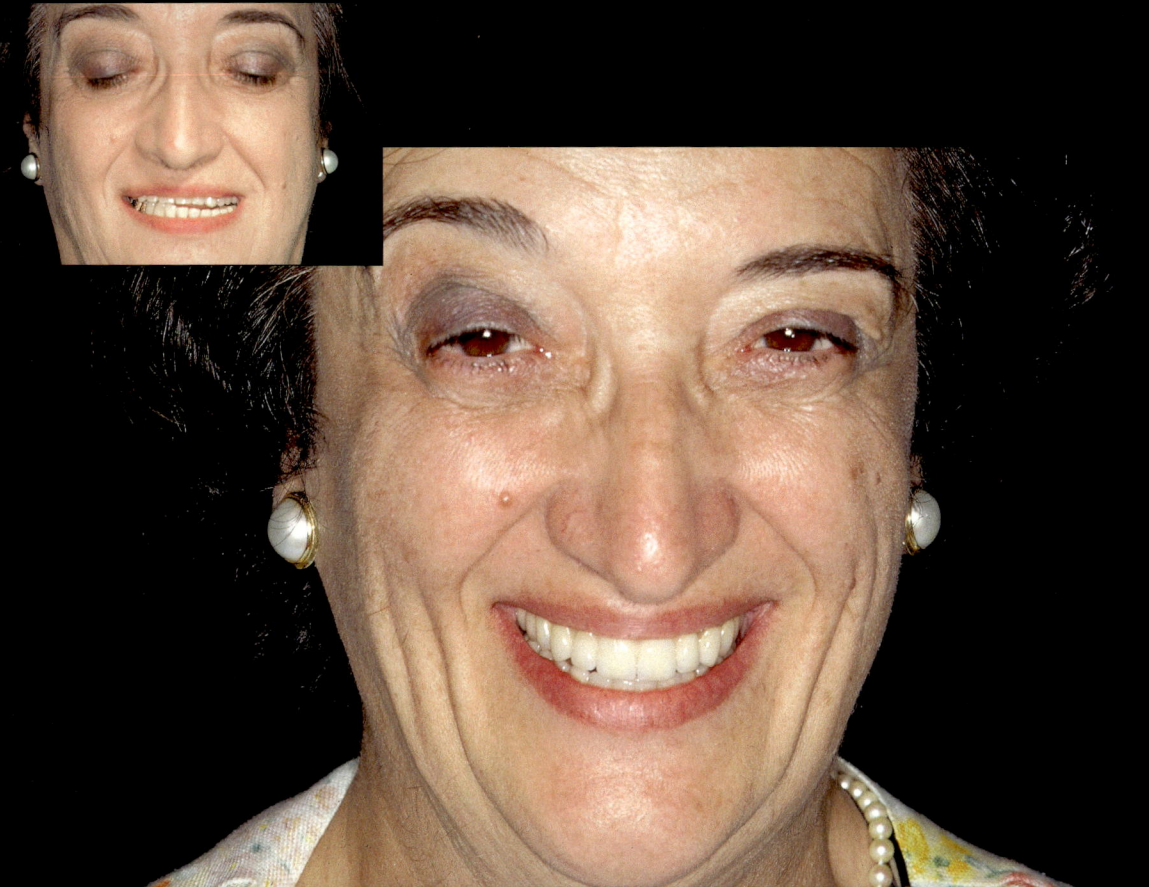

2007

533

Patient: T.P.   **Gender: F**   **Age: 44 years**

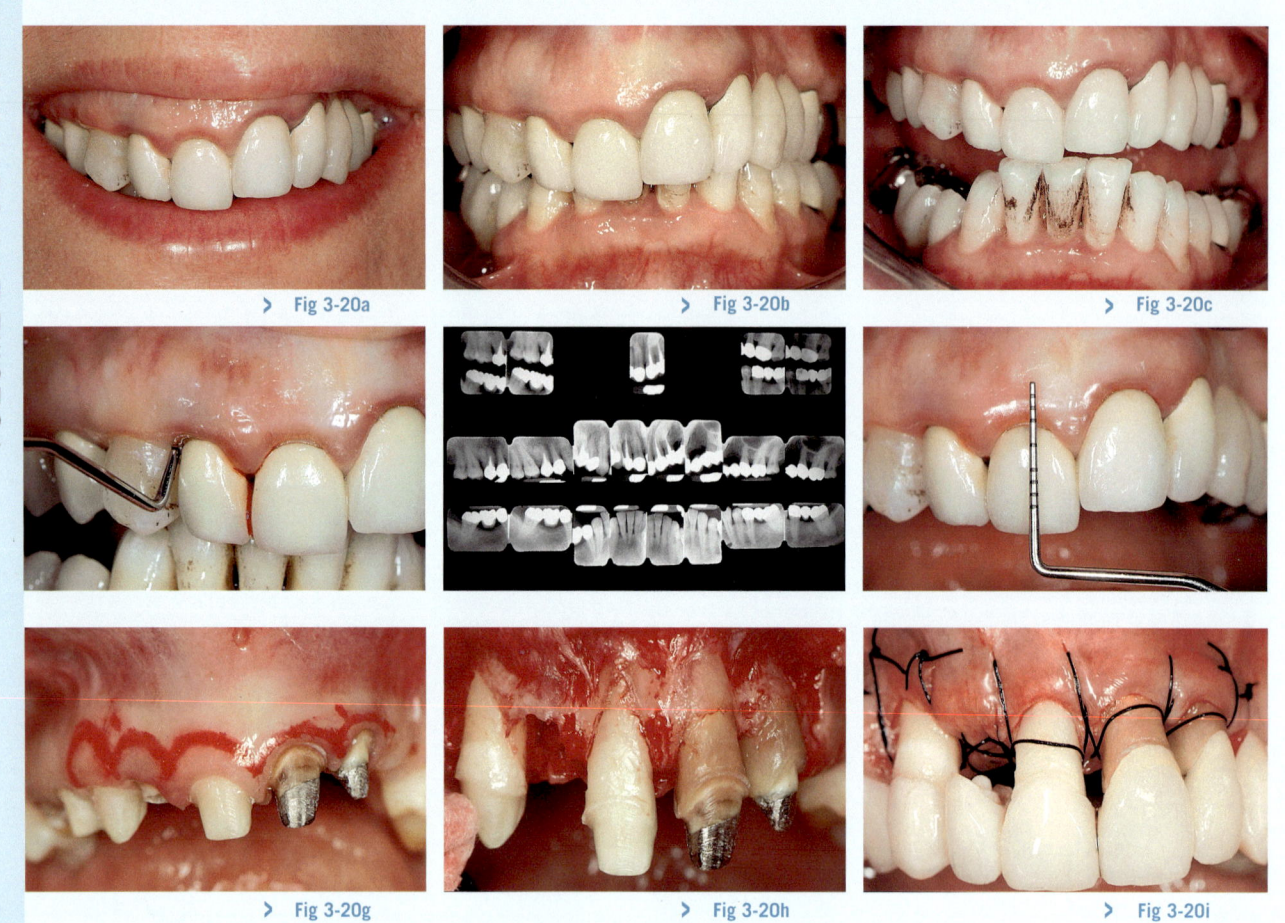

> Fig 3-20a

> Fig 3-20b

> Fig 3-20c

> Fig 3-20g

> Fig 3-20h

> Fig 3-20i

PAGES 534–535   The serious initial esthetic-functional compromise was remedied thanks to prosthetic-periodontal therapy that not only eliminated the defects, but also realigned the maxillary gingival levels and re-established the correct incisal outline. Only when maturation of the gingival tissues had been completely reached was it possible to create a second provisional restoration, which proved to be optimally integrated from the biologic viewpoint.

PAGES 536–537   Together with the impressions of the provisional restorations and those of the final preparations, all of the data necessary for cross-mounting the casts and for carrying out the preventive simulation (PS) were sent to the laboratory before we proceeded with finalizing the work with the help of the silicone indices.

PAGES 538–541   The definitive rehabilitation demonstrates the excellent biologic integration achieved thanks also to the presence of suitable spaces in the interproximal areas for cleaning these extremely delicate areas properly.

PAGES 542–543   The long-term maintenance of the excellent esthetic-functional integration achieved is demonstrated by the photos of the restorations taken more than 10 years after the treatment was completed.

537

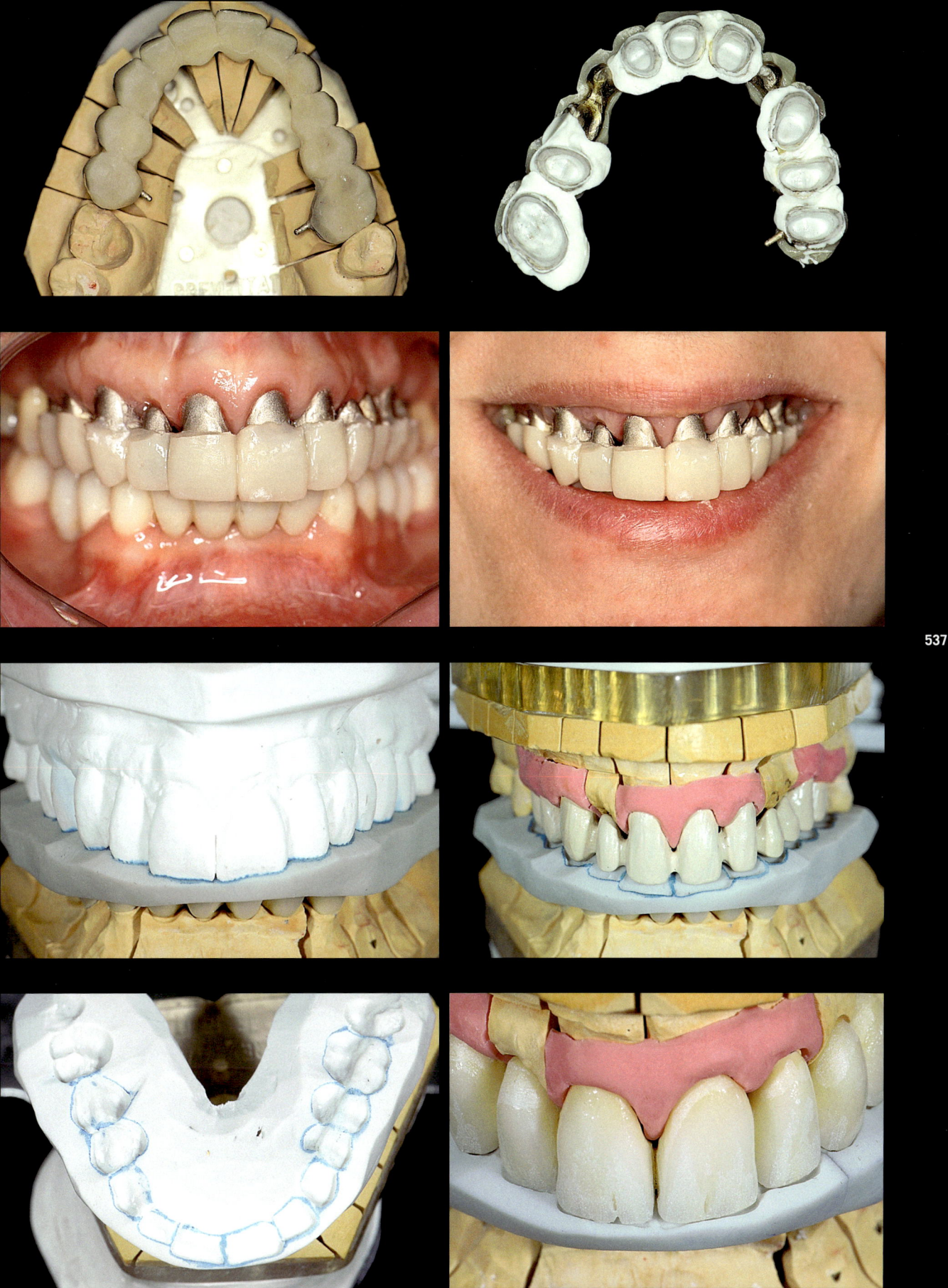

538

Prosthetic-periodontal therapy — Treatment: 1996–1997

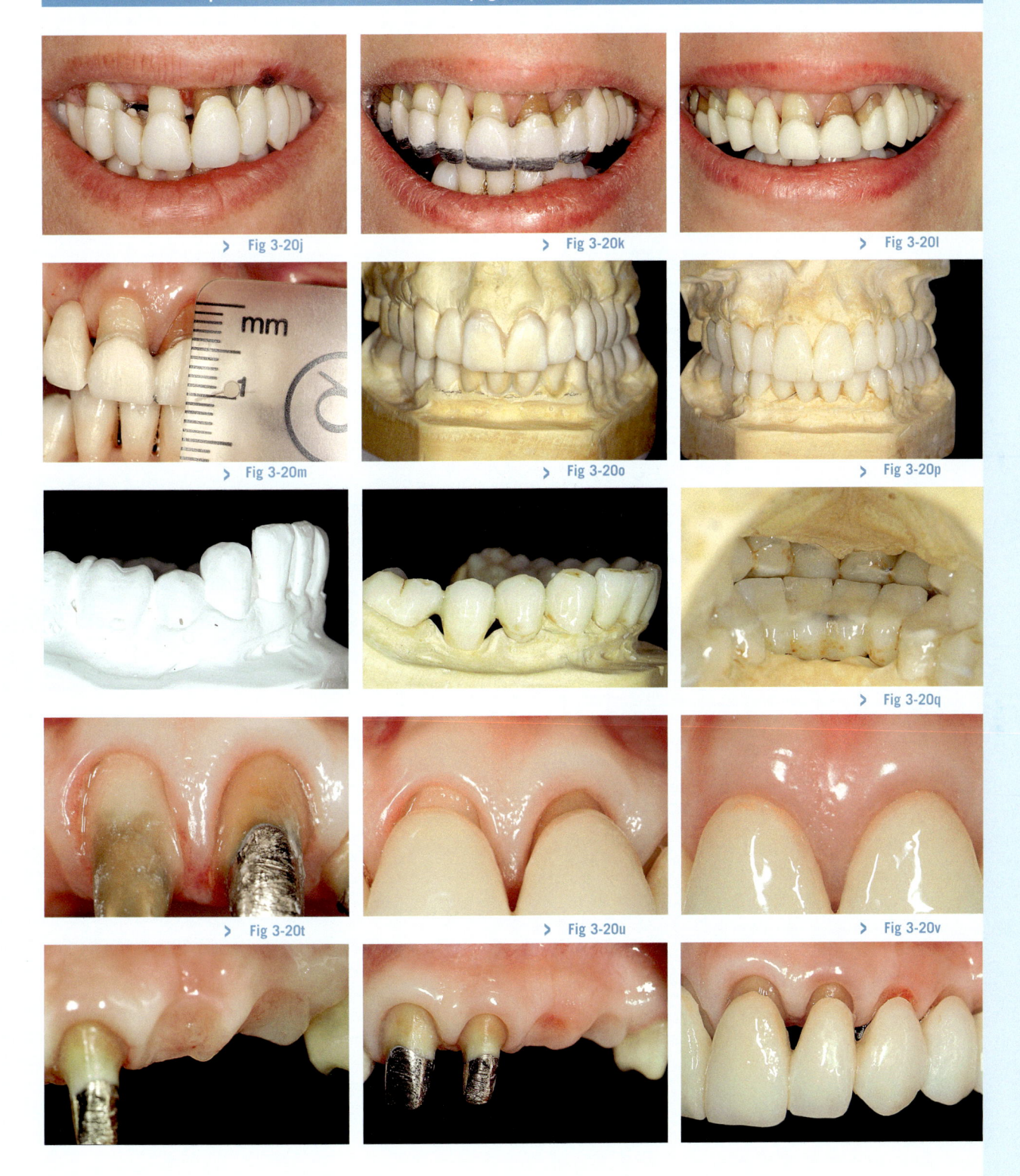

> Fig 3-20j

> Fig 3-20k

> Fig 3-20l

> Fig 3-20m

> Fig 3-20o

> Fig 3-20p

> Fig 3-20q

> Fig 3-20t

> Fig 3-20u

> Fig 3-20v

> Fig 3-20x

> Fig 3-20s

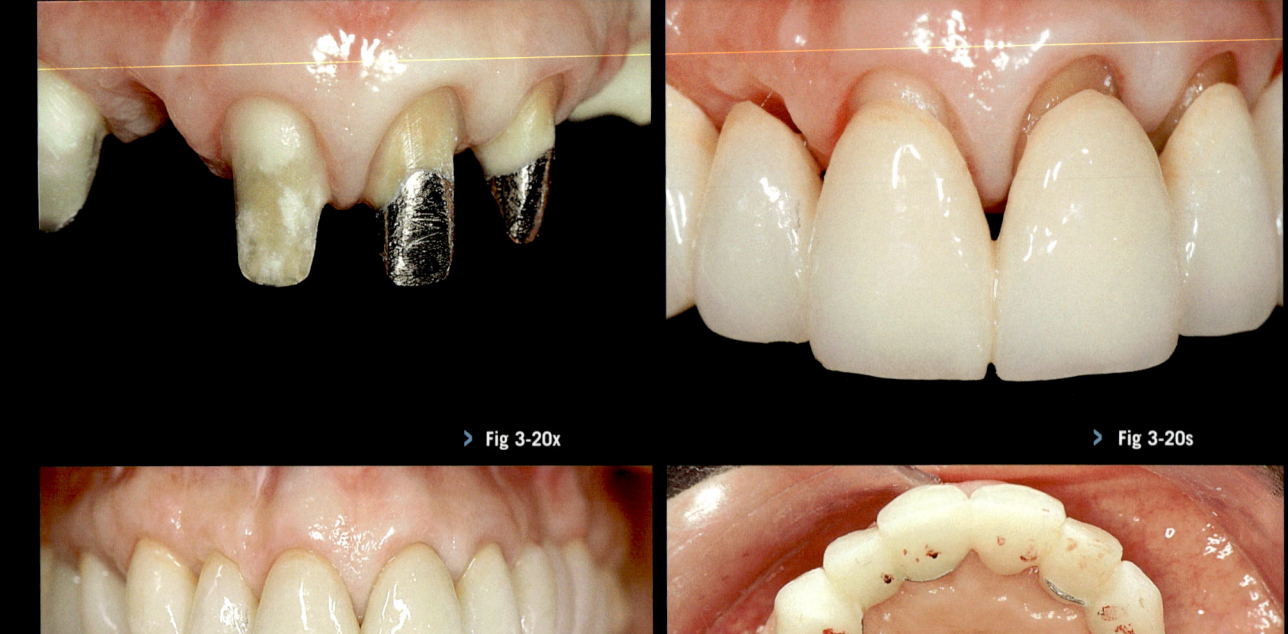

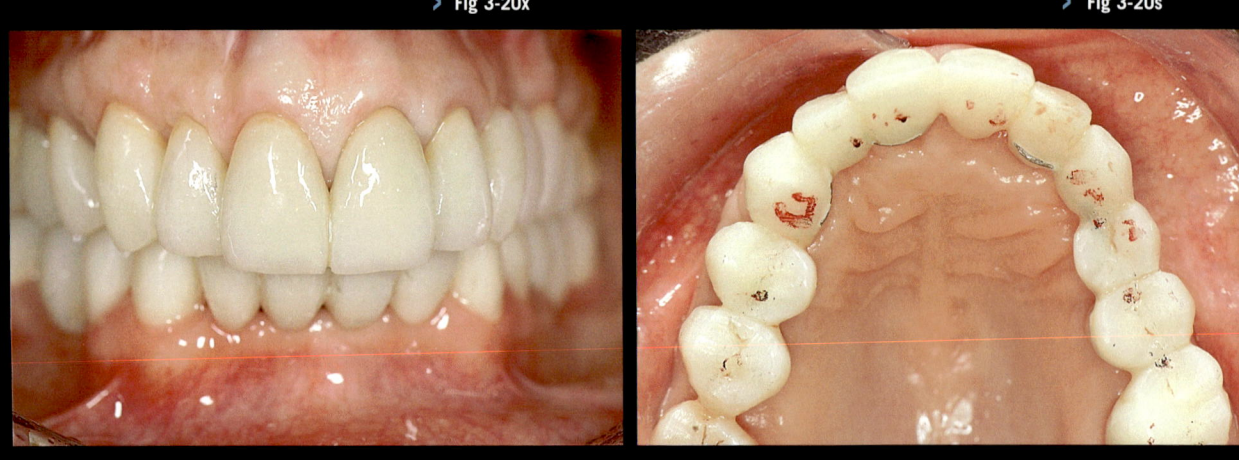

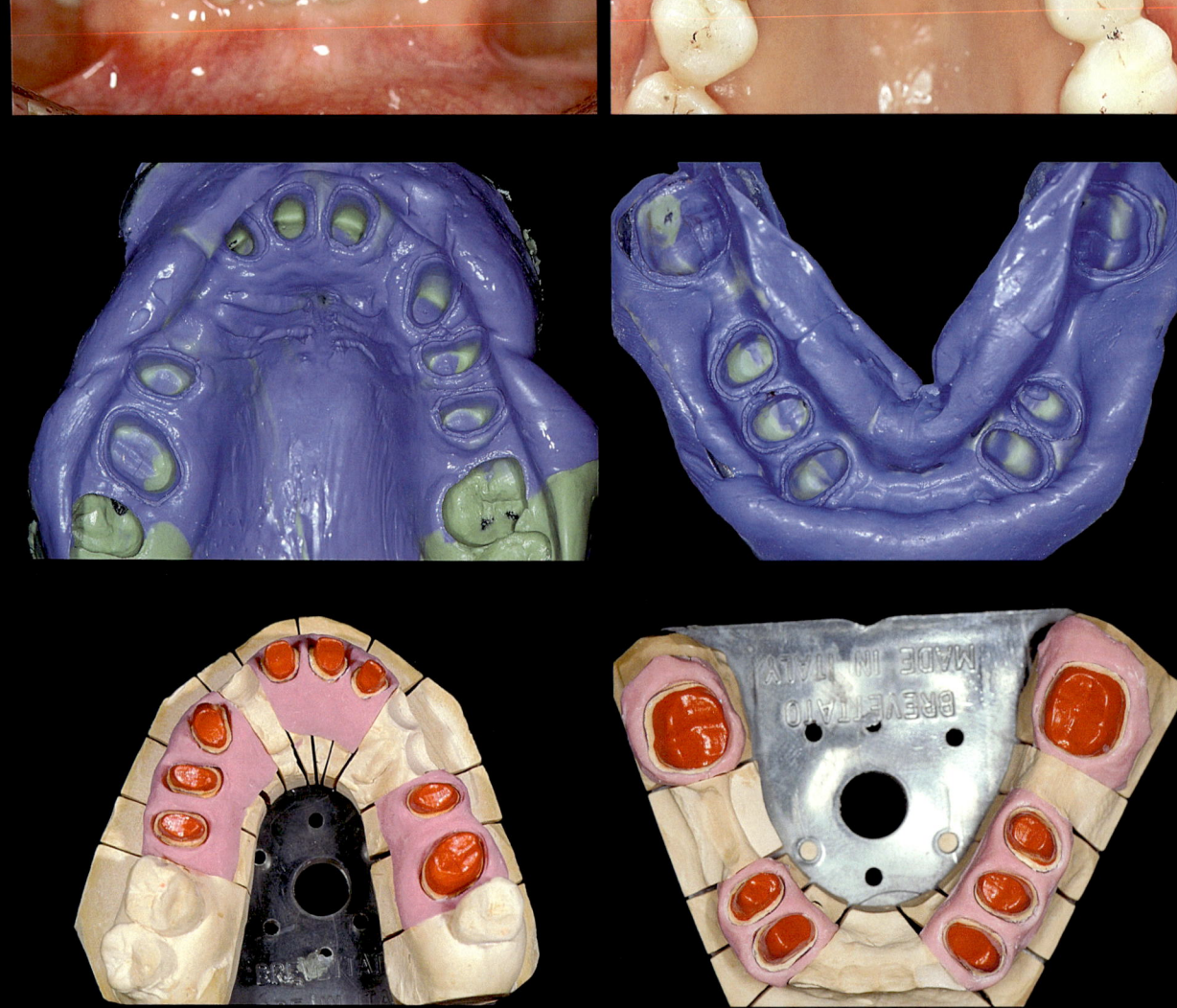

536

539

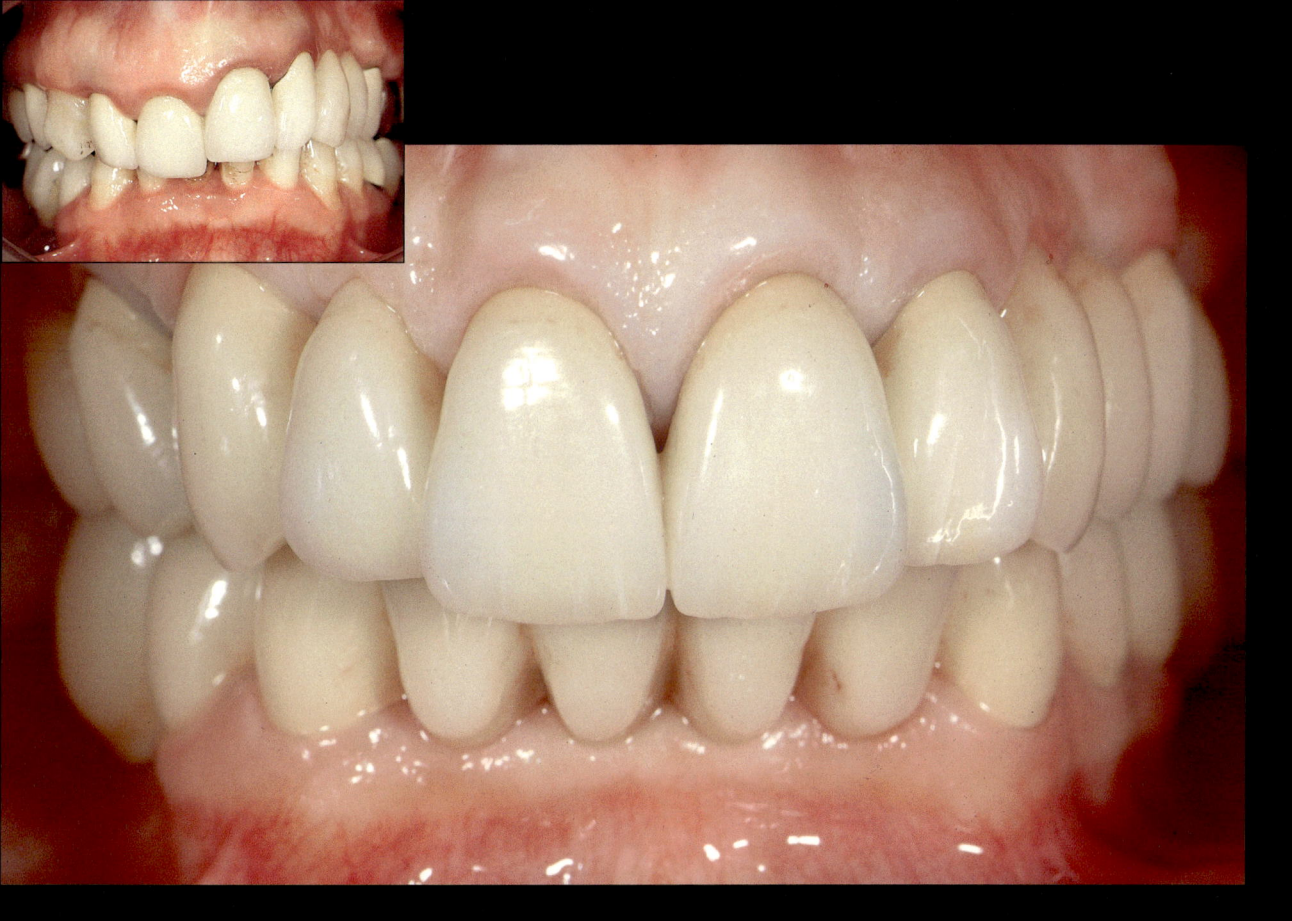

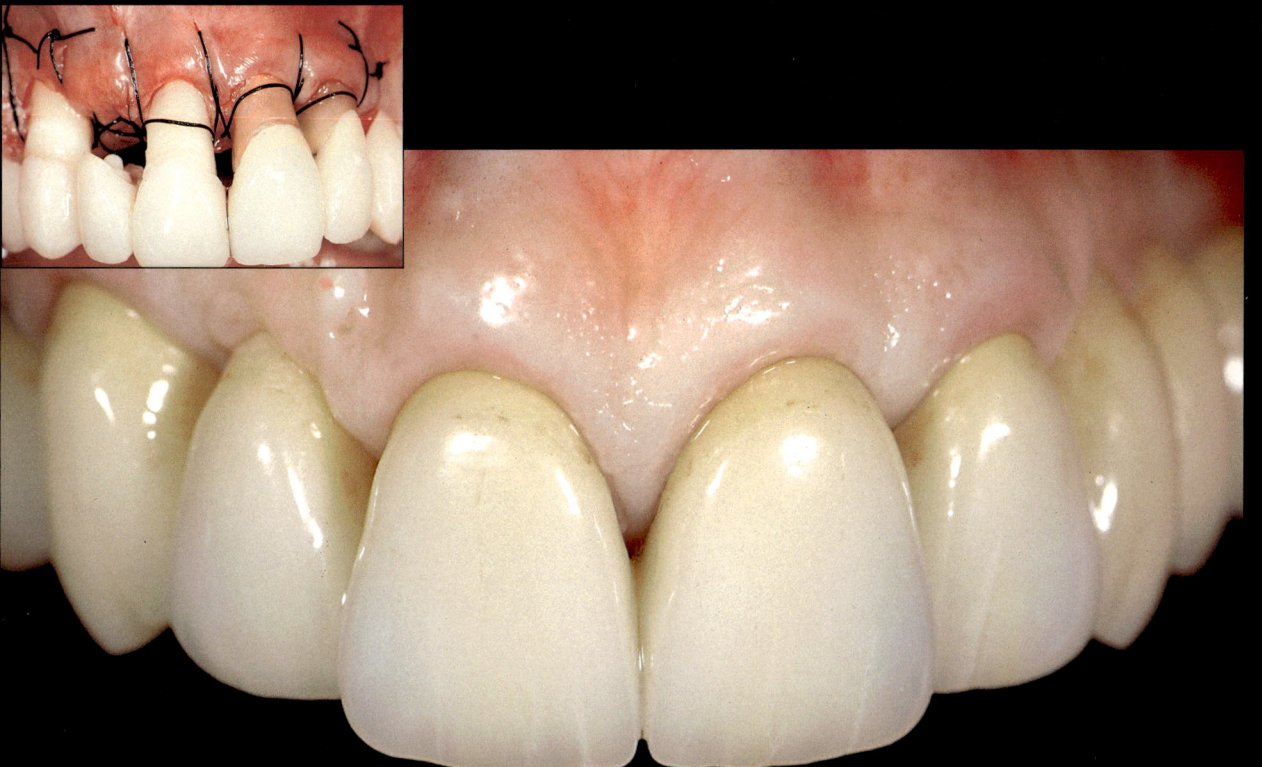

540

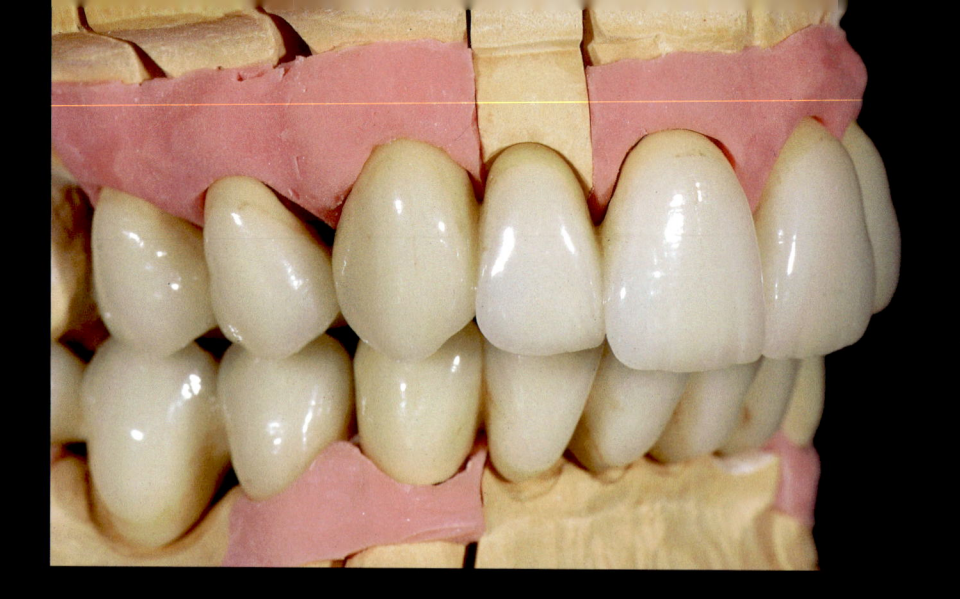

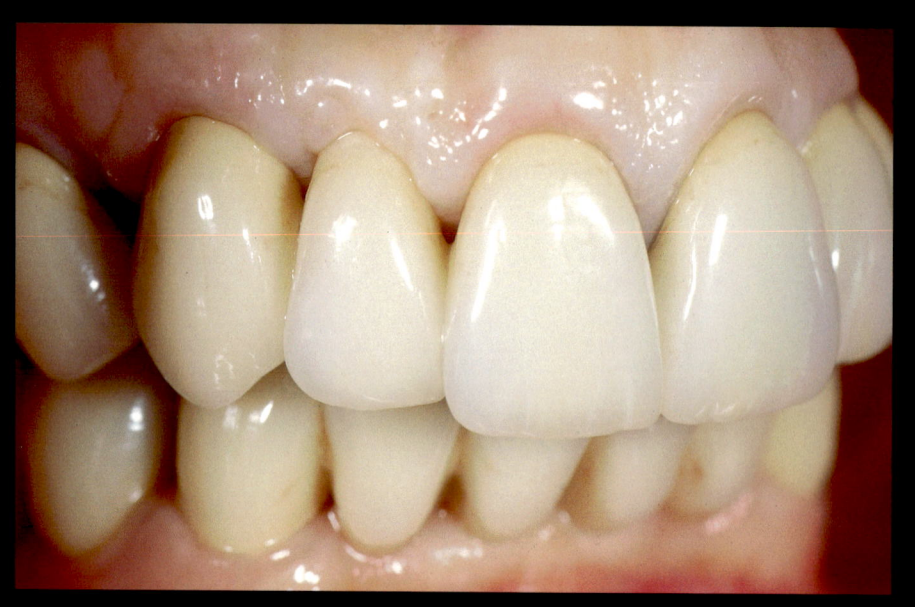

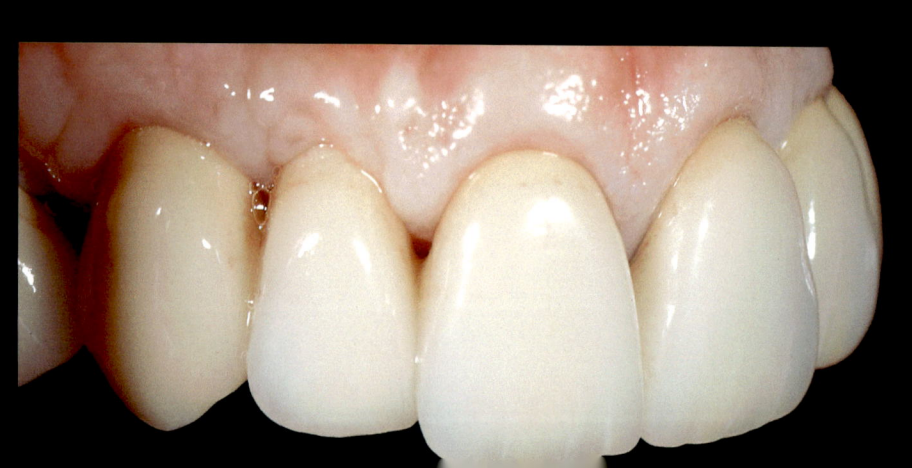

541

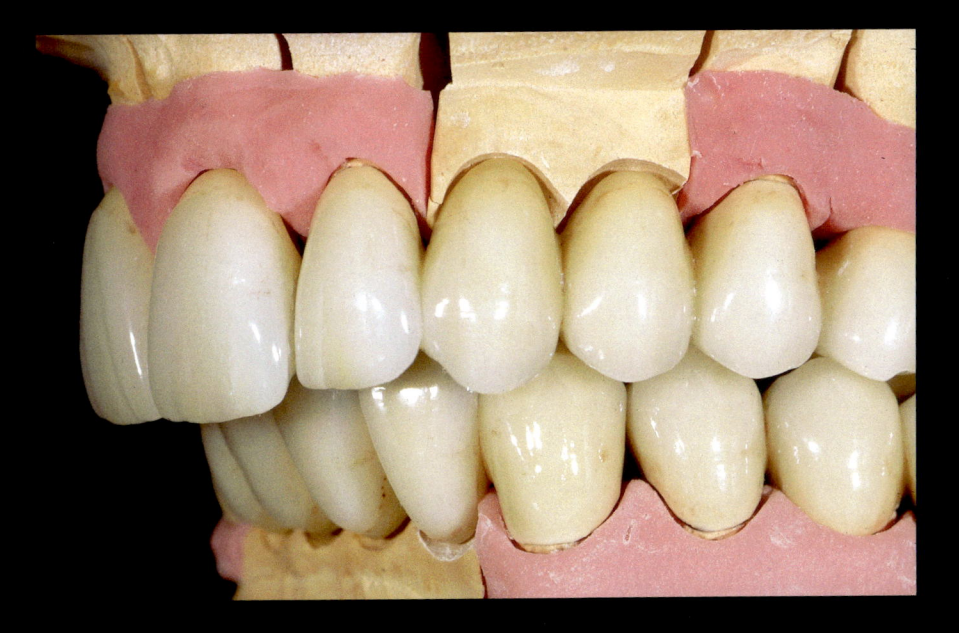

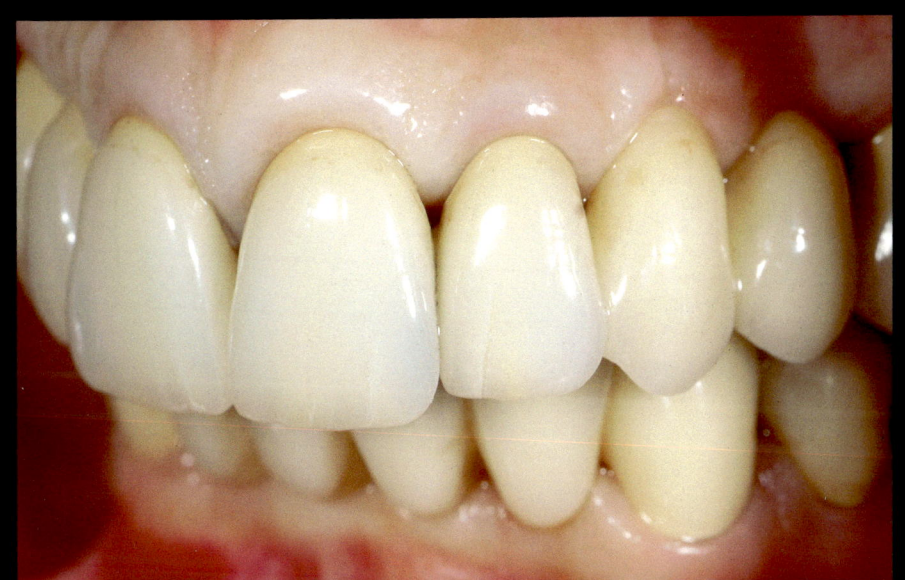

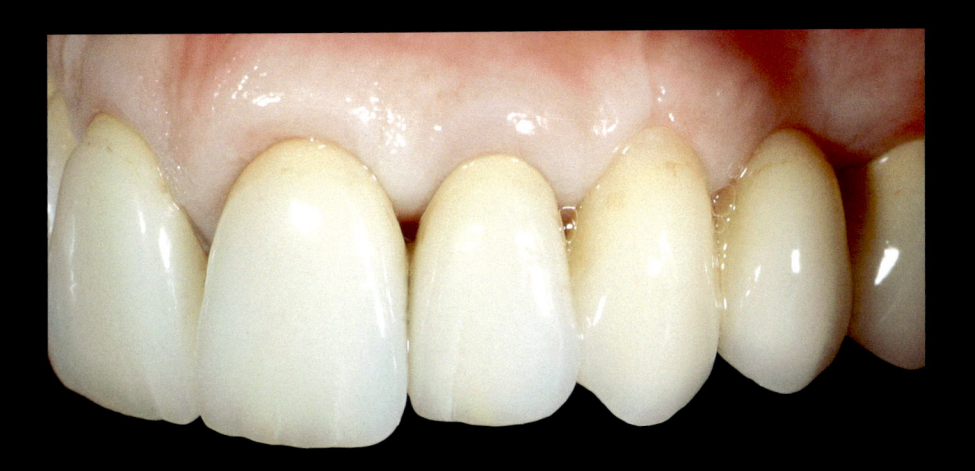

542

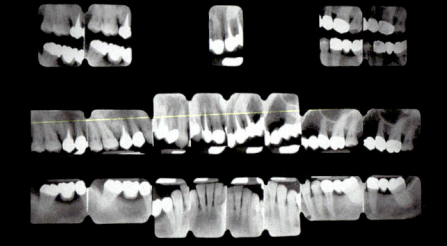

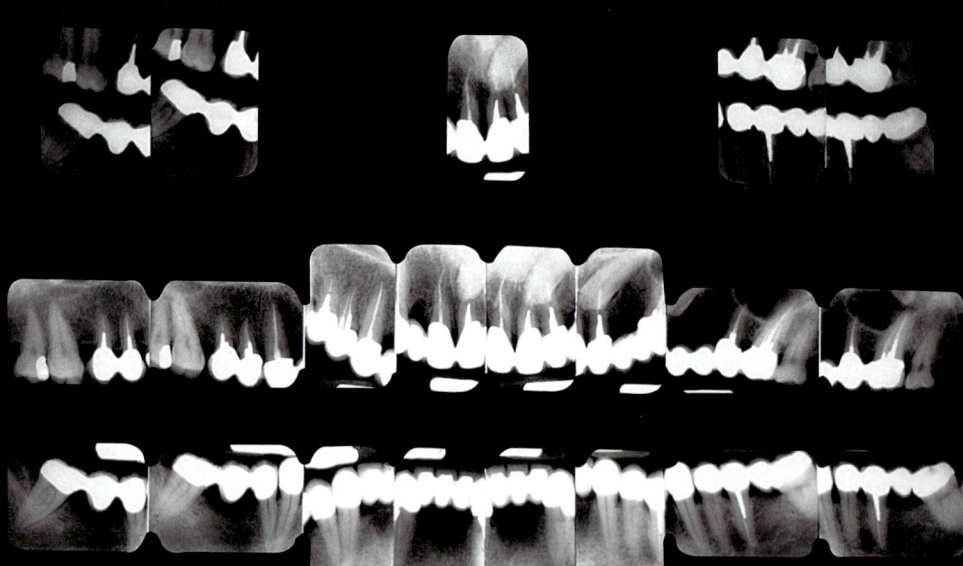

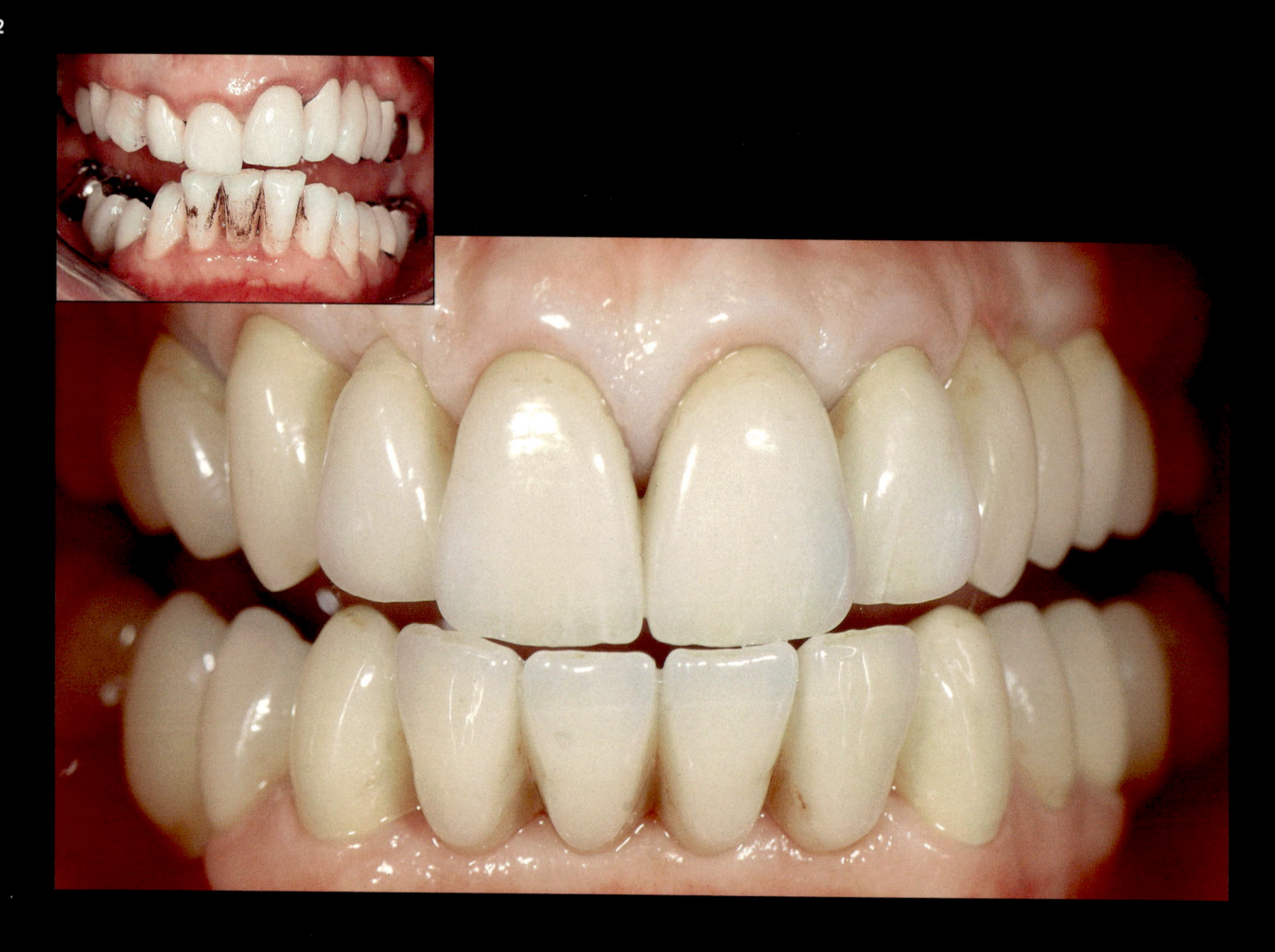

1997

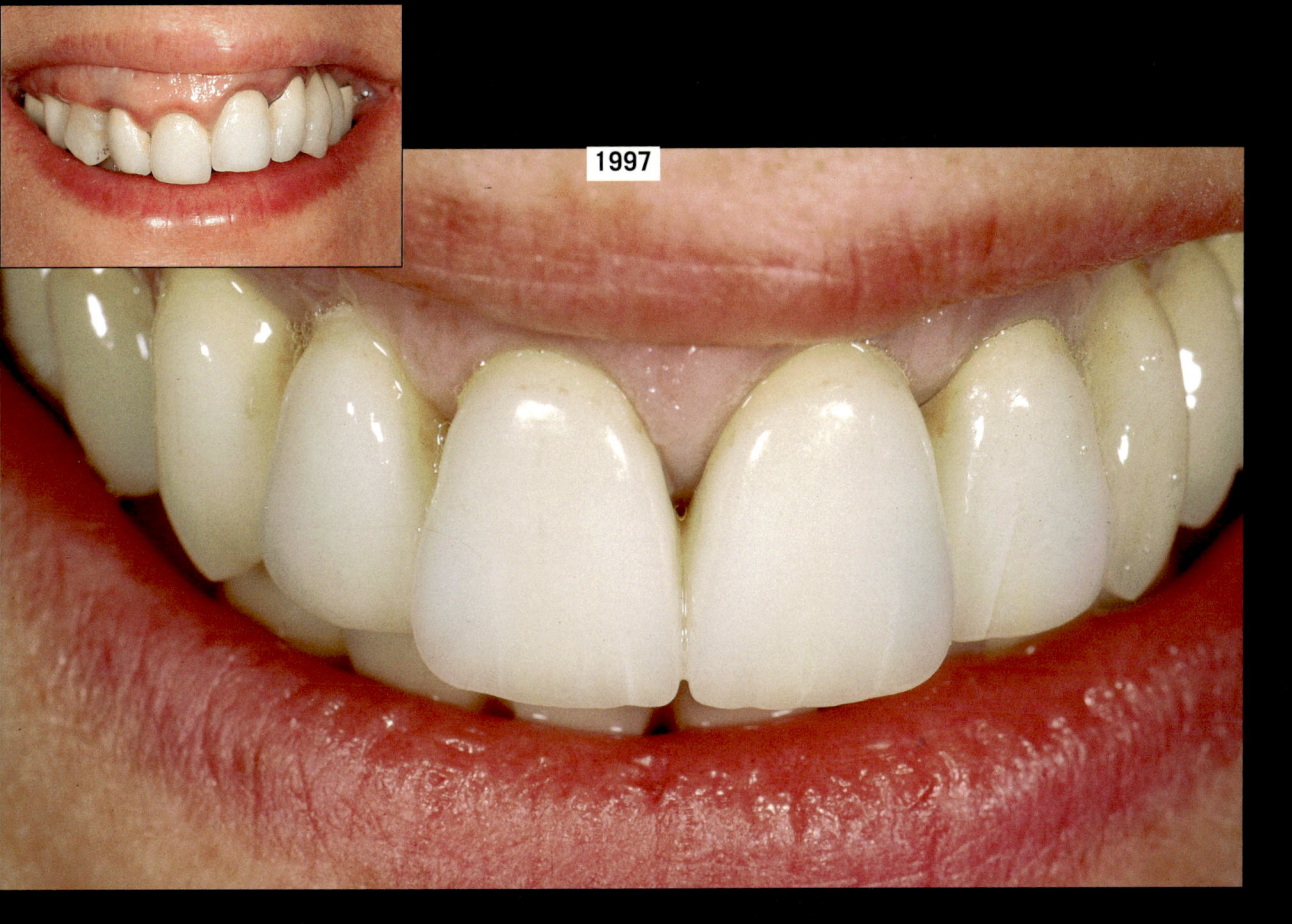

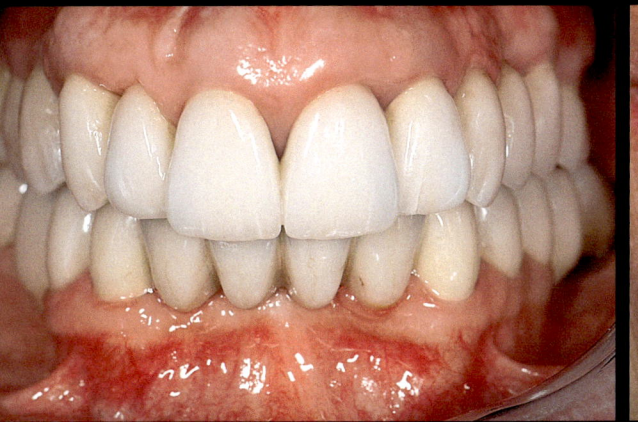

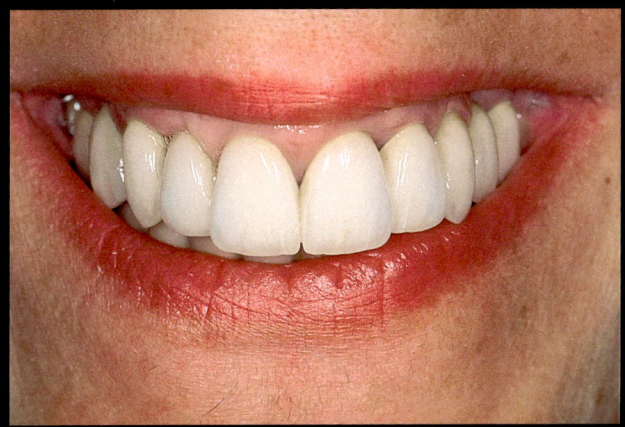

2007

| Patient: M.S. | Gender: M | Age: 55 years |

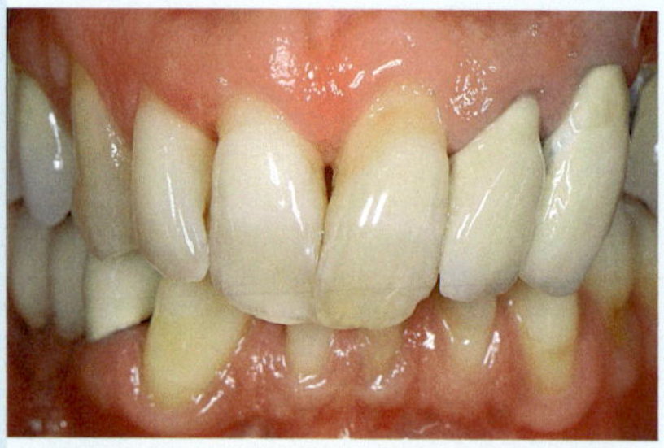

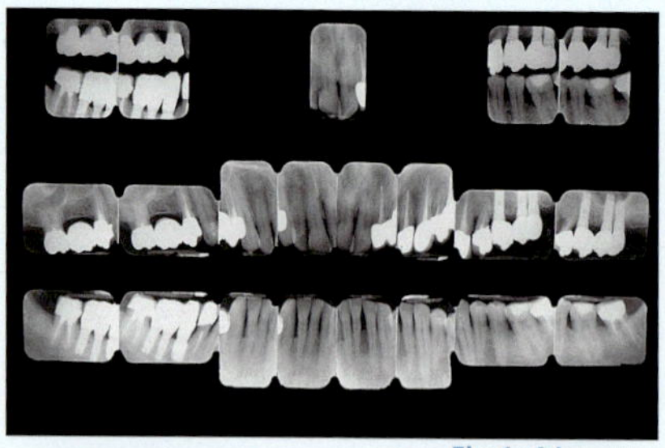

> Fig 1-4d
> Fig 1-4g 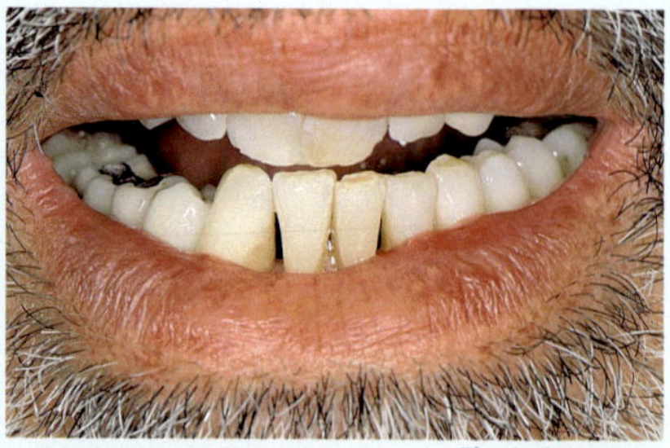
> Fig 1-22a 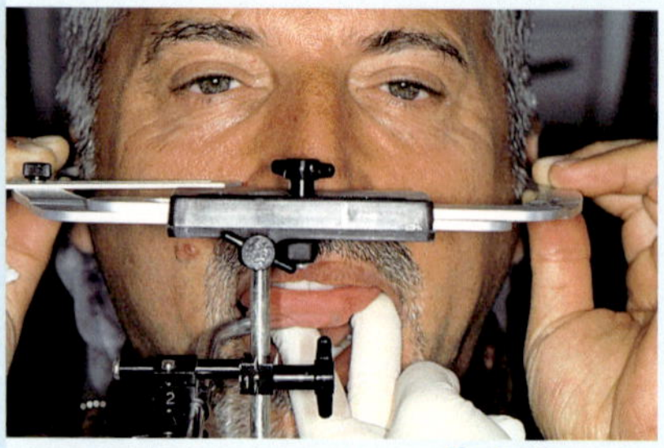
> Fig 1-6a 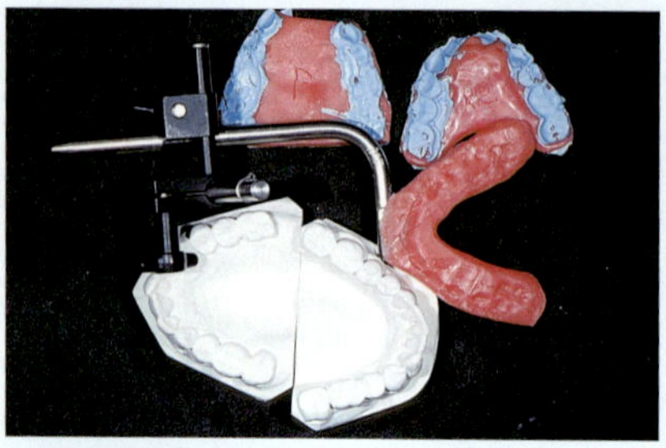
> Fig 1-24b 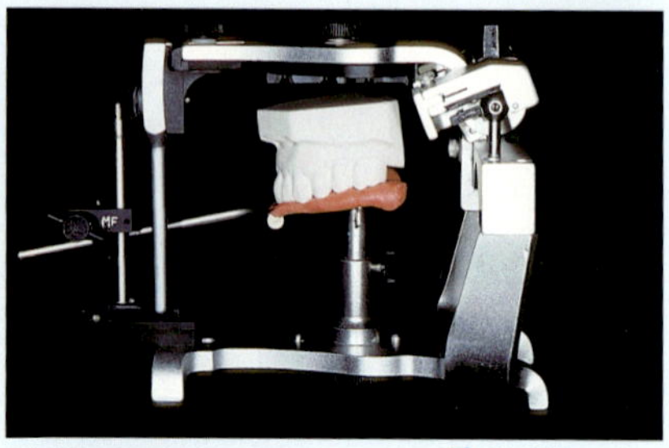
> Fig 2-9a 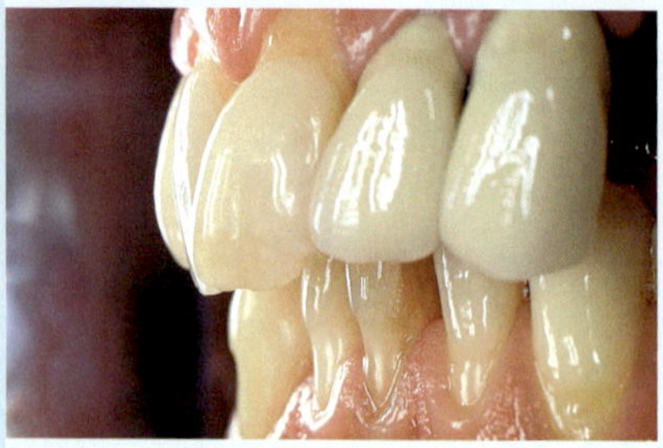 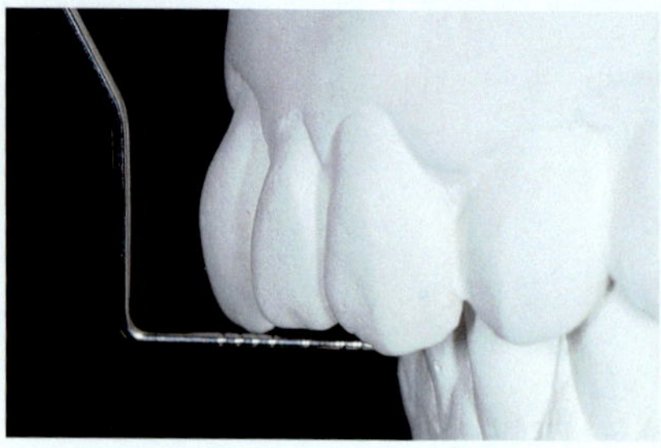
> Fig 2-9b 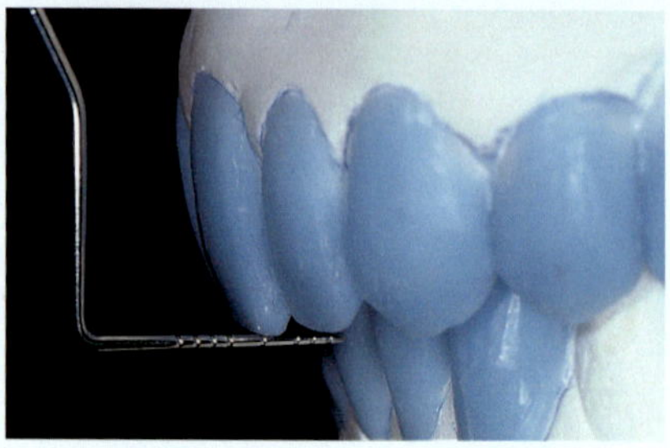

PAGES 544–545 After fabricating the stone casts and recording the facebow and the occlusal registration, the technician was given all the information necessary for finalizing the diagnostic wax-up. After a preliminary preparation of the abutments, the provisional restoration was put in place and relined in the mouth, checking the ideal esthetic and functional integration.

PAGES 546–547 The substructures were molded thanks to the guidance of the silicone indices derived from the functionalized provisional, which the technician will also make use of during the ceramic layering phase.

PAGES 548–551 The rehabilitation on natural teeth and implants (positioned at another office) was finalized using metal-ceramic in the posterior sectors, and glass-ceramic (Empress, Ivoclar Vivadent) in the anterior sector.

PAGES 552–553 A comparison of the before and after photos shows how, on completion of the treatment, the new orientation of the occlusal plane contributes strongly to the pleasant appearance of the smile.

Rehabilitation on natural teeth and implants   Treatment: 2003

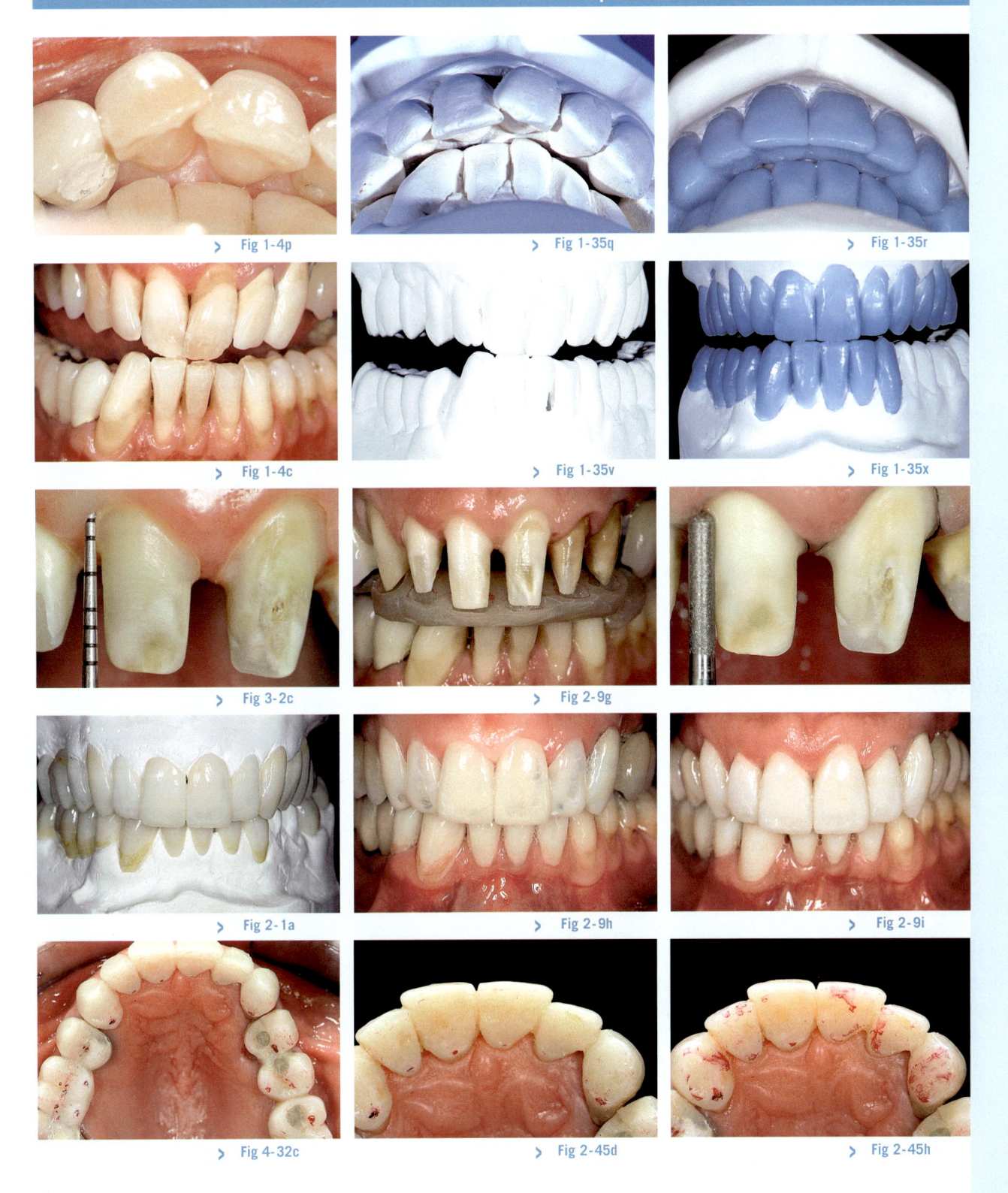

› Fig 1-4p

› Fig 1-35q

› Fig 1-35r

› Fig 1-4c

› Fig 1-35v

› Fig 1-35x

› Fig 3-2c

› Fig 2-9g

› Fig 2-1a

› Fig 2-9h

› Fig 2-9i

› Fig 4-32c

› Fig 2-45d

› Fig 2-45h

546

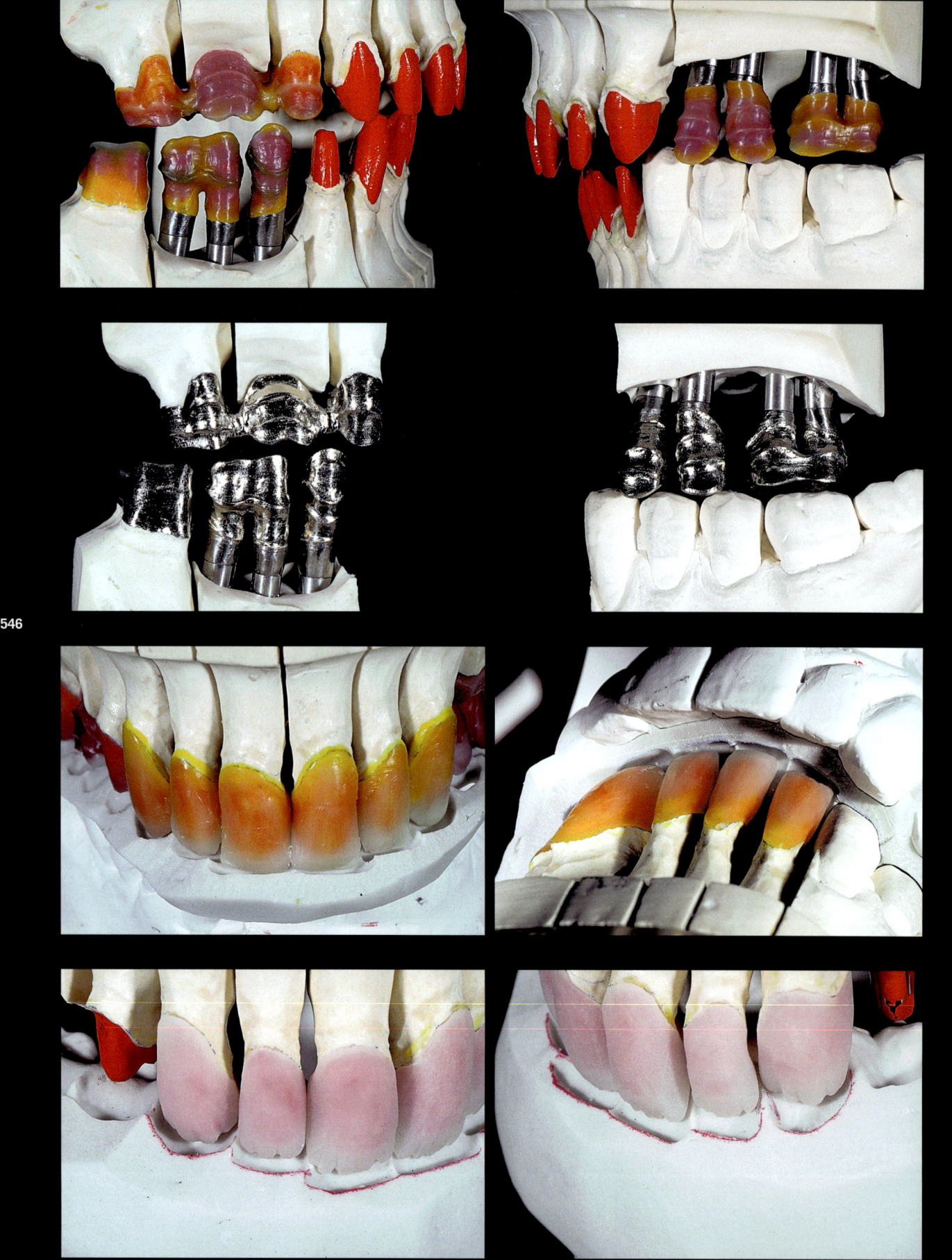

547

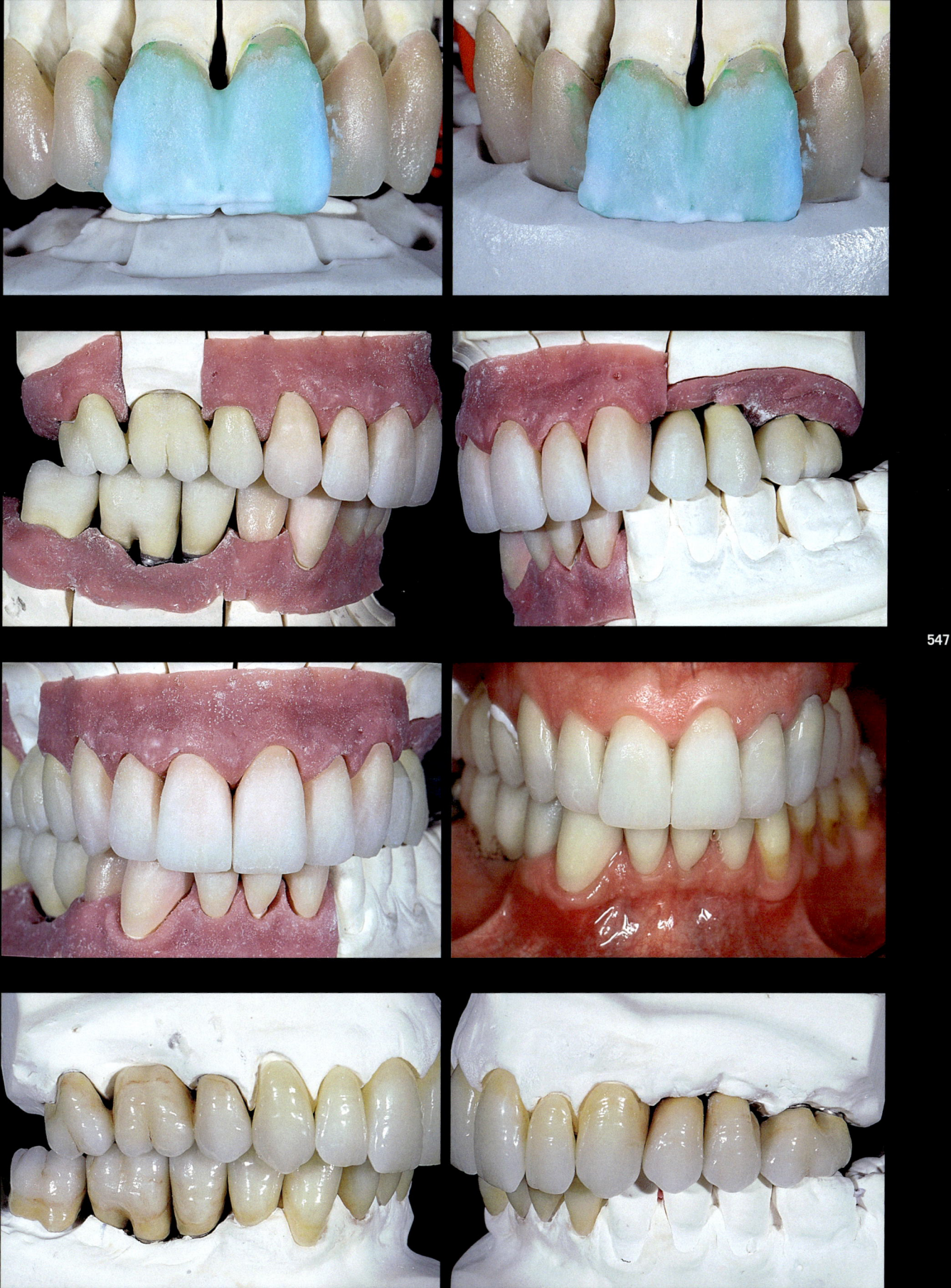

548

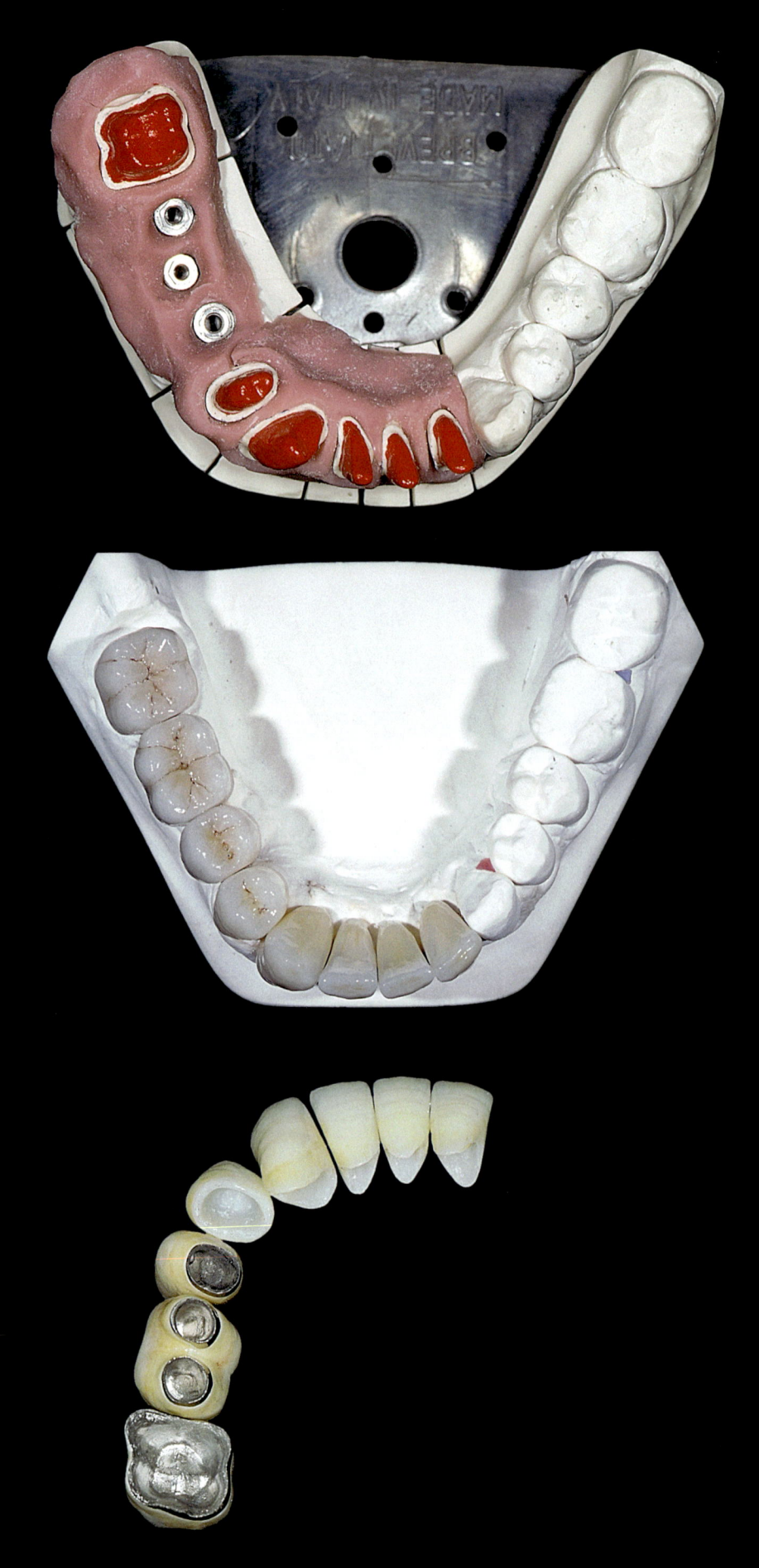

549

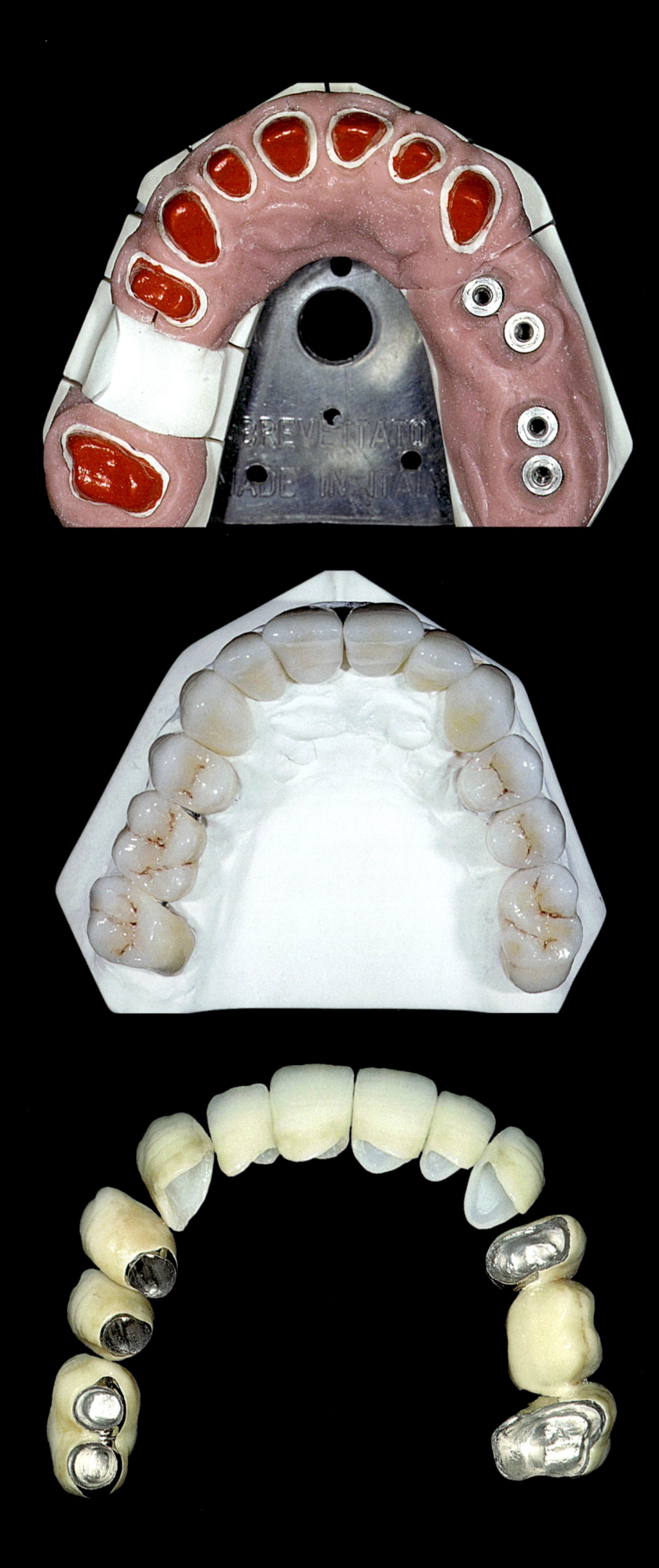

550

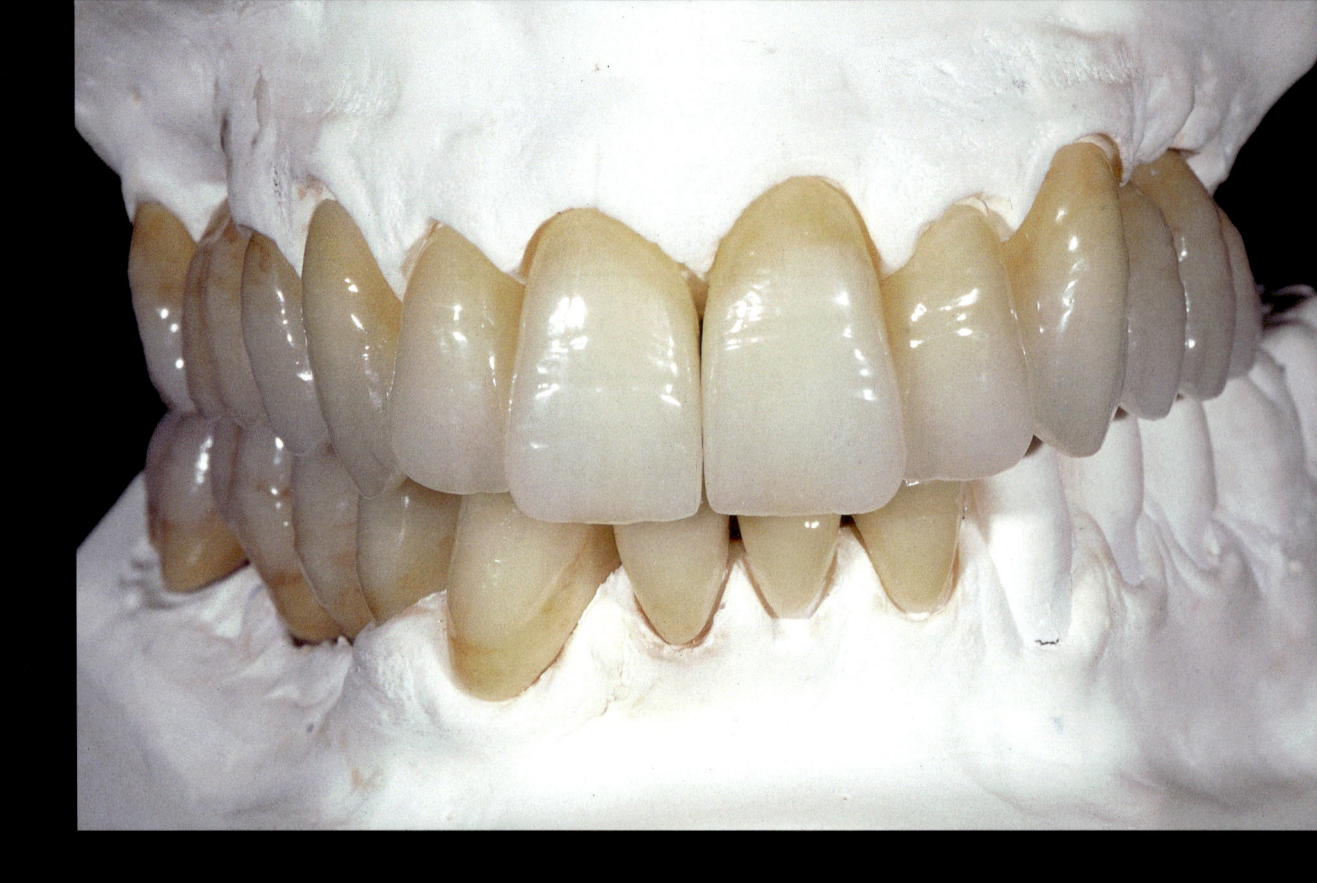

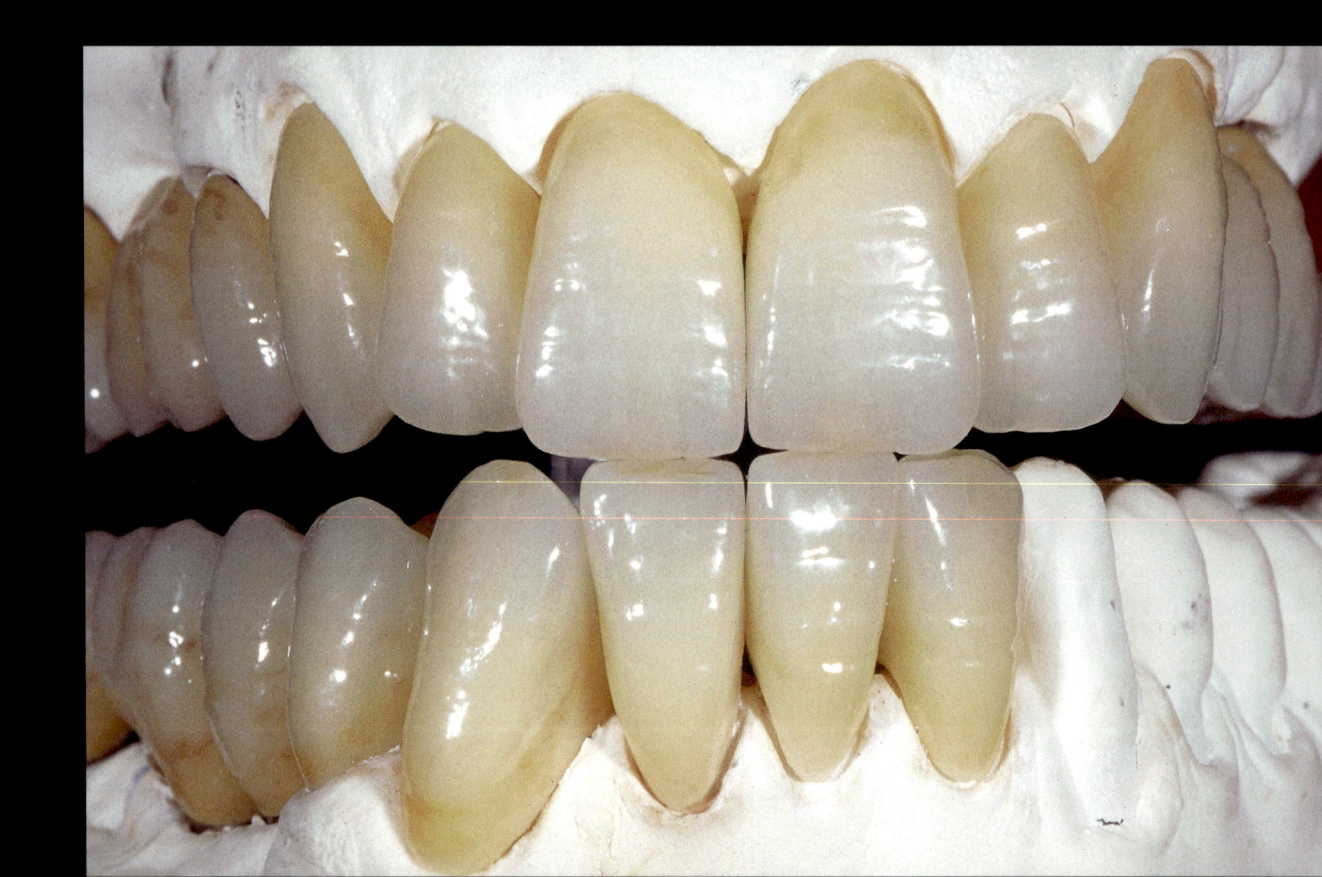

551

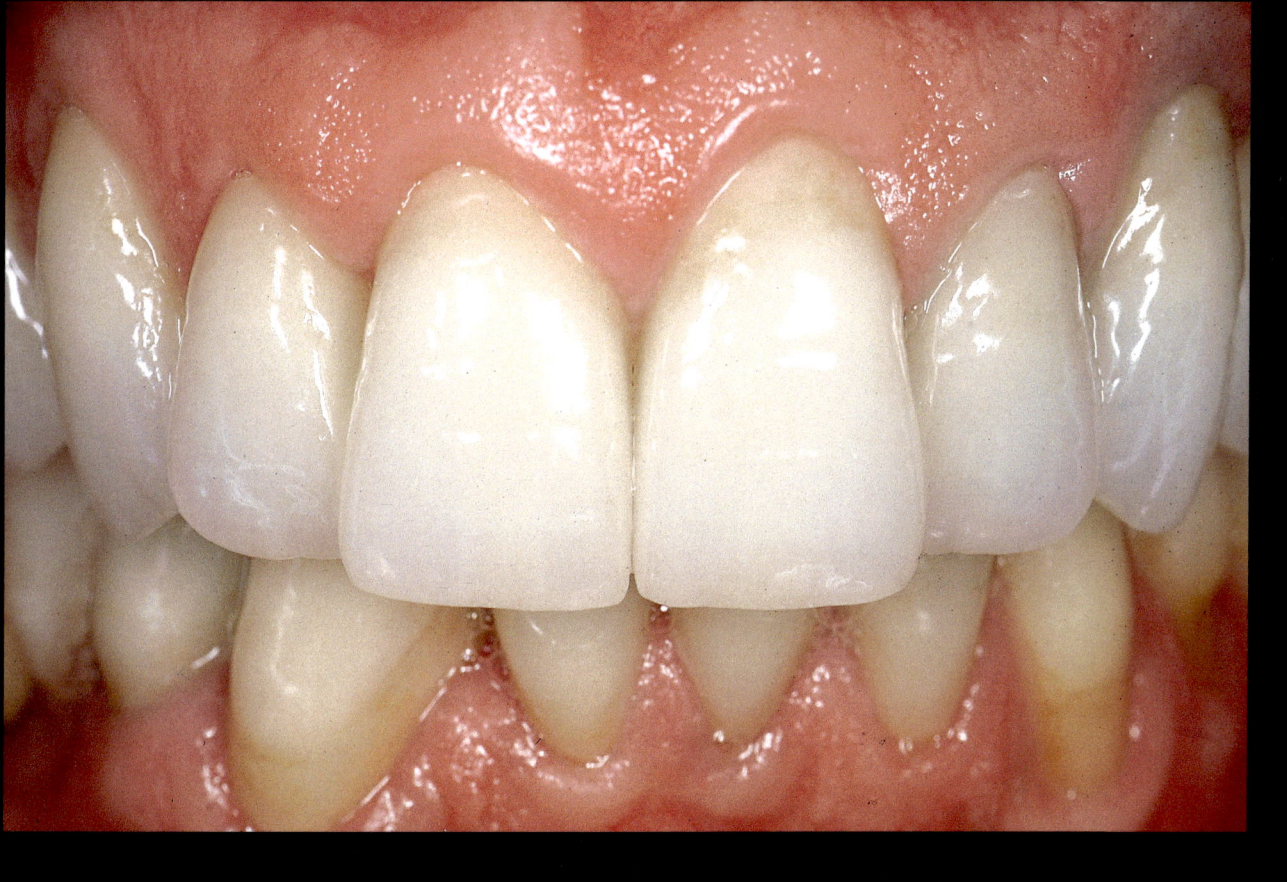

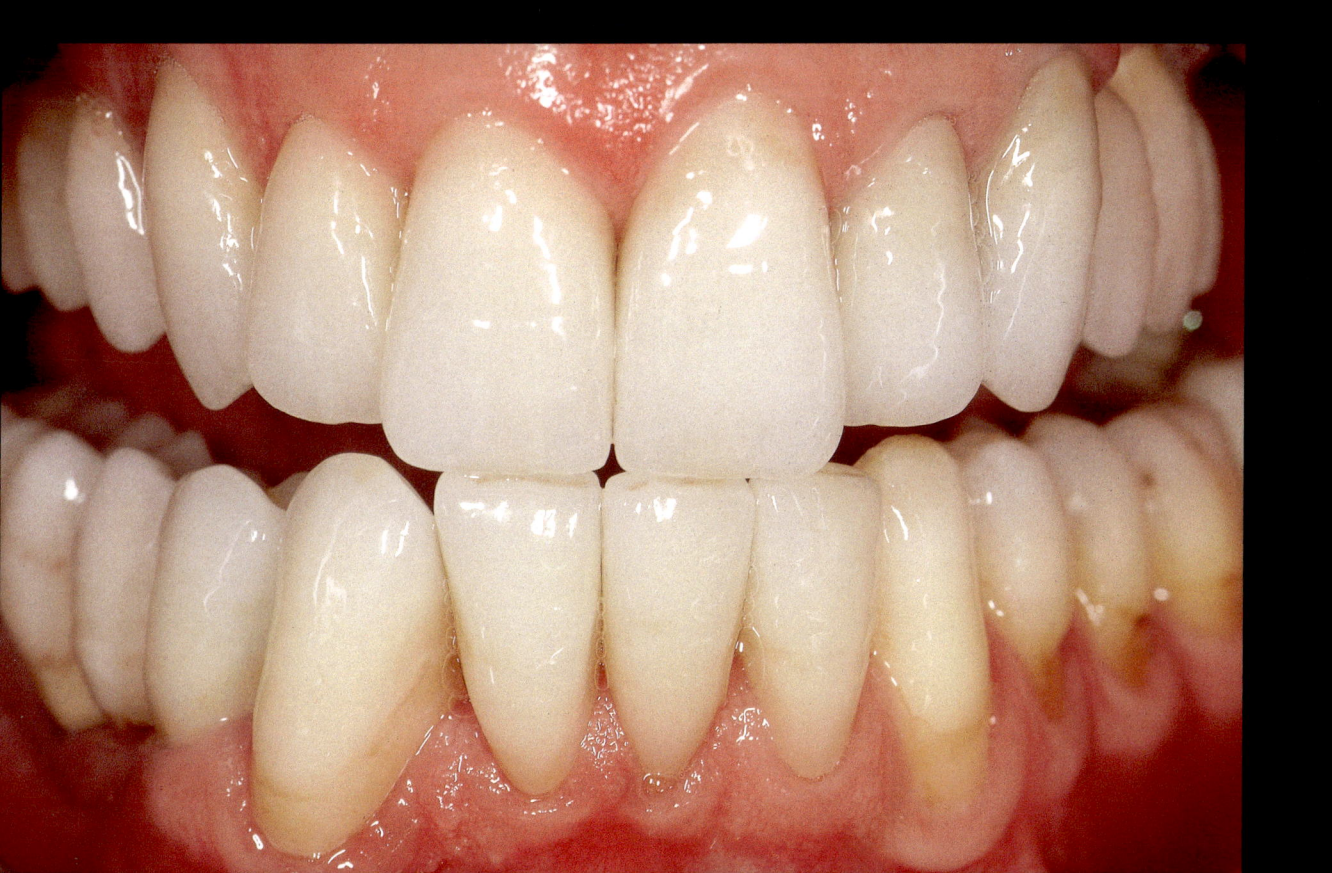

552

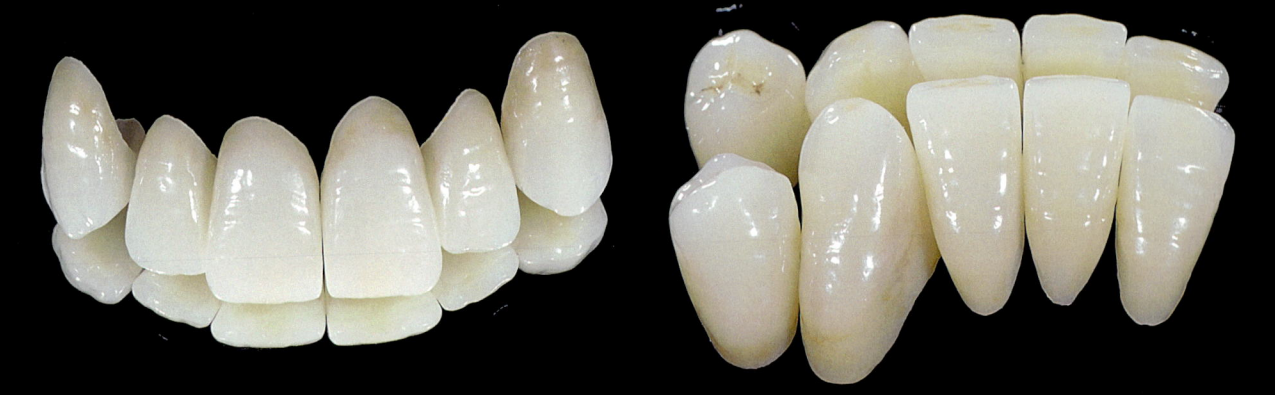

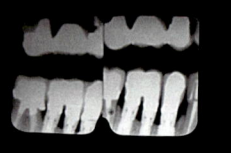

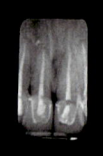

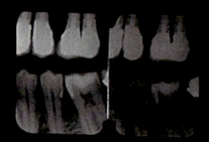

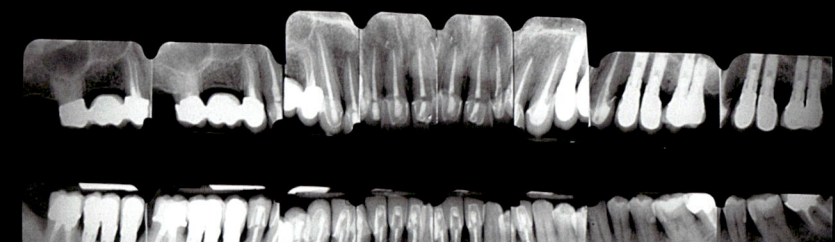

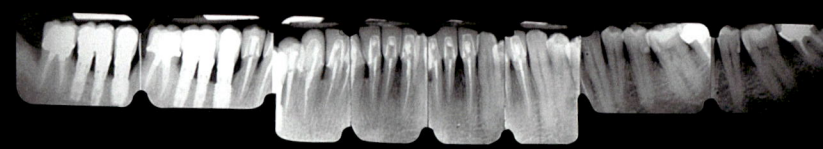

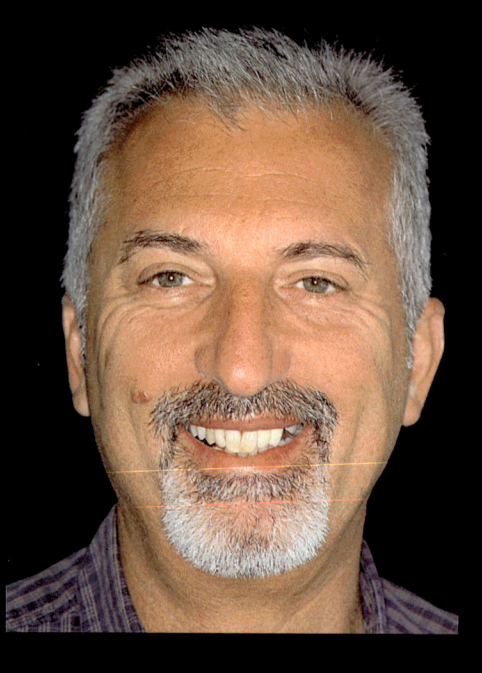

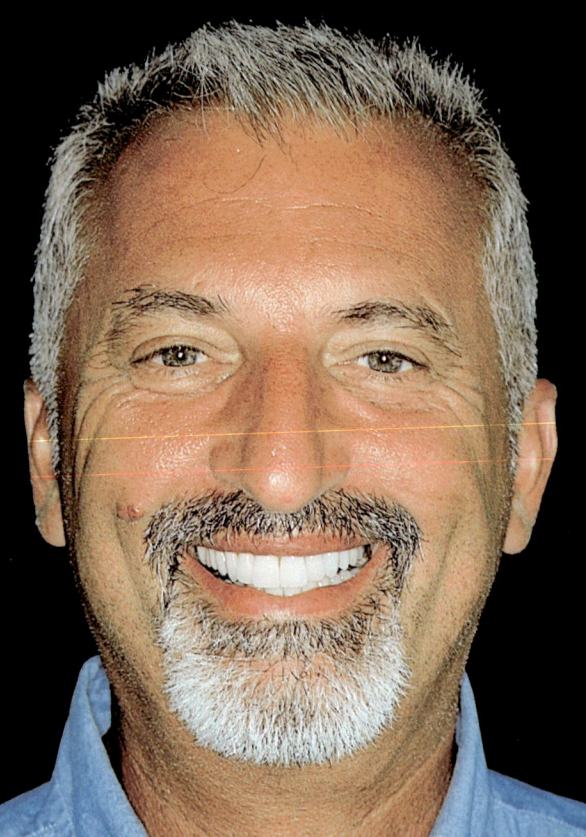

553

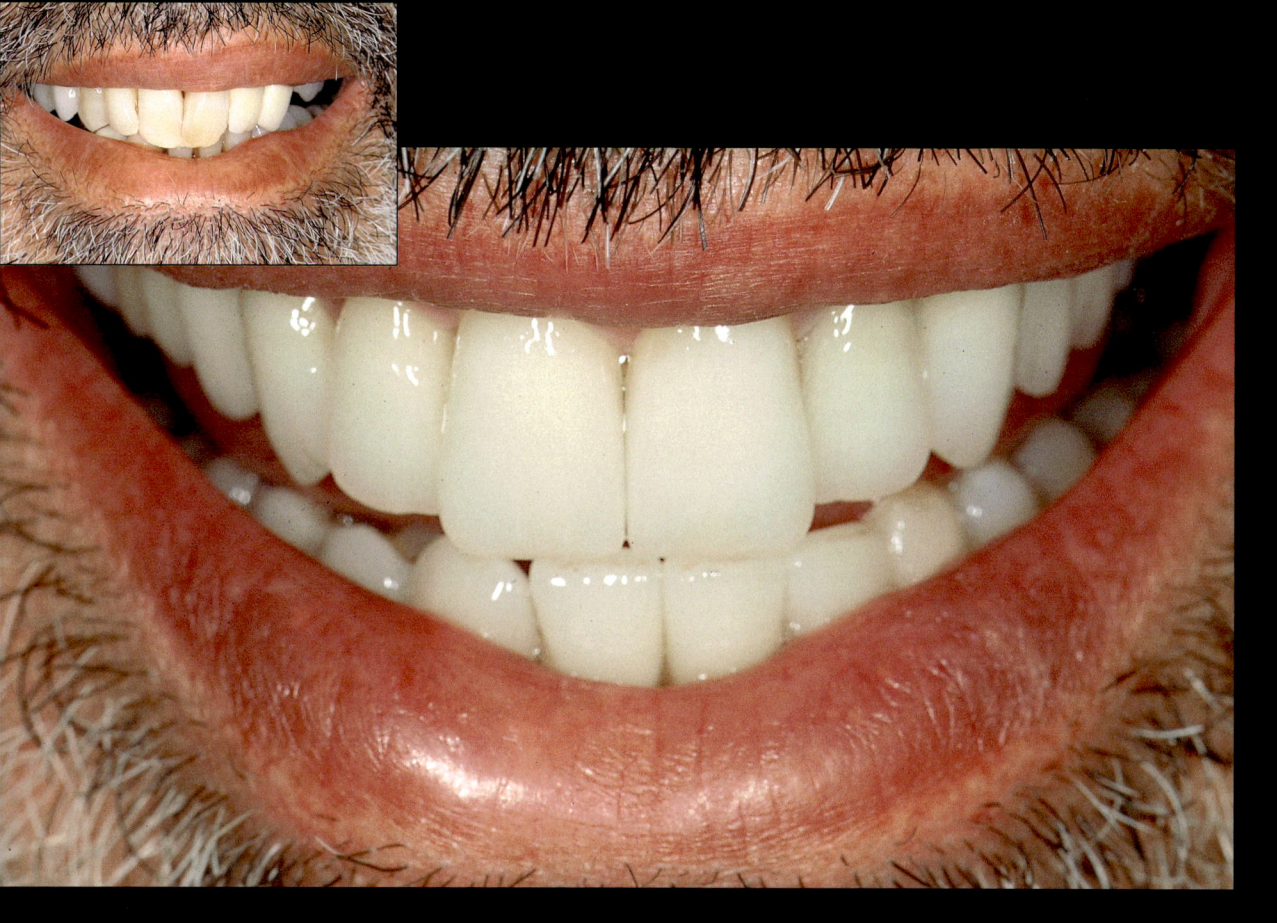

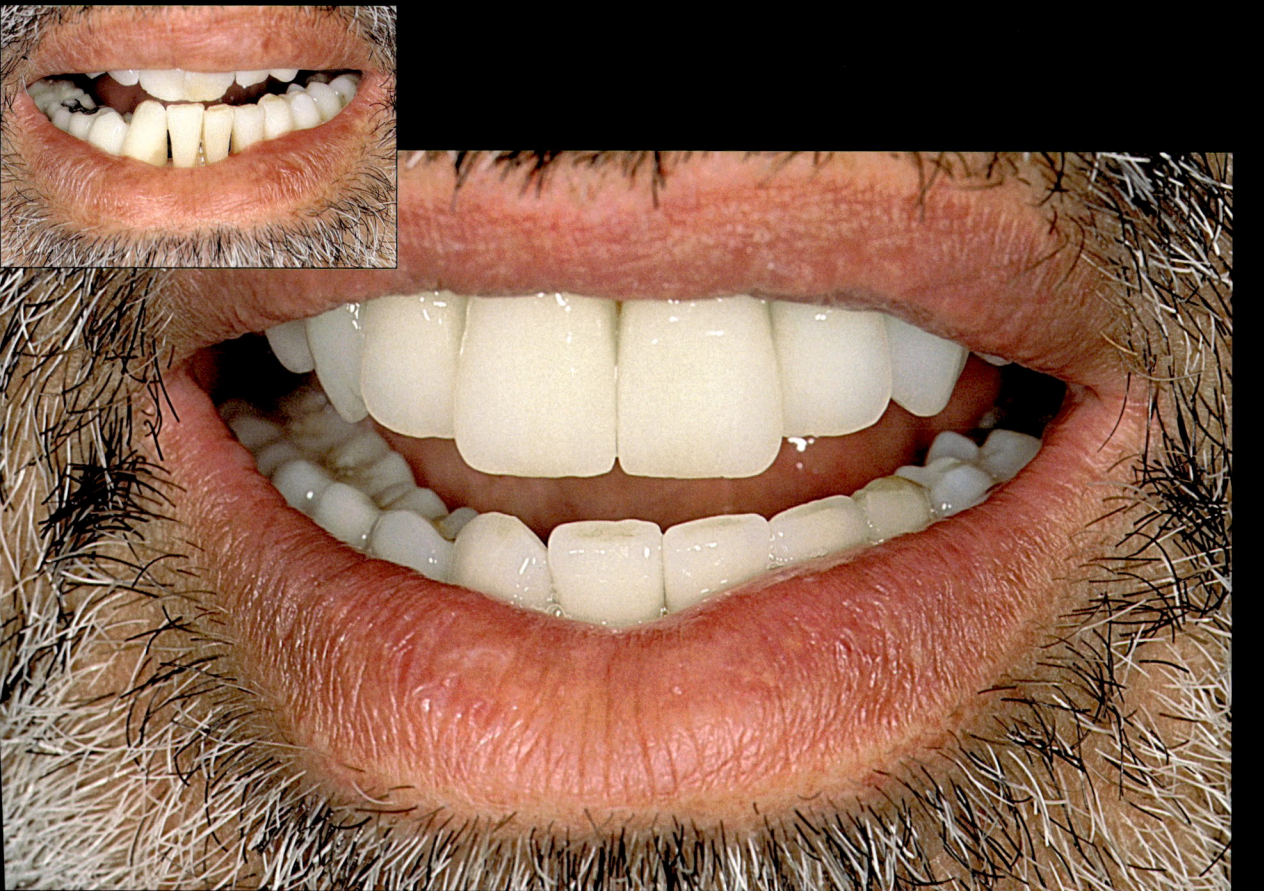

Patient: T.W.   Gender: M   Age: 55 years

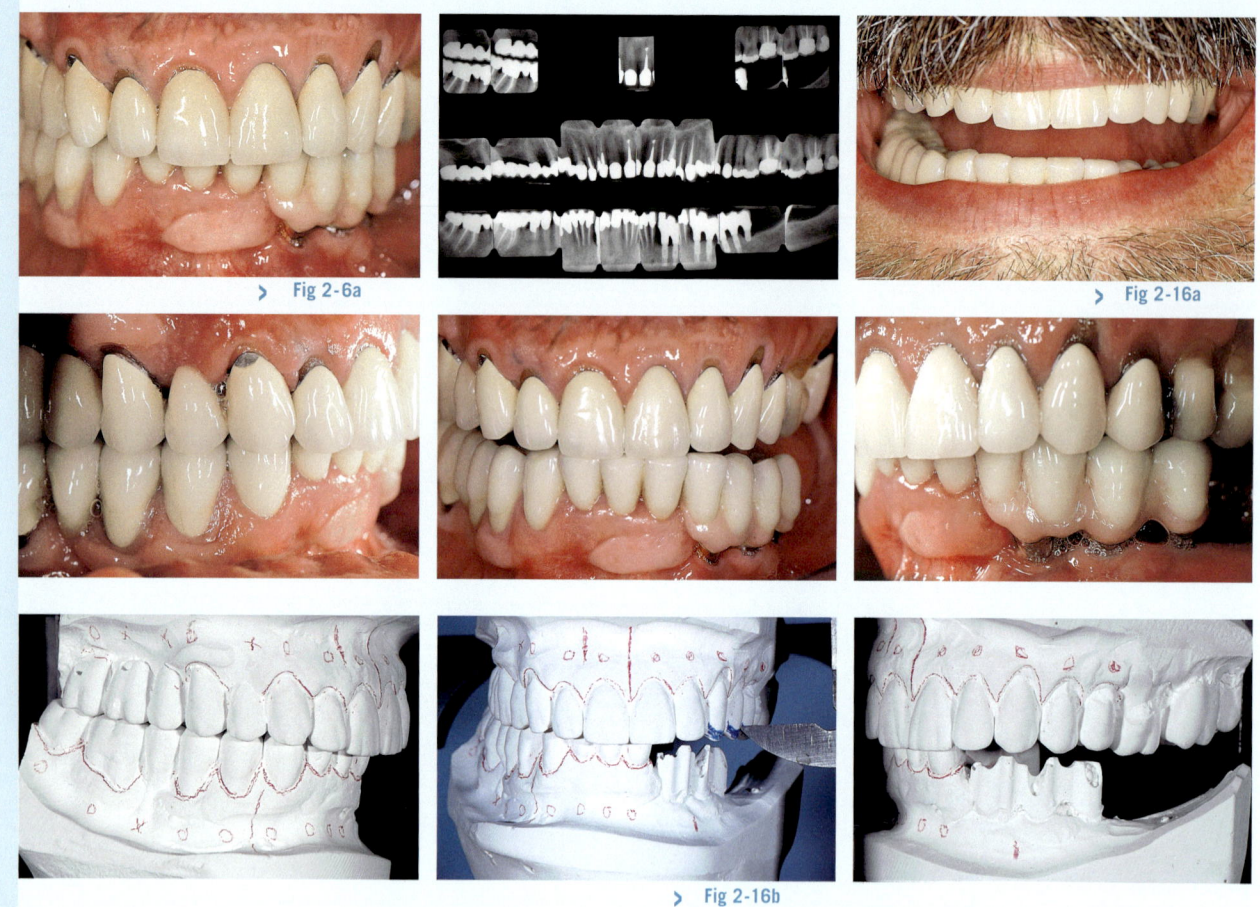

> Fig 2-6a

> Fig 2-16a

> Fig 2-16b

PAGES 554–555 After the old restorations were removed, the diagnostic wax-up and the provisional restoration were made, which, once fitted and relined, showed a substantial change of orientation in the mandibular occlusal plane.

PAGES 556–559 After suitably functionalizing the provisional restoration and taking all of the registrations necessary for transferring the relative esthetic-functional information to the technician, the substructures were made, using metal-ceramic in the posterior sectors and all-ceramic in the anterior sectors (Procera Alumina, Nobel Biocare). Preventive simulation (PS) allows the congruity of the cast cross-mounting to be checked; this was carried out before we proceeded with finalizing the work.

PAGES 560–561 Despite the presence of metal collars in the posterior sectors, the esthetic result was satisfactory thanks to the patient's low smile line. Note above all that a correct orientation of the mandibular occlusal plane, which was decidedly canted in the preoperative view, has been restored.

Rehabilitation on natural teeth and implants   Treatment: 2006

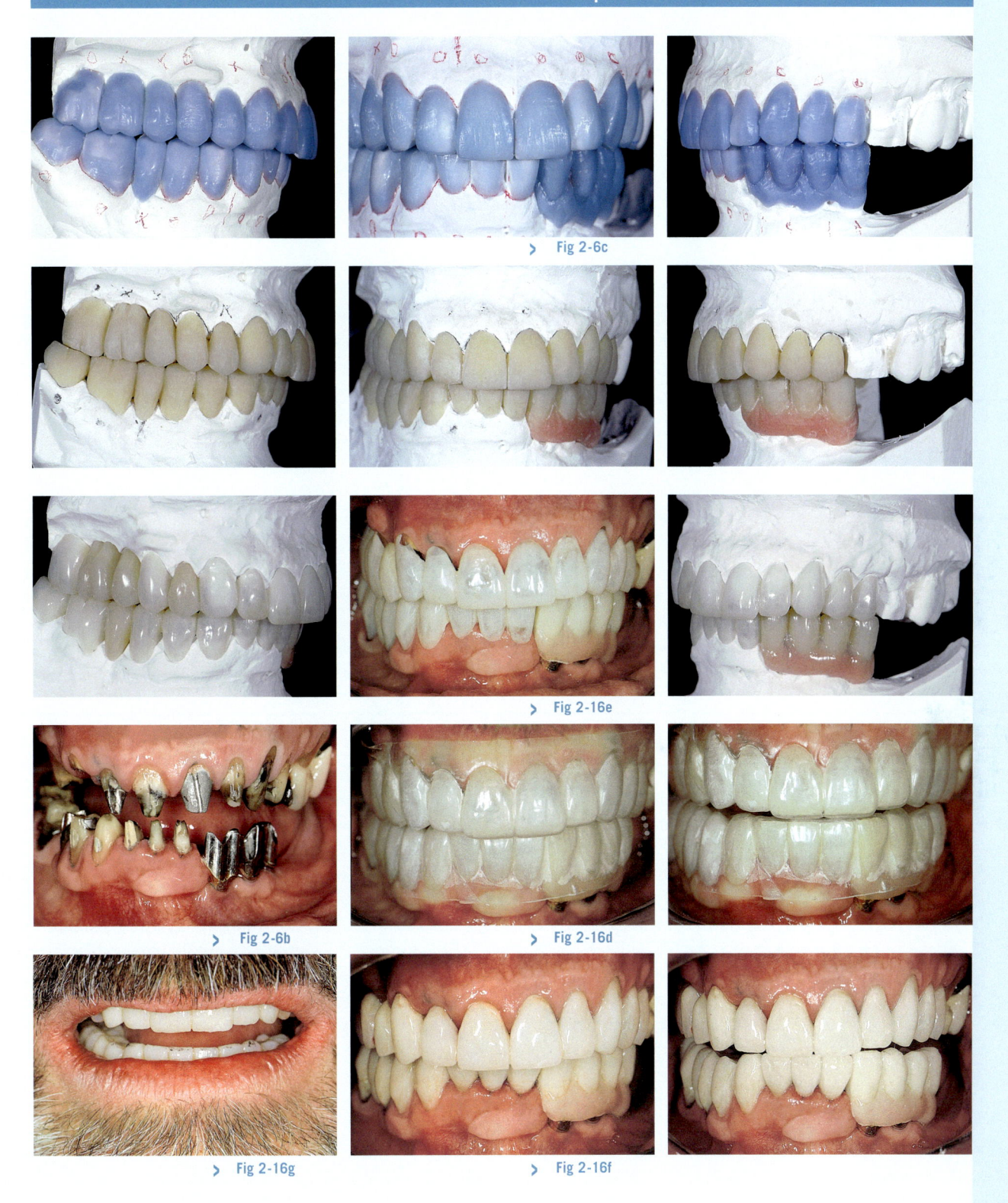

> Fig 2-6c

> Fig 2-16e

> Fig 2-6b

> Fig 2-16d

> Fig 2-16g

> Fig 2-16f

555

556

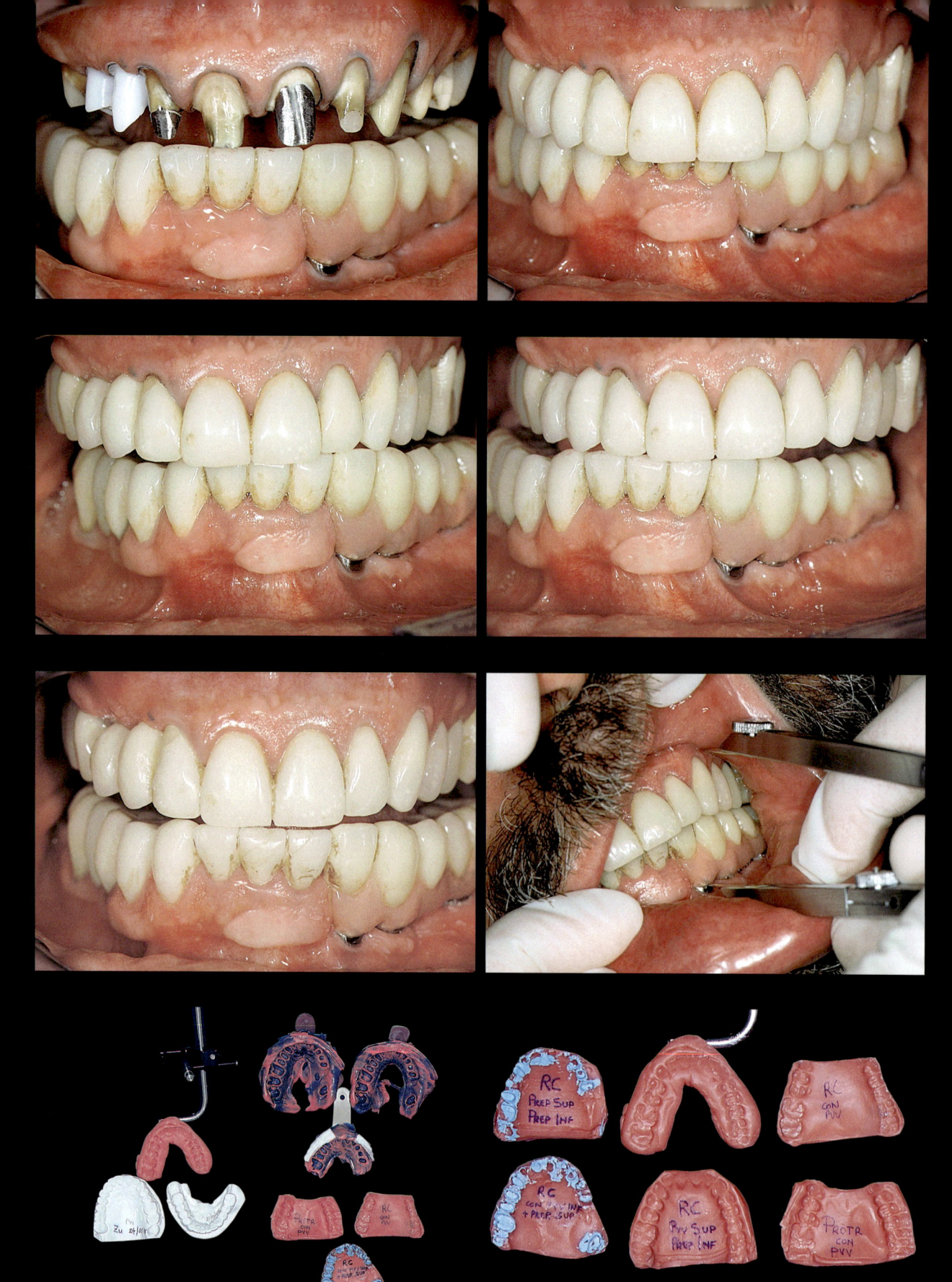

557

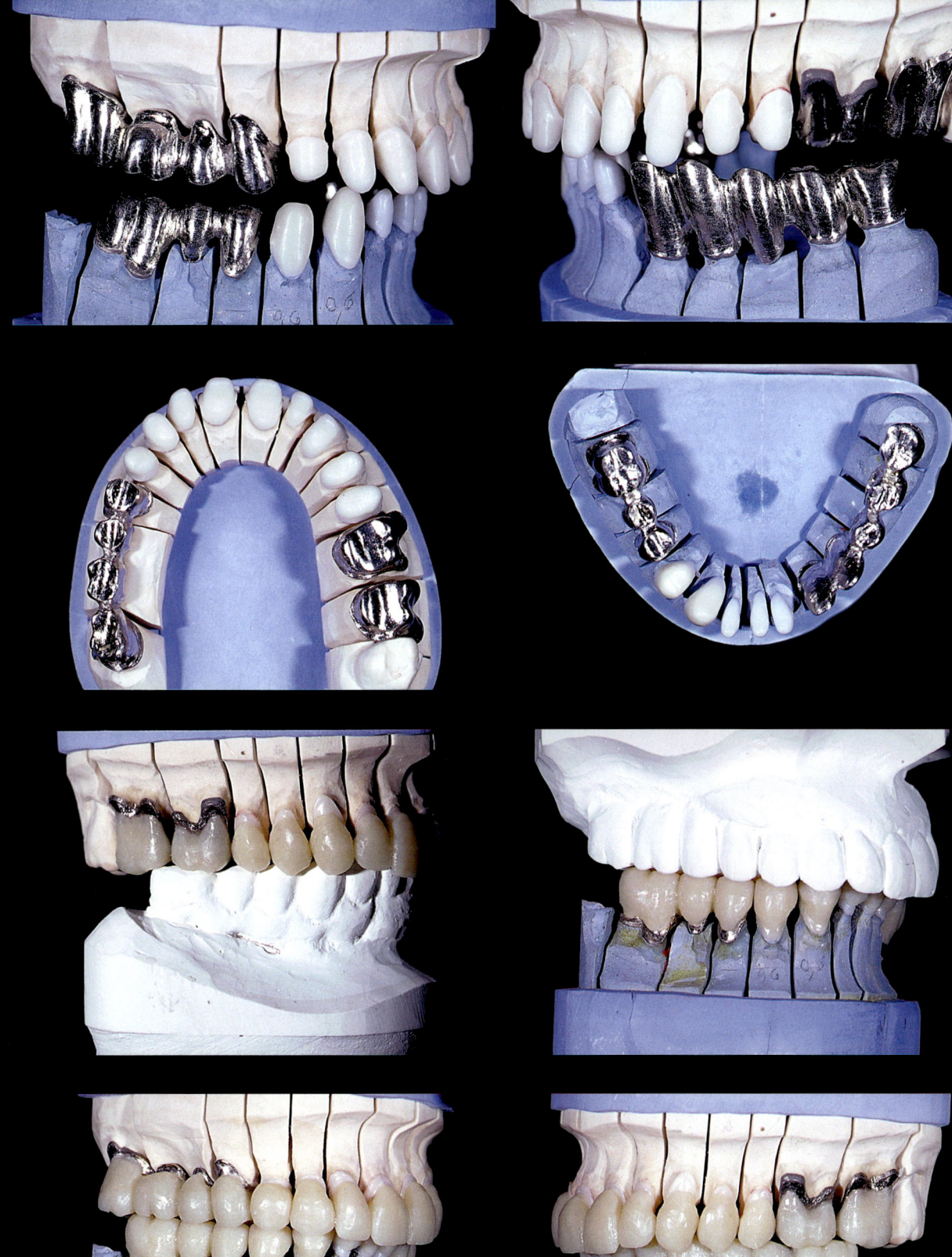

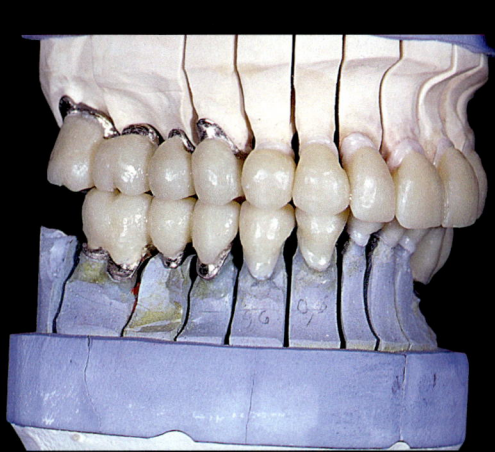

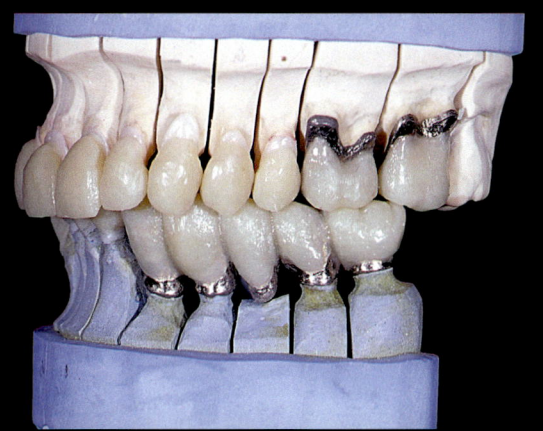

558

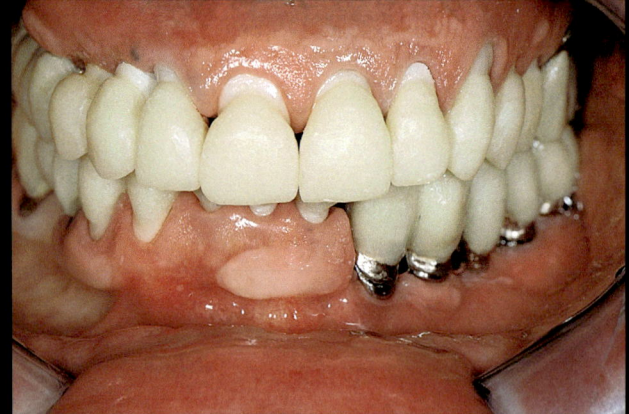

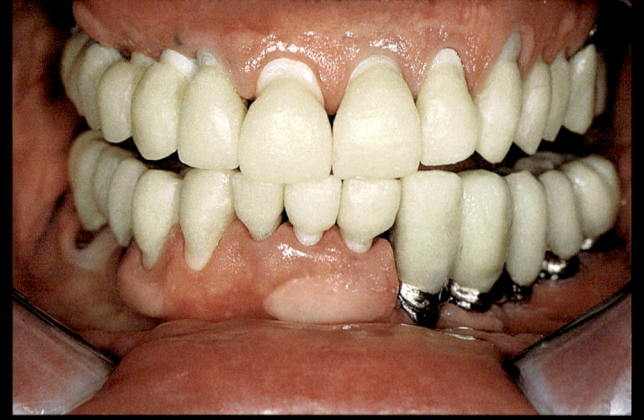

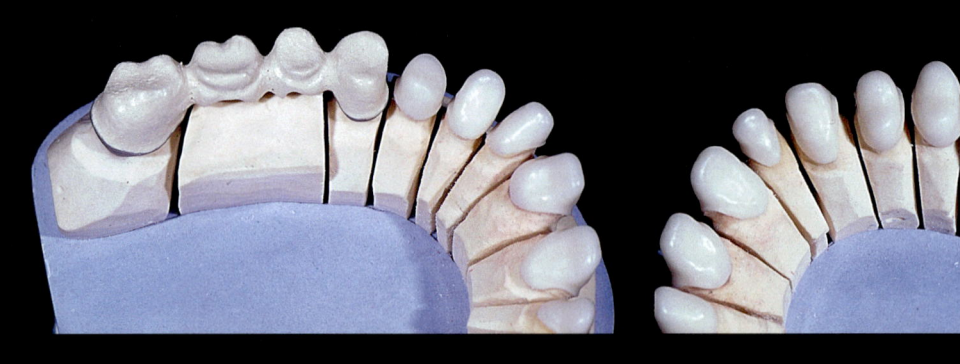

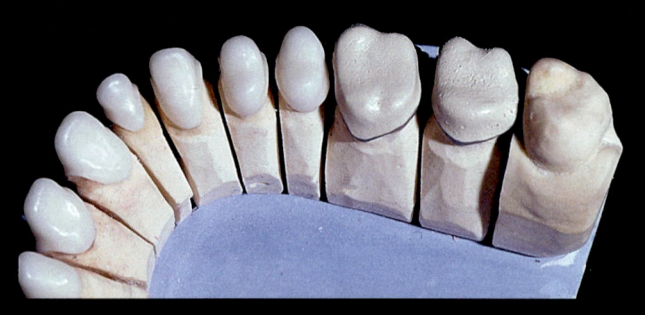

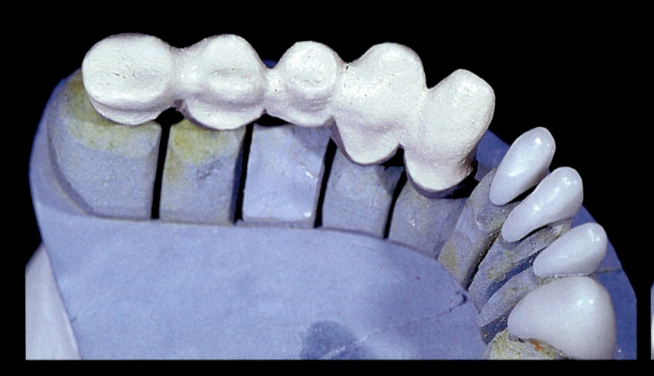

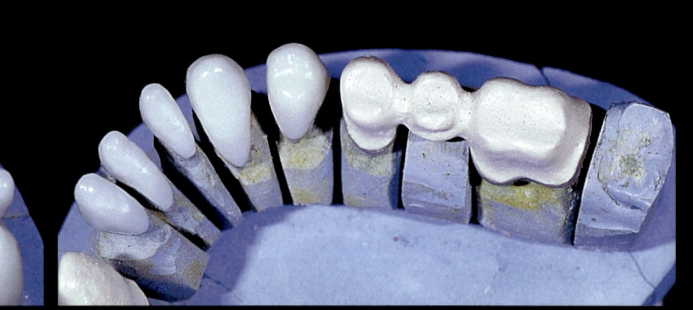

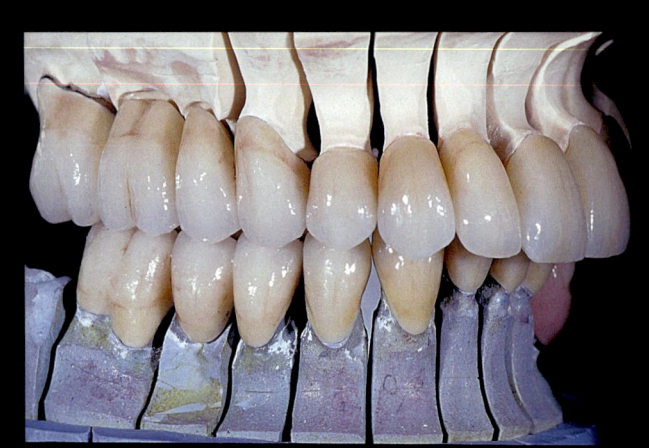

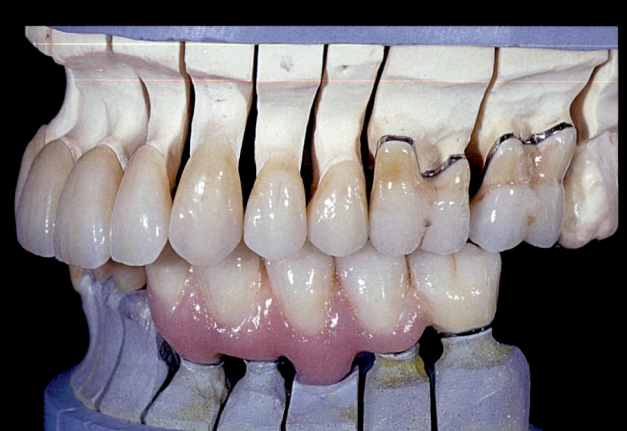

559

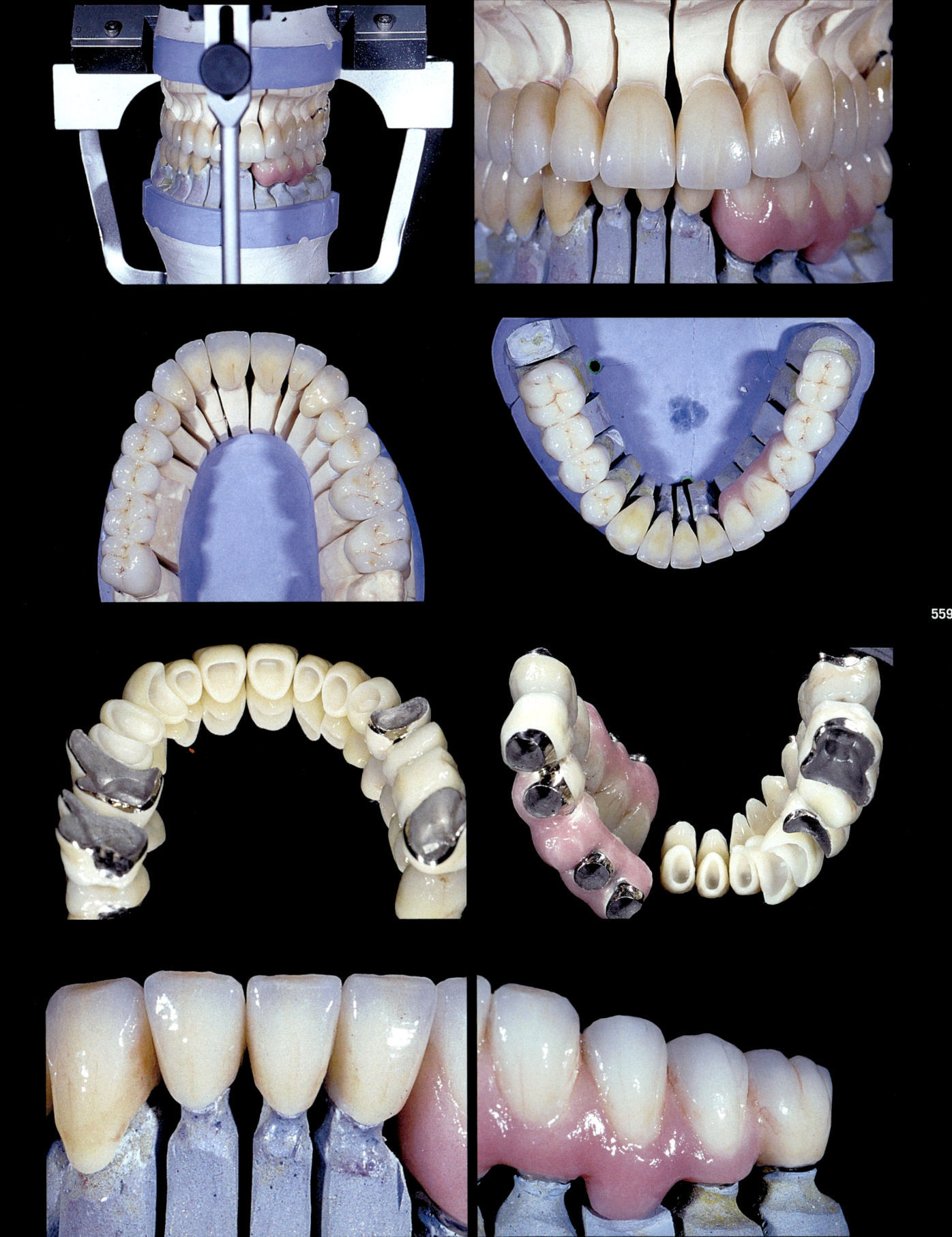

560

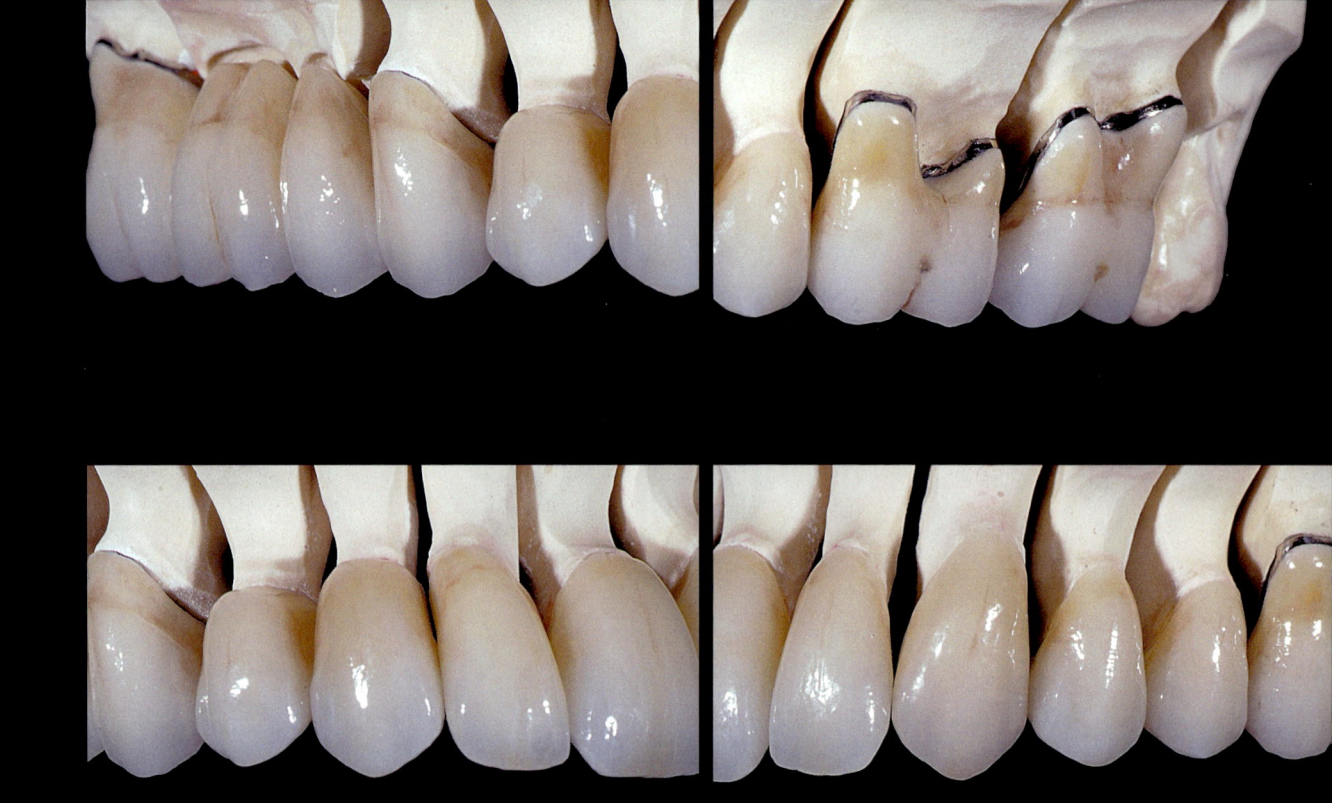

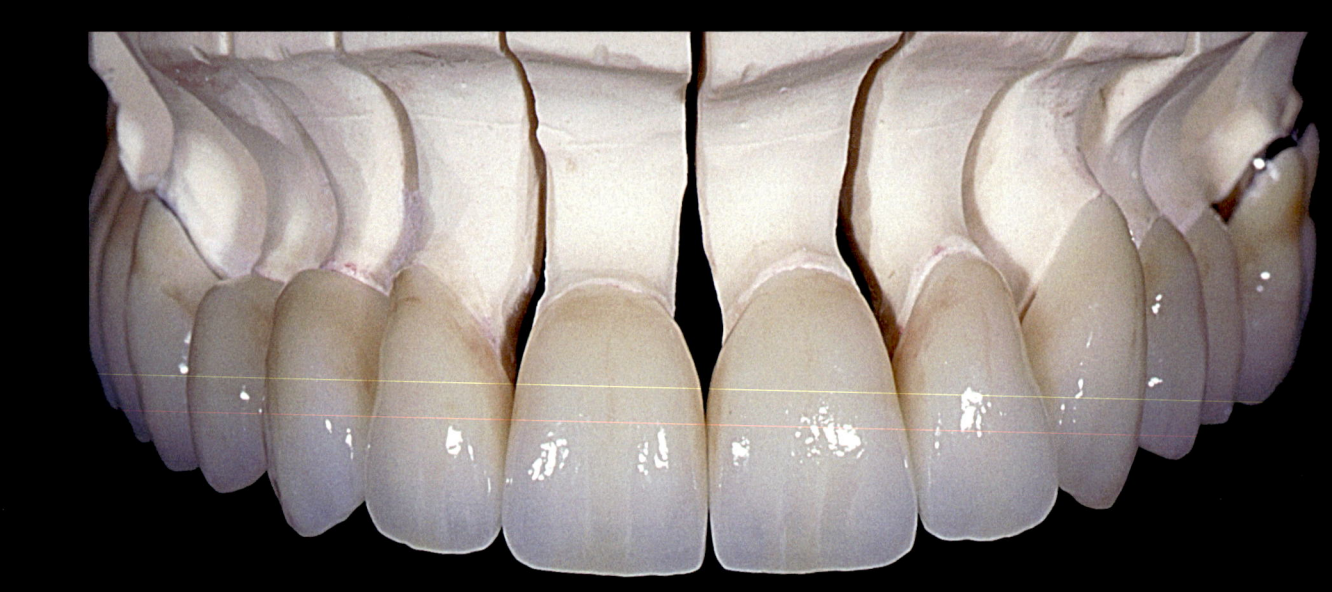

561

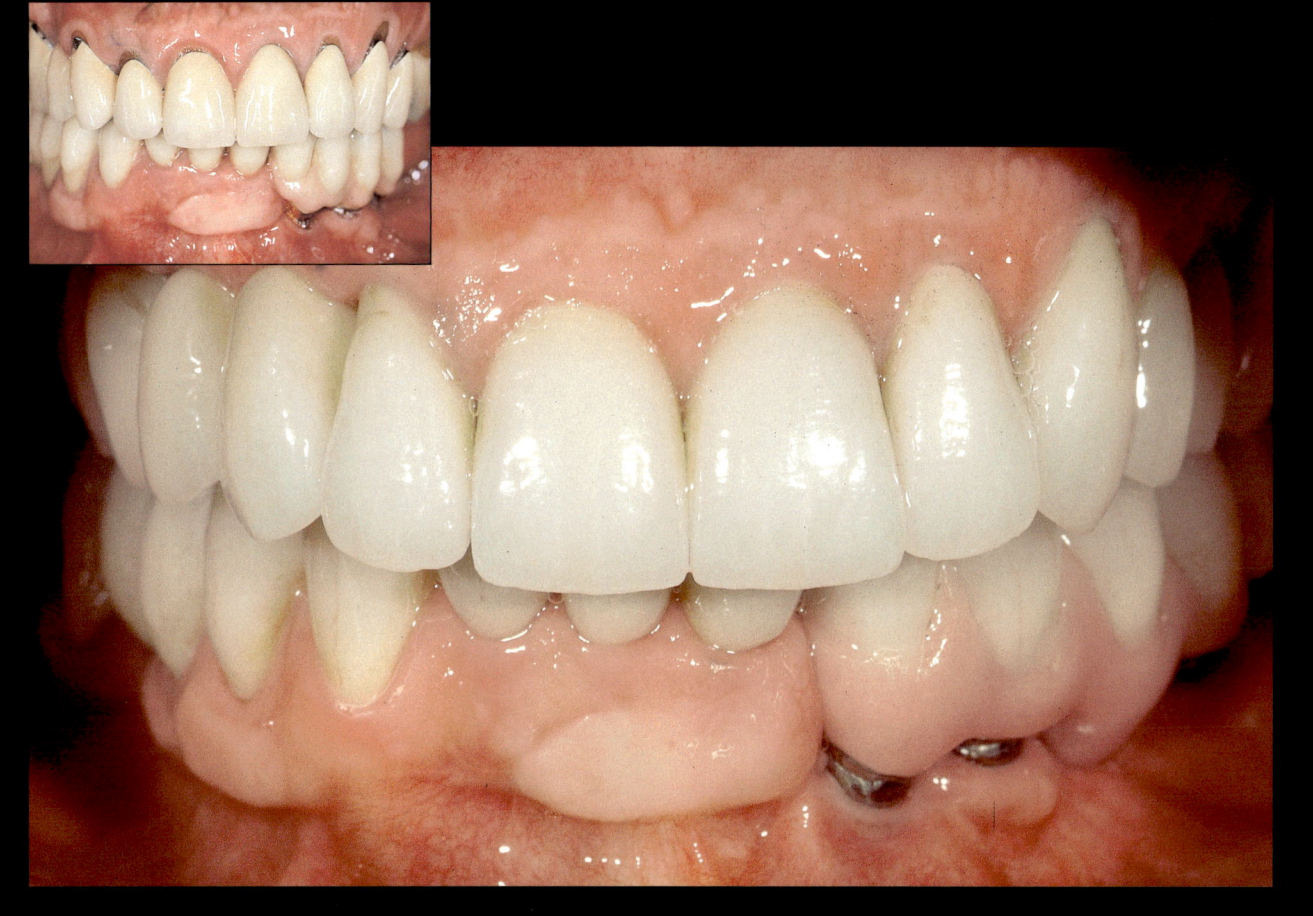

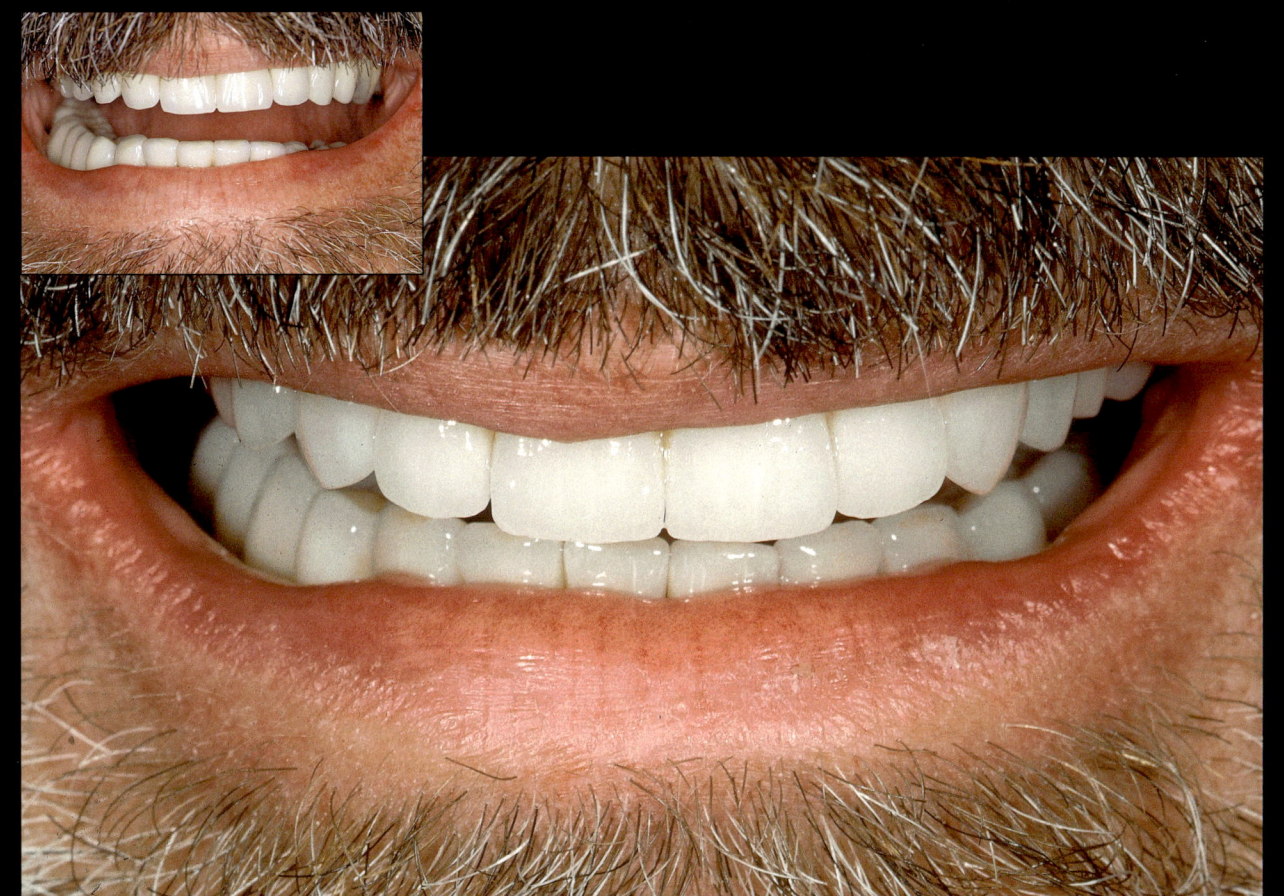

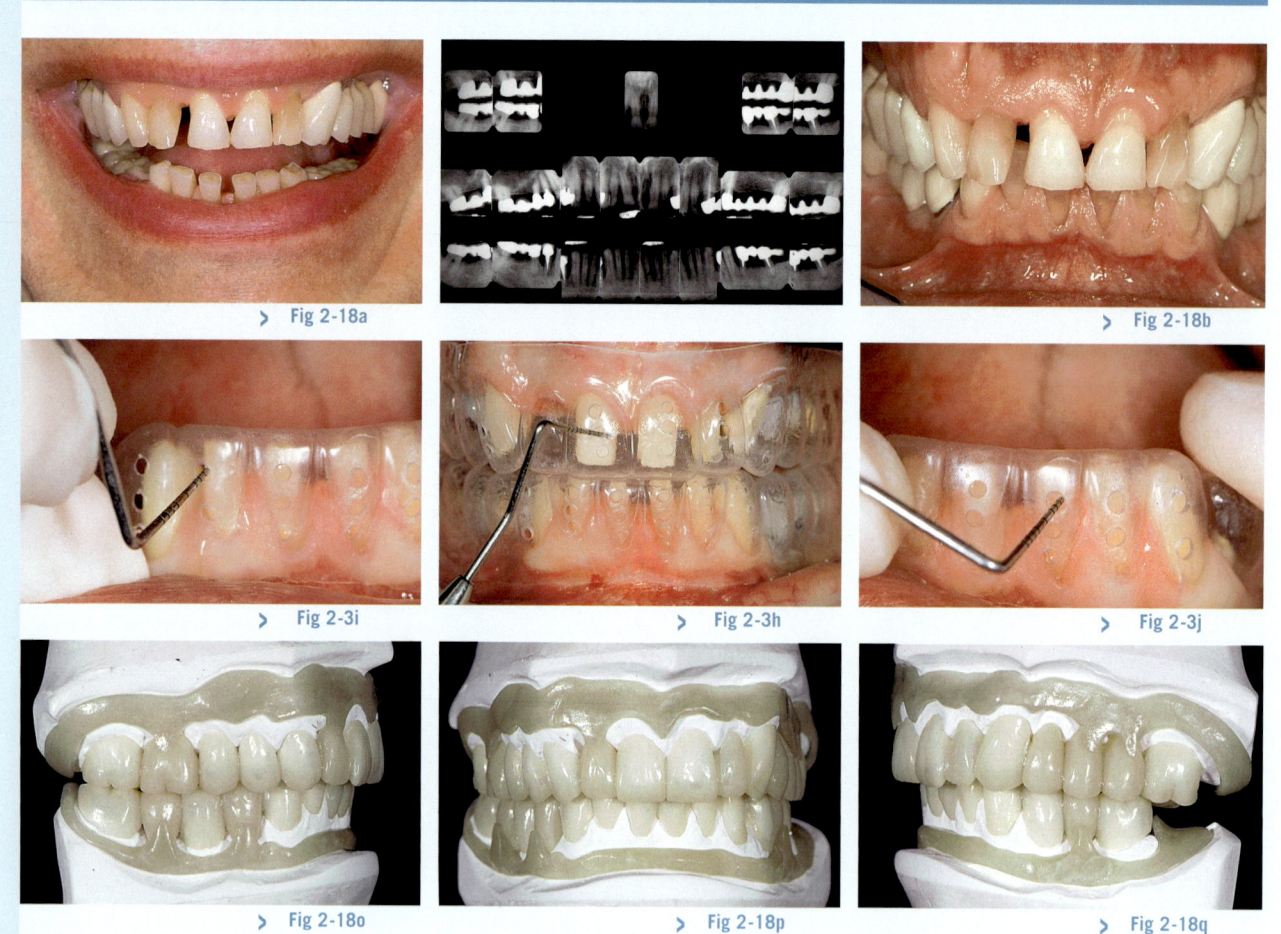

| Patient: R.A. | Gender: M | Age: 53 years |

> Fig 2-18a   > Fig 2-18b

> Fig 2-3i   > Fig 2-3h   > Fig 2-3j

> Fig 2-18o   > Fig 2-18p   > Fig 2-18q

PAGES 562–563   After receiving all of the indications regarding the modifications to be carried out, the technician first created the diagnostic wax-up and then the provisional restoration, which was subsequently fitted perfectly into the mouth by the clinician with the aid of the centering device. With the achievement of a satisfactory overall integration, the final impressions were taken of both arches, on natural teeth as well as implants.

PAGES 564–567   Complete recording of all the registrations indicated that the information necessary for cross-mounting the casts could be transferred to the laboratory. Preventive simulation (PS) was used to check the correctness before we proceeded with the ceramic layering.

PAGES 568–571   An ideal state of health of the gingival tissues is an indispensable condition if we intend to finalize the prosthetic rehabilitation with all-ceramics (anterior units: Procera Alumina; posterior units: Procera Zirconium, Nobel Biocare) especially if we intend to use a resinous cement to bond it (Unicem, 3M ESPE).

PAGES 572–577   The final result shows ideal esthetic, biologic, and functional integration of the prosthetic rehabilitation, especially compared with the patient's initial situation.

Rehabilitation on natural teeth and implants   Treatment: 2006

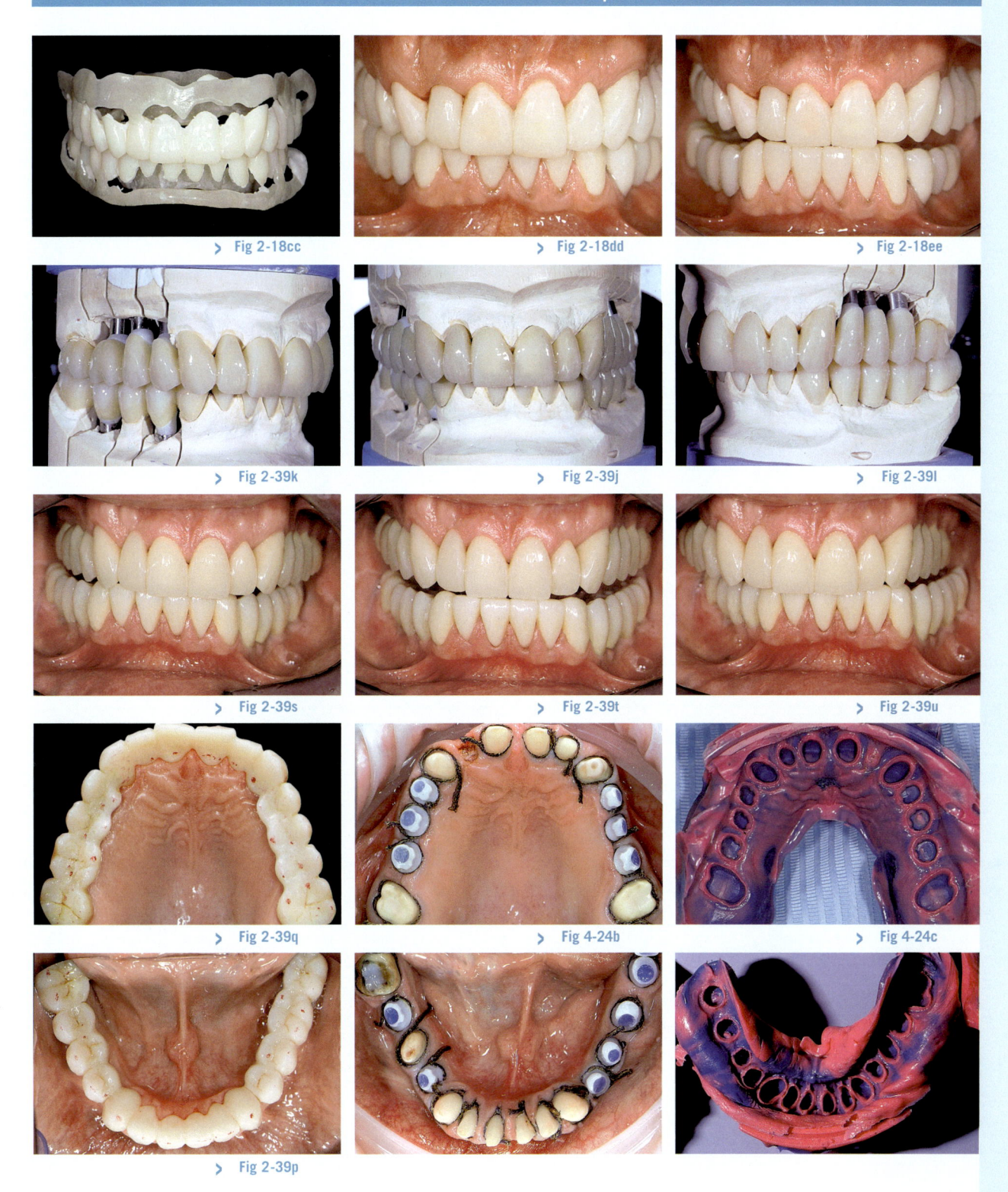

> Fig 2-18cc

> Fig 2-18dd

> Fig 2-18ee

> Fig 2-39k

> Fig 2-39j

> Fig 2-39l

> Fig 2-39s

> Fig 2-39t

> Fig 2-39u

> Fig 2-39q

> Fig 4-24b

> Fig 4-24c

> Fig 2-39p

563

564

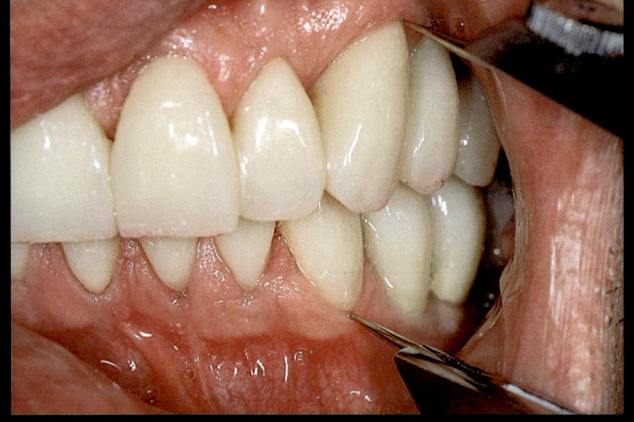

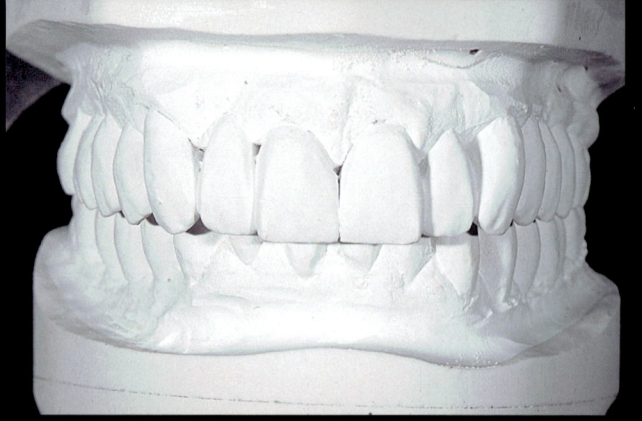

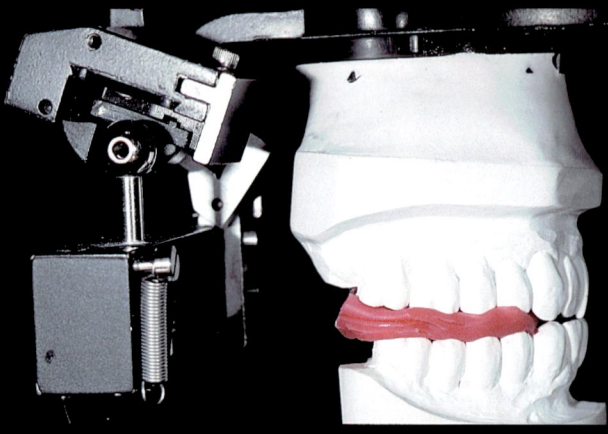

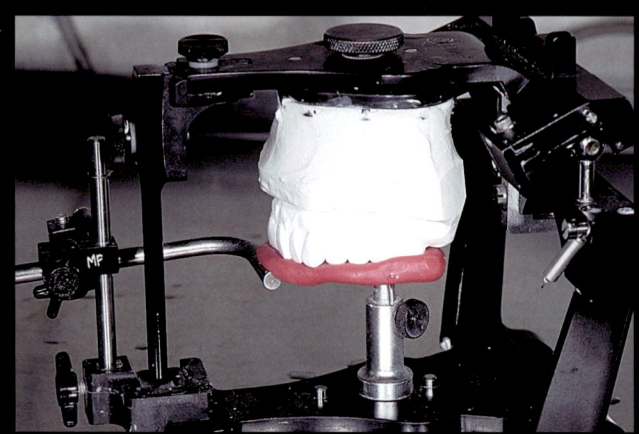

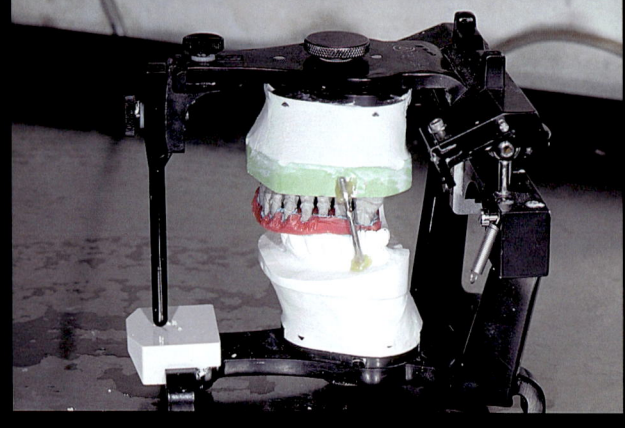

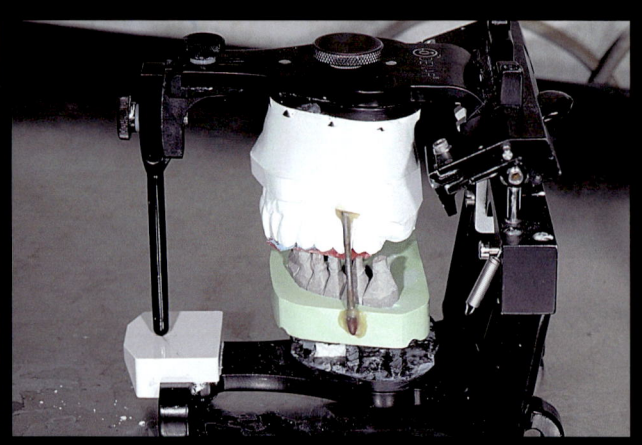

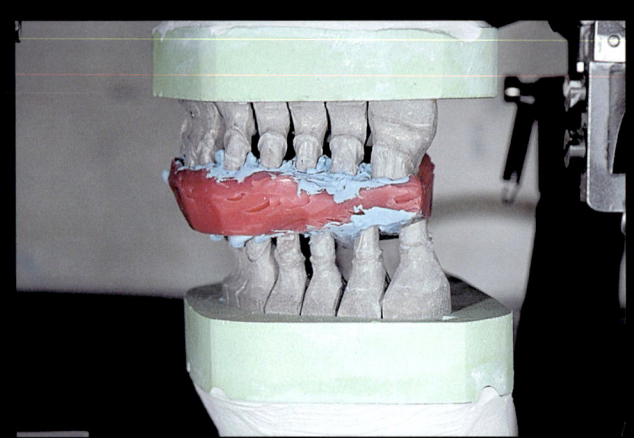

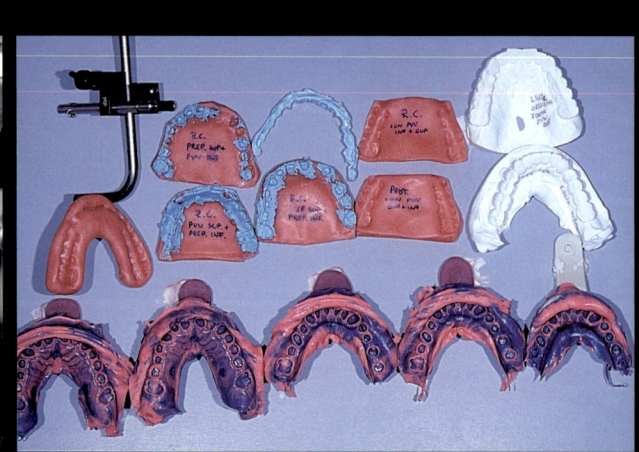

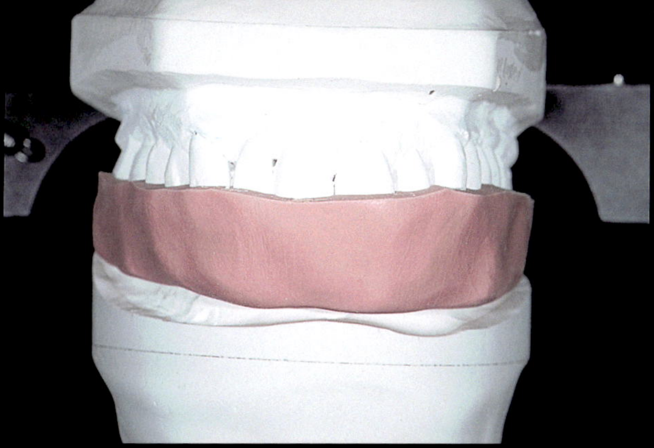
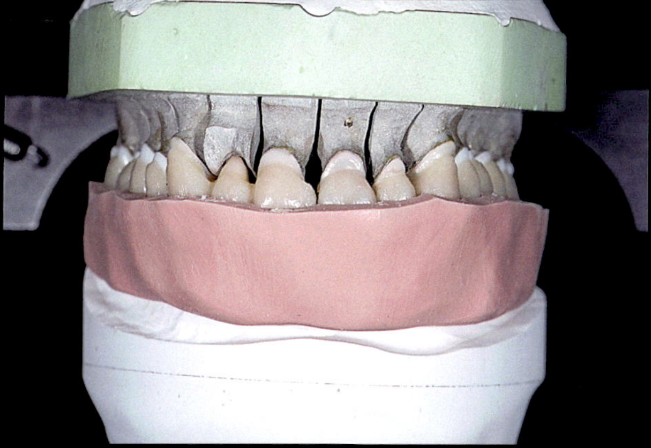
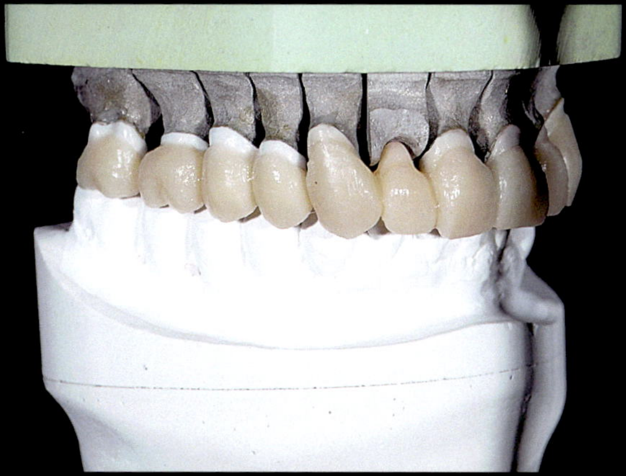
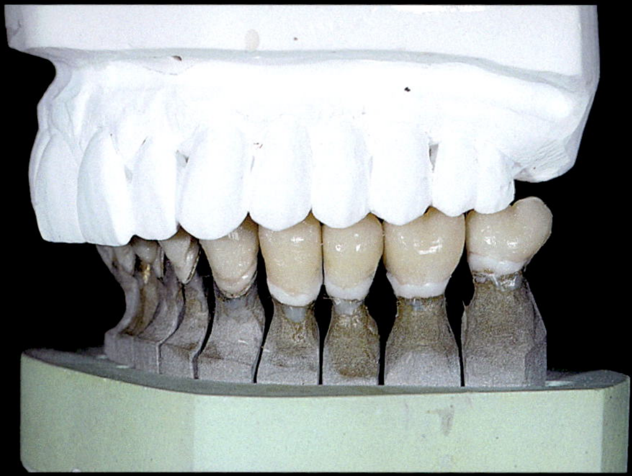
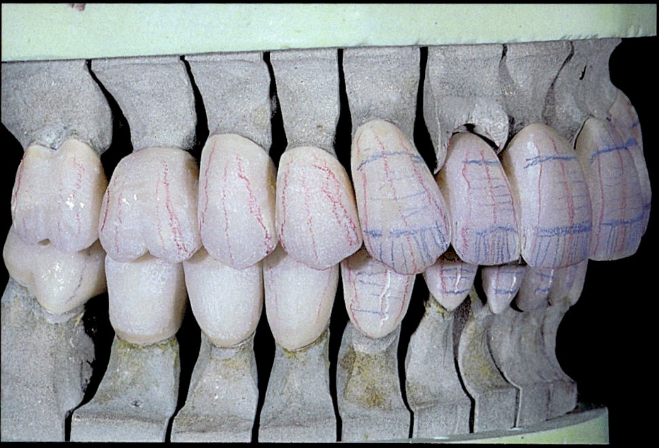
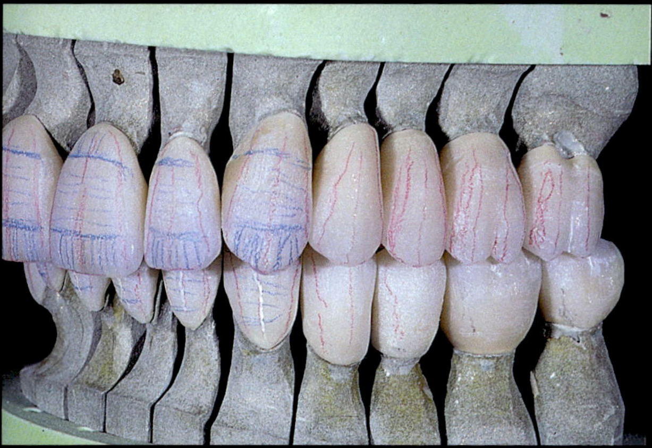
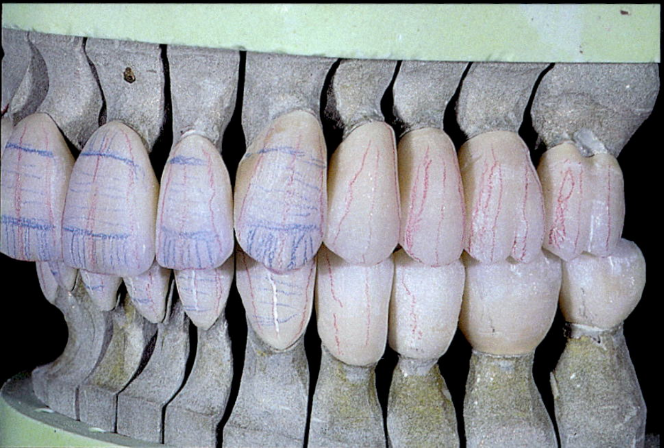
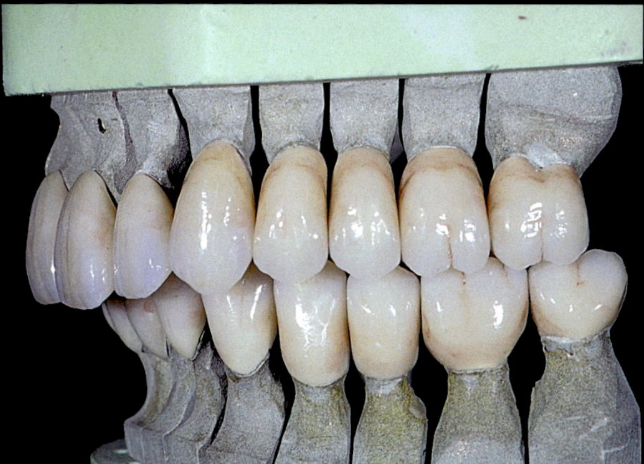

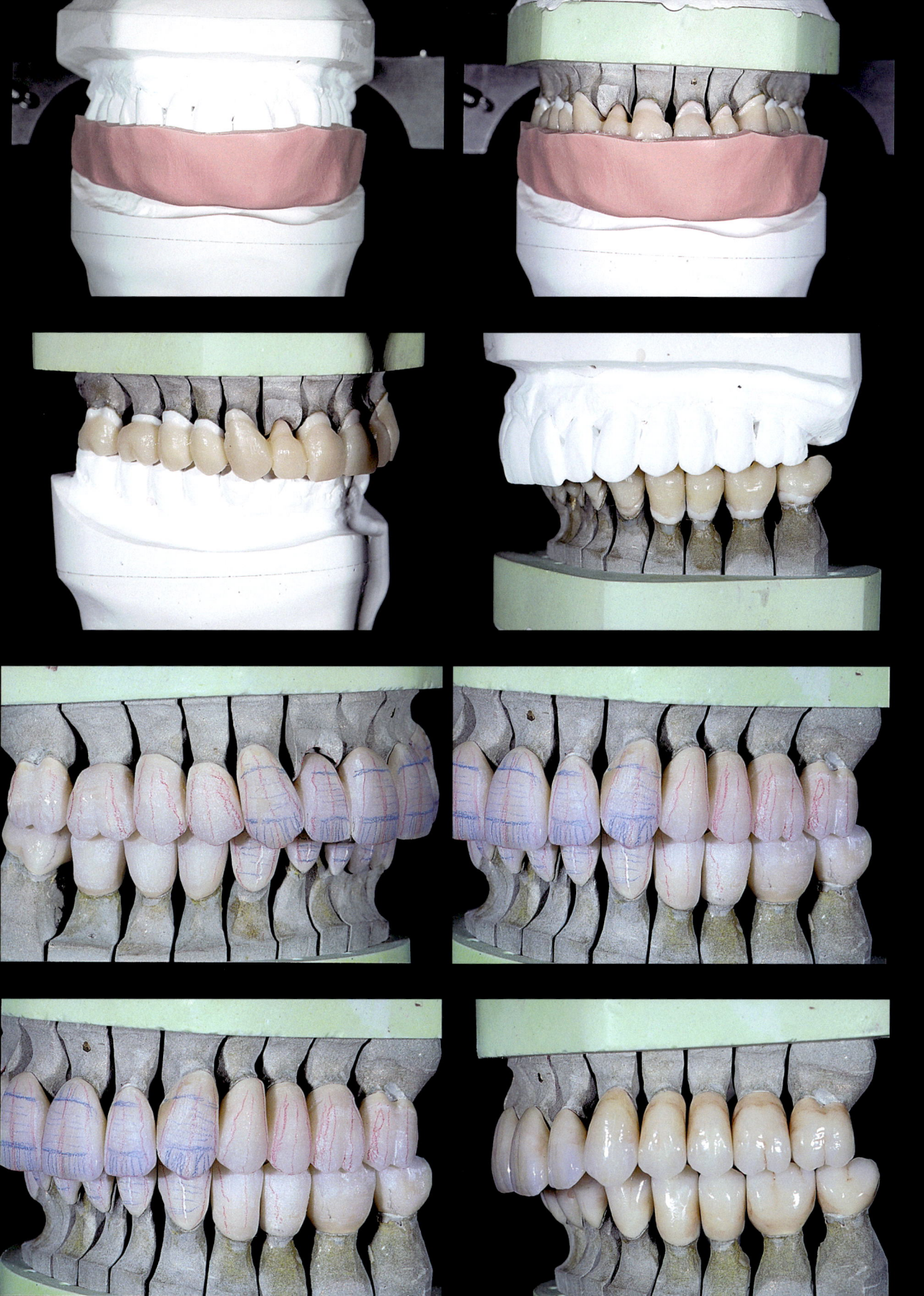

566

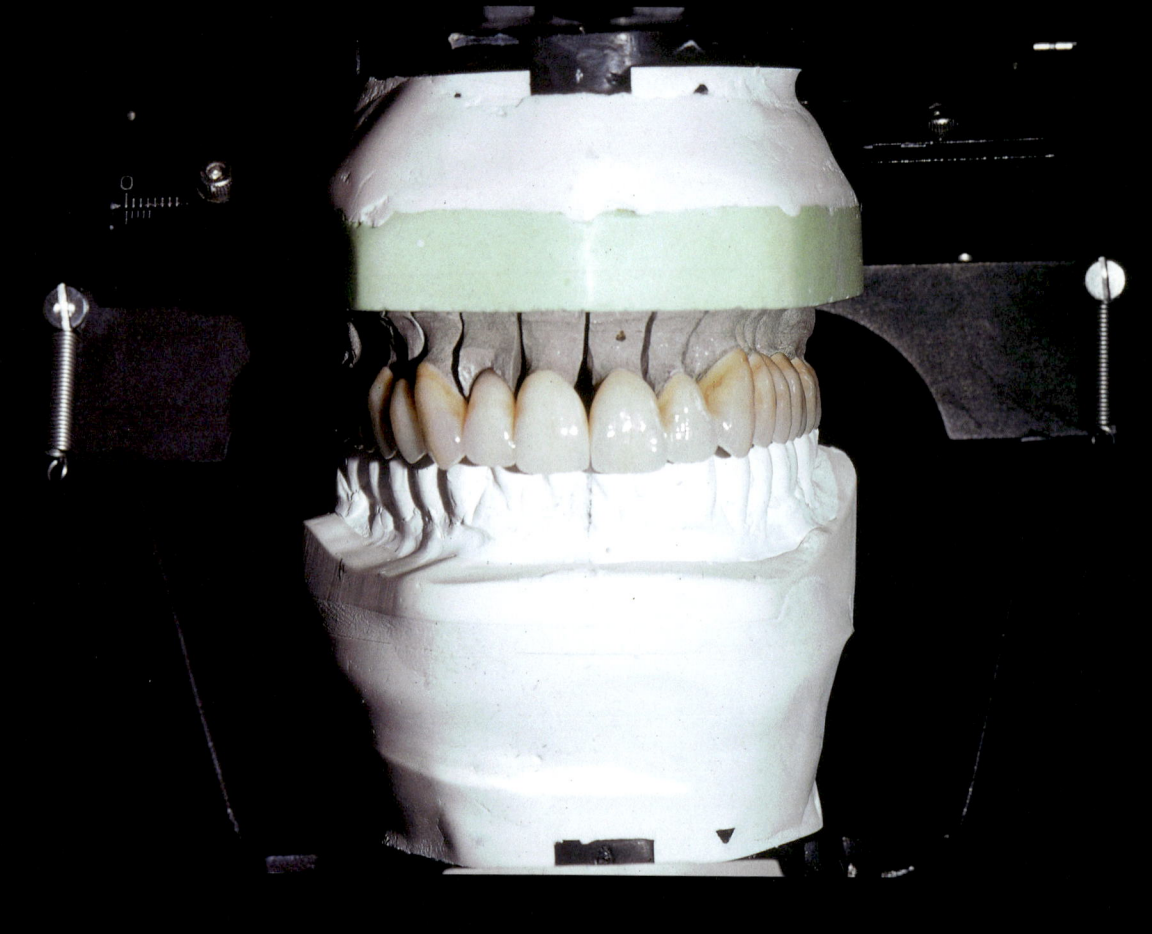

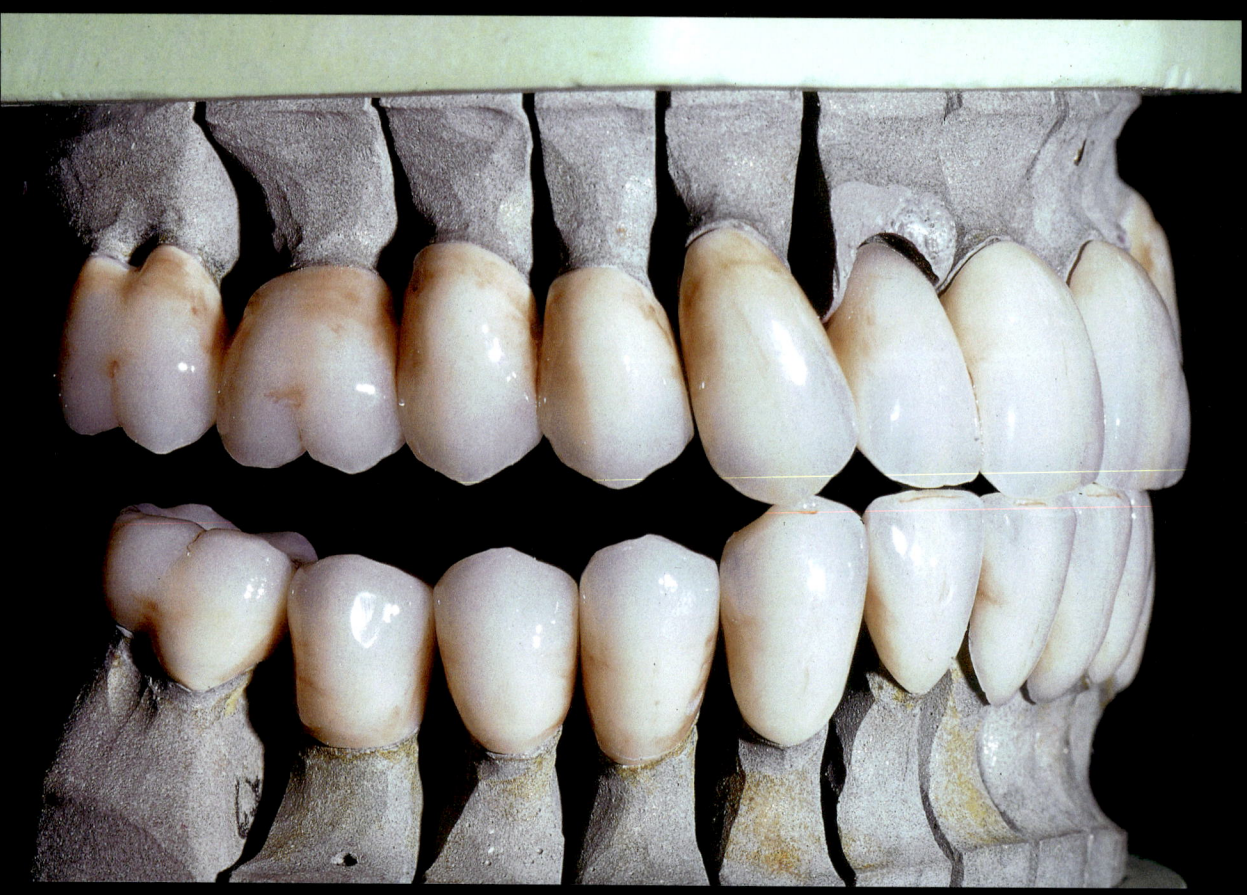

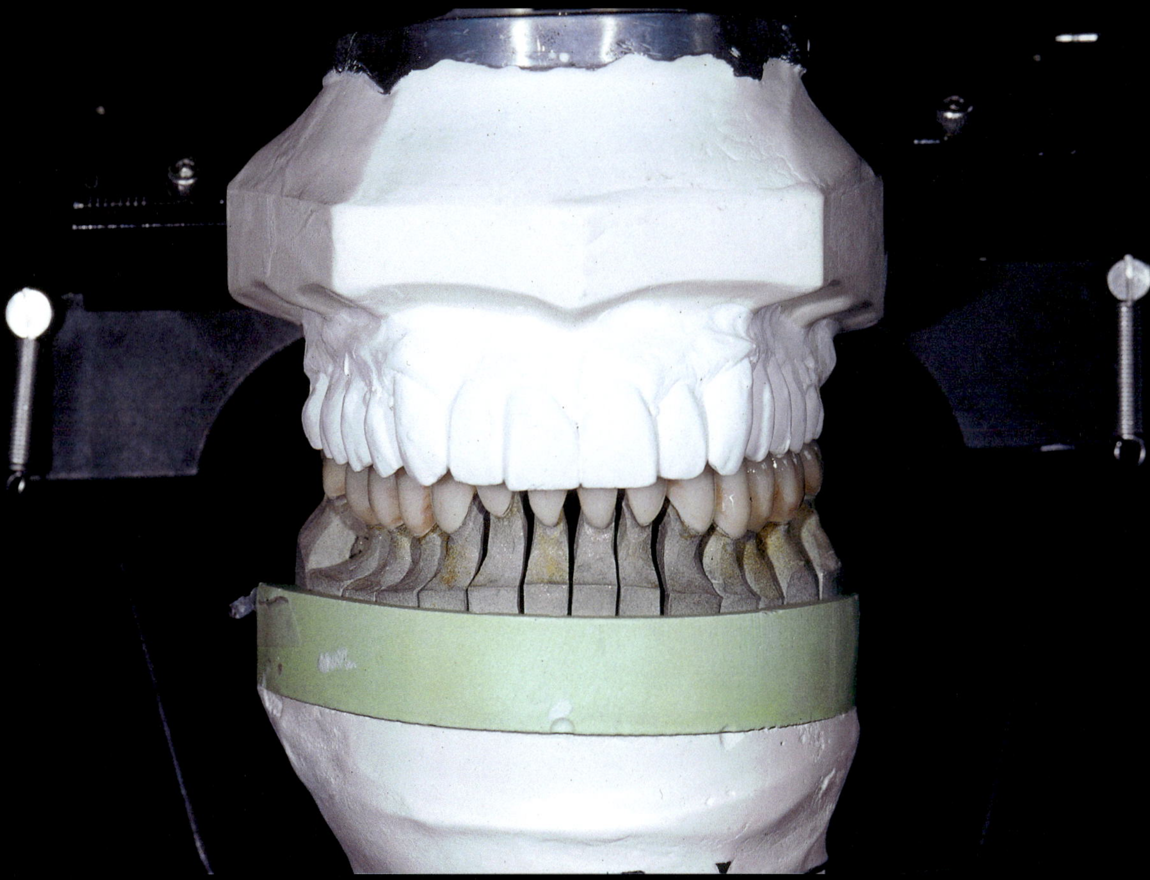

567

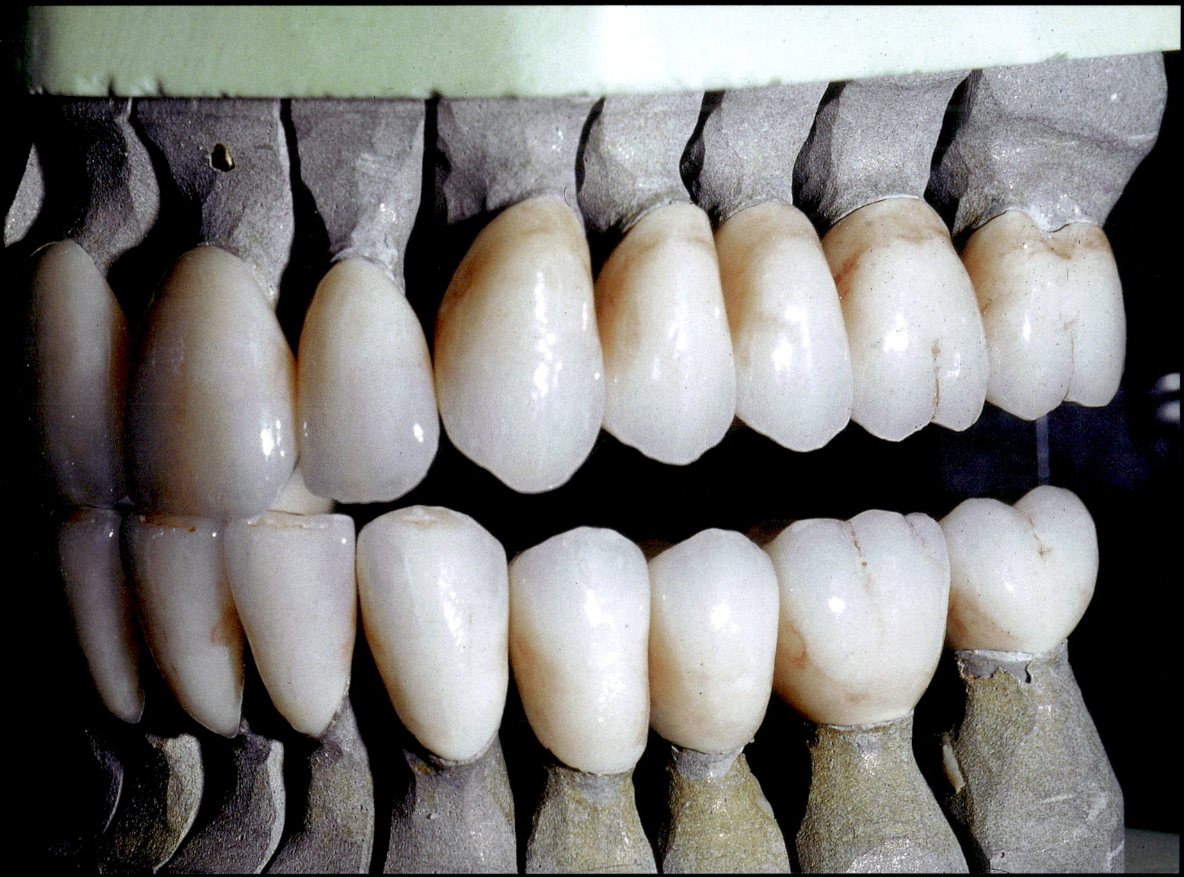

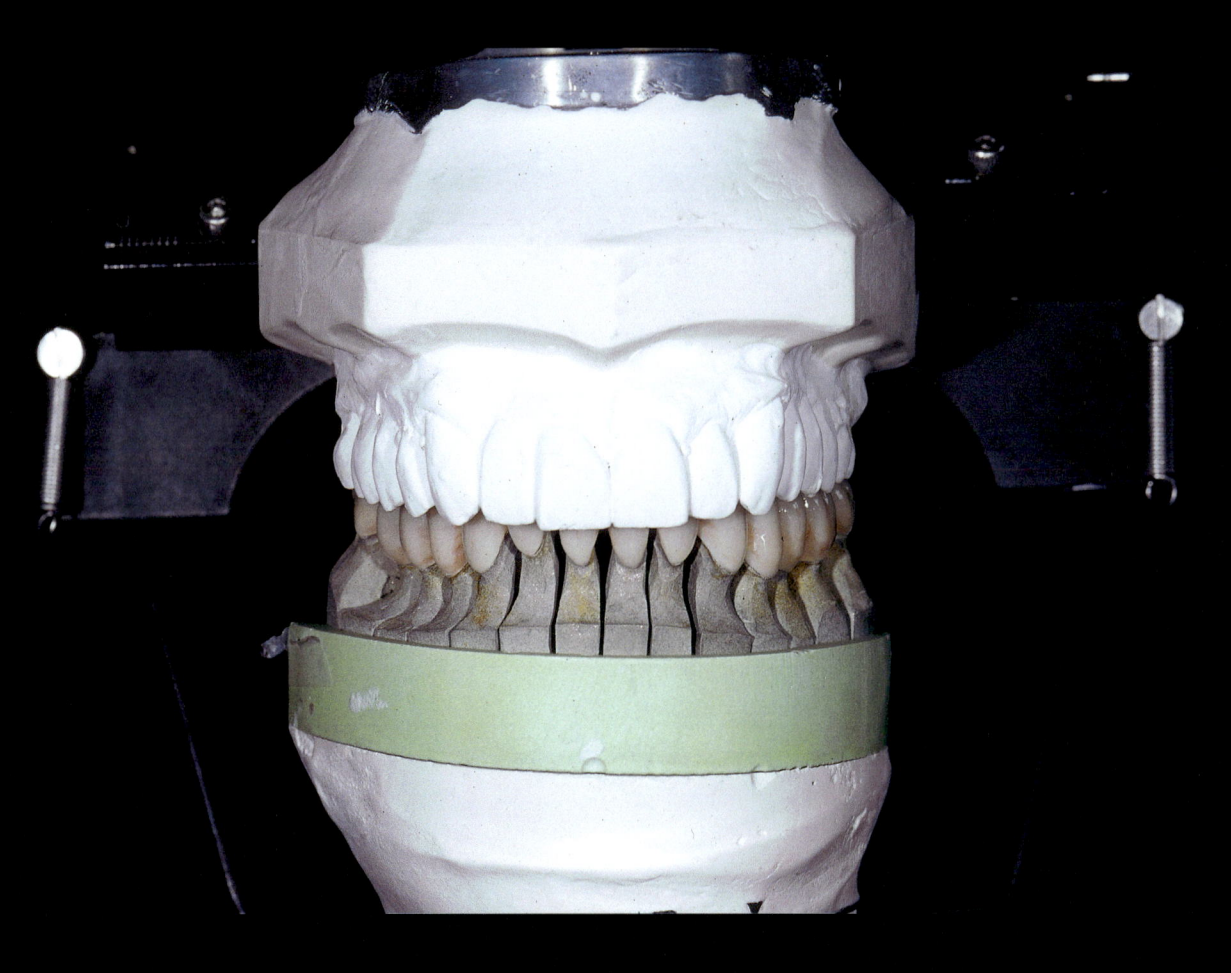

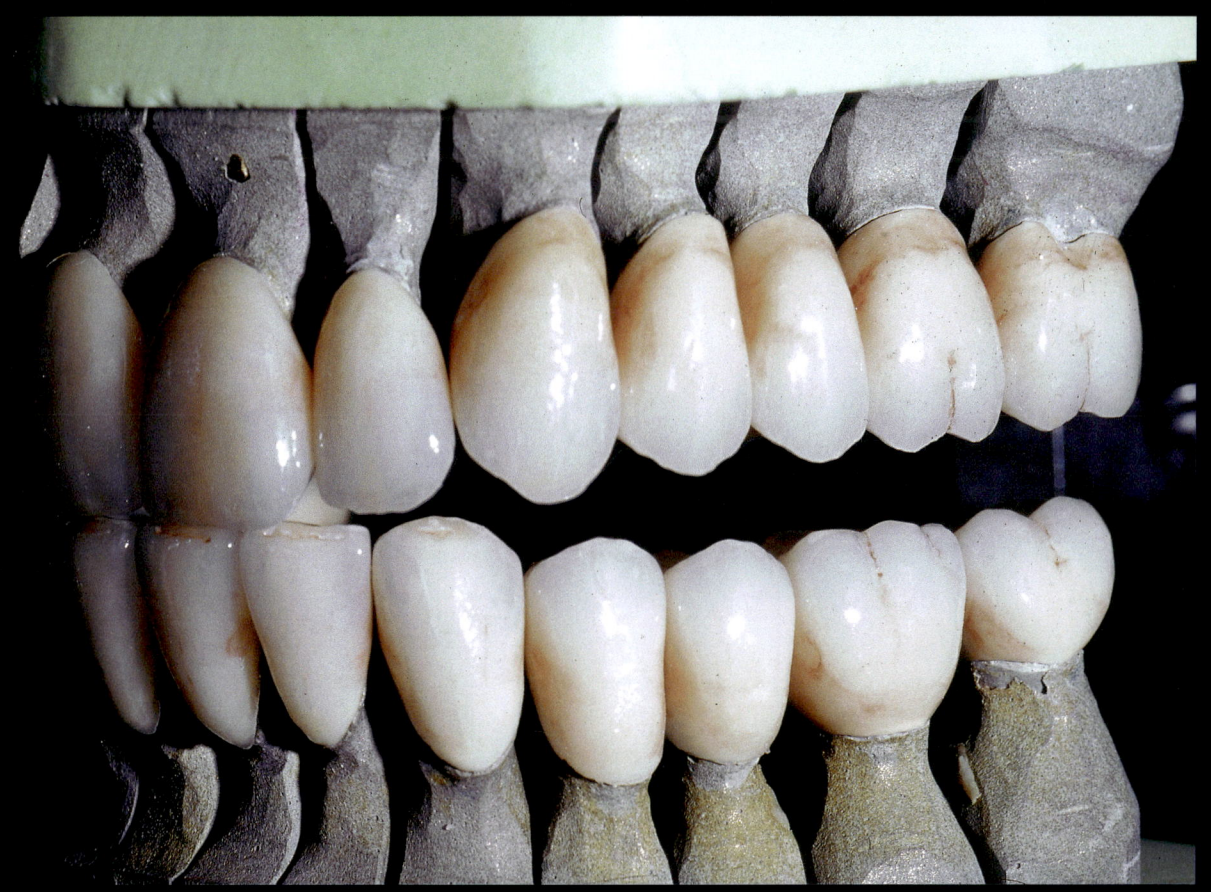

568

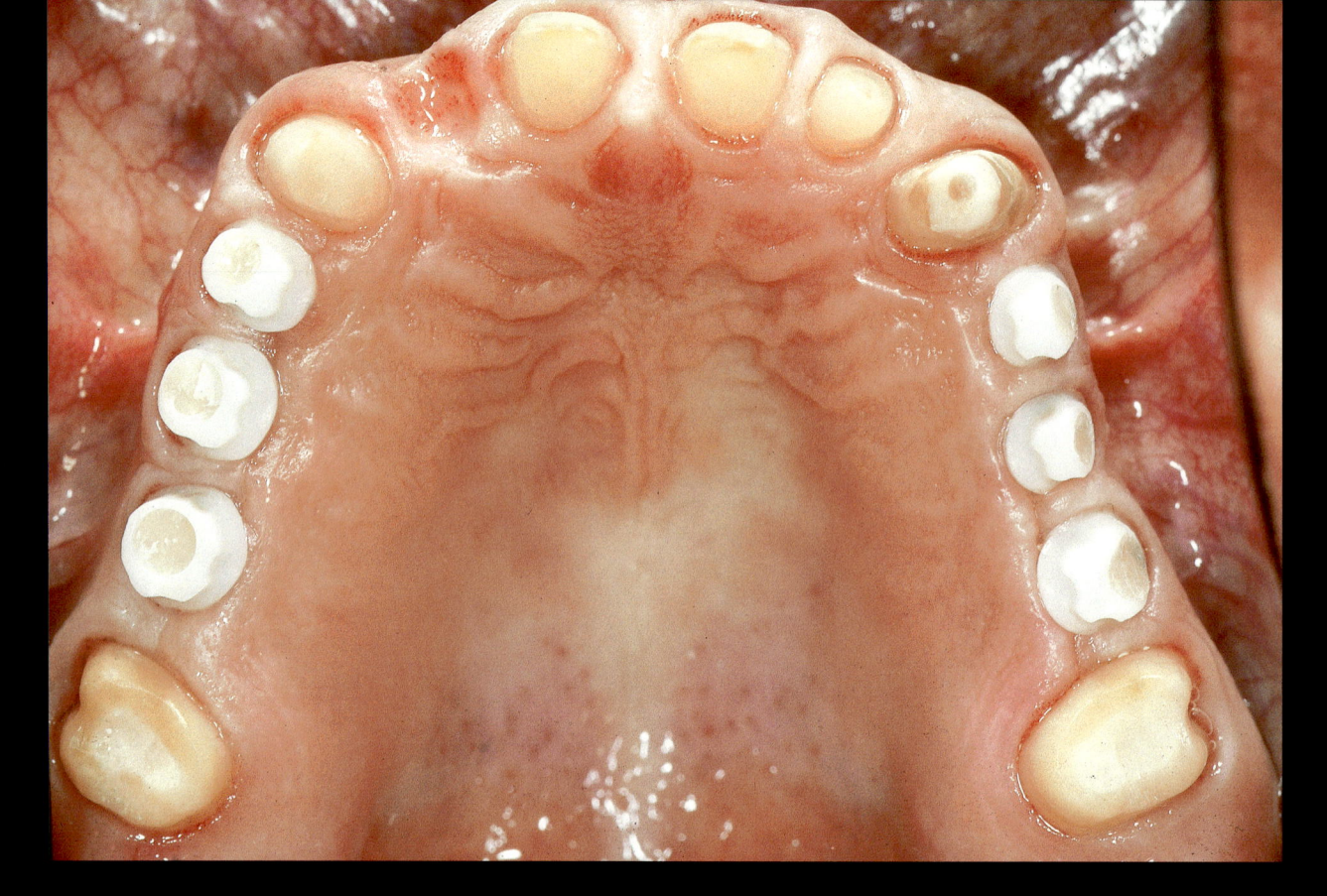

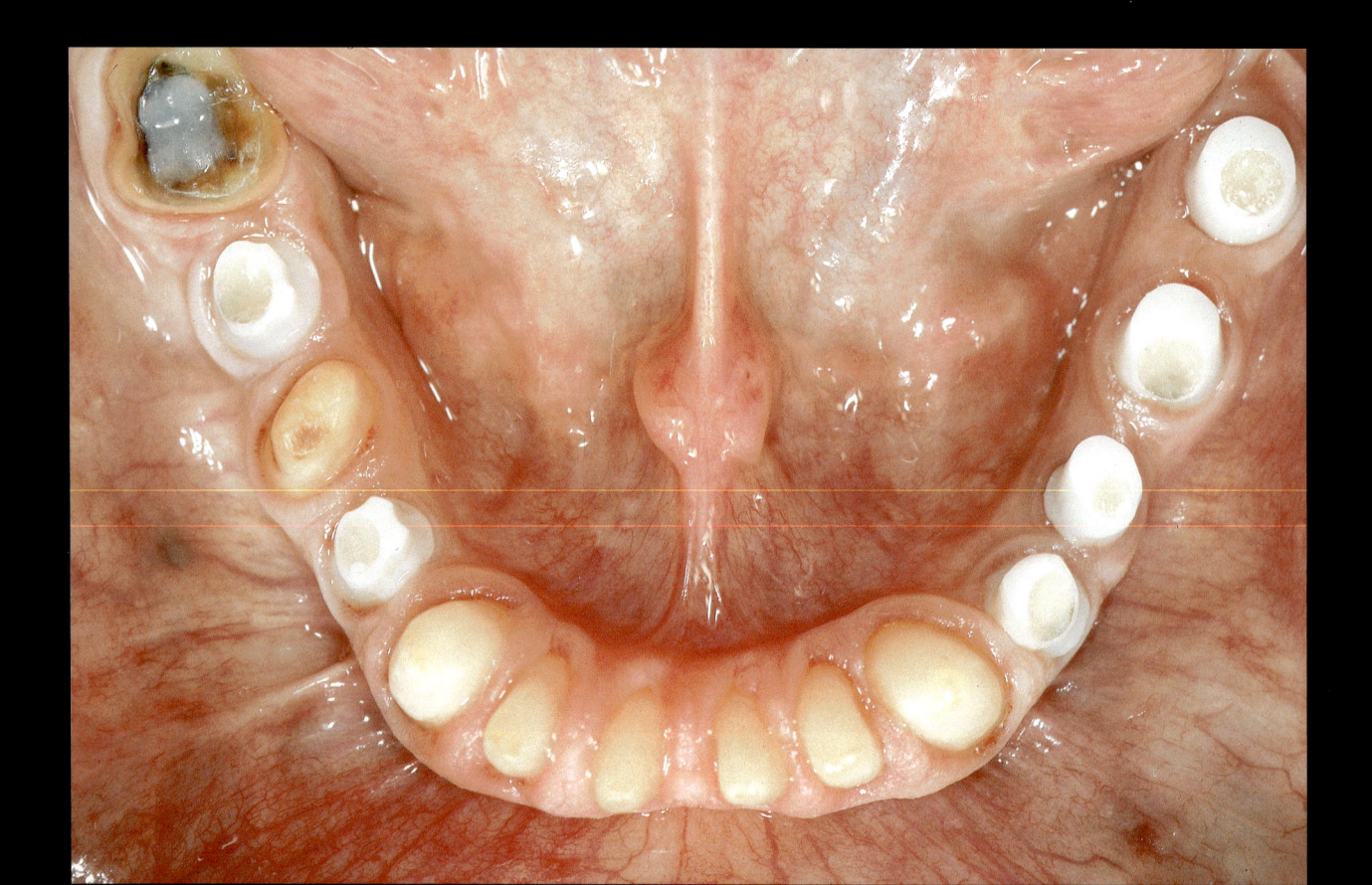

569

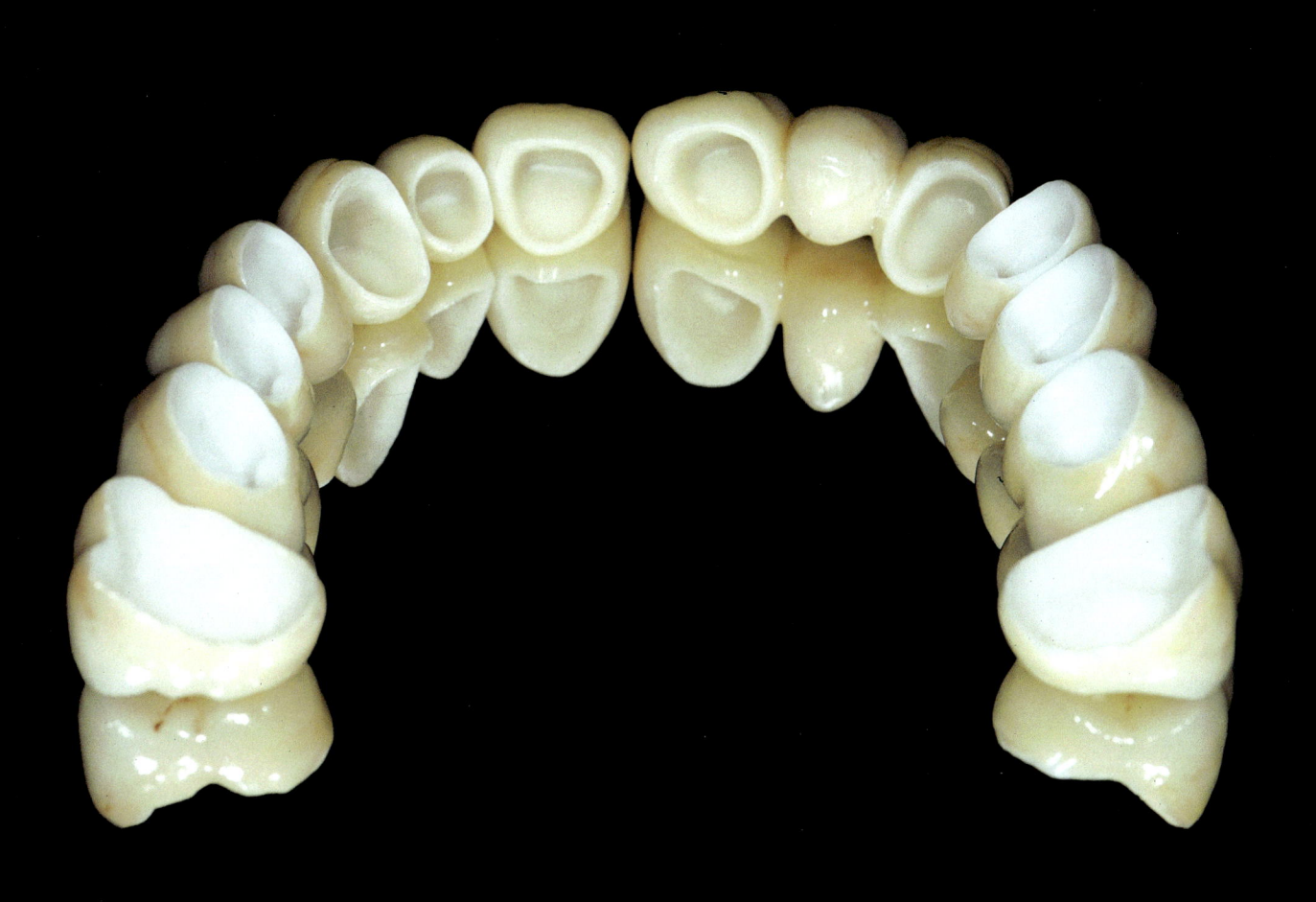

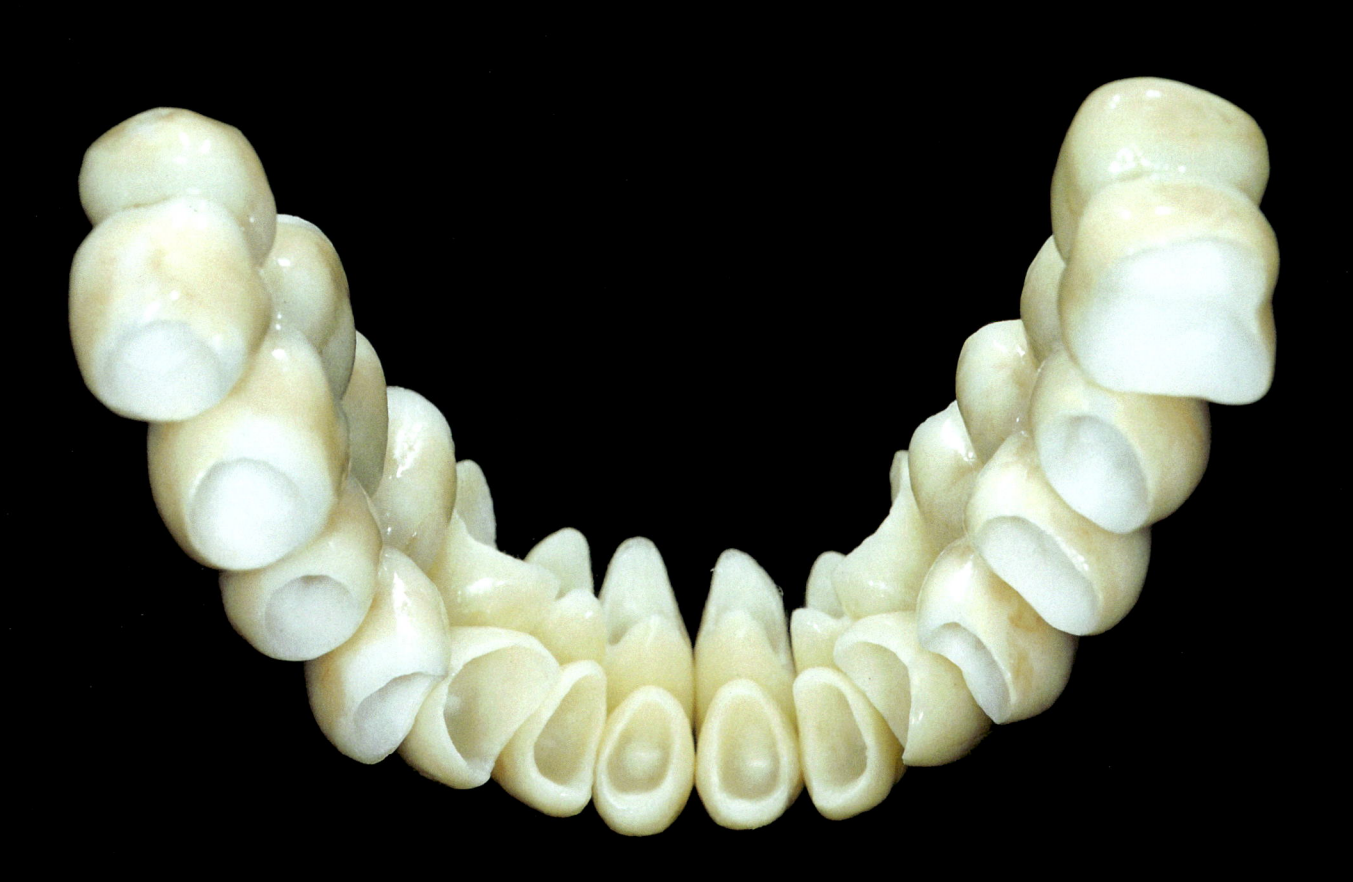

570

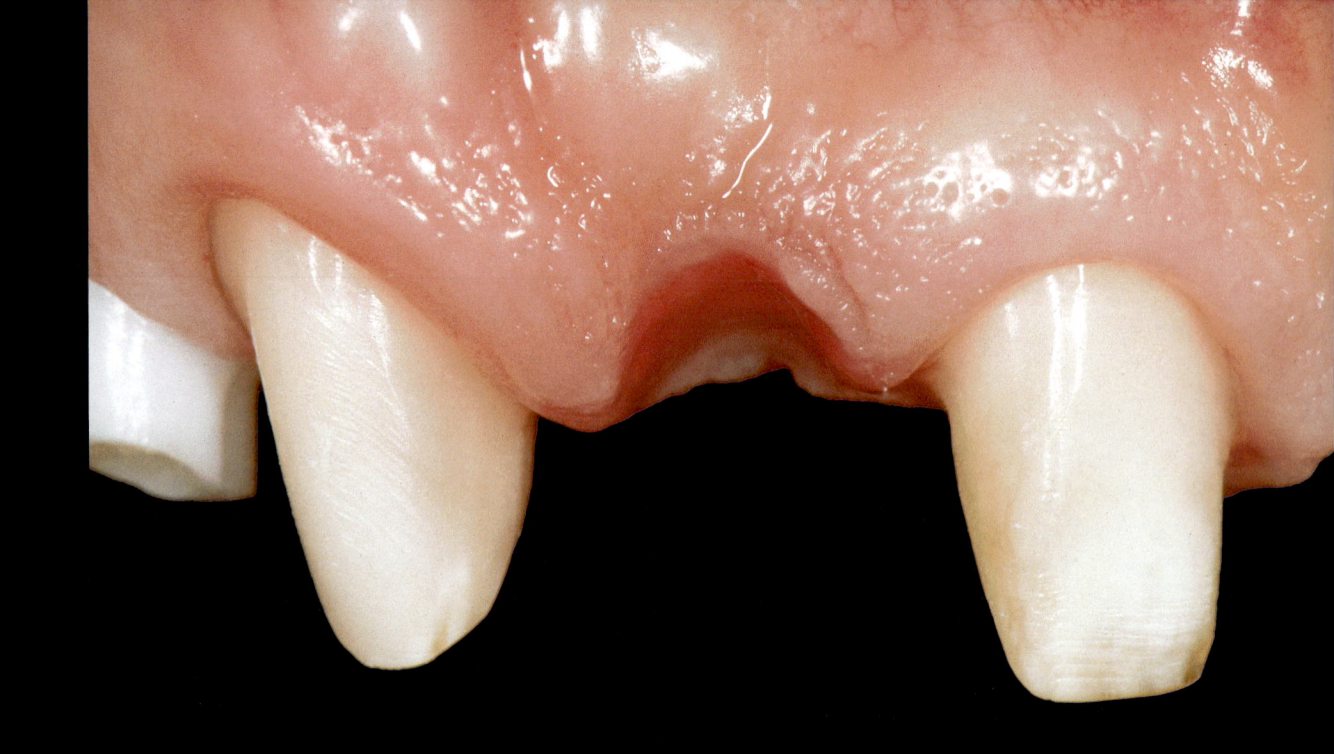

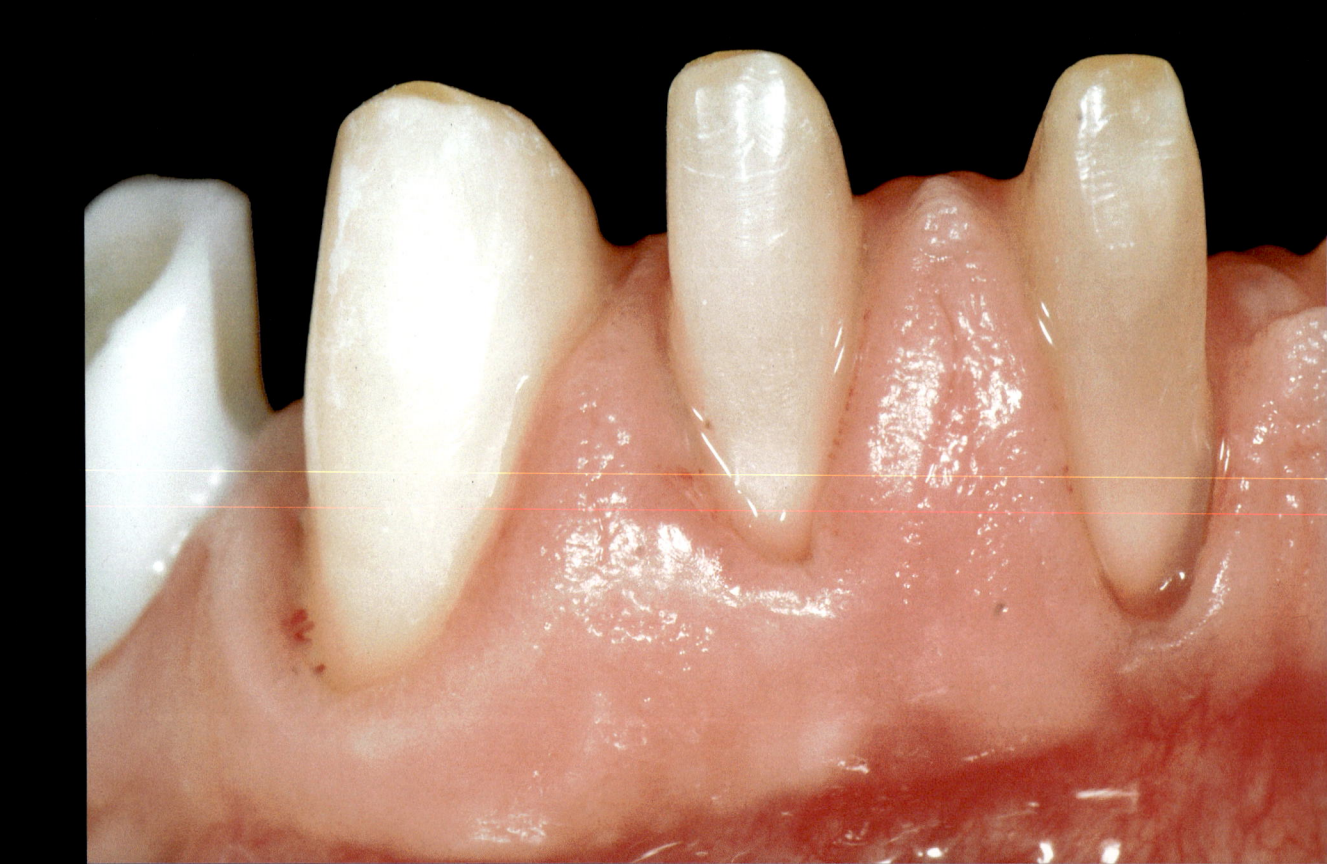

571

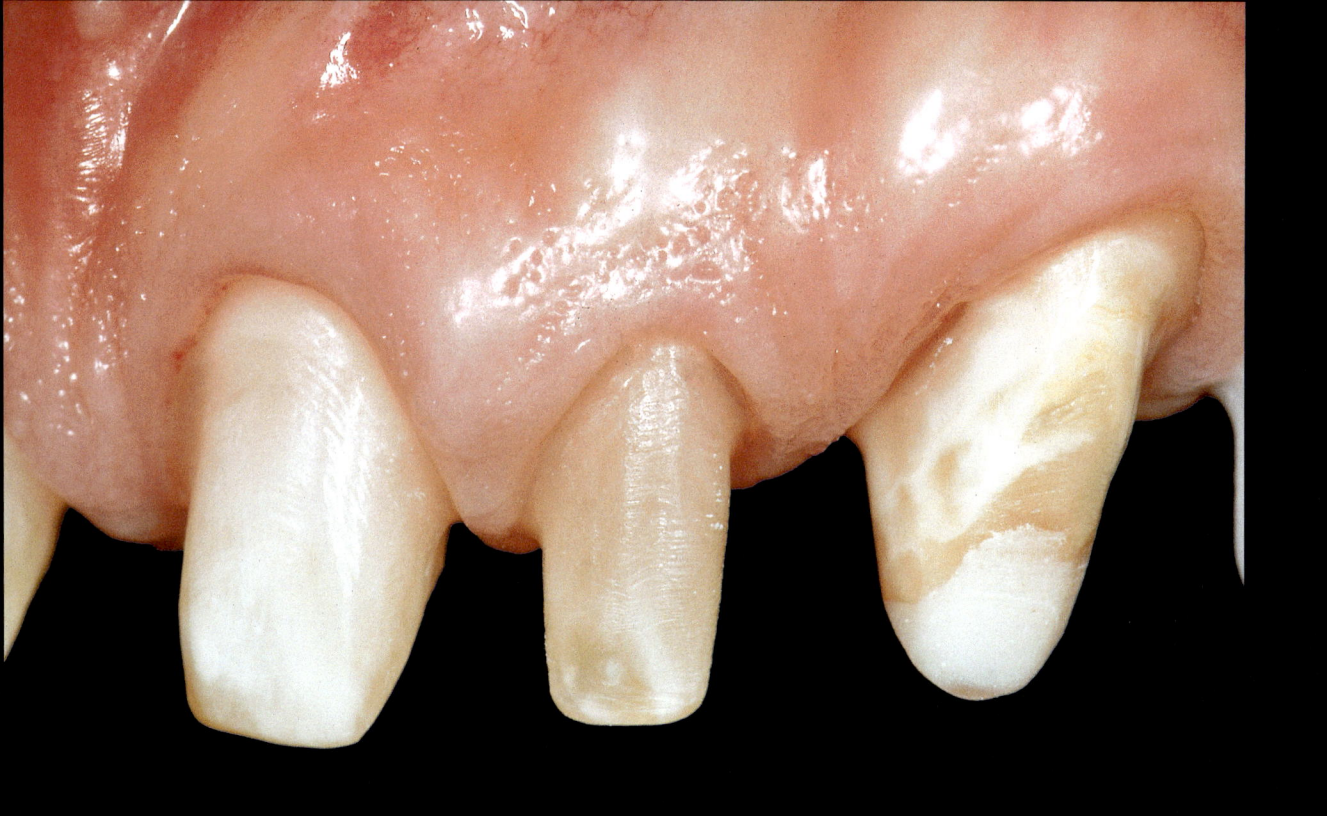

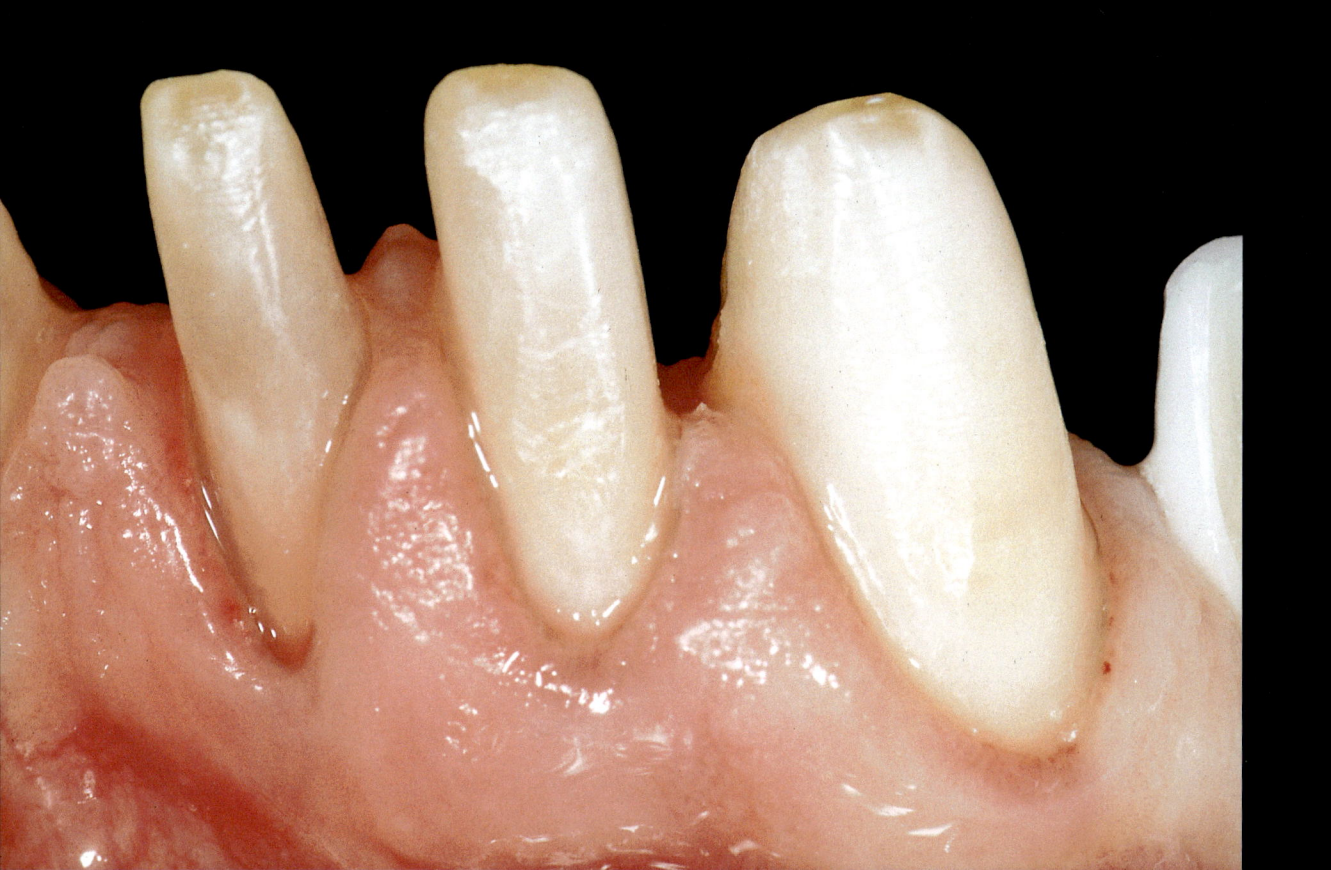

572

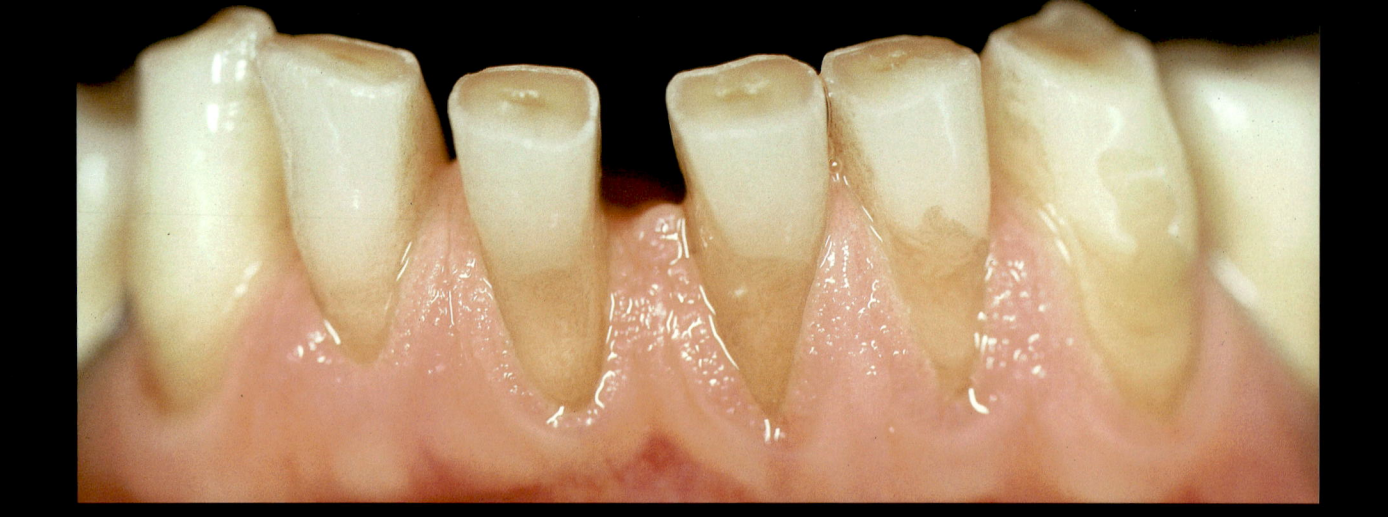

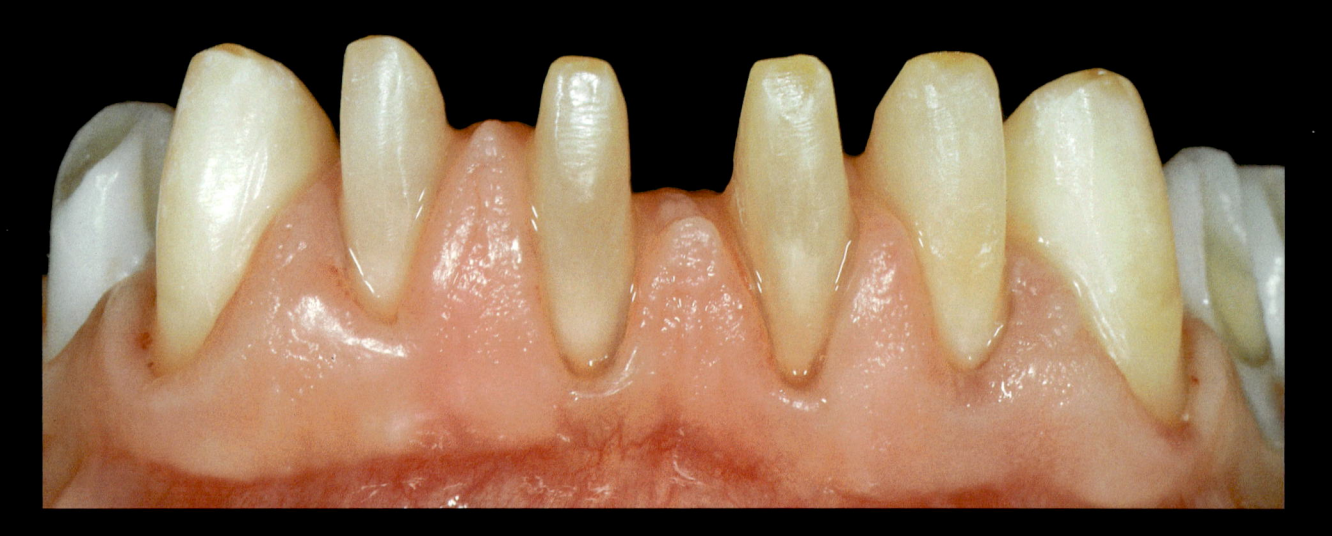

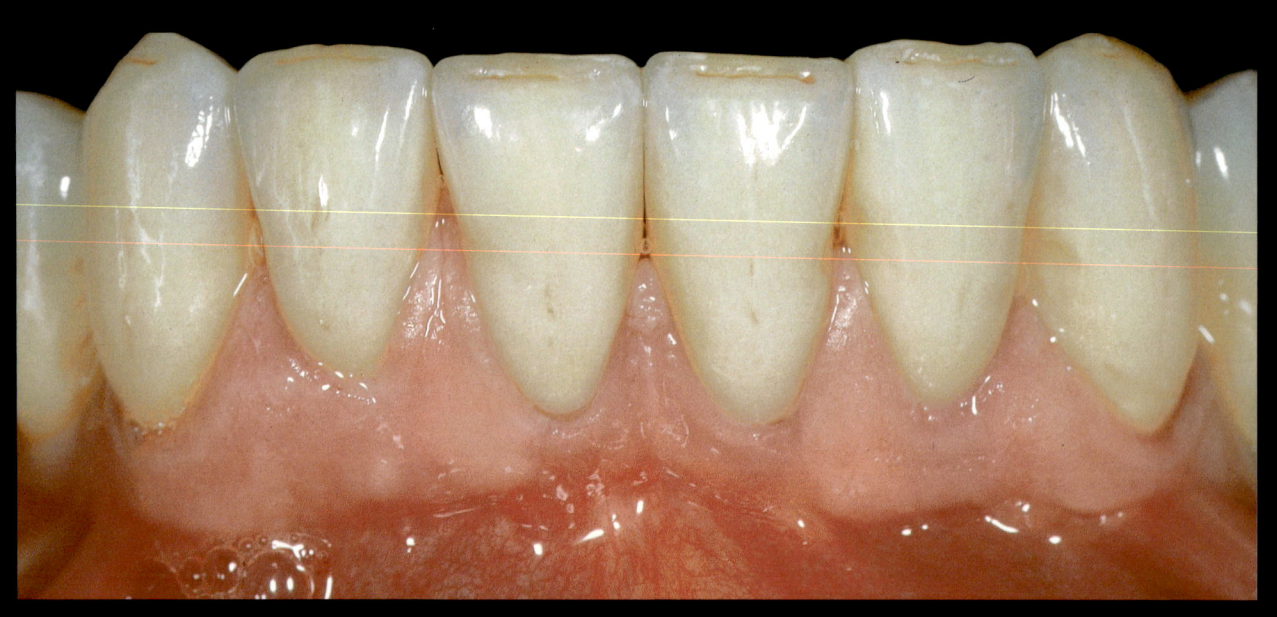

573

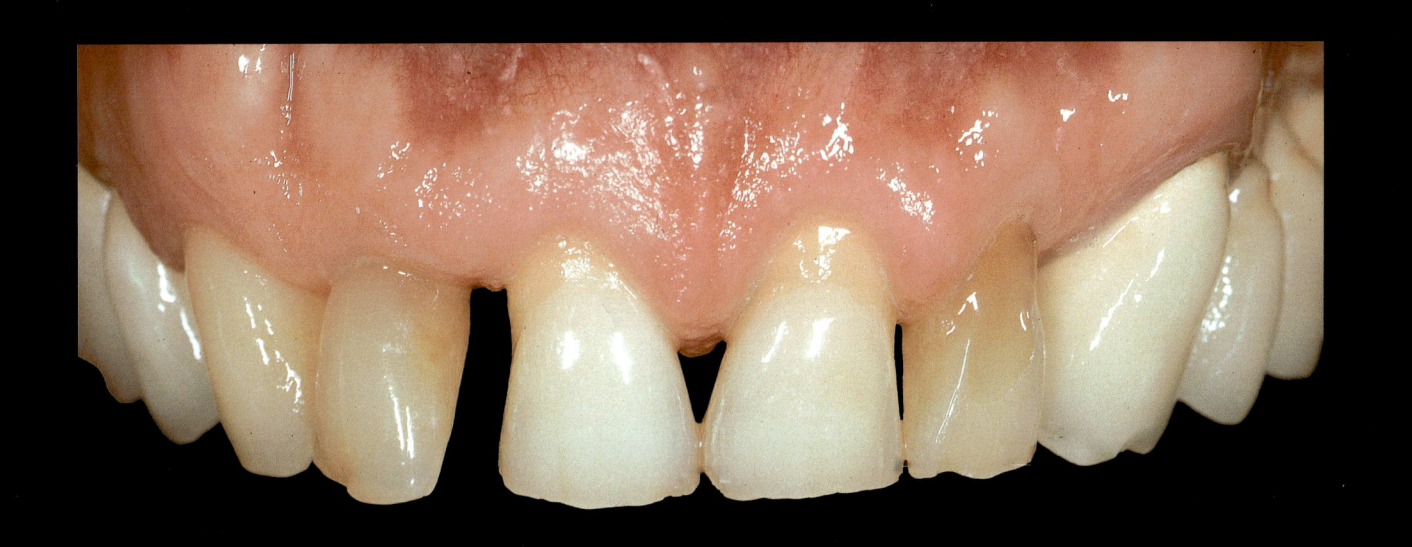

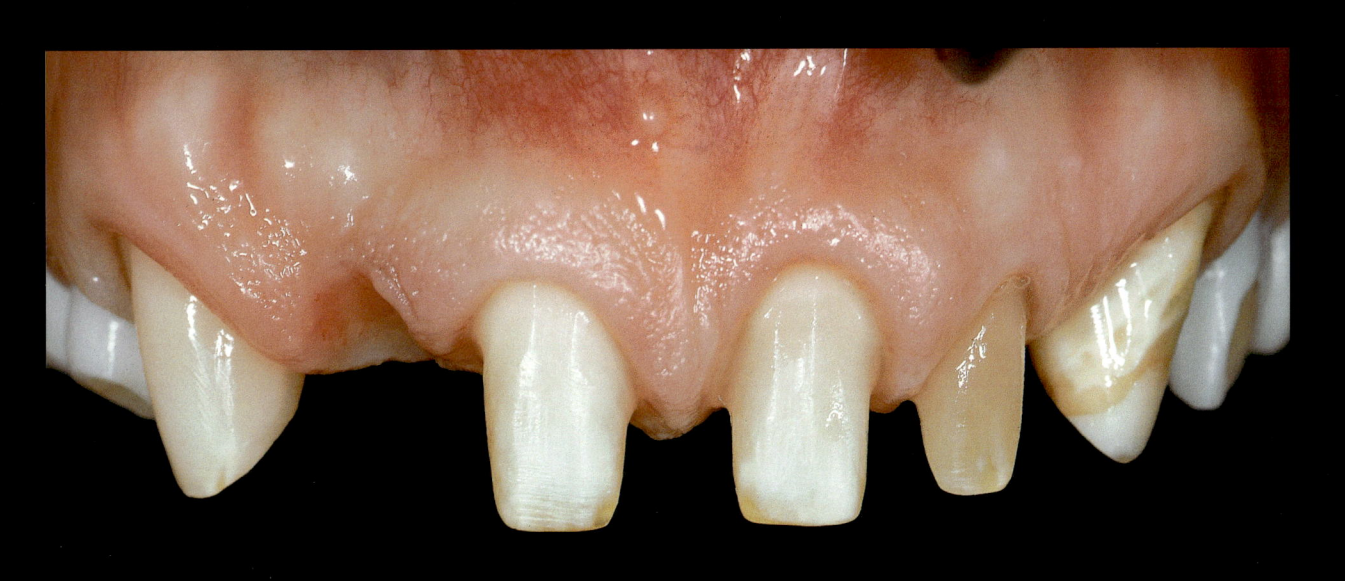

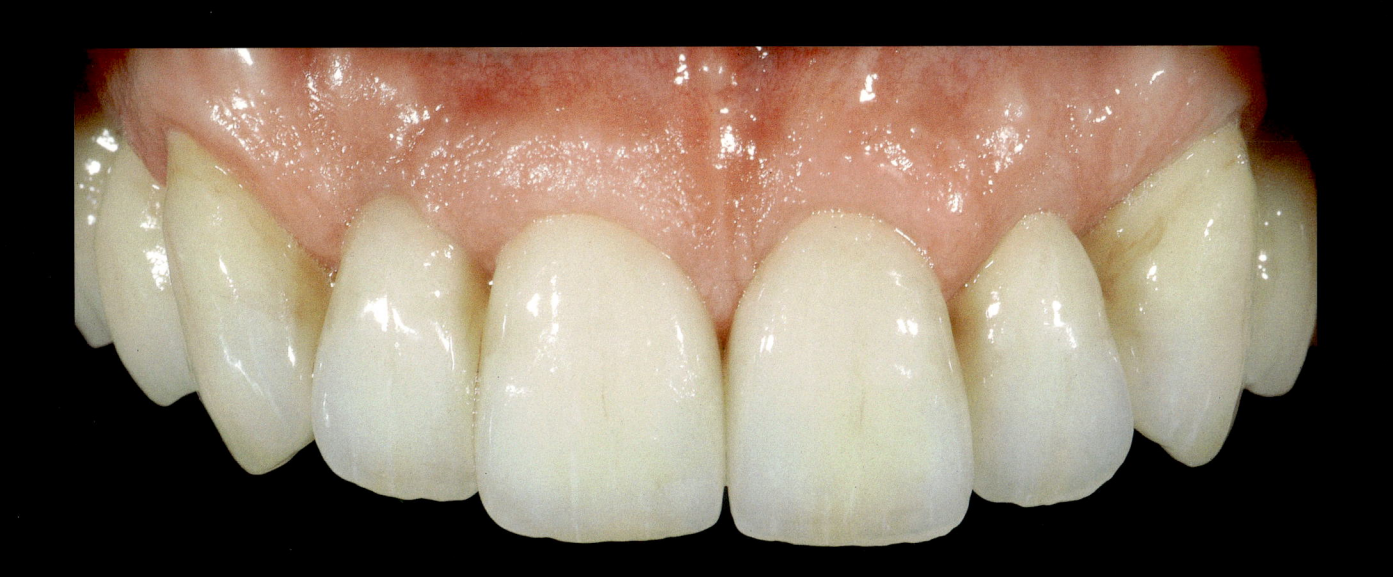

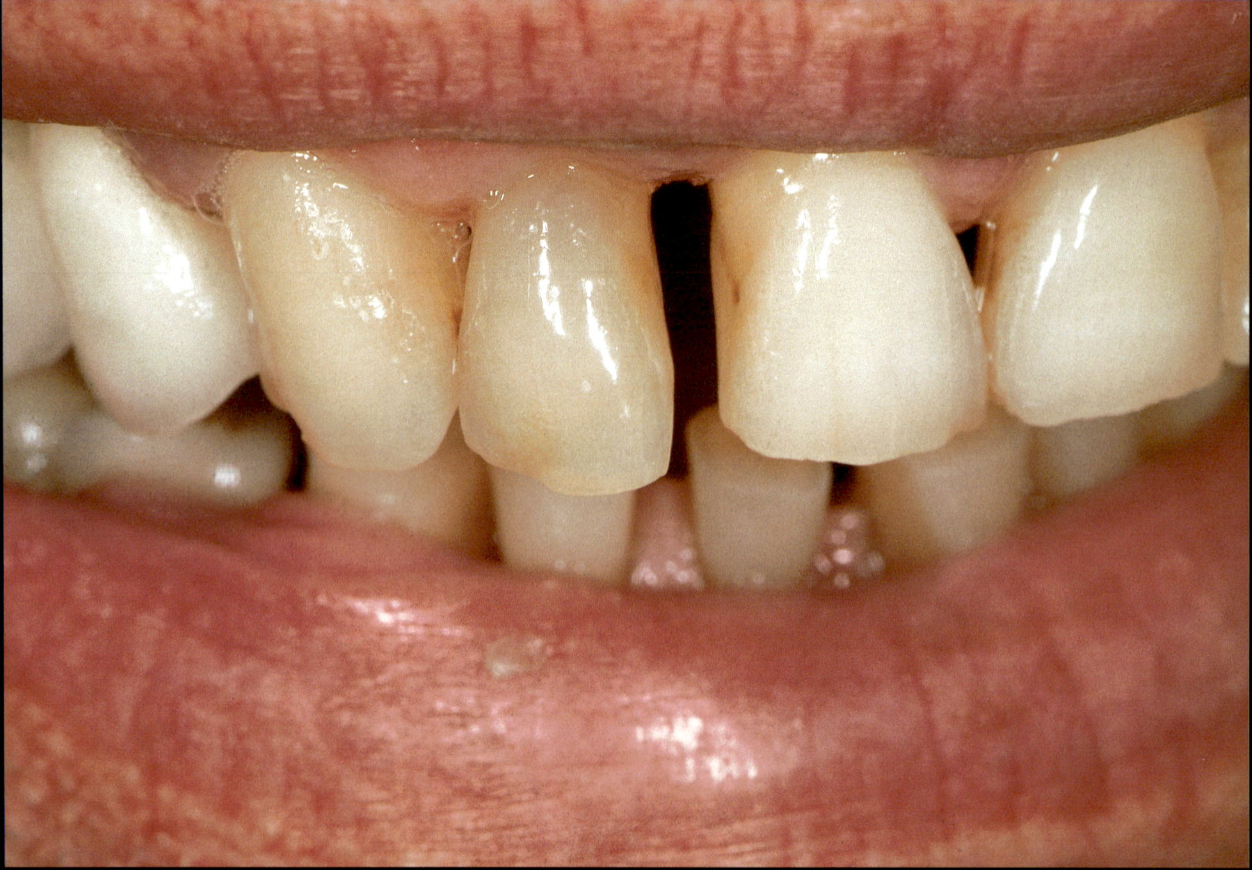

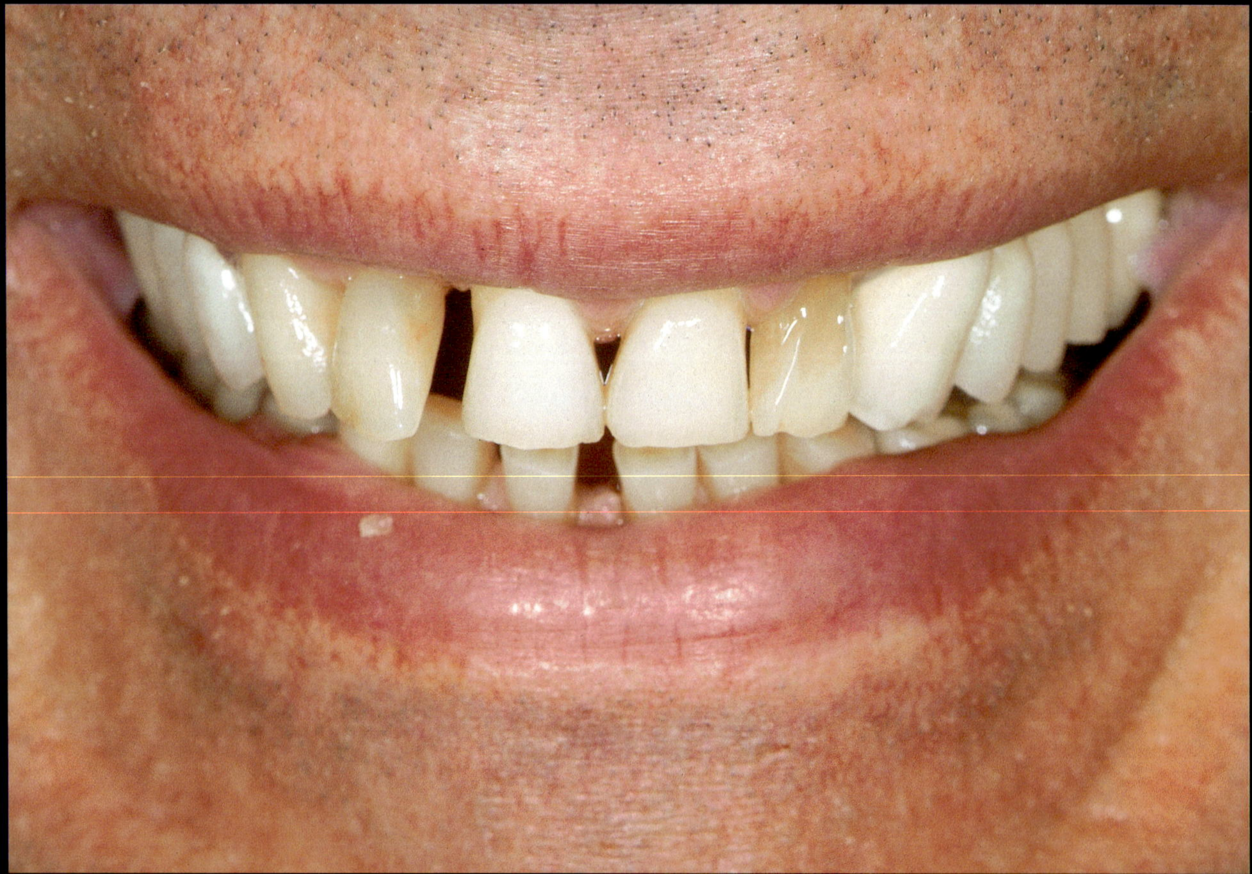

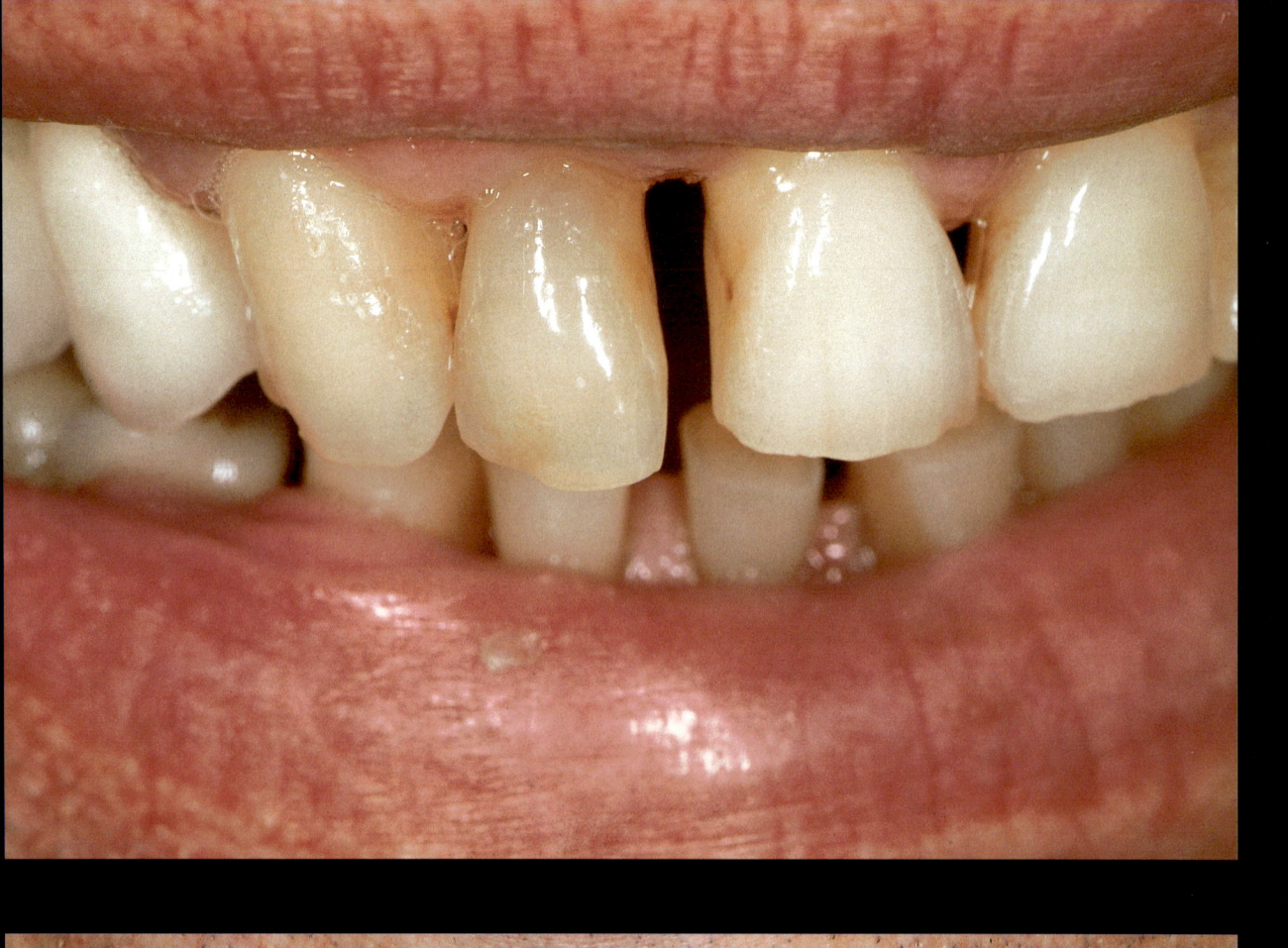

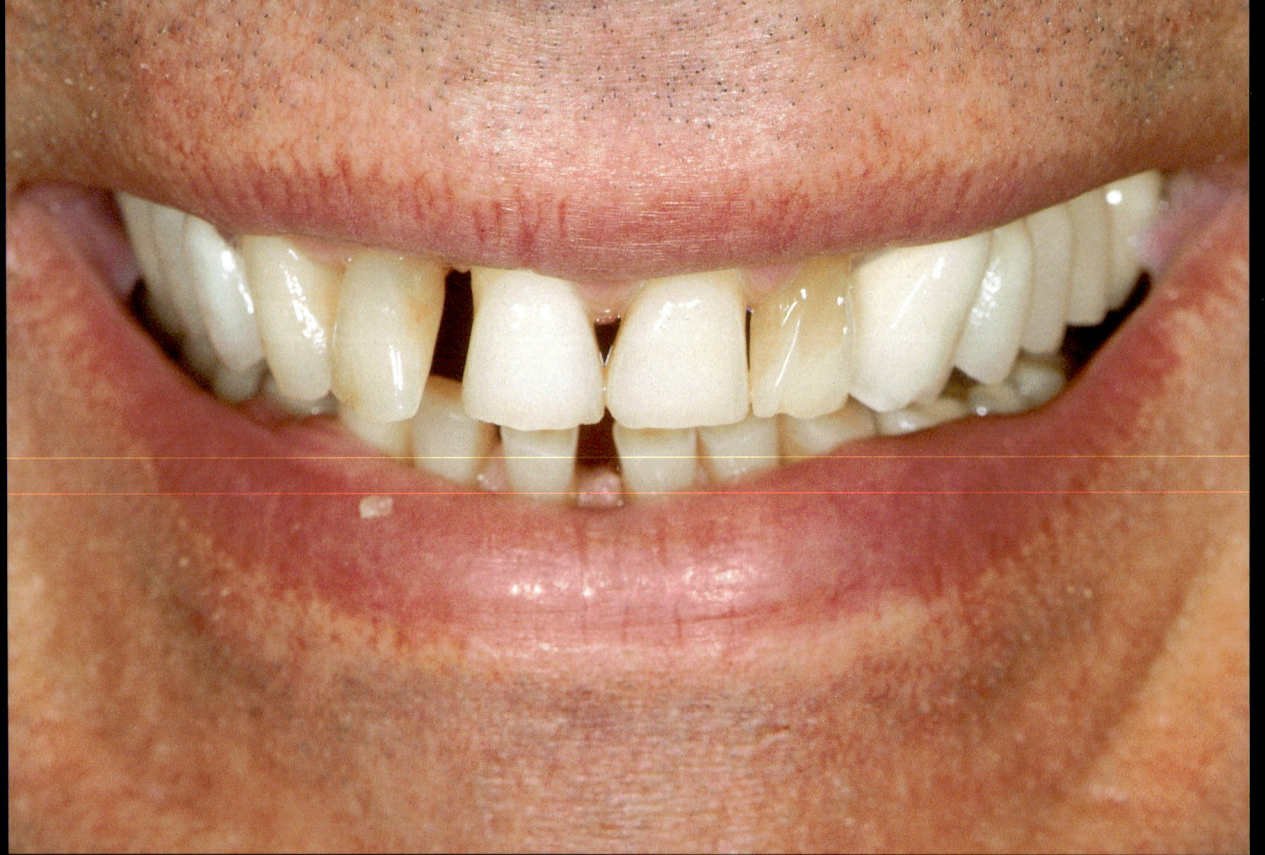

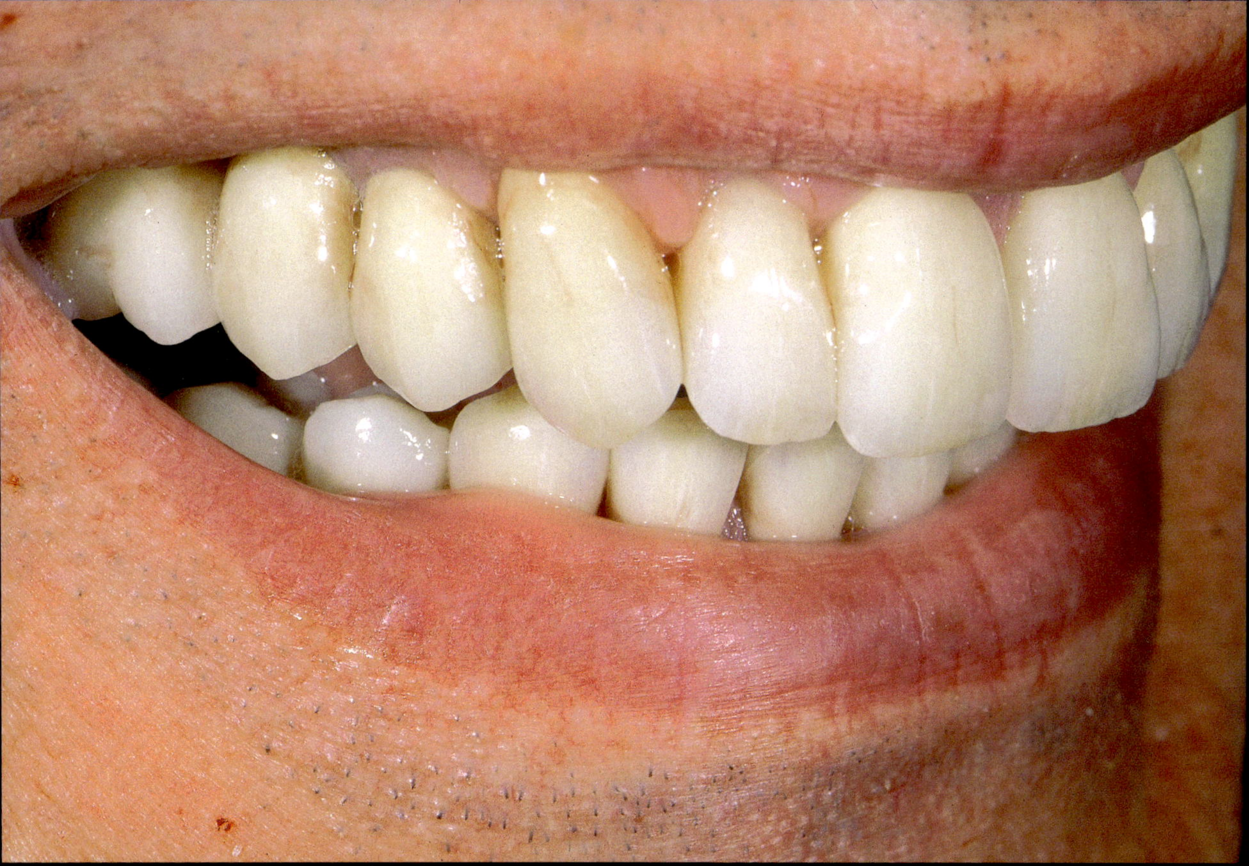

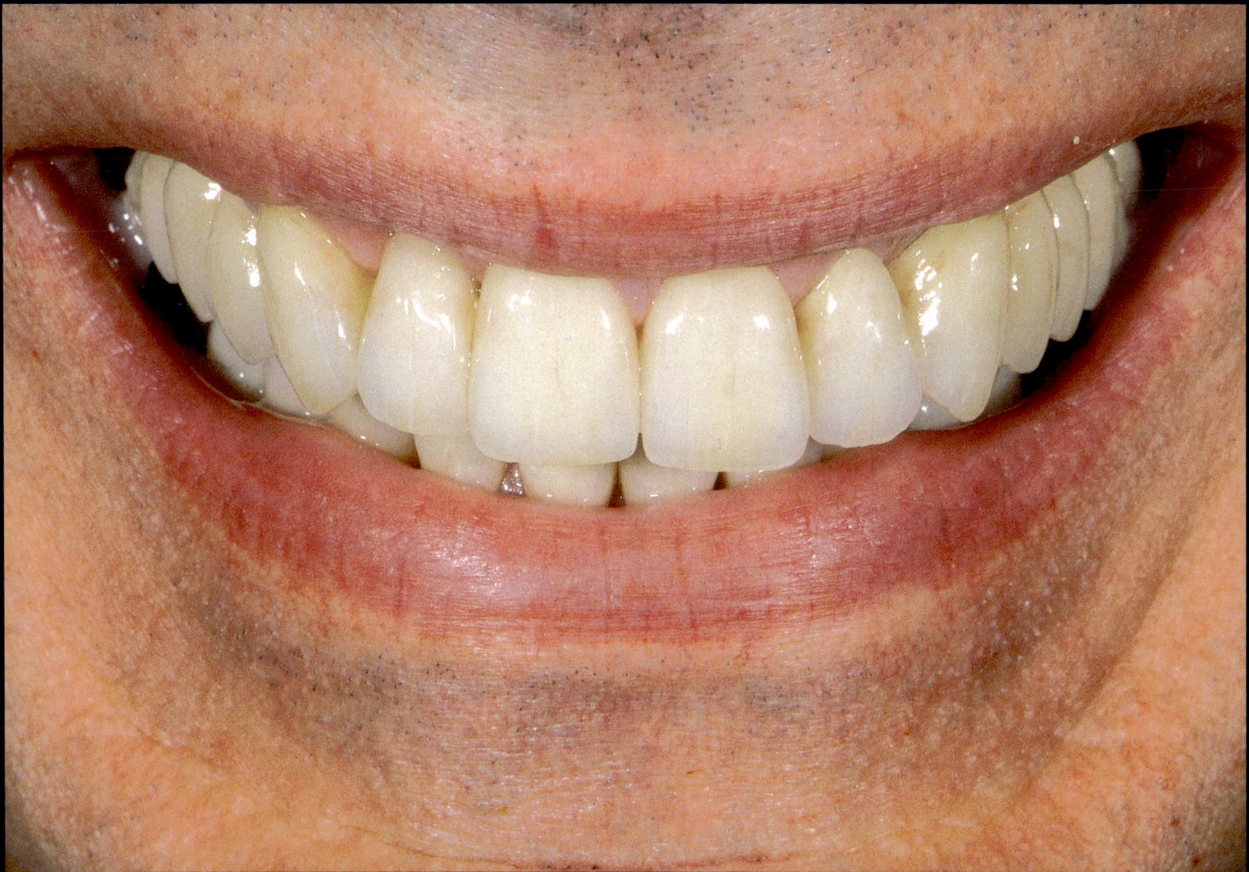

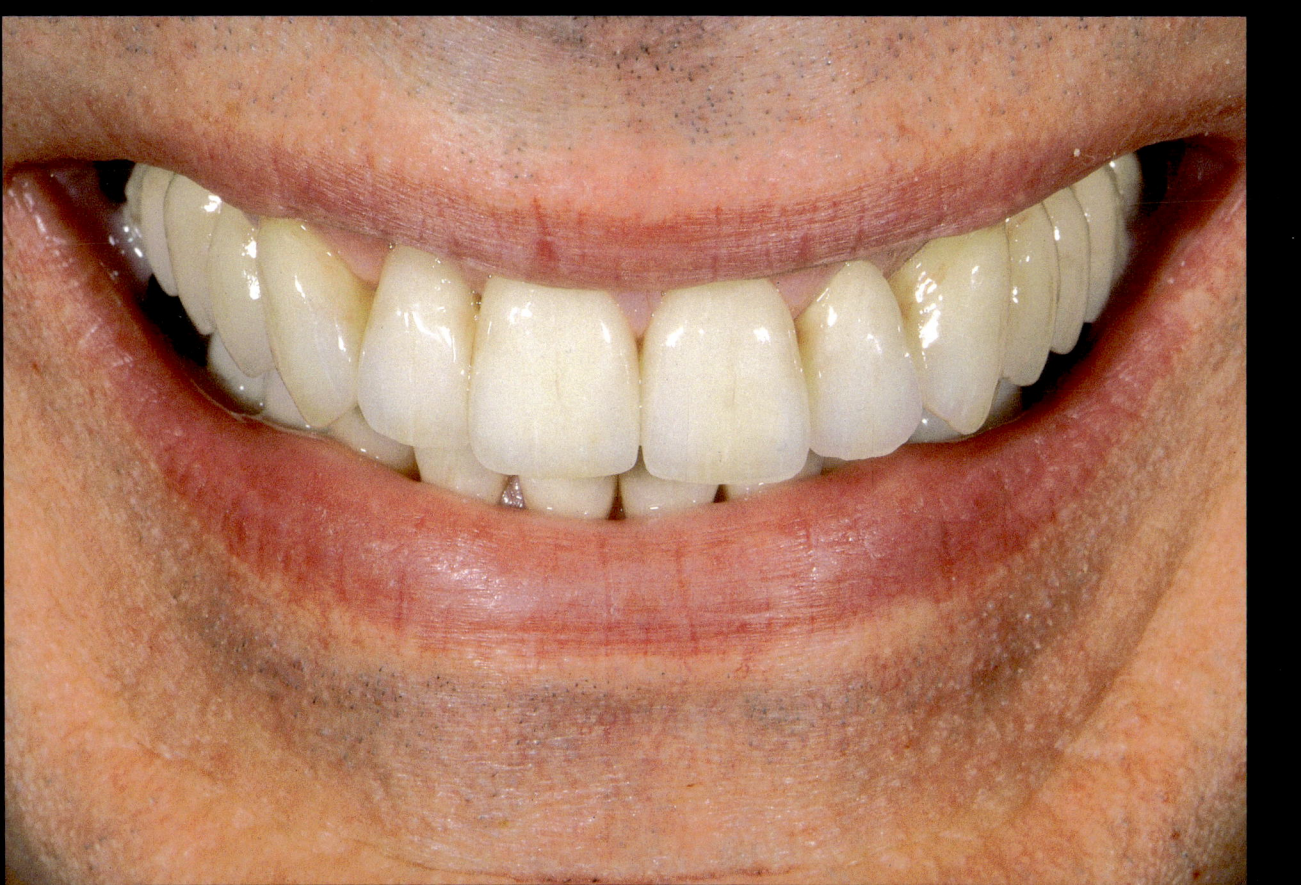

576

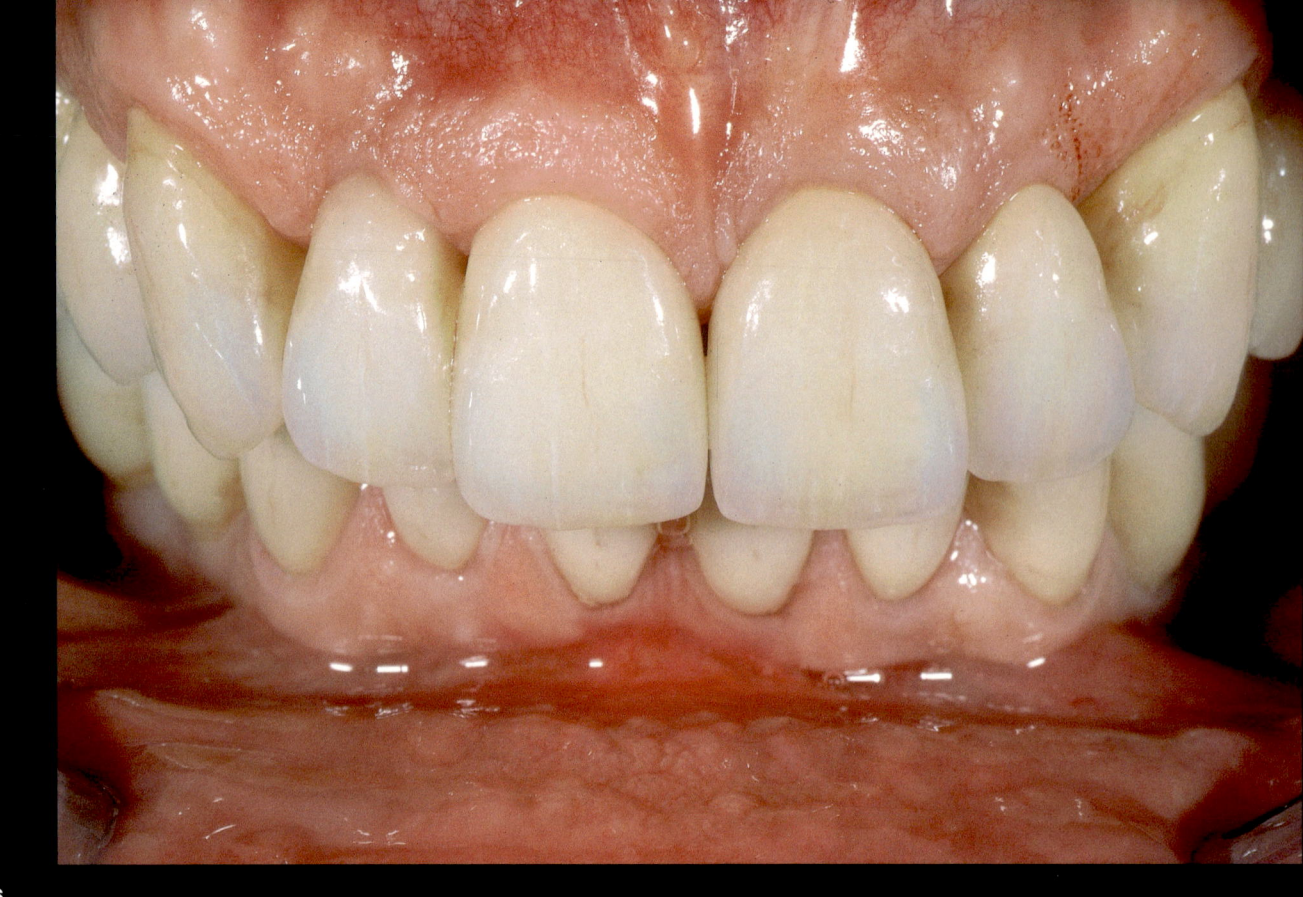

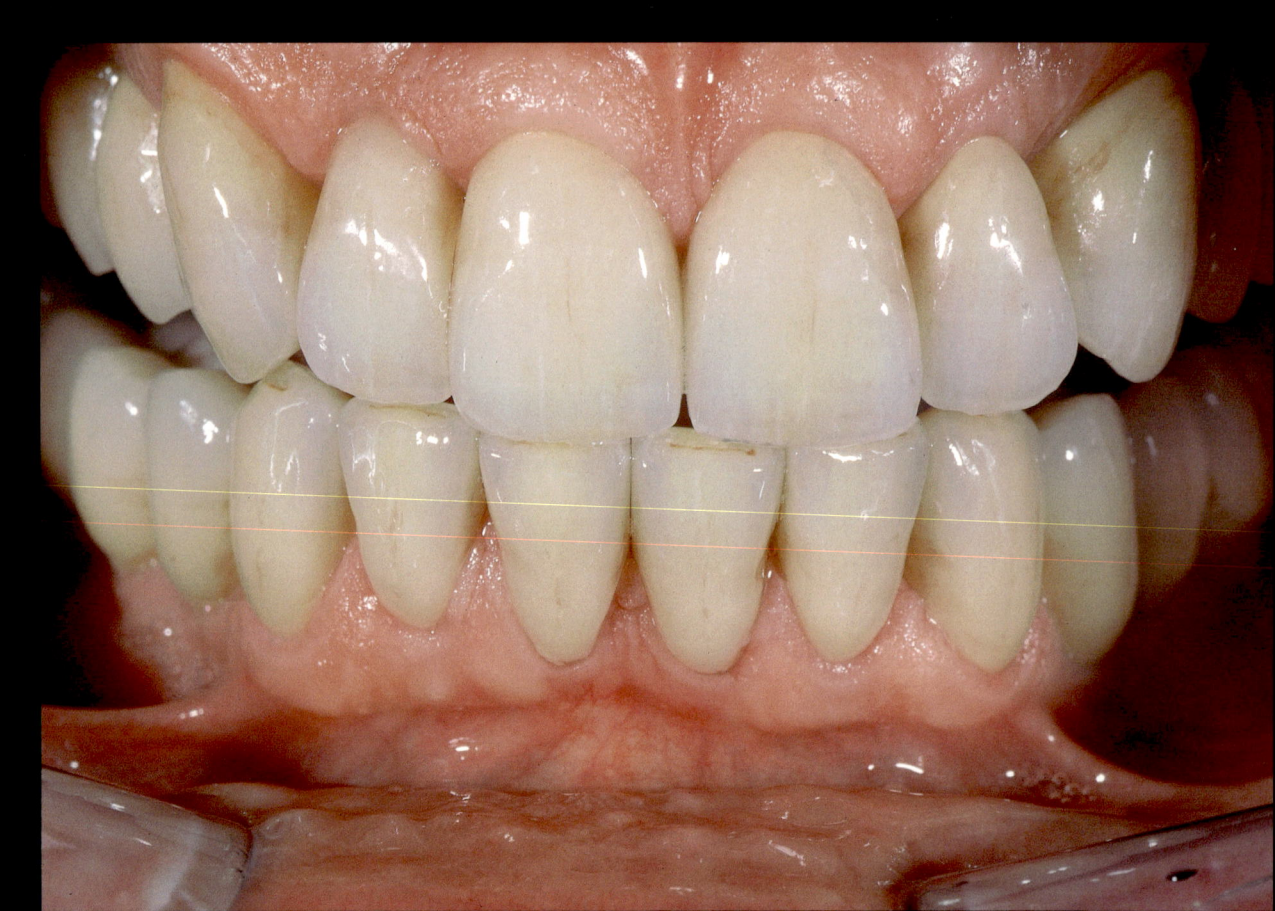

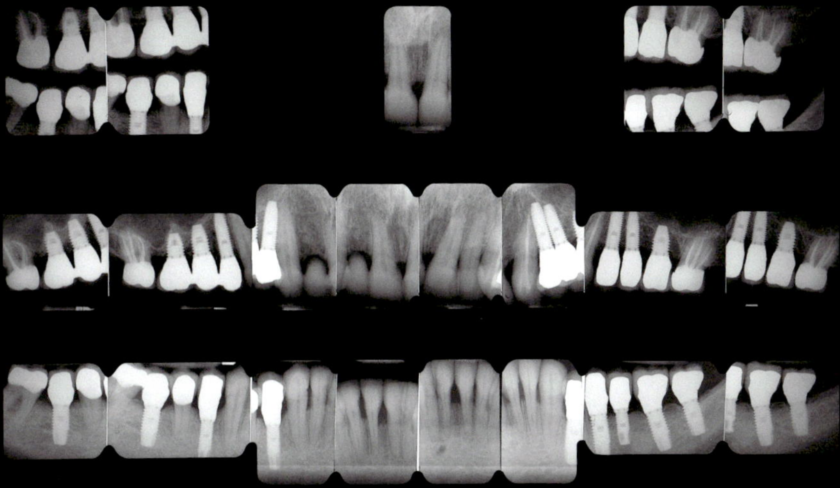

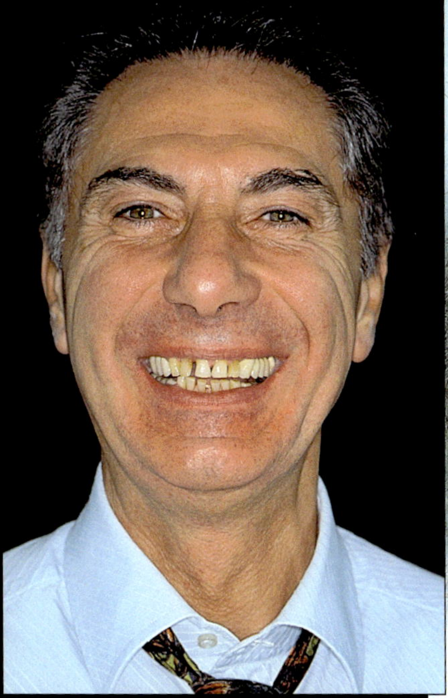

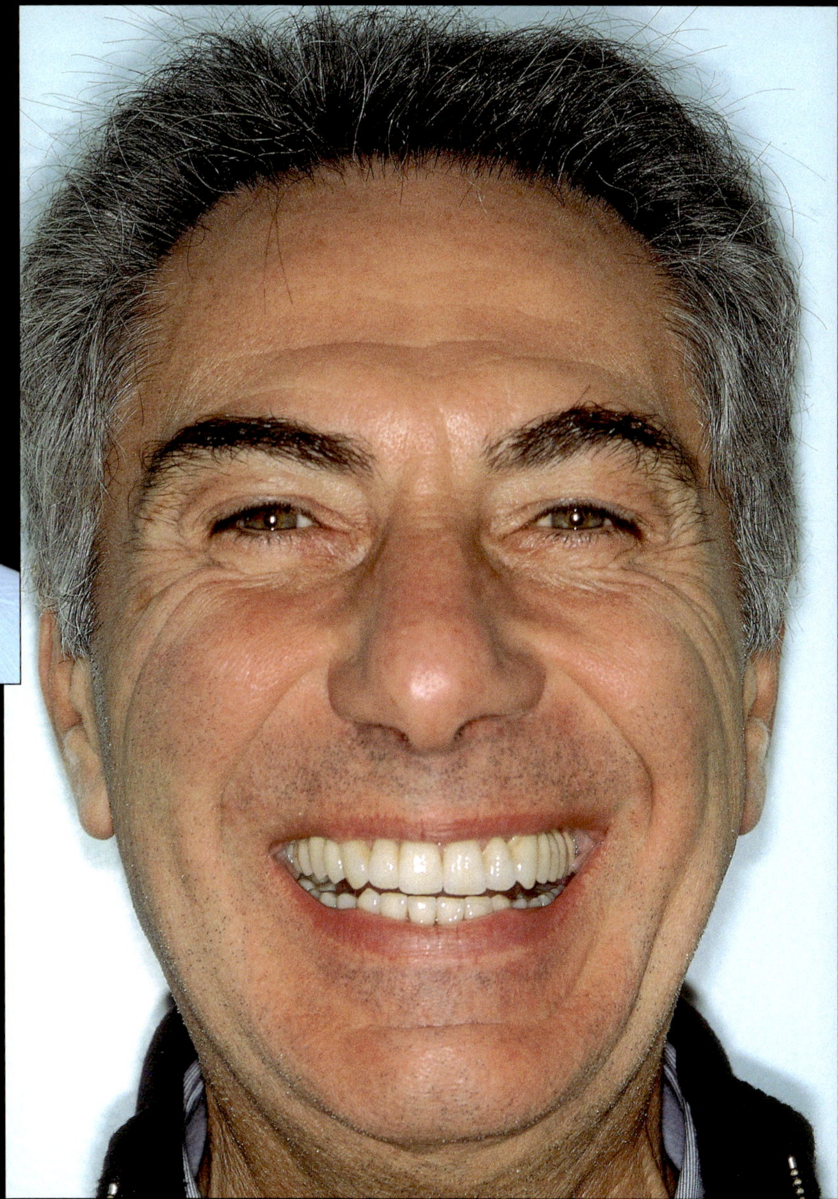

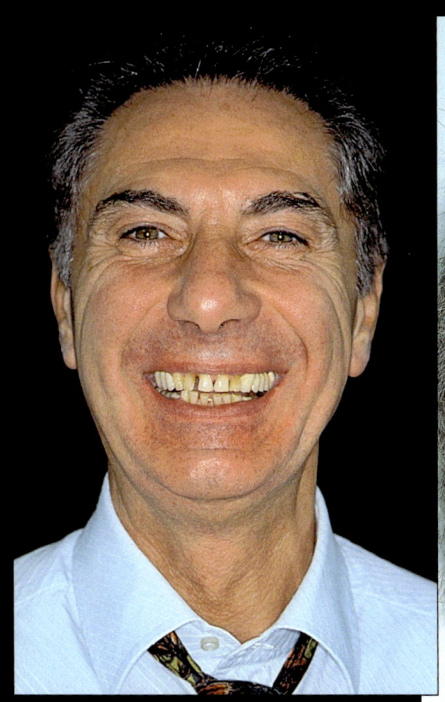

| Patient: N.S. | Gender: F | Age: 20 years |

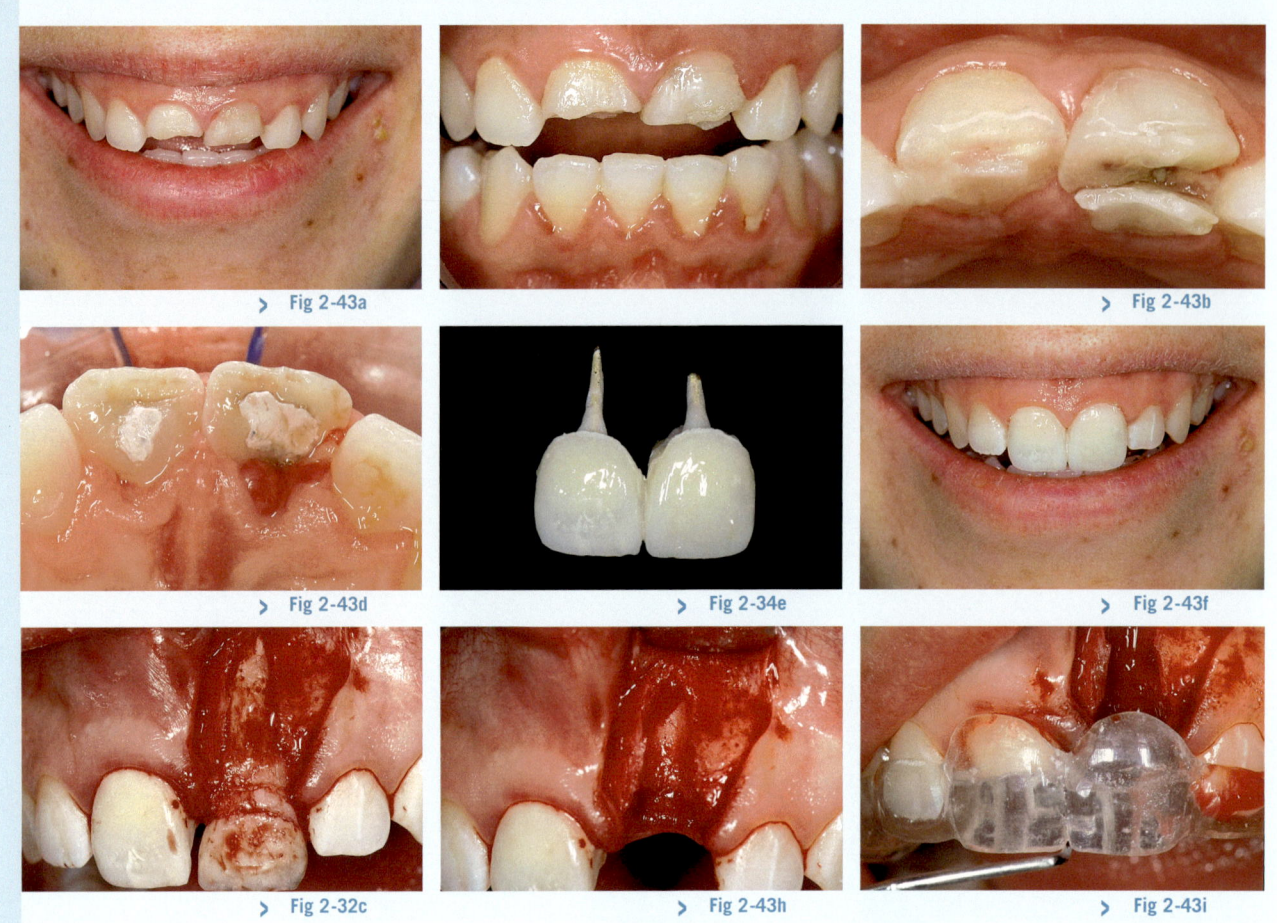

> Fig 2-43a

> Fig 2-43b

> Fig 2-43d

> Fig 2-34e

> Fig 2-43f

> Fig 2-32c

> Fig 2-43h

> Fig 2-43i

PAGES 578–579 Following a road accident, the young patient suffered fractures of the two maxillary central incisors. After a first provisional restoration was positioned, the left central incisor was extracted and replaced with an implant that was put into immediate function; a regenerative technique was used to fill the large buccal fenestration. A customized abutment coated in zirconium was then fabricated on the same unit.

PAGES 580–581 The final impressions of the two central incisors were then taken (right central incisor: natural tooth; left central incisor: implant). Under the guidance of the silicone index, which reproduces the shape and position of the functionalized provisional restoration, two all-ceramic crowns were created (Procera Alumina).

PAGES 582–585 The two definitive restorations appear to be adequately integrated, from both the biologic and esthetic viewpoints, thanks in part to the presence of the interdental papillae, which contribute to giving the restorations a particularly natural appearance.

Anterior rehabilitation　　　　　　　　　　Treatment: 2004–2005

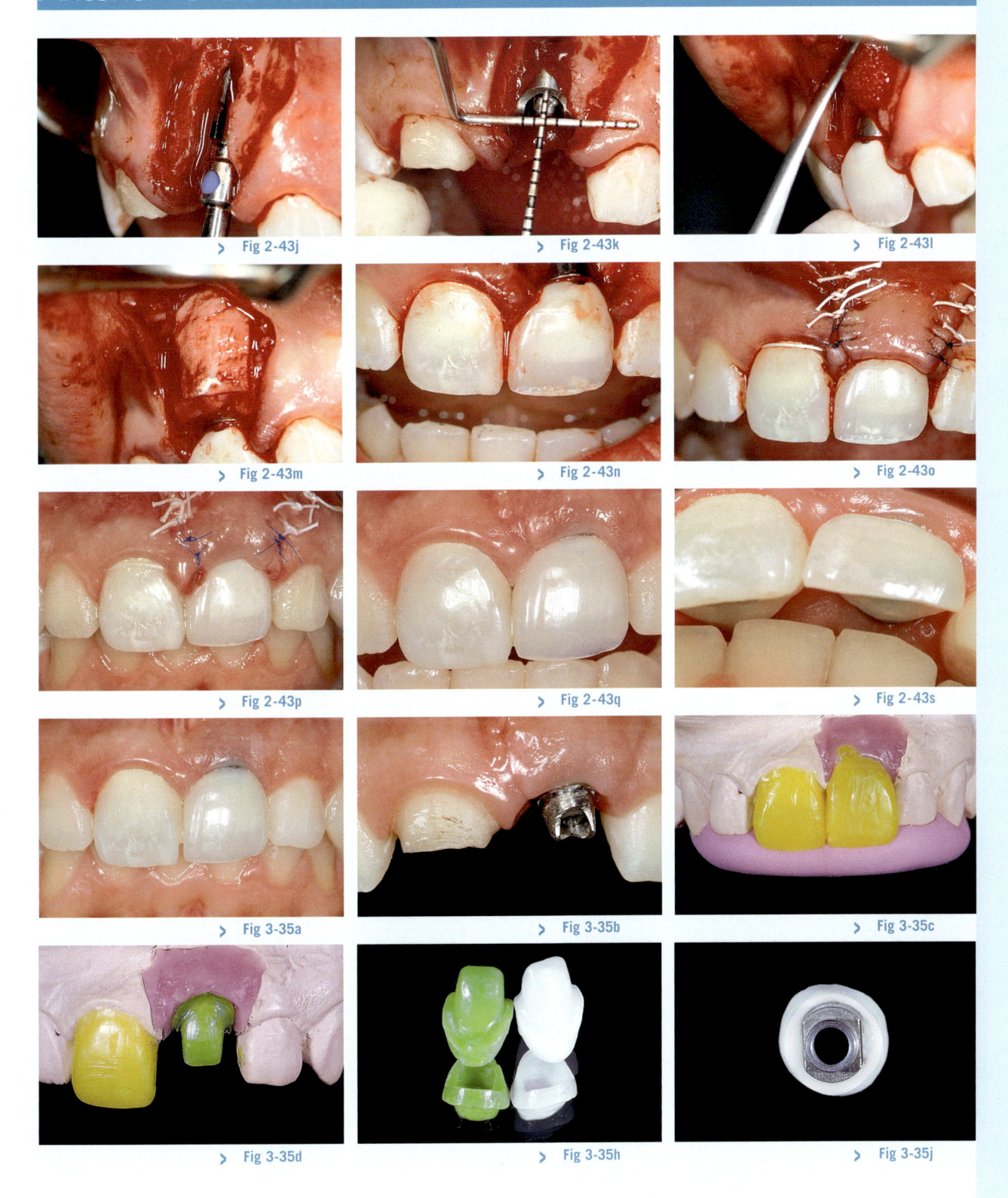

> Fig 2-43j

> Fig 2-43k

> Fig 2-43l

> Fig 2-43m

> Fig 2-43n

> Fig 2-43o

> Fig 2-43p

> Fig 2-43q

> Fig 2-43s

> Fig 3-35a

> Fig 3-35b

> Fig 3-35c

> Fig 3-35d

> Fig 3-35h

> Fig 3-35j

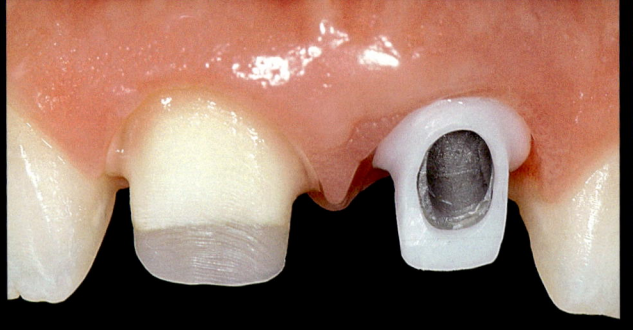

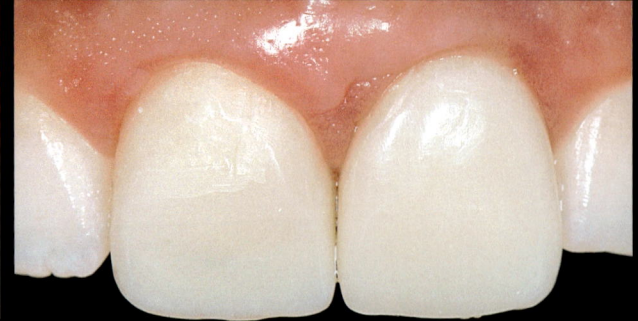

2_2 / 35n

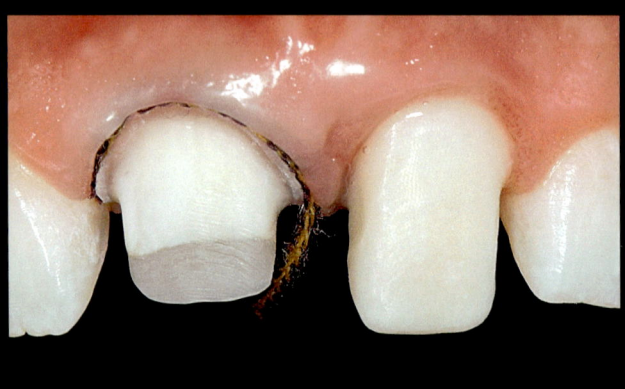

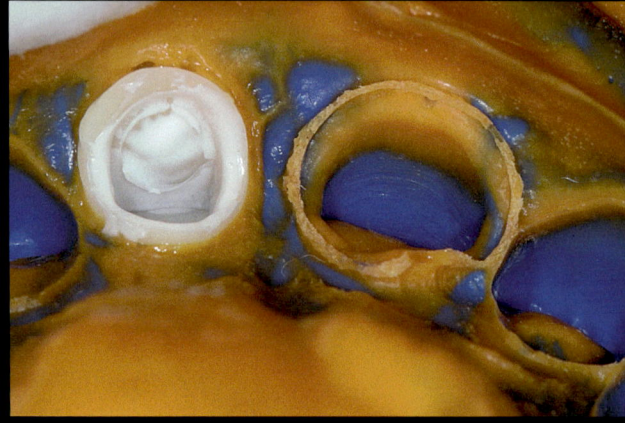

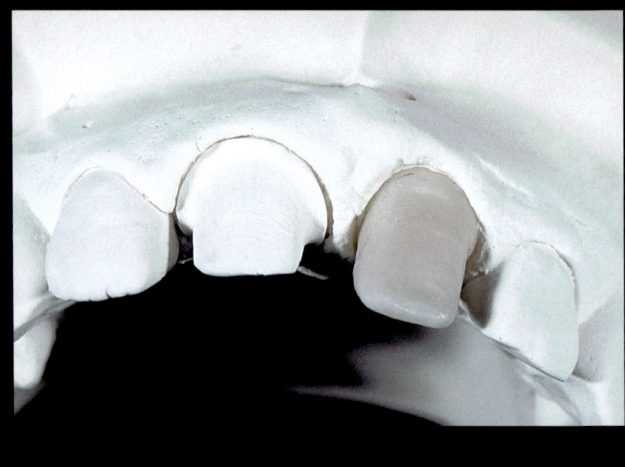

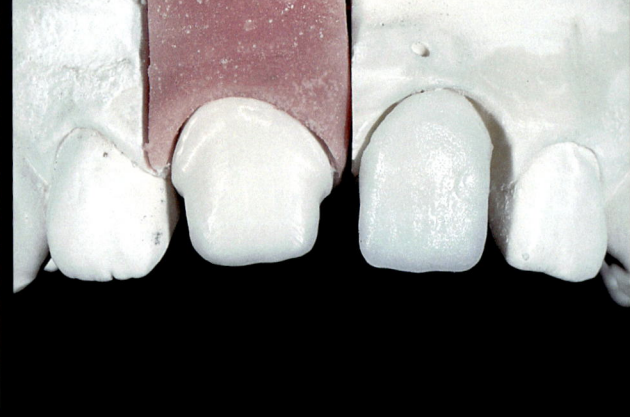

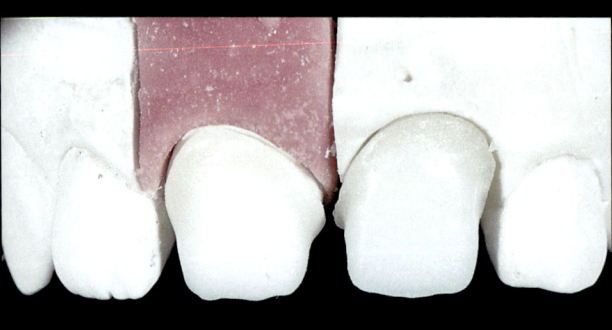

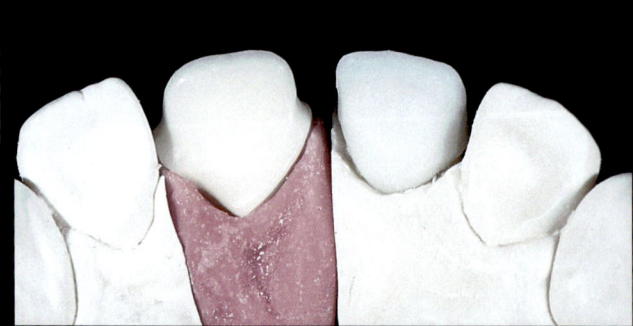

581

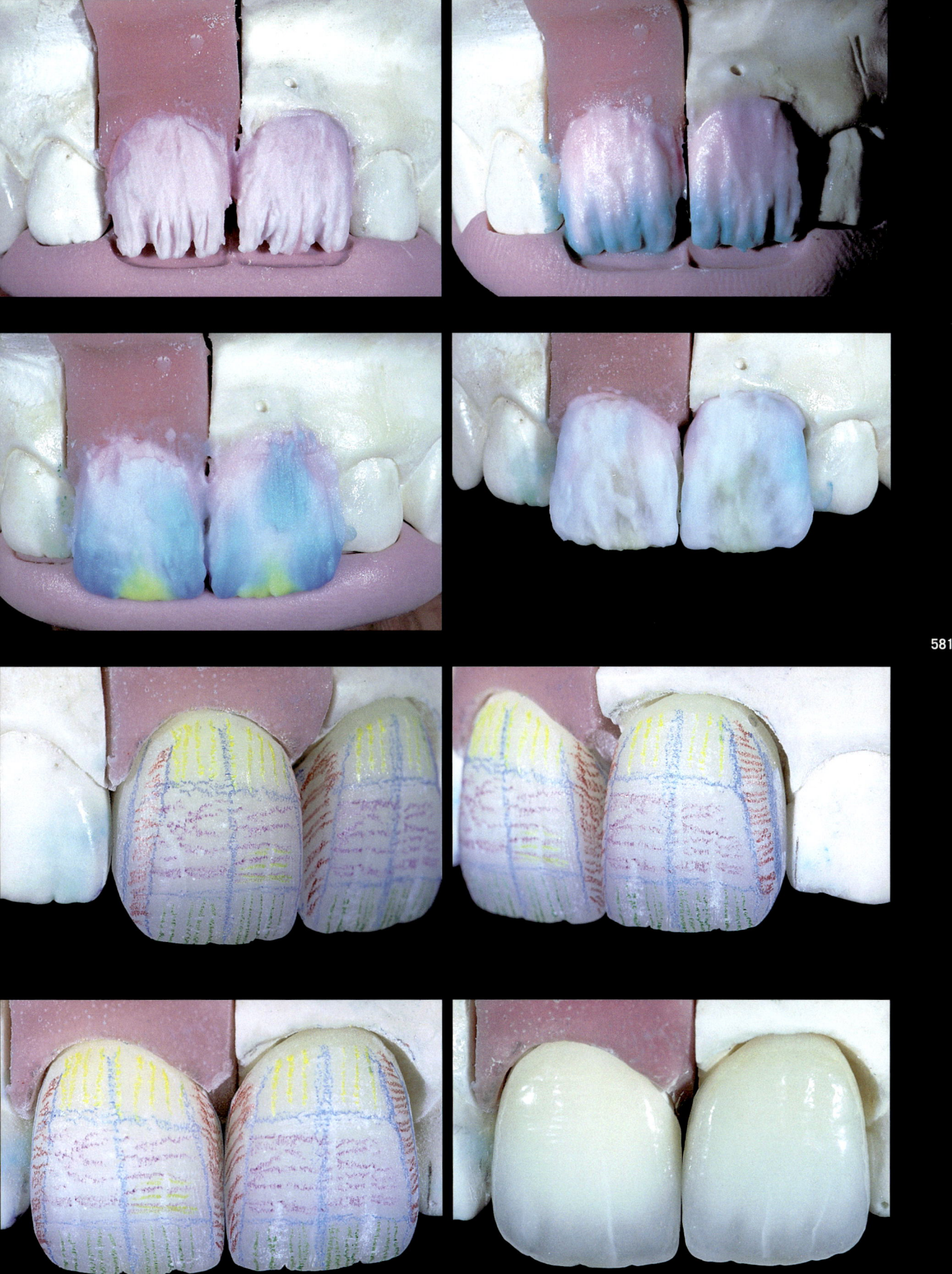

582

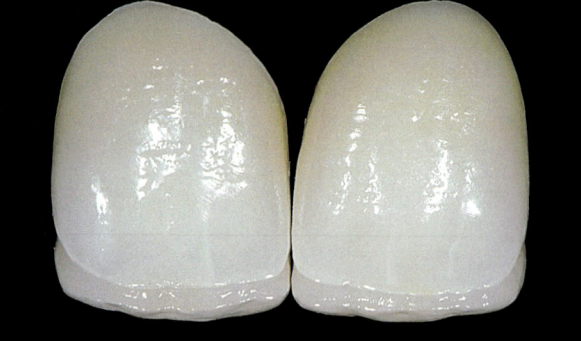

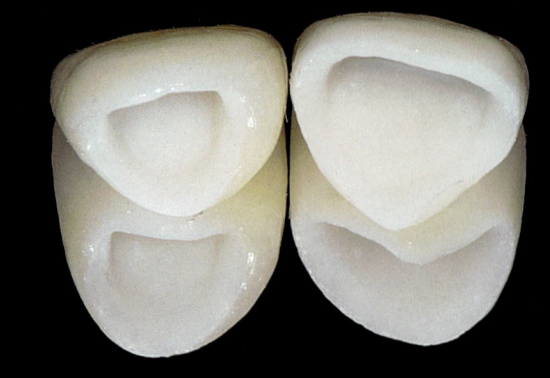

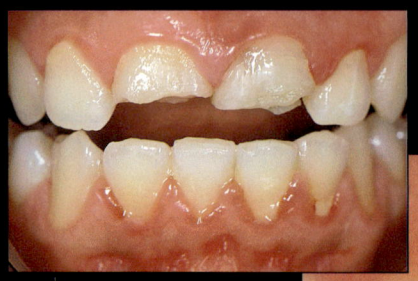

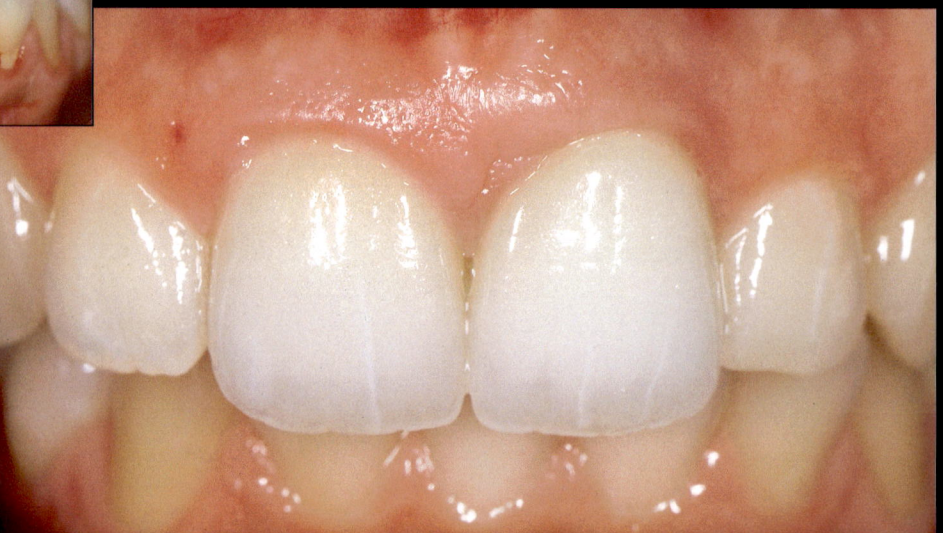

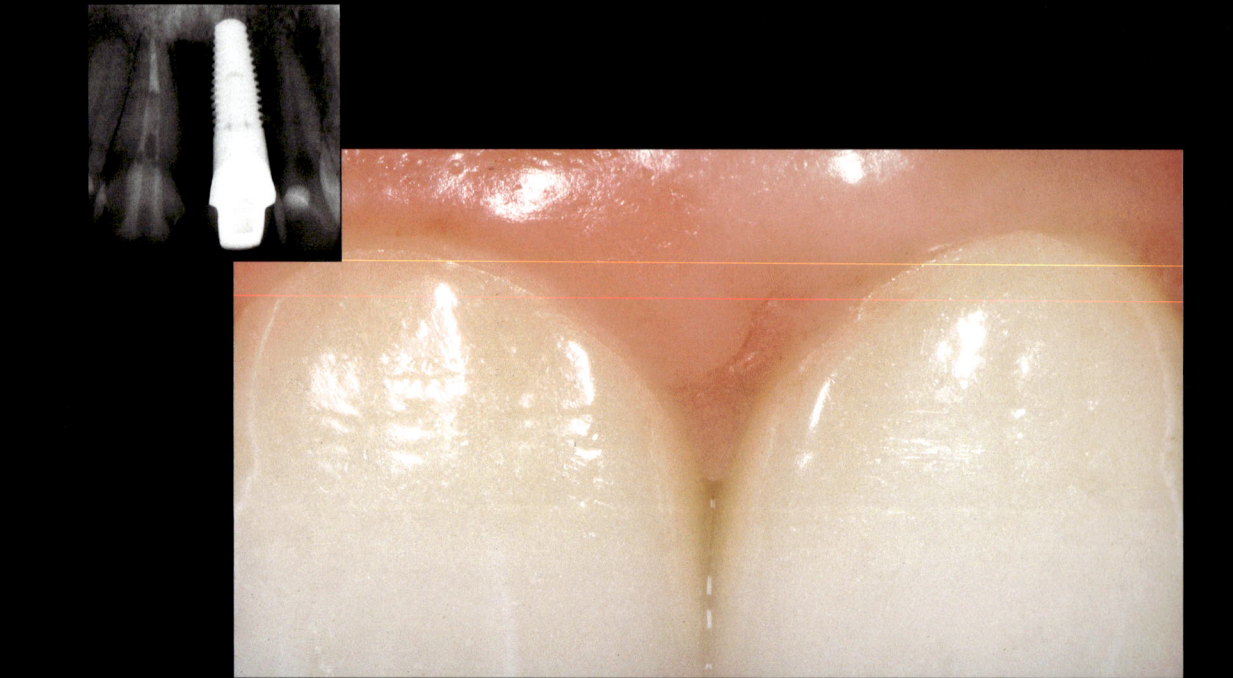

583

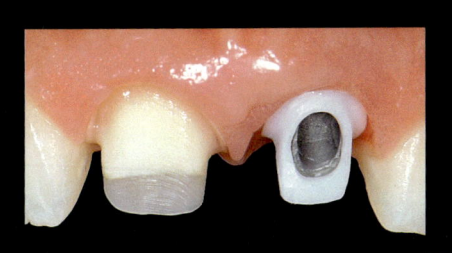

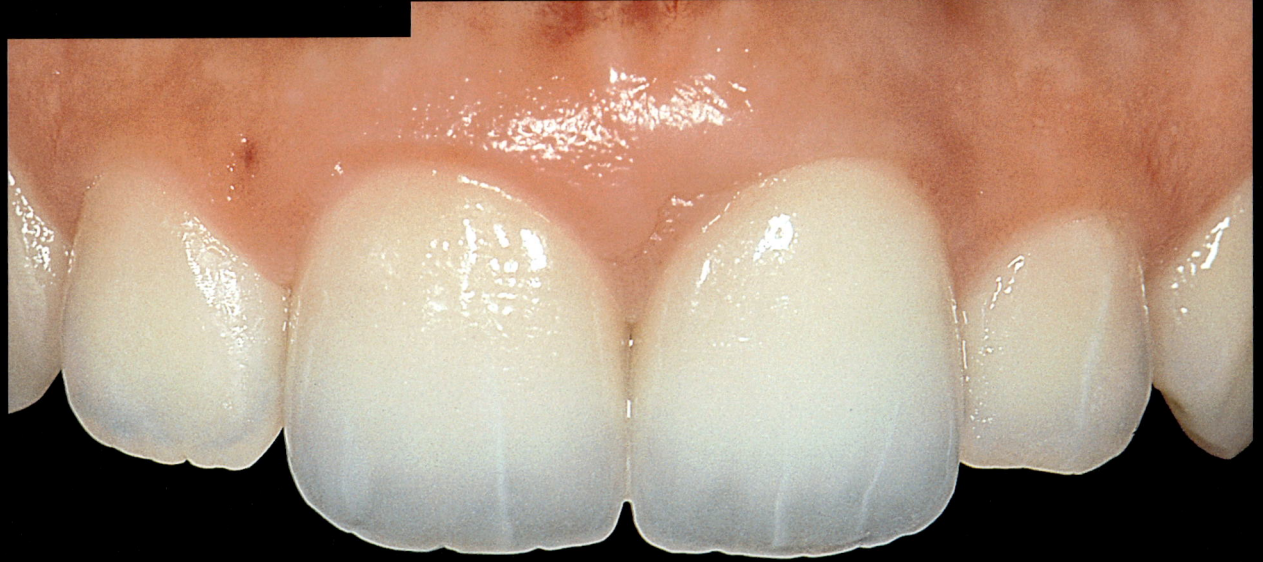

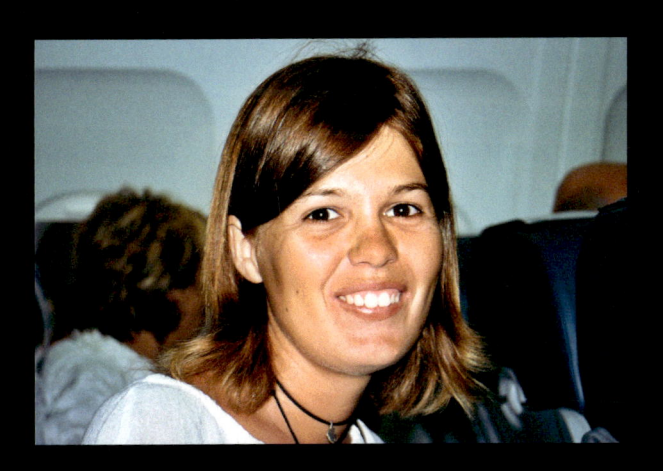

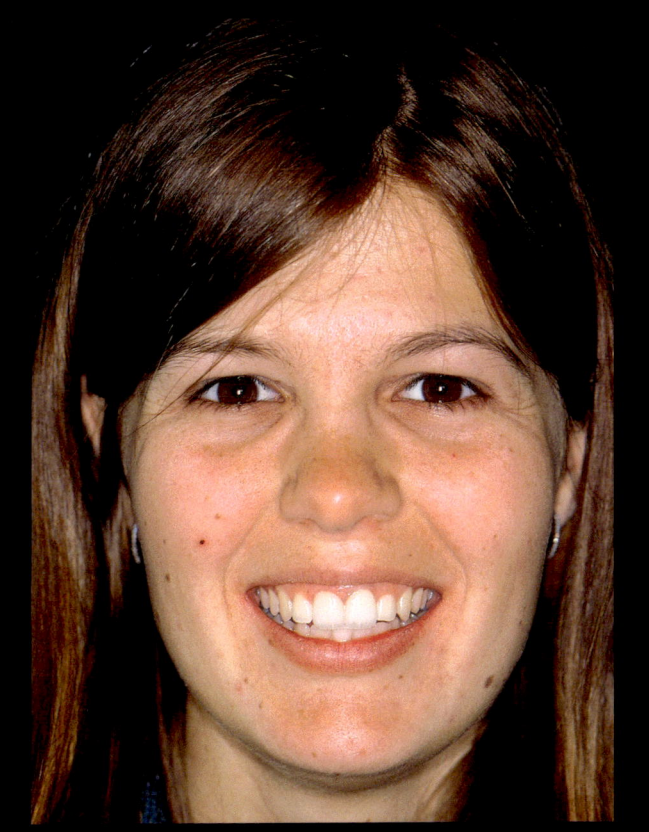

584

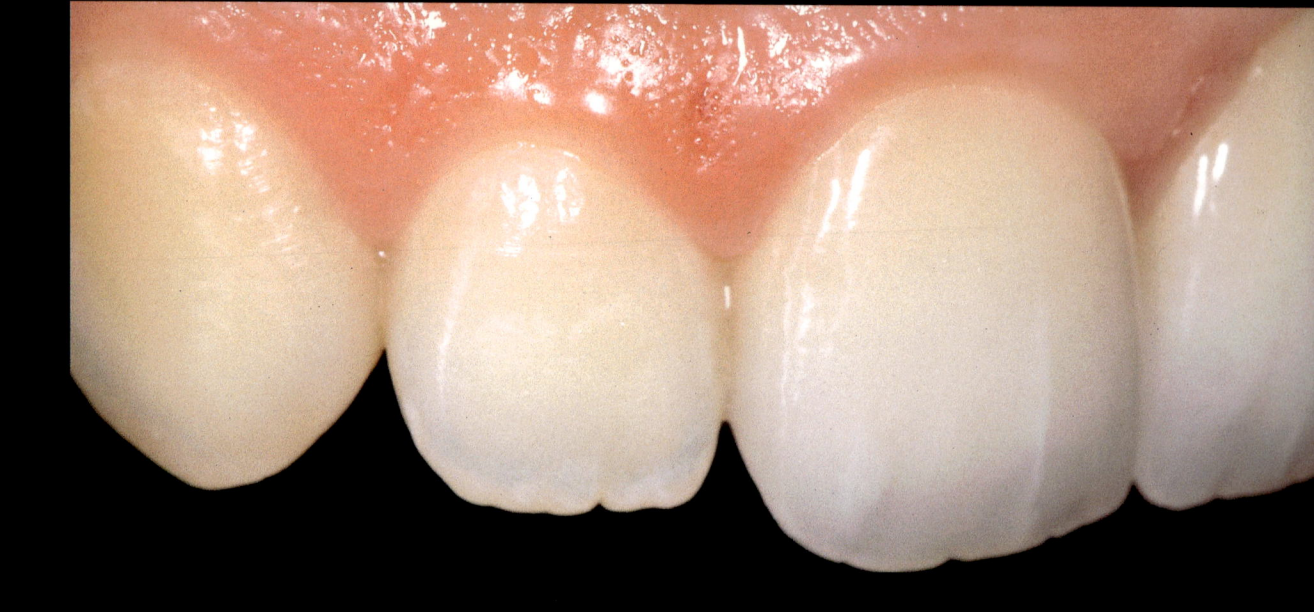

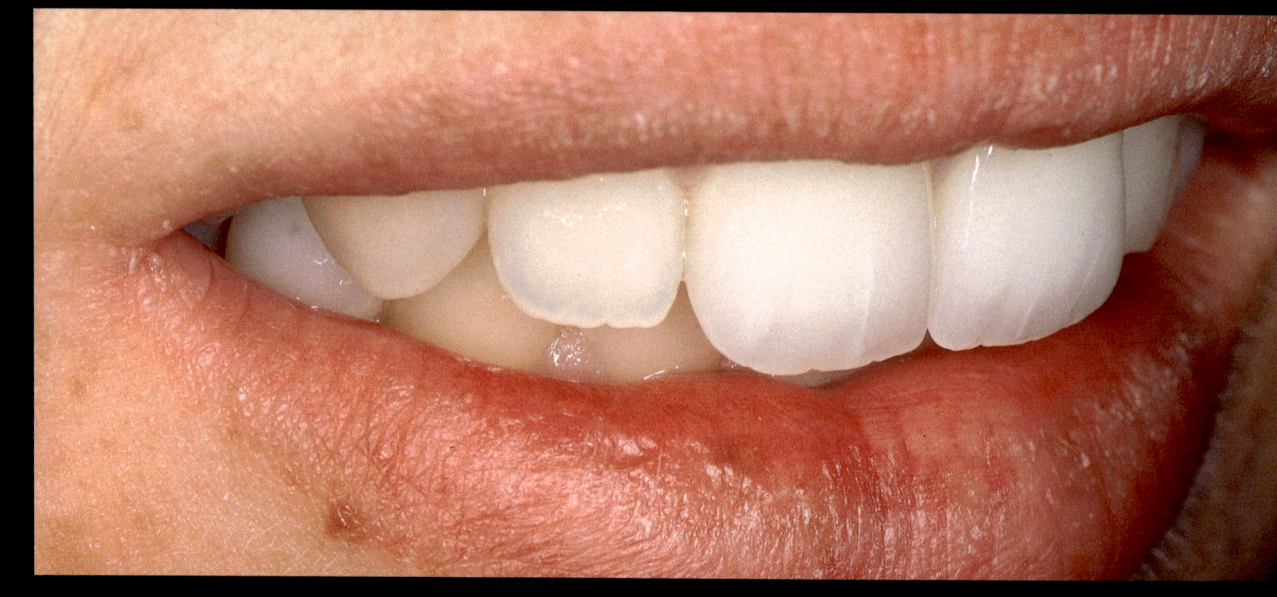

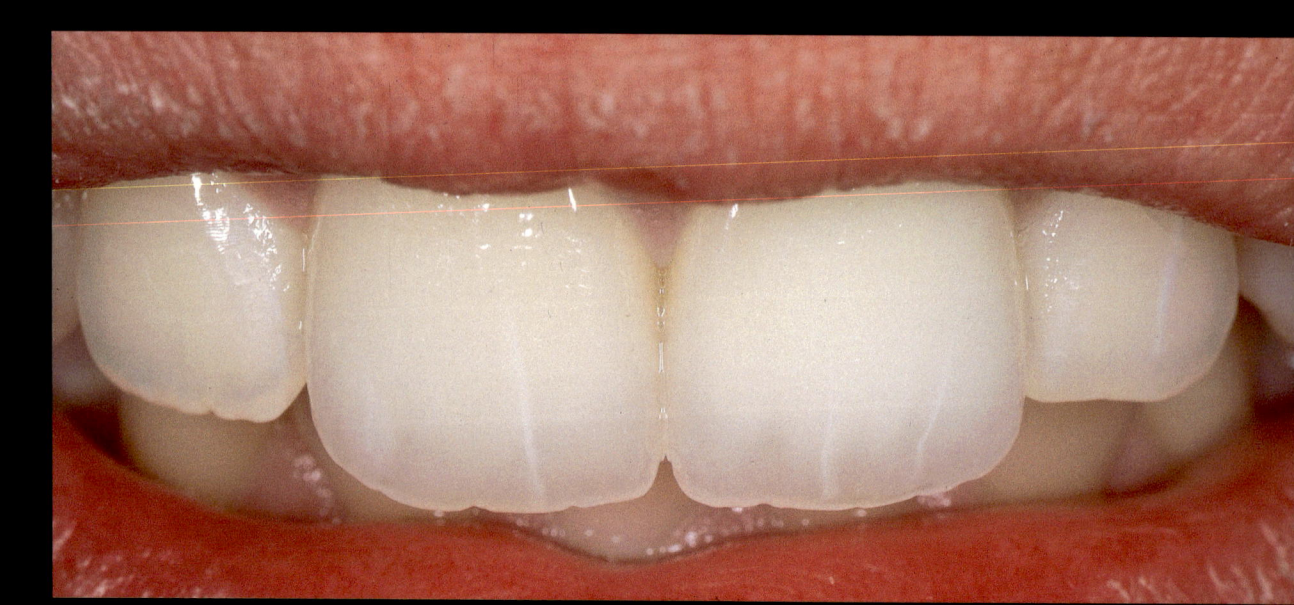

585

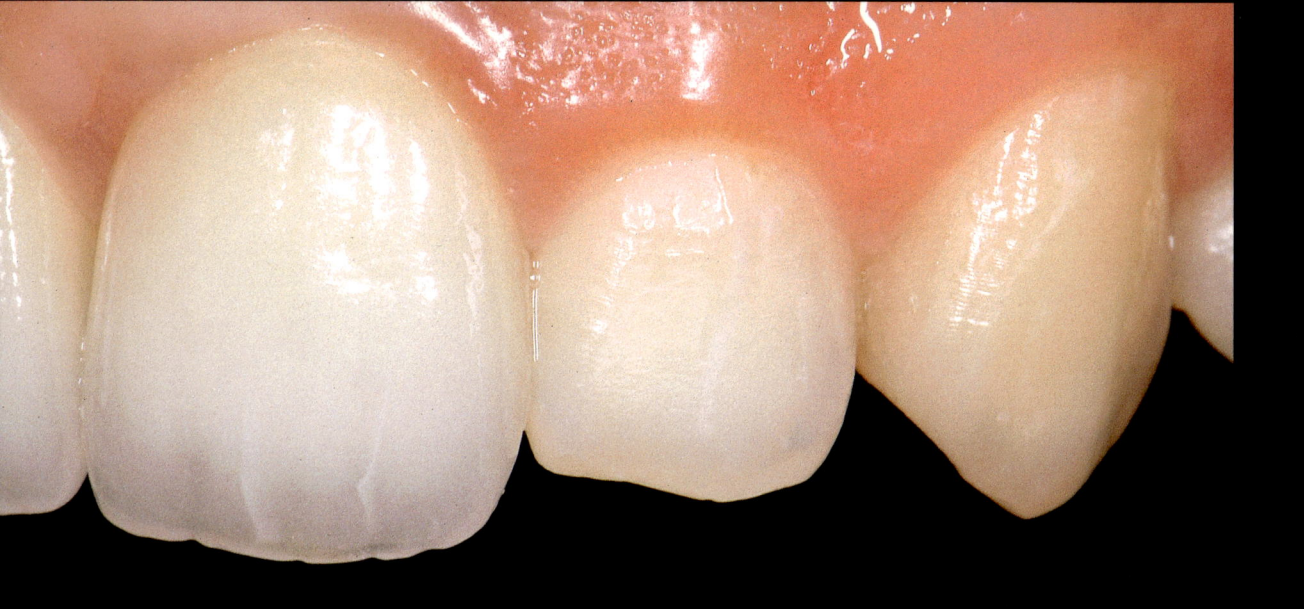

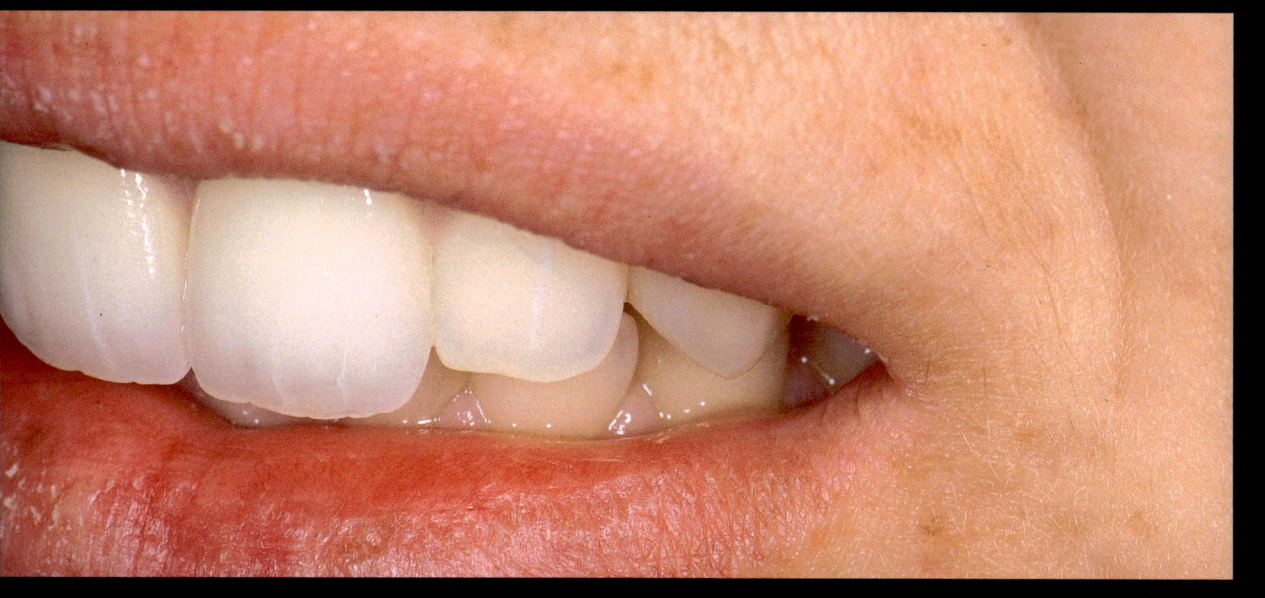

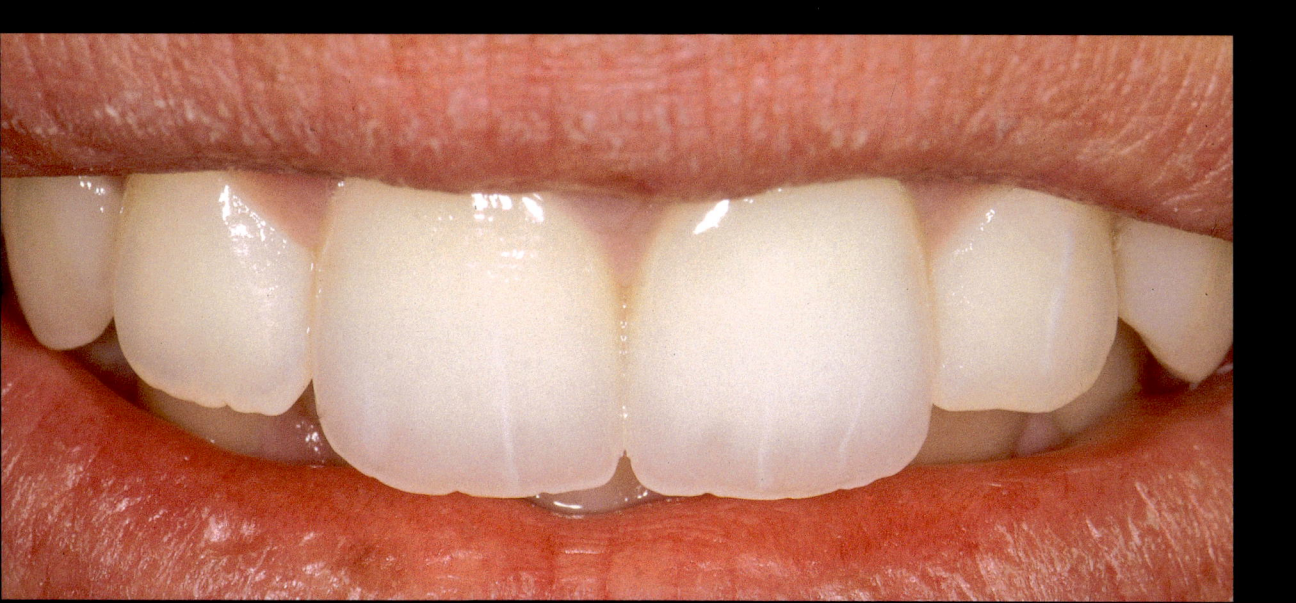

Patient: T.T.   Gender: M   Age: 23 years

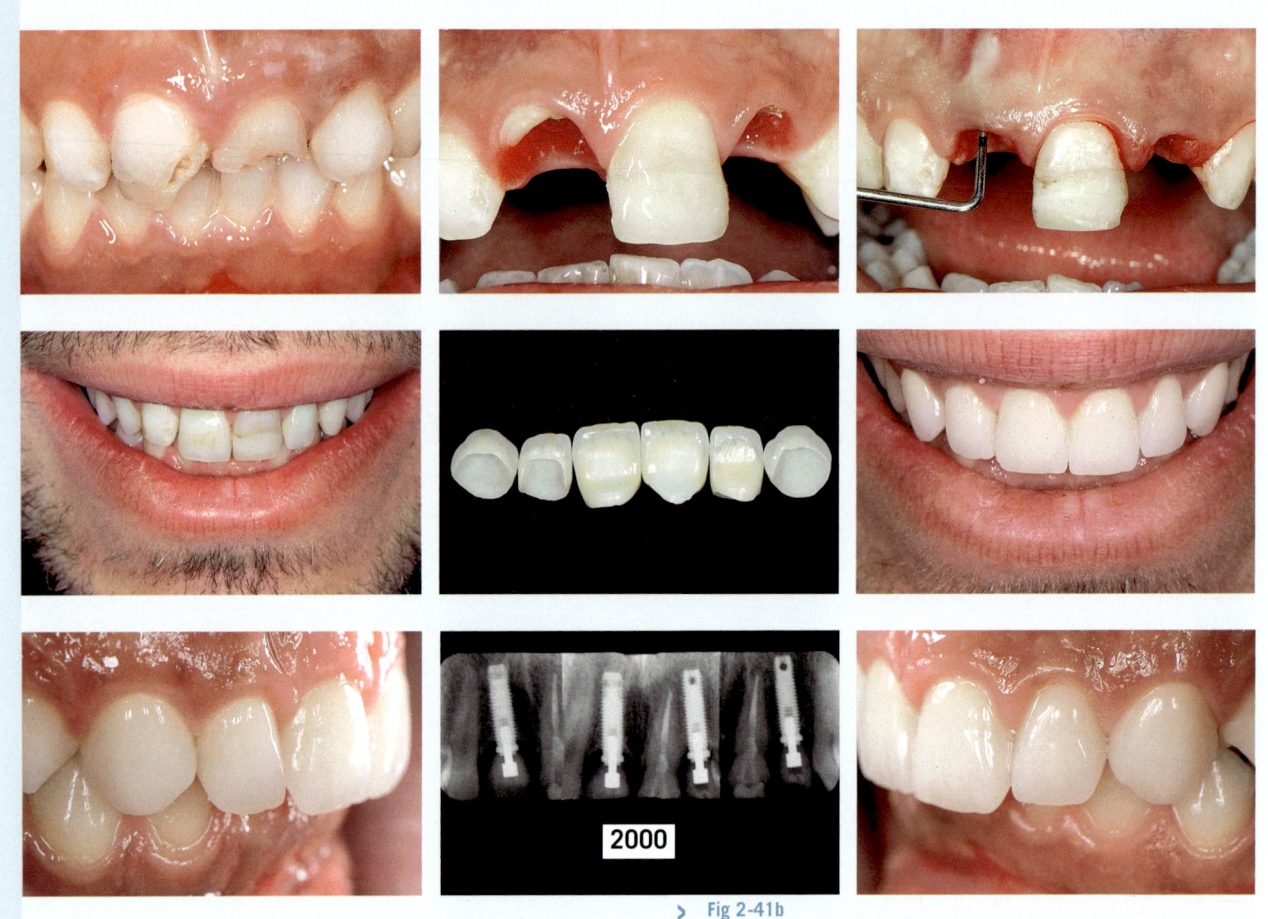

> Fig 2-41b

PAGES 586–587   Because of trauma suffered in a motorcycle accident in 2000, the patient had undergone treatment to receive two crowns on implants and four restorations on natural teeth (Procera Alumina). A second accident, which took place in 2004, made it necessary to extract the right lateral incisor and to replace it with an implant, in addition to the repair of the two fractured central incisors.

PAGES 588–589   After two zirconium abutments were positioned on implants, three all-ceramic restorations were carried out (Procera Alumina).

PAGES 590–593   The photos of the definitive restorations show the satisfactory result achieved even after the second treatment, despite the difficulty of having to finalize three new restorations to place next to those previously made. Furthermore, it is possible to notice a substantial stability of the esthetic result achieved over the course of the years, with particular reference to maintenance of the gingival levels and the interdental papillae, despite the presence of two adjacent implants.

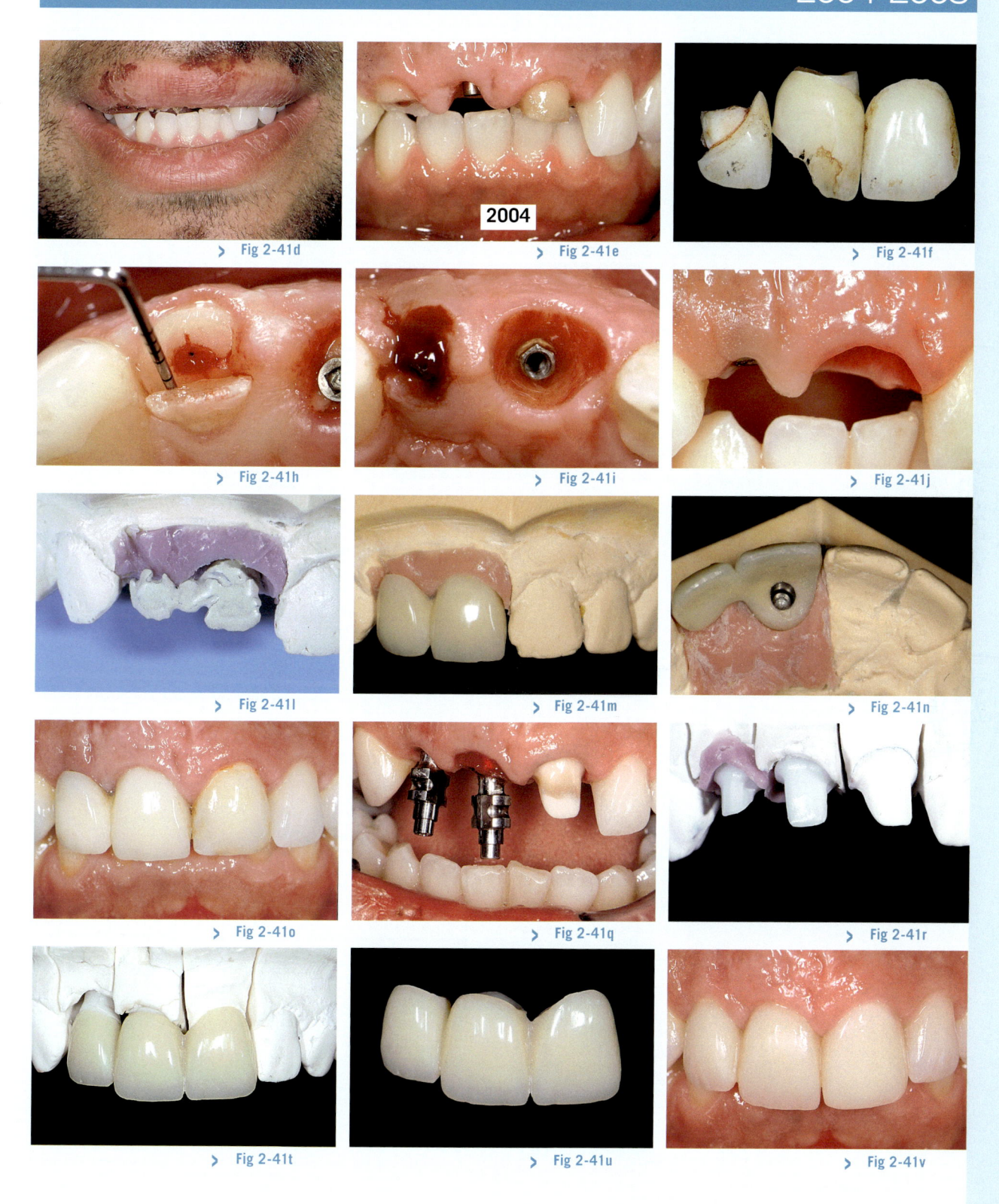

Anterior Rehabilitation

Treatments: 1999–2000 2004–2005

> Fig 2-41d

> Fig 2-41e

> Fig 2-41f

> Fig 2-41h

> Fig 2-41i

> Fig 2-41j

> Fig 2-41l

> Fig 2-41m

> Fig 2-41n

> Fig 2-41o

> Fig 2-41q

> Fig 2-41r

> Fig 2-41t

> Fig 2-41u

> Fig 2-41v

587

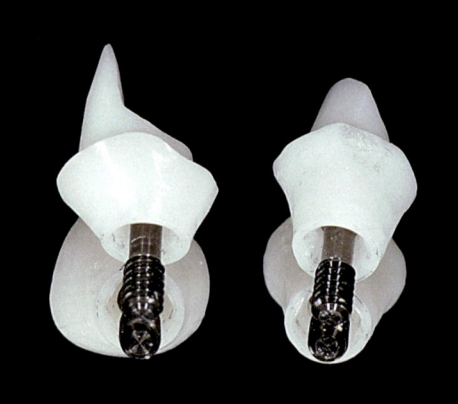

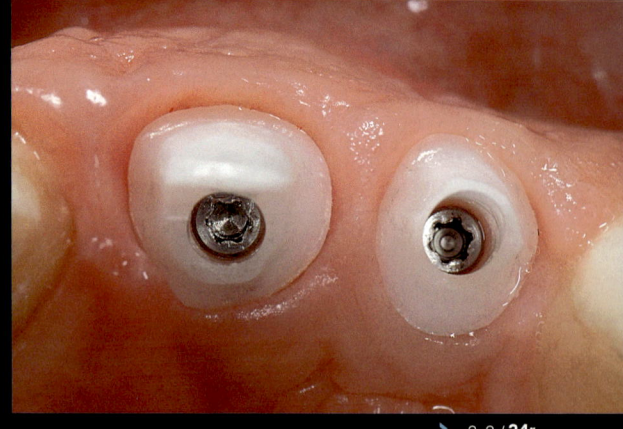

2_2 / **34p**

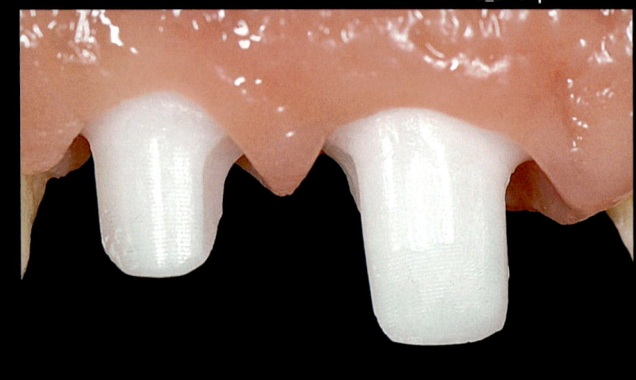

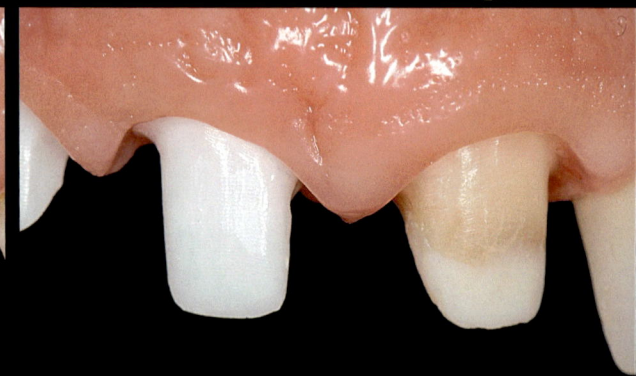

2_2 / **34r**

2_2 / **34q**

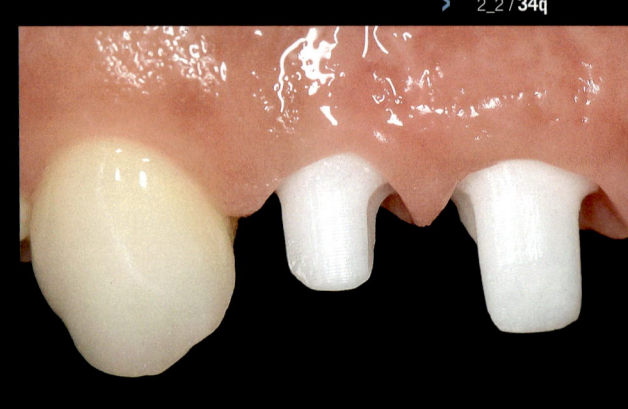

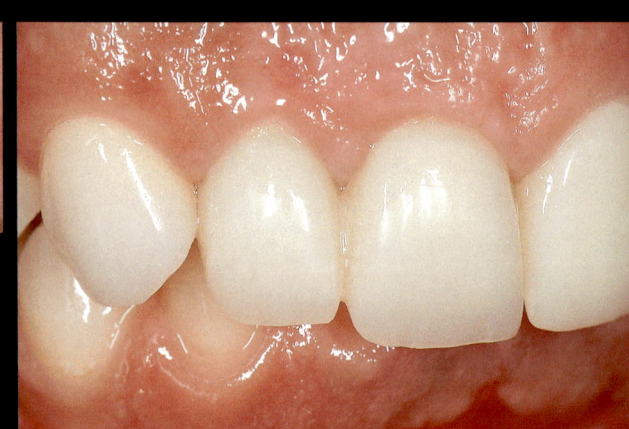

2_2 / **34s**

2_2 / **34u**

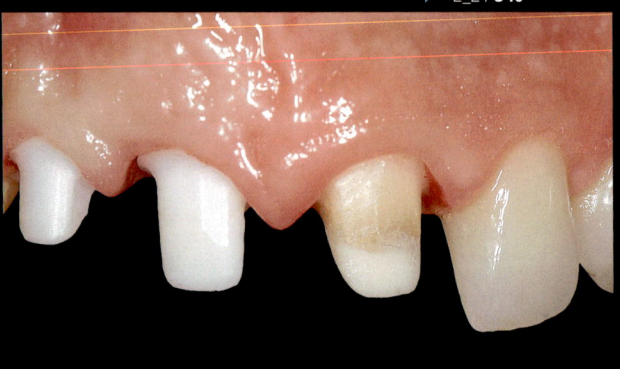

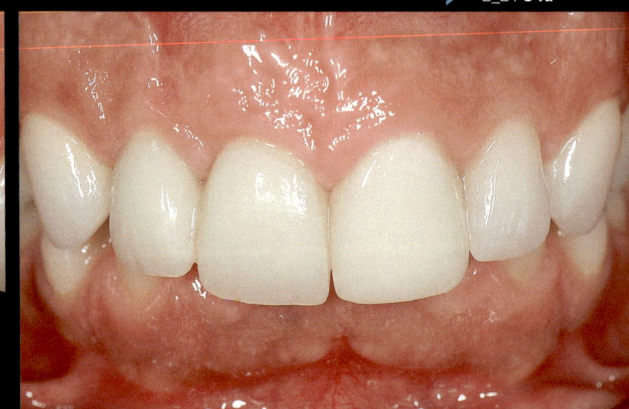

2_2 / **34t**

2_2 / **34v**

589

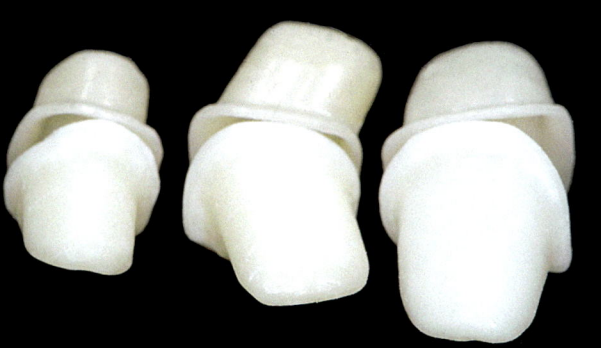

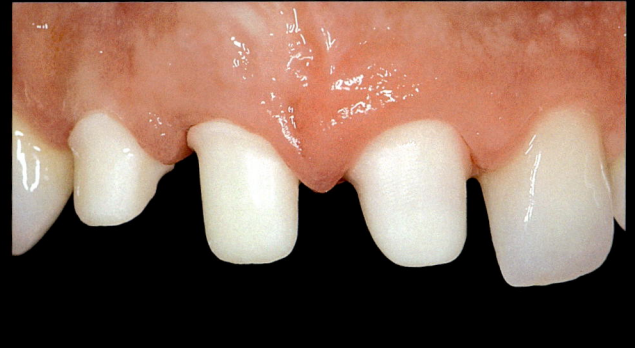

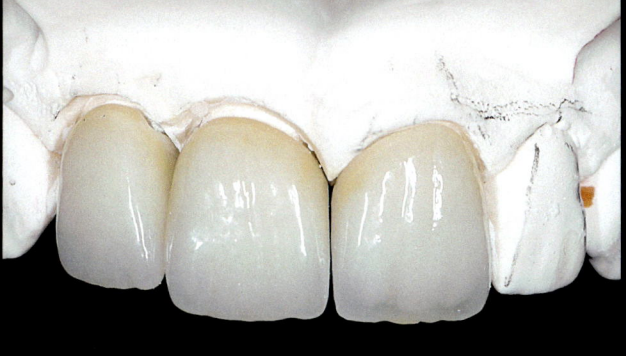

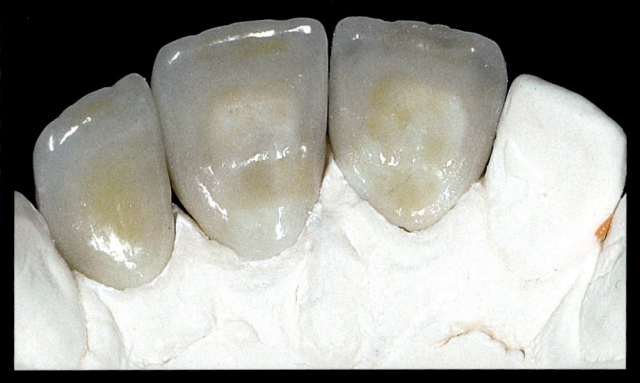

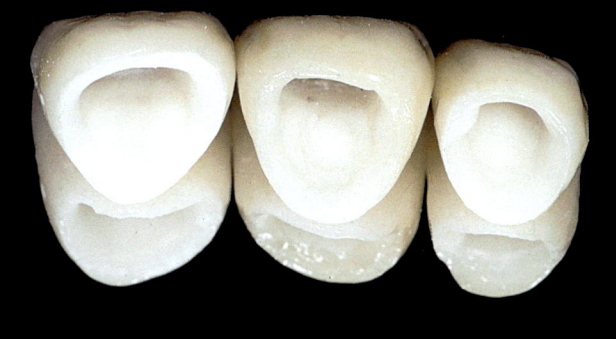

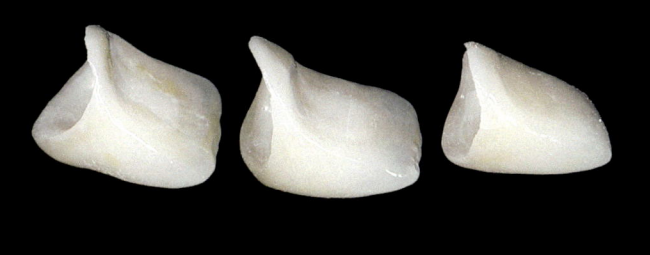

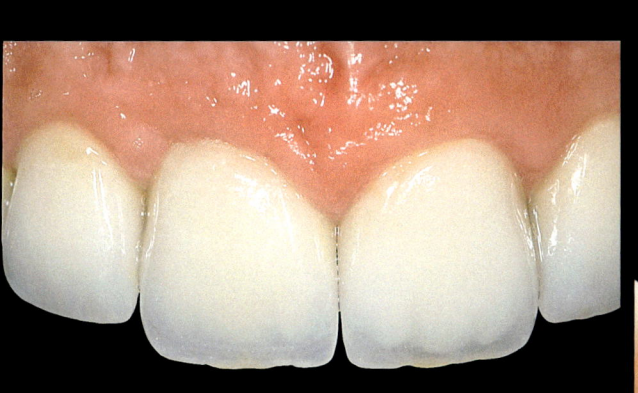

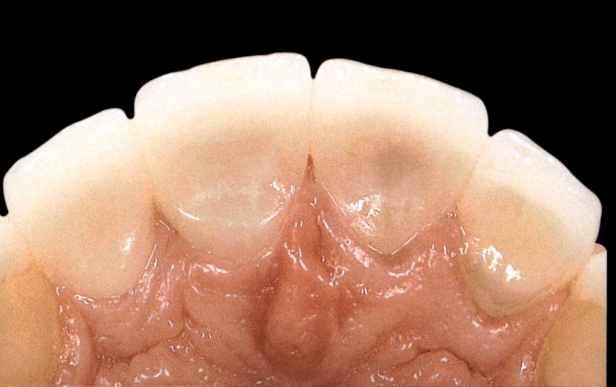

590

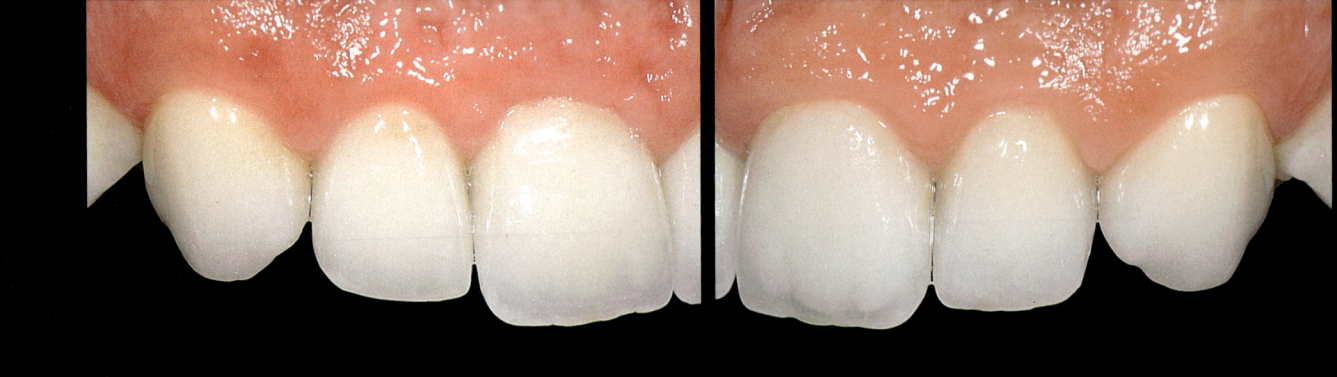

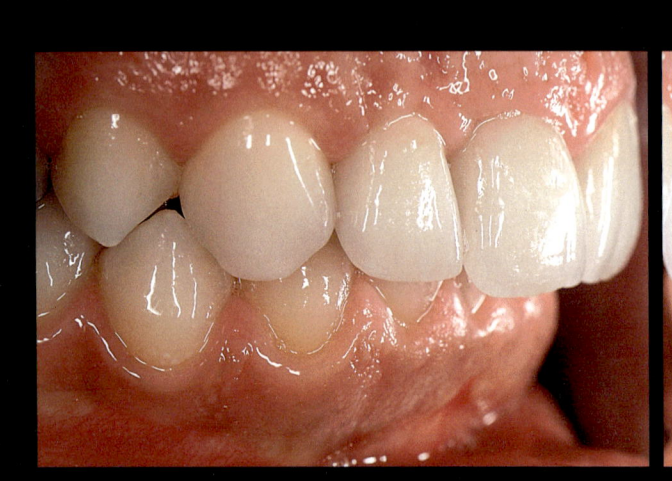

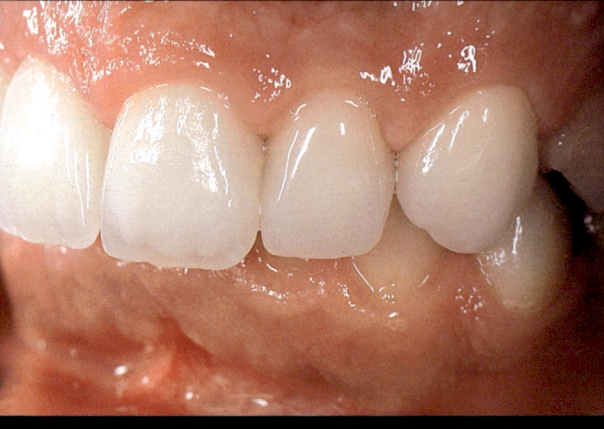

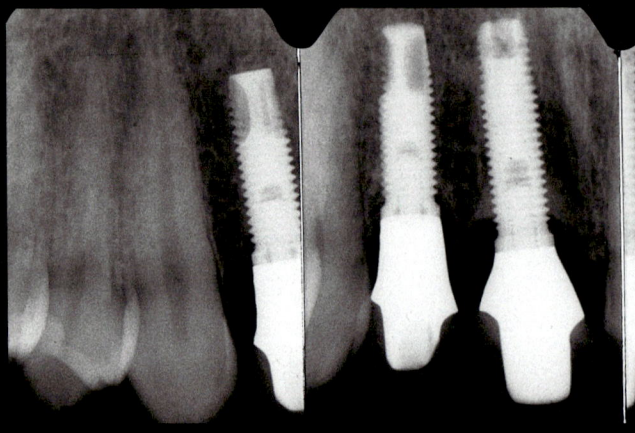

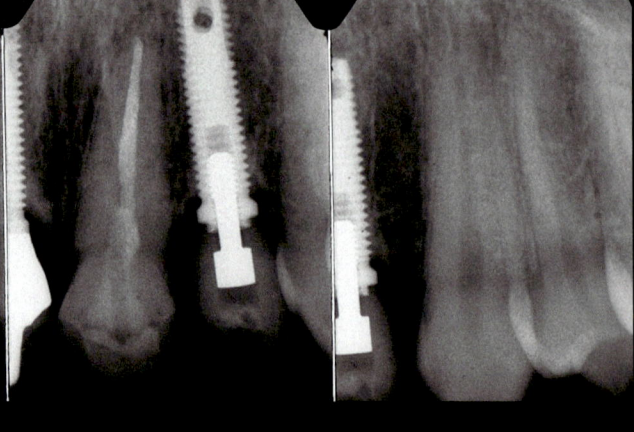

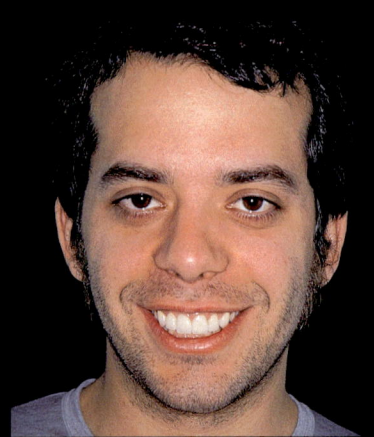

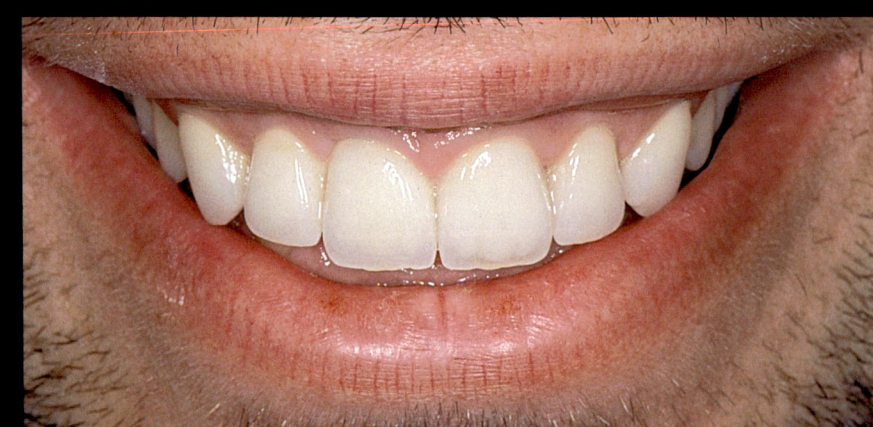

591

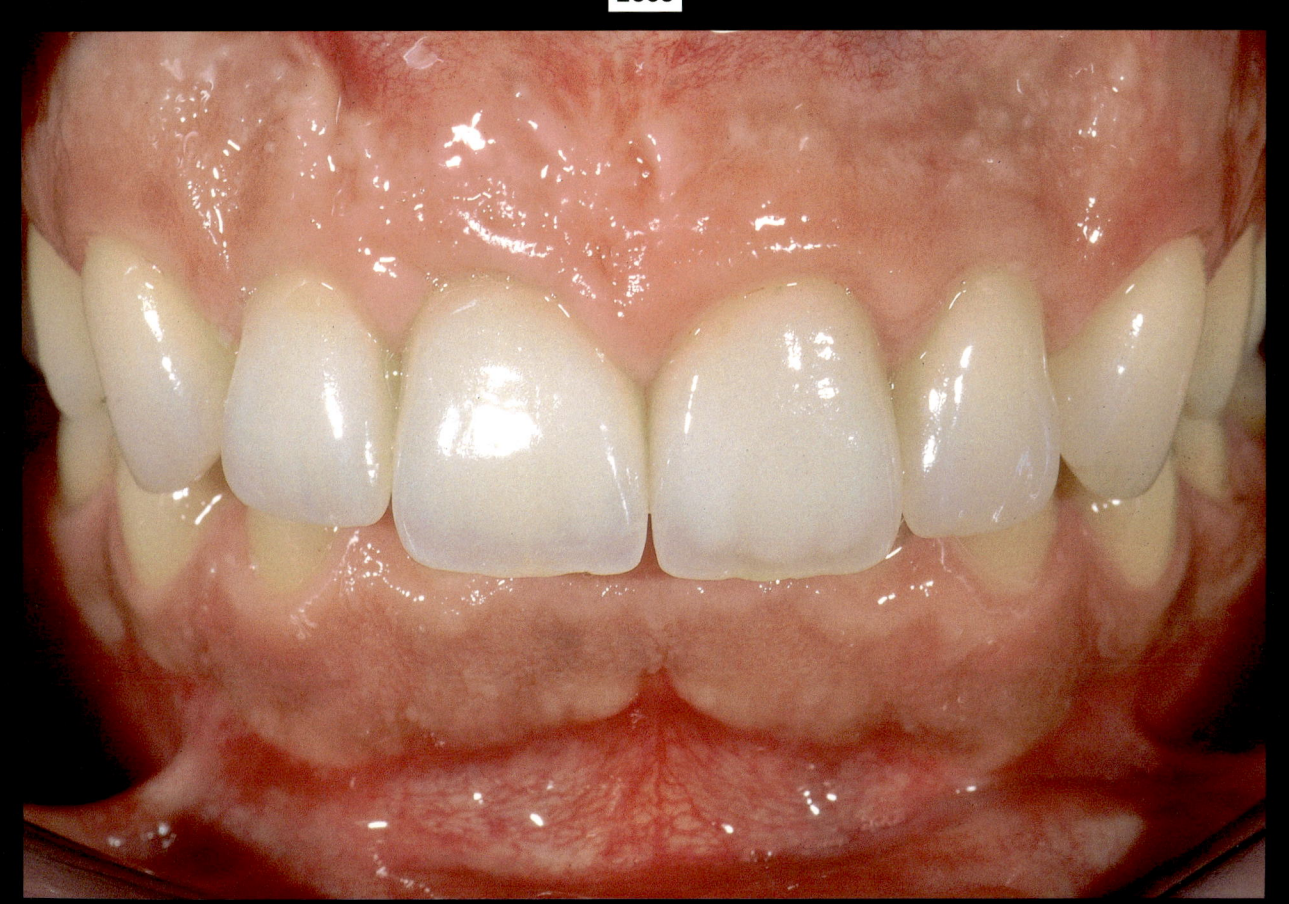

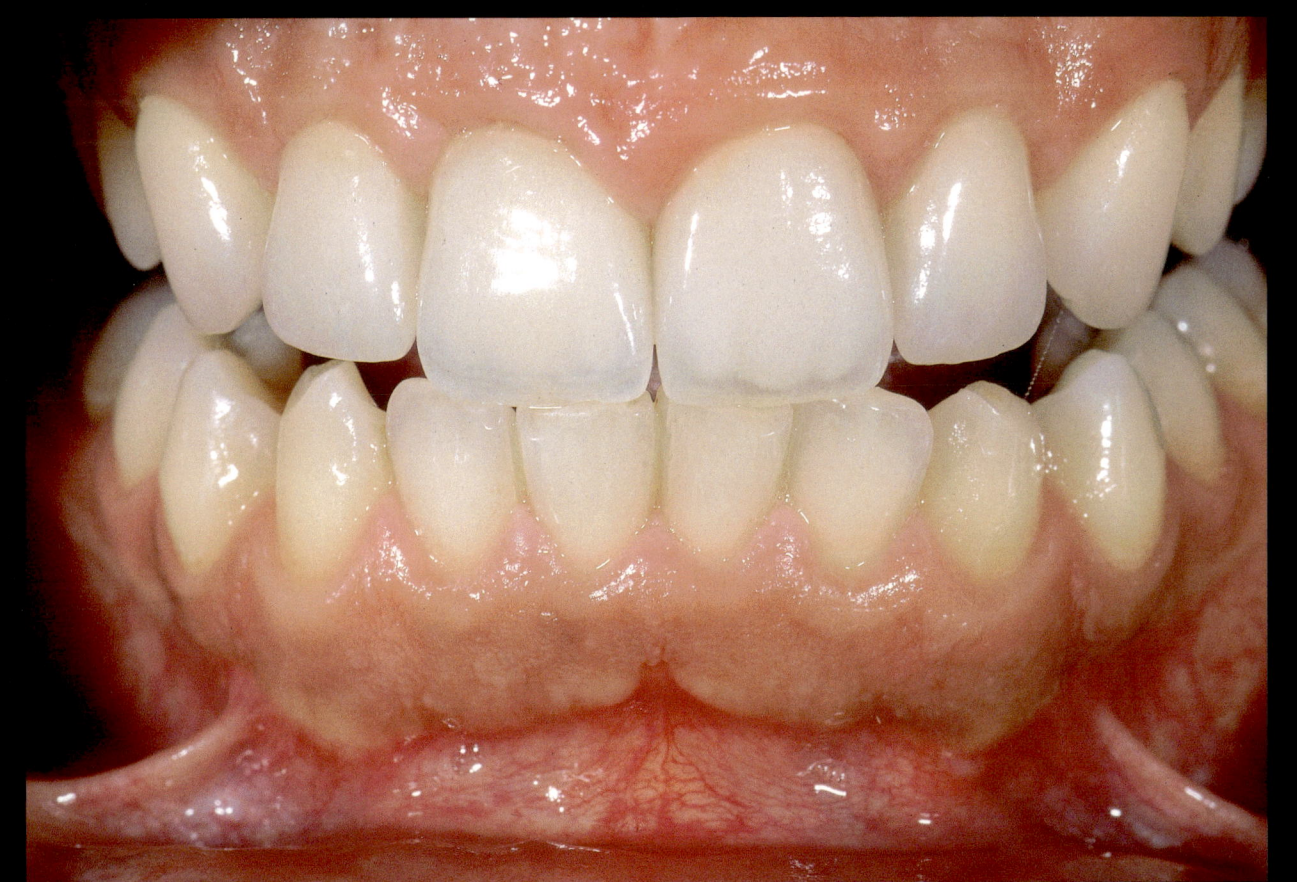

First treatment: 1999–2000

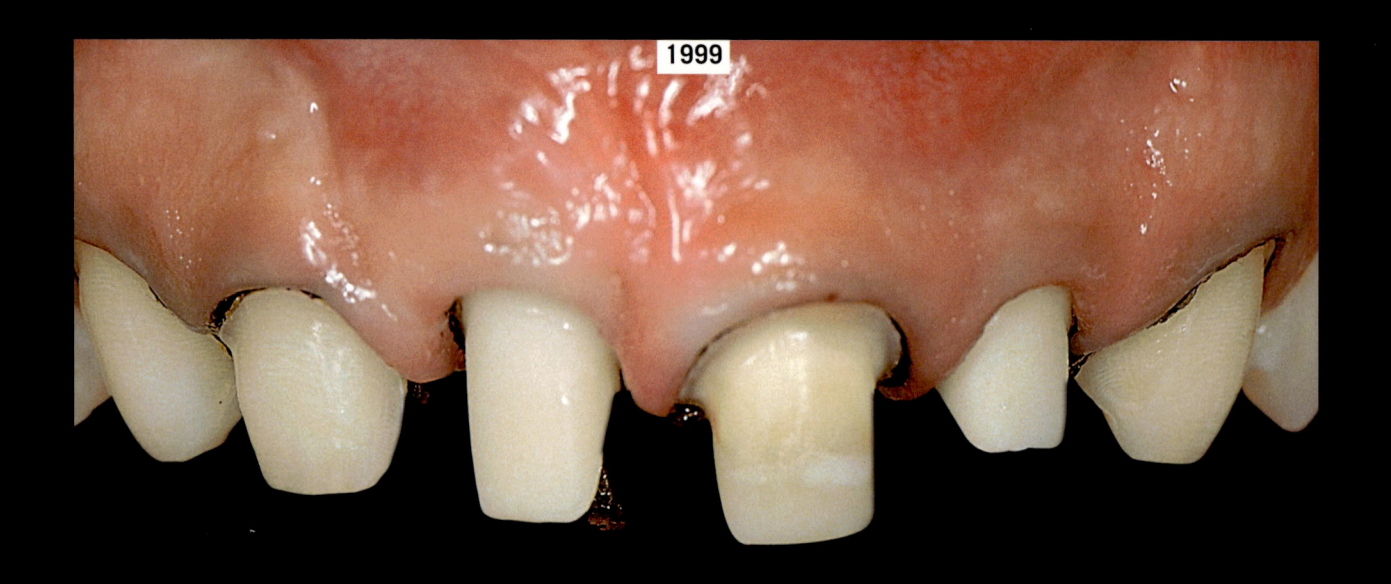

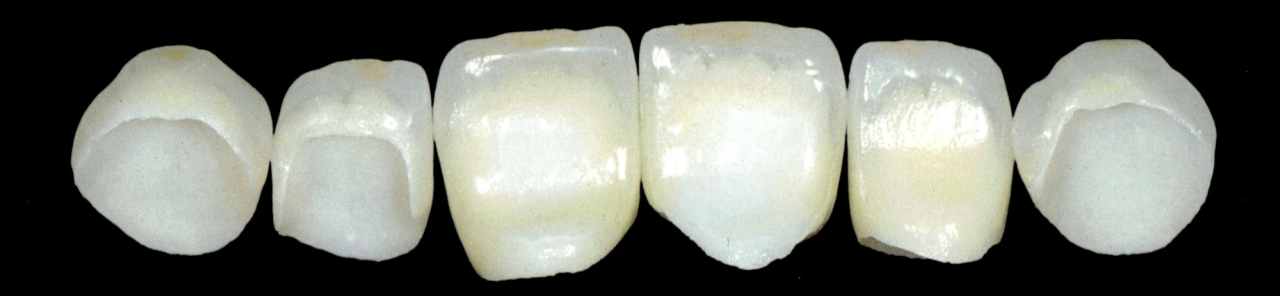

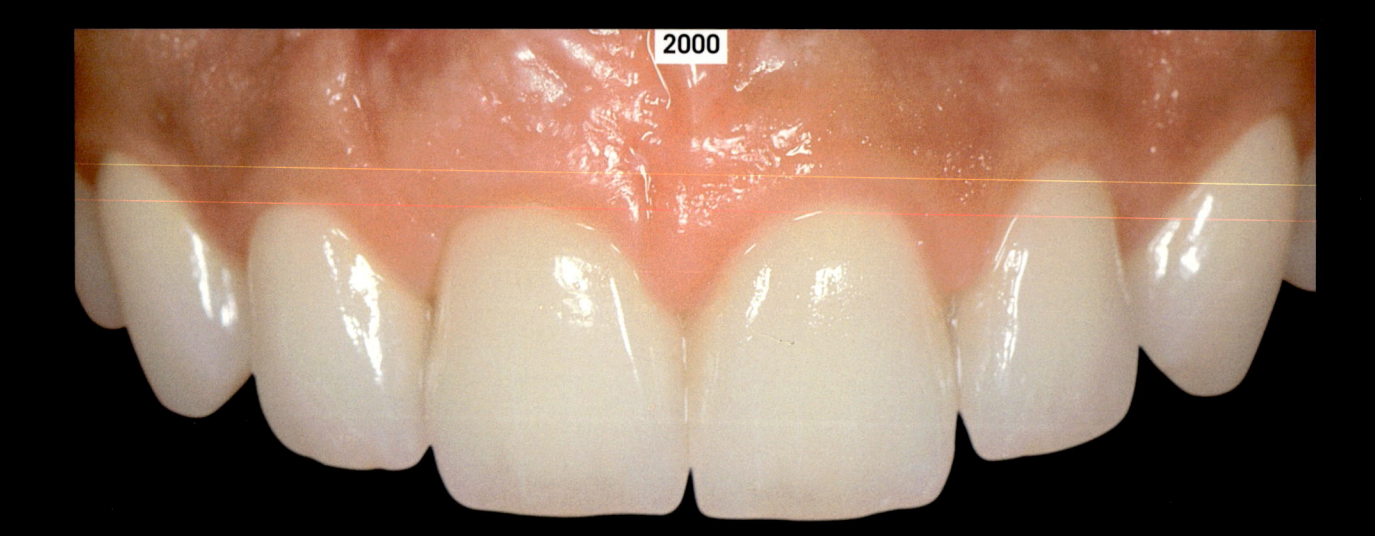

1999

2000

Second treatment: 2004–2005

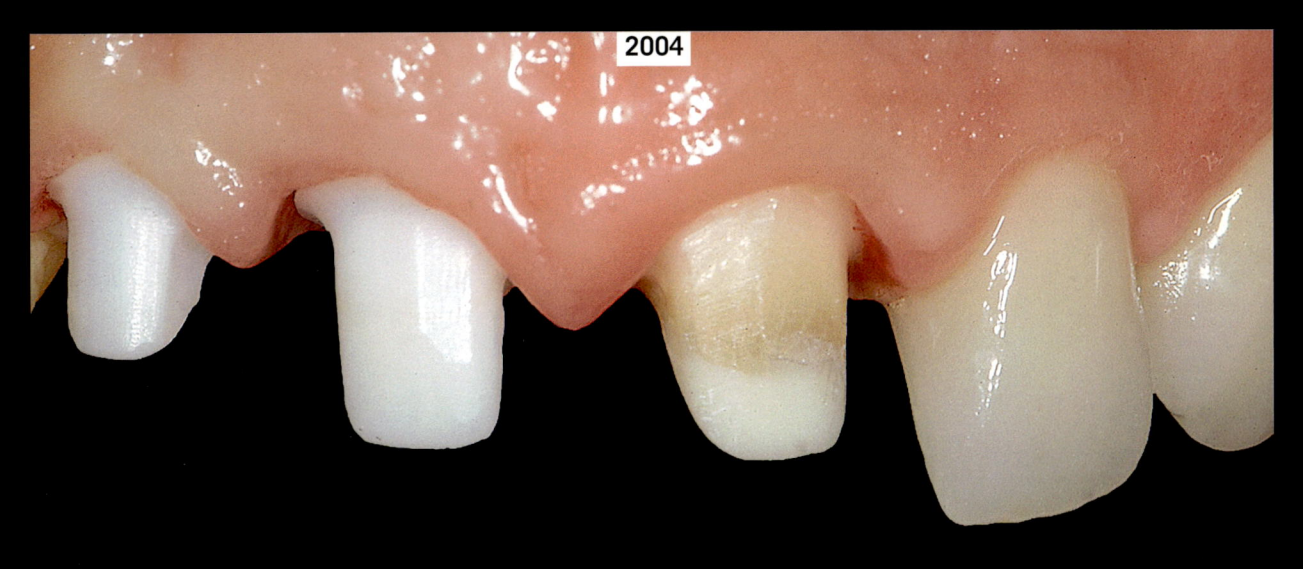

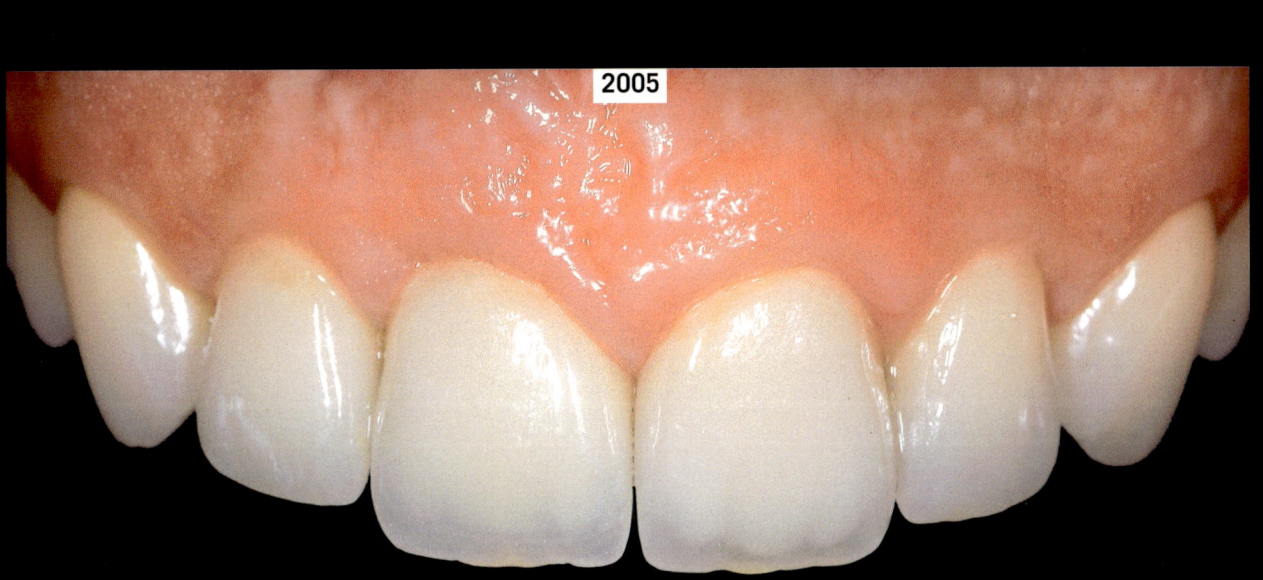

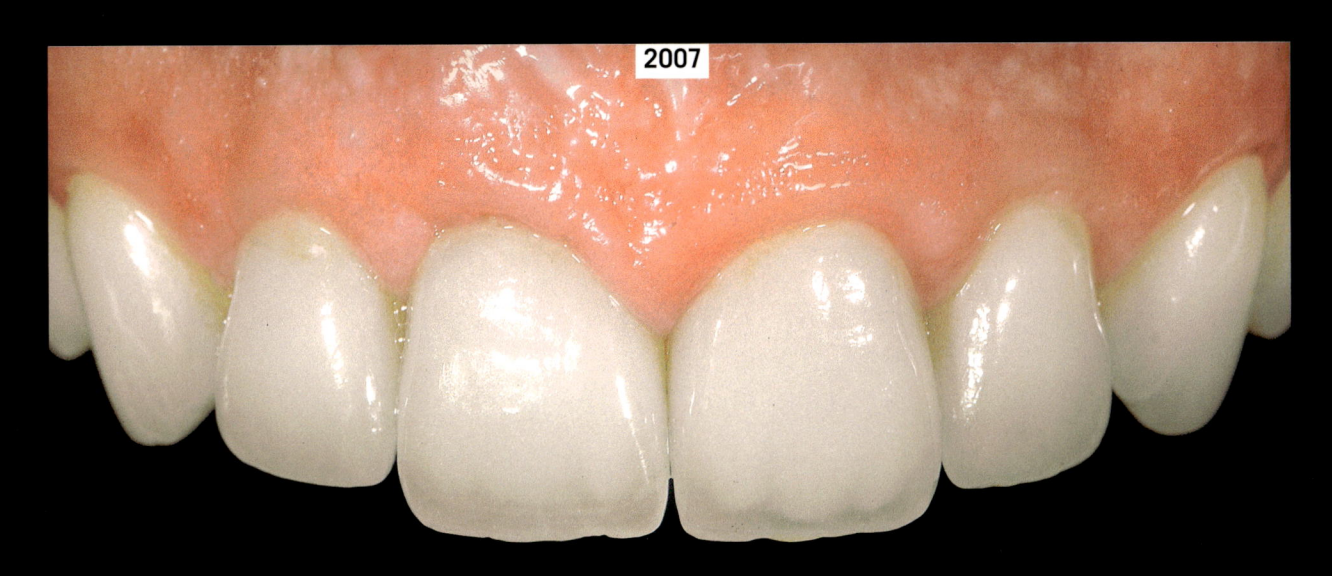

2004

2005

2007

ESTHETIC REHABILITATION
IN FIXED PROSTHODONTICS

PROSTHETIC TREATMENT VOLUME 2

A SYSTEMATIC APPROACH TO ESTHETIC, BIOLOGIC, AND FUNCTIONAL INTEGRATION

Page numbers followed by "f" denote figures; those followed by "t" denote tables

A

Abutments
  definitive
    creation of, 358, 359f
    provisional restoration on, 236, 236f–239f
    second provisional restoration on, 240, 243f–245f
  evaluation of, 40
  final preparation of, 324
  healing, 227f
  implants used as, 42, 43f
  impression taking on, 410, 411f
  irrigating of, 336, 337f
  maxillary and mandibular, 416, 416f–417f
  natural teeth as, 42–44, 43f
  onlays and overlays, 212
  opposing arch and, occlusal registration between, 412, 413f
  prosthetic
    countersinking, 358
    materials used for, 358, 359f
    preparation of, 346
    screw-retained, 356
    shape of, 358, 359f–365f
    transmucosal path replica used to create, 356, 357f
  provisional
    definitive abutments, 236, 236f–239f
    description of, 130, 131, 240, 241f–242f
  removable, 438
  titanium, 234f, 362f
Acetate matrix, 134–137, 135f–137f
Acetate mockup, 52, 53f
Acrylic resin mockup, 52, 53f
Acrylic-resin provisional restoration, 128, 129f, 202
Adapted centric posture, 68
Additive diagnostic wax-up, 112, 113f–115f
All-ceramics
  description of, 468
  fixed partial dentures constructed of, 474, 475f
  fracture modality, 478
  marginal adaptations, 482, 483f
  treating of, 488, 489f
Allergic stomatitis, 280
Alumina, 470, 471f, 476, 477f
Aluminum chloride, 394, 395f
Angle's class, 382
Anterior guidance, 378, 379f, 454, 455f–457f, 496
Anterior reference point, 72, 73f
Anterior sector
  cross-mounting techniques, 446, 447f
  occlusal registrations, 412
  provisional restorations in, 214–216, 215f–216f, 304, 305f–306f
  resective therapy, 316–323
  tooth preparation thickness, 326, 327f
Ante's law, 40
Arbitrary facebow, 72, 73f, 96
Arbitrary plane, 74
Arches
  opposing
    impression of, 382
    master cast mounting with cast of, 446, 447f, 448, 449f
  rehabilitation of
    immediate loading, 254, 255f–263f
    occlusal registrations, 412–417, 413f–417f
    one arch, 170–181, 171f–177f, 179f–181f, 414, 415f, 448, 449f
    oral cavity positioning, 178–181, 179f–181f
    pressing onto the stone cast, 170–177, 171f–178f
    two arches, 182f–187f, 182–187, 416, 417f, 450, 451f–453f
Articulator
  cast mounting on. *See* Stone casts, articulator mounting of.
  condylar inclination in, 70, 71f

definition of, 72
fully adjustable, 98, 99f
semi-adjustable, 98–100, 99f, 446
Axial inclination, 132, 133f

B

Biologic integration, 318
Biologic width, 352, 353f
Biscuit try-in
  biologic parameters, 498–501
  contours, 498
  edentulous ridges, 500
  esthetic parameters, 494, 494f–495f
  functional parameters, 496, 497f
  marginal closure, 498
"Black triangles," 338, 518
Bleeding during probing, 356
Buccal contour, 288f–289f, 288–290
Buccal index, 462, 463f–465f, 490

C

CAD/CAM systems, 470, 472
Camper's plane, 74
Caries, 296
Case histories, 30, 32
Case studies, 60–71, 480, 481f
Cast
  master, 438, 439f–441f
  secondary, 442, 443f–445f
  stone. *See* Stone casts.
Cementation, of provisional restoration, 206–209, 207f–209f
Cementoenamel junction, 302
Centric occlusion, 106
Centric relation
  biscuit try-in, 496
  description of, 66–68, 69f, 71f, 380
  mandibular position in, 448
  provisional restoration in, 268
Ceramics
  all-. *See* All-ceramics.
  layering, 490, 491f
  metal-. *See* Metal-ceramics.
Cervical thickness, 326
Chamfer margin, 331f
Chromatic map, 420
Clinical crown lengthening, 294, 295f
Clinical examination, 34, 35f
Clinician, 30
Color
  description of, 62
  provisional restoration, 202–205, 203f–205f
  recording the, 418–420, 419f
  transmitting the, 420, 421f–423f
Commissural line, 80, 81f, 90, 92f
Computed tomography, 32, 33f
Condylar eminence inclination, 100, 101f
Coronal restorations, 332
Craniofacial case history, 32
Craniofacial evaluation, 34
Cross-mounting techniques
  checking of, 450
  description of, 435
  one-arch rehabilitation, 448, 449f
  two-arch rehabilitation, 450, 451f–453f
Crown lengthening, 294, 295f
Curve of Spee, 132
Curve of Wilson, 132
Customized anterior guidance, 454, 455f–457f
Cyanoacrylate, 440f

D

Dawson's bimanaul manipulation method, 66, 69f
Definitive restorations
  delivering the, 502, 503f
  description of, 374

laboratory production of, 436, 437f
producing of, 436, 437f
Delayed loading, 232
Dental case history, 32
Dentolabial analysis, 34, 35f
Deprogrammer, 68
Diagnosis
clinical examination, 34, 35f
definition of, 38
dental case history used in, 32
direct mockup for, 48, 50f–51f
elements of, 39f, 45f
extraoral examination, 34, 35f
indirect mockup for, 52, 53f–55f
intraoral examination, 36–38, 37f
medical case history used in, 30
radiographic examination, 32, 33f
treatment plan created from, 40, 41f
Diagnostic wax-up
additive, 112, 113f–115f
clinical information necessary for, 52, 53f
esthetic information, 60–65
functional information for, 110f
laboratory checklist information, 56, 58f–59f
occlusal plane changes tested in patient, 110, 111f
overview of, 104–106
posterior teeth morphology, 110
provisional restoration and, 112, 114f–115f
stone casts of, 131f
Diamond burs, 196, 336
Die spacer, 438, 441f
Direct mockup, 48, 50f–51f
Disinfection, 390

E
Edentulous areas
fixed partial dentures in, 42
orthodontic provisional restorations for, 230, 230f–231f
Endodontic case history, 32
Endodontic treatment, 40
Esthetic checklist, 48, 49f, 56, 57f
Esthetic plane, 74
Esthetic preview
direct mockup, 48, 50f–51f
indirect mockup, 52, 53f–55f
Esthetic rehabilitation, 30
Esthetics
diagnostic wax-up, 60–65
facebow, 76, 77f–79f
incisal plane, 80, 81f
provisional restorations, 266, 267f, 376
Ethyl methacrylate, 128
Extraoral examination, 34, 35f

F
Face
oblique inclination of, 94f–97f, 94–97
photograph of, 60, 61f
Facebow
arbitrary, 72, 73f, 82, 96
arms of, 82, 83f, 85, 86f
data transfer, 382, 383f
definition of, 72
esthetic-functional implications, 76, 77f–79f
Frankfort plane as reference, 76, 77f–78f
incorrect positioning, 84, 85f–87f
kinematic, 72, 73f
recording of, 382, 446, 447f
reference points, 72, 73f
Facial analysis, 34
Facial harmony, 80, 81f
Feldspathic ceramics, 468
Ferrule, 40
Final impression, 384–388
Finish line, 392–395

Finishing
marginal, 348, 349f
provisional restoration, 196–199, 197f–199f
Fixed partial dentures
all-ceramics for, 474, 475f
alumina ceramics for, 476, 477f
in large edentulous spaces, 42
marginal adaptation, 482, 483f
metal-ceramics for, 474
rocking motion in, 478
temporary luting of, 504
zirconium-based ceramics for, 476, 477f
Fixed prosthesis, 226–231
Frankfort plane, 74, 75f, 76, 77f–78f
Full-mouth series, 32, 33f, 518, 519f
Furcations, 312, 313f

G
Gingival crest
margin, 338
retraction cords for preparation of, 396, 397f
Gingival integrity, 338, 339f–341f
Gingival margins, 284f–293f, 284–293
Gingival recession, 280
Gingival retraction cords
chemical agent–impregnated, 394, 395f
description of, 344, 346, 347f, 348, 349f
gingival crest preparation using, 396, 397f
gingival sulcus preparation using, 392, 393f, 394f
impression with cord inserted, 396, 397f, 400, 402f–403f
insertion of, 392, 394
intrasulcular preparation, 398, 399f–407f, 400
one-cord technique, 396, 397f
two-cord technique, 398, 399f–407f, 400
Gingival sulcus
cord preparation of, 392, 393f–394f
description of, 278, 344, 345f
mapping of, 392, 393f
Gingival tissue
apicalization of, 324
health of, 518
maturation indicators, 301f–303f, 302, 304
maturation times for, 298
periodontal biotype effects on, 300
regrowth of, 300, 301f
stability of, 282, 283f
surgical therapy for exposure of, 296, 297f
Gingivectomy, 296, 298
Glass ionomers, 505f
Glass-ceramics, 468, 469f, 474, 475f
Glazing, 202–205, 203f–205f, 500

H
Handpieces, 336, 337f
Heat pressing, 468, 469f
Heat-activated acrylic resin, 128, 129f
High-strength ceramics, 470
Horizontal incisal plane, 82–87, 83f, 85f–87f

I
Immediate implant function, 248
Immediate loading, 248–265, 254
Implants
as abutments, 42, 43f
delayed loading, 232
distance between, 354, 355f
hygienic maintenance of sites, 356
immediate loading of, 248–265
impression taking for, 410, 411f
provisional restorations used with, 226–235, 227f–231f, 233f–235f
single, 248–265
three-dimensional positioning of, 354, 355f
Impression
on abutments, 410, 411f

description of, 382, 383f
final
    description of, 384–388
    master cast created from, 438, 439f–441f
    with gingival retraction cords inserted in gingival crest, 396, 397f, 400, 402f–403f
for implants, 410, 411f
for inlays, 408
one step–double mix technique, 390, 391f
for onlays, 408
for partial restorations, 408
polyethers, 388, 389f, 391f
polyvinyl siloxanes, 388, 389f, 391f
for veneers, 408, 409f
Impression tray, 390
Incisal plane
esthetic considerations, 80, 81f
horizontal, 82–87, 83f, 85f–87f
inclined, 88, 88f–93f
Incisal thickness, 326
Indirect mockup, 52, 53f–55f
Inflammation, 282, 282f, 380
Inlays
impression for, 408
provisional, 210, 211f
tooth preparation for, 332, 333f
Interproximal cervical design, 162
Interproximal contours, 286, 287f
Interproximal undercuts, 408
Interpupillary line, 80, 81f, 90, 92f
Intraoral examination, 36–38, 37f
Intrasulcular margin, 341, 344
Intrasulcular preparation, 344–351, 345f–351f

J
Junctional epithelium, 352, 353f

K
Kinematic facebow, 72, 73f, 96, 96f–97f
Knife-edge margin, 330, 331f

L
Laboratory checklist, 56, 58f–59f, 424, 425f–427f
Loading
delayed, 232
immediate, 248–265
Lost-wax casting technique, 466, 467f
Luting
definitive, 504, 505f–517f
temporary, 504

M
Maintenance, 518, 519f
Mandible
centric relation positioning of, 66, 68
manipulation of, 68, 69f
movement of, during excursive movements, 378, 379f
retrusion of, 179f
Mandibular anterior sextant, 64, 64f
Mandibular arch
occlusolingual index of, 461f
rehabilitation of. See Arches, rehabilitation of.
Mandibular incisors, 108, 109f
Mandibular lateral translation, 102, 103f
Mandibular provisional restoration
master cast mounted on, 450, 452f
maxillary abutments and, 416
Margins
closure, 284, 285f
finish, 392–395
finishing of, 196–199, 197f–199f, 348, 349f
gingival crest, 284f–293f, 284–293, 338
intrasulcular, 344
marking of, 164f
precision concerns, 150, 151f–152f
re-margining, 200, 201f

subgingival, 342, 343f
supragingival, 338, 339f
tooth preparation, 330, 330f–331f
visibility of, 338, 339f
Master cast
description of, 438, 439f–441f
gingival matrices on, 512f
maxillary, 450, 452f
mounting of, with cast of opposing arch, 446, 447f, 448, 449f
Masticatory system, 72
Maxillary anterior sextant, 64, 64f
Maxillary arch
incongruities in, 31f
prosthetic-periodontal rehabilitation of, 316f
rehabilitation of. See Arches, rehabilitation of.
tooth abrasions in, 70
Maxillary incisors
agenesis of, 286, 287f, 333f
fracture of, 251f
Maxillary provisional restoration
mandibular abutments and, 416
mandibular master cast mounted on, 450, 452f
Maximum intercuspation, 66, 168, 380, 496
Medical case history, 30
Metal-ceramics
clinical considerations, 478, 479f
description of, 466, 467f
fixed partial dentures constructed from, 474, 475f
marginal adaptations, 482, 483f
postsoldering, 500, 501f
tooth preparation considerations, 478, 479f
treating of, 488, 489f
Methyl methacrylate, 128, 193f
Mockup
direct, 48, 50f–51f
indirect, 52, 53f–55f
Modified indirect technique, for provisional restorations, 154–159, 155f–159f, 188

N
Natural teeth
as abutments, 42–44, 43f
provisional restorations on, 226, 227f
Non–implant-supported provisional restorations, 226

O
Oblique facial inclination, 94f–97f, 94–97
Oblique transcranial radiographs, 32
Occlusal device, for parafunctional activity, 40
Occlusal evaluation, 38, 38f
Occlusal index, 490
Occlusal plane
description of, 62, 62f, 80, 81f
testing of, 110, 111f
Occlusal registrations
between abutments and opposing arch, 412, 413f
accuracy of, 66
centric relation, 66–68, 69f, 71f
description of, 38
maximum intercuspation, 66
for one-arch rehabilitation, 412, 413f
in partial restorations, 412
between prepared teeth and opposing arch, 412, 413f
protrusive movement, 70, 71f
for two-arch rehabilitation, 416, 417f
vertical dimension of occlusion, 70, 71f
Occlusal stability, 380, 381f
Occlusal trauma, 519f
Occlusion
provisional restoration fitting guided by, 168, 169f, 178, 184, 184f–187f, 268, 269f
provisional veneers and, 216
stone cast adjustments, 106f–111f, 106–111
vertical dimension of. See Vertical dimension of occlusion.

Occlusopalatal index, 458, 459f–461f, 490, 491f
One step–double mix technique, for impressions, 390, 391f
Onlays
  impression for, 408
  provisional, 212, 213f
Operational sequence, 44, 45f
Oral hygiene, 286
Orbital-axis plane, 74, 76
Orthodontic case history, 32
Orthodontic evaluations, 36, 37f
Orthodontic provisional restoration, 230, 230f–231f
Orthopantomography, 33f
Osseointegration, 248, 249f
Overbite, 64, 64f–65f, 378
Overjet, 64, 64f–65f, 108, 108f, 378
Overlays, 212, 213f
Oxyphosphate cement, 505f

P

Panoramic radiographs, 32, 33f
Parafunctional activity, 40
Peri-implant soft tissues, 352–365
Periodontal assessments, 36, 37f
Periodontal biotype, 278, 288, 290, 291f, 300
Periodontal case history, 32
Periodontal disease
  characteristics of, 40, 41f
  tooth extractions secondary to, 42
Periodontal tissue, 278, 279f
Phonetic analysis, 34
Phonetic tests, 378
Photographs, 60
Pick-up technique, 410, 411f
Polyethers, 388, 389f, 391f
Polymethyl methacrylate, 194
Polyvinyl siloxanes, 388, 389f, 391f
Posterior reference point, 72, 73f
Posterior teeth disocclusion, 70
Postsoldering, 500, 501f
Pouring in the silicone matrix technique, 160–166, 161f–165f, 174
Preprosthetic surgery, 294–311
Preventive simulation, 484, 485f–487f
Progressive mandibular lateral translation, 102, 103f
Prosthetic-periodontal therapy, 312
Protrusive movement, 70, 71f
Protrusive interocclusal record, 382, 383f, 454, 455f
Provisional restorations
  abutment for, 130, 131, 416, 416f–417f
  acetate matrix for, 134–137, 135f–137f
  acrylic resins, 128, 129f, 148, 202, 280
  arbitrary realignments, 142, 142f–143f
  arch rehabilitation. *See* Arches, rehabilitation of.
  buccal contour of, 288f–289f, 288–290
  cementation of
    description of, 206–209, 207f–209f
    excess cement removal, 290
  centering device, 188–191, 189f–191f
  in centric relation, 268
  chairside production of, 134–137, 135f–137f
  coloring of, 202–205, 203f–205f
  container effect, 156, 157f
  contour of, 286–290, 287f–289f
  coronal, 332
  description of, 123
  diagnostic wax-up and
    comparisons between, 112, 114f–115f
    oversizing of, 154
  direct technique for, 134–137, 135f–137f
  emergence profile of, 198f
  esthetics, 266, 267f, 376
  with facilitated insertion, 154–159, 155f–159f
  finalization of, 302, 303f–311f, 304, 318
  finishing of, 196–199, 197f–199f
  first
    description of, 220, 221f
    on provisional abutments, 240, 241f–242f
  fitting and insertion of
    description of, 132, 133f
    difficulty in, 148f–153f, 148–153
    facilitated insertion guide, 188–191, 189f–191f
    failed, 144–147, 145f–146f
    marginal fit, 194
    occlusion-guided, 168, 169f, 178, 184, 184f–187f
  fixed, 226–231
  friction considerations, 148, 148f–149f
  functional integration of, 268, 269f
  gingival margin stability, 284f–293f, 284–293
  gingival tissue for. *See* Gingival tissue.
  glazing of, 202–205, 203f–205f
  gold alloy reinforcement of, 224
  immediate loading of a single implant, 250, 251f–253f
  implant-supported, 232–235, 233f–235f
  indirect technique for
    description of, 138–139, 139f
    modified, 154–159, 155f–159f, 188
  inflammatory reactions, 282, 282f
  inlays, 210, 211f
  integrated, 374, 375f
  interferences, 166, 167f, 178, 180f, 182, 183f
  interproximal contour of, 286, 287f
  laboratory fabrication of, 138–139, 139f
  long-term, 220–225, 221f–225f
  margins. *See* Margins.
  materials, 128
  metallic reinforcement, 224
  on natural teeth, 226, 227f
  non–implant-supported, 226
  objective in creating, 124–126, 125f, 127f
  occlusal stability of, 268, 269f
  onlays, 212, 213f
  oral cavity positioning of
    for anterior rehabilitation, 166–169, 167f–168f
    for one arch rehabilitation, 178–181, 179f–181f
  oral hygiene, 286
  orthodontic, 230, 230f–231f
  overcontours, 198f
  overlays, 212, 213f
  periodontal biotype, 278, 288, 290, 291f
  phonetic tests for, 378
  positioning considerations, 280, 281f
  posterior sector, 210–213, 302
  pouring in the silicone matrix, 160–166, 161f–165f, 174
  preliminary preparation for, 130, 132, 133f
  for prepared teeth, 138, 139f
  preprosthetic surgery, 294–311
  pressing onto the stone cast, 170–177, 171f–178f
  recementing of, 208
  relining of. *See* Relining.
  re-margining of, 200, 201f
  removable, 226
  removal of, 220, 384
  requirements, 126
  resin composites, 128, 129f
  resin-bonded prosthesis, 228, 229f
  retention of, 208, 209f
  risk factors for, 280–283, 281f–283f
  second
    on definitive abutments, 240, 243f–245f
    description of, 220, 222
    on provisional abutments, 240, 243f–244f
    reinforcement of, 222–225, 223f–225f
  shortening of, 150
  short-term, 210–219, 211f–219f
  in situ verification of, 376–381, 377f
  surface characteristics of, 290
  thickness measurements, 328, 329f
  tooth preparation. *See* Tooth preparation.
  undercontouring of, 150, 151f
  for unprepared teeth, 138, 139f
  veneers, 214–216, 215f–216f
  vertical dimension of occlusion considerations, 268, 269f
Pulp integrity, 332, 336, 337f

R

Radiographic examination, 32, 33f
Reference planes
    description of, 74
    Frankfort plane, 74, 75f, 76, 77f–78f
    incisal plane, 80, 81f
    occlusal plane, 80, 81f
Registrations
    for inclined incisal plane, 88, 88f–93f
    occlusal. *See* Occlusal registrations.
Relining
    after gingival retraction cord removal, 348
    after tooth preparation, 376
    anterior sectors, 316–323
    posterior sectors, 302, 303f–311f, 304, 312
    procedure for, 152, 153f, 192–195, 250, 280
    in root amputations, 312, 313f–315f
Re-margining, of provisional restoration, 200, 201f
Removable denture, 44
Removable prosthesis, 226
Resective therapy
    in anterior sector, 316–323
    in posterior sector, 312, 313f–315f
Resin cements, 505f
Resin-bonded prosthesis, 228, 229f
Resin composite provisional restoration, 128, 129f
Resinous cement, 214
Restorations. *See* Definitive restorations; Provisional restorations.
Restorative case history, 32
Root amputations, 312, 313f–315f

S

Salt and pepper technique, 200, 201f
Screw-retained prosthetic abutments, 356
Secondary cast, 442, 443f–445f
Self-curing acrylic resin, 128, 129f, 214
Semi-adjustable articulator, 98–100, 99f, 446
Silicate-based ceramics, 468, 469f
Silicone index
    anchoring of, 492f
    buccal index, 462, 463f–465f, 490
    description of, 172f, 458
    occlusopalatal index, 458, 459f–461f, 490, 491f
    wax-up guided by, 466, 467f
Silicone matrix, 160–165, 161f–165f
Single restorations
    marginal adaptation, 482
    temporary luting of, 504
Smile, 60, 61f
Smile line, 56f
Spectrophotometer, 420, 423f
Spot-etching technique, 214
Stone casts
    analysis of, 38
    articulator mounting of
        adjustments, 100–103
        with arbitrary plane, 79f
        assessment of, 485f
        with cast of opposing arch, 446, 447f
        description of, 66, 71f
        with Frankfort plane, 78f
        mandibular lateral translation, 102, 103f
        procedure for, 98–103
    creation of, 52, 53f, 71f
    of diagnostic wax-up, 131f
    occlusal adjustment of, 106f–111f, 106–111
    occlusal instability in, 171f
    provisional restoration pressed onto, 170–177, 171f–178f
    reference points for orienting of, 72, 73f
Subgingival margins, 282, 342, 343f
Substructures
    all-ceramics, 468
    alumina, 470, 471f
    fixed partial dentures. *See* Fixed partial dentures.
    high-strength ceramics, 470
    metal-ceramics. *See* Metal-ceramics.
    preventive simulation, 484, 485f–487f
    silicate-based ceramics, 468, 469f
    treating of, 488, 489f
    try-in, 482, 483f
    zirconium, 472–474, 473f
Sulcular epithelium, 352, 353f
Supracrestal connective tissue, 352, 353f
Supragingival margin, 338, 339f

T

Teeth
    length reductions, 340f
    photograph of, 60, 61f
    preparation of. *See* Tooth preparation.
    as prosthetic abutments, 42–44, 43f
    supporting tissue of, 278, 279f
Temporomandibular joint examination, 34
Titanium abutments, 234f, 362f
Tooth abrasions, 70
Tooth extrusions, 228, 229f
Tooth preparation
    biologic integrity maintenance during, 332
    description of, 130–133, 131f, 133f, 144
    differentiated, 330
    final, 324–325, 325f
    horizontal, 330
    intrasulcular, 344–351, 345f–351f
    lingual area, 328, 329f
    marginal configuration, 330, 330f–331f
    for metal-ceramics, 478, 479f
    pulp integrity, 332, 336, 337f
    thickness, 326–329
    vertical, 330
Tooth preparation index, 144, 146f–147f
Tooth structure
    evaluation of, 36, 37f
    exposure of, 294, 296
    surgical therapy for exposure of, 296, 297f
Transmucosal path, 356, 357f
Treatment plan
    case study of, 46f–47f
    creation of, 40, 41f
    elements of, 45f
    multidisciplinary approach, 44
    operational sequence, 44, 45f
    patient's participation in, 44
Try-in
    biscuit. *See* Biscuit try-in.
    substructures, 482, 483f

V

Veneers
    impression for, 408, 409f
    provisional, 214–216, 215f–216f
    tooth preparation for, 332, 333f
Vertical dimension of occlusion
    description of, 34, 38, 70, 71f, 178, 184
    inaccuracies in, 450
    maxillary casts, 448, 449f
    provisional restoration considerations, 268, 269f, 380

W

Wax-up
    diagnostic. *See* Diagnostic wax-up.
    silicone index used for guidance of, 466, 467f

Z

Zinc oxide–eugenol cements, 206, 212
Zirconium, 472–474, 473f, 476, 477f

LABORATORY CHECKLIST

mf M. FRADEANI   Gb G. BARDUCCI

1/4

Patient _____   Age _____   Date __/__/__   ☐ Male   ☐ Female

ESTHETIC INFORMATION

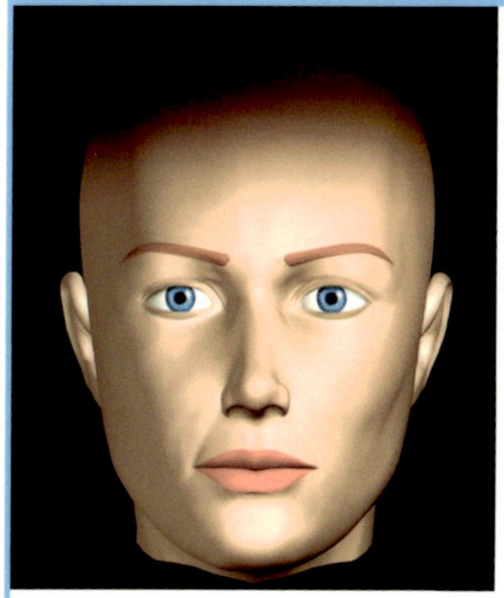

PATIENT'S PHOTOGRAPH 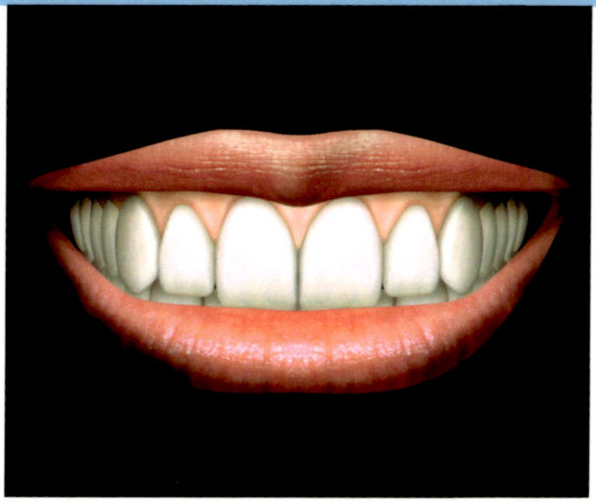   PATIENT'S PHOTOGRAPH 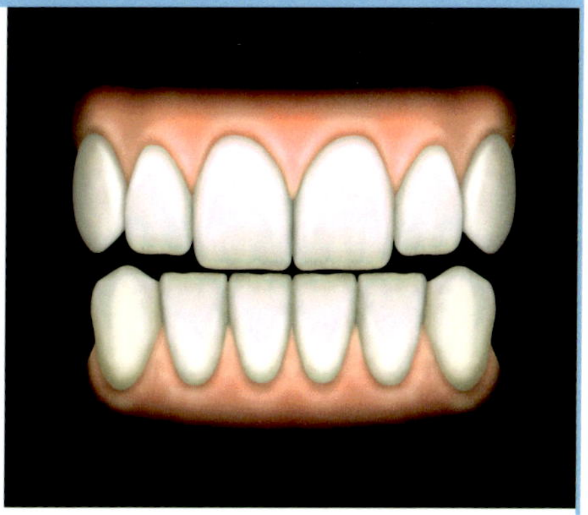   PATIENT'S PHOTOGRAPH

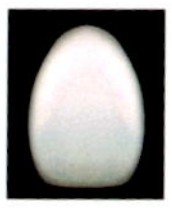

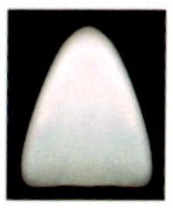

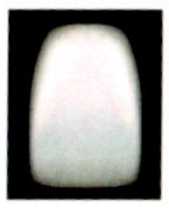

■ **PHOTOGRAPHS** ☐ Old ☐ New   ■ **SMILE LINE** ☐ Average ☐ Low ☐ High

■ **ALIGNMENT** ☐ Yes ☐ No   ■ **APPEARANCE** ☐ Youth ☐ Adult ☐ Mature

■ **TOOTH TYPE** ☐ Ovoid   ☐ Triangular   ☐ Square

■ **TEXTURE**   **Macro** ☐ None ☐ Slight ☐ Pronounced   **Micro** ☐ None ☐ Slight ☐ Pronounced

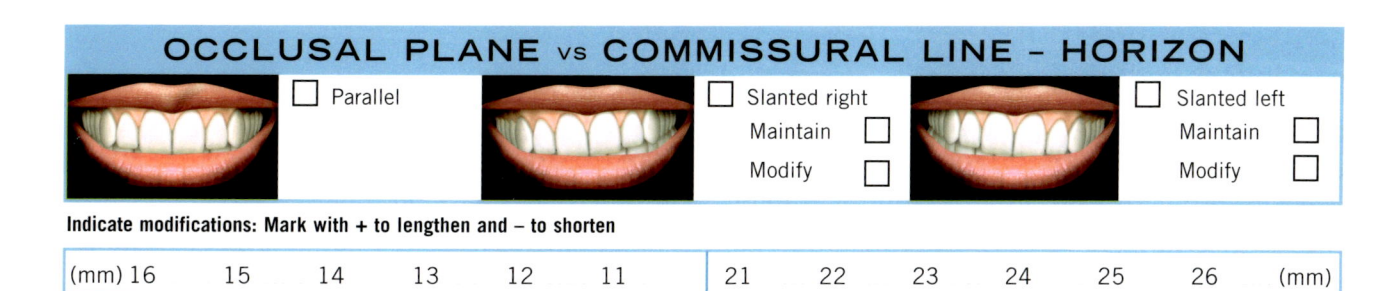

OCCLUSAL PLANE vs COMMISSURAL LINE – HORIZON

☐ Parallel   ☐ Slanted right   Maintain ☐   Modify ☐   ☐ Slanted left   Maintain ☐   Modify ☐

Indicate modifications: Mark with + to lengthen and − to shorten

(mm)	16	15	14	13	12	11	21	22	23	24	25	26	(mm)
(mm)	46	45	44	43	42	41	31	32	33	34	35	36	(mm)

Notes

COLOR

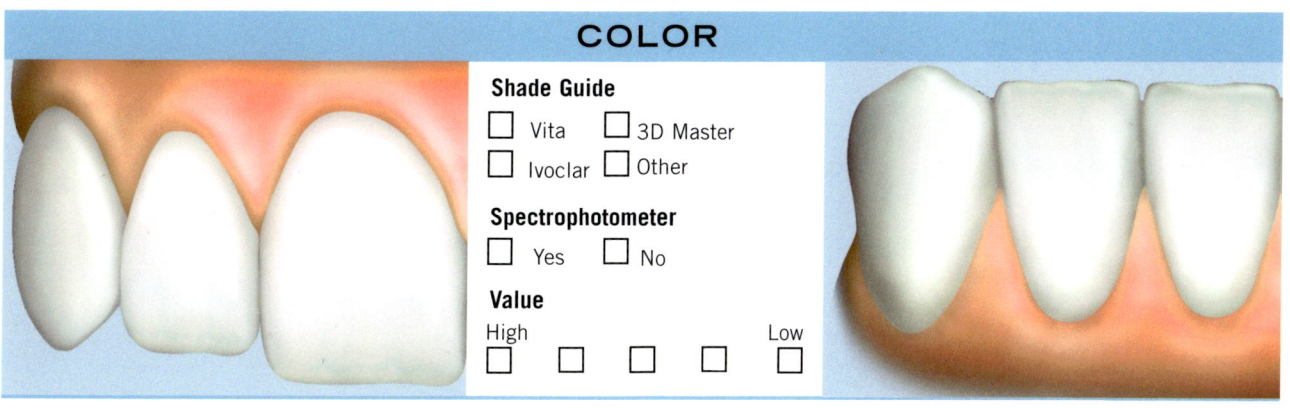

Shade Guide
☐ Vita   ☐ 3D Master
☐ Ivoclar ☐ Other

Spectrophotometer
☐ Yes ☐ No

Value
High ☐ ☐ ☐ ☐ Low

Notes

Copyright © 2008 by Quintessence Publishing Co. Inc

SHAPE	Modifications	POSITION
13 lengthen/shorten (mm)	widen/narrow (mm)	labial/palatal (mm)
12 lengthen/shorten (mm)	widen/narrow (mm)	labial/palatal (mm)
11 lengthen/shorten (mm)	widen/narrow (mm)	labial/palatal (mm)
21 lengthen/shorten (mm)	widen/narrow (mm)	labial/palatal (mm)
22 lengthen/shorten (mm)	widen/narrow (mm)	labial/palatal (mm)
23 lengthen/shorten (mm)	widen/narrow (mm)	labial/palatal (mm)

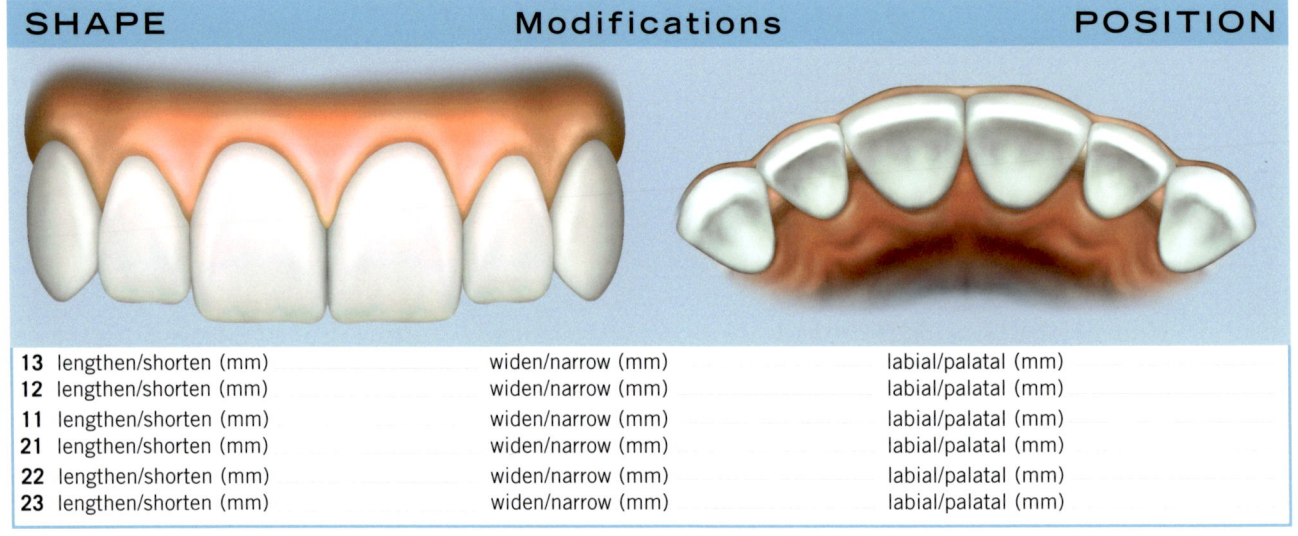

Notes

SHAPE	Modifications	POSITION
43 lengthen/shorten (mm)	widen/narrow (mm)	buccal/lingual (mm)
42 lengthen/shorten (mm)	widen/narrow (mm)	buccal/lingual (mm)
41 lengthen/shorten (mm)	widen/narrow (mm)	buccal/lingual (mm)
31 lengthen/shorten (mm)	widen/narrow (mm)	buccal/lingual (mm)
32 lengthen/shorten (mm)	widen/narrow (mm)	buccal/lingual (mm)
33 lengthen/shorten (mm)	widen/narrow (mm)	buccal/lingual (mm)

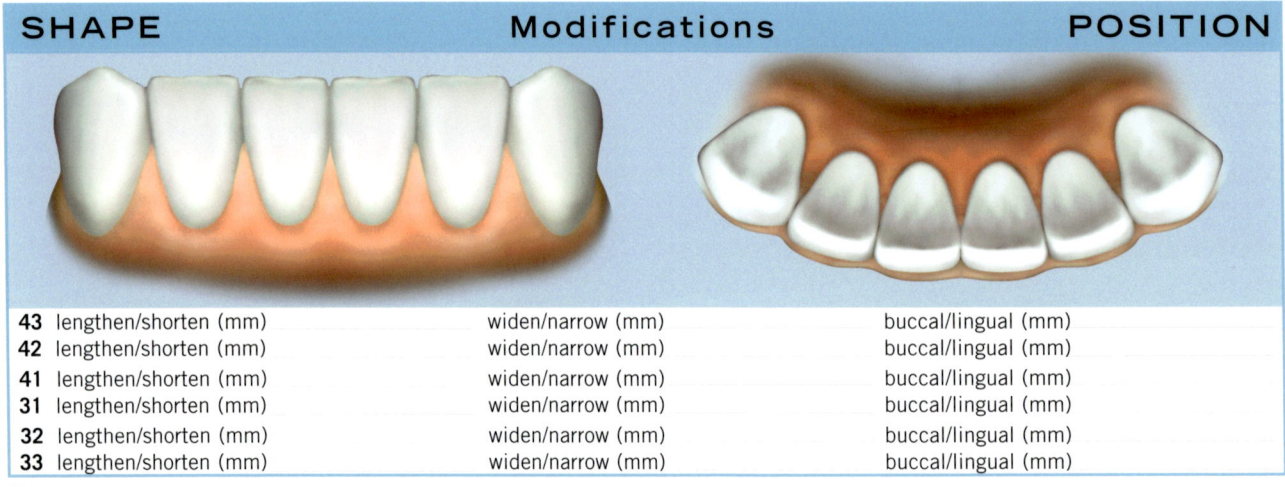

Notes

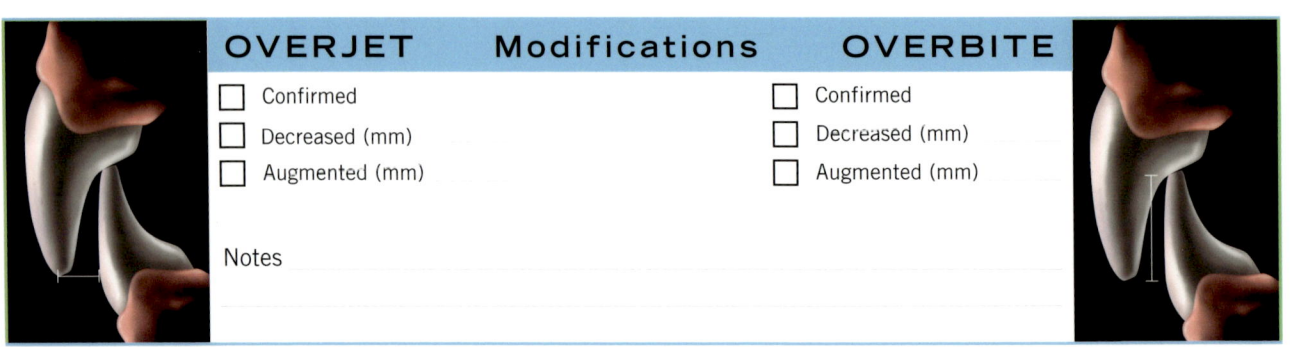

OVERJET	Modifications	OVERBITE
☐ Confirmed		☐ Confirmed
☐ Decreased (mm)		☐ Decreased (mm)
☐ Augmented (mm)		☐ Augmented (mm)

Notes

Copyright © 2008 by Quintessence Publishing Co. Inc

FUNCTIONAL INFORMATION

■ STONE CASTS

- [ ] **Previous**
  - [ ] Maxillary [ ] Mandibular
- [ ] **Diagnostic**
  - [ ] Maxillary [ ] Mandibular
- [ ] **Provisional**
  - [ ] Maxillary [ ] Mandibular

■ OCCLUSAL RECORDS

- [ ] MI
- [ ] CR
- [ ] Protrusive interocclusal record
- [ ] Lateral interocclusal records

■ VERTICAL DIMENSION

- [ ] Unchanged
- [ ] Increase (mm)
  - [ ] Maxillary (mm)
  - [ ] Mandibular (mm)
- [ ] Decrease (mm)
  - [ ] Maxillary (mm)
  - [ ] Mandibular (mm)

■ FACEBOW   ■ Reference lines

- [ ] Arbitrary
- [ ] Kinematic
- [ ] Horizon
- [ ] Interpupillary
- [ ] Commissural
- [ ] Other

■ ARTICULATOR SET-UP

- [ ] **Semi-adjustable**
  - [ ] Condylar inclination (degrees)   OR [ ] Protrusive interocclusal record
  - [ ] Progressive mandibular lateral translation (degrees)   OR [ ] Lateral interocclusal records
  - [ ] Immediate mandibular lateral translation (mm)
- [ ] **Fully adjustable**
  - [ ] Mechanical pantograph
  - [ ] Electronic pantograph

■ DISOCCLUSION

- [ ] Incisal guidance
- [ ] Canine guidance
- [ ] Group function
- [ ] Balanced occlusion

IMPRESSION

Recorded on ____/____/____ Time ____:____ Disinfected with _____

■ Impression materials

- [ ] **ALGINATE**
  - [ ] Maxillary [ ] Mandibular
- [ ] **POLYETHER**
  - [ ] Maxillary [ ] Mandibular
- [ ] **ADDITION SILICONE**
  - [ ] Maxillary [ ] Mandibular
- [ ] **POLYSULFUR**
  - [ ] Maxillary [ ] Mandibular
- [ ] **CONDENSATION SILICONE**
  - [ ] Maxillary [ ] Mandibular
- [ ] **OTHER**
  - [ ] Maxillary [ ] Mandibular

DOCUMENTATION

■ CASE HISTORY

- [ ] Contagious diseases
- [ ] Confirmed allergies
- [ ] Other medical device present
- [ ] Psychomotor handicap
- [ ] Bruxism
- [ ] Other

Notes

■ ATTACHMENTS

- [ ] Slides/Photographs
- [ ] Esthetic Checklist
- [ ] Other

LABORATORY WORK ORDER

Dr name Address City State Telephone	Dental lab name Address City State Telephone

Date____/____/____   Work order no._____

Patient/Code_____ Age_____ ☐ Male   ☐ Female

■ TYPE OF WORK

☐ Diagnostic waxing   ☐ Indirect mock-up   ☐ Provisional   ☐ Fixed prosthesis   ☐ Removable prosthesis

■ Description

■ SCHEMA

o = Natural abutment   ☐ = Implant   X = Missing tooth

❶
18	17	16	15	14	13	12	11	21	22	23	24	25	26	27	28
48	47	46	45	44	43	42	41	31	32	33	34	35	36	37	38
❹   ❸   ❷

PFM: *Porcelain-fused-to-metal*   **PS1:** *Presoldering*   **PS2:** *Postsoldering*   **MM:** *Metal margins*
MCM: *Metal-ceramic margin*   **CS:** *Ceramic shoulder*   **PC:** *Post and core*   **ABU:** *Abutment*
AC: *All-ceramic*   **RB:** *Resin-bonded*   **V:** *Veneer*   **IN:** *Inlay*   **ON:** *Onlay*

Alloy:
Ceramic:

COLOR

Shade Guide
☐ Vitapan
☐ 3D Master
☐ Ivoclar
☐ Other

Value
High   Low
☐   ☐   ☐   ☐   ☐

TRY-INS

Try-in	Date____/____/____ Notes:	☐ Attachment No.
Try-in	Date____/____/____ Notes:	☐ Attachment No.
Try-in	Date____/____/____ Notes:	☐ Attachment No.
Delivery	Date____/____/____ Notes:	☐ Attachment No.

Dentist's signature

Copyright © 2008 by Quintessence Publishing Co. Inc

DR. | **LABORATORY**

Patient/Code

TRY-IN

ATTACHMENT NR. | Try-In | date____/____/____

Notes

ATTACHMENT NR. | Try-In | date____/____/____

Notes

Copyright © 2008 by Quintessence Publishing Co. Inc

TRY-IN

ATTACHMENT NR. Try-In date____/____/____
Notes

ATTACHMENT NR. Try-In date____/____/____
Notes

3 3008 00591 1460

UMDNJ / Smith-Newark

UMDNJ-SMITH LIBRARY
30 12th Avenue
Newark, NJ 07103